Vinzenz Hombach
Nico Merkle
Volker Rasche

Cardiovascular Magnetic Resonance Imaging

Contributors

Jörg Barkhausen
Philipp Beerbaum
Peter Bernhardt
Axel Bornstedt
René Botnar
Horst Brunner
Loren Budge
Kieran Clarke
Christoph Galm
Bernhard L. Gerber
Mathias Goyen
Christina Heilmaier
Christoph U. Herborn
Volker Herold
Karl-Heinz Hiller
Martin Hoffmann
Cameron Holloway
Peter M. Jakob
Raymond Kim
Won Yong Kim
Oliver Klass
Igor Klem
Christopher M. Kramer
Markus Kunze
Gregory M. Lanza
Peter R. Luijten
Stefan Neubauer
Dipanjan Pan
Sandra Pauls
Maythem Saeed
Tobias Schäffter
Jeanette Schulz-Menger
Christian Schumann
Johannes Schwab
Jochen Spiess
Matthias Stuber
Florian Vogt
Ralf Wassmuth
Mark W. Wilson
Sabine Wuchenauer

Cardiovascular Magnetic Resonance Imaging

Textbook and Atlas

Editors

Vinzenz Hombach
Nico Merkle
Volker Rasche

Foreword by

Sebastian Kozerke and Peter Bösiger

With 846 Figures and 18 Tables

Schattauer

Vinzenz Hombach, MD
Cardiology – Angiology – Pneumology –
Sports and Rehabilitation Medicine
Department of Internal Medicine II
University Hospital of Ulm
Albert-Einstein-Allee 23
D-89081 Ulm, Germany
vinzenz.hombach@uni-ulm.de
vinzenz@hombach.us

Nico Merkle, MD
Gemeinschaftspraxis für Radiologie und Neuroradiologie
and Zentrum für minimal invasive Therapie
Heinz-Galinski-Straße 1
D-13347 Berlin, Germany
nico.merkle@ihre-radiologen.de

Volker Rasche, PhD
Experimental Cardiovascular Imaging (ExCaVI)
and Core Facility Small Animal MRI
Department of Internal Medicine II
University Hospital of Ulm
Albert-Einstein-Allee 23
D-89081 Ulm, Germany
volker.rasche@uni-ulm.de

Bibliographic information published by the Deutsche Nationalbibliothek. The Deutsche Nationalbibliothek lists this publication in the Deutsche Nationalbibliografie; detailed bibliographic data is available in the Internet at <http://dnb.d-nb.de>.

Important note: Medicine is an ever-changing science, so the contents of this publication, especially recommendations concerning diagnostic and therapeutic procedures, can only give an account of the knowledge at the time of publication. While utmost care has been taken to ensure that all specifications regarding drug selection and dosage and treatment options are accurate, readers are urged to review the product information sheet and any relevant material supplied by the manufacturer, and, in case of doubt, to consult a specialist. The publisher will appreciate – also in the public's interest – to be informed of possible inconsistencies. The ultimate responsibility for any diagnostic or therapeutic application lies with the reader.
No special reference is made to registered names, proprietary names, trade marks etc. in this publication. The appearance of a name without designation as proprietary does not imply that it is exempt from the relevant protective laws and regulations and therefore free for general use.

E-Mail: info@schattauer.de
Internet: www.schattauer.de
Printed in Germany

Jacket design: Reform-Design, 70565 Stuttgart,
www.reform-design.de
Composing: Stahringer Satz GmbH, 35305 Grünberg
Printing and binding: Mayr Miesbach GmbH,
Druck · Medien · Verlag, 83714 Miesbach
Printed on paper bleached without chlorine or acid.

ISBN 978-3-7945-2799-1

Foreword

Cardiovascular magnetic resonance has evolved at enormous pace over the last decades. Starting from early experiments to probe cardiac high-energy phosphate metabolism by spectroscopic methods in the 1970s, the development of zeugmatography led to first attempts producing pictures of the heart in 1982. The potential of magnetic resonance imaging started to emerge and the assessment of cardiac morphology and function gained momentum. Important methodological improvements have been added to the fundamental concept over the years enabling a steady growth of cardiovascular applications.

Among the various imaging modalities available to assess the cardiovascular system, magnetic resonance imaging stands out. Besides its fully non-invasive principle permitting imaging without the use of ionizing radiation, it is the great versatility that makes magnetic resonance so attractive. Various tissue-related properties including water concentration, composition, perfusion and diffusion can be imaged. Moreover, methods encoding quantitative information of the dynamics of cardiac function and blood flow are at hand. Further advances now even permit to interrogate aspects of microstructure including myofiber arrangement. And, the range of applications continues to grow with hyperpolarization methods enabling insights into cardiac metabolism in real-time. Alongside there is an increasing number of clinical indications and routine use of cardiovascular magnetic resonance imaging is spreading word-wide.

The ability to resolve high-resolution anatomical and functional detail and the option to perform repeated measurements and longitudinal studies in conjunction with the wealth of contrast options have also triggered significant progress in experimental applications. These include the use of magnetic resonance imaging to guide cardiovascular interventions. Beyond application in humans, imaging of animal models has attracted considerable attention as part of a bench-to-bedside approach to understanding disease onset, progression and therapeutic options.

Considering the complexity of the magnetic resonance principle, advances have been and continue to be the result of very close interaction between physicians and scientists. Adoption of new methods and their translation into clinical reality necessitate forward thinking, expertise and enthusiasm. It is not surprising that major contributors in the field speak both scientific and medical "language".

The present book exemplifies the interdisciplinarity of the field and the collaboration across disciplines bringing together contributions from physicists and clinical colleagues. Covering the fundamentals including the magnetic resonance principle, hardware and safety considerations, to the full portfolio of clinical applications, the book also addresses innovative techniques and experimental methods.

Acknowledging the steady development and progress in diagnostic modalities other than magnetic resonance imaging, an overview of the principles and applications of state-of-the-art computed tomography is part of the content.

The authors of the different chapters are world-experts in their respective fields. It is a challenge to bring together such expertise and it is even more challenging to form a congruent and consistent essay of the different topics. Thanks to the excellent work of the authors and the editors this task has been accomplished.

In view of other textbooks available, the present work is comprehensive and unique in that it also includes topics beyond the standard portfolio of applications of cardiovascular magnetic resonance. Areas such as the measurement of myocardial blood flow and myocardial oxygenation, heart failure and cardiac transplantation, follow-up of cardiovascular interventions, pulmonary circulation, incidental findings on routine examinations, experimental studies in animals, and the role of cardiac computed tomography in clinical routine are included.

The book will appeal to users new to the field and experienced researchers and clinicians alike. References to the relevant literature including the key and most recent publications make it easy to connect to the much wider spectrum that is impossible to cover in a single textbook.

We are convinced the reader will enjoy the clarity and quality of the text, the description of the many routine applications in patients with all types of cardiovascular disease and the outlook of the innovations ahead.

It is our pleasure to congratulate the editors and authors for their efforts in providing this comprehensive summary and review of the exciting and rapidly evolving field of cardiovascular magnetic resonance imaging.

Zurich, August 2012

Sebastian Kozerke, Peter Bösiger
Institute for Biomedical Engineering,
University and ETH Zurich

Preface

The first edition of this book was published in Germany in 2005 at a time when cardiac MRI (CMR) gained increasing interest for diagnosis of cardiovascular diseases. With the ongoing technical advances of MRI over recent years, CMR has rendered highly effective for clinical applications and proven unique performance in the evaluation of cardiovascular anatomy, physiology, and pathophysiology. The continuously increasing interest in CMR is mainly driven by its ability to provide high resolution anatomical, functional and structural information with unique soft tissue contrast without the need for any ionizing radiation.

Over the last years a huge number of scientific publications on CMR methods and its clinical application to the diagnosis of cardiovascular diseases has been published resulting in some major advances of MRI in the cardiovascular field. With the 2nd edition of this book, the current state of CMR including all relevant recent technical advances will be covered, and the publication in English will bring the fascinating CMR technique to a broader international readership.

We like to express our gratitude to all authors who did a tremendous job in providing a comprehensive and excellent state-of-the-art description of their topics. We are grateful to the international publishers of journals and books, who gave their permission to reproduce figures from original publications. Many thanks to Mrs. Lisa Leick and Dr. William Adamson, Ulm, who as native speaker carefully proofread the chapters. We appreciate very much the substantial financial support of the Rudolf and Clothilde Eberhardt Foundation Ulm. Without their grant this book could not have been realized and published. Finally, we are also indebted to the Publishers, particularly the readers Mrs. Eva Wallstein, Dr. Annett Gesien and Mrs. Ellen Sudholt, for their extremely valuable readership, and the management of Schattauer Publishers, Mr. Bergemann and Dr. Bertram, for their valuable and consistent support for publishing this book.

We hope that the interested reader will read this book with great pleasure and will take advantage of this information for his/her daily work in experimental research and/or clinical routine. We appreciate very much the reader's response to this book and look forward to receiving comments and suggestions for the upcoming editions of the book.

Ulm and Berlin, August 2012

Vinzenz Hombach
Nico Merkle
Volker Rasche

Contributors

Jörg Barkhausen, MD
Department of Radiology and Nuclear Medicine
University Hospital of Schleswig-Holstein, Campus Lübeck
Ratzeburger Allee 160, Zentralklinikum (Haus 40)
D-23538 Lübeck, Germany
joerg.barkhausen@uksh.de

Philipp Beerbaum, MD, PhD
Cardiac Imaging Group
Department for Radiology and Paediatric Cardiology
Radboud University Nijmegen Medical Centre
Geert Grooteplein zuid 10, Route 766
NL-6525 GA Nijmegen, The Netherlands
p.beerbaum@cukz.umcn.nl

Peter Bernhardt, MD
Cardiology – Angiology – Pneumology –
Sports and Rehabilitation Medicine
Department of Internal Medicine II
University Hospital of Ulm
Albert-Einstein-Allee 23
D-89081 Ulm, Germany
peter.bernhardt@uniklinik-ulm.de

Axel Bornstedt, PhD
Experimental Cardiovascular Imaging (ExCaVI)
and Core Facility Small Animal MRI
Department of Internal Medicine II
University Hospital of Ulm
Albert-Einstein-Allee 23
D-89081 Ulm, Germany
axel.bornstedt@uni-ulm.de

René Botnar, PhD
Division of Imaging Sciences
School of Medicine, King's College London
The Rayne Institute 4th Floor Lambeth Wing
St Thomas' Hospital
Lambeth Palace Road
GB-London SE1 7EH, Great Britain
rene.botnar@ kcl.ac.uk

Horst Brunner, MD
Department of Diagnostic and Interventional Radiology
University Hospital of Ulm
Steinhövelstraße 9
D-89079 Ulm, Germany
horst.brunner@uniklinik-ulm.de

Loren Budge, PhD
Cardiovascular Imaging Center
University of Virginia Health System
1215 Lee St., Box 800170
USA-Charlottesville, VA 22908
lbudge@virginia.edu

Kieran Clarke, PhD
Department of Physiology, Anatomy and Genetics
Centre for Clinical Magnetic Resonance Research
University of Oxford
GB-Oxford OX3 9DU, Great Britain
kieran.clarke@physiol.ox.ac.uk

Christoph Galm, MD
Section of Pediatric Cardiology
Department of Pediatrics
University Hospital of Ulm
Eythstraße 22
D-89079 Ulm, Germany
christoph.galm@uniklinik-ulm.de

Bernhard L. Gerber, MD
Departement Cardiovasculaire
Cliniques Universitaires St. Luc
Université Catholique de Louvain
Avenue Hippocrate 10
B-1200 Bruxelles, Belgique
bernhard.gerber@uclouvain.be
bernhard.gerber@clin.ucl.ac.be

Mathias Goyen, MD
University Medical Center Hamburg-Eppendorf
Martinistraße 52
D-20251 Hamburg, Germany
goyen@uke.de

Christina Heilmaier, MD
Institute of Diagnostic and Interventional Radiology and Neuroradiology
University Hospital of Essen
Hufelandstraße 55
D-45122 Essen, Germany
christina.heilmaier@uni-due.de

Christoph U. Herborn, MD, MBA
University Medical Center Hamburg-Eppendorf
Martinistraße 52
D-20251 Hamburg, Germany
herborn@uke.de

Volker Herold, PhD
Department of Experimental Physics 5 (Biophysics)
University of Würzburg
Am Hubland
D-97074 Würzburg, Germany
vrherold@physik.uni-wuerzburg.de

Karl-Heinz Hiller, PhD
Department of Experimental Physics 5 (Biophysics)
University of Würzburg
Am Hubland
D-97074 Würzburg, Germany
hiller@mr-bavaria.de

Martin Hoffmann, MD
Interventional Radiology
Department of Radiology
Kantonsspital Lucerne
CH-6000 Lucerne, Switzerland
martin.hoffmann@luks.ch

Cameron Holloway, MD
Department of Cardiovascular Medicine
Centre for Clinical Magnetic Resonance Research
John Radcliffe Hospital
University of Oxford
Headley Way
GB-Oxford OX3 9DU, Great Britain
cameron.holloway@dpag.ox.ac.uk

Vinzenz Hombach, MD
Cardiology – Angiology – Pneumology –
Sports and Rehabilitation Medicine
Department of Internal Medicine II
University Hospital of Ulm
Albert-Einstein-Allee 23
D-89081 Ulm, Germany
vinzenz.hombach@uni-ulm.de
vinzenz@hombach.us

Peter M. Jakob, PhD
Department of Experimental Physics 5 (Biophysics)
University of Würzburg
Am Hubland
D-97074 Würzburg, Germany
peja@physik.uni-wuerzburg.de

Raymond Kim, MD
Duke Cardiovascular Magnetic Resonance Center
DUMC, Box 3934 or Duke Clinic, Orange Zone, Rm 4231
Trent Drive
USA-Durham, NC 27710
rjkim@duke.edu

Won Yong Kim, MD, PhD
Department of Cardiology and MR Center
Aarhus University Hospital Skejby
Brendstrupgaardsvej 100
DK-8200 Aarhus, Denmark
yong.kim@ki.au.dk

Oliver Klass, MD
Department of Diagnostic and Interventional Radiology
University Hospital of Ulm
Steinhövelstraße 9
D-89079 Ulm, Germany
oliver.klass@uniklinik-ulm.de

Igor Klem, MD
Duke Cardiovascular Magnetic Resonance Center
DUMC, Box 3934 or Duke Clinic, Orange Zone, Rm 4231
Trent Drive
USA-Durham, NC 27710
iklem@duke.edu

Christopher M. Kramer, MD
Cardiovascular Imaging Center
University of Virginia Health System
1215 Lee St., Box 800170
USA-Charlottesville, VA 22908
ckramer@virginia.edu

Markus Kunze, MD
Cardiology – Angiology – Pneumology –
Sports and Rehabilitation Medicine
Department of Internal Medicine II
University Hospital of Ulm
Albert-Einstein-Allee 23
D-89081 Ulm, Germany
markus.kunze@uniklinik-ulm.de

Gregory M. Lanza, MD, PhD
Cardiovascular Division
Washington University School of Medicine
Campus Box 8215, 4320 Forest Park
USA-St. Louis, MO 63108
greg@cvu.wustl.edu
greg.lanza@mac.com

Peter R. Luijten, PhD
UMC Utrecht
Heidelberglaan 100 (P.O. Box 85500),
room Q 02.2.315 (E 01.132)
NL-3584 CX Utrecht (3508 GA Utrecht), The Netherlands
P.Luijten@umcutrecht.nl

Nico Merkle, MD
Gemeinschaftspraxis für Radiologie und Neuroradiologie
and Zentrum für minimal invasive Therapie
Heinz-Galinski-Straße 1
D-13347 Berlin, Germany
nico.merkle@ihre-radiologen.de

Stefan Neubauer, MD
Department of Cardiovascular Medicine
Centre for Clinical Magnetic Resonance Research
John Radcliffe Hospital
University of Oxford
Headley Way
GB-Oxford OX3 9DU, Great Britain
stefan.neubauer@cardiov.ox.ac.uk

Dipanjan Pan, MD
Cardiovascular Division
Washington University School of Medicine
Campus Box 8215, 4320 Forest Park
USA-St. Louis, MO 63108
dpan@ cvu.wustl.edu

Sandra Pauls, MD
Section of Radiology and Nuclear Medicine
Sana Kliniken Lübeck GmbH
Kronsforder Allee 71–73
D-23560 Lübeck, Germany
Sandra.Pauls@Sana.de

Volker Rasche, PhD
Experimental Cardiovascular Imaging (ExCaVI)
and Core Facility Small Animal MRI
Department of Internal Medicine II
University Hospital of Ulm
Albert-Einstein-Allee 23
D-89081 Ulm, Germany
volker.rasche@uni-ulm.de

Maythem Saeed, PhD
Department of Radiology and Biomedical Imaging
San Francisco General Hospital
School of Medicine
University of California, San Francisco
185 Berry Street, Suite 350, Campus Box 0946
USA-San Francisco, CA 94107-5705
Maythem.Saeed@ucsf.edu

Tobias Schäffter, PhD
Division of Imaging Sciences
School of Medicine, King's College London
The Rayne Institute 4th Floor Lambeth Wing
St Thomas' Hospital
Lambeth Palace Road
GB-London SE1 7EH, Great Britain
tobias.schaeffter@kcl.ac.uk

Jeanette Schulz-Menger, MD
Cardiac MRI Unit
Klinik und Poliklinik für Kardiologie und Nephrologie
HELIOS Klinikum Berlin and Charité Campus Buch
Universitätsmedizin Berlin
Schwanebecker Chaussee 50
D-13125 Berlin, Germany
jeanette.schulz-menger@charite.de

Christian Schumann, MD
Section of Pneumology
Cardiology – Angiology – Pneumology –
Sports and Rehabilitation Medicine
Department of Internal Medicine II
University Hospital of Ulm
Albert-Einstein-Allee 23
D-89081 Ulm, Germany
christian.schumann@uniklinik-ulm.de

Johannes Schwab, MD
Medical Clinic 8 – Cardiology and
Institute of Diagnostic and Interventional Radiology
Klinikum Nürnberg Süd
Breslauer Straße 201
D-90471 Nuremberg, Germany
Johannes.Schwab@klinikum-nuernberg.de

Jochen Spiess, MD
Cardiology – Angiology – Pneumology –
Sports and Rehabilitation Medicine
Department of Internal Medicine II
University Hospital of Ulm
Albert-Einstein-Allee 23
D-89081 Ulm, Germany
jochen.spiess@uniklinik-ulm.de

Matthias Stuber, PhD
Center for BioMedical Imaging (CIBM)
Centre Hospitalier Universitaire Vaudois (CHUV)
Rue de Bugnon 46, BH 8.80
CH-1011 Lausanne, Switzerland
matthias.stuber@chuv.ch

Florian Vogt, MD
Department of Radiology and Nuclear Medicine
University Hospital of Schleswig-Holstein, Campus Lübeck
Ratzeburger Allee 160, Zentralklinikum (Haus 40)
D-23538 Lübeck, Germany
florian.vogt@uksh.de

Ralf Wassmuth, MD
Cardiac MRI Unit
Klinik und Poliklinik für Kardiologie und Nephrologie
HELIOS Klinikum Berlin and Charité Campus Buch
Universitätsmedizin Berlin
Schwanebecker Chaussee 50
D-13125 Berlin, Germany
ralf.wassmuth@charite.de

Mark W. Wilson, MD
Department of Radiology and Biomedical Imaging
San Francisco General Hospital
School of Medicine
University of California, San Francisco
185 Berry Street, Suite 350, Campus Box 0946
USA-San Francisco, CA 94107-5705
mark.wilson@ucsf.edu

Sabine Wuchenauer, MD
Department of Diagnostic and Interventional Radiology
University Hospital of Ulm
Steinhövelstraße 9
D-89079 Ulm, Germany
sabine.wuchenauer@uniklinik-ulm.de

Abbreviations

Abbreviations in Clinical Cardiovascular Disease

AAA abdominal aortic aneurysm
ACA anterior cerebral artery
ACE arteria carotis externa (external carotid artery)
ACC American College of Cardiology
ACI arteria carotis interna (internal carotid artery)
ACS acute coronary syndrome
AF atrial fibrillation
AHA American Heart Association
AIE arteria iliaca externa (external iliac artery)
AII arteria iliaca interna (internal iliac artery)
AMI acute myocardial infarction
Ao aorta
AP anterior-posterior (orientation)
APAH associated pulmonary arterial hypertension
AR aortic regurgitation
ARVD arrhythmogenic right ventricular dysplasia
AS aortic stenosis
ASA atrial septal aneurysm
ASD atrial septal defect
$AVDO_2$ arteriovenous oxygen difference
AVM arteriovenous malformation
AVR aortic valve replacement (surgical)
AVSD atrioventricular septal defect

BMD Becker muscular dystrophy
BSA body surface area

C compliance
CABG coronary artery bypass graft (grafting)
CAC coronary artery calcium
CAD coronary artery disease
CBF coronary blood flow
CBF cerebral blood flow
CCA common carotid artery
cNC cardiac non-compaction
ccTGA congenitally corrected transposition of the great arteries
CHD congenital heart disease
CFR coronary flow reserve
CHF chronic heart failure
CI cardiac index
cMR congenital mitral regurgitation
cMS congenital mitral stenosis
CO cardiac output
CoA coarctation of the aorta
COPD chronic obstructive pulmonary disease
CPC cardiovascular progenitor cells
cPS congenital pulmonary stenosis
CRT cardiac resynchronization therapy
CS coronary sinus
CSF coronary sinus flow
CSS Churg-Strauss syndrome
CT computerized tomography
CTA CT angiography
CTED chronic thromboembolic disease
CTEPH chronic thromboembolic pulmonary hypertension
cTn cardiac troponin
CTO chronic total occlusion (of a coronary artery)

DILV double inlet left ventricle
DMD Duchenne muscular dystrophy
DORV double outlet right ventricle
DSA digital subtraction angiography
DVT deep vein thrombosis

ECA external carotid artery
ECG electrocardiogram
EDMD Emery-Dreifuss muscular dystrophy
EDV end-diastolic volume
EDVI end-diastolic volume index
EDWT end-diastolic wall thickness
EF ejection fraction
EPS electrophysiological study
ERO effective regurgitant orifice
ESC European Society of Cardiology
ESC embryonic stem cells
ESHLT European Society of Heart and Lung Transplantation
ESV end-systolic volume
ESVI end-systolic volume index
ET endothelin
EVAR endovascular aortic (stent graft) repair
EVCPP endoventricular circular patch plasty (Dor procedure)

FPP	first-pass perfusion (study)
GRE	gradient recalled echo (sequence)
HCM	hypertrophic cardiomyopathy
HFdEF	heart failure with depressed (left ventricular) ejection fraction
HFnEF	heart failure with normal (left ventricular) ejection fraction
HFpEF	heart failure with preserved (left ventricular) ejection fraction
HFrEF	heart failure with reduced (left ventricular) ejection fraction
HIV	human immunodeficiency virus
HLHS	hypoplastic left heart syndrome
HOCM	hypertrophic obstructive cardiomyopathy
ICA	internal carotid artery
ICD	implantable cardiac defibrillator
IDC(M)	idiopathic dilated cardiomyopathy
ICM	ischemic cardiomyopathy
IMH	intramural hematoma (of the aorta)
IS	infarct size
IVC	inferior vena cava (caval vein)
IVRT	isovolumetric relaxation time
IVS	interventricular septum
LA	left atrium
LAD	left anterior descendent (coronary) artery
LC	lung cancer
LCX	left circumflex (coronary artery)
LHAS	lipomatous hypertrophy of the (inter)atrial septum
LSVC	left superior vena cava (caval vein)
LV	left ventricle
LVEF	left ventricular ejection fraction
LVEDV	left ventricular end-diastolic volume
LVEDVI	left ventricular end-diastolic volume index
LVESV	left ventricular end-systolic volume
LVESVI	left ventricular end-systolic volume index
LVMM	left ventricular muscle mass
LVOT	left ventricular outflow tract
MBF	myocardial blood flow
MCA	medial cerebral artery
MD	muscular dystrophy
MI	myocardial infarction
MR	mitral regurgitation
MS	mitral stenosis
MTT	mean transit time
MVA	mitral valve area
MVO_2	myocardial oxygen consumption
MVR	mitral valve replacement
NC	non-compaction (of the ventricles) = ventricular non-compaction
NPV	negative predictive value
NSTEMI	non-ST-elevation myocardial infarction
nsVT	non sustained ventricular tachycardia
OR	original report
PA	pulmonary artery
PAH	pulmonary arterial hypertension
PAP	pulmonary arterial pressure
PAPVC(R)	partial anomalous pulmonary venous connection (return)
PAU	penetrating aortic ulcer
PCA	posterior cerebral artery
PCH	pulmonary capillary hemangiomatosis
PCI	percutaneous coronary intervention
PCR	percutaneous coronary revascularization
PDA	patent ductus arteriosus
PDA	posterior descendent (coronary) artery
PE	pulmonary embolism
PEA	pulmonary (thromb)endarterectomy
PH	pulmonary hypertension
PLV	posterior left ventricular branch of the RCA or LCX (coronary artery)
PPCM	post-partum (peri-partum) cardiomyopathy
PPV	positive predictive value
PPVI	percutaneous pulmonary valve implantation
PR	pulmonary regurgitation
PTCA	percutaneous transluminal coronary angioplasty
PVI	pulmonary vein isolation (for ablation of atrial fibrillation)
PVOD	pulmonary veno-occlusive disease
PVOD	peripheral vascular occlusive disease
PVR	pulmonary vascular resistance
PVR	pulmonary valve replacement
PWV	pulse wave velocity
Qp	pulmonary blood flow (quantitative blood flow through both lungs)
Qs	systemic blood flow (quantitative blood flow in the systemic circulation)
RA	right atrium
RCA	right coronary artery
RCM	restrictive cardiomyopathy
RFA	radiofrequency ablation
RV	right ventricle
RVEF	right ventricular ejection fraction
RVEDV	right ventricular end-diastolic volume

RVEDVI	right ventricular end-diastolic volume index
RVESV	right ventricular end-systolic volume
RVESVI	right ventricular end-systolic volume index
RVOT	right ventricular outflow tract
SCD	sudden cardiac death
SLE	systemic lupus erythematosus
SS	systemic sclerosis
STEMI	ST-elevation myocardial infarction
SV	stroke volume
SVI	stroke volume index
SVC	superior vena cava (caval vein)
sVT	sustained ventricular tachycardia
TAC	truncus arteriosus communis (common trunk)
TAPVC(R)	total anomalous pulmonary venous connection (return)
TASH	transcutaneous alcohol septal ablation
TAVI	transcutaneous aortic valve implantation
TCPC	total cavo-pulmonary connection
TDI	tissue Doppler imaging
TEE	transesophageal echocardiography
TEVAR	thoracic endovascular aortic repair
TGA	transposition of the great arteries
Tn	(cardiac) troponin
ToF	tetralogy of Fallot
TR	tricuspid regurgitation
TS	tricuspid stenosis
TT	transit time
TTE	transthoracic echocardiography
TVP	transplant (coronary) vasculopathy
Tx-CAD	(heart) transplant coronary artery disease
UA	unstable angina
VA	ventricular arrhythmias
VBA	vertebral artery
VF	ventricular fibrillation
V/Q scan	ventilation-perfusion scan
VSD	ventricular septal defect
VT	ventricular tachycardia

Abbreviations in (Cardiac) Magnetic Resonance Imaging

AIF	arterial input function
AP	anterior-posterior (orientation)
ASL	arterial spin labeling
B_0	static magnetic field
bFFE	balanced fast field echo = SSFP sequence
BOLD	blood oxygen level dependent (imaging)
BRISK	block regional interpolations scheme
CAC	coronary artery calcium
CE	contrast-enhanced
2-ch	two-chamber (view)
3-ch	three-chamber (view)
4-ch	four-chamber (view)
CHESS	chemical shift selective (prepulse)
CLIO	coated iron oxide (particles)
CMR	cardiac magnetic resonance
CMRI	cardiac magnetic resonance imaging
CNR	contrast-to-noise ratio
CSI	chemical shift imaging
CCTA	coronary computerized tomography angiography
CTA	computerized tomography angiography
DE-CMR	delayed enhancement cardiac magnetic resonance imaging
DENSE	displacement encoding with stimulated echoes (imaging of myocardial displacement and strain)
DIR	double inversion recovery (prepulse)
DNP	dynamic nuclear polarization
DRESS	depth-resolved surface (coil in vivo) spectroscopy
EBT	electron beam tomography
EPI	echo planar imaging
FARM	fast acquisition relaxation mapping
FAST	(image-guided) four-angle saturation transfer
FFE	fast field echo (synonym of GRE)
FH	foot-head (orientation)
FIESTA	fast imaging employing steady-state acquisitions = SSFP sequence
FISP	fast imaging with steady-state precession = SSFP sequence
FLASH	fast low angle shot
FOV	field of view
FSE	fast spin echo
Ga	gadolinium (-based contrast agent)
Gd	gadolinium
GE	gradient echo

GRAPPA	generalized autocalibrating partially parallel acquisition (parallel imaging in k-space)
GRASE	gradient and spin echo (synonym of spin echo-EPI)
GRE	gradient recalled echo (sequence)
HARP	harmonic phase (analysis)
HASTE	half-fourier acquisition single-shot turbospin echo
HOPE	hybrid ordered phase encoding
HU	Hounsfield unit
ICMR	interventional cardiovascular magnetic resonance (imaging)
IR	inversion recovery (pulse)
ISIS	image-selected in vivo spectroscopy
LAO	left anterior oblique (view)
LGE	late gadolinium enhancement
MDCT	multi detector computerized tomography
MEMRI	manganese-enhanced magnetic resonance imaging
MIO	micrometer (sized) iron oxide (particles)
MIP	maximum intensity projection
MO	microvascular obstruction
MOTSA	multiple overlapping thin slab acquisition
MPR	multiplanar reconstruction
MRA	magnetic resonance angiography
MRCA	magnetic resonance coronary angiography
MRI	magnetic resonance imaging
MRM	magnetic resonance microscopy
MRS	magnetic resonance spectroscopy
MSCT	multislice (multidetector) computerized tomography
MTC	magnetization transfer contrast
MTS	magnetization transfer saturation
NMR	nuclear magnetic resonance
PC	phase-contrast (flow mapping)
PCA	phase contrast angiography
PE	phase-encoding
PET	positron emission tomography
PEVM	phase-encoded velocity mapping
PILS	partially parallel imaging with localized sensitivities (parallel imaging in spatial domain)
PMO	persistent microvascular obstruction
pMRI	parallel magnetic resonance imaging
PSEM	pressure strain elastic modulus
RAO	right anterior oblique (view)
REST	regional saturation technique
RF	radiofrequency (pulse)
ROI	region of interest
ROPE	respiratory ordered phase encoding
sa	short axis (view)
SA	signal averaging (averaged)
SAR	specific absorption rate
SE	spin echo (sequence)
SE-EPI	spin echo EPI (echo planar imaging)
SENC	strain encoding (to measure strain)
SENSE	sensitivity encoding (parallel imaging in spatial domain)
SI	signal intensity
SLOOP	spectral localization with optimum point spread function
SMART	serial motion artefact reduction technique
SMASH	simultaneous acquisition of spatial harmonics (parallel imaging in k-space)
SNR	signal-to-noise ratio
SPAMM	spatial modulation of magnetization
SPECT	single photon emission computed tomography
SPGE	spoiled gradient echo
SPI	spiral planar imaging
SPIO	small superparamagnetic iron oxide (particles)
SPIR	spectral inversion recovery (prepulse)
SSFP	steady-state free precession (sequence) = bFFE, true FISP, FIESTA
STIR	short tau inversion recovery (prepulse)
T	Tesla
T1	longitudinal relaxation time
T2	transversal relaxation time
TE	echo time
TI	inversion time
TOF	time-of-flight (MR angiography)
TPM	tissue phase mapping
TR	repetition time
TrueFISP	true fast imaging with steady-state precession = SSFP sequence
TSE	turbospin echo (sequence)
TSI	tissue synchronisation index
UBO	unknown bright object (artefact)
USPIO	ultrasmall superparamagnetic iron oxide (particles)
VENC = Venc	velocity encoded (encoding)

Contents

Part III
Innovative and Experimental Imaging Techniques

Part I

Basic Technology

1 Basic Principles of Cardiac Magnetic Resonance Imaging

Volker Rasche and Tobias Schäffter

1.1 Nuclear Spin and Magnetic Moment

In clinical magnetic resonance imaging (MRI) the magnetic moment μ of the water- or fat-bound hydrogen (^1H) protons of the biological tissue is used for image formation. As a basic property, the proton has a so-called spin, which in the **classical picture** can be interpreted as a rotation of the proton around its central axis. The related rotating electrical charge of the proton causes a magnetic moment μ. After introduction of the proton into an external static magnetic field B_0, μ aligns with the direction of B_0. Due to the quantum mechanical properties of the spin, the orientation of μ relative to B_0 can only take two discrete angles of $\pm$ 54.7° called spin-up (parallel) or spin-down (anti-parallel) as

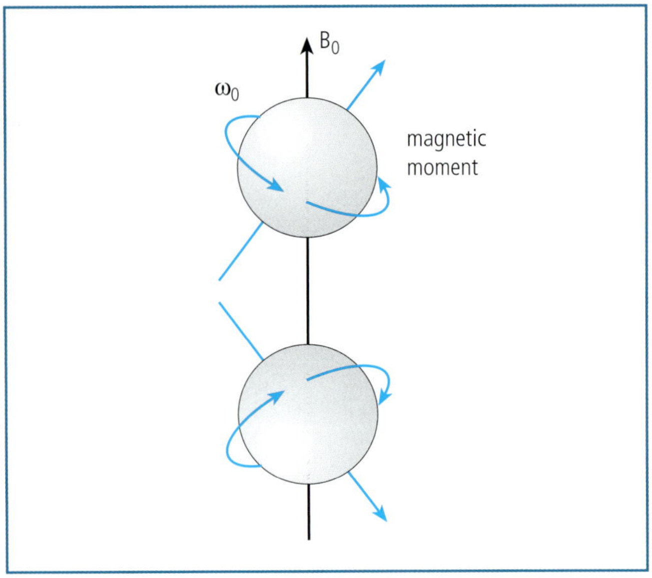

Figure 1-1 Possible orientations of the magnetic moment μ with the external static magnetic field B_0.

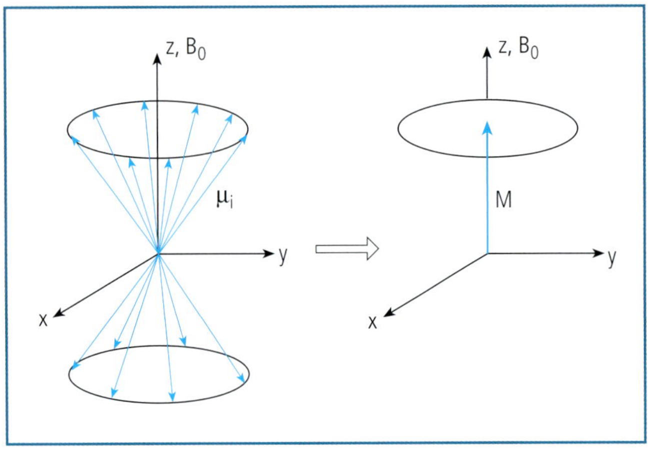

Figure 1-2 Formation of the macroscopic magnetic moment M after introduction of an ensemble of spins in a magnetic field.

shown in Figure 1-1. Similar to a gyroscope precessing around the axis of the gravitational field, μ starts precessing around the axis of B_0 with the **Larmor frequency** $\omega_0 = \gamma B_0$. For hydrogen nuclei, the gyromagnetic ratio is γ_H = 42.6 MHz/T, yielding ω_0 between 21 MHz (0.5 T) to 128 MHz (3 T) on conventional clinical MRI systems.

To explain final signal formation from biological tissue, an ensemble of protons must be considered. When the protons are introduced into the magnet field, the related spins are oriented arbitrarily in space. Each spin aligns either parallel or anti-parallel with B_0. After alignment their xy-component is distributed arbitrarily over a circle in the xy-plane (perpendicular to the B_0 axis) and each spin is precessing around the z-axis (aligned with B_0 axis) at the Larmor frequency. All microscopic magnetic moments μ_i sum up to a macroscopic magnetic moment M as shown in Figure 1-2. Since more spins are in the low-energy (spin-up) state than in the high-energy (spin-down) state, macroscopic magnetization M is formed, which is aligned along B_0. Due to the random distribution of the transversal components of the μ_i, in the **thermal equilibrium** state, the resulting transversal component of the macroscopic magnetic moment M_{xy} equals 0 and the longitudinal component M_z equals M_0, with M_0 being the available magnetization in the thermal equilibrium state. It can be shown that M behaves like a classical magnetic moment, the behavior, which can be described by the classical **Bloch equations.**

1.1.1 Excitation of the Spin System

In the *thermal equilibrium* state the magnetization M is static and no magnetic resonance (MR) signal can be measured by an external antenna (coil). For generation of a measurable signal, a magnetic component in the xy-plane has to be generated, meaning that M has to be rotated towards the xy-plane to generate a non-zero M_{xy} component. According to the *Bloch equations* rotation of M can be obtained by irradiation with electromagnetic waves (*RF-pulse*) at the Larmor frequency causing the formation of an M_{xy} component (Figure 1-3). This transversal magnetization M_{xy} precesses in the xy-plane with *Larmor frequency* and induces an MR signal into the external coil. The process of generating transversal magnetization is called *excitation* of the spin system. In a simplified picture (*rotating frame*) the excitation can be described as a simple rotation of M around the y-axis. Depending on the length of the RF excitation pulse, M is rotating around a certain *excitation angle* α (also called flip angle). In principle, α can more or less be chosen

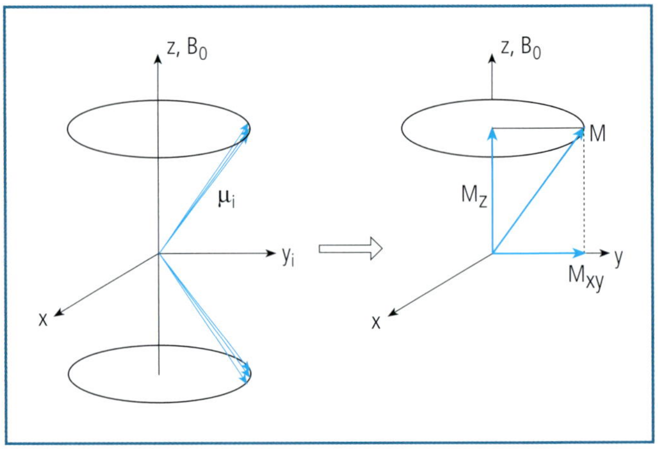

Figure 1-3 Formation of a measurable M_{xy} component by synchronization of the precessing spins and transfer of spins into the high energy state.

arbitrarily with typical values between 10° and 90° (depending on the acquisition technique). Special excitation pulses include a 90° excitation, in which the original magnetization M_0 is completely transferred to transversal magnetization and a 180° excitation, in which the magnetization is inverted.

1.1.2 Chemical Shift

The Larmor frequency is defined according to the magnetic field at the location of the nucleus. Since the electrons circulating around the nucleus may partially shield the external magnetic field, the resulting Larmor frequency is depending on the environment of the hydrogen atom and hence on the tissue.

In **biological tissue** there are **two main components** with **sufficiently high hydrogen content**:
- water (in which the hydrogen is bound in a H_2O) and
- fat (in which the hydrogen is bound in a CH_2 complex).

Due to different shielding, the differently bound hydrogen nuclei show different resonance frequencies. This effect is called *chemical shift*. The chemical shift is tissue dependent, and between water and fat the chemical shift results to 3.5 ppm or roughly 75 Hz (0.5 T), 150 Hz (1.0 T), 225 Hz (1.5 T), and 450 Hz (3.0 T). In MRI, the chemical shift is e.g. used for fat suppression. Since the chemical shift is characteristic for the type of hydrogen bounding, it can be applied for analysis in **nuclear magnetic resonance spectroscopy**.

1.1.3 Relaxation Processes

After the *excitation*, the rotating M_{xy} component of M causes a measurable RF signal at the *Larmor frequency* in the receive coil, which is decaying over time. The reason for this is that the magnetization returns to equilibrium due to relaxation.

Relaxation combines **two independent different mechanisms**:
- **longitudinal relaxation** (or T1-relaxation), which corresponds to recovery of longitudinal magnetization, and
- **transverse relaxation** (or T2-relaxation), which corresponds to transverse magnetization decay.

Longitudinal Relaxation

The longitudinal relaxation describes the return of the spin system to the *thermal equilibrium* state. After the *excitation*, the spin system is in an excited state. As in any system, the spin system tends back to *thermal equilibrium* by transferring energy to its environment (the lattice). Therefore this process is also called *spin-lattice relaxation*. The transfer of energy causes spins to go back to the low energy state and hence cause the spin system to build up longitudinal magnetization until it finally approaches the thermal equilibrium state. The temporal behavior of the relaxation is described by an exponential function according to $M_z(t) = M_0\left(1 - e^{-\frac{t}{T_1}}\right)$, with T_1 being a tissue-specific constant describing the time required until 63 % of the initial magnetization is being re-established after a 90° pulse (Figure 1-4).

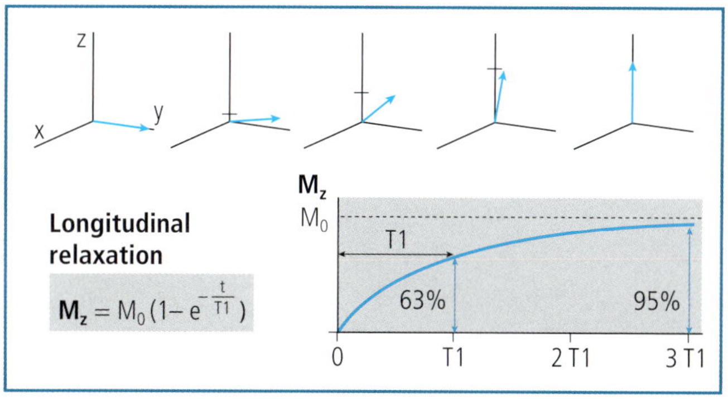

Figure 1-4 Return of the longitudinal magnetization M_z to the thermal equilibrium state after a 90° excitation.

Transversal Relaxation

The transversal relaxation describes the decay of the MRI signal after the excitation. The decay of the MRI signal after the excitation is caused by a loss of phase coherence between the spins. Directly after the excitation all spins are perfectly in phase (directed into the same direction). This results into the maximal possible transversal magnetization. In an ideal system, the spins would remain in-phase and the loss of transversal magnetization would be caused by the spin-lattice relaxation, only.

In a real system, however, the transversal magnetization decays much faster, caused by
- local **magnetic field fluctuations** due to spin-spin interactions (Figure 1-5), and
- local **magnetic field distortions** (inhomogeneities), which cause a loss of phase coherence and concomitant reduction of the transversal magnetization.

Local Field Fluctuations

The magnetic moment of each spin represents a tiny magnetic field (dipole field), which is superimposed to the main magnetic field B_0. Since the hydrogen atoms, and hence the related magnetic moments of the spins, are constantly moving, each spin is exposed to tiny rapidly fluctuating magnetic field changes caused by its neighboring spins. These fluctuating

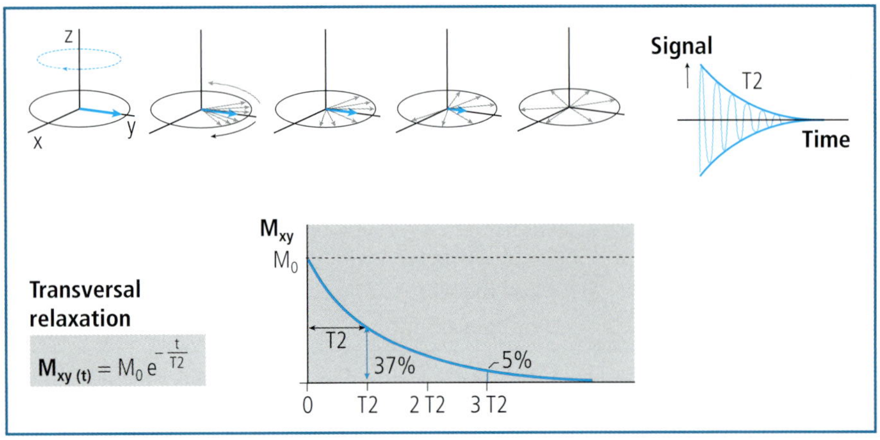

Figure 1-5 Decay of the transversal magnetization M_{xy} after a 90° excitation due to the loss of the phase coherence of the spins.

magnetic field distortions cause the spins to precess at locally fluctuating Larmor frequencies, which cause a loss of phase coherence.

Static Field Distortions

Decent MRI systems provide magnetic fields with excellent field homogeneity with less than 1 ppm deviation within the imaging volume. Slight field distortions are compensated by static *shimming* during installation of the system. The remaining source of local field variation is the object under investigation, caused by *susceptibility* differences of the different tissues. In contrast to the fluctuating field distortions introduced by the spin-spin interaction, the susceptibility introduced distortions are static.

The transversal relaxation due to the fluctuating magnetic fields causes an exponential decay of the transversal magnetization according to $M_{xy}(t) = M_0\, e^{-\frac{t}{T2}}$, with T2 describing the tissue-specific time period in which the transversal magnetization has decreased to 37 % of its initial value. The static field distortions cause a faster signal decay according to $M_{xy}(t) = M_0\, e^{-\frac{t}{T2^*}}$, with T2* being defined similar to T2.

In general, T2* < T2 << T1. Static off-resonance effects can be compensated by a *spin echo* experiment.

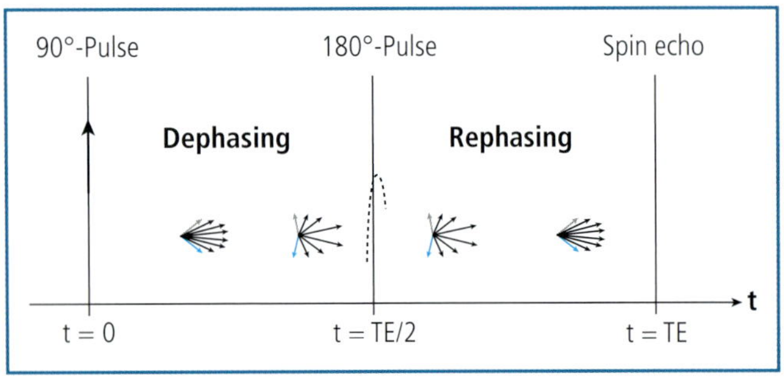

Figure 1-6 Principle of a spin echo experiment.

1.1.4 Spin Echo Experiment

The spin echo experiment is a sequence of rf-excitations, in which after the initial excitation pulse at TE/2 an additional 180° pulse (or *inversion pulse*) is applied and the signal is received at *echo time* TE (Figure 1-6).The spins loose phase coherence after excitation caused by the fluctuating magnetic fields and due to static perturbations of the main magnetic field. Spins experiencing a locally reduced static magnetic field precess with slightly reduced, those experiencing a slightly increased local static magnetic field with slightly increased rotation speed. Hence over time the spins accrue a magnetic field distortion ΔB_0 dependent phase. The loss of phase coherence causes a reduction of the transversal magnetization. The 180° inversion pulse at t = TE/2 causes an inversion of the phase of the spins. Thus spins rotating with lowest angular velocity change their position with those rotating at highest angular velocity (first gets last and vice versa). Since the local static magnetic field properties (and hence the rotation speed) do not change, the local angular velocities of the spins do not change (fastest is still fastest, slowest is still slowest). Hence, the spins gain the same phase over the following TE/2 interval and at t = TE all spins are in phase again. The spin echo principle relies on static magnetic field distortion. Fluctuating contributions still cause phase incoherence and the transversal magnetization will still decay with T2.

1.2 Contrast

In MRI the intrinsic and exogenic contrast mechanism have to be considered. Intrinsic contrast results from the intrinsic properties of the tissue, whereas exogenic contrasts are caused by injecting contrast giving compounds (contrast agents) into the human body, which alter the intrinsic contrast properties.

The contrast in medical imaging is based on the signal difference between adjacent tissues. The contrast C between two tissues is defined as the ratio of the signal difference and the signal sum according to $C_{1,2} = \frac{|S_1 - S_2|}{S_1 + S_2}$.

1.2.1 Intrinsic Contrast

The signal in MRI is governed by the differences in the transversal and longitudinal relaxation properties of the tissues (Table 1-1) and, to a less significant part, the local *spin density* in the tissue. The longitudinal relaxation property of the tissue depends on the main magnetic field strength with increasing T1 values with increasing field strength. T2 relaxation constants do normally less depend on the main magnetic field strength.

The influence of the relaxation properties of the tissue on the resulting MRI signal can be controlled by adequate selection of the MR sequence parameters. The important parameters here are the *repetition time* (TR) and the *echo time* (TE). TR is defined as the time interval between subsequent excitations of the spin system. Within this time longitudinal magnetization recovers due to the spin-lattice (longitudinal) relaxation. A short TR causes a non-complete return of the spin system to thermal equilibrium (Figure 1-7a). At the point of the subsequent excitation, only a fraction of the equilibrium magnetization can be transferred to transversal magnetization. Hence the available transversal magnetization (which is used for signal formation) strongly depends on the tissue T1 property (the available transversal magnetization is reciprocally proportional to the T1 relaxation time of the tissue). A long TR ($TR > 5 \times T1$) causes an almost complete return of the spin system to thermal equilibrium. Hence the transversal magnetization generated during the subsequent excitation (and hence the MRI signal measured) does not depend on the tissue T1 value (Figure 1-7b). Superimposed to the dependency of the resulting MR signal on the repetition time is its dependency on the echo time TE. TE is defined as the time between the actual excitation of the spin system and the time of the signal reception. In this time period, the generated transversal magnetization decays due to T2 relaxation (spin echo experiment) or T2* relaxation (non spin-echo experiment). The resulting MR signal is still proportional to the chosen repetition time and the respective T1-weighting, but additionally weighted by the T2(*) decay. A short TE reduces the impact of the T2(*) relaxation on the final MR signal, a long TE can be used for increasing the impact of the T2(*) relaxation. Furthermore, the MRI signal is proportional to the local spin density ϱ (or magnetization M_0), which defines the maximal available magnetization of the tissue. The resulting image contrast can be controlled by proper choice of the acquisition parameters (Table 1-2 and Table 1-3).

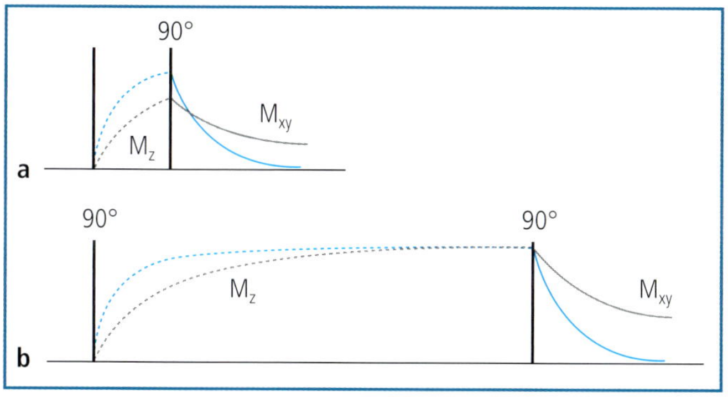

Figure 1-7 Available longitudinal magnetization in case of short TR (a) and long TR (b).

Table 1-1 Relaxation constants (T1, T2) and relative proton density (PD) for different human tissues.

Tissue	PD (%)	T1 (ms)		T2 (ms)	
		1.5 T	3 T	1.5 T	3 T
myocardium	80	1,030	1,470	45	
sceletal muscle	80	1,000	1,400	35	
oxygenated blood (100% O_2)	100	1,450	1,900	240	170
desoxygenated blood (35% O_2)	100	1,450	1,900	70	35
fat	100	280	365	165	133
kidney	81	700	1,200	55	

Table 1-2 Resulting image contrast depending on the sequence timing.

Weighting	TE	TR
T1-weighted	short	short
T2-weighted	long	long
PD-weighted	short	long

Table 1-3 Signal intensity of different tissues.

Tissue	T1-weighted	T2-weighted
fat	high	high
muscle	low	low
fluid	low	high
fibrous tissue	low/medium	low
air	no	no

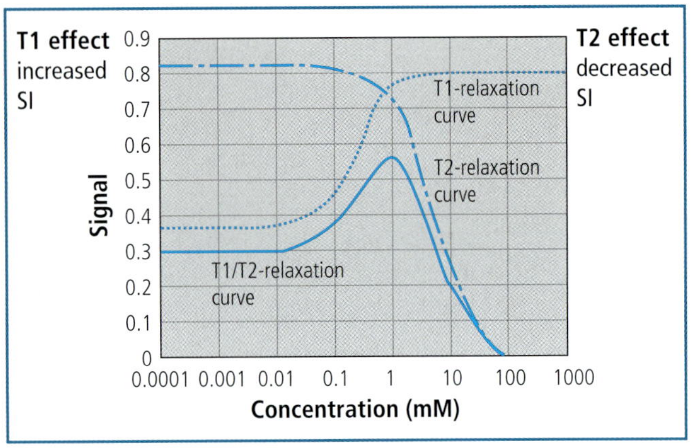

Figure 1-8 Dose efficiency curve of GD-DTPA.

1.2.2 Exogenic Contrast

The relaxation properties of tissues can be altered by the administration of contrast agents (CA) prior to scanning. CAs are defined as chemical compounds capable of markedly altering the local relaxation properties of e.g. the water protons in the tissue. In MRI, the absolute resulting changes in signal intensities are used as well as the dynamics of the changes caused by uptake and washout of the contrast agent by the body (pharmacokinetics). The efficiency of a contrast agent to change the relaxation rate is represented by the relaxivity r with r_1/r_2 describing the effeciency of altering the $T1/T2$ relaxation properties. With $T^{obs}_{1,2}$ being the observed relaxation time, $T_{1,2}$ the native relaxation constants, and $[M]$ the local concentration of the contrast agent, the observed relaxation constants can be calculated according to:

$$\frac{1}{T^{obs}_{1,2}} = \frac{1}{T_{1,2}} + r_{1,2}[M].$$

The relaxivity is measured in units of $mMol^{-1}s^{-1}$ and depends on the main magnetic field strength. In MRI, all CA have T1 as well as T2 effects. Thus, its efficiency does normally not show a simple linear relation on the signal intensities in the final image as used from e.g. X-ray imaging. A dose-efficiency curve is depicted in Figure 1-8 exemplarily for the commonly applied contrast agent Gd-DTPA. Here, at low doses, the T1 effect dominates resulting in an increase of signal intensity. With increasing dose, however, the signal reduction due to T2 shortening becomes dominant and the overall signal intensity decreases. Superposition of both effects results in a non-linear dose-efficiency curve usually showing a maximal effect for a certain dose.

MRI CAs do indirectly impact the signal intensity by local alteration of the relaxation properties. Thus, not the CA itself but its local changes to resonance properties are used for altering the MRI signal. Local changes are normally caused by interaction of the unpaired electron spins with the proton spins of the tissue. Efficient interactions occur by binding of the proton to the CA (inner-sphere water) as well as with unbound protons (outer-sphere water). Both effects significantly contribute to the overall efficiency of the CA by open up additional relaxation paths for the excited spins, which cause shortening of T1 as well as T2. Further mechanisms include the use of super paramagnetic iron oxides particles, which cause local magnetic field pertubations due to magnetic dipole moment of the particles. The fluctuating particles cause additional dephasing of the spins after excitation and significantly reduce T2 and T2* relaxation constants. With few exceptions (liver imaging), clinically approved CAs are based on Gadolinum (Gd^{3+}). Since Gd^{3+} itself is toxic, it has to be embedded in a complex. Commonly used complexes relevant for cardiovascular applications are summarized in Table 1-4.

CAs are administered intravenously either as bolus injection or as infusion. One has to distinguish between extracellular CAs, which extravasate quickly into the interstitial spaces (tissue perfusion) and intravascular CAs, which bind to albumin and are supposed to mainly remain in the bloodpool. Half-life time of extracellular CAs is usually in the order between 1 and 2 h and systemic clearance by the kidney is normally done after 24 h. Intravascular CAs re-

Table 1-4 Overview of most commonly used contrast agents. Relaxivity values are provided for 1.5 T.

Product	Active component	Concentration (mol/l)	Element	Relaxivity R1/R2	Comment
gadovist	gadobutrol	1.0	GD^{3+}	5.3/5.7	
magnevist	gadopentetat-dimeglumin	0.5	GD^{3+}	4.3/4.4	
multi-hance	gadobenat-dimeglumin	0.5	GD^{3+}	6.7/8.7	slight albumine binding
omniscan	gadodiamid	0.5	GD^{3+}	4.4/6.6	
prohance	gadoteridol	0.5	GD^{3+}	4.1/4.6	
vasovist	gadofosvesettrinatrium		GD^{3+}	21/46	binds to albumine ≥ blood pool

main in the blood stream for hours and systemic clearance can take up to 14 days.

Apart from intravascular agents, most CAs are unspecific and cannot be applied for specific targeting of structures of interests (with exception liver imaging). Future developments comprise specific targeted contrast agents, which can be used to specifically target molecular markers.

For more specific information on contrast agent-enhanced MRI, please see Chapter 3.

1.3 MR Imaging

With the current MR experiment, all magnetization generates a similar MRI signal independently on its origin. Assuming a perfectly homogeneous main magnetic field, after the excitation, each spin generates a signal S with constant frequency ω_L and its location cannot be extracted from the MRI signal. To resolve these ambiguities, the homogeneity of the static main magnetic field is disturbed by the superposition of small switchable magnetic fields, the strength of which linearly scales with increasing distance to the iso-center of the magnet. The linear magnetic fields are referred to as *gradient fields* or short *gradients* with abbreviation G (mT/m). Characteristic properties of the gradients include the gradient strength G_0 (mT/m), describing the maximal amplitude; its slew-rate dG/dt (mT/m × s), describing the speed a certain gradient can be switched; and its linearity.

The spatial encoding used in MR imaging can be separated in two subsequent steps, slice selection and spatial encoding of excited transversal magnetization, which will be described in the following two sections.

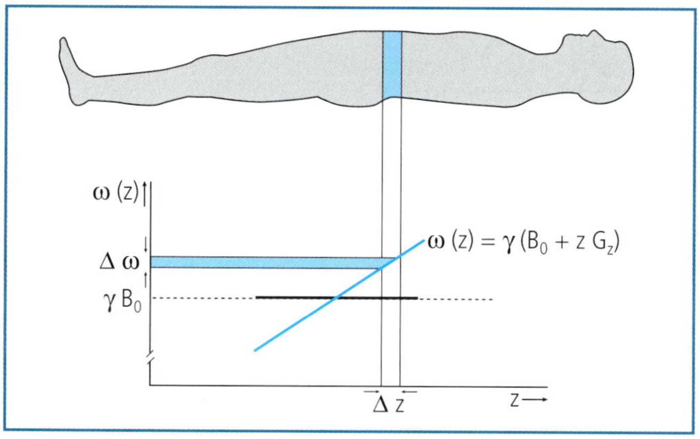

Figure 1-9 Superimposed linear magnetic fields cause a linear dependency of the resulting magnetic field and hence the local Larmor frequency from the location within the magnet.

1.4 Slice Selection

In most imaging applications not the entire object is of interest, but the imaging needs to be restricted to a certain slice/volume. This can be achieved by superposition of a spatially linear changing magnetic field G_z onto the main magnetic field B_0. This so-called gradient field causes a linear dependency of the local magnetic field along the z-direction according to $\bar{B}(z) = B_0 + zG_z$ (Figure 1-9). The modification of the local magnetic field causes a concomitant linear dependency of the Larmor frequency according to $\omega_0(z) = \gamma(B_0 + zG_z)$. So, spins located in a confined region Δz ranging from $z_0 - \frac{\Delta z}{2}$ to $z_0 + \frac{\Delta z}{2}$ can be identified according to their unique Larmor frequencies. In case the spins are irradiated with an RF pulse containing only Larmor frequencies within the respective range (bandwidth), only spins inside the slice/volume of interest are excited and will generate an MRI signal. Excitation of a certain frequency range can be achieved by applying an *RF excitation pulse with a sinc-shaped envelope*.

1.5 Spatial Encoding of the MR Signal

After selective excitation, three orthogonally oriented gradients are applied that enable variation of the main magnetic field in all spatial directions. Assuming a perfect linearity of the gradients, the resulting spatial dependency of the magnetic field $\bar{B}(r)$ yields $\bar{B}(r) = B_0 + \bar{r}\bar{G} = B_0 + xG_x + yG_y + zG_z$, causing a spatially dependent Larmor frequency. The different Larmor frequencies result in spatially dependent phase shifts of the measured MRI signal *S(t)*, which scale with time. It is important to note that the MRI signal of all spins is superimposed in the measured MRI signal. For the generation of the final image of the distribution of the magnetization $M_{xy}(r)$, the MRI signal has to be separated into the individual signals from the spatial locations under investigation, which is being done by applying a *Fourier transformation* to the measured MRI data *S(t)* (Figure 1-10). To resolve all ambiguities, the MRI signal has to be measured at as many different time points in each dimension as matrix elements (*pixel*) in the final reconstructed image. Since the gradients cause a phase, which is increasing linearly with space, the MRI signal is denoted to be measured in *k-space*, with the respective k-value *k(t)* describing the phase per meter at time t. The relation between k-value and the respective gradient is as $k = \gamma \times Gt$. At which positions in k-space the MRI signal has to be measured is defined by the acquisition

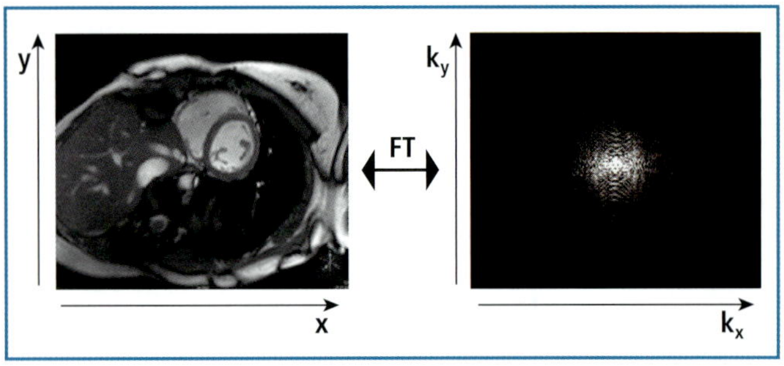

Figure 1-10 Image of the heart **(left)** and its respective representation in k-space **(right)**.

geometry (spatial resolution and spatial extent [*region of interest*]). The order of measurement (encoding of k-space) depends on the MRI acquisition technique chosen.

The spacing Δk of the measurement points in k-space is directly related to the coverage x_0 (*field of view*) in the spatial domain according to $x_0 \, \alpha \, \frac{1}{\Delta k}$, whereas the coverage in k-space k_0 defines the final spatial resolution Δx in the spatial domain according to $\Delta x \, \alpha \, \frac{1}{k_0}$.

1.5.1 k-Space Encoding

The direct relation between the gradient fields and the location in k-space implies that after the excitation of the spin system, the gradient fields have to be switched according to a function, which traverses the k-space dense enough and covers a sufficiently large volume, while simultaneous sampling of the MRI signal. In almost all MRI techniques, the k-space is not completely covered after a single excitation of the spin system. Main reason here is the resulting long acquisition time, which would be required for full coverage of k-space. Due to the T2 and T2* signal decay, the MR signal will be completely gone after some 100 ms. Therefore, the acquisition of all k-space data is normally split up into subsequent acquisitions of segments of the k-space, each acquired after an independent excitation of the spin system. In the majority of MRI techniques, the k-space is covered on a rectangular grid (*Cartesian grid*; Figure 1-13a). The acquisition is split up into a readout phase, in which normally one line in k-space (aligned with the x-axis) is acquired, and a phase encoding phase, in which the spin system is moved along the two remaining orthogonal axes before readout.

Readout Phase (Frequency-Encoding)

The readout phase can be interpreted as a one-dimensional MRI experiment (Figure 1-11). Directly after the excitation, the spin system is in the center of k-space (t_0, all spins in-phase). Application of a negative gradient in x-direction drives the spin system along the k_x-axis into negative direction until it reaches the minimal required k_x value at t_1 (spins gain increasing phase with increasing distance to the iso-center of the magnet and time, dephasing). By inverting the gradient sign, the spin system starts moving along the k_x-axis in positive direction (rephasing). At t_2, the spin system is back at the center of k-space (all spins in-phase). Continuation of the positive x-gradient enforces the spin system to continue moving along the positive direction until it reaches the maximal required k_x-value. The MRI signal is normally acquired from t_1 to t_3. The negative part of the gradient is called *pre-phasing gradient* and the positive part is called the *readout gradient*. The dephasing with subsequent rephasing causes the formation of a so-called gradient echo. Since the phase of the spins is not inverted as in the spin echo case (Figure 1-6), signal decay due to static off-resonances is not compensated (T2* decay). Compensation of static off-resonances can be achieved by incorporation of a spin echo in the readout phase by applying a 180° inversion pulse at TE/2 as shown in Figure 1-11.

Phase-Encoding

For covering the entire k-space, the spin system has to additionally be moved along the y-direction (two-dimensional imaging) or the y- and z-direction (three-dimensional imaging) in k-space. This is achieved by application of additional pre-phasing gradients in y- and z-direction (Figure 1-12). During the pre-phasing period, the spin system is additionally moved along the y- (2D) or y- and z- (3D) direction by application of additional *phase-encoding gradients* before applying the readout section. Each line in k-space has to be acquired with different y- and z-gradient amplitudes during subsequent excitations and is called a single *phase encoding step*. Different choices of gradient switching enables the coverage of k-space on different grids (*sampling pattern*) such as polar grids (radial sampling, FID sampling [UTE]) or spiral grids (Figure 1-13b, c). Where theoretically the image quality should be independent on the sampling pattern, rising image artifacts e.g. due to motion may be strongly dependent on the sampling pattern chosen.

> For acquiring an MRI image with $n_x \times n_y$ image pixel, in conventional imaging methods acquiring the MRI signal along a single line in k-space after each excitation, n_y excitations or basic MRI readout experiments have to be performed. Extension to 3D imaging with $n_x \times n_y \times n_z$ image voxel (voxel = 3D pixel) requires $n_y \times n_z$ excitations of the spin system.

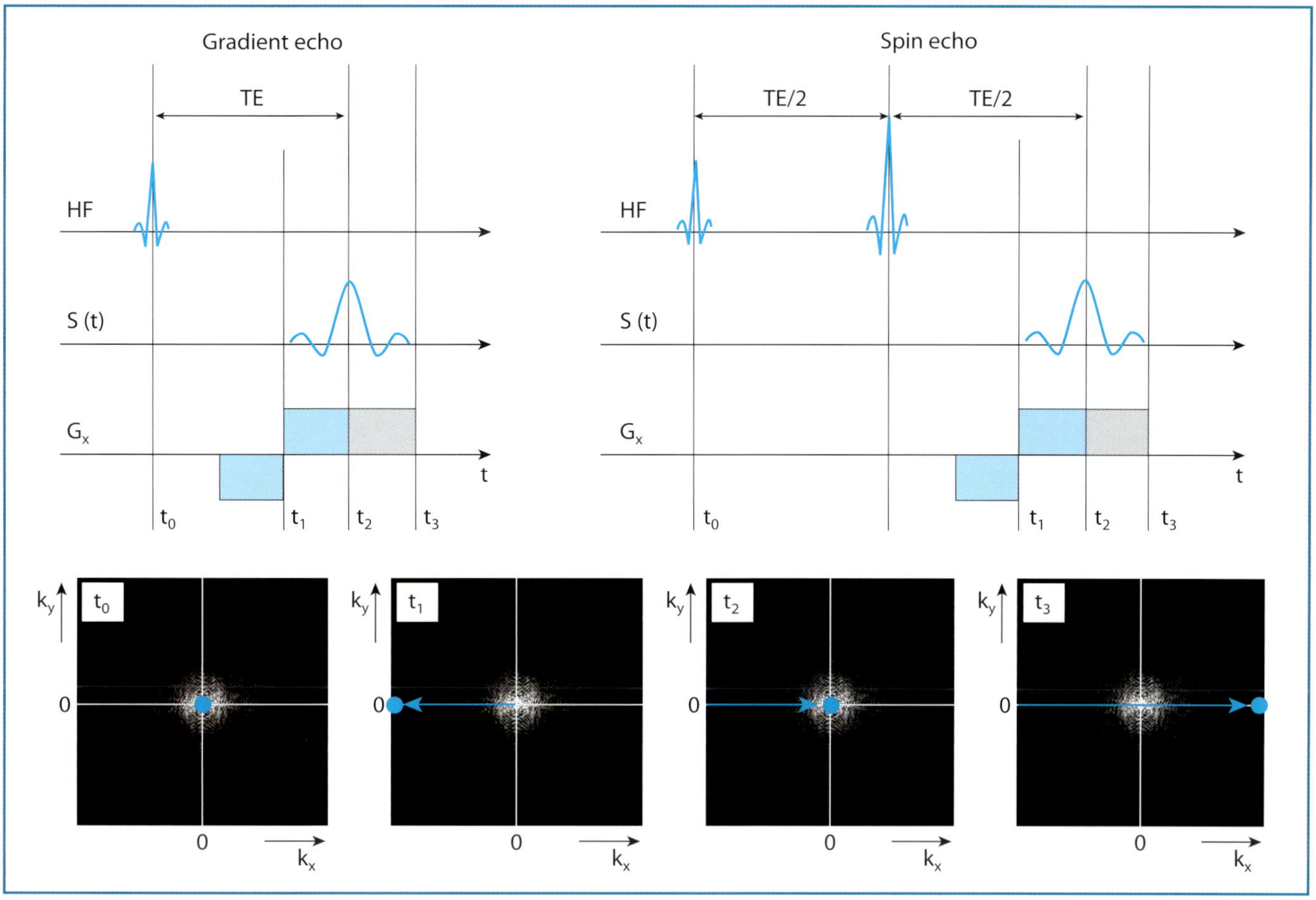

Figure 1-11 Principle of a single readout experiment covering a single x-line in k-space by a gradient echo or a spin echo technique. HF: excitation pulse; S(t): measured MRI signal; G_x: readout gradient in x-direction.

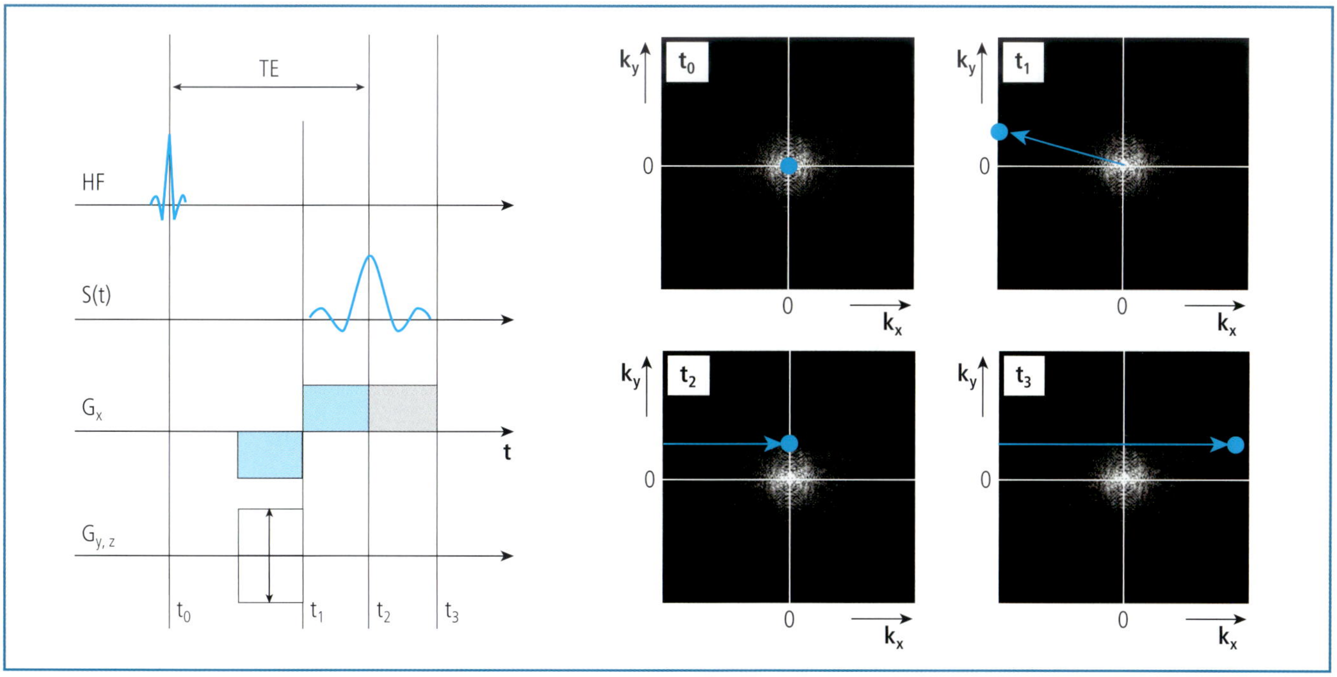

Figure 1-12 Application of additional phase-encoding gradients ($G_{y,z}$) enables the readout of k_x-lines located at different positions in y- and z-direction.

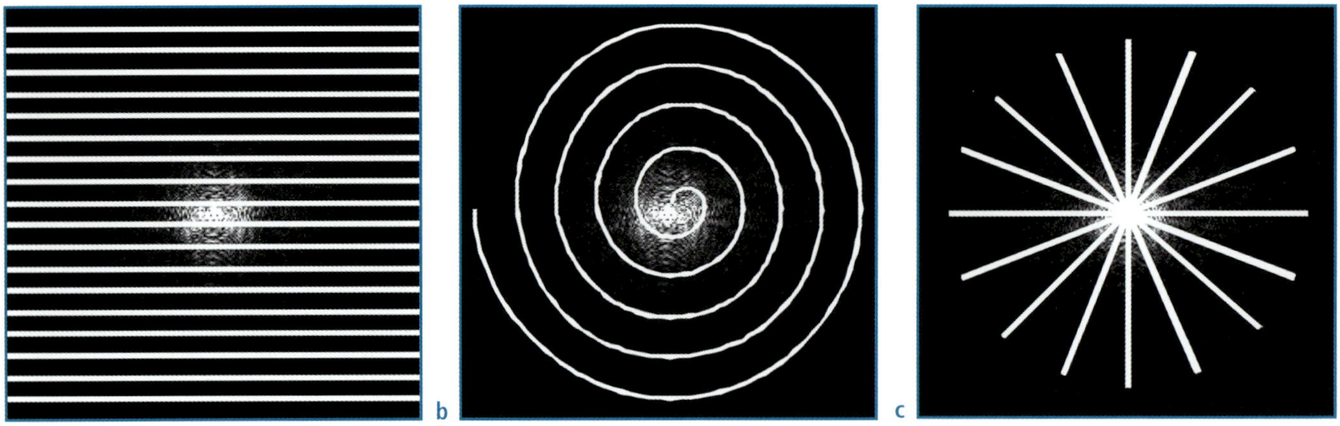

a b c

Figure 1-13 Encoding of k-space on a Cartesian grid (a), a spiral grid (b), and a radial grid (c).

1.6 Basic MRI Pulse Sequences

As described above, each point of the k-space has to be covered during an MRI experiment, which can basically be done based on a gradient echo or a spin echo-based technique. The respective switching of the gradient waveforms, HF-pulses and sampling of the MRI signal is called a *MRI pulse sequence*. A pulse sequence is meant to realize a certain coverage of k-space plus preparation of the spin system for providing dedicated image contrasts.

1.6.1 Spin Echo-Based Techniques (SE)

Spin echo-based techniques offer a larger variety in choosing the final image contrast by variation of the respective echo and repetition times. Their intrinsic low sensitivity to off-resonances normally provides excellent image quality. For cardiac applications, spin echo sequences are only of limited value due to the long acquisition times. In current clinical routine, SE-based techniques are almost limited to questions such as diagnosis of sarcoidosis or edema in which images of the myocardium with different image contrast or with strong T2-weighting are required. Furthermore, SE techniques are often applied together with a black-blood preparation pulse (see below) to assess vascular structures. This combination is also used in clinical research for the assessment of the coronary artery wall.

Since spin echo techniques are prone to flow artifacts, for cardiovascular applications, spin echo techniques are normally combined with black-blood preparation.

1.6.2 Gradient Echo-Based Techniques (GE)

GE techniques provide much shorter echo (TE) and repetition times (TR), which results in shorter image acquisition times. Due to the very short TR, the longitudinal magnetization can not sufficiently relax between subsequent excitation pulses. The frequent excitation of the spin system causes the magnetization to approach a steady state after a certain number of excitations. In a steady-state condition, the same amount of transversal magnetization is lost (by relaxation) as freshly generated (by excitation). The transversal steady-state magnetization is a fraction of the available equilibrium magnetization, which in comparison with the SE techniques results in a substantially lower SNR in GE-based imaging. In case of short TR (TR < T2), the transversal magnetization cannot fully relax between subsequent excitation pulses. This causes magnetization to contribute to the MR signal over a variety of subsequent excitation cycles. The contributions of the residual transversal magnetization may comprise spin echo components (the RF pulses partly act like inversion pulses on the residual transversal magnetization) as well as gradient echo components originating from freshly or previously excited spins. In cardiac applications, two different GE techniques, which mainly differ by the way the residual transversal magnetization is treated, are frequently used.

T1-Weighted or -Spoiled GE (T1w)

In many applications such as the imaging of contrast agent distribution the imaging target mainly comprises short T1 species. Short TR sequences have an intrinsic T1-weighting. The aim in T1w-GE-imaging is to almost completely suppress the contributions of the residual transversal magnetization for providing a pure T1w-contrast from the freshly generated

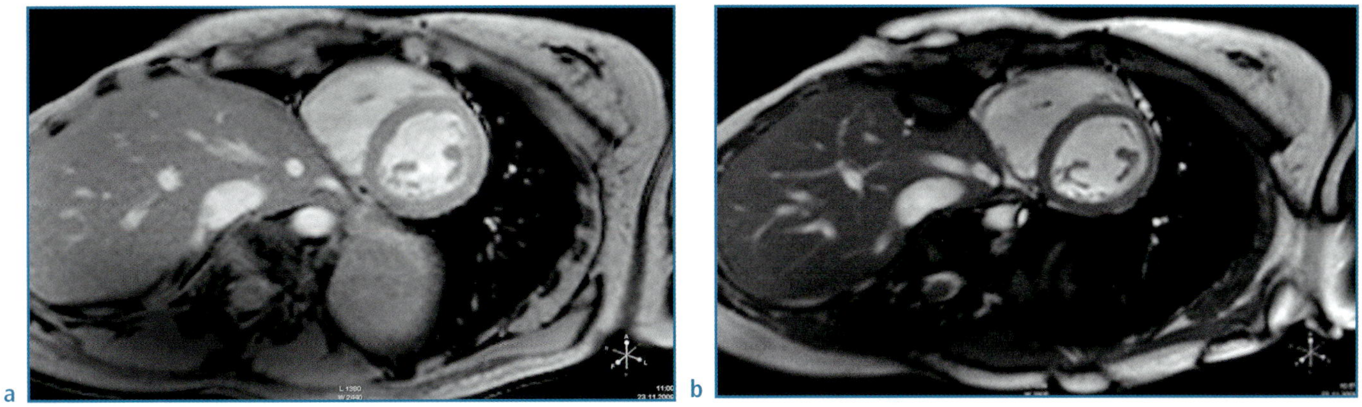

Figure 1-14 The blood-myocardium contrast in cine-MRI can be substantially improved by applying a SSFP imaging technique **(b)** instead of a conventional spoiled gradient echo technique **(a)**. Images acquired at 3 T, flip angle 10° **(a)** and 45° **(b)**.

transversal magnetization. This is achieved by applying a huge *de-phasing gradient* (so-called *spoiler gradient*) after the readout, which ensures almost zero MRI signal from the residual magnetization. Additionally or alternatively, subsequent excitation pulses and readouts are done with different RF phases, so that residual MRI signal does not constructively add to the sampled MRI signal. This technique is the workhorse for contrast agent-enhanced (reduction of T1) and inflow (see Angio) techniques.

Maximal steady-state signal is obtained with an excitation angle of $\alpha_{opt} = \arccos\left(e^{-\frac{T_R}{T_1}}\right)$, which is called the Ernst angle. For short TR, the Ernst angle results quite small (in the order of 10–20°), causing a significant reduction of the magnetization used for image formation.

Steady-State Free Precession (SSFP)

In the SSFP approach, all spins (residual transversal and freshly generated) are kept in-phase, meaning that all gradient and RF pulses are completely balanced (integral over all gradient waveforms and RF waveforms between two subsequent magnetic centers of the RF pulse equals zero). Since the residual transversal magnetization is kept in-phase, the residual signal results as a superposition of gradient and spin echo components, which are either freshly generated by the most recent excitation pulse or generated during prior excitation pulses. Neglecting off-resonance effects, the SSFP techniques generate a unique contrast, which depends on the fraction of the T1 and T2 tissue property, which is especially pronounced at higher excitation flip angles. The T1 and T2 properties of the different tissues (Table 1-1) reveal an almost unique property of oxygenated blood (long T2 and long T1), which causes SSFP techniques to provide excellent blood/myocardium contrast (Figure 1-14). However, since the SSFP gradient echo signal is a combination of two magnetization components, the sequence is quite off-resonant sensitive and resulting images show often black-band artifacts due to destructive interference of both magnetization components. Severe artifacts can be avoided if TR is kept below $1/\Delta\omega$, with $\Delta\omega$ being the bandwidth of the off-resonance. With the increasing power of recent gradient systems, this condition can normally be fulfilled on MR systems up to 1.5 T. On high-field systems ($\geq$ 3 T), the application of SSFP sequences is often limited by the increasing $\Delta\omega$ black-band artifacts rising inside the region of interest (ROI). The application of SSFP MRI is sometimes limited at higher field strengths due to the high RF energy depositions in the tissue (specific absorption rate, SAR) by using larger flip angles.

1.7 Motion Synchronization in CMR Imaging

In cardiac magnetic resonance imaging (CMRI) the data acquisition has to be synchronized with the heart and respiratory motion.

1.7.1 ECG-Triggered Data Acquisition

Synchronization with the heart motion is achieved by triggering of the data acquisition with the patient's ECG. A schematic representation of a typical cardiac MRI acquisition is given in Figure 1-15. The MRI sequence is normally triggered to the R-peak of the ECG. After the R-peak, MRI data is acquired for a certain period of time. To avoid motion artifacts, the acquisition is split up in the subsequent acquisition of several blocks, each of it representing data for a specific cardiac phase. To ensure insignificant motion blur,

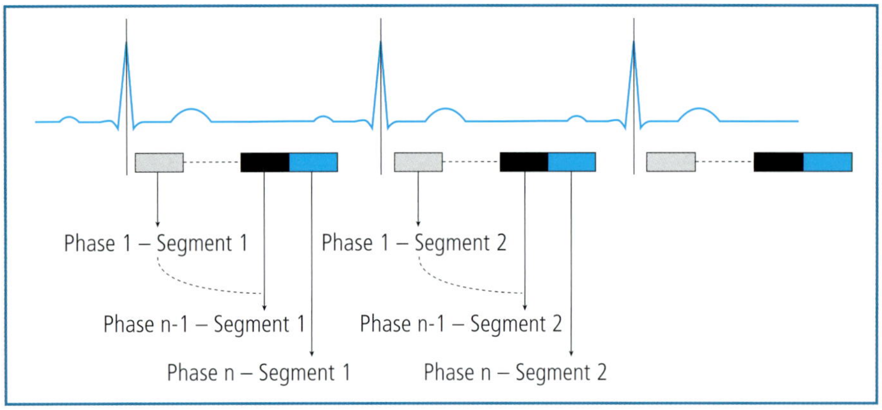

Figure 1-15 Multi-phase ECG triggered cardiac imaging.

each block/phase is normally kept below 40 ms. Since the length of a cardiac block is normally not sufficient for acquiring the data for a complete image, data has to be acquired over several cardiac cycles and only a segment of k-space is covered during a single heart beat. The final data is then composed from data acquired over multiple cardiac cycles, which demands reproducible contraction of the heart over multiple cardiac cycles. For coping with arrhythmia decent scanner provide arrhythmia rejection capabilities, in which data acquired in irregular heartbeats or during phases with substantially differing heart rates is not used for reconstruction. Please note that arrhythmia rejection prolongs the overall acquisition time since the neglected data has to be remeasured during subsequent heartbeats. The acquisition provides temporal snapshots of each cardiac phase and hence yields a movie representation (cine) of the beating heart. The technique described above is called prospective triggering, in which the data acquisition in each heartbeat starts triggered by the preceding R-peak. A major drawback of this technique rises from the required security gap at the end of the cardiac cycle, which is required to not miss the subsequent R-peak in case of a slightly increased heart rate. This hinders the coverage of the entire cardiac cycle and the end-diastolic function during the gap is not completely assessable. For full coverage of the heart cycle, *retrospective gating* has to be used. Here, the MR data are acquired continuously over several heart beats and the ECG is simultaneously recorded. Multi-phase data is generated after the acquisition by sorting the data according to the recorded ECG data.

For conventional cine imaging of the heart, retrospective triggering is the current standard. Prospective triggering is used in cases where either special spin preparation (see Chapter 1.8) is required or in cases where the data acquisition is restricted to a certain heart phase. This is typically been done for high-resolution anatomic imaging (e.g. coronary vasculature or *late enhancement* imaging). Here, data acquisition is normally restricted to the resting phases of the heart to enable longer data acquisition periods per heart cycle and hence completion of the data acquisition in less heartbeats.

1.7.2 Respiratory-Gated Data Acquisition

Superimposed to the heart motion, the respiratory motion introduces a further complication in cardiac MRI. Depending on the required scan time, different approaches are currently used in clinical routine. In most functional investigations, the acquisition time per image is restricted to few seconds. In this case, the patient is normally asked to stop breathing. Due to its better reproducibility, keeping the breath in end-expiratory position is preferred. For avoiding motion artifacts, the breath-hold time should be kept below 15 s. In case the patient is not compliant, resulting motion artifact due to respiration can be reduced by acquiring the image data multiple times with subsequent averaging (*signal averaging*).

For high-resolution scans, signal averaging is no real alternative. Here, the data acquisition has to be synchronized or gated with the breathing motion. Since external sensors such as respiratory belts or pillows do not provide sufficient accuracy in prediction of the position of the heart, on decent scanners a dedicated *navigator* MRI experiment is incorporated in the acquisition. The principle of a navigator is the monitoring of the position of the diaphragm prior to the actual data acquisition. This is achieved by using an additional one-dimensional MRI technique of a pencil-beam shaped volume, which is normally located at the dome of the right hemisphere of the diaphragm (Figure 1-16). The technique measures the diaphragm position prior to the actual data acquisition. Depending on the identified respiratory position, the data is either accepted or rejected. In the latter case, the data has to be remeasured. The rejection percentage depends on the user-defined acceptance window. Reduction of the acceptance window reduces the motion artifacts but increases the overall acquisition time since more

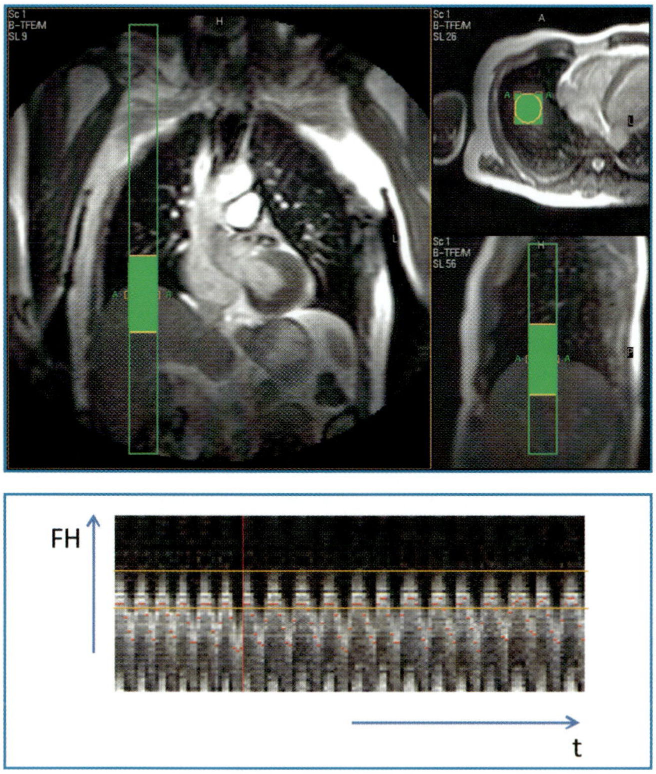

Figure 1-16 Navigator position in coronal, axial and sagittal orientation (a) and the respective one-dimensional MRI signal along FH position over time, clearly indicating the respiratory movement of the liver/lung interface (b). The yellow lines indicate a user-defined acceptance window.

data is rejected. To enable larger acceptance windows, the position of the imaging slice can be adapted to the measured respiratory position and so follow the respiratory motion. Normally the motion of the heart due to breathing is less pronounced than the motion of the diaphragm, and a factor between 0.4–0.6 has to be used for proper slice following. Since respiration-induced motion of the heart cannot be modeled by a simple translation along FH direction, slice following does not work properly in all patients and in up to 30% patients other motion components will still hinder the use of larger acceptance windows.

1.8 Spin Preparation

The resulting image contrast in MRI is governed by the basic MR sequence chosen for data acquisition. In many cases, the imaging sequence cannot be freely chosen, since certain constraints like measurement time demand compromises. For improving or altering the imaging contrast, several dedicated MRI techniques have been introduced, many of them applying dedicated *preparation pulses* (or short *prepulse*). Spin preparation can be obtained by various strategies (Figure 1-17).

1.8.1 Preparation per Heart Beat

A single preparation step per heartbeat is a quite common technique applied for a variety of special contrast manipulations.

Most frequently used techniques comprise:

- inversion recovery,
- black-blood contrast (double inversion recovery),
- T2-preparation,
- saturation,
- tagging.

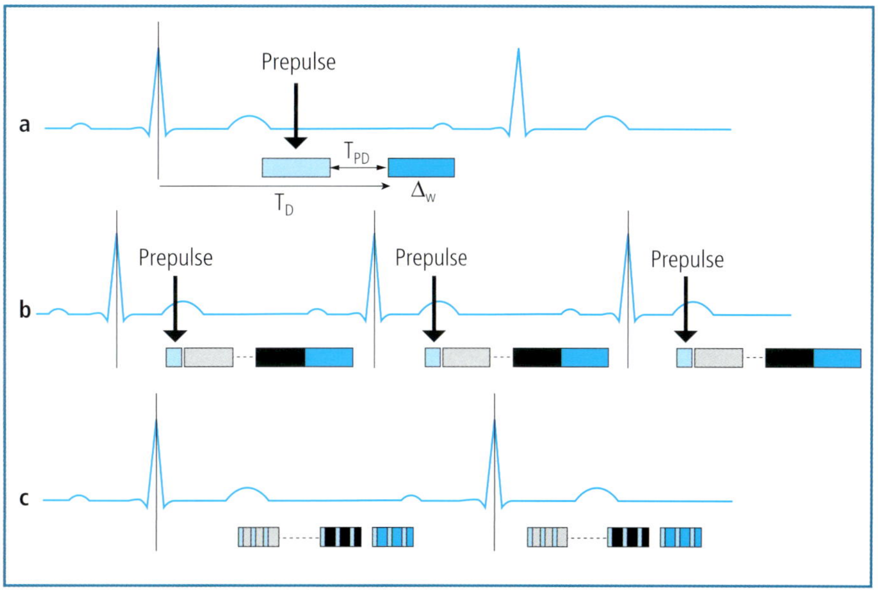

Figure 1-17 Spin preparation can be obtained by applying different preparation strategies such as (a) one preparation per heart beat in combination with a single phase or multi-phase readout; (b) one preparation per heart phase; or (c) a preparation per excitation.

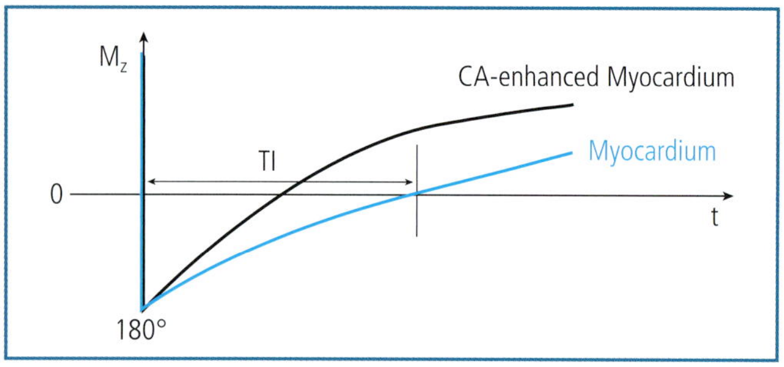

Figure 1-18 Principle of signal nulling by an inversion recovery spin preparation exemplarily for late enhancement imaging.

Inversion Recovery

In inversion recovery (IR) techniques (Figure 1-18), an 180° or inversion pulse is applied prior to the conventional MR sequence causing the longitudinal magnetization M_z being aligned antiparallel with the axis of the main magnetic field. Due to the longitudinal relaxation, the M_z starts building up again and depending on the tissue's T1 value crosses the x-axis ($M_z = 0$) at TI. If the acquisition is synchronized with TI, the respective tissue will not contribute to the MRI signal, since no longitudinal magnetization is available ($M_z = 0$!) as shown in Figure 1-19 for late enhancement imaging and Figure 1-22a, d for fat/water-only images. With the knowledge of the tissue's T1 value, the IR technique can be applied for nulling its MRI signal. Typically IR techniques are used for fat- or water-only images and in *late enhancement* imaging for suppression of the myocardium.

Black-Blood Contrast (Double Inversion Recovery)

A dedicated variant of the IR technique is used for the generation of black-blood contrast. In a preparation step the longitudinal magnetization M_z of the entire object is inverted by a non slice selective 180° excitation pulse. Immediately after the inversion the magnetization in the *volume of interest* (VOI) is restored by the subsequent slice selective 180° pulse (Figure 1-20). All magnetization outside the VOI is not affected by the restore pulse and starts relaxing according to the longitudinal relaxation. Since the blood flow through the VOI causes replacement of the restored

a

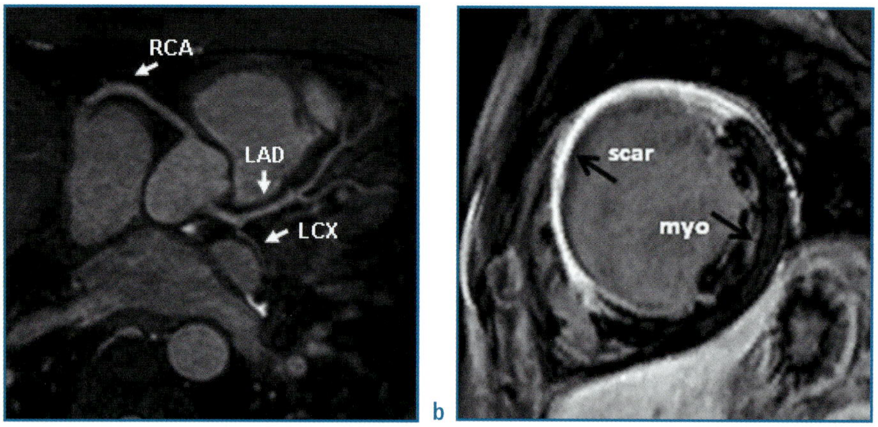

b

Figure 1-19 Inversion recovery technique applied to late enhancement imaging. By proper choice of the inversion recovery time TI, the signal from the myocardium (myo) can be completely suppressed and the scar can be nicely delineated.

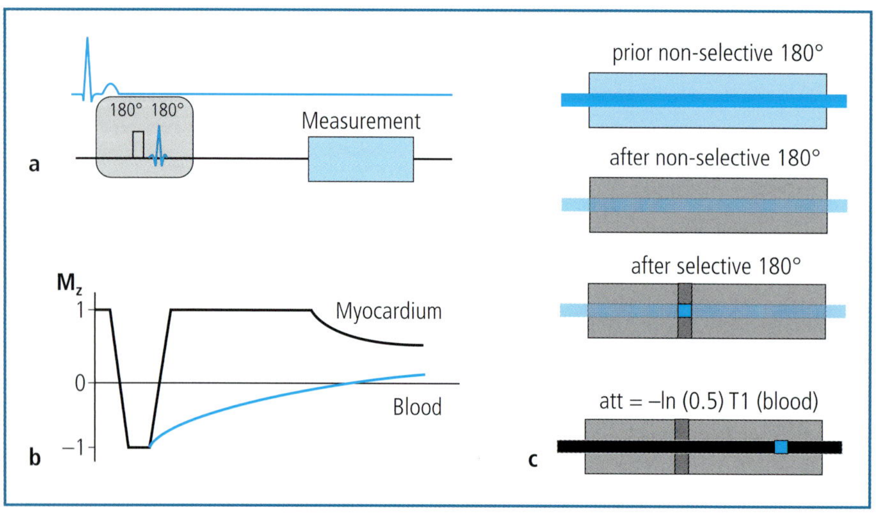

Figure 1-20 Principle of a black-blood preparation. **(a)** MR pulse sequence; **(b)** longitudinal magnetization over time, and **(c)** resulting contrast in the respective slice (restored by the slice selective 180° pulse).

blood by non-restored blood, the M_z of the blood in the VOI crosses the x-axis ($M_z = 0$), which can be used for blood signal suppression as already discussed for the inversion recovery preparation.

T2-Preparation

The underlying idea in the **T2-preparation techniques** (T2-prep) is to utilize the different T2 values of the tissue for increasing the intrinsic T2 contrast of the imaging technique. The T2-prep pulse sequence is depicted in Figure 1-21. In principle, the preparation consists of a 90° excitation pulse, followed by a certain period of time (T2-preparation echo time) to allow the spins some transversal relaxation with a subsequent −90° restore pulse flipping back the remaining transversal magnetization to the longitudinal axis. Since between the excitation and restore pulse M_{xy} decays according to the respective relaxation constant of the tissue, the longitudinal magnetization after the restore pulse is weighted accordingly and for the subsequent imaging experiment, the M_z is pre-weighted according to the tissues' T2 properties, causing a T2-weighting in the final image, which is almost independent on the imaging technique applied. To avoid decay of the M_{xy} according to T2*, 180° refocusing pulses are interwoven. Typically the T2-prep technique is applied for enhancing the contrast between blood and myocardium, but can also be applied for acquiring a T2-weighted image of the myocardium.

Saturation

A saturation preparation is similar to the inversion recovery technique, but instead of applying a 180° inversion pulse, preceding to the imaging experiment, a 90° excitation (or saturation) pulse followed by a spoiler gradient is applied. By adding a delay (saturation recovery time) between saturation pulse and imaging experiment, it can be used for providing a very strong T1 contrast in the image, since only magnetization with a very short T1 property can sufficiently build up longitudinal magnetization in-between the saturation pulse and the imaging experiment. Typically this technique is applied in combination with contrast agents such as in myocardial perfusion imaging. Typical delay times are in the order of 100 ms.

Tagging

In tagging, a certain saturation pattern is printed on the myocardium, the deformation of which can be followed over the cardiac cycle allowing the visualization and assessment of myocardial strain. Since tagging is based on local spin saturation of the tag pattern, the contrast between the pattern and the myocardium is decreasing with increasing heart phase due to the buildup of longitudinal relaxation. Especially at 1.5 T, the tag pattern is significantly fading during diastole. At the expense of a doubled acquisition time, a modified tagging approach based on the subtraction of two images with complementary signed tagging modulation can be used to reduce tagline intensity fading and consequently allows observation of the heart motion throughout the entire heart cycle.

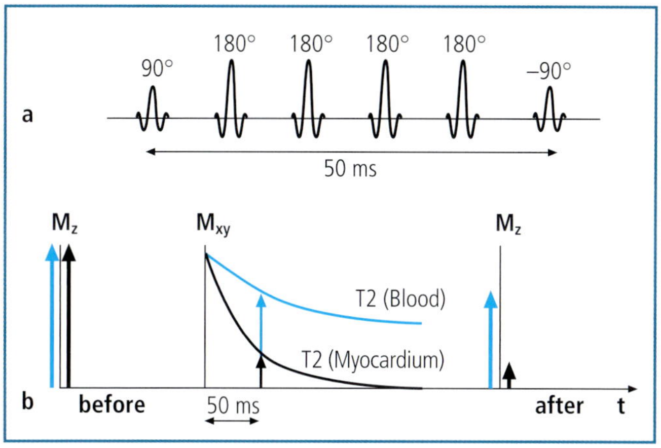

Figure 1-21 T2-preparation pulse **(a)** and the respective M_z and M_{xy} over time **(b)**.

1.8.2 Preparation per Heart Phase

For maintaining the preparation effect over multiple heart-phases, a single preparation step per heartbeat is often not sufficient and the preparation has to be applied once per heart phase.

> **Most frequently used techniques** using a single application of the preparation per heart phase comprise:
> - fat/water separation,
> - black-blood contrast,
> - spatial presaturation.

Fat/Water Separation

Due to the chemical shift (see Chapter 1.1.2), water-bound and fat-bound protons have different resonance frequencies. In case a saturation pulse is selectively applied on the fat or water frequency with direct subsequent image data acquisition, fat or water protons will not substantially contribute to the final image (Figure 1-22).

Since the system cannot separate between frequency shifts introduced by the chemical shift or by magnetic field distortions, the saturation may be incomplete or even the

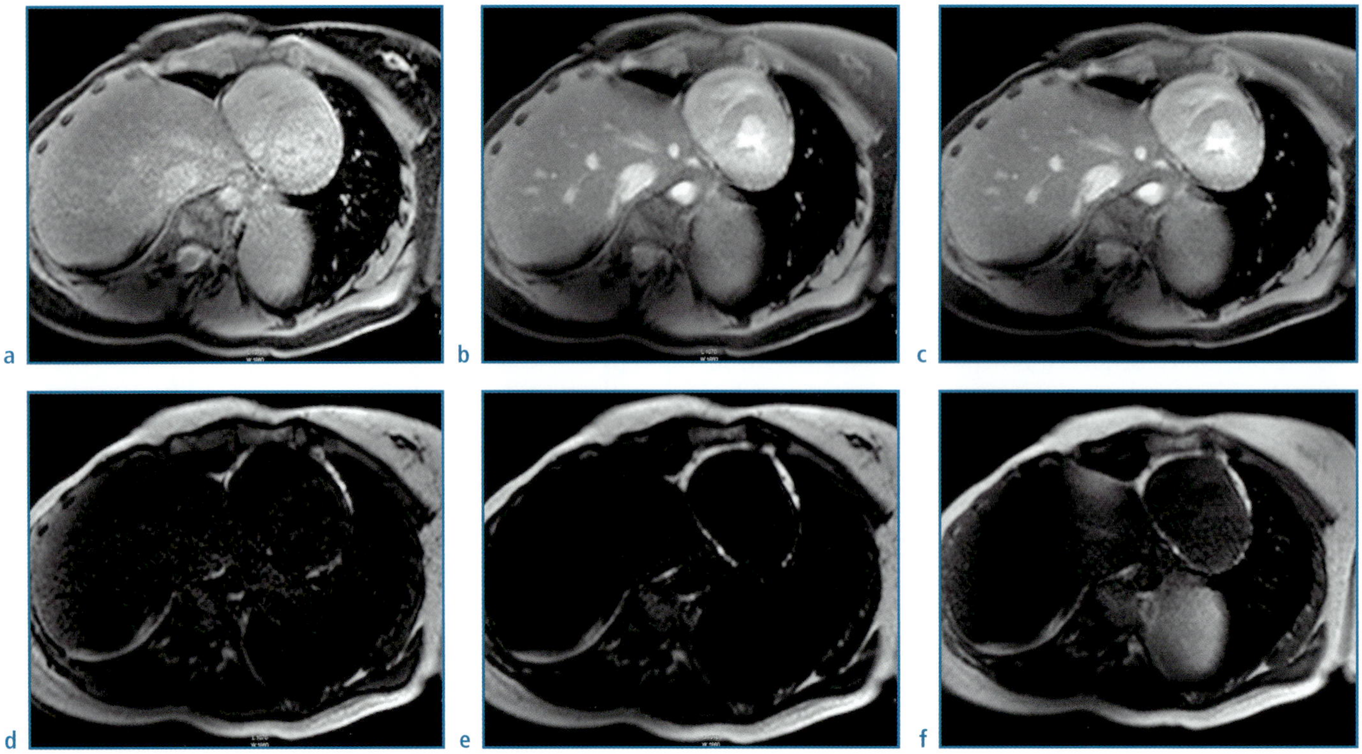

Figure 1-22 Water-only (a–c) and fat-only (d–f) images generated by inversion recovery (a, d), spectral saturation (b, e), and spectral selective excitation (c, f).

signal from the wrong tissue can be affected in areas of magnetic field distortions.

Black-Blood Contrast

Since the black-blood contrast prepulse introduced earlier is based on an inversion recovery experiment, perfect cancelation of the blood signal can only be achieved at a single phase within the cardiac cycle. Recently, two alternative approaches applicable to multi-phase imaging have been introduced either based on placing saturation slabs in the neighboring slices or by applying a diffusion preparation type prepulse (motion sensitized) but with stronger gradients, which cause complete dephasing of the signal from moving spins.

Spatial Presaturation

In many applications cancelation of the signal in certain regions is advantageous e.g. for the reduction of the volume of interest (VOI) or to avoid artifacts introduced by the strong signal of the thoracic fat during respiration. Where in the saturation recovery prepulse the entire imaging slice is being saturated prior to data acquisition, spatial presaturation is achieved by selective saturation e.g. in a para-coronal slab positioned at the position of the fat layer of the breast. The number of saturation slabs and their location and orientation can normally be freely controlled by the operator during geometry planning.

1.8.3 Preparation per Excitation

Some techniques require modification of the magnetization for each excitation and hence have to be applied once for each data acquisition.

> **Most important** here are:
> - fat/water suppression,
> - motion encoding.

Fat/Water Suppression

The previous approaches to fat/water suppression were based on prepulses. Due to the longitudinal relaxation, the magnetization of the saturated component will partly recover during the data acquisition after applying the saturation pulse. The application of spectral excitation pulses can be used for fat/water only excitation. The principle is depicted in Figure 1-23 for a 90° excitation pulse. After an initial 45° excitation of the spin system the magnetization is allowed free precession for 2.3 ms (1.5 T) or 1.15 ms (3 T). In this interval, the frequency difference between fat- and water-

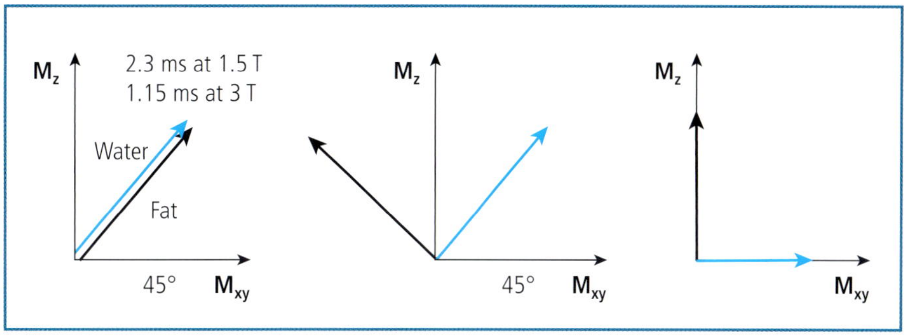

Figure 1-23 Principle of a 11 binominal 90° excitation pulse comprising a 45° excitation followed by a field strength dependent idle time with subsequent second 45° excitation.

Table 1-5 Advantages and disadvantages of the different fat suppression techniques.

Technique	Advantages	Disadvantages
inversion recovery	• off-resonance insensitive	• long preparation time • no cine acquisition
spectral selective saturation	• short preparation time • cine acquisition possible	• off-resonance sensitive • distortion of steady-state
spectral selective excitation	• cine acquisition possible • no steady-state disturbance	• prolongation of spin excitation • off-resonance sensitive

Table 1-6 Advantages and disadvantages of the different black-blood techniques.

Technique	Advantages	Disadvantages
double inversion recovery	• excellent blood signal reduction independent on the flow direction	• long preparation time • complete exchange of blood required • no cine acquisitions
motion sensitized	• significant blood signal reduction • no complete blood exchange required	• reduced SNR • suppression efficiency may depend on flow direction • could also suppress moving structures (e.g. ventricle) • cine acquisitions compromised preparation time
spatial saturation	• significant blood signal reduction • cine acquisition possible	• limited for long-axis geometries • complete exchange of blood required • high SAR

bound protons will cause a 180° phase between the magnetization of fat and water. The subsequent second 45° pulse causes final rotation of the water magnetization into the xy-plane, while the magnetization from the fat-bound protons (180° phase) will be flipped back onto the z-axis.

Please note that as in the saturation approach, the quality of the resulting suppression is heavily depending on the homogeneity of the main magnetic field and non-optimal suppression will occur at locations of magnetic field distortions (Figure 1-22).

Advantages and disadvantages of the different fat suppression techniques are described in Table 1-5, and of the different black-blood techniques in Table 1-6.

Motion Encoding

Motion encoding can be achieved according to the phase contrast angiography technique (see Chapter 1.10.3). Encoding of the motion of the myocardium is often called tissue phase mapping (TPM). In direct comparison to conventional cine imaging or tagging approaches, TPM has the advantage of enabling full access to the three-dimensional motion vector.

1.9 Rapid MR Imaging Techniques

A major limitation in cardiac MRI is the rather long acquisition time required to completely acquire all k-space data. For following dynamic processes such as the contrast agent dynamic but also for reduction of the motion sensitivity, fast data acquisition is required. Over recent years several approaches have been introduced for improving the acquisition speed.

Most commonly used approaches include:
- partial k-space coverage,
- acquisition of larger k-space segments per excitation,
- parallel imaging and k-t acceleration techniques.

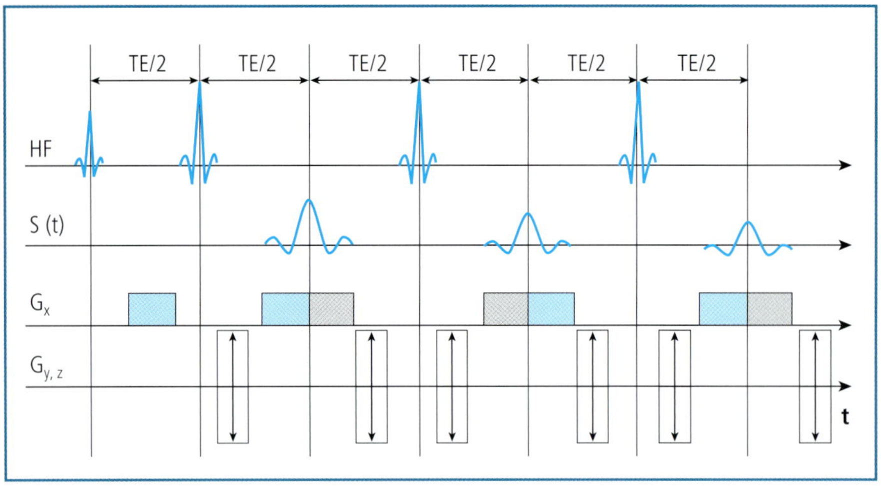

Figure 1-24 Multi-spin echo imaging.

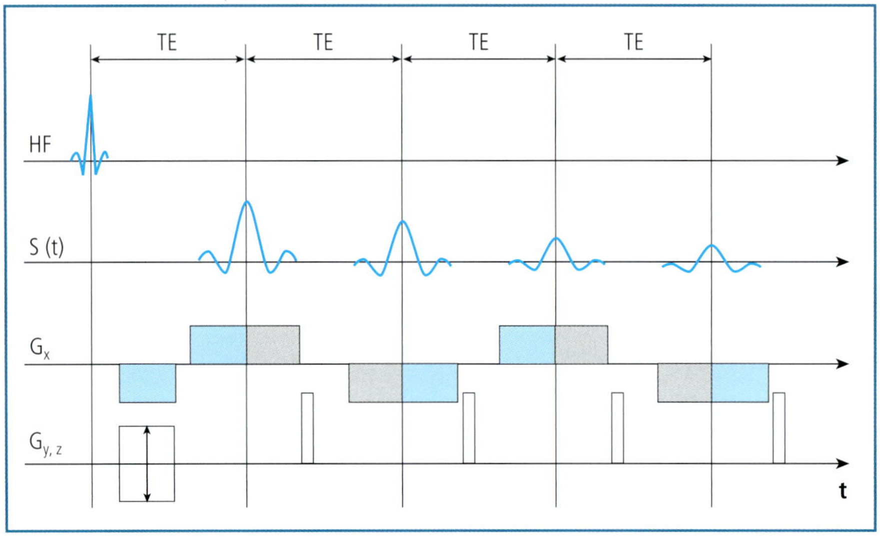

Figure 1-25 Multi-gradient echo imaging (EPI).

1.9.1 Partial k-Space Coverage

Since the object in MRI is described by a real function, the respective k-space representation shows a hermitian symmetry and $S(-k) = S^*(k)$. Due to this property, redundant data is acquired in case of full k-space sampling. Theoretically, the acquisition of one half of k-space is sufficient for reconstruction of the image data. *Partial k-space* techniques exploit the hermitian symmetry for significant reduction of the measurement time. The theoretical improvement of 50 % cannot be achieved in reality due to B_0 inhomogeneities, which may cause phase errors, the correction of which requires complete coverage of at least the central part of k-space. Partial k-space method can be applied in almost all applications, when some compromises in *signal-to-noise ratio* (SNR) can be accepted.

Partial k-space imaging along the phase-encoding direction is denoted as half-scan technique. Partial k-space imaging along the readout direction is denoted asymmetric or partial echo technique. Where in half-scan techniques the measurement time can be substantially reduced due to the reduced number of phase-encoding steps, the main advantage of partial echo techniques is the possible reduction of the echo and repetition time.

1.9.2 Acquisition of Larger k-Space Segments per Excitation

The basic MRI sequences discussed earlier acquire a single line of k-space (phase encoding step) per excitation of the spin system. The number of excitations, however, has a substantial influence on the overall acquisition time (time of the excitation plus required waiting time for allowing relaxation of the longitudinal magnetization). Acquisition of more than just a single line of k-space per excitation is often applied for acquisition acceleration.

The turbo-spin echo (TSE) technique is a variant of the conventional spin echo approach in which after the 90° excitation pulse multiple spin echoes are formed by a train of 180° inversion pulses as shown in Figure 1-24. After each inversion pulse the spin system is pre-phased to a different k_y-position and the data of the respective k_y-line is acquired.

Similar to TSE in multi-gradient echo techniques (echo planar imaging, EPI) multiple lines of k-space are acquired after a single excitation. However, in EPI no inversion pulses are applied and a train of gradient echoes is formed by applying a train of readout gradients with alternating polarity (Figure 1-25). Between subsequent readouts, small blip gradients are applied for driving the spin system to the subsequent k_y-line. The alternating readout gradients cause an inversion of the readout direction between even and odd echo numbers.

The acceleration of the acquisition for either technique is directly proportional to the number of readouts acquired after a single excitation pulse.

Compromises have to be made regarding:

- **image contrast:** Since the k-space data is acquired at different echo times, the contrast in the resulting image is not as well defined as in the conventional approaches. Instead of a well defined echo time TE, the multi-echo sequences show an effective echo time TE_{eff}, which is the echo time at which the central part of k-space (contrast defining) is acquired.
- **image blur:** Over the course of the echo train, the MR signal is decaying due to the transversal relaxation. This decay causes an increasing attenuation of the MR signal with increasing echo number. The uneven weighting of the different frequency components cause blurring in the reconstructed image.

In multi-gradient echo techniques, the alternating readout direction can likely additionally cause *ghosting artifacts* and the increasing phase accrual due to the off-resonances often causes severe degradation of the image.

Alternative to multi-echo techniques, dedicated trajectories through k-space such as spiral imaging (Figure 1-13) can be applied for measuring larger portions of k-space after each excitation of the spin system.

1.9.3 Parallel Imaging and k-t Acceleration Techniques

Parallel Imaging (pMRI)

In conventional imaging, the k-space data are acquired subsequentially, and only a single k-space point is acquired per time interval. Recently, new parallel imaging (pMRI) methods have been introduced. The approach is based on a dedicated RF receive unit, which comprises multiple independent receive units (coil elements *and* receiver, Figure 1-26), which independently sample the MRI signal. During the pMRI acquisition, the MRI signal is undersampled causing aliasing in the images reconstructed independently from each coil.

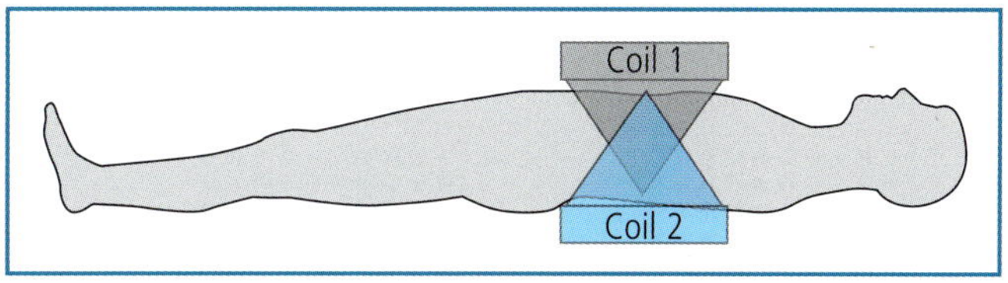

Figure 1-26 The use of multiple independent receive coils with knowledge of the respective coil sensitivity pattern can be applied for pMRI (schematic example using 2 coils).

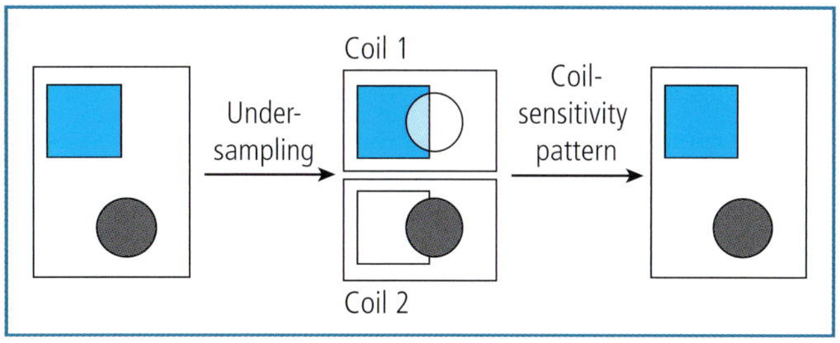

Figure 1-27 Undersampling of the MRI data causes aliasing (ghosting), which can be mathematically resolved under consideration of the coil sensitivity pattern.

By combination of the signal from the different receive units the entire FOV can be covered. The gain in image acquisition time in pMRI is achieved by undersampling of the data in k-space. Due to the undersampling, ghosting (aliasing) artifacts appear in the reconstructed image. pMRI methods use the sensitivity pattern of the receive coils for aliasing correction. Depending on the location r_i of a certain coil element i relative to the location r in the ROI, the signal $S_i(r)$ measured by the coil is proportional to $M_{xy}(r)$ weighted by its sensitivity profile $p_i(r)$. For simplicity, a 2-fold undersampling in k-space (every other y-line in k-space is not measured) is assumed. The undersampling causes aliasing as shown in Figure 1-27. The appearance of the aliasing artifacts depends on the coil sensitivity pattern and their position in the image is well known, which can be used to reconstruct an artifact free image. In case of more than two receive coils, higher acceleration factors R can be achieved. The correction must not necessarily be applied in the spatial domain as demonstrated (SENSE, PILS, …), but can also be done in k-space (SMASH, GRAPPA, …).

Theoretically, the gain in acquisition speed is directly proportional to the number of independent receive coils. However, in clinical practice possible R values are limited by

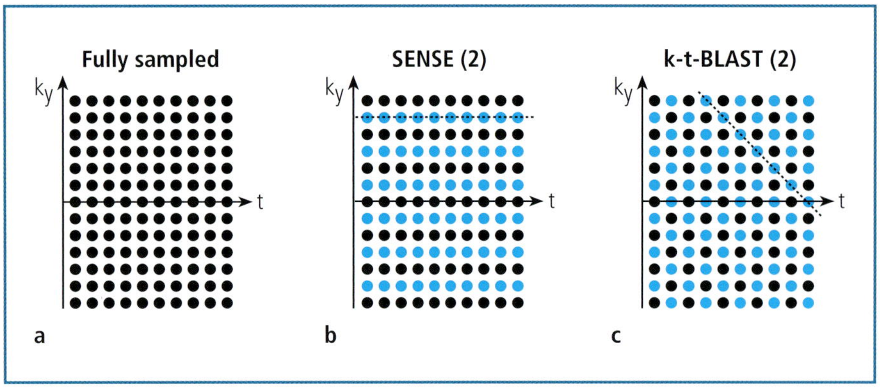

Figure 1-28 Fully sampled kt-space (a); 2-fold under sampled kt-space (pMRI) (b); 2-fold under sampled kt-space (k-t acceleration) (c). Please note that in this representation each point represents one line (readout) along the k_x-direction.

the concomitant reduction in SNR and the g-factor noise. The g-factor noise originates from the non-ideal data measured in MRI. Since all data is contaminated with noise, the identification of tiny differences in the MRI signal as well as in the coil sensitivity pattern is impossible, which leads to a limited accuracy of the numerical calculations. The g-factor and the decreasing SNR are the biggest limits for using higher *R* values in clinical routine. Parallel imaging can normally only be performed along the phase-encoding direction and, in case of three-dimensional imaging, the slice direction. Since in cardiac imaging the phase-encoding direction is often chosen along the anterior-posterior axis, even in case of 32 channel coils the maximal acceleration factor is limited to about 2–3 in two-dimensional imaging and about 5–6 in three-dimensional imaging.

k-t Acceleration

In case of imaging of dynamic processes such as contraction of the heart or blood flow, the dynamics are often confined to a certain region of the object. For contraction of the heart e.g. the motion is restricted to the area of the heart, while other structures such as the thorax wall, spine and lung do not move. In conventional imaging techniques the static part of the image is unnecessarily also measured completely over time. The basic idea of k-t acceleration (*k* stands for the frequency domain, *t* for the time) is to exploit the redundancy of the data and thus not completely measure all k-space points at each temporal snapshot but to skip sampling of certain k-space points along the time axis. In principle, all k-space data is completely measured, but not at all time points. A typical acquisition scheme with a k-t-factor of 2 is shown in Figure 1-28. Different sampling pattern can be used for achieving acceleration factors of up to 8. Similar to pMRI, the undersampling causes aliasing. However, aliasing occurs along the time domain and is non static, which usually appears in the images as intensity flickering. For removing of the aliasing artifacts, knowledge about the dynamic behavior of the object is required. This knowledge is provided by a low-resolution fully sampled trainings dataset. The need of a trainings dataset reduces the absolute gain in acquisition speed. The k-t reconstruction is based on the knowledge of the dynamic behavior of the object and hence does *not* require the reception of the signal with multiple coils as in pMRI.

1.10 MR Angiography (MRA)

The visualization of vessel (angiography) is of paramount importance in multiple applications. In its simplest form, enhancement of oxygenized blood-filled structures can be achieved applying a SSFP sequence. Caused by the unique T1/T2 properties of oxygenated blood, arterial blood signal will be enhanced by the intrinsic properties of the acquisition technique.

Furthermore, in MRI **three dedicated angiography techniques** are widely used:
- inflow techniques,
- contrast-enhanced techniques (CE-MRA),
- phase contrast techniques (PCA).

1.10.1 Inflow Techniques

The underlying idea in inflow angiography techniques is to utilize the replacement of blood by the blood flow as contrast property (Figure 1-29). Steady-state gradient echo techniques with as short as possible repetition times in combination with flip angles substantially above the Ernst angle of the static tissue are used. This combination causes a rather low steady-state signal from the static tissue. However, since the blood flow provides fresh (non-steady-state) spins to the vessels, the acquired signal from the vessels results substantially above the signal from the static tissue providing an excellent delineation of the vessels.

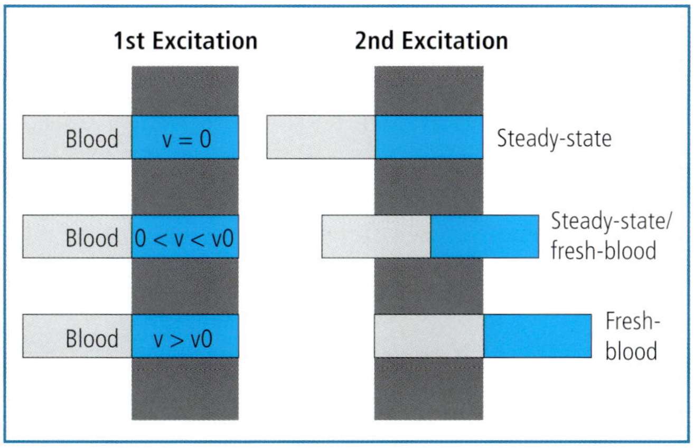

Figure 1-29 Depending on the blood velocity v, the spins of the blood see a different number of excitation pulses. Over a certain threshold velocity v0, the blood is replaced completely between subsequent excitation pulses.

Limitations from the inflow techniques arise in cases, where large sections of the vessel run in-plane or where the covered volume is too large. In both cases blood spins experience a significant number of excitation pulses causing a reduction of the steady-state signal of the blood with concomitant contrast reduction between the blood and the static tissue.

1.10.2 Contrast-Enhanced Techniques (CE-MRA)

In MRA, contrast agents (CA) can be applied for enhancing the contrast between blood and the surrounding tissue. After intravenous injection of the CA, a substantial reduction of the T1 relaxation constant of blood well below 100 ms can be achieved. The strong reduction of the T1 value yields a substantial enhancement of the blood signal in T1-weighted imaging techniques. Please note that the signal enhancement is caused by the CA and no inflow of blood is required. This enables the homogeneous visualization of large vessel segments even if the vascular structure is aligned with the imaging plane. CE-MRA is often much more efficient than inflow techniques, since the readout direction can be aligned with the main orientation of the vascular structure and the required coverage along the two phase-encoding directions can be kept minimal. Main limitation in CE-MRA is the only limited duration of the CA in the vascular bed. If no blood-pool contrast agents are used, the scan has to be finished during the first passage of the CA, since extravasation of the CA into the interstitial spaces occurs rapidly, causing additional signal enhancement of non-vascular structures.

1.10.3 Phase Contrast Techniques (PCA)

In PCA, the velocity of the blood is directly encoded. The encoding is achieved by applying a **bipolar gradient**, which comprises a pair of gradients with similar area but opposite sign (Figure 1-30a). Neglecting all non-idealities such as eddy currents, the bipolar gradients do not affect static tissues. For moving magnetization, however, the phase gained during the negative gradient is different from the phase gained during the positive gradient, since the spin magnetization experiences different B values depending on its location. The resulting phase can be calculated to $\Phi\,(t, \bar{v}) = \int_0^T \gamma\bar{G}(\bar{r} + \bar{v}t)dt - \int_T^{2T} \gamma\bar{G}(\bar{r} + \bar{v}t)dt = \gamma\bar{G}\bar{v}^2$, and is hence directly proportional to the velocity of the magnetization.

To compensate for artifacts caused by non-flow induced phase errors, normally an additional *flow-compensated image* has to be acquired and the components of the velocity vector are calculated from the phase difference between flow-encoded and flow-compensated image. Compared to the other angiography techniques, PCA has the advantage of providing quantitative information on the blood flow, including velocity and direction. Since the PCA technique encodes motion, its application is not restricted to imaging of flow, but it is more and more applied to the quantitative assessment of cardiac motion. Here the PCA technique is often referred to as *tissue phase mapping* (TPM).

Major drawback of the PCA techniques is the prolonged acquisition time. For each flow encoding direction one additional image has to be acquired resulting in a 4-fold measurement time in case the full flow vector into all three dimensions is acquired.

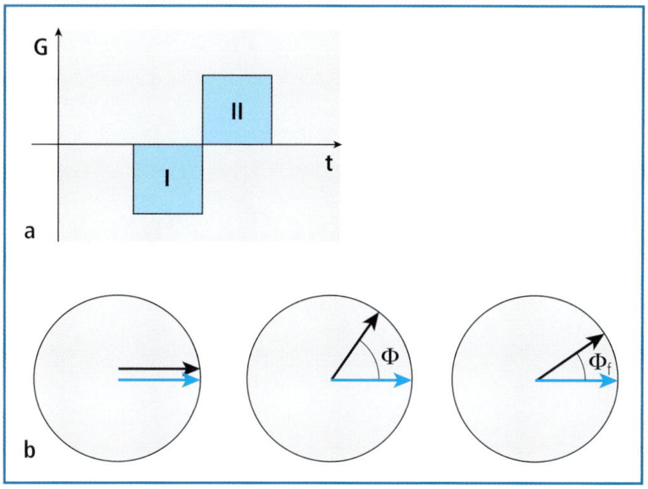

Figure 1-30 A bipolar gradient waveform (a) and its impact on the magnetization (b); static magnetization (blue arrow) do not accrue any phase, whereas moving magnetization (black arrow) accrue a phase shift, which is directly proportional to the velocity.

1.11 Signal-to-Noise Considerations

In all MRI measurements a substantial contribution to the final signal stems from noise. For magnetic fields applied in medical imaging, the main source of noise is fluctuating charges in the human body. These generate electromagnetic fields, which are superimposed to the MR signals as noise. The ratio between MR signal and noise is called the *signal-to-noise ratio*, or short SNR. The final SNR in a MR image is depending on multiple factors, the most important of which will be briefly discussed in the following.

1.11.1 MRI Sequence

The MRI sequence and its parameters and timing chosen for the acquisition has a substantial impact on the final SNR. In general spin echo techniques tend to have more SNR than gradient echo techniques. Sequences with long echo time show less SNR than the same sequence with shorter echo time, since T2 (spin echo) or T2* (gradient echo) decay significantly impacts the MRI signal. Increasing the repetition time normally improves the SNR, since the longitudinal magnetization has more time to build up again. Increasing the flip angle in gradient echo sequences may cause reduction of the SNR if flip angles are larger than the Ernst angle (see Chapter 1.6.2) are chosen.

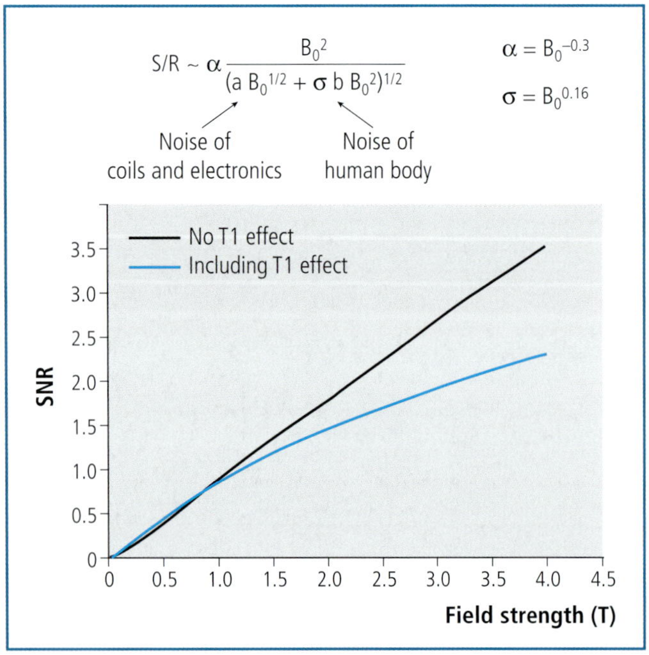

Figure 1-31 SNR dependency on the main magnetic field strength.

1.11.2 Main Magnetic Field Strength

The resulting magnetization is directly proportional to the main magnetic field strength B_0. Since other effects such as inductivity, conductivity in the human body, T1 relaxation properties, also depend on B_0, the dependency of the SNR on B_0 is somehow more complicated and increases slightly less than linear with B_0 as shown in Figure 1-31.

1.11.3 Pixel Voxel Size

The geometrical resolution of an MRI experiment directly defines the magnetization per *voxel* and hence its MRI signal. Changing the resolution in the image has a substantial impact on the SNR, which is linearly proportional to the voxel size. Reduction of the voxel size by a factor of two into one spatial direction, halves the resulting SNR. Consequently, halving the voxel size in all spatial directions results in a reduction of the SNR by a factor of 8.

1.11.4 Acquisition Time

An important component for the resulting SNR is the measurement time per voxel. Since the noise increases with the square root of the measurement time and the signal linearly, the SNR increases proportional to the square root of the measurement time per voxel.

> There are **several parameters/techniques in MRI** impacting the measurement time per voxel and hence the resulting SNR:
> - signal averaging,
> - partial Fourier imaging,
> - acquisition bandwidth,
> - parallel imaging techniques.

Signal Averaging

For improving the SNR, the same data can be acquired multiple times and the final image be reconstructed from the average signal of the multiple acquisitions. Since the signal adds up synchronously and the noise only with the square root (statistical process), the gain in SNR is proportional to $\sqrt{n}$, with n being the number of averages. Please note that for compensating the loss in SNR due reduction of the voxel by a factor of n, n^2 signal averages have to be acquired.

Partial Fourier Imaging

The partial Fourier imaging techniques introduced in Chapter 1.9.1 cause a reduction in the measurement time, since less points in k-space are covered. This results in a

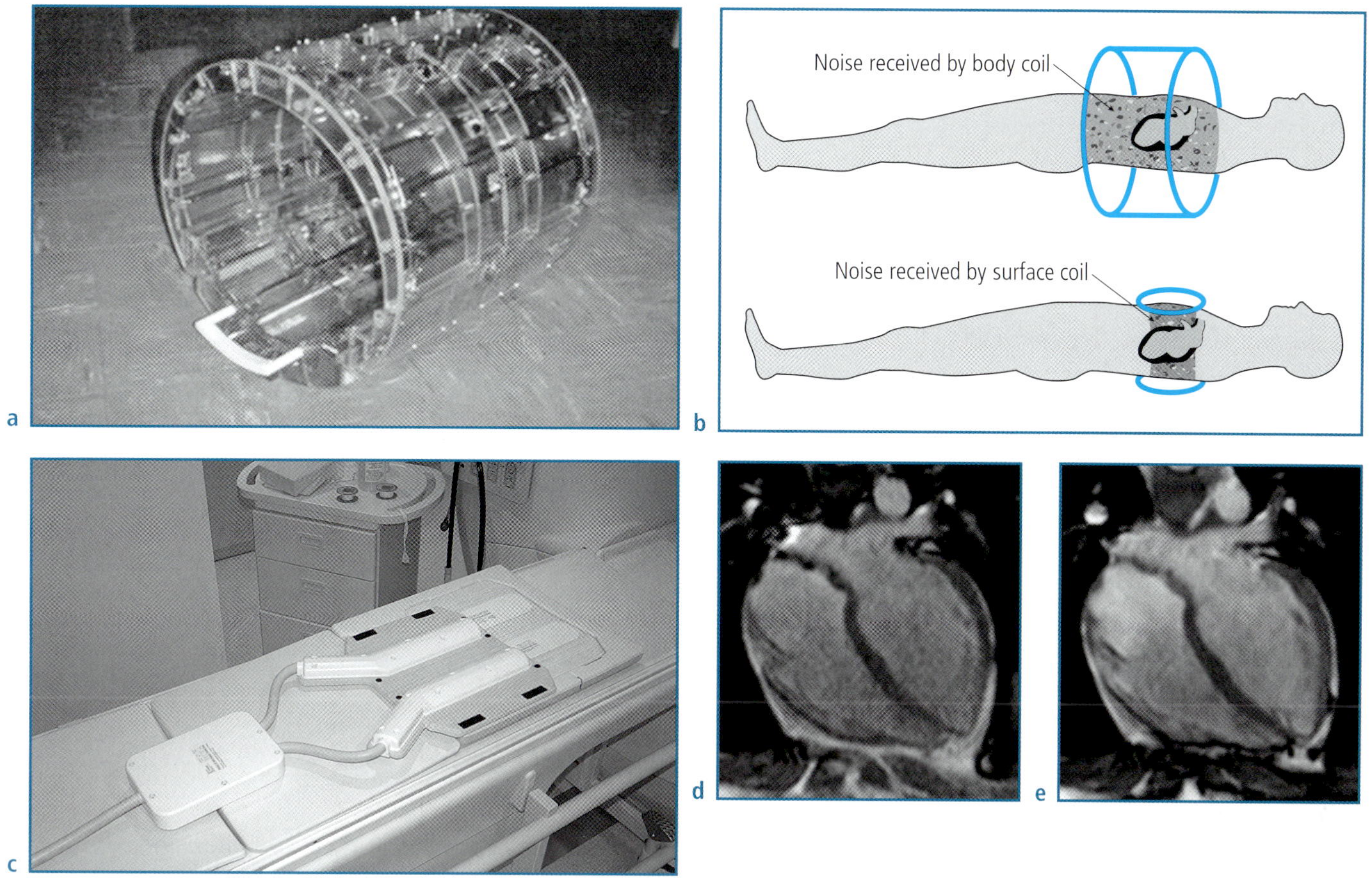

Figure 1-32 Signal-to-noise improvement by coil arrays (b). In cardiac imaging 32-channel receive coils (c, e) are used providing significant improvements in SNR as compared to the inbuilt whole-body coil (a, d).

reduction of the SNR by a factor of $\sqrt{\alpha}$, with α being the relative reduction in measurement time.

Acquisition Bandwidth

The acquisition bandwidth defines the time spend for the acquisition of a single readout (line in Cartesian acquisitions) in k-space. Since the k-space properties are defined by the geometrical settings of the experiment, increasing the speed requires increase of the readout gradients (integral of the gradients defined by the geometrical setting). Since the frequency spectrum (= *bandwidth*) over the field of view is directly proportional to the gradient strength, the bandwidth scales with the strength of the readout gradient and hence with the readout length. Since the noise is white, increasing the bandwidth of the signal simultaneously increases the bandwidth of the noise and hence its contribution to the readout. Since the MR signal remains constant, the overall SNR drops.

Parallel Imaging Techniques

Since the SNR is proportional to the time spent for acquisition of the entire data set, reduction of the measurement time by applying parallel imaging techniques reduces the final SNR by at least $\sqrt{R}$, with R being the acceleration factor. Often, the loss in SNR appears to be higher, since poor geometry factors (describing the possible quality of the pMRI reconstruction at a certain position) may add background signal, which appears very similar to noise.

1.11.5 Receive Coils

The application of dedicated MRI receive coils, which are optimized for the anatomy under investigation is a very efficient option for SNR improvement. While the in-build body coils receive noise from a large portion of the patients, the local sensitivity of the dedicated coils acquire noise from a much smaller region. Since the MRI signal remains the same, the respective SNR improves substantially (Figure 1-32). For cardiac applications, dedicated receive coils with up to 32 channels are currently in use in clinical routine.

Table 1-7 Impact of the different imaging parameter on the measurement time, the resolution and the SNR.

Parameter	Measurement time	Resolution	SNR
field of view (FOV) +	=	–	+
matrix size +	+	+	–
slice thickness +	=	–	+
averages +	+	=	+
bandwidth +	=/–*	=	–
half scan/half Fourier	–	=	–
partial echo	=/–*	=	–
p-MRT	–	=	–

+ = increase; – = decrease; = = equal; * = shorter echo times possible.

1.11.6 SNR Optimization

The final SNR in the MR image results from a complex interplay of the above described properties. Where certain parameters such as the main magnetic field strength or the receive coils cannot be adjusted, the operator has some freedom in optimizing the MR sequence parameters regarding SNR performance. Due to the linear relationship between voxel size and SNR, compromising the spatial resolution is the most efficient mean for SNR improvement. Alternatively, the reduction of the imaging bandwidth often also results in substantial improvement of SNR with only moderate prolongation of the echo and repetition times. Increasing the number of averages can be applied for SNR improvement, but due to acquisition time constraints is often not a valid option. Table 1-7 describes the impact of different imaging parameters on measurement time, resolution, and SNR.

References

Further Readings

Magnetic resonance imaging (MRI) is a quite complex technique and this chapter is only meant to provide some superficial insights in the basic imaging techniques. For further reading, several textbooks on basic principles of MRI can be found. Some interesting textbooks available are:

Ax PD, Weishaupt D, Kochli V. How does MRI work? An Introduction to the Physics and Function of Magnetic Resonance Imaging. Berlin, Heidelberg: Springer Verlag 2006.

Bernstein MA, King KF, Zhou XJ. Handbook of MRI Pulse Sequences. Academic Press 2004.

Chavhan GB. MRI Made Easy. Anshan Ltd. 2007.

Haacke EM, Brown RW, Thompson MR, Venkatesan R. Magnetic Resonance Imaging: Physical Principles and Sequence Design. Wiley & Sons 1999.

Liang ZP, Lauterbur PC. Principles of Magnetic Resonance Imaging: A Signal Processing Perspective. Wiley & Sons 1999.

Neri E, Cossottini M, Caramella D (eds). MR Angiography of the Body: Technique and Clinical Applications (Medical Radiology: Diagnostic Imaging). Berlin: Springer Verlag 2009.

Prince MR, Grist GM. 3D Contrast MR Angiography. Berlin: Springer Verlag 2002.

Vlaardingerbroek MT, den Boer JA. Magnetic Resonance Imaging: Theory and Practice (Physics and Astronomy Online Library). Berlin: Springer 2002.

Waedock W, Chenevert T, Chenevert TL. Emerging Concepts in MR Angiography, an Issue of Magnetic Resonance Imaging Clinics. W. B. Saunders 2009.

Further Readings in Relevant Topics

Over the last 20 years, an enormous amount of technical and clinical papers on the different topics in MRI has been published. It appears impossible to reference all relevant literature here. In the following we will restrict the referenced literature to some review articles and related textbooks nicely summarizing the state of the art in the relevant topics. For more detailed information, please refer to the references in the review articles.

Contrast Modification

Botnar RM, Stuber M, Danias PG et al. Improved coronary artery definition with T2-weighted, free-breathing, three-dimensional coronary MRA. Circulation 1999; 99: 3139–48.

Brittain JH, Hu BS, Wright GA et al. Coronary angiography with magnetization-prepared T2 contrast. Magn Reson Med 1995; 33: 689–96.

Delfaut EM, Beltran J, Johnson G et al. Fat suppression in MR imaging: techniques and pitfalls. Radio Graphics 1999; 19: 373–82.

Myocardial Function

Axel L. Biomechanical dynamics of the heart with MRI. Annu Rev Biomed Eng 2002; 4: 321–47.

Delfino JG, Johnson KR, Eisner RL et al. Three-directional myocardial phase contrast tissue velocity MR imaging with navigator-echo gating: in vivo and in vitro study. Radiology 2008; 246: 917–25.

Haacke EM, Tkach JA. Fast MR imaging: techniques and clinical applications. AJR 1990; 155: 951–64.

Jung B, Markl M, Föll D, Hennig J. Investigating myocardial motion by MRI using tissue phase mapping. Eur J Cardiothorac Surg 2006; 29: 150–7.

Masood S, Yang GZ, Pennell DJ, Firmin DN. Investigating intrinsic myocardial mechanics: the role of MR tagging, velocity phase mapping, and diffusion imaging. J Magn Reson Imaging 2000; 12: 873–83.

Osman NF, Kerwin WS, McVeigh ER, Prince JL. Cardiac motion tracking using CINE harmonic phase (HARP) magnetic resonance imaging. Magn Reson Med 1999; 42: 1048–60.

Petersen SE, Jung BA, Wiesmann F et al. Myocardial tissue phase mapping with cine phase contrast MR imaging: regional wall motion analysis in healthy volunteers. Radiology 2006; 238: 816–26.

Parallel Imaging and KT

Blaimer M, Breuer F, Mueller M et al. SMASH, SENSE, PILS, GRAPPA: how to choose the optimal method. Top Magn Reson Imaging 2004; 15: 223–36.

Kozerke S, Tsao J. Reduced data acquisition methods in cardiac imaging. Top Magn Reson Imaging 2004; 15: 161–8.

Niendorf T, Sodickson DK. Parallel imaging in cardiovascular MRI: methods and applications. NMR Biomed 2006; 19: 325–41.

Ohliger MA, Sodickson DK. An introduction to coil array design for parallel MRI. NMR Biomed 2006; 19: 300–15.

Pruessmann KP. Encoding and reconstruction in parallel MRI. NMR Biomed 2006; 19: 288–99.

Pruessmann KP, Weiger M, Scheidegger M, Boesiger P. SENSE: Sensitivity encoding for fast MRI. Magn Reson Med 1999; 42: 952–62.

Robin M, Heidemann RM, Özsarlak Ö et al. A brief review of parallel magnetic resonance imaging. Eur Radiol 2004; 13: 2323–37.

Sodickson DK, Manning WJ. Simultaneous acquisition of spatial harmonics (SMASH): ultrafast imaging with radiofrequency coil arrays. Magn Reson Med 1997; 38: 591–603.

Tsao J, Boesiger P, Pruessmann KP. k-t BLAST and k-t SENSE: dynamic MRI with high frame rate exploiting spatiotemporal correlations. Magn Reson Med 2003; 50: 1031–42.

Wilson GJ, Hoogeveen R, Willinek W et al. Parallel imaging in MR angiography. Top Magn Reson Imaging 2004; 15: 169–85.

2 Cardiac Magnetic Resonance Imaging Laboratory

Nico Merkle and Axel Bornstedt

2.1 Introduction

Since the advent of whole-body, high-field MRI scanners, fast imaging techniques and dedicated receive coils, the spectrum of clinical MRI applications has widened substantially. Further progress in the field of computational effectiveness in hard and software has even enabled cardiovascular MRI (CMRI), which poses high demands on the technique due to the specific physiological and anatomical requirements, mostly related to the intrinsic and extrinsic motion of the heart. The technique as of today (2012) is mature, however, for optimal security and image quality and a smooth workflow some important issues have to be considered for site planning and regular operation.

2.2 Site Planning

The measurement principle is very susceptible to external environmental influences, as it can have detrimental effects on the environment itself, thus several aspects have to be taken into account during planning. Depending on the field strength and the design of the installed magnet, the three-dimensional stray fields extend differently into the spatial directions. Each magnetic object in the zone of the stray field of a magnet will be magnetized itself and its generated field will in reverse have an impact on the homogeneity of the main magnet. In the case of static objects, these inhomogeneities can be mostly compensated by individual static optimization of the magnetic field during installation (shimming). Problems can arise if large moving (partly) magnetic objects such as elevators or streetcars are located in the vicinity of the scanner. The introduced non-static magnetic field inhomogeneities cannot be compensated for and the functionality or operational safety of the moving objects could be affected. The effects on the scanner and, in reverse, the magnetic effects on technical equipment like computers, pacemakers and implantable cardioverter defibrillators (ICDs) can be avoided by ensuring a sufficient distance between the objects and the magnet. A static magnetic field of 0.5 mT or 5 Gauss, respectively, is considered safe for humans, even with implanted devices. Considering the rapid decay of the main magnetic field with the third power of the distance (Figure 2-1) in combination with active shielding (specially designed counter coils, which minimize the stray field), the maximal extent of the restricted area is approximately 8 m by 5 m for a typical whole-body 1.5 T actively shielded system and 10 m by 6 m for a 3 T system, respectively. This borderline, where the magnetic field approaches 5 Gauss (5-Gauss line), is not necessarily enclosed in the scanner room. Thorough site planning has

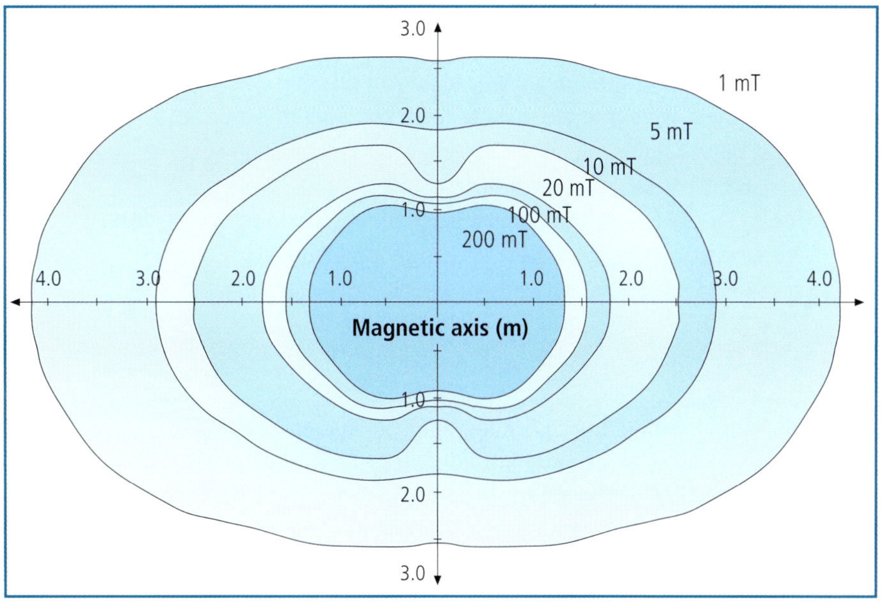

Figure 2-1 Typical stray field distribution of a commercial magnet of a 1.5 T scanner; it should be kept in mind that the magnetic field strength decays with the third power of the distance between object and magnet and that the magnet field acts in all three spatial domains. m: meter; mT: milli Tesla.

to ensure that no public accessible area reaches inside this 5-Gauss line. Sometimes additional shielding measures have to be taken.

External electromagnetic fields or radiofrequencies (RF), which can originate from all electrical devices or broadcasting systems (TV, radio, mobile phones) pose a further problem. To prevent interference with the MR signal, the scanner has to be efficiently shielded against external signals. This can be accomplished by setting up the scanner inside a Faraday cage. Walls, floor and ceiling have to be lined with highly conductive material like copper meshes and foils. The doors and a window, which allows the visual surveillance of the patient and the scanner room, are also framed RF secure and the glass contains a copper mesh. The necessary electrical connections for the system electronics, but also for lighting etc., have to go through a RF shielded filter plate to minimize interference, which could lead to artifacts in the images. Other non-conducting lines like infusion tubings or optical data fibers can be fed into the Faraday cage through copper conduits with a specific length-diameter ratio depending on the Larmor frequency of the system. This special design inhibits external RF fields effectively, unless ordinary conducting wires acting as RF antennas are fed through the conduit.

A high quality power supply system is needed and sufficient air conditioning must be provided to keep the engineering room as well as the scanner room in an acceptable temperature range for equipment and patients.

Generally the vendor of the MR system is involved in site planning and knows exactly the requirements for the system to be installed and ensures their adherence and the compliance with the regulations.

2.3 CMR-Facility Room Configuration

A **typical MRI suite for cardiovascular imaging** could be configured as follows:

- scanner zone:
  - examination room with magnet,
  - control room with operator console and workstations,
  - engineering room,
- patient zone:
  - reception,
  - waiting room,
  - patient dressing,
  - restrooms,
- personnel zone:
  - reporting room,
  - recreation room,
- service zone:
  - storage for medical equipment and drugs,
  - misc storage.

Typically, **the MRI system is spread over three separate rooms**:

- The **Faraday shielded examination room** accommodates the magnet, the patient bed and offers storage space for equipment, which is required at patient side during the examination: coils, support pillows, positioning aids, injection system and medical disposables like ECG electrodes, syringe kits et cetera. It should provide wall mount sockets for medical gases.

- The **control room** with the operator console and workstations for online patient monitoring and reporting. It often contains or gives a gateway to patient dressing and preparation. Access to the scanner room and patient bed must be designed with quick and safe patient evacuation in mind, because resuscitation measures cannot be taken inside the 5-Gauss line due to the magnetic equipment of the emergency teams; the patient's bed should be oriented towards the door. A trolley with the patient table could be used to bed handicapped people outside the magnetic field. The doorway must be wide enough to support this procedure.
- The **engineering room** provides space for the spectrometer, RF- and gradient amplifiers and cooling devices, thus completing the MRI suite.

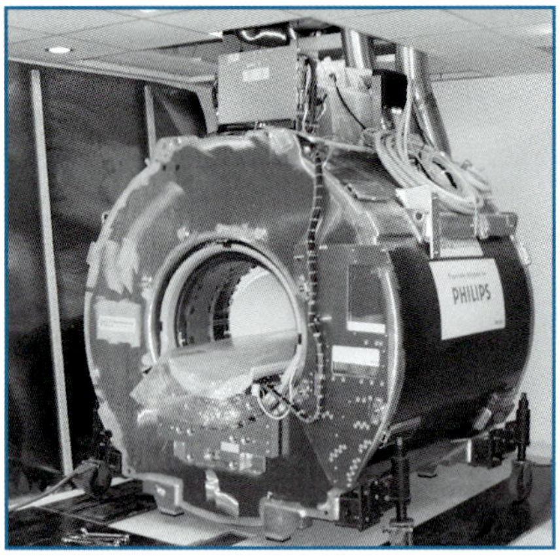

Figure 2-2 Superconducting MR magnet with cryostat (from Hombach et al. "Kardiovaskuläre Magnetresonanztomographie", Schattauer Verlag 2005; with permission of Philips Medical Systems, Best, The Netherlands).

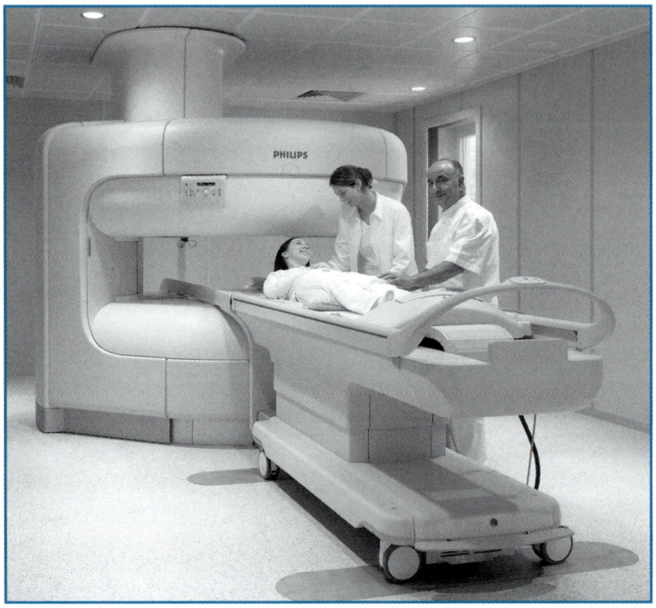

Figure 2-3 Open MR scanner for general imaging or cardiovascular interventions (with permission of Philips Medical Systems, Best, The Netherlands).

2.4 Hardware

2.4.1 Magnet

For a CMR laboratory, actively shielded whole-body superconducting magnets with a magnetic field strength B_0 between 1.5 and 3.0 T are mainly used. This is 30,000 to 60,000 times stronger than the earth's magnetic field of ~ 0.05 mT. Mainly for research purposes higher field strengths up to 7 T are used. They can deliver a higher signal-to-noise ratio (SNR), but also increase image artifact levels due to magnetic and RF field homogeneity difficulties, which scale with the resonance frequency. The improved SNR is either used to increase the spatial resolution, or to shorten acquisition times. A more thorough field strength discussion can e.g. be found in Rutt and Lee (1996) and Niendorf et al. (2010).

The commonly used superconducting magnet, weighing 3–5 t, is a special type of electromagnet, using coils wrought from niobium alloys as e.g. niobium-titanium (Nb-Ti, T_c = 10 K), which have to be kept below their critical temperature T_c to lose their ohmic resistance, thus being superconductive. Once energized, the coils in their superconducting state enable a very high and constant current flow, independent from an external power supply and generate very high and stable magnetic fields of excellent homogeneity. Typically 4–8 coil elements are used. The coil windings are made from fine filaments (~ 20 µm) of the superconducting material. To add mechanical stability and to protect the filaments against fusing in case of a quench, they are embedded in a copper envelope. The coils, together with 1,200–2,000 l of liquid helium at 4.2 K as a coolant, are contained in a thermally insulated housing called cryostat (Figure 2-2). During installation the magnetic field is initialized by an external power supply and ramped up to the desired field strength. After this the coil is short circuited to a closed loop and will maintain its current and magnetic field as long as it is kept constantly below the critical temperature. The inevitable loss of the expensive helium through boil off can be reduced to nearly zero by a coldhead as recuperation equipment, so that replenishment is scarcely necessary. For active shielding, additional superconducting coils in the magnet can be used to minimize the fringe field. Nearly all superconducting magnets are of cylindrical design, which hinders their application to interventional procedures. Only recently have high-field open designs, starting at 1.0 T and granting lateral access to the patient, been introduced, which should be considered for these purposes (Figure 2-3).

Quench

In rare cases the superconductivity in a part of the coil breaks down and it becomes resistive again; a magnet quench is triggered. This can be caused by a failing cooling system, mechanical vibrations or by a defective magnet. The affected part is rapidly heated, in a chain reaction the complete system makes a transit to normal conductivity in a few seconds, leading to a rapid helium boil off. The burst disc, an overpressure protection, is blown out by the expanding helium, which evaporates similar to an explosion through the quench pipe to a restricted access area outside of the building, thus minimizing the danger of frostbite and asphyxiation for patients and personnel.

2.4.2 Gradients

Three gradient coils, assembled typically in a cylindrical configuration inside the magnet of a whole-body scanner, produce the small temporally varying magnetic fields (G_x, G_y, G_z) needed to spatially encode the position of spins in a magnetic resonance imaging experiment. They can make the resonance frequency spatially dependent. The origin of the gradient system is put in the center of the magnet and called isocenter. The horizontal direction along the body axis of the patient is defined as z-axis, left-right and up-down are defined as x- and y-axis.

The **relevant parameters** to describe a gradient system are:
- gradient strength in mT/m and
- slew rate in mT/m/s or rise time in ms, respectively.

The first describes how fast the magnetic field changes in spatial dependency, while the latter is a measure for the switching speed from zero to maximum amplitude. The coils are powered by highly linear amplifiers, which permit rapid and accurate adjustment of their output currents and are able to deliver gradients of up to 100 mT/m with maximum slew rates in the range of 100–200 mT/m/s leading to rise times below 1 ms. Scan speed is dependent on the performance of the gradient system. Stronger gradients allow for faster imaging or for higher resolution; similarly, gradient systems capable of faster switching can also permit faster scanning, which is quite important for some CMR applications. However, the applicable gradient performance is restricted by safety concerns about peripheral nerve stimulation. The high performance gradient systems necessary for CMR produce a significant amount of waste heat, which necessitates water cooling for the gradient coils and sometimes also for the gradient amplifiers.

2.4.3 Radiofrequency (RF) System

The radiofrequency (RF) system is a further important part of the scanner hardware. It emits and receives RF signals with the device specific resonance or Larmor frequency.

Transmitter

The transmitter can generate RF signals with adjustable frequency, amplitude, and phase to excite the spins contained in a well defined slice. In combination with the slice selection gradient, the frequency defines the position of the slice in relation to the isocenter, while the bandwidth of the signal controls the thickness of the slice. The excitation angle is controlled by the RF amplitude, while the phase of the signal defines the rotation axis. The envelope of the RF signal is digitally generated, while phase and amplitude are modulated by special filters and mixers. The result is converted by a DAC (digital analog converter) to a low power analogous waveform. The final signal, used for excitation, is linearly amplified afterwards by RF amplifiers of up to 25 kW maximum power output.

Transmit/Receive or Body Coil

To accomplish a homogeneous RF field for the spin excitation (B_1 field), a big volume coil is required which is invisibly integrated as a quadrature body coil into the bore of the scanner below the plastic covers. In addition to its function as transmitter, the body coil can also be used as receive coil or antenna for big regions of interest (ROI).

Dedicated Receive Coils

Optimal image quality is not solely dependent on signal strength; moreover, the SNR is the determining quality factor. Receive coils have to collect the maximal required signal, while keeping the noise signal low. Noise is generated by the thermal motions of the electrons in the receiving hardware, but the strongest source of noise signal is the patient itself. The design of the coil is important to optimize the SNR: the bigger the volume of the coil, the better the homogeneity and penetration depth, but the worse the SNR. As a rule of thumb the coil should be as big as necessary, while also staying as small as possible. Of course this cannot always be accomplished and compromises have to be accepted concerning homogeneity, penetration depth, and SNR.

Two basic types of coils can be distinguished:
- volume coils,
- surface coils.

a
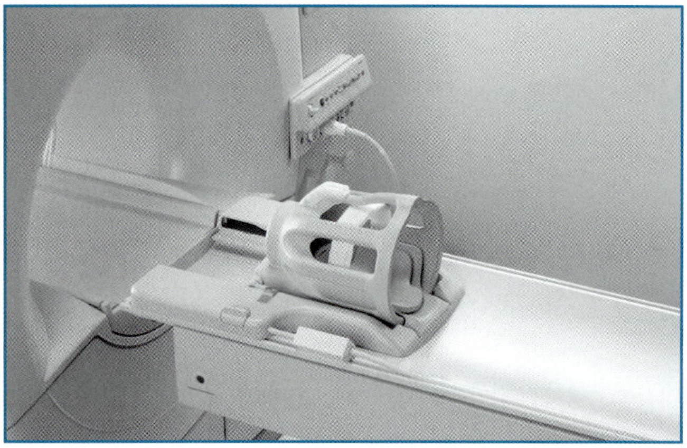
b
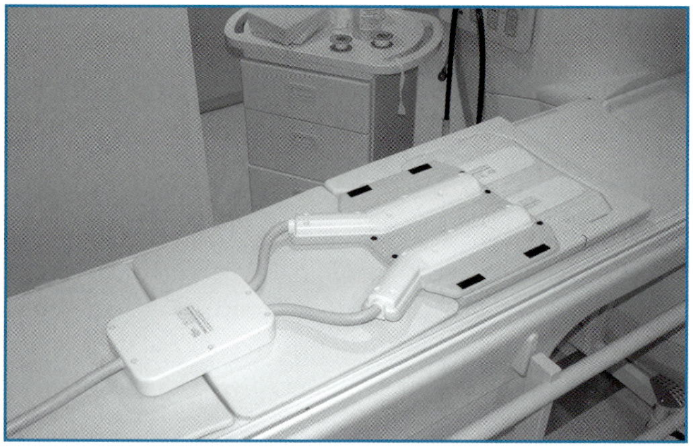

Figure 2-4 Volume coil for examining the head **(a)** (from Hombach et al. "Kardiovaskuläre Magnetresonanztomographie", Schattauer Verlag 2005; with permission of Philips Medical Systems, Best, The Netherlands). Surface phased array coil (32 channels) for imaging of the heart and the great vessels **(b)**.

Volume Coils

Volume coils (Figure 2-4a) cover a certain volume as e.g. the head, a knee, a wrist, or the whole-body coils and certain head coils can work in transmit and receive mode.

Surface Coils

Surface coils are almost exclusively used as receive coils, while the integrated body coil is necessary as transmitter. With their flexible design and their small coil diameters, they are very well suited for the depiction of small anatomical structures in the vicinity of the body surface and deliver very good SNR. A single wire loop can be sufficient to build a linear surface coil, while two orthogonal wire loops can form a quadrature coil with improved SNR. The disadvantage of the surface coils is the restricted field of view (FOV), signal homogeneity, and penetration depth.

Phased Array Coils

In CMR dedicated cardiac phased array coils are mandatory. A phased array coil is a group of linked surface coil elements, typically 4 to 32, with a complete and independent receive channel for each single coil. It is able to combine advantages of the surface coils with some properties of the volume coils. The arrays can have a very flexible design, are adapted to specifically fit the target anatomy and cover a much bigger ROI compared to a single surface coil, while maintaining the excellent SNR properties of the small coils (Figure 2-4b). An additional advantage of the multi-coil design is its capability for parallel imaging. Parallel imaging techniques exploit the redundancy in local coil information and sensitivity to speed up the imaging process, which can be used to either increase the spatial or temporal resolution of the CMR sequences. A disadvantage of the phased array coils is the added computational overhead. The data of each coil has to be received and reconstructed separately before it can be combined to the final image, but this fact is being mitigated as fast as computer hardware and software development progresses.

2.4.4 Computer Control Systems, Operator Console and Workstations

The computer system in the spectrometer unit controls and synchronizes all hardware devices, which are necessary for the generation and acquisition of the MR signals. These are the RF and gradient amplifiers as well as coils, receiver channels, and analog to digital converters (ADC). The reconstruction computer, the most computational powerful system in the setup, handles the reconstruction of the digitized image data from the spectrometer, which is finally delivered to the console computer for storage and review. The operator console allows interactive planning of the imaging sequences, low level image processing, and data handling. Usually the images are processed and reviewed afterwards at dedicated workstations, which also offer higher level image processing capabilities.

2.5 Software

The scanner software comprises patient data administration, an interactive planning mode and basic viewing functionality to review the acquired images. In the case of CMR, some specialized acquisition software options, such as respiratory navigators, black-blood imaging and advanced cardiac triggering methods should be available on the system as well as dedicated reviewing workstations, which provide specialized cardiac and vascular analysis software.

2.6 Safety Aspects

MRI has its own specific risks, and precautions have to be taken to avoid potentially hazardous situations. The most important consideration is attraction of ferromagnetic objects to the static magnetic field. However, the potential unwanted effects of peripheral nerve stimulation or tissue heating must be considered, as well. This is particularly important for investigating patients with permanent pacemakers, automatic implantable cardiac defibrillators (ICD), metallic stents, prosthetic valves (older types), and with lengthy temporary cardiac pacing wires. Though MRI is safe when all precaution measures are observed, particularly since the patient is not exposed to radiation during the imaging procedure, the MRI system is potentially dangerous to patient and staff if safety issues are neglected. This relates to the static magnetic field, the alternating magnetic field gradients, and the radiofrequency energy.

2.6.1 Static Magnetic Field

The static magnetic field of a 1.5 T scanner with its strength 30,000 times the earth's magnetic field will pull all ferromagnetic objects in the near vicinity to the bore of the magnet (Figure 2-5). Such objects (e.g. scissors, coins etc.) can become fast-moving projectiles within the magnetic field, which can cause severe injury to an individual inside the magnet, in rare instances with fatal outcome. Therefore all ferromagnetic items should be removed from the MR suite, including objects associated with patient management such as monitors, injection systems, drips stands, and oxygen cylinders. The physical boundary up to which ferromagnetic objects can be safely manipulated is indicated by the 5-Gauss line that in most MRI suites is visually indicated on the floor to prevent accidental movement of these objects. In addition, the magnetic field can also impair or destroy the proper function of electronic devices (monitors, CT scanners, gamma cameras, computer hard disks) and can destroy magnetic storage media, e.g. diskettes, credit cards, magneto-optical discs etc. There are threshold values of magnetic field scatter for a safe distance of different electronic devices (Table 2-1).

Similar forces have an effect on ferromagnetic material, implants, or foreign objects (e.g. shrapnel) inside the individuals being imaged. These forces can pull on or torque these objects, thereby cutting or compressing healthy tissue. Therefore individuals with such foreign metal objects are

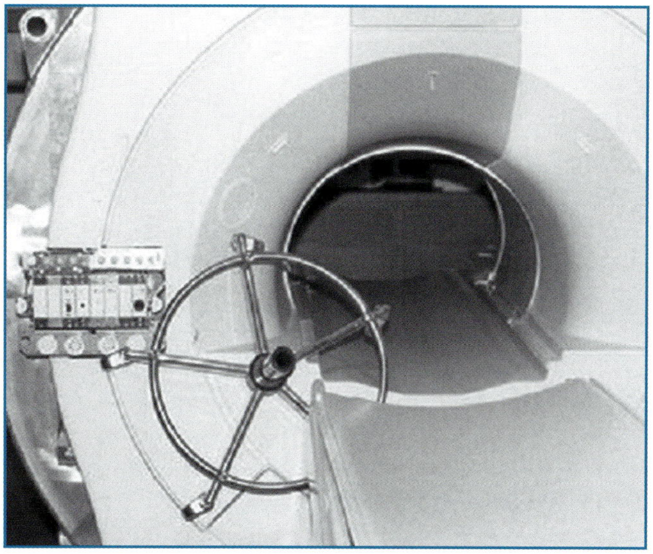

Figure 2-5 Accidental attraction of the support of an office chair shooting like a projectile onto the magnet (from Hombach et al. "Kardiovaskuläre Magnetresonanztomographie", Schattauer Verlag 2005; with permission of Philips Medical Systems, Best, The Netherlands).

Table 2-1 Threshold values of magnetic field scatter for electronic devices.

Scatter field (mT)	Object
3	magnetic storage media
1	computer hard disk, X-ray tube
0.5	pacemaker, intracardiac defibrillator
0.1	monitor, computer tomography
0.05	gamma camera, linear accelerator

generally not suitable for MRI studies. Biological side effects, e.g. nausea, vertigo, or retinal lightnings, or psychophysiological alterations, e.g. fatigue or loss of concentration, may be observed only with long investigation times (several hours) and high-field magnets (Schenck 2000, De Voch 2003). Moreover, flow- or motion-dependent current induction with consecutive nerve or muscle excitations have been reported (Kinouchi 1996). Yet, due to the weak interactions of biological tissues with static magnetic fields, and lack of reproducibility, these biological effects are judged controversial and negligible with currently available modern MR scanners (Schenck 1998, Kangarlu 1999, Shellock 2003).

The International Electro-Technical Commission (IEC) has elaborated **three different operational modes**:

- the **"normal operating mode"** (up to 2.0 T) for routine examinations without danger of exceeding threshold values,

- the **"first controlled operating mode"** (2–4 T) with visual and verbal control of the patient when departing from normal imaging programs, and
- the **"second controlled operating mode"** (> 4 T) only for investigational studies.

2.6.2 Alternating Magnetic Field Gradients

Rapid switching of the gradient magnetic fields is necessary for spatial encoding. The high power gradients may induce small currents in biological tissue, which may induce peripheral nerve stimulation. The United States FDA has issued recommendations for gradients powers (expressed as dB/dt) for each MRI system to be at a level less than that required to produce peripheral nerve stimulation. In addition, the switching of these magnetic gradients produces high acoustic noise levels sometimes beyond 100 dB (A). Since the threshold of acute damage to the human inner ear is at 140 dB (A), the FDA has limited the noise level in MRI scanners to this level. It is both recommended and mandatory that all patients should be provided with hearing protection using earplugs or headphones. Ongoing development and improvement of new coil and hardware design and imaging sequences (e.g. using fast imaging techniques) will further reduce the noise level during MRI examinations (Mansfield 2001, Edelstein 2002).

2.6.3 Radiofrequency Energy

The great majority of radiofrequency energy, a non-ionizing electromagnetic radiation in a high frequency range, is dissipated as heat into the patient's tissues due to resistive losses. Such temperature changes are commonly not recognized by the patient, but if certain energy levels are exceeded, significant heating of body tissues will occur. The transfer of RF energy to heat into the tissue is called "specific absorption rate" (SAR), expressed in watts per kg body weight (W/kg BW), and special attention should be paid for temperature sensitive organs like eyes or testes. Table 2-2 and Table 2-3 show threshold values that should not be exceeded. Furthermore, RF energy may heat metallic and nonferromagnetic implants, e.g. pacemaker leads, or external cable loops of malpositioned ECG leads and cables, or loops built up by closed hands or feet. Though the latter side effect is relatively uncommon, hands and feet should be separated from each other during MR imaging.

Table 2-2 Whole-body threshold values for SAR (W/kg BW) according to IEC 60601-2-33.

normal mode	2
first control level	4
second control level	> 4

Table 2-3 Local threshold values for SAR (W/kg BW) averaged over 6 s measurement time according to IEC 60601-2-33.

Mode	Head – Trunk	Extremities
normal mode	10	20
first control level	10	20
second control level	> 10	> 20

The level of SAR with consecutive increase of body temperature depends on the different scan modes, the RF application time, and the environmental conditions (room temperature, humidity), and **some measures may be applied** for SAR reduction:

- use of quadrature- or multi-transmit coils,
- short repetition times (TR),
- imaging fewer slices,
- using a low turbo factor in fast-echo sequences.

2.7 MRI Safety and Compatibility

The United States FDA has issued **safety declarations** that are helpful for the investigator when using medical devices or implants within the 5-Gauss (0.5 mT) area of the MRI suite:

- MR safe:
  - investigations have to verify that the presence of a given object within the scanner or MR suite will not give rise to potential danger or safety risks to the patient or personnel,
  - absence of corresponding research data requires a scientific rationale, why a device or object was not tested for MRI safety,
- MR compatible:
  - investigations have to verify that a given object or device within the scanner or MR suite will not give rise to danger, will function properly, and will not disturb the function of the scanner,
  - absence of corresponding research data requires a scientific rationale, why a device or object was not tested for MRI safety,
  - at the same time specific data on the test environment (type of scanner, field strength) and test conditions (investigational protocols, MR sequences) should be documented to enable a more precise risk calculation.

2.8 Emergency Management

In distinct situations, e.g. scanner defect (quench), dislocation of metallic implants, or burns as well as circulatory collapse, the patient has to be removed quickly out of the scanner in order to initiate adequate emergency management of the patient. For those situations or in case of fire, "Emergency Plans" have to be available in the MR suite, which have to be discussed and rehearsed with the personnel in regular time intervals. In addition, resuscitation equipment and medication including an external defibrillator should be in the immediate vicinity of the MRI suite to be administered by experienced staff in case of an emergency. Special care must be taken with individuals taking part in emergency treatment of the patients (e.g. staff of intensive care units) or are present during emergency situations (technicians, firemen, or policemen), who are not familiar with the special requirements of working in a scanner room. Therefore, regular training of the MRI staff as well as of all persons who are in regular contact with the MRI suite is mandatory.

Table 2-4 Absolute and relative contraindications to an MRI study.

Absolute contraindications	Relative contraindications
• cardiac pacemaker and implantable defibrillator (ICD) • carotid artery vascular clamp/clip • post-surgical intracranial artery clip • aneurysm clip (in general) • prosthetic cardiac valves (only first series, e.g. Starr-Edwards etc.) • metal splinter or shrapnel in patient's body • cochlear, otological, or ear implant • insulin or infusion pump • implanted drug infusion pump • neurostimulator • bone growth/fusion stimulator • corpus cavernosum implant • patients with unstable angina or NYHA class IV heart failure	• severe claustrophobia • massive obesity • dyspnea at rest • patients with pollakisuria • restlessness patients or those with pain in the back or pruritus • intrauterine pessary • pregnancy

2.9 Contraindications to MRI

Before positioning a patient in an MRI scanner, a potential danger to the patient from the static magnet field or radiofrequency energy has to be definitively excluded. A list of absolute and relative contraindications, as given in Table 2-4, may be helpful for assessing the individual risk of a given patient. Patients with ferromagnetic implants (pacemakers, ICDs, clips etc.), metal splinter or shrapnel in their body, or electronic implants (insulin pumps, neurostimulators, cochlea or other implants) should definitively not be placed in an MRI scanner. Patients after surgical revascularization with bypass clips and sternal cerclage can be examined after 2 weeks post-operatively without additional risk, and patients with intracoronary stents do not carry a relevant risk when investigated with MRI. The same applies for patients with prosthetic heart valves, only two manufacturers warned against MRI studies in patients with the Starr-Edwards model Pre-1,000 and Pre-6,000 (implanted from 1960 to 1964), and the Jomed Monodisc with a metal ring in the occluder. Patients with modern artificial cardiac valves do not carry any additional risk when studied by MRI, as aplies also for orthopedic implants (hip or knee implants). Be aware that MR-safe equipment and implants are often tested for up to 1.5 T magnetic field strength, only.

As regards safety aspects of pregnancy, pregnant health care practitioners are allowed to work in and around the MR unit throughout their entire pregnancy, including positioning of the patient, injecting contrast material, and entering the MR room. Pregnant MR operators should not enter the scanner room during actual data acquisition. For pregnant patients, the actual recommendation is to avoid MR examinations within the first trimester. Thereafter MRI studies can be performed if the patient's clinician and the performing cardiologist/radiologist concur that the patient's risk-benefit ratio warrants the study to be performed. This means that the information provided by the MR investigation cannot be acquired by other non-invasive and non-ionizing techniques, e.g. by echocardiography, and that the information from this study has therapeutic consequences during the period of pregnancy. If the indication for an MRI study is confirmed, MR contrast agents should not be administered to pregnant patients, since there is insufficient data regarding the pharmacokinetics of MR contrast agents passing through the placenta, as well as into the mother's milk after delivery when patients are studied at this time point.

References

De Vocht F. Enviromental and Occupational Health Group. Temporal neurobehavioral effects among subjects exposed to high static and dynamic fields from MRI systems. ISMRM Workshop on Current Issues in MR Safety, Munich: February 23–24, 2003.

Edelstein WA, Hedeen RA, Mallozzi RP et al. Making MRI quieter. Magn Reson Imaging 2002; 20: 155–63.

Kangarlu A, Burgess RE, Zhu H et al. Cognitive, cardiac and physiological safety studies in ultra high-field magnetic resonance imaging. Magn Reson Imaging 1999; 17: 1407–16.

Kinouchi Y, Yamaguchi H, Tenforde TS. Theoretical analysis of magnetic field interaction with aortic blood flow. Bioelectromagnetics 1996; 17: 21–32.

Mansfield P, Haywood B, Coxon R. Active acoustic control in gradient coils for MRI. Magn Reson Med 2001; 46: 807–18.

Niendorf T, Sodickson DK, Krombach GA, Schulz-Menger J. Toward cardiovascular MRI at 7 T: clinical needs, technical solutions and research promises. Eur Radiol 2010; 20: 2806–16.

Rutt BK, Lee DH. The impact of field strength on image quality in MRI. J Magn Reson Imaging 1996; 6 (1): 57–62.

Schenk JF. Safety of strong, static magnetic fields. J Magn Reson Imaging 2000; 12: 2–19.

Schenk JF. MR safety at high magnetic fields. Magn Reson Imaging Clin N Am 1998; 6: 715–30.

Shellock FG. Reference Manual for Magnetic Resonance Safety. 3rd ed. Salt Lake City, UT: Amirsys Inc. 2003.

3 Contrast Agents for Magnetic Resonance Imaging – Recent Advances

Dipanjan Pan and Gregory M. Lanza

3.1 Introduction

The end of the nineteenth century witnessed the discovery of X-rays which brought a powerful tool for the non-invasive study of human organs. However, it soon became quite evident that the technique was not truly non-invasive due to its destructive effect on tissues caused by ionizing radiation. Today's X-ray-based imaging technologies employ sophisticated means to improve patient safety, but radiation can still be involved and poses similar inherent health risks as decades ago.

In 2003, Paul Lauterbur from the University of Illinois in Urbana and Peter Mansfield from the University of Nottingham were awarded the Nobel Prize for jointly inventing Magnetic Resonance Imaging. Dr. Lauterbur discovered how to create a two-dimensional image by introducing gradients into the magnetic field. By processing the data from emitted radio waves, he demonstrated two-dimensional images of structures that had not been previously visualized. This seminal breakthrough was further developed by Peter Mansfield who showed how the signals could be mathematically reconstructed based on differences in resonances and processed extremely fast into useful images; these now serve as pillars for radiological medical diagnosis of soft-tissue disease. The improved safety of MRI over techniques requiring ionizing radiation remains a milestone of enormous proportions in medicine.

Molecular imaging is an emergent technology at the interface of biological and physical science that extends the utility of MRI imaging toward understanding the components, processes, dynamics and therapeutic response of disease from a biochemical and functional perspective. Novel molecular agents are integrated with traditional imaging tools to visually describe the cellular event and capture specific molecular pathways in the body that are key targets in disease progression. The numerous opportunities of this research are applicable to the diagnosis of diseases such as cancer and cardiovascular to name a few (Weissleder 2001, Massoud 2003, Doubrovin 2004, Thakur 2005, Mankoff 2007). The tremendous potential of this technology to identify pre-clinical pathology has resulted in a surge in the contrast agent's research. In this chapter, we will particularly emphasize these contrast agents for MRI-based application.

3.2 Contrast Materials for MRI – General Consideration

3.2.1 Contrast Materials and Broader Classifications

Magnetic resonance imaging (MRI) is a non-invasive diagnostic technique based on the interaction of nuclei with each other and with surrounding molecules in a tissue. Although the sensitivity of MR is low in comparison to nuclear and optical modalities, the absence of radiation (transmitted or injected) and high spatial resolution (e.g. sub-millimeter) makes it advantageous over the techniques involving radioisotopes. There are many medically relevant nuclei, but the

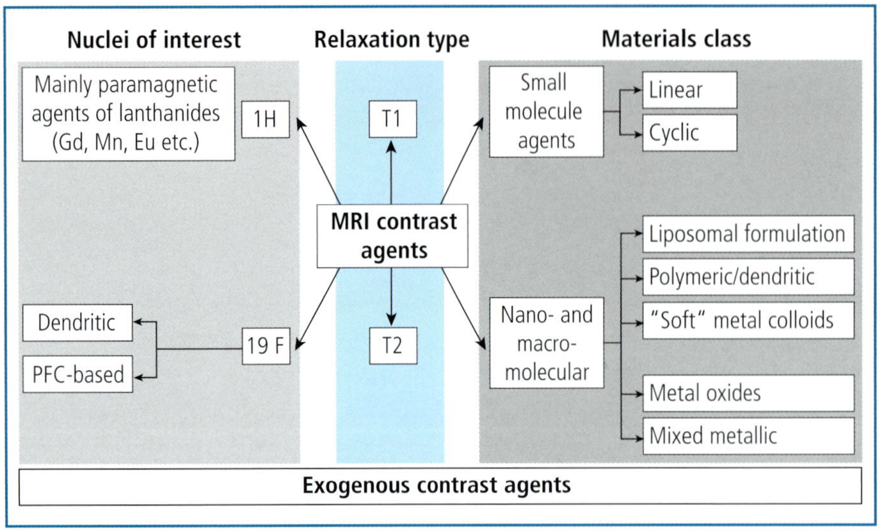

Figure 3-1 Classifications of MRI contrast agents based on materials class, relaxation type and nuclei of interest.

^{1}H-nucleus (i.e. proton) has been the most widely studied in clinical practice due to its high gyromagnetic ratio, high abundance in nature and biological tissues. ^{19}F has a similar high gyromagnetic ratio as proton and a very high (~ 100%) natural occurrence, which also makes it an interesting choice for MR imaging (Longmaid 1985, Damadian 1971). At constant field strength and with equivalent number of nuclei, ^{19}F has a sensitivity of about 83% compared to ^{1}H.

In MRI, the protons in different tissues have different relaxation times, which can result in endogenous image contrast (Damadian 1971). Inherent image contrast can be enhanced using exogenous contrast agents to preferentially shorten the T1 (longitudinal, spin-lattice) or T2 (transverse, spin-spin) relaxation times. Relaxivity is defined as the ability of contrast agents to increase the relaxation rates of the surrounding water proton spins. Gadolinium and iron oxide-based agents have dominated the MR contrast agent scenario and have been used to increase the T1- and T2-weighted image contrast (de Roos 1988, Prince 1993, Kaufman 1996, Thorek 2006). T1 agents influence protons within their proximity and are highly dependent on local water flux (Lanza 2004) to predominantly shorten T1 relaxation, thus producing bright signals on T1-weighted images.

The signal intensity in MRI depends not only on the concentration of free-water in a location, but also upon the magnetic relaxation times T1 and T2. Because the proton density within tissues differs, the MR relaxation times are inherently altered resulting in unique appearances. MR contrast agents further accentuate inherent tissue signal differences, which greatly increases the diagnostic power of the technology.

Typically, in terms of the materials class, MR contrast agents can be classified into two broad categories i.e. small molecule agents and nanoparticulate agents (Figure 3-1). These agents are mainly paramagnetic and superparamagnetic in nature. Paramagnetic species contain unpaired electrons e.g. molecular oxygen, a stable radical (i.e. nitroxide radical) or metal ions (i.e. transition metals). Radicals are not typically suitable agents for MRI application, since they can exert adverse effects on the living tissues. Molecular oxygen produces a very weak paramagnetic effect. Transition metal ions, however, exhibit suitable effect owing to the presence of a number of unpaired electrons in their outer most d or f orbitals. Several transition and lanthanide metals are available with unpaired electrons, but their spin-relaxation times must match the Larmor frequency of the protons. Typically, Fe^{3+}, Mn^{2+} and Gd^{3+} ions have adequate Larmor frequencies of about 10^{-8}. This chapter will mainly discuss contrast agents-based on these metal ions. Some paramagnetic metals (e.g. manganese) have been used in both ionic and chelated forms as blood pool contrast. The fundamental drawback of paramagnetic metals is their intrinsic toxicity as free ions. Studies have focused on the development of stable paramagnetic ion complexes by generating a thermodynamically and kinetically stable compound. Complexation of the metal ion with organic ligand (i.e. DTPA, EDTA, BMA etc.), has been used extensively to limit the bioavailability of free metal. Particulate entities such as liposomes or nanoparticles have been used to enhance the magnitude of contrast effect and to control the distribution and localization by entrapping or binding increased payloads of paramagnetic metal.

Iron oxide-based agents, on the other hand, are generally considered as T2 agents, which exhibit high magnetic susceptibility inherently and produce local disturbances in the field (Nelson 1995). Signal dephasing in tissues resulting from magnetic susceptibility heterogeneity disturbances leads to signal loss through T2* decay, especially with gradient versus spin echo image pulse sequences.

3.2.2 T1 Small Molecule Contrast Agents

Gadolinium

Gadolinium (III)-based agents dominate the small molecule-based MR contrast agents area (Krasnow 1972, Wiegers 1992, Spanoghe 1992, Carollo 1990). Gd (III) is an attractive choice due to the presence of seven unpaired electrons. Interestingly Gd (III) retains its number of unpaired spins when bound to an organic chelate (Figure 3-2). Several Gd complexes are very stable and exhibit low toxicity. Magnevist® is a DTPA complex of Gd [([Gd(DTPA)(H_2O)]$^{2-}$], which has been approved for clinical use. This extracellular contrast agent is relatively inexpensive to synthesize and provides excellent safety in patients with all but severe renal dysfunction. The allowed doses can be as high as 0.3 mmol/kg for angiography and other clinical applications. At high Magnevist® dose, T1 is much shorter than in any other tissue and contrast is excellent.

Several other Gd complexes have been tested which include the use of ligands e. g. DTPA-BMA (diethylenetriamine-pentaacetic acid bis[methylamide]), DTPA-BP (N,N'-bis [2-pyridylmethyl] diethylenetriamine N,N'N"-triacetic acid), CDTA (trans-1,2-diaminocyclohexane-N,N'N"N'"-tetraacetic acid), DOTA (1,4,7,10-tetraazacyclododecane N,N',N",N'"-tetraacetic acid). The role of chelates in MRI studies with gadolinium has been reviewed by Low et. al. (1998) as well as Tripathi et. al. (2009), who describe the current uses of gadolinium chelates for clinical MRI.

Highly stable Gd (III) complexes were prepared as coordination cages. These agents were responsible for increasing relaxivity through enhanced hydration of the gadolinium ion. Examples of these agents are macrocyclic heptadentate PCTA and AAZTA ligands (Aime 1997, Tircso 2009, Elemento 2009). Raymond and coworkers reported similar hexadentate macrocyclic HOPO-based ligands (Thompson 2003, Datta 2009). These complexes offer highly hydrated Gd complexes with high relaxivity and high stability against transmetallation.

For most of the biological targets, the presence of more than one gadolinium ion is desired to produce the necessary relaxation rate changes. Different constructs have been proposed for increasing relaxivity. Synthesizing polymers in a linear fashion increases the number of Gd per molecule but due to the flexibility or internal motion the net relaxivity is somewhat diminished. Casali and coworkers reported a modified dextran polymer carrying DO3A-monoamide chelates. The relaxivity has been reported to be 10.6 $mM^{-1}s^{-1}$ at 37 °C, 0.47 T on a per gadolinium basis (Casali 1998).

Dendrimers on the other hand carrying multiple gadolinium ions have a tendency to exhibit higher relaxivity by introducing a more globular structure and thereby slowing the internal rotation. Gadomer-17 (MW = 17 kDa) is an example of this kind of dendritic molecule appending 24 gadolinum chelates as compared to its linear counterpart. Gadomer-17 shows a relaxivity of 16.5 $mM^{-1}s^{-1}$ at 37 °C, 0.47 T on a per gadolinium basis (Rohrer 2005).

The effect of motion can also be optimized in another approach. This time, the gadolinium ion is placed as a monomer at the barycenter of a molecule. In this way, the non-gadolinium containing moieties are free to have rotation, however the metal at the barycenter can only rotate at the rate of the entire molecule resulting in a very high relaxivity. This approach has been exemplified by the Gurbet group in a molecule called Vistarem (gadomelitol) (Port 2001). Gadomelitol is a compound incorporating Gd-DOTA which exhibits a relaxivity of 39.0 $mM^{-1}s^{-1}$ at 37 °C, 0.47 T on a per gadolinium basis.

Desreux and coworkers proposed a metal template self-assembly approach to control the rotation flexibility of these molecules carrying multiple gadolinium ions. Bis-gadolinium DTPA complexes were synthesized with pendant bidentate ligands to assemble around a transition metal (i. e. Fe^{2+}) to increase the molecular weight and hence the relaxivity. The per gadolinium relaxivity was found to be 12.5 $mM^{-1}s^{-1}$ at 37 °C, 40 MHz as compared to 3.8 $mM^{-1}s^{-1}$ for Gd-DTPA under the similar condition (Jacques and Desreux 2002).

Zhang and coworkers (2005) showed that the relaxivity can be further improved by restricting internal motion upon binding to a biological target. They exemplified in a model system comprising a compound carrying four Gd-DTPA units coupled to a targeting vector. This compound is quite flexible in the absence of serum albumin but in the presence of the protein the relaxivity is increased by a factor of three.

Non covalently bound Gd (III) complexes to human serum albumin (HSA) have been shown to alter the residence lifetime of the water protons at the metal sites. High relaxivity has been reported for the complexes interacting with macromolecules. A markedly diminished lability of the water molecule at the metal sites has been observed, which can be attributed to the formation of H-bonding of the metal with the polar groups of the protein. The concept has been confirmed with complexes carrying non coordinating polar groups (Zech 2007).

Stimuli responsive agents are another class of contrast materials that are of considerable interest. Meade and coworkers reported a Gd (III) agent (a- and b-EGadMe) containing a galactopyranosyl functionality responsive to enzyme β-galactosidase (Urbanczyk-Pearson 2008). A similar agent has been reported by Weissleder's group responsive to the myeloperoxidase enzyme, an important marker for inflammation (Breckwoldt 2008). Novel pH responsive system has also been reported recently (Morawski 2004, Gianolio 2009). However, most of these examples have been con-

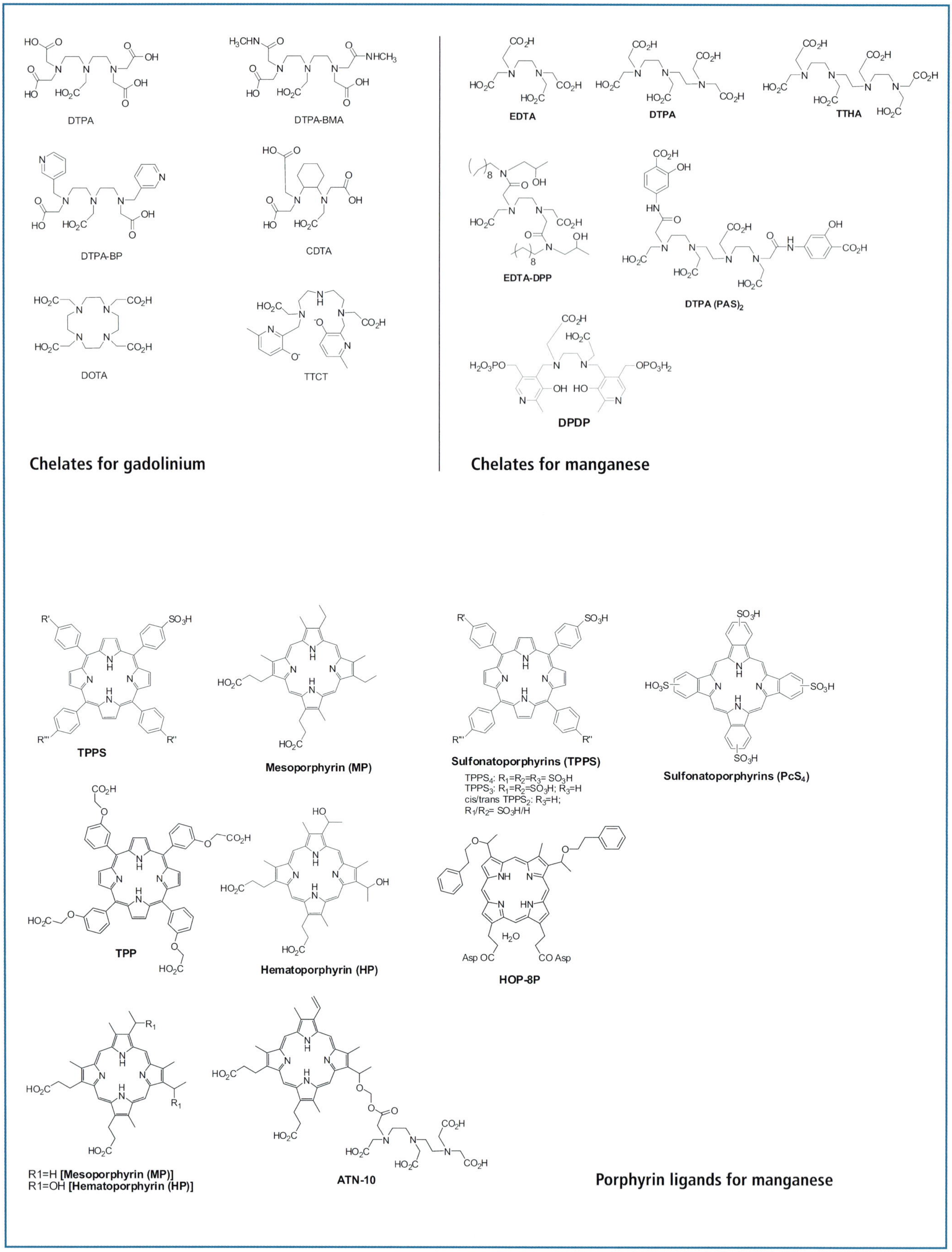

Figure 3-2 Examples of small molecule chelates for gadolinium and manganese.

ducted *in vitro* and only a very few *in vivo* studies have been published.

Nephrogenic Systemic Fibrosis

In recent years concern about the safety of gadolinium came to the fore forcing regulatory agencies to constrain the use of these chelates in patients with severe renal disease. The discovery of nephrogenic systemic fibrosis (NSF) began with a San Diego, CA hospital over a three-year period noting that a small subset of renal transplant patients had developed joint contractures, brawny induration and hyperpigmentation of the skin in their extremities. Skin biopsies revealed fibrosis and elastosis with mucin deposition, dermal spindle cells, histiocytes, dendrocytes, and increased type1 procollagen (Cowper 2001). Although initially referred to as "nephrogenic fibrosing dermopathy", subsequent recognition of visceral involvement led to the renaming of the condition to "nephrogenic systemic fibrosis" or NSF. The number of cases increased from the original 8 to over 250 in some registries, with all affected individuals noted to have chronic kidney disease (CKD). Clinical observation by Grobner et al. (2006), an Austrian nephrologist, led to the association of gadolinium-enhanced magnetic resonance angiography and the development of NSF. Subsequently, others confirmed this finding (Todd 2008). Gadolinium has been detected in skin and other tissues obtained from patients with NSF, further supporting this causal association.

> In response, the US FDA and other regulator agencies have issued a boxed warning of gadolinium blood pool agents that stipulates that gadolinium-based contrast agents (GBCAs) increase **the risk for NSF** in patients with:
> - acute or chronic severe renal insufficiency (glomerular filtration rate < 30 ml/min/1.73 m²),
> - acute renal insufficiency of any severity due to the hepatorenal syndrome, or
> - in the peri-operative liver transplantation period.

The agency suggested that the use GBCAs be avoided unless the diagnostic information was essential and unavailable with non-contrast-enhanced magnetic resonance imaging (MRI) (Mazhar 2009). They recommended screening all patients for renal dysfunction by obtaining a history and/or laboratory tests, not exceeding the recommended dosage on the product labeling (e.g. prior practice for myocardial scar imaging), and allowing adequate time for complete elimination before any readministration. Although dialysis of patients may be considered promptly following GBCA administration, there is no evidence that hemodialysis prevents NSF (Marckmann 2008).

The FDA noted that post-marketing reports suggested that the most commonly reported agent was Omniscan®, followed by Magnevist® and OptiMARK®. These gadolinium chelates are in a chemical class known as linear molecules, which differentiates them from another category of gadolinium chelates, i.e. the macrocyclic molecules discussed above. In general, the kinetic, thermodynamic and conditional stability of the macrocyclic chelates to transmetallation with zinc and cations is known to be superior to the linear forms (Port 2008a, b). In normal patients, the distribution phase of gadolinium chelates lasts 4 min and the elimination half-life is around 5 h (Abraham 2008). Over 24 h, virtually all of the metal has been excreted through the urine. Of course, with increasing degrees of renal insufficiency, this clearance rate is prolonged. Fortunately, since the relabeling restriction of the approved use of gadolinium agents, no further incidences of NSF have been highlighted.

Manganese

One of the earliest examples of manganese contrast agents was a solution of manganese(II)chloride (Lauterbur 1978). The measured r1 value is $8.0 \pm 0.1\ mM^{-1}s^{-1}$ at 20 MHz and 37 °C (Chen 1984) and $6.0\ mM^{-1}s^{-1}$ at 40 MHz and 40 °C (Kreft 1993). However, it was revealed that both i.p. and i.v. injected aquo manganese(II) impart neurotoxicity. The LD_{50} in mice for manganese(II) is 0.3 mmol kg^{-1} injected intravenously and 1.0 mmol kg^{-1} injected intraperitoneally.

Toxicity can be lowered by chelation of the free manganese with dipyridoxaldiphosphate (DPDP) (Figure 3-2), which also provides selective tissue uptake. Mn-DPDP has been approved for liver imaging. It has an LD_{50} of 540 mmol kg^{-1}, which is much higher in comparison to gadolinium diethylenetriaminepentaacetic acid (Gd-DTPA) ($LD_{50} = 60-100$). The relaxivity of Mn-DPDP in aqueous solutions was found to be $r1 = 2.8\ mM^{-1}\ s^{-1}$, $r2 = 3.7\ mM^{-1}\ s^{-1}$ and the highest tissue r1 value was found in kidney ($r1 = 276.6\ mM^{-1}\ s^{-1}$).

Manganese(II) ions encapsulated within liposomes have been reported to have r1 value of 35.34 $mM^{-1}\ s^{-1}$ at 20 MHz. Liposomes encapsulating chelated Mn(II) to various polycarboxylic acid ligands, e.g. EDTA (Schwendener 1990), EDTA-DPP (Unger 1993), DTPA, $DTPA(PAS)_2$ (Schwendener 1990) and TTHA (Rongved 1991) have been reported. Porphyrins are common chelators for manganese (Figure 3-2). Examples of such chelators include sulfonatoporphyrins, where it undergoes rapid oxidation to Mn(III) (Buchler 1979). Manganese(III)tetra-(4-sulfonatophenyl)porphyrin ($TPPS_4$) was one of the earliest examples of sulfonatoporphyrins followed by analogues with progressively fewer sulfonate functionalities ($TPPS_3$, $TPPS_2$) (Fiel 1990, Place 1992). Additional closely related manganese complexes include UROP-1 (Schmiedl 1993), mesoporphyrin, hematoporphyrin (Fawwaz 1969, Fawwaz 1971) and ATN-10

(Fujimori 1997). A potentially tumor-seeking MR agent α-Aqua-13,17-bis(1-carboxypropionyl)carbamoylethyl-3,8-bis(1-phenethyloxyethyl)-β-hydroxy-2,7,12,18-tetramethyl-porphyrinato manganese(III) (HOP-8P) has been studied in a tumor bearing mouse model (Takehara 2002).

3.2.3 Nanoparticle-Based Agents

Organization of the components at the nanometric scale creates unique chemical and biological properties based on interaction over their increased functional surface areas. Over the past decade, nanomaterials have been the subject of vast interest. Due to their extremely small feature size, they have the potential for wide-ranging biomedical applications as contrast agents alone and as image-based drug delivery systems. Research at nanometric scale has shown that particle size and character govern circulatory half-life, reticuloendothelial clearance rate, protein-binding and blood contact compatibility, as well as accessibility to pathological target receptors. From a material science perspective, nanoparticles are in the 100 nm and below range, which corresponds to a size at which the physical properties of matter can be altered. However, for biomedical applications the definition of nanoparticle in the biological sciences is dynamic and much more liberal, typically < than 300 nm in the US and < 500 nm in Europe. In this context the longer circulating half-lives and greater surface-to-volume ratio of these minute particles offer the principle advantages. Typically, particles below 100 nm, dependent upon chemical design have better extravasation potential, while agents greater than 100 nm are best suited for intravascular applications. The often reported enhanced permeability and retention (EPR) phenomenon of particles with wide ranging sizes refers to an extravasation effect predominantly associated with subcutaneous tumor grafts implanted in mice. However, similar tumors implanted into tissues in mice, such as a fat pad, or in any location in larger animals have considerably less inherent extravascular transport due to "leakage".

The high surface area to volume ratio on nanoparticles allows functionalization to accommodate targeting moieties and contrast agents on the surface. This way, the number of ligands per nanoparticle is increased and thereby decreases the rate of dissociation and improves their binding affinity. This "stick-and-stay" effect is referred to as avidity. Towards this goal, well-defined nanoscale materials are being developed involving classical and advanced techniques to carry paramagnetic metals and other constructs are, themselves, the imageable agent, but are functionalized for targeting (e.g. carbohydrate coated superparamagnetic iron oxides). Molecular agents must be clinically translatable and must possess specific properties e.g. tolerable toxicity, long circulating half-life, excellent contrast-to-noise ratio enhancement, and high binding efficacy.

Of late there has been a surge in the development of nanoparticle platforms in the literature directed towards active and passive targeting mechanisms. Iron oxides, in magnetite (Fe_3O_4) and maghemite (Fe_2O_3) forms have dominated the superparamagnetic nano-sized contrast agent field. Superparamagnetic iron oxides (SPIO) constitute iron oxide, coated with hydrophilic agents e.g. polymers (PMMA, PVA, PLGA, PEG, PEG-lipid), dextrans, starch, oleic acid etc. Standard SPIO (SSPIO) can be categorized as particles having sizes ranging from 300 nm to micron level. The examples of the smallest candidates of iron oxide family come from the ultrasmall SPIO (USPIO) and monocrystalline iron oxide nanoparticles (MION) within the size range from 10–40 nm. Superparamagnetic iron oxide particles represent one of the earliest known applications for MR imaging in healthy hepatocytes (Saini 1995), prostate cancer (Harisinghani 2003) and even in atherosclerotic rabbit models (Ruehm 2001).

There has been significant research in the development of other nano-sized constructs such as dendrimers (Quintana 2002, Kobayashi 2003), shell-crosslinked polymers (Turner 2005), nanocages (Loo 2004, Cang 2005, Agrawal 2006), magneto-micelles (Byeong 2005), virus particles (Wang 2002, Manchester 2006), and ultra small superparamagnetic iron oxide (USPIO) (Josephson 1999, Dodd 2001, Kang 2002, Schellenberger 2002, Artemov 2003). Star polymers (Moffat 2003, Kobayashi 2002, Kobayashi 2004, Dear 2005) and other hyperbranched polymers (Kobayashi 2001, Stiriba 2002, Hisataka 2005) have demonstrated that dynamic high-resolution micro-MRI combined with a novel dendrimer-based macromolecular renal MRI contrast agent ("dendrimer-enhanced MRI") can be a powerful tool for *in vivo* observation of renal structure, function, and injury and also can be used as a novel marker for diagnosis and prognosis of sepsis-induced acute renal failure in aged mice. An avidin-conjugated, gadolinium-loaded dendrimer has been efficiently internalized into SHIN3 ovarian adenocarcinoma cells *in vitro* and shown to be accumulated in the intraperitoneally disseminated ovarian tumor (SHIN3) in a mouse model (Kobayashi 2001). Recently dendrimer-based MR contrast agents have been successfully employed *in vivo* for articular cartilage assessment by MR imaging (Winalski 2008) and in angiogenesis (Quido 2005).

Liposomes (Navon 1986, Grant 1989, Koenig 1992, Sipkins 1998, Fossheim 1999, Hood 2002, Moffat 2003) and nanoemulsions (Lanza 1996, Flacke 2001, Schmieder 2005, Winter 2005, Winter 2008) represent other classes of nanoparticles that have been studied extensively *in vivo* for targeted imaging. The perfluorocarbon (PFC) nanoparticle is a unique platform technology, which may be applied to

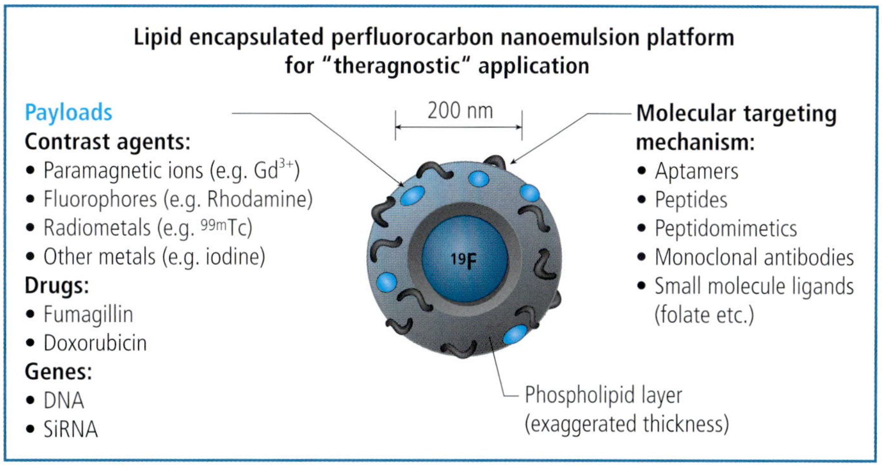

Figure 3-3 Lipid encapsulated perfluorocarbon nanoemulsion carrying high payload of contrast agents and drugs, which represents an extremely versatile platform for molecular imaging and drug delivery application. PFC nanoparticle carries contrast agents, drugs etc. as a constituent of phospholipid layer. For ligand-directed molecular imaging, aptamers, peptides, small molecule ligands and monoclonal antibodies are used.

clinically relevant modalities. Ligand directed, phospholipid-encapsulated PFC nanoparticles are vascularly constrained (~ 250 nm) and fluidic in nature (Figure 3-3). The surface of a paramagnetic nanoparticle may present more than 100,000 contrast metals and several hundreds of homing ligands per particle, which provides high signal amplification and avidity i.e. "stick and stay" quality. Therefore the surface area to volume ratio allows an even greater concentrating effect to deliver massive amounts of contrast agent per binding site and per volume, which allows them to be non-invasively detected by clinically relevant modalities.

More recently imaging of nanoparticles has been extended to include therapeutic agents for image guided drug delivery application. These theragnostic agents allow confirmation and quantification of local delivery for the response to be serially monitored for targeted agent. The utility of perfluorocarbon nanoparticle technology as a potential theragnostic agent (i.e. a targeted therapeutic delivery agent that can also be imaged for diagnostic or dose quantification purposes) is being explored (Lanza 1996).

The challenge to overcome the sensitivity and partial volume effect that is normally faced by T1- and T2-weighted MR contrast agents, prompted the development of T1-weighted paramagnetic PFC particles. Typically, for a 200-nm diameter particle, more than 100,000 gadolinium atoms per particle can be incorporated within the outer surface of the lipid membrane where they influence the surrounding water for maximum T1 relaxation effect (Lanza 1996, Flacke 2001, Winter 2003). In doing so, high payload of gadolinium is incorporated to produce adequate MR signal. The relaxivity of reported Gd^{3+}-chelates (4.5 $mM^{-1}sec^{-1}$) is lower than Gd^{3+} bound to the surface of the particle (33.7 $mM^{-1}sec^{-1}$) as measured at 1.5 T (Stanisz 2000). The particulate relaxivity (i.e. the relaxivity on a per particle basis, rather than per concentration of Gd) has also been found to be very high (~ 2,000,000 $mM^{-1}sec^{-1}$) since each particle carries a heavy payload of paramagnetic metal atoms, making them an effective agent for targeted molecular imaging but a poor blood pool contrast agent. This relationship ensures that the accumulating increase in targeted signal at a desired pathology is not confounded by blood pool contrast signal (i.e. background noise). This property was exploited to quantitatively image and successfully predict a range of sparse concentrations in experimental phantoms and targeted smooth muscle cell (SMC) monolayers expressing "tissue factor" (Parmelee 1997, Lauffer 1998).

Unlike paramagnetic gadolinium-based particles carrying high payload of metals, gadofosveset trisodium (MS-325) is a small molecule contrast agent, which has a strong affinity towards albumin and it is highly protein bound after injection providing vascular signal enhancement superior to other agents. Notably, MS-325 is the first gadolinium-based blood pool magnetic resonance (MR) "targeted" imaging agent (Moody 1999).

Molecular Imaging Opportunities with PFC Nanoparticle

Magnetic resonance imaging (MRI) has emerged as a particularly sensitive, non-ionizing modality to non-invasively visualize thromboses within the carotid artery (Moody 1999). High-resolution MRI detection and characterization of atherosclerotic lesions (including advanced lesions, such as the fibrous cap, the lipid core, and even plaque fissuring) with serial imaging over time has been used to assess lesion progression or regression (Yuan 1994, Skinner 1995, Toussaint 1996). High-resolution MRI can be used to distinguish intact, thick fibrous caps from intact thin and disrupted caps in atherosclerotic human carotid arteries *in vivo* (Hatsukami 2000, Fayad 2000a). Advances in high spatial resolution black-blood techniques further improved

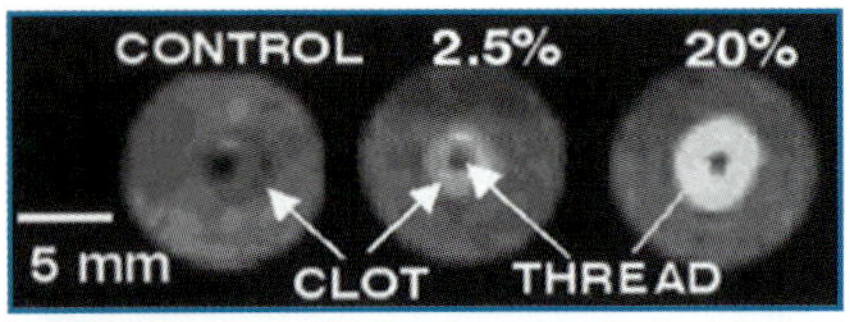

a

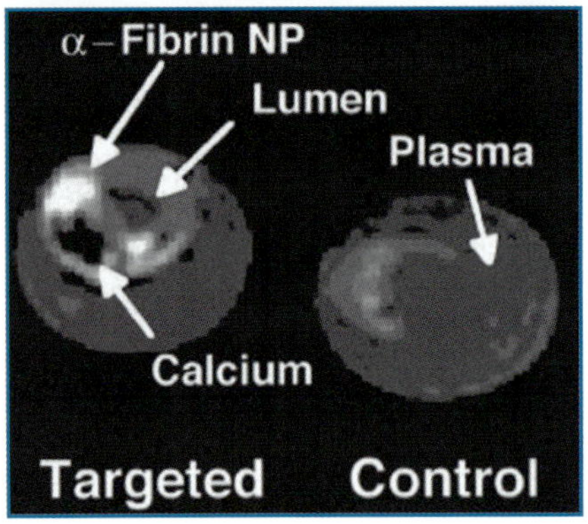

b

Figure 3-4 MR images of plasma clots (in vitro) and carotid endarectamy specimen (ex vivo) pre-targeted with antifibrin monoclonal antibody and exposed to control or biotinylated PFC nanoparticle. **(a)** Low-resolution images (three-dimensional T1-weighted) of control and fibrin-targeted clot with paramagnetic nanoparticles presenting a homogeneous, T1w-enhancement. **(b)** Magnetic resonance imaging of fibrin-targeted and control carotid endarterectomy specimens revealing contrast enhancement (white) of a small fibrin deposit on a symptomatic ruptured plaque, calcium deposit (black) (from Winter PM, Caruthers SD, Yu X et al. Improved molecular imaging contrast agent for detection of human thrombus. Magn Reson Med 2003; 50: 411–6; with permission of Wiley & Sons, USA).

non-invasive imaging of human coronary and carotid arteries and facilitate the early assessment of atherosclerotic disease (Fayad 2000b). Although cardio-respiratory motion has complicated coronary imaging with MRI, rapid advancements in motion correction are being reported, which will likely limit or resolve this issue in the not-too-distant future (King 2008, Odille 2008, Maclaren 2008).

Sensitive and fibrin-specific contrast agents-based on PFC-nanoemulsions (Lanza 1996, Botnar 2004) and peptides (Yu 2000) have recently been developed that are capable of detecting and quantifying microthrombus. As briefly discussed before, perfluorocarbon nanoparticle have been used in conjunction with paramagnetic metals as a bifunctional contrast agent that can be used as a paramagnetic MRI agent separately and in combination with fluorine imaging. A targeted MRI agent (Winter 2003), was developed by incorporating a lipid-conjugated gadolinium-DTPA complex into the surfactant layer for targeting clots in dogs *in situ* (Figure 3-4). Subsequently, the MRI agent was refined to optimize the concentration of gadolinium borne on the particle surface (Yu 2000, Morawski 2004, Winter 2003, Winter 2005) to overcome the partial volume effects that have negated so many previous attempts at targeted MRI agents. In this experiment using MRI, the gadolinium-enriched nanoemulsions provided outstanding contrast properties and overcame the partial volume effects expected with routine imaging at 1.5 T when targeted to artificially prepared fibrin clots.

Morawski et al. (2004) have demonstrated the utility of fibrin-targeted nanoparticles to delineate intravascular thrombus in dogs and conceptually on vulnerable plaque using human carotid endarterectomy (CEA) specimens from diseased human patients. These data indicate that small, perhaps even microscopic, deposits of human fibrin in microfissures of vulnerable carotid plaques can be detected with the contrast agent.

Winter et al. (2003) reported quantitative MR molecular imaging with $\alpha v\beta 3$-targeted gadolinium incorporated paramagnetic nanoparticles. In this study, $\alpha v\beta 3$-targeted fumagillin loaded nanoparticles were used to suppress the neovasculature and inhibit Vx-2 adenocarcinoma development using minute drug doses. With the help of MR imaging and high-resolution three-dimensional neovascular maps, tumor size and neovascularity was assessed. Authors illustrated the asymmetric, patchy pattern of angiogenic expression that diminished by $\alpha v\beta 3$-targeted fumagillin nanoparticles. Results also revealed that the neovasculature was predominantly located in the peripheral aspects of the tumor, which was corroborated by the colocalization of $\alpha v\beta 3$-targeted rhodamine nanoparticles with FITC-lectin exclusively in the tumor periphery (Figure 3-5).

The high fluorine content of the PFC nanoparticles was further exploited for ^{19}F MR imaging and spectroscopy. Using the ^{19}F signal Morawski et al. (2004) quantified the number of nanoparticles bound to the fibrin clot. Additional study revealed that two perfluorocarbon cores i.e. perfluorooctyl bromide (PFOB) and crown ether (CE) can be differentiated, for targeting clot phantoms. On a 4.7 T imaging system, the cores exhibited two distinct ^{19}F spectra with the signal strength of each unique spectral signature correlating well with the ratio of the two emulsions used. These findings could lead us to quantitatively image two separate nanoparticles for targeting two distinct biomarkers.

The feasibility of ^{19}F imaging of both PFOB and CE nanoparticle-labeled stem/progenitor cells was shown. Several MRI-based agents e.g. gadolinium (Kraitchman 2003, Hill 2003), superparamagnetic iron oxides (Yeh 1993, Ahrens 2003, Kirchner 2003, Kraitchman 2003, Hill 2003, Bulte 2004, Stroh 2005) and few others (Cunningham 2005) find significant use to visualize immune cells and others *in vivo*. However, contrast agents based on protons suffer from high background signal from water, which complicates unequivocal identification of transplanted cells *in vivo*. Ahrens et al. (2005) reported efficient intracellular uptake of the perfluoropolyether (PFPE)-based agents by phenotypi-

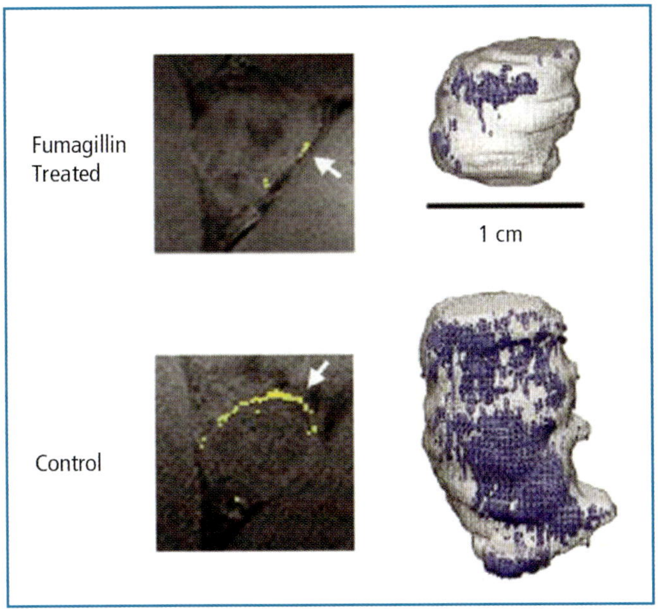

Figure 3-5 MR molecular imaging of Vx-2 tumor in rabbits. **Left**: Diminished αvβ3-integrin contrast enhancement in T1-weighted, fat-suppressed, three-dimensional (3D) gradient echo MR single slice images (enhancing pixels, color coded in yellow) in rabbits treated with αvβ3-targeted fumagillin-loaded nanoparticles **(top)** vs. αvβ3-targeted nanoparticles without drug **(bottom)**. **Right**: 3D neovascular maps of example Vx-2 tumors on day 16 following treatment with αvβ3-targeted fumagillin nanoparticles **(top)** vs. αvβ3-nanoparticles without drug **(bottom)**. Neovessel dense islands and the interspersed fine network of angiogenic proliferation over the tumor surface are diminished in rabbits receiving the targeted fumagillin treatment (from Winter PM, Caruthers SD, Kassner A et al. Molecular imaging of angiogenesis in nascent Vx-2 rabbit tumors using a novel alpha(nu)beta3-targeted nanoparticle and 1.5 T magnetic resonance imaging. Cancer Res 2005; 63: 5838–43; with permission of the American Association for Cancer Research).

cally defined dendritic cells (DCs) ex vivo into tissue or intravenously in mice and then tracked the cells *in vivo* using ^{19}F MRI. Along the same line, Partlow et al. (2007) recently demonstrated that PFC nanoparticles provide an unique signature for stem/progenitor cells, enabling spatial cell localization with ^{19}F MRI, and permit quantification and detection of multiple fluorine signatures with fluorine MR imaging and spectroscopy. PFC-labeled cells were detectable rapidly not only *in vitro*, but also in liver tissue *in vivo* with 11.7 T spectroscopy and at potential target sites *in situ* using both experimental (11.7 T) and clinical (1.5 T) field strengths. Similar methods previously performed using iron oxide particles can potentially lead to significant losses in cell viability (Arbab 2004). The resultant intracellular fluorine levels were readily detectible at both 11.7 T and 1.5 T, considering the relatively low number of cells utilized and the reasonably short imaging times (under 7 min) (Partlow 2007). The ability to quantify fluorine levels present and to differentiate distinct PFC signals with MR spectroscopy could provide additional advantages such as the type and number of cells accumulating at target sites.

PARACEST Agents

PARACEST (paramagnetic chemical exchange saturation transfer) agents represent a new class of MRI contrast agents that has been recently introduced, where the bulk water signal intensity is altered via chemical exchange saturation transfer (CEST), which was later extended to paramagnetic systems (Ward 2000, Zhang 2003). The contrast can be switched on and off as desired simply by adjusting the pulse sequence parameters avoiding the extra need to record pre- and post-injection images to define contrast agent binding. Liposome-based chemical exchange saturation transfer (lipoCEST) agents have shown great sensitivity and potential for molecular magnetic resonance imaging (MRI) (Stancanello 2008, Zhao 2008, Terreno 2007, Terreno 2008).

A PARACEST chelate has been used in conjunction with PFC-nanoparticle and produced > 10 % signal enhancement and a bound water peak at 52 ppm, in spectroscopy (4.7 T) of PARACEST nanoparticles. This result stands in agreement with results from the water-soluble chelates. PARACEST nanoparticles were targeted to artificially prepared plasma clots via antifibrin antibodies producing a contrast-to-noise ratio (CNR) of 10 at the clot surface (Winter 2006).

Manganese Nanoparticle-Based Approach

Shapiro and Koretsky (2008) reported on insoluble, inorganic manganese oxide particles (i.e. MnO, MnO_2, and Mn_3O_4) and manganese carbonate ($MnCO_3$) as convertible contrast agents for molecular and cellular MRI agents. These water insoluble Mn particles are formulated into nano- or microparticles. They have high magnetic susceptibilities and produce dark contrast when using T2*-weighted MRI pulse sequences. However, after cellular internalization and localization within endosomes and/or lysosomes, the particles are degraded by the abundant proteolytic enzymes in the predominantly acidic environment, releasing Mn^{2+} ions, which are strong T1 MRI contrast agents (Shapiro and Koretsky 2008).

One-dimensional Mn-Fe oxide composite nanostructures have been reported with 400–1,000 nm sizes in needles, rods, and wires form. *In vitro* studies showed the transport of the nanostructures into the cells of monocyte/macrophage cell line (RAW264.7) with negligible impact on cell viability at labeling concentration < 50 µg/ml. The results from 1.5 T MR were not satisfactory and indicated that the T2 relaxivities (r2) for nanoneedles, nanorods, and nanowires were 20.81 ± 0.58, 8.10 ± 0.31, and 6.62 ± 0.42 mM^{-1} s^{-1}, respectively, which were lower than the corresponding iron oxide nanoparticle derivatives (e.g. VSOP-C184 and SHU-555C [Supravist]). It was hypothesized that the formation of the larger nanostructures led to lower MR relaxivities (Leung 2009).

Manganese-doped superparamagnetic iron oxide (Mn-SPIO) nanoparticles were developed as ultrasensitive MRI contrast agents for liver imaging. At room temperature Mn-SPIO nanoparticles exhibited superparamagnetism. At the 1.5 T, the clustering micelles had a T2 relaxivity of 270 (Mn + Fe) mM^{-1} s^{-1}, which was much higher than single Mn-SPIO nanoparticle in a lipid-PEG micelle. This resulted in significant liver contrast with signal intensity decreased of ~ 80% in 5 min after intravenous administration. The strongly enhanced-MRI negative contrast liver images were highly prolonged and offered sensitive detection of minute liver lesions (Lu 2009). Similarly, multi-functional magneto-polymeric nanohybrids (MMPNs) have been synthesized using ultrasensitive $MnFe_2O_4$ nanocrystals, chemotherapeutic agents, and encapsulating amphiphilic block copolymers for targeted MR detection and treatment of breast cancer (Yang 2007).

Manganese-based oxo clusters (e.g. $Mn_{12}O_{12}(O_2CCH_3)_{16}(H_2O)_4$) are another class of important contrast agents of inorganic nature. Typically they are considered as prototypical "single molecule magnet" (SMM) since at low temperature the high spin state (S = 10) and anisotropy results in favorable magnetic properties (Sessoli 1993). Stoll and co-workers showed that manganese-oxo clusters had promise as an MRI contrast agent. Moreover, their MR and water solubility properties improved when incorporated onto the surface of polymer (e.g. polystyrene) beads (Figure 3-5) (Mertzman 2009).

Li et al. (2007) reported the synthesis and MR evaluation of two Mn(II)-monosubstituted polyoxometalates (MnPOMs), $MnSiW_{11}$ and MnP_2W_{17}. These agents were evaluated by *in vivo* and *in vitro* experiments as the candidates of tissue-specific MRI contrast agents. The measured relaxivities exhibited improved relaxation ability in comparison with Gd-DTPA. *In vivo* MR imaging in healthy rats demonstrated signal enhancement in liver and kidney, suggesting that with appropriate chemical modification, these two agents could be used as promising liver- and kidney-specific MRI contrast agents.

Wenbin Lin's group synthesized manganese-based core-shell nanoscale metal-organic frame works (NMOFs) (Taylor 2008). Mn-NMOFs comprised of terephthalic acid (BDC) and trimesic acid (BTC) bridging ligands. Rhodamine B and C (RGDfK) coupled particles demonstrated effective target-specific MR imaging to cancer cells *in vitro,* which was supported by optical imaging data. Although the r1 values exhibited by the Mn-NMOFs were unexceptional, their high water solubility delivered large doses of Mn^{2+} ions inside cells. *In vitro* and *in vivo* results both suggested that the silica-coated particles could deliver Mn^{2+} to sites of interest for high T1-weighted contrast enhancement.

Biocompatible MnO nanoparticles were prepared for MR imaging to elicit bright signal enhancement and fine anatomic detail in the T1-weighted MR image of a mouse brain. These particles were shown to target breast cancer cells in a metastatic tumor in brain (Na 2007). In another relevant work (Shin 2009), the relaxivity of MnO nanoparticles was altered by manipulating the size and curvature of the particles. Manganese oxide nanoparticles (20 nm) stabilized by oleic acid (MONs) as well as water-dispersible manganese oxide nanoparticles (WMONs) were prepared as encapsulated with poly(ethylene glycol) phospholipids. The selective removal of the MnO phase from the WMONs created hollow manganese oxide nanoparticles (HMONs). These hollow manganese oxide nanoparticles were incorporated with drugs and they retained efficient cellular uptake illustrating the potential of bifunctional theragnostic approach.

Organic or Polymeric Nanoparticle-Based Approach

Manganese(III)-labeled nanobialy, a "soft-type" toroidal biconcave particle, has potential as targeted MR theragnostic agent (Pan 2008). Nanobialys are formed through spontaneous self-assembly of amphiphilic hyperbranched polyethylenimine particle size (180–200 nm) with low polydispersity. The "Bialys" presented Mn(III) in a kinetically stable, manganese protoporphyrin coupled complex directly exposed to the surrounding water producing ionic r1 and r2 relaxivities of 3.7 ± 1.1 (s × mmol $[Mn])^{-1}$ and 5.2 ± 1.1 (s × mmol $[Mn])^{-1}$ and particulate relaxivities of 612,307 ± 7,213 (s × mmol $[nanobialy])^{-1}$ and 866,989 ± 10,704 (s × mmol $[nanobialy])^{-1}$, respectively. The theragnostic potential of nanobialys was illustrated through targeted Mn MR imaging *in vitro* using antifibrin monoclonal targeting to fibrin-rich clots with efficient (98%) synthetic incorporation and *in vitro* dissolution retention (80%) of chemotherapeutic compounds (doxorubicin and camtothecin).

Another "soft-particle" approach included manganese oxide and manganese oleate nanocolloids (Pan 2009) (particle size ~ 120 nm). These colloidal particles were developed by incorporating manganese(II) oxide (~ 10 nm) particles (ManOC) or manganese(II) oleate (ManOL) within a hydrophobic core matrix encapsulated by phospholipids. MR experiments (3.0 T) revealed the ionic r1 relaxivities of ManOC and ManOL as 4.1 ± 0.9 (s × mmol $[Mn])^{-1}$ and 20.4 ± 1.1 (s × mmol $[Mn])^{-1}$, while the particulate relaxivities were 85,099 (s × mmol $[ManOC])^{-1}$ and 631,208 (s × mmol $[ManOL])^{-1}$, respectively. The ionic r2 relaxivities of ManOC and ManOL were 18.9 ± 1.1 $(s \times mmol [Mn])^{-1}$ and 65.6 ± 0.9 $(s \times mmol [Mn])^{-1}$, and the r2 relaxivities were 395,410 $(s \times mmol [ManOC])^{-1}$ and 2,028,925 $(s \times mmol [ManOL])^{-1}$, respectively. The specific relaxivities were found to be unexpectedly higher for the ManOL as compared to the ManOC. Fibrin-rich clots targeted in vitro with fibrin-specific monoclonal antibodies revealed increased T1w-images of the targeted specimens, yielding signal intensities (75 ± 20 a.u. and 95 ± 19 a.u., respectively) versus the control nanocolloids (32 ± 7 a.u.), and background air (7 ± 4 a.u.). These results suggest that ManOL has potential for imaging intravascular microthrombus associated with ruptured atherosclerotic plaque, and may provide adequate contrast to detect the sparse biosignatures of angiogenesis in cancer and vascular diseases.

3.3 Conclusions

While MRI contrast agents universally enhance the discrimination of tissues by shortening the T1 and or T2 relaxation properties, the approaches used to accomplish this feat are highly varied. In some instances, particularly for the T1-weighted variety, small molecules containing paramagnetic agents are driving the influence on local protons e.g. in blood pool discriminiation. In other situations where targeted molecular imaging is sought, nanoparticles of various forms are used to amplify the amount of metal concentrated at a specific receptor in order to overcome partial volume dilution effects, which diminish the signal. Among T2-weighted agents, iron oxide-based particles with high magnetic susceptibility dominate the field.

Although only alluded to in this chapter, MR molecular imaging agents can be combined with therapeutics and localize to distinctive biomarkers to achieve higher target drug concentrations with lower overall body exposure. In both instances, the local drug dose delivered can be quantitatively confirmed with imaging, allowing therapeutic response prediction. In this manner, image guided drug delivery is an individualized therapy where imaging techniques are utilized in quantitative assessments of tumor-targeted therapeutic delivery, distribution, uptake and response.

References

Abraham JL, Thakral C. Tissue distribution and kinetics of gadolinium and nephrogenic systemic fibrosis. Eur J Radiol 2008; 66: 200–7.

Agrawal S, Huang S, Wei Haw Lin A et al. Quantitative evaluation of optical coherence tomography signal enhancement with gold nanoshells. J Biomed Opt 2006; 11: 041121.

Ahrens ET, Feili-Hariri M, Xu HY et al. Receptor-mediated endocytosis of iron-oxide particles provides efficient labeling of dendritic cells for in vivo MR imaging. Magn Reson Med 2003; 49: 1006–13.

Ahrens ET, Flores R, Xu H, Morel PA. In vivo imaging platform for tracking immunotherapeutic cells. Nat Biotechnol 2005; 23: 983–7.

Aime S, Botta M, Geninatti Crich S et al. Synthesis and NMR studies of three pyridine-containing triaza macrocyclic triacetate ligands and their complexes with lanthanide ions. Inorg Chem 1997; 36: 2992.

Ali MM, Woods M, Caravan P et al. Synthesis and relaxometric studies of a dendrimer-based pH-responsive MRI contrast agent. Chemistry 2008; 14 (24): 7250–8.

Arbab AS, Yocum GT, Wilson LB et al. Comparison of transfection agents in forming complexes with ferumoxides, cell labeling efficiency, and cellular viability. Mol Imaging 2004; 3: 24–32.

Artemov D, Mori N, Okollie B, Bhujwalla ZM. MR molecular imaging of the Her-2/neu receptor in breast cancer cells using targeted iron oxide nanoparticles. Magn Reson Med 2003; 49: 403–8.

Botnar RM, Perez AS, Witte S et al. In vivo molecular imaging of acute and subacute thrombosis using a fibrin-binding magnetic resonance imaging contrast agent. Circulation 2004; 109: 2023–9.

Breckwoldt MO, Chen JW, Stangenberg L et al. Tracking the inflammatory response in stroke in vivo by sensing the enzyme myeloperoxidase. Proc Natl Acad Sci U S A 2008; 105 (47): 18584–9.

Buchler JW. Synthesis and properties of metalloporphyrins. In: Dolphin D (ed). The Porphyrins, Vol I. New York: Academic Press 1979; 389–483.

Bulte JW, Arbab AS, Douglas T, Frank JA. Preparation of magnetically labeled cells for cell tracking by magnetic resonance imaging. Meth Enzymol 2004; 386: 275–99.

Bulte JW, Kraitchman DL. Monitoring cell therapy using iron oxide MR contrast agents. Curr Pharm Biotechno 2004; 5: 567–84.

Byeong-Su K, Jiao-Ming Q, Jian-Ping W, Taton TA. Magnetomicelles: composite nanostructures from magnetic nanoparticles and cross-linked amphiphilic block copolymers. Nano Lett 2005; 5: 1987–91.

Cang H, Sun T, Li Y et al. Gold nanocages as contrast agents for spectroscopic optical coherence tomography. Opt Lett 2005; 30: 3048–50.

Carollo BR, Runge VM, Price AC et al. The prospective evaluation of Gd-DTPA in 225 consecutive cranial cases: adverse reactions and diagnostic value. Magn Reson Imaging 1990; 8 (4): 381–93.

Casali C, Janier M, Canet E et al. Evaluation of Gd-DOTA-labeled dextran polymer as an intravascular MR contrast agent for myocardial perfusion. Acad Radiol 1998; 5: S214.

Chen C-W, Cohen JS, Myers CE, Sohn M. Paramagnetic metalloporphyrins as potential contrast agents in NMR imaging. FEBS Lett 1984; 168: 70–4.

Cowper SE, Su LD, Bhawan J et al. Nephrogenic fibrosing dermopathy. Am J Dermatopathol 2001; 23: 383–93.

Cunningham CH, Arai T, Yang PC et al. Positive contrast magnetic resonance imaging of cells labeled with magnetic nanoparticles. Magn Reson Med 2005; 53: 999–1005.

Damadian R. Tumor detection by nuclear magnetic resonance. Science 1971; 171: 1151–3.

Datta A, Raymond KN. Gd-hydroxypyridinone (HOPO)-based high-relaxivity magnetic resonance imaging (MRI) contrast agents. Acc Chem Res 2009; 42: 938.

Dear JW, Kobayashi H, Jo SK et al. Dendrimer-enhanced MRI as a diagnostic and prognostic biomarker of sepsis-induced acute renal failure in aged mice. Kidney Int 2005; 67: 2159–7.

De Roos J, Doornbos D, Baleriaux HL, Bloem TH. In: Kressel HY (ed). Magnetic Resonance Annual. Raven Press 1988; 113–45.

Dodd CH, Hsu HC, Chu HW et al. Normal T-cell response and in vivo magnetic resonance imaging of T cells loaded with HIV transactivator-peptide-derived superparamagnetic nanoparticles. J Immunol Methods 2001; 256: 89–105.

Doubrovin M, Serganova I, Mayer-Kuckuk P et al. Multi-modality in vivo molecular-genetic imaging. Bioconjugate Chem 2004; 15: 1376.

Elemento EM, Parker D, Aime S et al. Variation of water exchange dynamics with ligand structure and stereochemistry in lanthanide complexes based on 1,4-diazepine derivatives. Org Biomol Chem 2009; 7: 1120.

Fawwaz RA, Hemphill W, Winchell HS. Potential use of ^{109}Pd-porphyrin complexes for selective lymphatic ablation. J Nucl Med 1971; 12: 231–6.

Fawwaz RA, Winchell HS, Frye F et al. Localization of ^{58}Co and ^{65}Zn-hematoporphyrin complexes in canine lymph nodes. J Nucl Med 1969; 10: 581–5.

Fayad Z, Fuster V. Characterization of atherosclerotic plaques by magnetic resonance imaging. Ann N Y Acad Sci 2000a; 902: 173–86.

Fayad Z, Fuster V, Fallon J et al. Non-invasive in vivo human coronary artery lumen and wall imaging using black-blood magnetic resonance imaging. Circulation 2000b; 102: 506–10.

Fiel RJ, Musser DA, Mark EH et al. Comparative study of manganese meso-sulfonatophenyl porphyrins: contrast-enhancing agents for tumors. J Magn Reson Imaging 1990; 8: 255–9.

Flacke S, Fischer S, Scott J et al. Novel MRI contrast agent for molecular imaging of fibrin: implications for detecting vulnerable plaques. Circulation 2001; 104: 1280–5.

Fossheim S, Fahlvik A, Klaveness J, Muller R. Paramagnetic liposomes as MRI contrast agents: influence of liposomal physicochemical properties on the in vitro relaxivity. Magn Reson Imaging 1999; 17: 83–9.

Fujimori H, Matsumura A, Yamamoto T et al. Tumor specific contrast enhancement study of Mn-metalloporphyrin (ATN-10) – comparison of rat brain tumor model, cytotoxic and vasogenic edema models. Acta Neurochir 1997; 70: 167–9.

Gianolio E, Napolitano R, Fedeli F et al. Poly-beta-cyclodextrin based platform for pH-mapping via a ratiometric ^{19}F/^{1}H MRI method. Chem Commun 2009; 40: 6044–6.

Grant CW, Karlik S, Florio E. A liposomal MRI contrast agent: phosphatidylethanolamine-DTPA. Magn Reson Med 1989; 11: 236–43.

Grobner T. Gadolinium – a specific trigger for the development of nephrogenic fibrosing dermopathy and nephrogenic systemic fibrosis? Nephrol Dial Transplant 2006; 21: 1104–8.

Harisinghani MG, Barentsz JF, Hahn PF et al. Non-invasive detection of clinically occult lymph-node metastases in prostate cancer. N Engl J Med 2003; 348: 2491–9.

Hatsukami T, Ross R, Polissar N et al. Visualization of fibrous cap thickness and rupture in human atherosclerotic carotid plaque in vivo with high-resolution magnetic resonance imaging. Circulation 2000; 102: 959–64.

Hill JH, Dick AJ, Raman K et al. Serial cardiac magnetic resonance imaging of injected mesenchymal stem cells. Circulation 2003; 108: 1009–14.

Hisataka K, Brechbiel MW. Nano-sized MRI contrast agents with dendrimer cores. Advanced Drug Delivery Reviews 2005; 57: 2271–86.

Hood JD, Cheresh DA. Targeted delivery of mutant Raf kinase to neovessels causes tumor regression. Cold Spring Harb Sym 2002; 67: 285–91.

Jacques V, Desreux JF. New classes of MRI contrast agents. Top Curr Chem 2002; 221: 123–64.

Josephson L, Tung CH, Moore AR, Weissleder R. High-efficiency intracellular magnetic labeling with novel superparamagnetic-tat peptide conjugates. Bioconj Chem 1999; 10: 186–91.

Kabalka G, Davis M, Holmberg E et al. Gadolinium-labeled liposomes containing amphiphilic Gd-DTPA derivatives of varying chain length: targeted MRI contrast enhancement agents for the liver. Magn Reson Imaging 1991; 9: 373–7.

Kang HW, Josephson L, Petrovsky A et al. Magnetic resonance imaging of inducible E-selectin expression in human endothelial cell culture. Bioconj Chem 2002; 13: 122–7.

Kaufman A, Geller C, Waltman AC. Renal insufficiency: gadopentetate dimeglumine as a radiographic contrast agent during peripheral vascular interventional procedures. Radiology 1996; 198: 579–81.

King AP, Boubertakh R, Rhode KS et al. A subject-specific technique for respiratory motion correction in image guided cardiac catheterisation procedures. Med Image Anal 2009; 13 (3): 419–31.

Kircher MF, Allport JR, Graves EE et al. In vivo high resolution three-dimensional imaging of antigen-specific cytotoxic T-lymphocyte trafficking to tumors. Cancer Res 2003; 63: 6838–46.

Kobayashi H, Brechbiel MW. Dendrimer-based macromolecular MRI contrast agents: characteristics and application. Mol Imaging 2003; 2: 1–10.

Kobayashi H, Kawamoto S, Brechbiel MW et al. Micro-MRI methods to detect renal cysts in mice. Kidney Int 2004; 65: 1511–6.

Kobayashi H, Kawamoto S, Jo SK et al. Renal tubular damage detected by dynamic micro-MRI with a dendrimer-based magnetic resonance contrast agent. Kidney Int 2002; 161: 1980–5.

Kobayashi H, Kawamoto S, Saga T et al. Avidin dendrimer-(1B4M-Gd)(254). Bioconjug Chem 2001; 12: 587–93.

Koenig SH, Ahkong QF, Brown RD et al. Permeability of liposomal membranes to water: results from the magnetic field dependence of T1 of solvent protons in suspensions of vesicles with entrapped paramagnetic ions. Magn Reson Med 1992; 23: 275–86.

Kraitchman DL, Heldman AW, Atalar E et al. In vivo magnetic resonance imaging of mesenchymal stem cells in myocardial infarction. Circulation 2003; 107: 2290–3.

Krasnow N. Effects of lanthanum and gadolinium ions on cardiac sarcoplasmic reticulum. Biochem Biophys Acta 1972; 282: 187–94.

Kreft BP, Baba Y, Tanimoto A et al. Orally administered manganese chloride: enhanced detection of hepatic tumors in rats. Radiology 1993; 186: 543–8.

Lanza GM, Wallace KD, Scott J et al. A novel site-targeted ultrasonic contrast agent with broad biomedical application. Circulation 1996; 94: 3334–40.

Lanza GM, Winter PM, Caruthers SD et al. Magnetic resonance molecular imaging with nanoparticles. J Nucl Cardiol 2004; 11: 733–43.

Lauffer RB, Parmelee DJ, Dunham SU et al. MS-325: albumin-targeted contrast agent for MR angiography. Radiology 1998; 207: 529–38.

Lauterbur PC, Mendonça-Dias HM, Rudin AM. Augmentation of tissue water proton spin-lattice relaxation by in vivo addition of paramagnetic ions. In: Dutton PL, Leigh JS, Scarpa A (eds). Frontiers of Biological Energetics. Vol 1. Academic 1978; 752–9.

Leung KC, Wang YX, Wang H et al. Biological and magnetic contrast evaluation of shape-selective Mn-Fe nanowires. IEEE Trans Nanobioscience 2009; 2: 192–8.

Li KC, Bednarski MD. Vascular-targeted molecular imaging using functionalized polymerized vesicles. J Magn Reson Imaging 2002; 16: 388–93.

Li Z, Li W, Li X et al. Mn(II)-monosubstituted polyoxometalates as candidates for contrast agents in magnetic resonance imaging. J Inorg Biochem 2007; 101: 1036–42.

Longmaid 3rd HE, Adams DF, Neirinckx RD et al. In vivo ^{19}F NMR imaging of liver, tumor, and abscess in rats. Preliminary results. Invest Radiol 1985; 20: 141–5.

Loo C, Lin A, Hirsch L et al. Nanoshell-enabled photonics-based imaging and therapy of cancer. Technol Cancer Res Treat 2004; 3: 33–40.

Low RN. Current uses of gadolinium chelates for clinical magnetic resonance imaging examination of the liver. Top Magn Reson Imaging 1998; 9: 141–66.

Lu J, Ma S, Sun J et al. Manganese ferrite nanoparticle micellar nanocomposites as MRI contrast agent for liver imaging. Biomaterials 2009; 30: 2919–28.

Maclaren JR, Bones PJ, Millane RP, Watts R. MRI with TRELLIS: a novel approach to motion correction. Magn Reson Imaging 2008; 26: 474–83.

Manchester M, Singh P. Virus-based nanoparticles (VNPs): Platform technologies for diagnostic imaging. Adv Drug Deliver Rev 2006; 58: 1505.

Mankoff DA. A definition of molecular imaging. J Nucl Med 2007; 48: 18N.

Marckmann P, Nielsen AH, Sloth JJ. Possibly enhanced Gd excretion in dialysate, but no major clinical benefit of 3–5 months of treatment with sodium thiosulfate in late stages of nephrogenic systemic fibrosis. Nephrol Dial Transplant 2008; 23: 3280–2.

Massoud TF, Gambhir SS. Molecular imaging in living subjects: seeing fundamental biological processes in a new light. Genes DeV 2003; 17: 545.

Mazhar SM, Shiehmorteza M et al. Nephrogenic systemic fibrosis in liver disease: a systematic review. J Magn Reson Imaging 2009; 30: 1313–22.

Mertzman JE, Kar S, Lofland S et al. Surface attached manganese-oxo clusters as potential contrast agents. Chem Commun 2009; 21: 788–90.

Moffat BA, Reddy GR, McConville P et al. A novel polyacrylamide magnetic nanoparticle contrast agent for molecular imaging using MRI. Mol Imaging 2003; 2: 324–32.

Moody AR, Allder S, Lennox G et al. Direct magnetic resonance imaging of carotid artery thrombus in acute stroke. Lancet 1999; 353: 122–3.

Morawski AM, Winter PM, Crowder KC et al. Targeted nanoparticles for quantitative imaging of sparse molecular epitopes with MRI. Magn Reson Med 2004; 51: 480–6.

Morawski AM, Winter PM, Yu SX et al. Quantitative "magnetic resonance immunohistochemistry" with ligand-targeted $^{(19)}$F nanoparticles. Magn Reson Med 2004; 52: 1255–62.

Na HB, Lee JH, An K et al. Development of a T1 contrast agent for magnetic resonance imaging using MnO nanoparticles. Angew Chem Int Ed Engl 2007; 46: 5397–401.

Navon G, Panigel R, Valensin G. Liposomes containing paramagnetic macromolecules as MRI contrast agents. Magn Reson Med 1986; 3: 876–80.

Nelson KL, Runge VM. Basic principles of MR contrast. Top Magn Reson Imag 1995; 7: 124–36.

Odille F, Cindea N, Mandry D et al. Generalized MRI reconstruction including elastic physiological motion and coil sensitivity encoding. Magn Reson Med 2008; 59: 1401–11.

Pan D, Caruthers SD, Hu G et al. Ligand-directed nanobialys as theragnostic agent for drug delivery and manganese-based magnetic resonance imaging of vascular targets. J Am Chem Soc 2008; 130: 9186–7.

Pan D, Senpan A, Caruthers SD et al. Sensitive and efficient detection of thrombus with fibrin-specific manganese nanocolloids. Chem Commun (Camb) 2009; 14: 3234–6.

Parmelee DJ, Walovitch RC, Ouelle HS, Lauffer RB. Preclinical evaluation of the pharmacokinetics, biodistribution, and elimination of MS-325, a blood pool agent for magnetic resonance imaging. Invest Radiol 1997; 32: 741–7.

Partlow KC, Chen J et al. ^{19}F magnetic resonance imaging for stem/progenitor cell tracking with multiple unique perfluorocarbon nanobeacons. FASEB J 2007; 21: 1647–54.

Place DA, Faustino PJ, Berghmans KK et al. MRI contrast-dose relationship of manganese(III)tetra(4-sulfonatophenyl) porphyrin with human xenograft tumors in nude mice at 2.0 T. Magn Reson Imaging 1992; 10: 919–28.

Port C, Corot I, Raynal J-M et al. Physicochemical and biological evaluation of P792, a rapid-clearance blood-pool agent for magnetic resonance imaging. Invest Radiol 2001; 36: 445.

Port M, Idee JM, Medina C et al. Stability of gadolinium chelates and their biological consequences: New data and some comments. Br J Radiol 2008a; 81: 258–9.

Port M, Idee JM, Medina C et al. Efficiency, thermodynamic and kinetic stability of marketed gadolinium chelates and their possible clinical consequences: A critical review. BioMetals 2008b; 21: 469–90.

Prince MR, Yucel EK, Kaufman JA et al. Dynamic gadolinium-enhanced three-dimensional abdominal MR arteriography. J Magn Reson Imaging 1993; 3: 877–81.

Quido G, Sander L, Regina GH et al. Dynamic contrast-enhanced MR imaging kinetic parameters and molecular weight of dendritic contrast agents in tumor angiogenesis in mice. Radiology 2005; 235: 65–72.

Quintana A, Raczka E, Piehler L et al. Design and function of a dendrimer-based therapeutic nanodevice targeted to tumor cells through the folate receptor. Pharm Res 2002; 19: 1310–6.

Rohrer M, Bauer H, Mintorovitch J et al. Comparison of magnetic properties of MRI contrast media solutions at different magnetic field strengths. Invest Radiol 2005; 40: 715.

Rongved P, Klaveness J. Water-soluble polysaccharides as carriers of paramagnetic contrast agents for magnetic resonance imaging: synthesis and relaxation properties. Carbohydr Res 1991; 214: 315–23.

Ruehm SG, Corot C, Vogt P et al. Magnetic resonance imaging of atherosclerotic plaque with ultrasmall superparamagnetic particles of iron oxide in hyperlipidemic rabbits. Circulation 2001; 103: 415–22.

Saini S, Edelman RR, Sharma P et al. Blood-pool MR contrast material for detection and characterization of focal hepatic lesions: initial clinical experience with ultrasmall superparamagnetic iron oxide (AMI-227). AJR 1995; 164: 1147–52.

Schellenberger EA, Bogdanov Jr. A, Hogemann D et al. Annexin V-CLIO: a nanoparticle for detecting apoptosis by MRI. Mol Imaging 2002; 1: 102–7.

Schmieder AH, Winter PM, Caruthers SD et al. Molecular MR imaging of melanoma angiogenesis with alpha(nu)beta3-targeted paramagnetic nanoparticles. Magn Reson Med 2005; 53: 621–7.

Schmiedl UP, Nelson JA, Robinson DH et al. Pharmaceutical properties, biodistribution, and imaging characteristics of manganese-mesoporphyrin. A potential hepatobiliary contrast agent for magnetic resonance imaging. Invest Radiol 1993; 28: 925–32.

Schwendener RA, Wüthrich R, Duewell S et al. A pharmacokinetic and MRI study of unilamellar gadolinium-, manganese-, and iron-DTPA-stearate liposomes as organ-specific contrast agents. Invest Radiol 1990; 25: 922–32.

Sessoli R, Gatteschi D, Caneschi A, Novak M. Magnetic bistability in a metal-ion cluster. Nature 1993; 365: 141.

Shapiro EM, Koretsky AP. Convertible manganese contrast for molecular and cellular MRI. Magn Reson Med 2008; 60: 265–9.

Shin J, Anisur RM, Ko MK et al. Hollow manganese oxide nanoparticles as multi-functional agents for magnetic resonance imaging and drug delivery. Angew Chem Int Ed Engl 2009; 48: 321–4.

Sipkins DA, Cheresh DA, Kazemi MR et al. Detection of tumor angiogenesis in vivo by v3-targeted magnetic resonance imaging. Nat Med 1998; 4: 623–6.

Skinner M, Yuan C, Mitsumori L et al. Serial magnetic resonance imaging of experimental atherosclerosis detects lesion fine structure, progression and complications in vivo. Nat Med 1995; 1: 69–73.

Spanoghe M, Lanens D, Dommisse R et al. Proton relaxation enhancement by means of serum albumin and poly-L-lysine labeled with DTPA-$Gd3^+$: relaxivities as a function of molecular weight and conjugation efficiency. Magn Reson Imaging 1992; 10: 913–7.

Stancanello J, Terreno E, Castelli D et al. Development and validation of a smoothing-splines-based correction method for improving the analysis of CEST-MR images. Contrast Media Mol Imaging 2008; 3: 136–49.

Stanisz GJ, Henkelman RM. Gd-DTPA relaxivity depends on macromolecular content. Magn Reson Med 2000; 44: 665–7.

Stiriba SE, Frey H, Haag R. Dendritic polymers in biomedical applications: from potential to clinical use in diagnostics and therapy. Angew Chem Int Ed 2002; 41: 1329–34.

Stroh A, Faber C, Neuberger T et al. In vivo detection limits of magnetically labeled embryonic stem cells in the rat brain using high-field (17.6 T) magnetic resonance imaging. Neuroimage 2005; 24: 635–45.

Takehara Y, Sakahara H, Masunaga H et al. Assessment of a potential tumor-seeking manganese metalloporphyrin contrast agent in a mouse model. Magn Reson Med 2002; 47: 549–53.

Taylor KM, Rieter WJ, Lin W. Manganese-based nanoscale metal-organic frameworks for magnetic resonance imaging. J Am Chem Soc 2008; 130: 14358–9.

Terreno E, Barge A, Beltrami L et al. Highly shifted LIPOCEST agents based on the encapsulation of neutral polynuclear paramagnetic shift reagents. Chem Commun (Camb) 2008; 5: 600–2.

Terreno E, Cabella C, Carrera C et al. From spherical to osmotically shrunken paramagnetic liposomes: an improved generation of LIPOCEST MRI agents with highly shifted water protons. Angew Chem Int Ed Engl 2007; 46: 966–8.

Terreno E, Castelli DD, Milone L et al. First ex-vivo MRI co-localization of two LIPOCEST agents. Contrast Media Mol Imaging 2008; 3: 38–43.

Thakur M, Lentle BC. Report of a summit on molecular imaging. Radiology 2005; 236: 753.

Thompson MK, Botta M, Nicolle G et al. A highly stable gadolinium complex with a fast, associative mechanism of water exchange. J Am Chem Soc 2003; 125: 14274–5.

Thorek DL, Chen AK, Czupryna J, Tsourkas A. Superparamagnetic iron oxide nanoparticle probes for molecular imaging. Ann Biomed Eng 2006; 34: 23–38.

Tircso G, Benyo ET, Suh EH et al. (S)-5-(p-nitrobenzyl)-PCTA, a promising bifunctional ligand with advantageous metal ion complexation kinetics. Bioconjugate Chem 2009; 20: 565.

Todd DJ, Kay J. Nephrogenic systemic fibrosis: an epidemic of gadolinium toxicity. Curr Rheumatol Rep 2008; 10: 195–204.

Toussaint J, LaMuraglia G, Southern J et al. Magnetic resonance images lipid, fibrous, calcified, hemorrhagic, and thrombotic components of human atherosclerosis in vivo. Circulation 1996; 94: 932–8.

Tripathi L, Kumar P, Singh R. Role of chelates in magnetic resonance imaging studies. J Cancer Res Ther 2009; 5: 148–53.

Turner JL, Pan D et al. Synthesis of gadolinium-labeled shell-crosslinked nanoparticles for magnetic resonance imaging applications. Adv Func Mat 2005; 15: 1248–54.

Unger E, Fritz T, Shen DK, Wu G. Manganese-based liposomes. Comparative approaches. Invest Radiol 1993; 28: 933–8.

Unger EC, Porter T, Culp W et al. Therapeutic applications of lipid-coated microbubbles. Adv Drug Deliv Rev 2004; 56 (9): 1291–314.

Urbanczyk-Pearson LM, Femia FJ, Smith J et al. Mechanistic investigation of beta-galactosidase-activated MR contrast agents. Inorg Chem 2008; 47: 56.

Wang Q, Lin T, Tang L et al. Icosahedral virus particles as addressable nanoscale building blocks. Angew Chem Int Ed 2002; 41: 459–62.

Ward KM, Aletras AH, Balaban RS. A new class of contrast agents for MRI based on proton chemical exchange dependent saturation transfer (CEST). J Magn Reson 2000; 143 (1): 79–87.

Weissleder R, Mahmood U. Molecular imaging. Radiology 2001; 219: 316.

Wiegers CB, Welch MJ, Sharp TL et al. Evaluation of two new gadolinium chelates as contrast agents for MRI. Magn Reson Imaging 1992; 10: 903–11.

Winalski CS, Shortkroff S, Schneider E et al. Targeted dendrimer-based contrast agents for articular cartilage assessment by MR imaging. Osteoarthr Cartilage 2008; 16: 815–22.

Winter PM, Athey P, Kiefer G et al. Improved paramagnetic chelate for molecular imaging with MRI. J Magn Magn Mater 2005; 293: 540–5.

Winter PM, Cai K et al. Targeted PARACEST nanoparticle contrast agent for the detection of fibrin. Magn Reson Med 2006; 56: 1384–8.

Winter PM, Caruthers SD, Kassner A et al. Molecular imaging of angiogenesis in nascent Vx-2 rabbit tumors using a novel alpha(nu)beta3-targeted nanoparticle and 1.5 tesla magnetic resonance imaging. Cancer Res 2005; 63: 5838–43.

Winter PM, Caruthers SD, Yu X et al. Improved molecular imaging contrast agent for detection of human thrombus. Magn Reson Med 2003; 50: 411–6.

Winter PM, Schmieder AH, Caruthers SD et al. Minute dosages of β3-targeted fumagillin nanoparticles impair Vx-2 tumor angiogenesis and development in rabbits. The FASEB J 2008; 22: 2758–67.

Yang J, Lee CH, Ko HJ et al. Multi-functional magneto-polymeric nanohybrids for targeted detection and synergistic therapeutic effects on breast cancer. Angew Chem Int Ed Engl 2007; 46: 8836–9.

Yeh W, Zhang ST, Ildstad CH. Intracellular labeling of T-cells with superparamagnetic contrast agents. Magn Reson Med 1993; 30: 617–25.

Yu X, Song SK, Chen J et al. High-resolution MRI characterization of human thrombus using a novel fibrin-targeted paramagnetic nanoparticle contrast agent. Magn Reson Med 2000; 4: 867–72.

Yuan C, Tsuruda JS, Beach KN et al. Techniques for high-resolution MR imaging of atherosclerotic plaque. J Magn Reson Imaging 1994; 4: 43–9.

Zech SG, Eldredge HB, Lowe MP, Caravan P. Protein binding to lanthanide(III) complexes can reduce the water exchange rate at the lanthanide. Inorg Chem 2007; 46: 3576–84.

Zhang S, Merritt M, Woessner DE et al. PARACEST agents: modulating MRI contrast via water proton exchange. Acc Chem Res 2003; 36: 783–90.

Zhang Z, Greenfield MT, Spiller M et al. Multilocus binding increases the relaxivity of protein-bound MRI contrast agents. Angew Chem Int Ed Engl 2005; 44 (41): 6766–9.

Zhang Z, Nair SA, McMurry TJ. Gadolinium meets medicinal chemistry: MRI contrast agent development. Curr Med Chem 2005; 12: 751–78.

Zhao JM, Har-el YE, McMahon MT et al. Size-induced enhancement of chemical exchange saturation transfer (CEST) contrast in liposomes. J Am Chem Soc 2008; 130: 5178–84.

Part II

Clinical Applications

4 Cardiac Magnetic Resonance Examination of the Patient

Nico Merkle and Vinzenz Hombach

4.1 Introduction

Magnetic resonance imaging is intrinsically based on the use of a strong magnet that requires special precaution measures and patient preparations. Many practical aspects have to be taken into consideration and a successful image acquisition and interpretation requires a sound knowledge of adequate patient preparation, ECG lead placement, breath-hold instructions, and contrast media injection. In addition, knowledge of safety issues and precautions in the MRI environment is required, related to the use of strong magnetic fields, radiofrequency energy, magnetic field gradients, and cryogenic liquids. Thus, the most important theoretical and practical issues are described in this chapter for the benefit of those aiming to perform cardiovascular MRI (CMR) studies in daily clinical practice.

4.2 Patient Informed Consent

Careful patient information and instruction on the course and aim of the study is an essential part of a successful CMR examination, because potential anxiety of the patient and dangerous situations may be avoided, the compliance of the patient improved, and shorter scan time and better image quality achieved. For safety and completeness reasons a standardized patient information sheet should be used that contains patient data, weight and height, and questions about metallic implants or splinter (shrapnel) residues, surgical interventions, and known allergies. After completing the sheet, the patient should be informed in detail by the physician about the special features of a CMR investigation, e.g. the narrow bore of the magnet including illumination and ventilation, noise of the gradient system, cooperation of the patient, i.e. absolutely calm behavior, breath-hold instructions, interaction and communication with the physician/technician, pressing alarm button in emergency situations, motion of the scanner table, and duration of the examination.

In addition, **possible risks** should be explained to the patient regarding the technique itself, e.g. static and alternating magnetic field, radiofrequency energy, noise level, as well as possible side effects of the drugs used at the CMR study:

- **gadolinium-based contrast media**:
  - metallic taste,
  - allergic reactions,
  - allergic shock (very uncommon),
  - renal insufficiency (e.g. systemic nephrogenic sclerosis),
- **dobutamine**:
  - tachycardia (palpitations),
  - complex ventricular arrhythmia (ventricular fibrillation: very uncommon),
  - acute myocardial ischemia (unknown coronary artery disease),
- **adenosine**:
  - headache,
  - acute dyspnea, asthmatic attack,
  - acute chest pain (angina pectoris),
  - tachycardia or bradycardia (less common than on dobutamine),
- **sedatives, anxiolytics**:
  - impaired compliance during breath-holding,
  - side effects of the individual substances.

Regarding special procedures, e.g. stress testing with adenosine, patients should be asked about ingestion of substances containing methylxanthines (chocolate, black tee, Coca Cola, medications with theophylline), as these substances will completely inhibit the vasodilatatory effect of adenosine. Moreover, patients should be asked about bronchopulmonary diseases, e.g. bronchial asthma, because adenosine may provoke or exaggerate an attack of bronchial asthma. Thereafter the patient should give his written informed consent.

Before placing the patient in the scanner, the physician/technician should ascertain whether the patient has a pacemaker or other implanted devices, retained pacemaker wires, or other foreign material inside the body, e.g. postsurgical subarachnoidal hemorrhage clips or metallic splinters. Jewellery, watches, rings, coins, hearing aids, removable dentures, piercings etc. should be removed, as well as make-up, since small metallic residues in cosmetics (as well as in tattoos) may cause artifacts in the images and/or may induce local burnings. The patient should be disrobed and wear a hospital gown, preferably without pockets, which avoids the accidental retention of materials in trouser or shirt pockets. Patients should also be asked to urinate before the CMR examination, because a full urinary bladder may result in impaired image quality due to tachycardia and restlessness of the patient.

4.3 General Patient Preparation

4.3.1 Positioning and ECG Electrode Placement

The patient should be placed in the scanner in a comfortable recumbent position with foamed material placed under his knees. The MR compatible ECG electrodes should be attached in a cross-shaped or triangular pattern, depending on the number of electrodes in the system (Figure 4-1). Before placing the electrodes, the skin should be cleaned and/or abraded with alcoholic pads and excess gel be removed. In general, nonmetallic, pregelled electrodes should be used for an optimal ECG recording. During positioning,

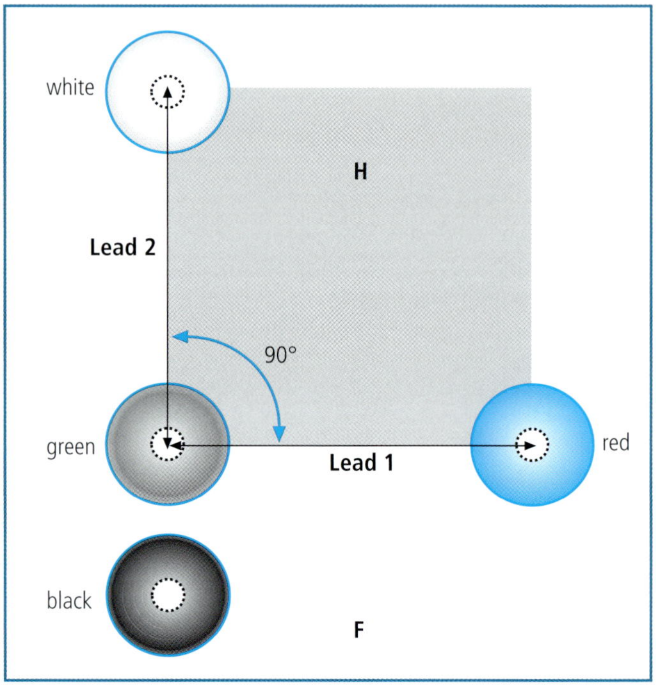

a

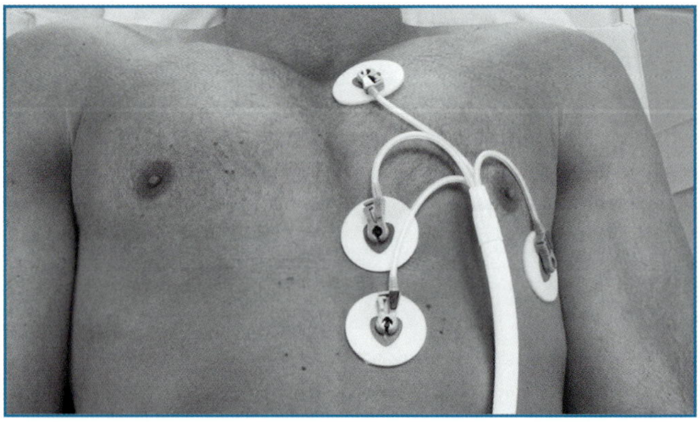

b

Figure 4-1 Placement of the ECG electrodes for a CMR examination: schematic of electrode placement for recording a vector electrocardiogram with two leads (a); recording of the vector cardiogram with position of the electrodes on the surface of the patient's chest (b). F: foot; H: head.

the quality of the ECG trace should be checked, and a constant, high-amplitude R-wave and low T-wave and low baseline noise be identified. If the ECG tracing is unsatisfactory, the electrodes should be repositioned in order to achieve an optimal result. Sometimes several attempts for optimal lead positioning are necessary, when baseline artifacts due to magneto-hydrodynamic effects and/or gradient pulses in the scanner occur. Most vendors use a vectorcardiogram as the ECG trigger because of an improved R-wave detection in relation to the T-wave, and much less influence of the magneto-hydrodynamic effect. The patient should also be fitted with a breathing belt to control patient compliance during breath-hold maneuvers, and to give the investigator the chance to entrain his breathing commands into the spontaneous breathing cycle of the patient.

In special situations, e.g. in patients at high risk, in children, or patients with impaired consciousness, and during stress testing additional monitoring measures are mandatory, e.g. pulse oximetry, blood pressure monitoring, temperature assessment, visual and verbal control via video camera and intercom, and if necessary, general anesthesia with artificial ventilation using MR compatible equipment.

4.3.2 Breath-Hold Instructions

Prior to the placement of the cardiac or torso coil and introduction into the magnet bore, the patient should be given instructions about the breath-hold commands. These instructions should be explained in detail and, if necessary, briefly rehearsed. Breath-holding can be performed in end-inspiration or endexpiration. If performed during expiration, the reproducibility among different MR views is higher and the chance of partial volume effects due to slice misregistration decreased. Some patients and physicians prefer breath-hold studies in inspiration for greater convenience of the patients, because patients feel less air during expiration and feel better with inspiration. When sequences with navigator gating are to be used, the patient should be asked not to move and to breathe as regularly as possible, and to avoid deep inspirations and falling asleep.

4.3.3 Coil Placement and Positioning in the Scanner

Phased-array coils should be generally used for CMR examinations; only in neonates or children small body coils (e.g. bird cage coils) are adequate. The number of elements in such dedicated coils ranges from 4–32 channels. These coils have anterior and posterior elements, which require accurate positioning that is critical for adequate signal acquisition. Phased-array coils offer the advantages of a high signal-to-noise ratio (SNR), a large field of view (FOV), and the application of parallel imaging (SMASH, SENSE) to significantly reduce scan time. The coils should always be centered over the organ of interest (Figure 4-2). When the heart is imaged the coil placement should be lower than when the aortic arch is imaged (e.g. in aortic coarctation). At the beginning of each CMR examination, visual inspection of the localizer or the scout images may indicate whether coil placement was performed correctly.

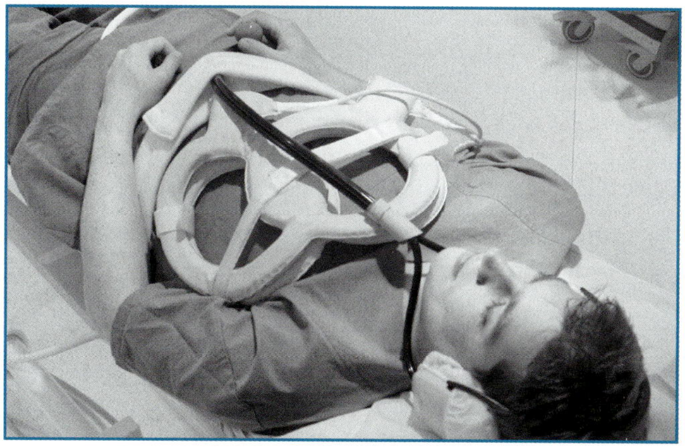

Figure 4-2 Patient fully fitted up for CMR examination with ECG electrodes (not visible), phased-array surface coil, breathing belt, and earphones.

Before moving the patient into the bore of the scanner, the patient receives headphones for noise reduction and proper communication with the investigator. A microphone is integrated in the headphones so that the patient can communicate with the investigator and vice versa. In addition, in case of problems during the MR examination, the patient can press an "alarm ball", that is given to him before moving into the scanner. After putting an i.v.-line (preferably in the cubital vein; in the case of stress testing both arms for adenosine or dobutamine infusion via one cubital vein, and contrast infusion and subsequent flushing via the second cubital vein), the patient is moved into the bore and centered using a weak laser beam that should be ultimately positioned within the region of interest, i.e. the heart. The final adjustment of the patients heart to the isocenter of the magnet is performed automatically by the scanner.

4.4 Specific Patient Preparation

4.4.1 Stress Testing

CMR imaging offers several clinically useful approaches to assess coronary heart disease, including stress testing with dobutamine to detect ischemia-induced wall motion abnormalities, or perfusion studies with adenosine stress to unravel regional perfusion defects, as well as viability studies using the late gadolinium enhancement technique. When performing stress CMR studies, a specific practical approach is required to address potential adverse effects of the substances used, because access to the patient is more limited than e. g. in stress echocardiography. The MR unit should be equipped with facilities to allow rapid extraction of the patient such as a removable tabletop, to enable rapid clinical assessment and treatment in case of an emergency situation. In addition, further safety measures are required when scanning patients with cardiovascular disease during stress testing, e. g. availability of emergency medication and a defibrillator and resuscitation equipment in the immediate vicinity of the scanner room. One should be aware that ST segment changes indicating myocardial ischemia are not reliable within the magnet, because magnetic field effects may alter the ST segment and the T-wave morphology, and thus, the ECG can only be used for monitoring of cardiac rhythm. In consequence, a physician has to supervise the whole stress procedure for online assessment of global and regional myocardial performance and early recognition of severe myocardial ischemia. Furthermore, audiovisual contact with the patient should be maintained throughout the examination, to be aware of any adverse symptoms that may occur during infusion of dobutamine or adenosine.

> Physicians performing stress studies should be aware of the patient's medical history and strictly observe the known contraindications of the individual stress test and substances used. Contraindications for use of sympathomimetics, e. g. dobutamine, are unstable angina, acute coronary syndromes, severe arterial hypertension, severe aortic stenosis, severe obstruction of the left ventricular outflow tract, high grade ventricular arrhythmias, and acute inflammatory cardiac disease. Contraindiactions for the use of adenosine are overt COPD or bronchial asthma, high-grade AV blocks, sinus node dysfunction, unstable angina, acute coronary syndromes, and severe arterial hypotension.

For further details see Chapter 6.

4.4.2 Pediatric and Neonatal CMR

CMR studies in children or young adolescents with congenital heart disease are increasingly performed; in our institution about 10% of all CMR studies (more than 2,000 per year) are used in this patient group to elucidate complex cardiac anatomy and abnormal cardiac function. The requirements of complete immobility and the ability to follow breathing instructions may be often not obtainable, at least in neonates and very young children. Therefore prolonged sedation or general anesthesia are often necessary to overcome these limitations and to complete the examination successfully. In this case MR compatible respirators and monitoring devices are mandatory. For further details see Chapter 14.

4.5 Practice of CMR Measurements

4.5.1 Imaging of Cardiac Position

Survey

For assessing both anatomy and function of the heart, special imaging planes along the different heart axes are mandatory. The first step of determining the position of the heart is acquisition of a scout or survey that forms the basis of all further measurements and includes the three main imaging planes of the heart, i. e. acquisition of several transversal, coronal and sagittal nonangulated planes. Axial planes of the whole heart have to be imaged from the diaphragm to the aortic arch, and the sagittal slab may be somewhat shifted to the left, and the coronal slab slightly anterior for reproducible anatomic reproduction and depiction of paracardiac structures in the thorax. Scout images are acquired during diastole with or without breath-holding with optimal results if the acquisition time is below 300 ms for each single slice.

> The following **CMR protocol** may be used for the survey:
> - SSFP sequence,
> - transversal, coronal, and sagittal nonangulated slices,
> - slice thickness 8–12 mm without gap,
> - field of view (FOV): 430 mm,
> - fold-over: a. p. for transversal and sagittal or right-left for coronal orientation,
> - prospective triggering in diastole; occasionally without triggering,
> - breath-hold (not always necessary; triggering is much more important).

Following acquisition of the survey, an optional scan may be performed if the use of parallel imaging (SMASH, SENSE) is planned for assessing the sensitivities of the elements of the phased-array coils used. Two scans each are acquired at maximal inspiratory breath-hold and free breathing, that does not take too much time because of the scan's low resolution; moreover, this data will not be used later on for any reconstruction purposes. The further scan procedures and determinations of the heart axes is shown in Figures 4-3a to c.

Survey (scout): SSFP, 24 transversal, 13 coronal, 15 sagittal, slice thickness: 8–10 mm, FOV: 430 mm, 2.2 × 3.2 mm

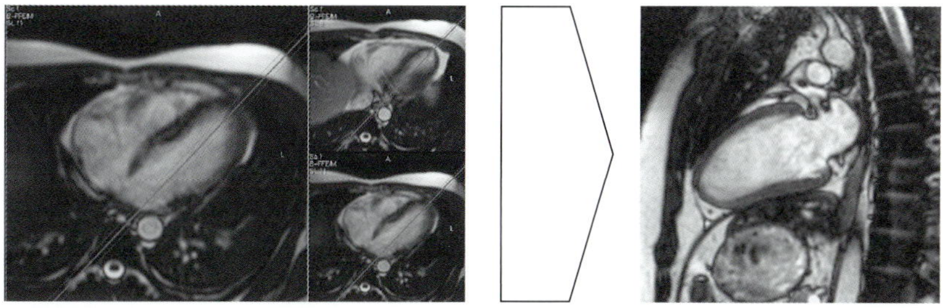

1: RAO-Equivalent (rao 2-ch)
- transversal survey through mid-mitral valve region and LV apex
- multi-phase cine-SSFP imaging
- final imaging for structure and function

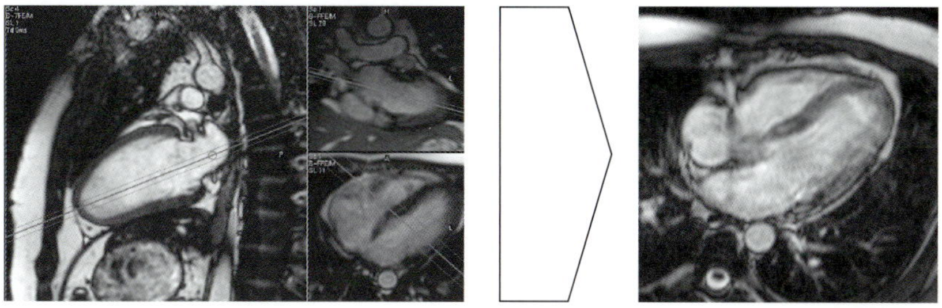

2: Transversal heart axis (2.tra)
- 90°-RAO (double-angulated)
- support plane for s. a. view

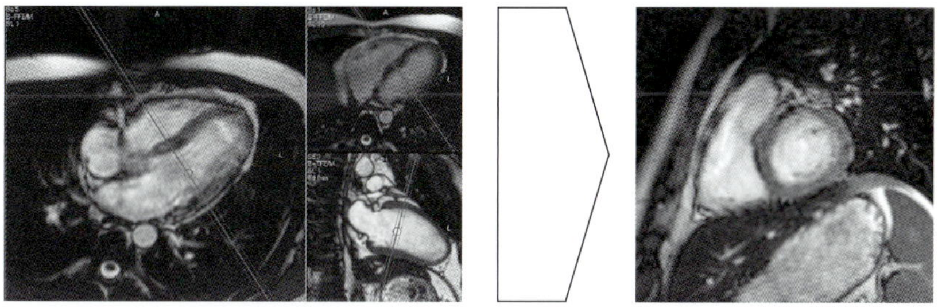

3: Short-axis (s. a.)
- 90° to 2.tra (3-fold angulated)
- about 1 cm apically parallel to valve area
- support plane for 4-ch view

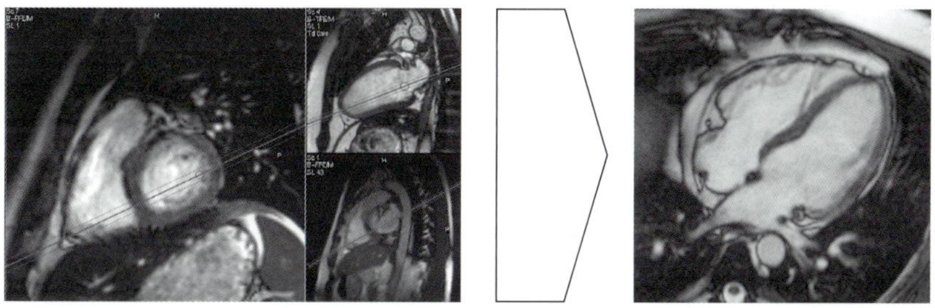

4: 4-chamber view (4-ch)
- short-axis basal slice orientation through LV and RV to achieve the largest longitudinal extension (area) of the LV and RV
- multi-phase cine-SSFP imaging
- final imaging for structure and function

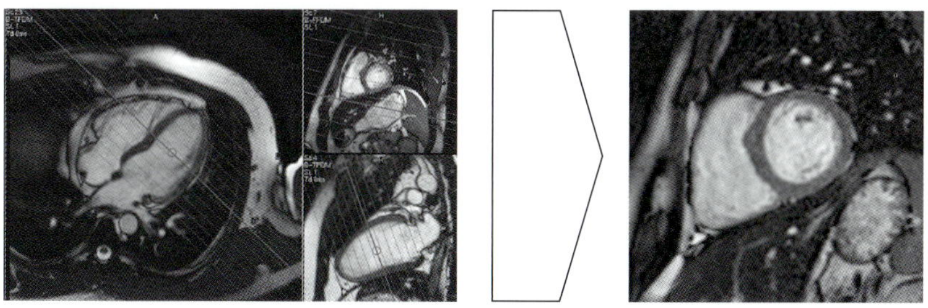

5: Short-axis stack (s. a.-10sl)
- 10–12 slices without gap
- 1–3 slices per breath-hold
- 32-phase cine-SSFP imaging
- final imaging for structure and function

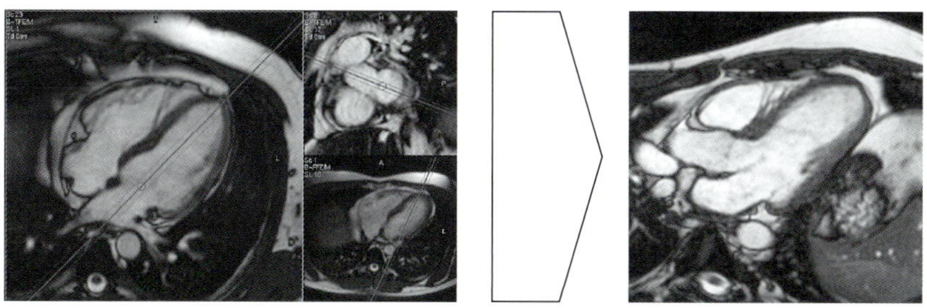

6: 3-chamber view (3-ch)
- on 4-ch view slice orientation 90° through mitral valve and LV apex tilted into LVOT
- 32-phase cine-SSFP imaging
- final imaging for structure and function
- plan scan for aortal flow measurement

Figure 4-3a

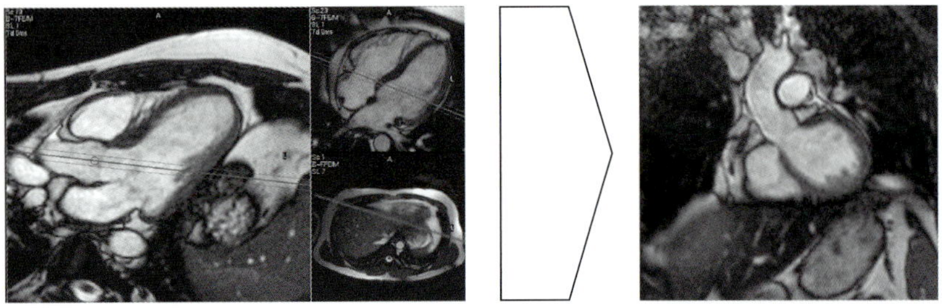

7: Left ventricular outflow tract (LVOT)

- coronal LVOT slice orientation with 90° 3-ch view (angulated through LVOT)
- geometry for imaging HOCM structure or flow mapping in LVOT

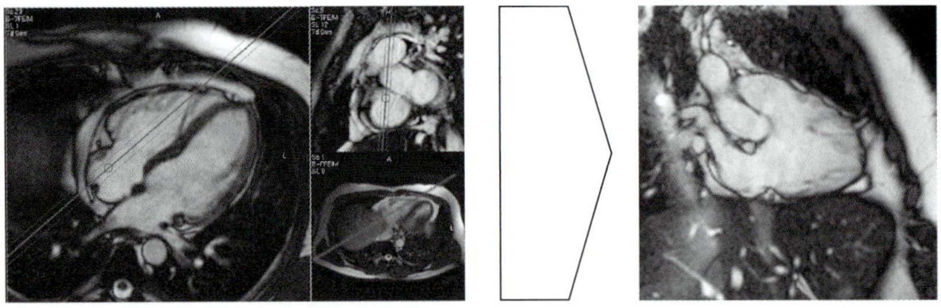

8: Right ventricular inflow/outflow tract (RVIT/RVOT)

- 4-ch plus s. a.-10sl, slice orientation through tricuspid valve (TV) and RV apex tilted into 4-ch plus TV/RVOT/ pulmonary trunk
- 32-phase cine-SSFP imaging
- plan scan for pulmonary flow measurement

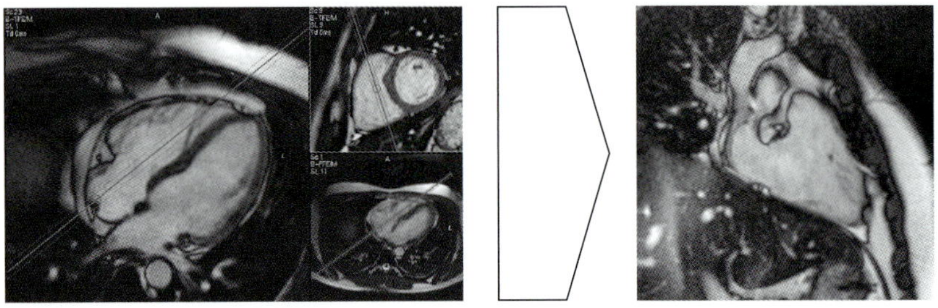

9: Right ventricular outflow tract (RVOT)

- RV to pulmonary valve (PV) tilted by 90° and 4-ch RV apex
- 32-phase cine-SSFP imaging
- abnormal structure and function of RVOT (e.g. ARVCM, RVOT tachycardia)

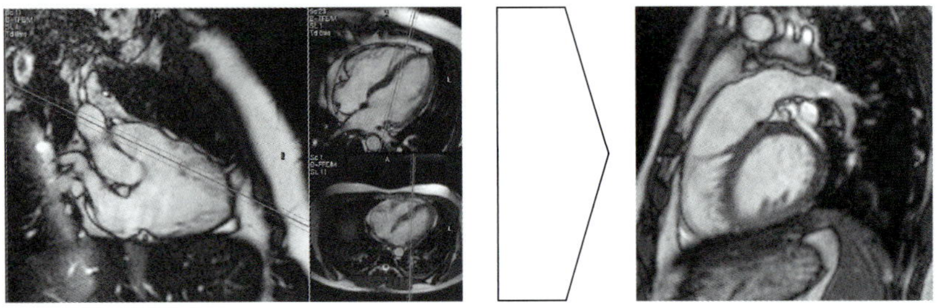

10: Right ventricular 2-chamber view (2-ch RV)

- 4-ch tricuspid valve and RV apex 90° parallel to the interventricular septum
- 32-phase cine-SSFP imaging
- abnormal structure and function

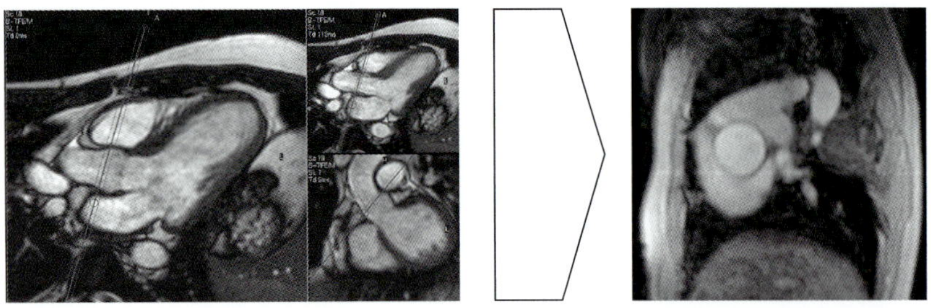

11: PC-flow mapping in the aorta (pc-ao)

- coronal survey plus 3-ch view perpendicular to aortic root 2–3 cm distal to aortic valve
- PC-GRE flow mapping sequence

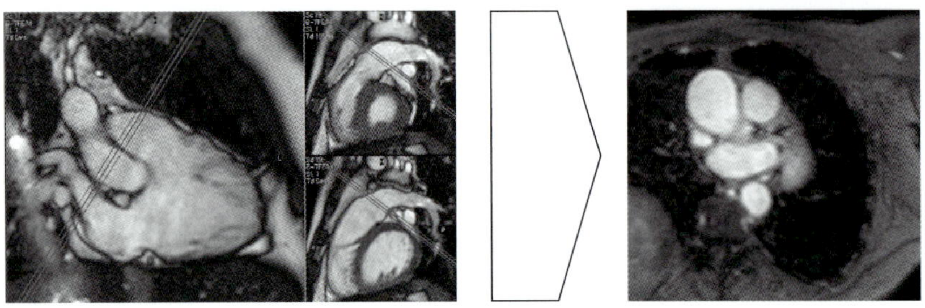

12: PC-flow mapping in the pulmonary artery (pc-pa)

- sagittal survey (pulmonary valve and trunk) plus RV plane perpendicular to pulmonary trunk 2–3 cm distal to pulmonary valve
- PC-GRE flow mapping sequence

Figure 4-3b

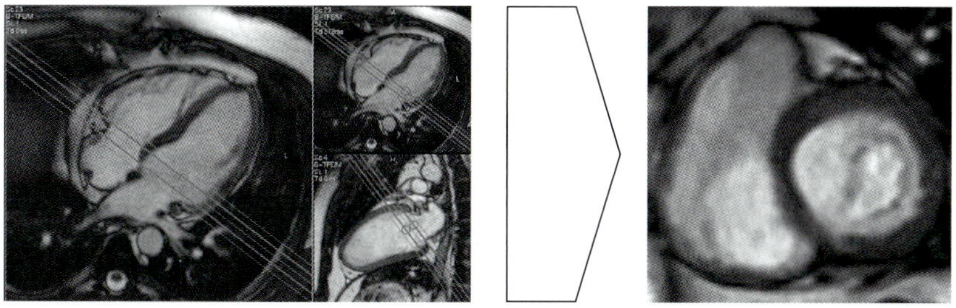

13: Mitral valve imaging (mv)
- 4-ch and 2-ch orientation perpendicular through valvular annulus
- single- and multi-phase imaging
- 32-phase cine-SSFP imaging
- structure and function (effective mitral valve orifice)

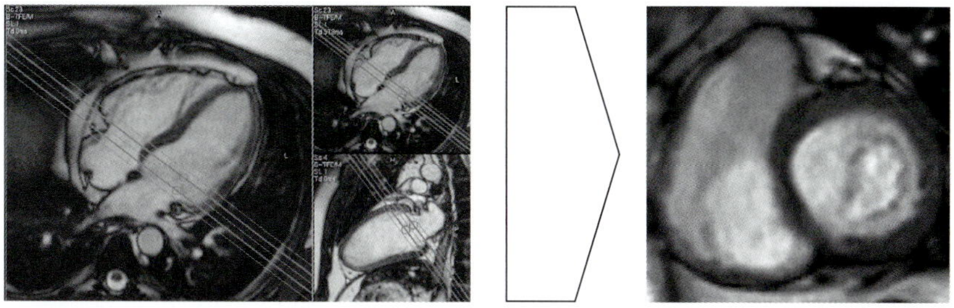

14: Tricuspid valve imaging (tv)
- 4-ch and RV-plane and 2-ch orientation perpendicular through valvular annulus
- single- and multi-phase imaging
- 32-phase cine-SSFP imaging
- structure and function (effective tricuspid valve orifice)

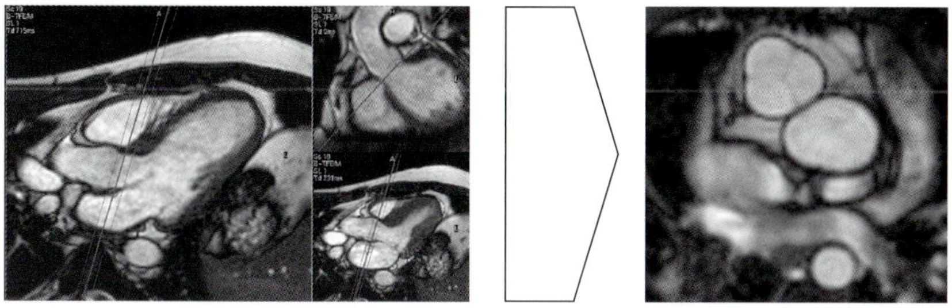

15: Aortic valve imaging (aov)
- coronal survey and 3-ch orientation perpendicular through valvular annulus
- single- and multi-phase imaging (8–14 mm)
- 32-phase cine-SSFP imaging
- structure and function (effective aortic valve orifice)

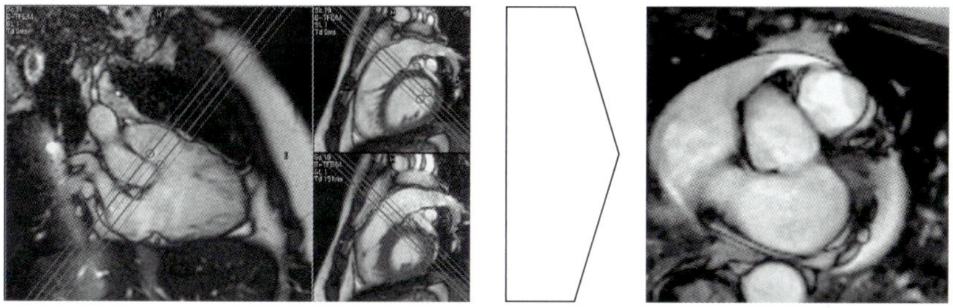

16: Pulmonary valve imaging (pav)
- sagittal survey and RV orientation perpendicular through valvular annulus
- single- and multi-phase imaging (8–14 mm)
- 32-phase cine-SSFP imaging
- structure and function (effective pulmonary valve orifice)

Figure 4-3c Standardized sequence of planning the different imaging planes relative to the long-axis of the heart for a CMR examination, starting with the scout and finishing with the pulmonary valve **(a–c)** (for further details see text).

RAO-Equivalent Plane

This single-angulated scan is used for determining the maximal length of the left ventricle, and corresponds approximately to apical 2-chamber (2-ch) view in echocardiography or RAO projection at cardiac catheterization and coronary angiography.

Plan scan is placed on the transversal survey through the center of the mitral valve orifice and left ventricular apex including left atrial appendage, using the following **CMR protocol**:
- SSFP sequence,
- single slice acquisition,
- FOV: 330–400 mm, in-plane resolution 1.6 × 1.6 mm,
- multi-phase cine-acquisition with 32 cardiac phases, temporal resolution < 50 ms,
- slice thickness 6–8 mm,
- fold-over: a.p. for sagittal or right-left for coronal orientation,
- retrospective triggering,
- end-expiratory breath-hold.

Second Transversal Plane Through Heart Axis (2.tra)

This is a double-angulated single slice acquisition in diastole and end-expiratory breath-hold (2.tra). The scan is planned on the RAO equivalent through left ventricular apex and center of the mitral valve orifice (Figure 4-3a), using a SSFP sequence, single slice single phase acquisition, retrospective triggering, and end-expiratory breath-hold.

Short-Axis View (s. a.)

This is a triple-angulated single slice acquisition in diastole and end-expiratory breath-hold (s. a.), planned orthogonal to the second transversal plane approximately 1 cm basal and parallel to the valvular plane with a cut through left ventricular outflow tract (LVOT); the protocol includes a SSFP sequence, single slice single phase acquisition, prospective triggering, and end-expiratory breath-hold (Figure 4-3a).

4.5.2 Functional Analysis of the Heart

4-Chamber View (4-ch)

The next step is assessment of left and right ventricular function as well as of atrial and valvular anatomy and function in the 4-chamber view (4-ch). Slice direction should be oriented so that the left and right ventricular chambers are imaged at their maximal orthogonal and longitudinal dimensions without a cut through the LVOT. Slice orientation is adjusted in the short axis using the most lateral point of RV wall and a point somewhat dorsal to the middle of LV (Figure 4-3a). If the atria are partly out of imaging plane or the LVOT is partly cut, a second plan scan may be performed later on using the short-axis stack.

The **CMR protocol for 4-ch view** includes:
- SSFP sequence,
- single slice acquisition,
- FOV: 330–400 mm, in-plane resolution 1.6 × 1.6 mm,
- multi-phase cine-acquisition with 32 cardiac phases, temporal resolution < 50 ms,
- slice thickness 6–8 mm,
- fold-over: a. p. for transversal or feet-head (FH) for coronal orientation,
- retrospective triggering,
- end-expiratory breath-hold.

2-Chamber View (2-ch)

Plan scan is derived from the 4-ch view through the center of the mitral valve orifice and left ventricular apex, i. e. by 90° tilting to the left ventricular long-axis. This view compares well with the 2.tra view as described above, and if this RAO equivalent view has been planned as cine-acquisition with the image plane projecting through left ventricular apex and the dorsal third or center of the mitral valve orifice, a second acquisition can be omitted.

Short-Axis View (s. a.)

Short-axis geometry is derived from the 2-ch and 4-ch view orthogonal to the longitudinal axis of the heart (Figure 4-3a). For volumetric measurements, the whole left and right ventricular volumes have to be covered using 10–12 slices with no gap (slice distance 0 mm) and a slice thickness of 8–10 mm. Using retrospective triggering and acquisition of 32 cardiac phases, the complete cardiac cycle can be scanned, which is essential for correct assessment of LV and RV volumes and function parameters.

The **CMR protocol** includes:
- SSFP sequence,
- 3D multi-slice stack,
- FOV: 330–400 mm, in-plane resolution 1.7 × 1.9 mm,
- multi-phase cine-acquisition with 32 cardiac phases, temporal resolution 120 ms, using phase interpolation acquisition time can be reduced by 50 %,
- slice thickness 8–10 mm,
- fold-over: a. p. for transversal or feet-head (FH) for coronal orientation,
- retrospective triggering,
- end-expiratory breath-hold; acquisition time 4–5 s per slice.

3-Chamber View (3-ch)

Plan scan is derived from 4-ch view and s. a. stack with slice direction similar to 2-ch view, i. e. through the center of the mitral valve orifice and left ventricular apex, but tilted through the LVOT (Figure 4-3a). This view shows the left atrium, left ventricle, and LVOT including the aortic root; the function of the mitral and aortic valve can also be assessed in this view. In addition, the 3-ch view forms the basis for planning PC flow mapping in the aorta. The CMR protocol is identical to that used for 2-ch view (see Chapter 4.5.1), only fold-over is different: a. p. for transversal or feet-head (FH) for coronal orientation.

Left Ventricular Outflow Tract (LVOT) View

This slice is derived from the 3-ch view with 90° angulated orientation through the LVOT, i. e. it represents the second plane 90° angulated to the 3-ch view (Figure 4-3b). This slice allows a precise assessment of the LVOT and relevant anatomic or functional abnormalities, e. g. in hypertrophic obstructive cardiomyopathy (HOCM), complex congenital or adult valvular diseases etc. Moreover, it is regularly used for planning PC flow measurements in the aortic root.

Right Ventricular Imaging Including Outflow Tract (RVOT) and Right Ventricular 2-Chamber View (RV 2-ch)

To assess structure and function of both the pulmonary and tricuspid valve, and to plan PC flow mapping in the pulmonary trunk, it is always necessary to acquire a longitudinal slice through the right ventricular inflow (RVIT) and outflow tract (RVOT). This is derived from 4-ch view and s.a. stack by taking a plane through the tricuspid valve and the right ventricular apex in the 4-ch view that is turned through the center of the tricuspid valve orifice and RVOT and pulmonary trunk in the s.s. stack (Figure 4-3b). The CMR protocol is identical to that used for 4-ch view imaging. To assess RVOT, the plan scan is constructed on the RV view by placing the scan through the pulmonary valve turned by 90° and corrected through the RV apex in the 4-ch view (Figure 4-3b). This view is used to asses abnormal structure and function of the RVOT and pulmonary valve, e.g. in patients with RVOT tachycardias, or with arrhythmogenic right ventricular dysplasia (ARVD). Plan scan for RV 2-ch view is derived from 4-ch view by positioning the plane through the center of the tricuspid valve orifice and the RV apex almost in parallel to the interventricular septum (Figure 4-3b).

4.5.3 Specially Adapted Imaging Planes

In some instances specially adapted imaging planes have to be used in different geometries, and as a rule, a second plane, usually perpendicular to the first one, should be acquired if abnormalities of structure (e.g. tumors or masses), regional myocardial function (e.g. after myocardial infarction), or blood flow (e.g. valvular regurgitation, shunt flow) are observed. Usually SSFP sequences are well-suited to assess these abnormalities due to the high blood to myocardial contrast, and if desired, the structure in question can be covered by additional single or multi-sclice acquisitions.

4.5.4 Flow Measurement (PC Flow Mapping)

In every CMR examination maximal flow rate (ml/s) and maximal flow velocity (m/s) should be determined in the aortic and pulmonary trunk, using PC flow mapping (see Chapter 1 for technical details). This allows quantitative assessment of valvular regurgitations (AV valves, aortic or pulmonary valves) or stenoses (aortic, pulmonary), as well as of shunt flow. In special situations flow measurements can be performed in every arterial or venous portion, either using through-plane or in-plane technique. The measurement plane should be placed approximately 2–3 cm distal to the valve to avoid false results due to turbulent flow within the valve area. In patients with distinct cardiac anatomy, the aortic and pulmonary trunk may be cut almost orthogonally in one plane, so that simultaneous measurements of flow in both vessels can be performed, which provide reliable results.

Flow in the Aorta

PC flow mapping scan in the aorta is planned on a coronal survey and from 3-ch view (Figure 4-3b) a few millimeters cranial to the aortic valve. Use of these two planes guarantees that the aortic root is imaged orthogonally and flow values will not be the underestimated. Moreover, choosing a priori the correct velocity encoding (VENC) factor is critical to avoid aliasing; in general practice a value of 150 cm/s is recommended. If flow voids are recognized in prior cine sequences, a flow rate 180–200 cm/s may be adequate, while lower VENC factors may be chosen in patients with severely reduced LV function.

The **CMR protocol** includes:
- gradient echo sequence in phase contrast technique,
- through-plane technique,
- flow rate (VENC factor) 150 cm/s,
- no breath-holding.

Flow in the Pulmonary Trunk

Planning PC mapping in the pulmonary trunk slice position is derived from the sagittal survey and the RV in a second perpendicular plane a few millimeters cranial to the pulmonary valve (Figure 4-3b). The CMR protocol is identical to that for aortic flow measurement, except the VENC factor should be set at 100 cm/s.

4.5.5 Imaging of Cardiac Valves

In patients with known or newly detected valvular dysfunctions, e.g. during the actual CMR examination, additional imaging planes are necessary to assess abnormal structure and function more adequately. In routine LV and RV imaging planes AV, aortic, and pulmonary valves are imaged along their longitudinal axes. For a more detailed analysis of a diseased valve, cross-sectional planes are necessary, and because of through-plane movement of the valves slice number and thickness have to be adapted to the position of the valve area in systole and diastole. Because of the extensive movements of both the aortic and pulmonary valve, in most instances several slices have to be acquired (multi-slice technique), yet sometimes a repeat acquisition is necessary to obtain an adequate imaging result.

The **CMR protocol** includes:
- SSFP sequence,
- single or multi-slice acquisition,
- slice thickness 8–14 mm,
- multi-phase cine imaging,
- retrospective triggering,
- end-expiratory breath-hold.

Mitral Valve

Plan scan is derived from 4-ch and 2-ch view perpendicular to the valvular ring (Figure 4-3c). The position is controlled in systole and diastole and slice number and thickness is adapted. In addition to quantify increased diastolic flow to asses mitral stenosis, mitral valve area (cross-section of mitral valve area) can be determined by planimetry as well (for details see Chapter 13).

Tricuspid Valve

Plan scan is derived from 4-ch across the tricuspid valve ring and controlled from the RV plane and RV 2-ch view (Figure 4-3c).

Aortic Valve

Plan scan may be derived similar to PC mapping, i. e. from a coronal survey and 3-ch view (Figure 4-3c). In addition, maximal systolic flow must be quantified in order to assess aortic stenosis. Aortic valve area (cross-section of aortic valve area) can be determined by planimetry as well (for details see Chapter 13).

Pulmonary Valve

Plan scan is derived similar to PC flow mapping from sagittal survey and the RV in a second perpendicular plane (Figure 4-3c). If necessary, correct positioning of the plane may be controlled from the RVOT view.

4.5.6 Imaging of Cardiac Anatomy

For a more detailed assessment of cardiac structure, high-resolution single-phase scans (spatial resolution at sub-millimeter level, slice thickness 3–4 mm) in black-blood technique with a dual-inversion-recovery (DIR) prepulse are recommended. This technique provides a maximal contrast between flowing blood or air (black) to myocardial tissue (bright signal), and these scans are less sensitive to turbulent flow or metallic artifacts than when using the "white blood technique". Images can be acquired in single slice technique using previous scan planes of the current examination, or taking new planes specifically directed through the anatomic area of interest, and if abnormalities are present another slice in a second (perpendicular) plane should be acquired. In addition to image larger volumes of tissue a 3D stack of slices may be used; this of course prolongs the scan time accordingly.

Imaging data is preferentially acquired during mid-diastole at the time of a relative standstill of the heart, the trigger delay has to be determined from a prior cine sequence, e. g. in 4-ch view, and adapted to the patient's actual heart rate. Acquisition may be done with breath-holding or using navigator techniques; the latter may be used in elderly or very sick patients, who cannot sustain the whole period of breath-holding. Navigator triggered data acquisition with prospective triggering allows free breathing of the patient combined with a high spatial resolution and suppression of breathing induced artifacts. Potential disadvantages of the navigator technique are the long acquisition time and baseline drifts of breathing depth and frequency that may prevent proper function of the navigator. Alternatively, fast high-resolution SSFP (balanced FFE) sequences with parallel imaging that provide an excellent blood-myocardial tissue contrast, may be used to overcome these problems.

Additional information on tissue characteristics may be obtained by different weighting, every MR sequence can be imaged with proton density (PD)-, T1- or T2-weighting. Also, fat suppression sequences, most frequently combined with T2-weighting, are useful to detect fatty components of a given tissue, i. e. to facilitate a differentiation between e. g. pericardial effusion from pericardial fat, or to characterize myocardial fat deposition, lipomas, or edema.

4.6 Computing and Report

After completion of the CMR examination, the patient can be removed from the scanner, detached from the coils, ECG leads and i.v. linings, and be slowly raised from the recumbent to the standing position. The operator/physician may have a first check of the reconstructed images that can be processed thereafter using the appropriate scanner software. Every single examination step has to be analyzed, and image and functional data assessed and stored on hard disk. A detailed report has to be produced including all personal data of the patient (short history, symptoms etc.), the MR sequences used, the description of structural and functional abnormalities including α-numeric data (e.g. ventricular volumes, cardiac index, ejection fraction, regurgitation fraction of valvular incompetence etc.), as well as incidental findings outside the heart, if present, and finally a comprehensive diagnosis has to be made.

5 Topographic Anatomy, Structure and Function of the Heart

Vinzenz Hombach

5.1 Topographic Anatomy of the Heart and Great Vessels

The heart as a muscle pump consists of two serial systems joined in one organ, enveloped by the pericardium, located in the mediastinum and extending obliquely from the second rib to the fifth intercostal space. The heart rests on the upper surface of the diaphragm just above the liver and is flanked and partially covered by the lungs. Its broad base is directed towards the right shoulder, and the apex towards the left hip, i.e. its long axis is rotated about 45° to both the sagittal and coronal planes. It has four chambers, two superiorly located atria and two inferiorly located ventricles. The heart described in terms of "right-sided" and "left-sided" chambers has its right chambers positioned more anteriorly in the chest and the left chambers more posteriorly. The left ventricle forms the inferoposterior; the right ventricle the most anterior part of the heart. The pulmonary trunk is the most anterior vessel.

The aorta arises from the center point of the base of the heart on the right posterior site of the pulmonary trunk, and curves upwards medially posterior to the aortic arch, giving rise to the brachiocephalic vessels. The junction between the aortic root with the sinuses of Valsalva and the ascending aorta is called the sinotubular junction. The normal anatomic feature of the aorta is a left-sided aortic arch running over the main stem bronchus and branching into the right brachiocephalic trunk, the left common carotid artery, and the left subclavian artery. The pulmonary trunk originates from the muscular pulmonary infundibulum on the left side and anteriorly to the aorta, and bifurcates into the right and left pulmonary arteries. Two of the pulmonary sinuses are always next to the aorta ("facing sinuses"), the third one is "non-facing". A fibrous remnant of the "Ductus arteriosus Botalli", the ligamentum arteriosum, extends from the pulmonary trunk into the descending aorta. The segment between the left subclavian artery and the aortic insertion of the ligamentum arteriosum is defined as the aortic isthmus, which is the typical location of an aortic isthmus stenosis (aortic coarctation).

The superior and inferior caval veins (vena cava superior, vena cava inferior) mediate the systemic venous return to the heart from the upper and lower parts of the body. The superior caval vein is formed by the confluence of the left and right innominate veins, which lie anterior to the brachiocephalic artery (arteria brachiocephalica). The inferior caval vein receives its blood from the hepatic veins; it crosses the diaphragm and enters the right atrium at its posterior part after a short intrathoracic portion. The two right and left pulmonary veins join the posterior part of the left atrium. The right pulmonary veins enter close to the atrial septum, while the two left pulmonary veins frequently join the left atrium as a common trunk.

The great vessels of the heart are usually examined by a combination of black-blood and bright-blood MRI sequences in different adapted imaging planes that provide a good visualization of the vessel lumen and wall and the para-aortic tissue. In addition, velocity-encoded flow studies are performed to visualize and quantitate flow patterns and volumes in blood vessels.

5.2 Structural Characteristics of Atria, Ventricles, Coronary Arteries and the Pericardium on CMR Imaging

Using CMR imaging special morphological criteria for the structures of the heart can be detected that are characteristic for the atria, ventricles and the great vessels, including the anatomical connections between these structures (Table 5-1).

Table 5-1 Structural characteristics of the heart on CMR imaging.

right atrium	• always connected with SVC and IVC • receives the coronary sinus • contains a fibro-muscular network • has an Eustachian valve (at the IVC) • has a Thebesian valve (at the coronary sinus) • has a crista terminalis (dissecting the venous component from the atrial component) • atrial appendage broad and triangular with broad connection to the right atrium
left atrium	• receives the four pulmonary veins • located posterior-superior • atrial appendage of long cylindrical shape with narrow connection to the left atrium
right ventricle	• thin walled and pyramid-shaped • course trabecularization • no connection between inflow and outflow tract (only connective tissue) • infundibulum present • septal tricuspid cusp inserts with the septum together with its chorda tendinea • moderator band present (trabecula septo-marginalis) • tricuspid valve attachment located more apically compared with mitral valve • fills the pulmonary artery
left ventricle	• thick walled and of oval to ellipsoid shape • fine trabecularization • inflow and outflow tract connected (muscle) • no visible infundibulum • smooth septal surface • mitral valve without chordal attachment to the ventricular septum • fills the aorta
pulmonary artery	• typical pulmonary artery bifurcation
aorta	• typical branching of the coronary arteries • typical branching of supra-aortic arteries (truncus brachiocephalicus, left carotid artery, left subclavian artery)

5.2.1 Atria

Both atria can be divided anatomically into a venous inflow, the vestibule of the atrioventricular valve, a septal component, and an atrial appendage. Both atria are separated by the atrial septum. The **right atrium** forms the border of the right side of heart, and inside the remnants of embryology, the sinus venosus and primitive auricle can be seen in the adult heart; both parts are separated by the terminal crest (crista terminalis), and outside by a groove, the sulcus terminalis. The former sinus venosus forms the venous component with a smooth interior, while the primitive auricle with a rough trabecular interior forms the appendage. Pectinate muscles branch from the crest at right angles and run into the appendage. The venous component of the right atrium receives the superior and inferior vena cava on its posterior surface, and the coronary sinus at the inferior junction with the septal component. The Eustachian valve attaches to the terminal crest near the opening of the vena cava inferior, and the Thebesian valve at the orifice of the coronary sinus. The coronary sinus runs through the left or posterior atrioventricular groove and opens into the right atrium above

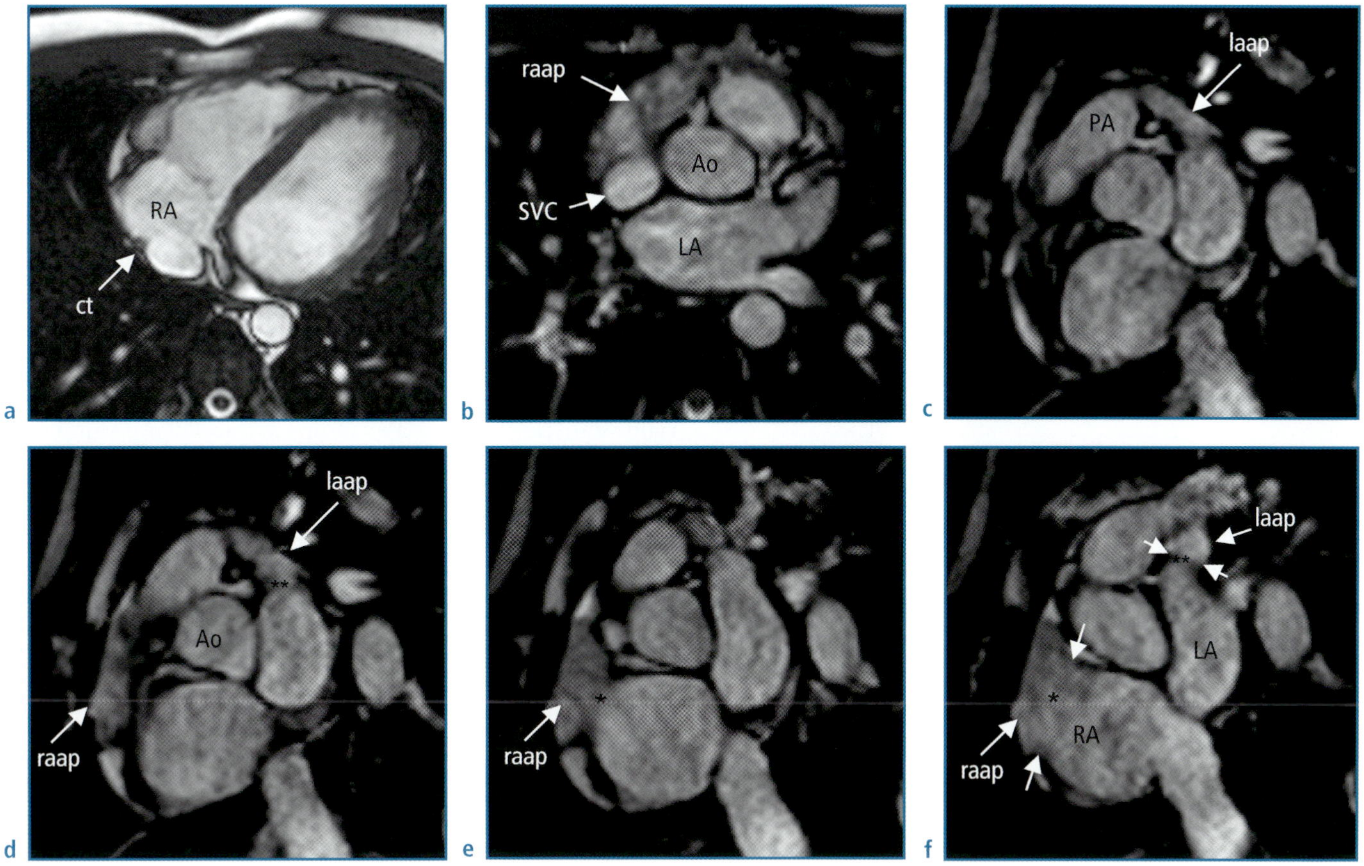

Figure 5-1 MR imaging of the right and left atrium in 4-ch and short-axis views using SSFP sequences of sub-millimeter spatial resolution. The right atrial appendage (raap) (b, e, f) has a triangular shape with broad communication to the right atrium (RA) and a visible crista terminalis (ct) (a). The left atrial appendage (laap) (c, d, f) has a tubular shape and a narrow communication to the left atrium (LA). The raap is located dorsal to the right coronary artery, the laap lies superior to the AV ring (sulcus) and to the left circumflex artery. Ao: aorta; PA: pulmonary artery; SVC: superior vena cava.

the posterior-inferior interventricular groove. The junction between the appendage and the venous component is particularly wide, the appendage has a broad, triangular appearance and is positioned ventrally to the entrance of the superior vena cava in the right atrium (Figure 5-1). The vestibule has a smooth wall and supports the attachments of the leaflets of the tricuspid valve. The crista terminalis (terminal crest) is routinely visible on black-blood and bright-blood MRI as a mural nodular or triangular structure adjacent to the lateral wall which connects both caval veins. Sometimes this muscular structure may be misinterpreted as an abnormal intra-atrial mass. The pectinate muscle in the right atrial appendage can also be imaged by bright-blood MRI.

The **left atrium** forms the upper posterior border of the heart; it lies beneath the carina and anterior to the esophagus and extends cranially behind the aortic root and the proximal part of the ascending aorta. Its appendage extends anteromedially. The remnants of the embryological parts of sinus venosus and primitive auricle may be differentiated in the adult heart, as well, and both form the same anatomical components as in the right atrium. The posteriorly located and smooth walled venous component receives the four pulmonary veins, one at each corner. The smooth walled vestibule supports the leaflets of the mitral valve. The pectinate muscles confined in the appendage are much less prominent compared to the right atrium and never extend around the atrioventricular junction. The left atrial appendage, which overlies the left atrioventricular groove and left circumflex artery, has a narrow junction with the body of the left atrium and has a long, tubular-shaped appearance (Figure 5-1).

The inter-atrial septum shows an oval depression on the right side, the fossa ovalis. While the floor of the fossa ovalis is the remains of the septum primum, the superior rim of the fossa, the so-called septum secundum, is an infolding of the atrial wall between the superior vena cava and right pulmonary veins. From the left atrial aspect, the septal surface is roughened, as is the flap of the fossa ovalis, and the flap valve overlaps the septum secundum, i.e. the infolded atrial wall. As long as the left atrial pressure exceeds that in the right atrium there will be no shunting across the inter-atrial septum. On SE-MRI the atrial septum can be seen as a thin line separating the two atria, but may be too thin at the level of the foramen ovale to be imaged. This finding should not be misinterpreted as an atrial septal defect. In contrast, bright-blood imaging depicts this thin part of the septum very well in most cases. Sometimes fatty infiltration of the inter-atrial septum is detected that can be easily differentiated from pathological masses by the characteristic signal intensity corresponding to the subcutaneous fat and by fat suppression sequences.

5.2.2 Ventricles

The **right ventricle** sits on the diaphragm above the liver and forms the anterior and inferior border of the heart except the apex. The right ventricle is characterized externally by its pyramidal shape and by its typical and distinctive coronary distribution pattern. The left anterior descending coronary artery (LAD) demarcates the left from the right ventricle. The right ventricle has an inlet component, an apical trabecular component, and an outlet tract. The inlet component with the tricuspid valve and interventricular septum surrounds and supports the leaflets and the subvalvular apparatus of the tricuspid valve. The leaflets can be divided into septal, anterosuperior, and inferior or mural locations within the atrioventricular junction. The characteristic feature of the tricuspid valve is the presence of tendinous chords (chordae tendineae) that attach its septal leaflet to the ventricular septum. Such chordal attachments to the septal surface are never seen in the left ventricle. A junction between the infundibulum and the right ventricle is composed of the parietal band, the septomarginal band (trabecula septomarginalis), and the moderator band. The moderator band containing the continuation of the right bundle branch passes from the interventricular septum to the anterior wall and is an essential characteristic of the right ventricle (Figure 5-2). The apical trabecular portion of the right ventricle shows characteristic coarse trabeculations. The infundibulum is incorporated into the right ventricle and forms the outflow tract (RVOT), the right ventricle proper forms the inflow tract. The RVOT forms a muscular ring between the tricuspid and pulmonary valve. Both valves are separated by the supraventricular crest (crista supraventricularis), which is caused by an infolding of the roof of the ventricle and is separated from the aorta by extracardiac space. Inside the right ventricle the muscular trabeculations are relatively coarse, few and straight, and tend to run parallel to the right ventricular inflow and outflow tracts. The papillary muscles of the right ventricle are relatively small and numerous and attach both to the septal and to the free wall

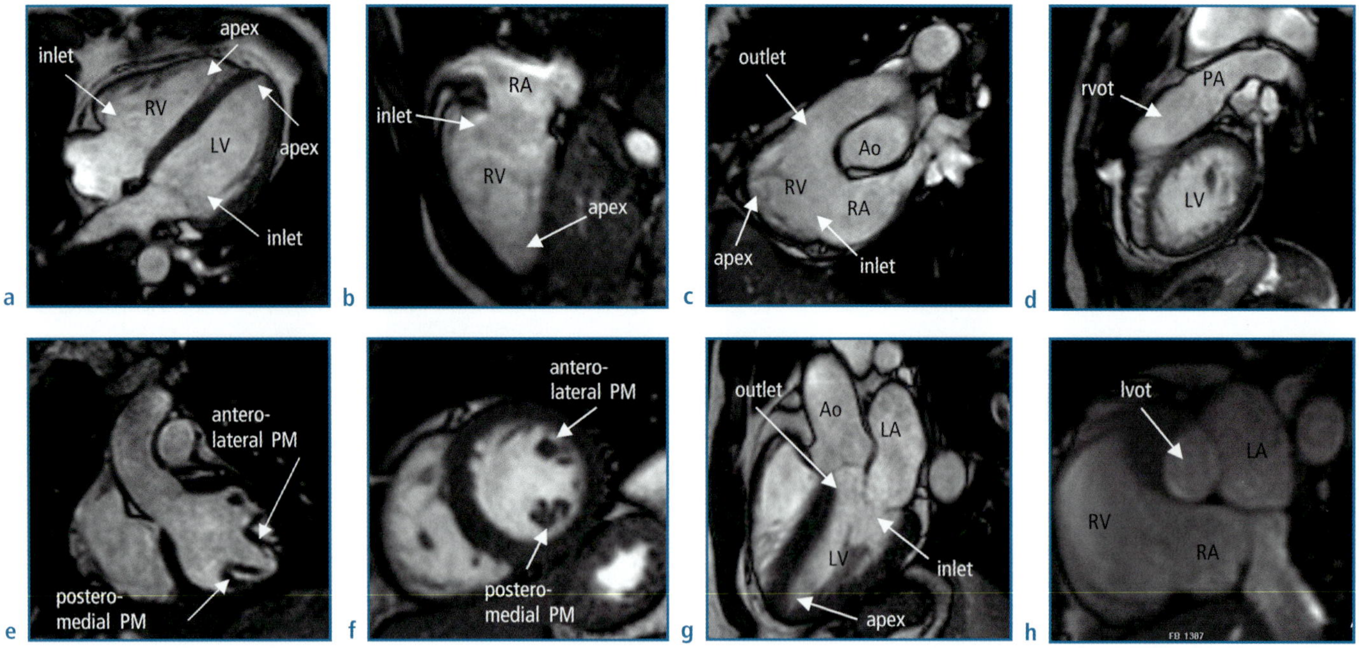

Figure 5-2 Morphological components of the right (a–d) and left ventricle (e–h). (a) 4-ch view; (b) short axis; (c) RV inflow and outflow tract; (d) cross-section of the infundibulum (rvot) and muscular ring between the tricuspid and pulmonary valve; (e) vertical long coronal axis with papillary muscles; (f) short axis with papillary muscles; (g) vertical long sagittal axis with LV inflow and outflow tract and aortic-mitral fibrous continuity; (h) cross-section of LV outflow tract and fibrous connection between mitral and aortic valve. Ao: aorta; LA: left atrium; LV: left ventricle; lvot: left ventricular outflow tract; PA: pulmonary artery; PM: papillary muscle; RA: right atrium; RV: right ventricle; rvot: right ventricular outflow tract.

surfaces. The lining of the chamber becomes smooth in the infundibulum, a funnel leading to the exit from the chamber which forms the pulmonary trunk. In the 4-chamber view there is a further characteristic of the tricuspid valve, whose valvular attachment is located more apically compared to the mitral attachment (under normal conditions < 8 mm/m^2 body surface). The normal right ventricle is a relatively thin walled chamber with an end-diastolic wall thickness of 3–4 mm, it is thicker than the wall of the right atrium but thinner compared to the wall of the left ventricle.

The normal **left ventricle** is a thick-walled chamber that forms the apex and the lower part of the left and posterior heart border. The oval to ellipsoid-shaped left ventricle shows numerous fine trabeculae with a smooth subtle surface. The left ventricle also possesses an inlet, an apical trabecular, and an outlet portion (left ventricular outflow tract = LVOT). The inlet portion contains the mitral valve and extends from the atrioventricular junction to the attachments of the prominent papillary muscles (Figure 5-2). The most important anatomic difference to the right ventricle is that the mitral valve does not have chordal attachments to the ventricular septum. The left ventricle possesses two papillary muscles, the anterior lateral and the posterior medial, and the papillary muscles do not attach to the septum. The outflow tract with the aortic valve is in direct continuity with the inlet portion, since normally there is little or no conal musculature beneath the aortic valve, but rather there is an aortic-mitral fibrous continuity. Part of the two or three leaflets of the aortic valve has muscular attachments to the outlet tract. The remainder of the leaflet originates from the fibrous tissue of the aortic root with extensive areas of fibrous continuity with the aortic leaflet of the mitral valve.

Wall thickness is not uniform throughout the left ventricle. In the longitudinal direction most pronounced differences are found with a gradual wall thinning toward the LV apex. Wall thickness of the septum is 8–10 mm, and of the LV left lateral wall segments 8–9 mm in men and 7–8 mm in women. Left ventricular apex can be extremely thin down to 3 mm in diameter, whereas less pronounced variations in wall thickness are seen around the LV circumference.

The **interventricular septum** separates the left from the right ventricle. It is mainly thick-walled except in the subaortic region, where it becomes very thin, the so-called membranous septum. In unloaded conditions the ventricular septum has a flat appearance, whereas in normal loading conditions it has a convex shape towards the right ventricle, which is maintained during the whole cardiac cycle. Enhanced filling of the right ventricle may lead to a flattening of the ventricular septum during early diastolic filling (so-called ventricular coupling).

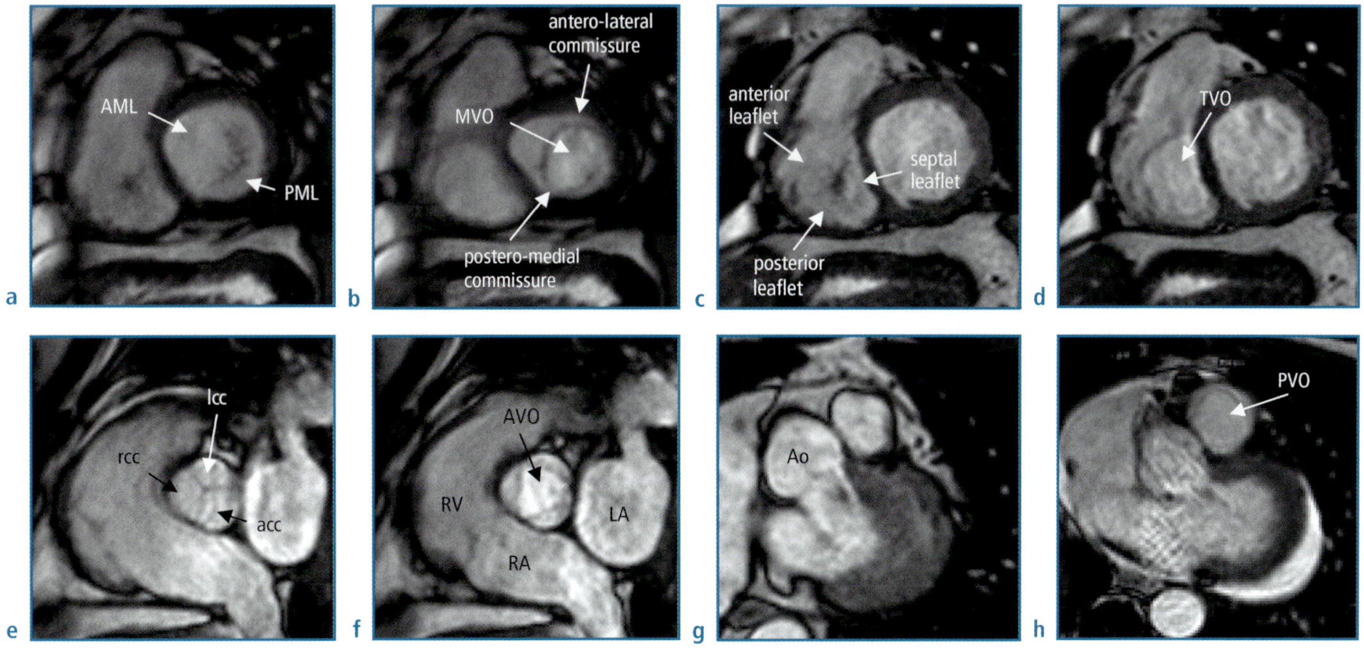

Figure 5-3 Cross-sectional plane through the AV valves (mitral and tricuspid valves) in open and closed position **(a–d)**, and cross-sectional plane through the semilunar valves (aortic and pulmonary valves) in open and closed position **(e–h)**. AML: anterior mitral leaflet; PML: posterior mitral leaflet; Ao: aorta; MVO: mitral valve orifice; TVO: tricuspid valve orifice; AVO: aortic valve orifice; PVO: pulmonary valve orifice; LA: left atrium; lcc: left coronary cusp; rcc: right coronary cusp; acc: acoronary cusp; RA: right atrium; RV: right ventricle.

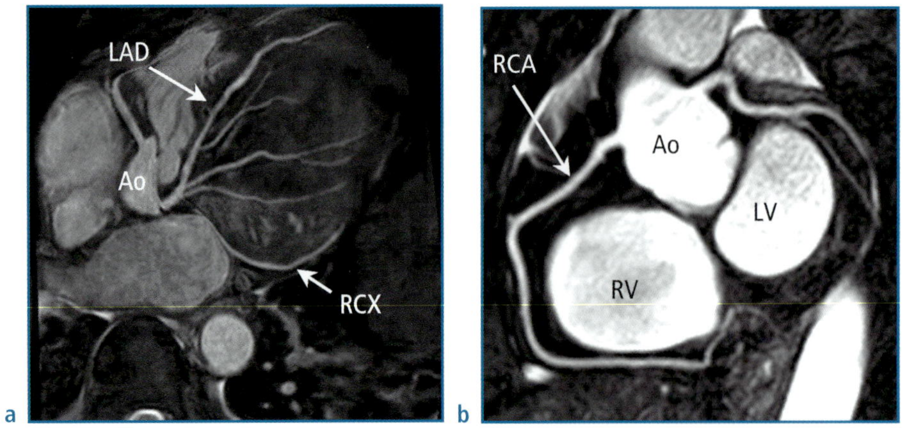

Figure 5-4 MR imaging of the left **(a)** and right **(b)** coronary arteries in adapted imaging planes. Ao: aorta; LAD: left anterior descendent artery; LV: left ventricle; RCX: left circumflex artery; RCA: right coronary artery; RV: right ventricle.

5.2.3 Cardiac Valves

The **atrioventricular valves** connect the atria with the ventricles, embryologically the mitral valve is always connected with the left and the tricuspid valve is connected with the right ventricle. Along the longitudinal cardiac axis, the tricuspid valve is always somewhat more apically positioned than the mitral valve (normally < 8 mm/m^2 body surface area). The tricuspid valve has three cusps, the septal, the inferior, and the anterosuperior cusp, whereas the mitral valve has an aortic and mural cusp. The muscular support for the septal cusp of the tricuspid valve comes from the trabeculae out of the septum, for the anterosuperior cusp from the medial papillary muscle, which is part of the trabecula septomarginalis, and for the inferior cusp from several smaller papillary muscles. The muscular support for the aortic mitral cusp comes from the anterior papillary muscle and for the mural cusp from the posterior papillary muscle.

The **semilunar valves** of both great arteries attach across the ventriculoarterial junction without chordal attachments, and lack a fibrous supporting annulus such as seen with the atrioventricular valves. The pulmonary artery normally arises from the infundibulum of the right ventricle, and the leaflets of the pulmonary valve and the leaflets of the tricuspid valve are widely separated by the infundibular musculature. The aortic valve cusps are described according to the origin of the coronary arteries as left, right and non-coronary cusps. Each valve cusp has a small nodule of connective tissue at its mid-point that facilitates firm aortic valve closure (Figure 5-3). The valve leaflets of the aorta and pulmonary artery are very thin and fibers may be best imaged by bright-blood MRI techniques for demonstrating valve leaflet morphology, leaflet motion, normal valve opening, and valvular flow pattern.

5.2.4 Coronary Arteries

The right coronary artery (RCA) arises from the right sinus of Valsalva from an ostium located just below the sinotubular junction (Figure 5-4). The RCA runs within the right atrioventricular groove and provides side branches to the infundibulum (conal branch) and to the free wall of the right ventricle. In the case of RCA dominance, the RCA branches at the crux cordis into the right posterior descending artery (supply for the inferoseptal part of the left ventricular myocardium) and into the posterolateral branch. In the case of left circumflex artery (LCx) dominance (5% of individuals), the LCx continues as posterior descending artery, while in 10% of individuals RCA and LCx supply the inferior wall in a balanced pattern.

The left coronary artery (LCA) arises from the middle portion of the left anterior sinus of Valsalva just below the sinotubular junction (Figure 5-4). The proximal part of LCA is the left main stem (LM) or trunk of a variable length ($\pm$ 1 cm), from which the LAD and LCx arteries normally arise. The LAD courses in the anterior interventricular groove, the LCx in the left posterior atrioventricular groove. The LAD provides branches to the interventricular septum (perforator branches) and side branches to the anterolateral wall of the left ventricle (diagonal branches), while the LCx provides branches to the posterolateral wall of the left ventricle, including the posteromedial papillary muscle. The LAD terminates at the cardiac apex or 1–2 cm before or after the apex of the left ventricle.

5.2.5 Pericardium

The pericardium envelops the heart and the origin of the great vessels; it consists of an outer fibrous layer, the fibrous pericardium, and an inner serous sack, the serous pericardium. The fibrous part is attached to the sternum and diaphragm, the serous pericardium consists of an inner visceral layer, the epicardium, which is intimately connected to the heart and the epicardial fat, while the outer parietal layer lines the fibrous pericardium. The pericardium contains two serous tunnels, the sinus transversus posterior to the great arteries and anterior to the atria and the vena cava superior, and the sinus obliquus posterior to the left atrium. The sinus transversus is divided into four recesses, the superior and inferior aortic recess and the left and right pulmonic recess. Normally the pericardial space contains 20–25 ml of serous fluid; the amount of fluid may vary considerably among different individuals.

On MR imaging the normal pericardial sack is visible as a very thin curvilinear structure of low signal intensity surrounded by the high-intensity mediastinal and subepicardial fat. Normally the pericardium has a thickness of 1.2 ± 0.5 mm in diastole and 1.7 ± 0.5 mm in systole (Sechtem 1986). On SE-MR sequences the pericardium may reach a thickness of 3 mm. This overestimation is caused by partial volume effects, by motion-dependent signal loss of the pericardial fluid, and by cardiac and pericardial motion. On SSFP gradient echo sequences the pericardium appears with low signal intensity. Minimal fluid accumulations together with epicardiac and pericardiac and mediastinal fat are imaged without high signal intensity and thereby add to the thickening of the pericardial structure within the CMR images.

5.3 CMR Projection Planes

5.3.1 Body Axes Oriented Imaging Planes

To assess structure and function of the heart and the great vessels it is essential to know the different imaging planes and the corresponding topographic anatomy.

> To provide an initial survey, or for imaging distinct congenital heart disease abnormalities, as a first step **2D imaging planes in the three orthogonal axes** are performed:
> - **coronal** (= frontal) imaging plane,
> - **sagittal** imaging plane,
> - **transversal** (= horizontal or axial) imaging plane.

The corresponding anatomical details within these three imaging planes are shown in Figure 5-5, Figure 5-6, and Figure 5-7, using T2-black-blood-TSE sequences.

5.3.2 Cardiac Oriented Imaging Planes

The morphological and functional analysis of the heart itself demands special heart oriented imaging planes in the main cardiac axes (see Chapter 4), similar to those used in echocardiography. After determining the anatomical cardiac axis (RAO equivalent, transversal imaging plane and short axis) axis-specific views are produced through the heart such as 2-chamber view, 4-chamber view, short-axis view of left ventricle and 3-chamber view. For special diagnostic purposes an adapted view through the left or right ventricular outflow tract or a special 2-chamber view through the right ventricle is used. Further adapted imaging views are used for imaging the ascending aorta or the pulmonary trunk, as well as to assess altered morphology and function of the four cardiac valves. In the case of cardiac masses or other altered structures of the heart imaging planes other than heart axis-specific may be used in multiple angulations, whereby a cardiac specific structure, e.g. cardiac apex or base, should be included in the imaging plane for better anatomic orientation.

5.4 Ventricular Performance

The heart with its thick-walled musculature serves as the central circulatory pump. After complete end-diastolic filling, electrical stimulation by the heart's intrinsic pacemaker (the sinus node plus the special conduction system = AV node, His-Purkinje system and bundle branches) leads to an increase in fiber tension and fiber shortening that is translated into a myocardial deformation or "strain", and at the ventricular level myocardial deformation and motion is translated into a rise of ventricular pressure and subsequent volume reduction and ejection of blood into the great arteries (aorta and pulmonary artery). After electrical stimulation, ventricular contraction starts accompanied by mitral and tricuspid valve closure followed by isovolumetric contraction, opening of the aortic and pulmonary valve, and early ejection as long as ventricular pressure is higher than aortic and pulmonary pressure.

The high efficiency of left ventricular pump function, i.e. the usual ejection of 65% ventricular end-diastolic volume by 10–15% myofiber shortening, may be explained by the unique myocardial fiber array. The individual myocardial fibers are grouped into fiber bundles, and the direction of these fiber bundles throughout the myocardial wall is highly variable. Three types of fiber bundles can be differentiated, the midwall fibers with a circumferential course and both the endo- and epicardial fiber bundles with a progressively oblique orientation, though towards a completely opposite

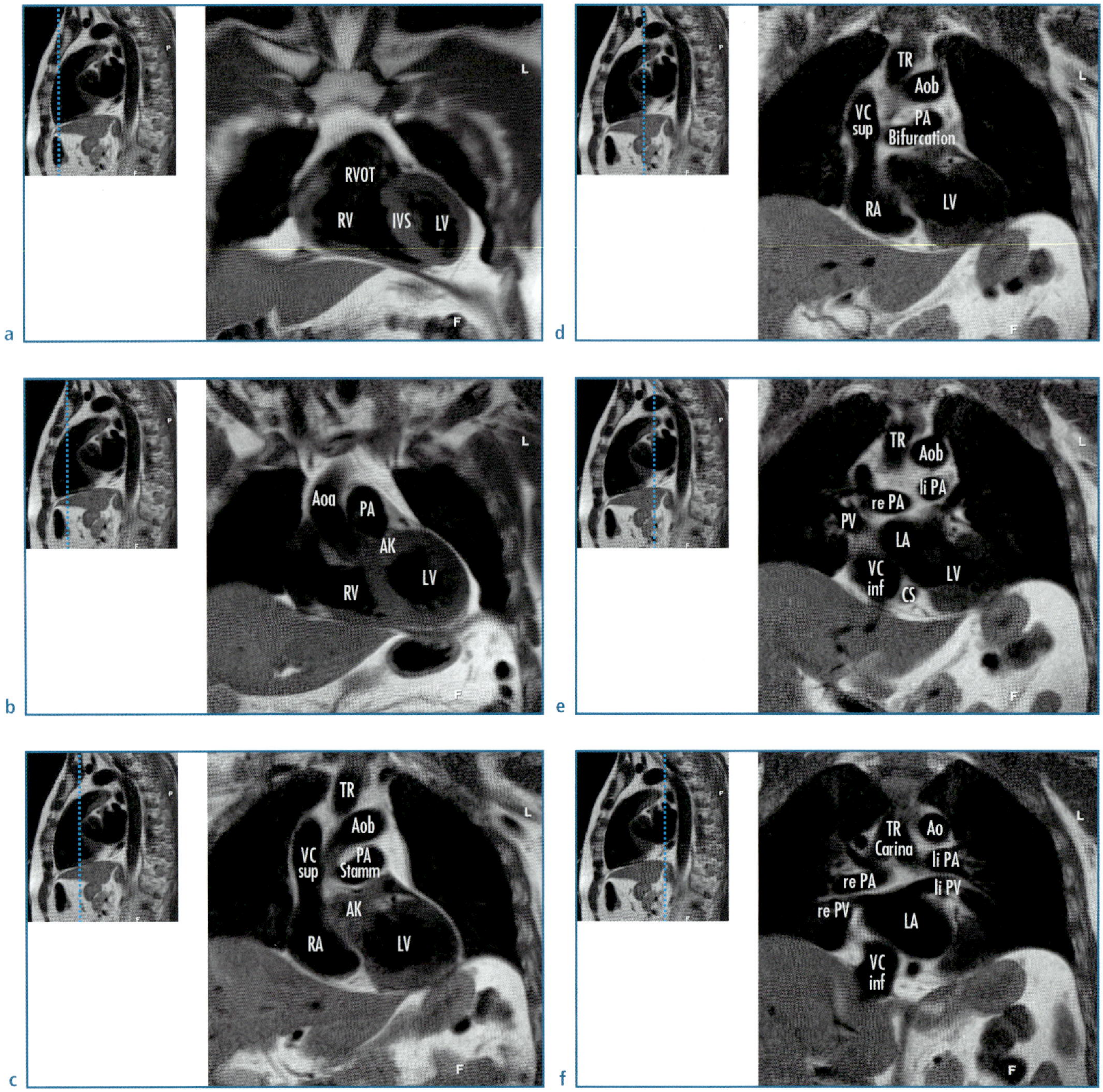

Figure 5-5 Standard image planes relative to the body position with representative MR images in the coronal planes from ventral (a) to dorsal (f). The small images (left columns) show the corresponding imaging planes in the sagittal direction. AK: aortic valve; Ao: aorta; Aoa: ascending aorta; Aob: aortic arch; Aod: descending aorta; CS and SC: coronary sinus; F: foot; IVS: interventricular septum; LA: left atrium; L: left; li: left; LV: left ventricle; MK: mitral valve; P: posterior; PA: pulmonary artery; PV: pulmonary vein; RA: right atrium; re: right; RV: right ventricle; RVOT: right ventricular outflow tract; Stamm: trunk; TR: trachea; V: vein; VC: vena cava; VC inf: inferior caval vein; VC sup: superior caval vein.

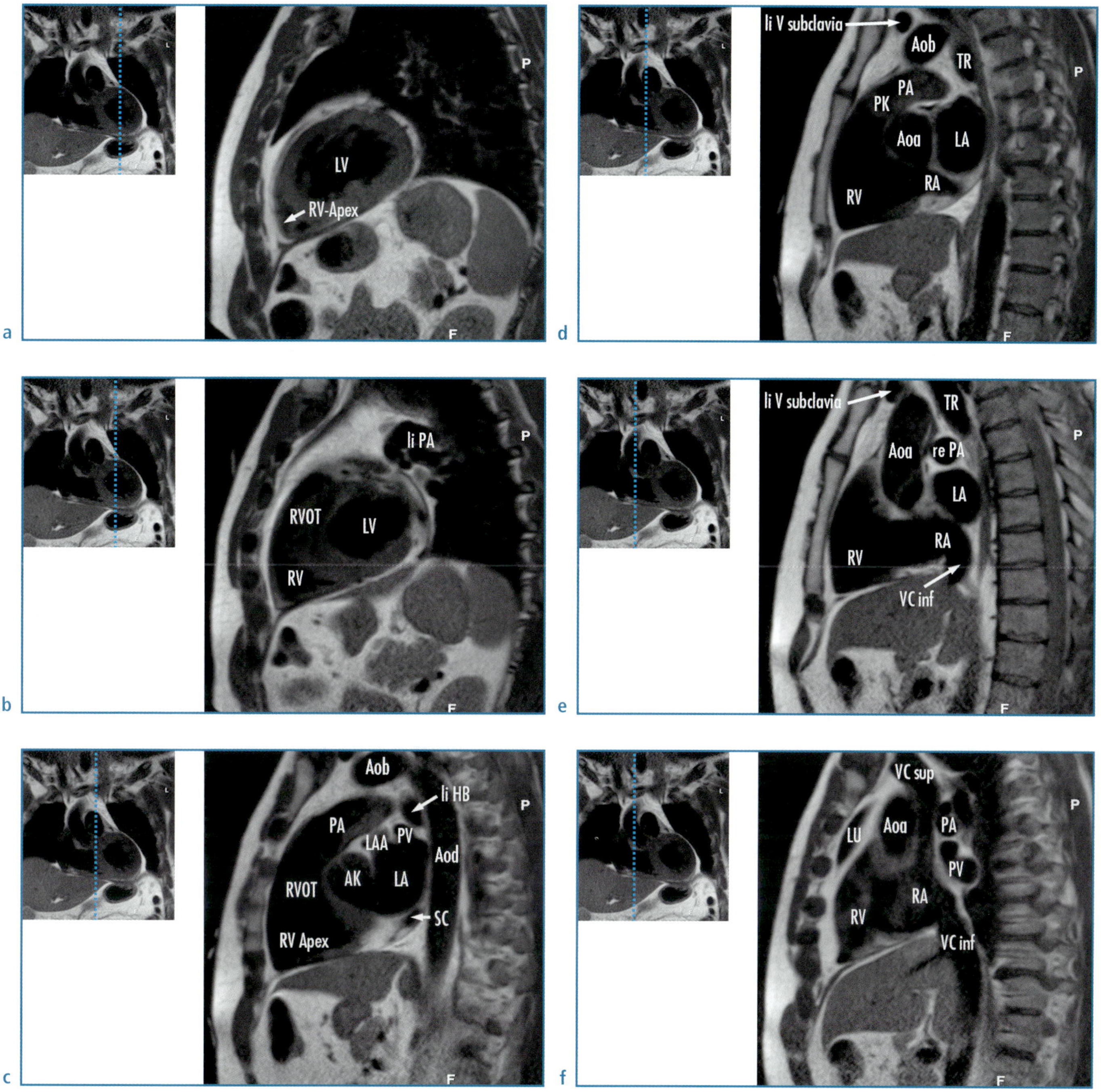

Figure 5-6 Standard image planes relative to the body position with representative MR images in the sagittal planes from left **(a)** to right **(f)**. The small images (left columns) show the corresponding planes in the coronal direction. AK: aortic valve; Ao: aorta; Aoa: ascending aorta; Aob: aortic arch; Aod: descending aorta; F: foot; HB: main bronchus; IVS: interventricular septum; L: left; LA: left atrium; LAA: left atrial appendage; li: left; LU: lung; LV: left ventricle; LVOT: left ventricular outflow tract; MK: mitral valve; P: posterior; PA: pulmonary artery; PK: pulmonary valve; PV: pulmonary vein; RA: right atrium; re: right; RV: right ventricle; RVOT: right ventricular outflow tract; SC: coronary sinus; TR: trachea; V: vein; VC: vena cava; VC inf: inferior caval vein; VC sup: superior caval vein.

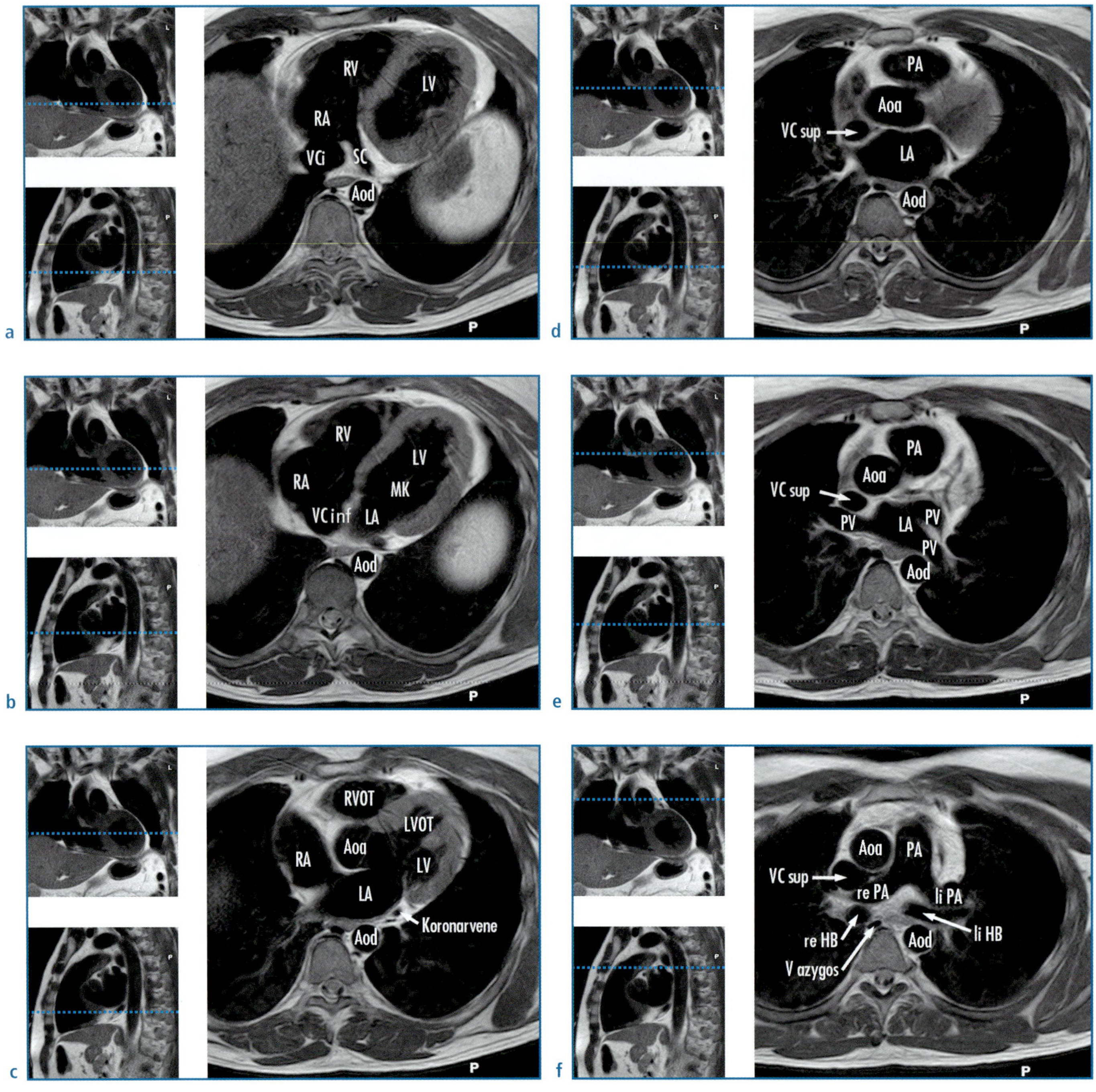

Figure 5-7 Standard image planes relative to the body position with representative MR images in the transversal (horizontal = axial) planes from caudal **(a)** to cranial **(f)**. The small images (left columns) show the corresponding planes in the coronal (top) and sagittal (bottom) direction of each image pair of the column. Aoa: ascending aorta; Aod: descending aorta; HB: main bronchus; Koronarvene: coronary vein; L: left; LA: left atrium; li: left; LV: left ventricle; LVOT: left ventricular outflow tract; MK: mitral valve; P: posterior; PA: pulmonary artery; PV: pulmonary vein; RA: right atrium; re: right; RV: right ventricle; RVOT: right ventricular outflow tract; SC: coronary sinus; V azygos: azygos vein; VC inf and VCi: inferior caval vein; VC sup: superior caval vein.

direction. Thus, the endo- and epicardial oblique fibers are almost perpendicularly oriented towards each other. This complex fiber orientation results in a complex myocardial deformation and contraction pattern: contraction of the midwall fibers results in circumferential shortening with centripetal wall motion, while shortening of the longitudinal fiber bundles results in shortening of the long axis of the ventricle. There is an intrinsic interaction between the contraction of the epicardial and endocardial fiber bundles, called "myocardial tethering", which is based on a predominance of the torque of the epicardial on the torque of endocardial fibers. Shortening of the epicardial fibers forces the endocardial fibers to reorder passively and to shorten along the epicardial fiber direction nearly perpendicular to the endocardial fiber orientation. The magnitude of this "cross fiber" endocardial shortening exceeds the endocardial fiber shortening, and together with the centripetal contraction of the midwall fibers this produces thickening of ventricular wall in the radial direction. The complex integrated mechanism of myocardial contraction and ejection can be easily studied using cine-MRI by imaging of systolic wall thickening by 40–50 % in both the short and long axes, circumferential shortening by 35–45 % in short-axis views, and longitudinal ventricular shortening by up to 20 % in the 4-chamber view.

A second mechanism may further support ventricular function, the torsion or twisting mechanism of myocardial fibers. The left ventricle shows a counterclockwise rotation when viewed from the apex, and this wringing or rotational motion increases the longer the distance from the base with a maximum of up to ± 28° of rotation, however, the spread is fairly homogenous from base to apex. This mechanism is probably produced by an imbalance between the contraction of fibers with a left-hand and right-hand oblique course with a dominance of epicardial over endocardial fiber bundles. This torsion mechanism not only improves and supports wall thickening and ejection, but also induces active ventricular relaxation by an effective untwisting motion in the early ventricular relaxation period. This results in a clear dissociation between ventricular untwisting and diastolic filling and may be a potent mechanism in the suction of blood from the atrium to the ventricle early in diastole. This twisting and untwisting movement of the heart can be easily assessed by MR myocardial tagging techniques (Rüssel 2008).

5.5 Quantitative Assessment of RV and LV Function and Muscle Mass

Ventricular function includes a repetitive process of ejection and filling, and changes in ventricular volumes and velocity of these changes should ideally be assessed over the whole cardiac cycle. Though this was recently realized by deriving RV pressure-volume loops during interventional CMR imaging in patients with congenital heart disease and pulmonary hypertension (Kühne 2004), in clinical practice ventricular volumes are measured at maximal filling (end-diastole) and maximal ejection (end-systole).

> From both end-diastolic (EDV) and end-systolic volumes (ESV) all other hemodynamic parameters such as stroke volume (SV), ejection fraction (EF), and cardiac output (CO) and their corresponding indices (I) through dividing by body surface area (BSA) can be derived:
> - SV (ml) = EDV – ESV,
> - EF (%) = SV × 100 / EDV,
> - CO (ml/min) = SV × heart rate,
> - EDVI (ml/m^2) = EDV / BSA,
> - ESVI (ml/m^2) = ESV / BSA,
> - CI (l/m^2) = CO / BSA.

In addition, RV and LV ventricular muscle mass (RVMM, LVMM) can also be measured by determining the volume of outer border of the RV or LV and subtracting the volume of the inner contours (i.e. blood volume) at end-diastole, whereby the interventricular septum is counted to the LV mass. LV mass can then be obtained by multiplication of the net volume (epicardial minus endocardial volume) with the specific density of the myocardium, 1.05 g/cm^3. In clinical practice, two principal techniques are used for volumetric measurements, geometric models (or assumptions), and volumetric ventricular quantification.

5.5.1 Geometrical Models

Geometric assumptions compare the ventricular cavity with a geometrical model, and using a limited number of standardized measurements of the ventricular cavity the corresponding volumes are calculated. For the left ventricle either long-axis views (e.g. bi-plane ellipsoid and single-plane ellipsoid models), or short axis views (e.g. hemisphere-cylinder model, Teichholz model), or a combination of long and short axis views is used for calculations of ventricular volumes (Figure 5-8). Geometric models are used in planar imaging and have the advantage of rapidly obtaining ventricular volumes and LV mass, but they are only reliable as long

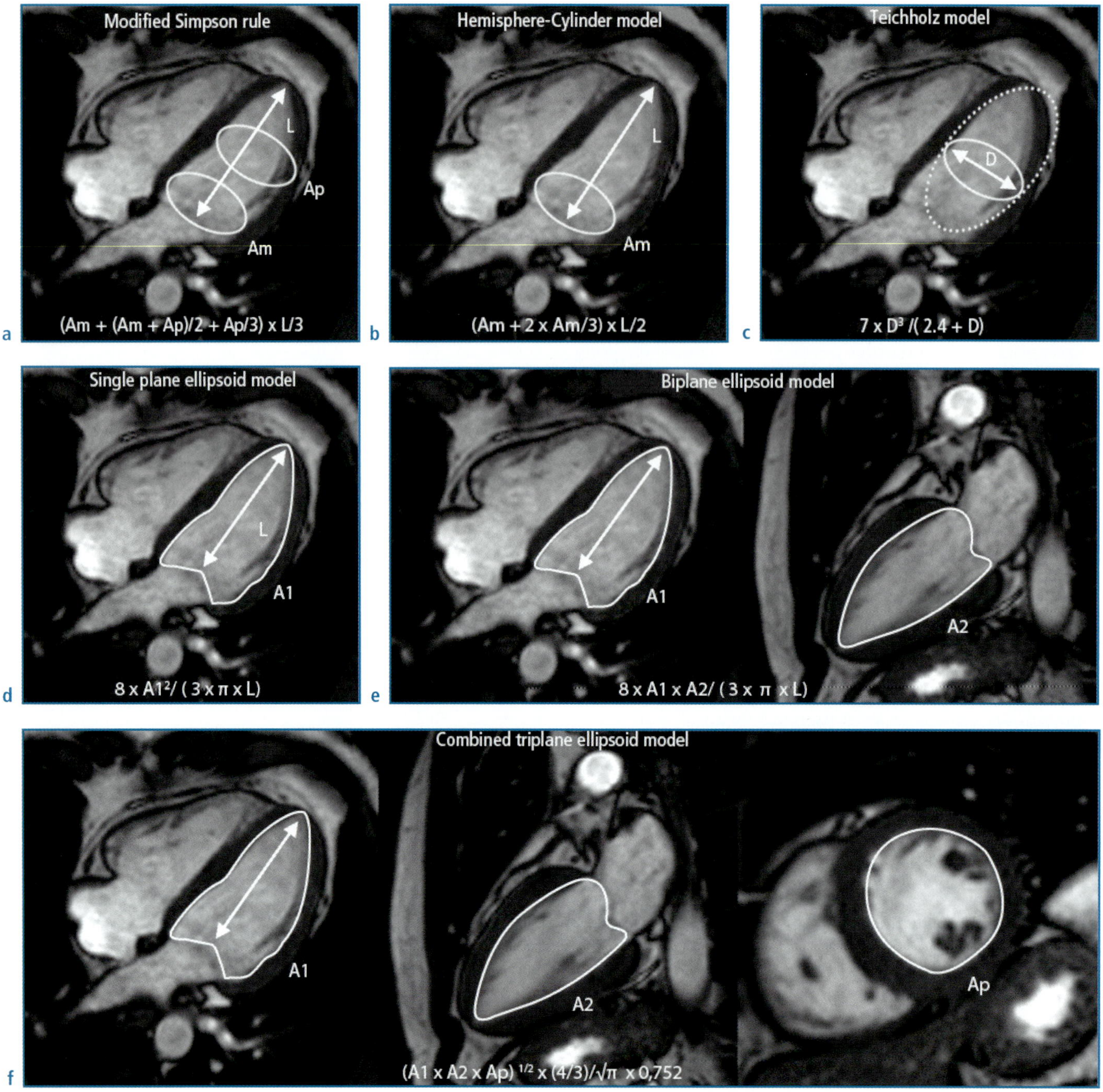

Figure 5-8 Schematic of left ventricular volume measurements according to geometric assumptions (modified Simpson's rule, hemisphere-cylinder model, Teichholz model, single-plane ellipsoid model, bi-plane ellipsoid model, combined tri-plane model). A: area; Am: area at mitral level; Ap: area at papillary muscle level; D: diameter; L: length (modified from Bogaert et al. 2005).

as the geometrical model corresponds to the true ventricular cavity or myocardial wall. This of course may not be the case in focally diseased ventricles, e.g. after myocardial infarction or severely remodeled ventricles, e.g. in dilated cardiomyopathy. Moreover, their role is limited in assessing small but significant changes in global ventricular function. An interesting new combined tri-plane geometric model, using a combination of short axis, and vertical and horizontal long axis to estimate LV volumes, has been proposed by Thiele et al. (2002). They were able to show that in comparison with the volumetric data set this geometric model combined with the b-FFE technique yielded the best accuracy and reproducibility even in patients with regional ventricular dysfunction. Though geometric models in general are not as reliable as volumetric measurements in clinical practice, their use is appropriate e.g. if something goes wrong with the volumetric data acquisition, or it may be used as a fast check for the validity of results obtained by the volumetric approach. For these purposes a simple geometric formula may be recommended: $(L1 \times L2 \times L3 \times \pi)/6$, where L1 represents the long-axis diameter of the LV on vertical or horizontal long-axis images, and L2 and L3 represent the maximal short axis diameters in two perpendicular views. It should be stressed that this type of measurement should be made from MR images with recent SSFP sequences (b-FFE), in contrast to spin echo or spoiled-GRE techniques. The reason is the excellent high contrast between myocardium and blood-filled ventricular cavities with the b-SSFP sequence that allows a precise delineation of the inner contours of the ventricular cavities.

5.5.2 Volumetry Using Simpson's Rule

With the advent of 3D MRI imaging, true volumetric quantification is now feasible. According to Simpson's rule, the volume of a complex structure such a ventricle can be quantified by dividing this structure into several smaller, less complex sub-volumes, and volume quantification of all sub-volumes yields the total volume of the complex structure. In clinical practice ventricular volumes are calculated from a stack of contiguous short axis slices that encompass the entire left and right ventricles. After delineation of the endocardial contours of each slice, multiplication of the area by the thickness of each slice and the interslice distance (if used), and addition of these sub-volume slices yields the total ventricular volume (Figure 5-9). With ultra-fast imaging the whole short axis stack can be now acquired in just one breath-hold of about 12 s, using the most modern b-SSFP GE sequences (Nagel 2000a).

The accuracy of volumetric measurements from multi-slice short axis acquisition is mainly determined by the accurate identification of the most basal slice level and the accurate definition of the endocardial and epicardial contours in this slice level. Through-plane motion represents a major challenge as the position of the heart towards a fixed imaging plane will continuously change during the cardiac cycle, and different parts of the heart will be visualized on consecutive images in this fixed imaging plane. Such through-plane motion is most obvious on cardiac short-axis images and the base of the heart, at the interface of the atria and ventricles. The through-plane movement of the heart at its base is the result of pronounced longitudinal shortening of the ventricles, whereby the base of the heart moves toward the cardiac apex (motion of the LV annulus towards the apex is about 1.3 cm in the normal heart). As a result, a short-axis slice positioned through the base of the left ventricle at end-diastole will be located in the left atrium during systole. Therefore one has to correct for through-plane motion, otherwise end-systolic volumes are significantly overestimated and stroke volumes underestimated. If the mitral valve cannot be accurately identified, the mitral valve ring plane may be used, which slightly overestimates LV volumes.

To compensate for through-plane motion a slice-omission technique is used that omits the slices being atrially located at end-systole. Based on LV morphology, short-axis slices with a complete muscular ring are considered as ventricular, while incomplete muscular rings with less than 75% myocardium or thin-walled rings are regarded as atrial. This slice-omission approach is not entirely correct, since the mitral valve anatomy is not taken into account. Another approach is to measure the longitudinal LV-shortening on a

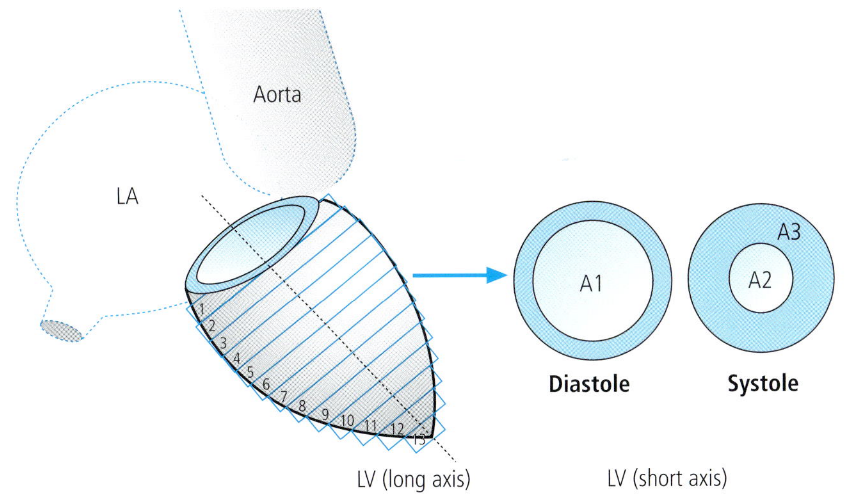

Figure 5-9 Schematic of volumetric measurement of left ventricular end-diastolic and end-systolic volumes by the slice-summation method; each of the 10–14 slices is acquired as one cine image, and the whole ventricular volume is calculated by assessing the area of each slice times the thickness of the slices and adding up the 10–14 slice volumes at both end-diastole and end-systole. A1: end-diastolic endocardial area; A2: end-systolic endocardial area; A3: myocardium; LA: left atrium; LV: left ventricle.

vertical or horizontal long-axis view and use this information to correct the short-axis images at end-systole. A third more difficult approach is using a priori knowledge about cardiac morphology during delineation of the images, e.g. excluding the mitral valve area but including the left ventricular outflow tract region into the ventricular cavity. In summary, a consistent approach for through-plane correction is definitely necessary for repeated studies, because the calculated values have a major impact on the calculated ventricular volumes.

To overcome the problem of through-plane movement of basal slices, Bloomer et al. (2002) used multiple radial long-axis views for quantification of left ventricular volumes and mass using a SSFP sequence. With a radial long-axis acquisition, multiple long-axis views are acquired sharing a common axis of rotation at equi-angular intervals. This orientation takes advantage of a short-axis imaging because of its clear visualization of the mitral and aortic valve planes, and in addition long-axis views have less partial volume effect near the apex. The authors could show a good agreement between multi-slice short-axis and radial long-axis acquisition, and as a result of the improved visualization of the myocardial boundaries and definition of the base, inter-observer agreement was better using the radial long-axis method.

Accuracy and Reproducibility

> CMR has the best accuracy of all imaging techniques for the measurement of left and right ventricular volume and muscle mass.

This has been proven ex vivo by comparing CMR measurements of left ventricles with water displacement volume of casts of the ventricles (Longmore 1985, Rehr 1985), as was also found for the right ventricle (Jauhainen 1998). In vivo the accuracy of volume measurement has been demonstrated in normal subjects by comparison of left and right ventricular stroke volumes, which have to be equal in normal circulation (Salm 2006, Sechtem 1987). Right and left stroke volumes have been demonstrated to be comparable to stroke volumes from pulmonary arterial and aortic flow mapping (Firmin 1987, Kondo 1991). Measurements of LV mass by CMR have been validated in human autopsy hearts and in animals (Myerson 2002, Katz 1988), and RV mass against ex vivo animal hearts (Bloomgarden 1997, Katz 1993). Excellent accuracy of CMR measurements have also been demonstrated for abnormally shaped hearts, e.g. in patients after myocardial infarction (Shapiro 1989), with left ventricular hypertrophy or dilated cardiomyopathy (Semelka 1990), or with congenital heart disease (Helbeing 1995).

Up to now, CMR has revealed the best interstudy reproducibility of any imaging technique for both volume and mass in the left (Grothues 2002) and right (Grothues 2004, Mooij 2009) ventricles, and is considered superior to that of 2D echocardiography (Semelka 1990). Reproducibility of an imaging technique is critical for calculating sample size in patients in whom changes may be expected, e.g. on a maintenance drug therapy. Interstudy reproducibility is determined by the standard deviation (SD) of the differences in two measured parameters over a time period with no clinical change expected and no recollection made by the operator. A power calculation for determining sample size for a trial can be made from interstudy SD, whereby low SDs are important as a reduction of SD leads to a squared reduction in sample size: i.e. half the SD equals one-quarter the sample size. For example, Bottini et al. (1995) showed that for a study to show a 10 g decrease in left ventricular mass with antihypertensive treatment, with a 90% power and a p-value of 0.05, the sample size would be 505 patients with 2D echo, but only 14 patients using CMR.

Influence of Imaging Sequences and Papillary Muscles and Trabeculations

Recent studies have shown that SSFP sequences provide the best endocardial border visualization compared with older spin echo or spoiled gradient echo sequences (Moon 2002). Due to the improved endocardial border visualization and absence of saturation effects with SSFP sequences, these authors found significantly larger ventricular volumes and decreased myocardial mass, compared with the spoiled-GRE technique. As a consequence, automated image segmentation techniques should also benefit from this increased discrimination of the blood-endocardium interface with the modern SSFP technique. Another issue is the question whether endocardial trabeculations and papillary muscles should be included or excluded from the measurements, since they have a significant impact on ventricular volume and mass. Trabeculations and papillary muscles may "pollute" regional morphological and functional data, and therefore exclusion of these structures from these measurements may best guarantee to provide homogeneous data throughout the ventricle. On the other hand, it may be advisable to include at least papillary muscles in the myocardium, particularly in patients with hypertensive diseases, hypertrophic cardiomyopathy, or myocardial storage diseases, because of concomitant hypertrophy of the papillary muscles, and hence this approach yields the best quantification of exact myocardial mass.

Imaging Protocol and Image Analysis

CMR ventricular assessment is performed in a highly standardized manner producing two long-axis cine images (vertical and horizontal) and a stack of 10–14 short-axis cines. A cine image can be acquired in one breath hold of about 10 s, and a typical set of ventricular images can be acquired within 5 min. The vertical and horizontal planes are used to plan the short-axis, and the first short-axis should be placed using the end-diastolic image at the base of the heart covering the most basal portion of the left and right ventricles just forward of the atrioventricular ring. The basal slice has to be acquired in a consistent and standardized manner in order to achieve optimal reproducibility. Further short-axis images are acquired every 1 cm along the long axis to the cardiac apex, and all cines should be acquired at end-expiration as this is more reproducible than held inspiration.

Cine images are now generally acquired using steady-state free precession (SSFP, b-FFE) sequences. The typical in-plane resolution is 1.4 × 1.8 mm (or 1.7 × 1.9 mm) and a slice thickness of 6–8 mm, and temporal resolution is 50 ms. Using the b-FFE technique together with parallel imaging, the breath-hold period can be reduced down to 6 s per slice while maintaining sufficient spatial resolution, and with latest generation of ultrafast imaging techniques real-time sequences during free-breathing are becoming available (Nagel 2000). This is particularly important for patients e.g. with heart failure, who cannot tolerate longer breath-hold periods.

In our institution the following **routine protocol for RV-LV volumetry** is used:

- SSFP sequence, possibly combined with parallel imaging (SENSE),
- 2D multi-slice stack,
- FOV: 330–400 mm, in-plane resolution 1.7 × 1.9 mm,
- multi-phase-cine images, 32 cardiac phases, temporal resolution 120 ms, possible phase interpolation with 50 % reduction of acquisition time,
- slice thickness 8–10 mm,
- fold-over AP with transversal and FH with coronal slice orientation,
- segmented k-space filling,
- retrospective triggering to span the whole systole and diastole,
- end-expiratory breath-hold,
- acquisition time 4–5 s/slice.

Retrospective gating and improvements in temporal resolution down to 26 ms have also allowed the assessment of diastolic function by CMR. In CMR LV volume is measured at each phase of the cardiac cycle including diastole, and a time-volume curve can be produced, from which the peak filling rate and the ratio of early and active filling rates can then be calculated (Maceira 2006). Recommendations on standardized CMR imaging protocols have recently been published (Kramer 2008).

In manual contouring, the long- and short-axis cines are used to measure the volumes and mass of the ventricles, whereby the operator traces the blood-endocardium border at end-diastole and end-systole for each slice. With modern software packages this process is substantially supported by automated contour tracking after setting contour makers by the operator. The end-diastolic and end-systolic volumes are calculated by adding the volume of blood in each slice that will be performed by the computer program. The left ventricular mass is typically measured at end-diastole by tracing the epicardial border in each slice of the short-axis. The area of the epicardium minus the area of endocardium indicates the area of myocardium in each slice, and the volume of mass can be determined by summing up these (net) areas. The true mass can be calculated from the volume and the myocardial density (1.05 mg/cm^3). Papillary muscles and endocardial trabeculae should be excluded from LV volume and included in the LV mass.

Computer-assisted evaluation tools may greatly increase the speed of image analysis and can potentially improve accuracy (Keenan and Pennell 2007). These approaches generate a three-dimensional model of the myocardium and blood pool. Their advantages are first that the operator does not need to trace the endocardium, which with its trabeculations is the most time-intensive part of analysis. But rather the operator can adapt the value of signal intensity-based thresholding until the anatomic border appearances correlate with a visual assessment. And second using the long-axis views the valve plane can be tracked and hence the software can compensate more accurately for atrioventricular valve descent in systole (Keenan and Pennell 2007). Recently Corsi et al. (2009) reported on excellent results of automated computer-based contour finding for LV volumes, compared with manually-traced endocardial boundaries. Analysis time for one cardiac cycle was < 15 min, intertechnique comparison resulted in high correlation (r > 0.96), small biases (volumes −6 ml, EF: 4.6 %), and narrow limits of agreement (volumes: 17.6 ml, EF: 9.2 %). Significant intergroup (14 patients with normal LV function, 12 patients with systolic dysfunction from DCM, and 10 patients with diastolic dysfunction secondary to LV hypertrophy) differences in multiple quantitative indices in systolic and diastolic function were found. The conclusion was that fast automated dynamic detection of LV cardiac boundaries is feasible and allows accurate quantification of LV size and function.

5.6 Assessment of Regional Ventricular Function

Clinically useful parameters for assessing regional ventricular function are circumferential and longitudinal wall motion or shortening, myocardial wall thickness, and systolic wall thickening in both the long- and short-axis planes. In clinical practice visual analysis is mainly used for regional wall motion assessment, and different types for wall motion abnormalities are used such as normokinesis (normal wall motion), hypokinesis (decreased wall motion), akinesis (absent wall motion), dyskinesis (outward wall motion), and hyperkinesis (increased wall motion). Hypokinesis can be further subdivided according to the severity, i.e. slight, moderate, and severe. For semiquantitative assessment of regional contraction abnormalities a 17-segment model (Cerqueira 2002) may be used to determine the so-called wall motion score, i.e. numbering the type of local contraction with normokinesis given the number 1, hypokinesia 2, akinesia 3, and dyskinesia number 4 (Figure 5-10).

5.6.1 Regional Wall Thickness

Regional wall thickness at end-diastole is a second important parameter, since preserved wall thickness is a good indicator of the presence of viable myocardium, e.g. after an acute myocardial infarction (cut-off value > 5.5 mm). Systolic thickening provides a powerful parameter of regional LV performance, which is independent of any external reference point, and may be used for visual analysis to score regionally systolic wall thickening: normal, diminished, absent, wall

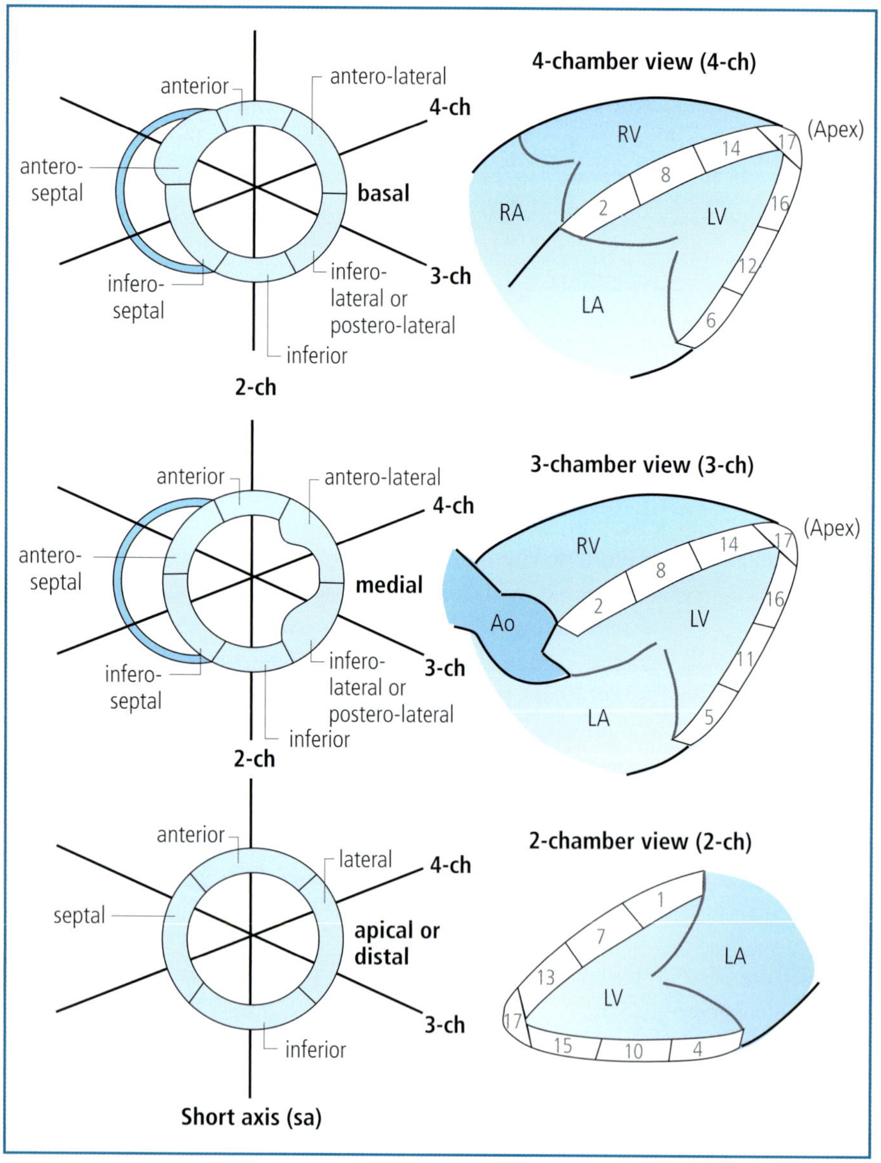

Figure 5-10 Schematic of the 17-segment model to localize regional (segmental) anomalies like contraction abnormalities or myocardial ischemia etc. in the four standard imaging planes (short-axis view, 4-ch view, 3-ch view, 2-ch view). Plan scans should be localized such that all segments are represented in the short- and long-axis planes (modified from Cerqueira et al. 2002).

thinning, or increased wall thickening. Systolic wall thickening > 2 mm is considered a good clinical sign of viability, e.g. in the region of infarcted myocardium. However, a quantitative approach is preferable since influences of exercise testing or pharmacological interventions can be assessed more reliably than by mere visual analysis. The optimal slice orientation is the short-axis plane, as in this orientation the major part of the myocardial wall is perpendicular to the imaging section. The best approach is to draw epicardial and endocardial contours in each short-axis image, and either use perpendicular lines between the two contours with an approximate center point in the LV cavum, or use segmental areas divided by the length of the segment, thereby yielding mean thickness values. Radial wall thickness quantification techniques use an approximate center point in the LV to measure the distance between endocardial and epicardial contours along radial lines starting from this center point. However, this method may result in significant overestimation of wall thickness when the ventricular cross-section deviates considerably from a circular shape. The centerline method has the advantage over radial methods, because it can be applied for a variety of LV shapes. This technique uses a path in between the endocardial and epicardial contours, the centerline, starting at a clearly visible anatomic reference point chords are constructed from the endocardium to epicardium. The length of such a chord represents the local wall thickness, the ratio between end-systolic and end-diastolic chord length equals the local end-systolic wall thickening.

5.6.2 Myocardial Tagging

While wall thickening and wall motion analyses are prone to errors of through-plane motion and allow only quantification of radial myocardial deformation, 3D myocardial tagging is a powerful technique that allows quantification of myocardial deformation (strain) in all three dimensions. In general, CMR methods to assess strain or strain rate, classified as tissue tracking techniques, include myocardial tagging, harmonic phase analysis (HARP), displacement encoding with stimulated echoes (DENSE), strain-encoded imaging (SENC), and velocity-encoded phase contrast. When using myocardial tagging, cine-MR images are acquired with a superimposed parallel, rectangular or radial grid of dark saturation lines, which are generated by a special prepulse sequence immediately after the R-wave of the ECG and can be followed subsequently over the cardiac cycle. The movements of the intersecting points of the grid (point tracking) in three directions can be analyzed by a computer algorithm, the HARP (Harmonic Phase) analysis software (Osman 1999), that enables rapid tracking with minimal manual intervention to assess myocardial strain. Myocardial strains are a measurement of local tissue deformation and represent myocardial regional contractile function. Strains express the fractional change in length in percent from a resting state (end-diastole) to one achieved following myocardial contraction. Problems with the tag technique include tag fading at least during diastole (careful adjustment of image parameters may make the tags long enough to cover early diastole), need for careful adjustment of sharpness of tags particularly related to computer analysis (blurred sinusoidal tag patterns are preferred), and adequate spacing between the tags (a rule of thumb is that tag spacing should be close to the slice thickness).

Harmonic Phase (HARP) Analysis

In clinical routine, short-axis tagged images are used to track myocardial strains in 2-dimensions. Epicardial and endocardial contours are manually traced on the images corresponding to a single cardiac phase, and HARP then automatically segments the LV myocardium in 12 equally sized regions, each with three layers (subepicardium, midwall, and subendocardium). This is visualized by the computer program as a circular grid and also tracked automatically along the remaining cardiac phases within a few seconds. The anterior attachment of the right ventricular wall to the LV is chosen as the landmark of reference for clockwise numbering of the segments. HARP computes several strain parameters, e.g. circumferential shortening (E_{cc}), radial thickening (E_{RR}), maximal elongation (Lamda 1 or E_1), maximal shortening (Lamda 2 or E_2), and angle β between the direction of E_{cc} and that of Lamda 2, for every layer in each segment. From E_{cc} strain curves strain rate patterns can be derived that demonstrate peak SRS at end-systole, peak E' wave in early diastole, and peak A' wave close to the end of diastole (Figure 5-11).

In a recent publication from the MESA cohort, Castillo et al. (2005) showed an excellent reproducibility of HARP analysis by three independent observers evaluating two separate quantitative strain analyses. For both peak and pooled systolic data on 24 participants, HARP yielded an excellent inter- and intra-observer agreement, that showed a direct relationship to the image quality of the myocardial tagged images; for diastolic pooled data, R values were lower due to tag fading, and both inter- and intra-observer agreement were better in the anterior and septal myocardial regions, and in the midwall layer. Recently Rutz et al. (2008) showed the feasibility of accelerated whole-heart 3D CSPAMM myocardial motion quantification that allows the measurement of myocardial deformations of the entire LV in three short breath-holds. The acceleration is achieved by splitting the acquisition into three orthogonally motion-encoded 3D measurements, and by applying a localized

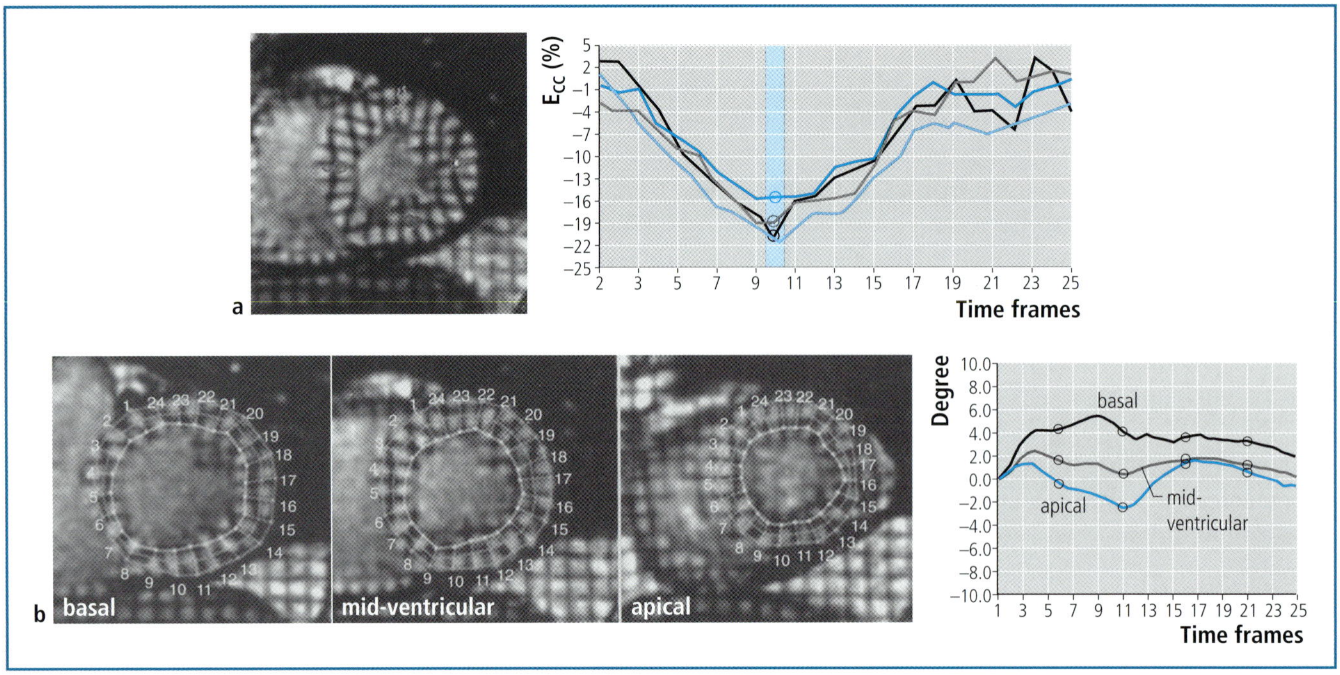

Figure 5-11 Principle of HARP-analysis of tagged left ventricular MR images **(upper row, left)** in a short-axis view. In this example HARP **(upper row, right)** analyses the parameter of circumferential shortening (E_{cc}) at the anterior, lateral, posterior, and mid-septal areas during one cardiac cycle (in systole downward movement = negative strain; in diastole upward movement = positive strain) **(a)**. Alternatively, in the same examination a circular mesh of 24 points may be created in the basal, mid-ventricular, and apical segments of the left ventricle. The movement of these points is analyzed by HARP, resulting in 3 displacing lines that represent the average rotation of each mesh during systole and diastole **(b)**.

tagging preparation in combination with a hybrid multi-shot, segmented EPI sequence. Circumferential shortening (E_{ss}) at end-systole ranged from 14.1% (base) to 20.1% (apex) in 5 healthy volunteers, and hypokinetic regions in patients with myocardial infarction corresponded well with regions exhibiting hyperenhancement (myocardial scar); time to maximal E_{ss} varied more significantly over the left ventricle in patients than in volunteers ($p > 0.01$). Whether or not this elaborate technique will become a clinical routine remains uncertain.

Limited experience exists also with RV strain (SENC) analyses. Recently Youssef et al. (2008) measured peak systolic circumferential strain rates in 21 healthy volunteers at six equidistant points along the RV free wall. The strain values were −20 ± 2.9%, −18.8 ± 3.9%, and −16.5 ± 5.7% of the basal, mid, and apical regions of RV free wall. They also found a good intra- and inter-observer agreement. The conclusion was that SENC CMR allows for rapid and reproducible quantification of RV regional function with the perspective of accurate quantification of regional strain in patients with RV dysfunction.

Displacement Encoding with Stimulated Echoes (DENSE)

This is a new technique for quantitative MR imaging of myocardial displacement and strain. In DENSE a precise set of radiofrequency and gradient pulses are used at end-diastole to tag (encode) the myocardial tissue longitudinal magnetization. Subsequently, a sequence of images is generated with the use of the encoded longitudinal magnetization, whereby the phase of each image pixel is directly proportional to the tissue displacement which occurred from the time of the application of the pulses. The specific signal generated by the radiofrequency and gradient pulses is called the stimulated echo, whereby the phase of the signal is proportional to the tissue displacement. The stimulated echo, like signals acquired at conventional tagging, fades with time, and therefore about 75% of the cardiac cycle can typically be captured by DENSE before the SNR becomes too low to assess tissue motion accurately. More recently the DENSE technique was combined with cine-SENC imaging in 6 healthy volunteers and showed good correlation to conventional 3D tagging (Hess 2009). Also the reliability of a newly developed navigator-gated 3D spiral DENSE technique was compared in 5 healthy volunteers with conventional 2D DENSE and

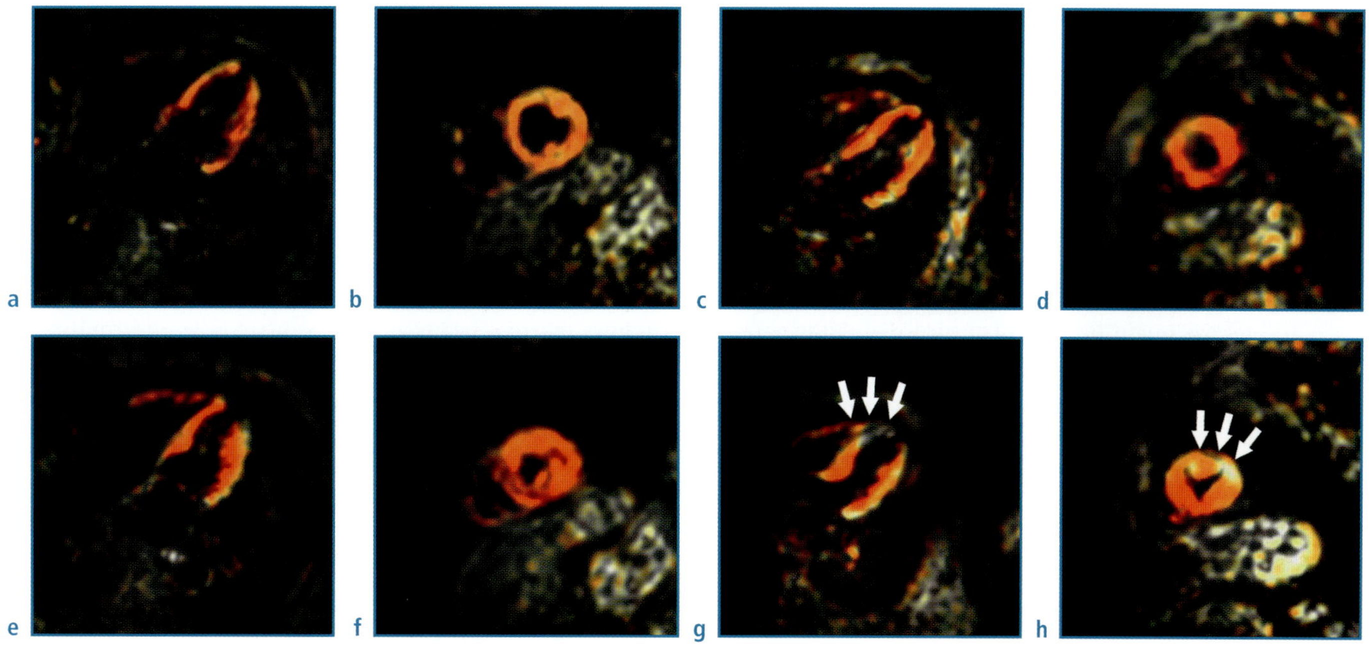

Figure 5-12 Strain-ENCoded (SENC) analysis during high-dose dobutamine MR stress testing. Corresponding 4-ch view and short-axis SENC images are presented at baseline (a–d) and during peak dobutamine stress (e–h) in a normal volunteer (a, b, e, f) and in a patient with coronary artery disease (c, d, g, h). Here, peak systolic images are presented, where active myocardial contraction is coded red and reduced or absent myocardial strain is coded yellowish/white. Normal strain response can be seen in the first subject (overall homogenous myocardial strain response in 4-ch view (a, e) and short-axis images (b, f)). Conversely, in the second subject strain is normal at baseline (c, d), while inducible strain defects can be depicted both in 4-ch view (yellow), arrows in the mid and apical septal wall in (g) and in short-axis images (yellow), arrows in the apical anterior wall in (h) (courtesy PD Dr. G. Korosoglu, University Hospital, Cardiology, Heidelberg, Germany).

historical 3D myocardial tagging with good correlations (Zhong 2010). The advantages of DENSE include a relatively high spatial resolution compared with conventional tagging, and a relatively automated analysis similar to HARP. The limitations of DENSE include a relatively low SNR compared with conventional tagging (because of the acquisition of the displacement-encoded stimulated echo that is generated from only half of the spin population that normally contributes to other commonly acquired echoes), its sensitivity to poor ECG gating (artifacts produced by an irregular heart rhythm or poor R-wave detection), and the lack of a fully automated analysis of displacement and strain analysis of DENSE images.

> The DENSE technique may be applied to assess abnormal regional strain (or contractility) in patients with CAD, ischemic cardiomyopathy, non-ischemic cardiomyopathy, restrictive cardiomyopathy, or pericardial constriction.

However, at present studies on larger patient populations to demonstrate the clinical value of this technique are not available.

Sensitivity Encoded (SENC) Tagging

The SENC pulse sequence is a modified SPAMM tagging pulse. To produce the tagged images, the SENC gradient is applied in the slice-selection direction, orthogonal to the imaging plane, in contrast to conventional tagging, with the modulation gradient applied in the phase- or frequency-encoding direction. By combining SENC magnitude images at two different frequency modulations ("tunings") – low-tuning = LT and high-tuning = HT images –, a SENC strain map is computed which is then overlaid pixel-by-pixel on the anatomical image. In this way, color-coded SENC functional images (maximum contraction illustrated as red, and lack of contraction illustrated as white) are generated. Such SENC images are usually acquired in the 4-, 2-chamber, and three short-axis views for regional contraction and strain analysis.

> This technique has been recently applied for CMR-dobutamine stress testing (Korosoglu 2009) that supports better visualization of regional contraction abnormalities due to stress induced myocardial ischemia (Figure 5-12).

5.6.3 Velocity-Encoded Tissue Imaging (Wall Velocity Mapping)

Myocardial wall deformation is characterized by both the amount of deformation and the velocity of deformation ("strain rate"). Using the phase-information from PC mapping the 2D or 3D myocardial motion and velocity can be quantified (Constable 1994). In contrast to tagging, phase imaging has a better persistence throughout the cardiac cycle and allows quantification of myocardial deformation in the entire wall, compared with fading of tagging pulses in diastole or analysis of deformation feasible only in regions with tagging pulses. PC tissue velocity mapping is at present a research tool and has been used for analysis of LV dyssynchrony (see Chapter 12.9) or for analysis of diastolic function (see Chapter 5.7.3).

5.7 Assessment of Diastolic Function

Diastolic function regarding LV and RV filling and compliance can be measured by CMR in a basic way using ventricular time-volume curves, mitral inflow velocities, pulmonary vein flow, and tissue Doppler similar to SPECT- or echocardiographic techniques. The complex strategy without any echocardiographic equivalent includes the diastolic untwisting rate or torsion recovery rate, and the diastolic myocardial strain rate.

5.7.1 Time-Volume Relationship

Time-volume curves as a measure of relative left ventricular volume change over time are assessed by tracing LV endocardial borders for each cardiac phase, which provide temporally resolved 3D volumes in systole and diastole. From these curves, peak filling rate and time to peak filling rate are commonly derived parameters computed by fitting third-order polynomial functions to the systolic ejection and rapid diastolic filling portions of the time-volume curves. Due to two main disadvantages of this method – it does not provide any information on LV filling characteristics, and is only partially representative of compliance with no distinction between RV and pericardial contributions – it is only rarely used nowadays.

5.7.2 Mitral Valve Inflow and Pulmonary Vein Phase Velocity Mapping

Phase contrast (PC) imaging is able to assess mitral valve inflow and pulmonary vein flow velocity profiles, similar to color Doppler echocardiography (Figure 5-13). CMR-PC imaging is highly accurate and reproducible and can be applied routinely in every patient without restrictions, seen with Doppler echocardiography such as limited imaging windows, narrow beam angle, eccentric flow and multiple velocity directions. CMR-PC can acquire the three direction velocity profiles across the 2D imaging plane, and its precision has been convincingly shown by Chatzimavroudis et al. (2001) with excellent correlation with aortic phantom measurements. The velocity data can be used to calculate pressure gradients using Bernoulli equation. Using CMR-PC various grades of diastolic dysfunction can be classified such as normal, impaired relaxation, pseudo-normal flow, and restrictive flow pattern (Figure 5-14).

Older studies with limited CMR technology (low field-strength, 16 phases per cardiac cycle etc) have shown good correlations between E and A waves with PC-CMR compared with Doppler. A recent study by Rathi et al. (2008) demonstrated the direct correlation of PC-CMR mitral (MV) and pulmonary vein (PV) diastolic function parameters with those of Doppler (TTE) in 31 subjects and 10 controls. Blood flow in the MV and PV were successfully imaged with CMR in all cases, while with TTE MV flow was also imaged in all, but PV in only 21/31 individuals. As a result, velocities of MV flow (E and A) measured by CMR correlated well with TTE ($r = 0.81$, $p < 0.001$), but demonstrated a systematic underestimation by CMR compared to TTE (slope 0.77). Bland-Altman analysis of the E: A ratio and deceleration time calculated from each modality showed excellent agreement. When assessing morphology using TTE, CMR correctly identified patients as having normal or abnormal inflow conditions (impaired relaxation, pseudo-normal, or restrictive). The PC-CMR step added an average of only 4 min to the total patient imaging time, and PC-CMR proved to be useful and accurate for the assessment of diastolic function as a routine practice for CMR similar to echocardiography. To overcome some limitations of current technique and speed up imaging by rarified sampling of the k-space (to reduce scan time by 2- to 4-fold, while maintaining SNR, spatial and temporal resolution), using e. g. block regional interpolations scheme (BRISK), flow data can be acquired within one breath-hold of 15–17 s (Rathi and Biederman 2009). Comparison of BRISK PC-CMR with conventional PC-CMR techniques on phantom studies have shown excellent correlation ($r = 0.98$–0.99), and BRISK sequences can be ported into conventional scanners with only software upgrading.

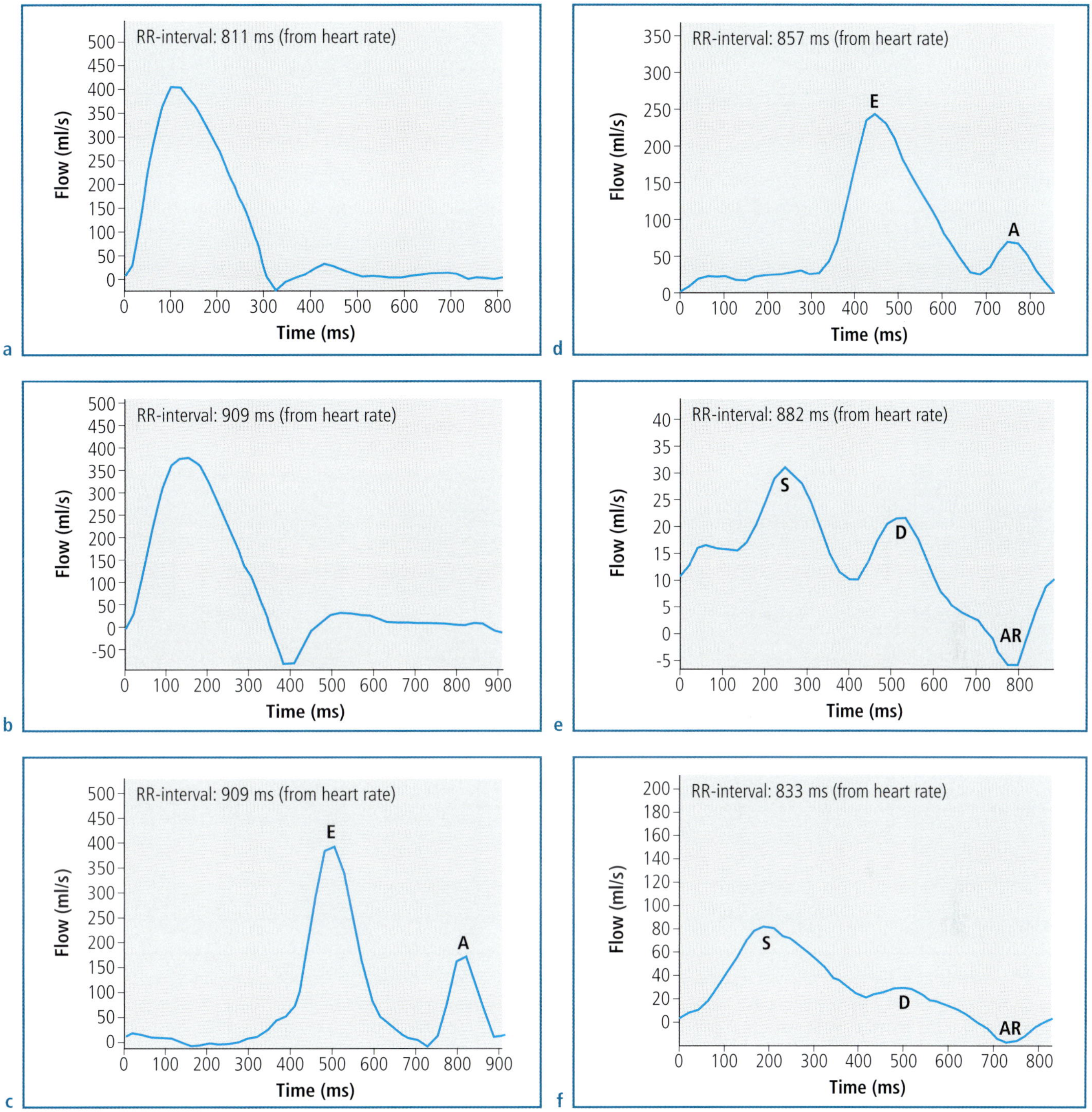

Figure 5-13 Flow profiles in the heart of a healthy volunteer as assessed by PC flow mapping (velocity-time profiles): systolic flow profiles in the aorta (a) and pulmonary artery (b), diastolic inflow profiles via the mitral valve (c) and the tricuspid valve (d), and within the pulmonary vein (e) and the caval vein (f). E: early diastolic filling phase; A: atrial diastolic filling phase; S: systolic antegrade pulmonary venous flow; D: diastolic antegrade pulmonary venous flow; AR: pulmonary venous or caval vein atrial reversal flow.

5.7.3 Myocardial Tissue Velocity Mapping

The PC-CMR technique can also be used to evaluate myocardial motion velocity similar to tissue Doppler imaging by echocardiography. The advantage of PC-CMR is the ability of acquiring images in multiple planes, so that the operator can choose in-plane or through-plane velocity acquisitions. An initial study of Karwatowski et al. (1994) showed significantly lower maximal early diastolic myocardial velocities in 26 patients with MI compared with 21 CAD patients without MI and compared with 19 controls. In a further study,

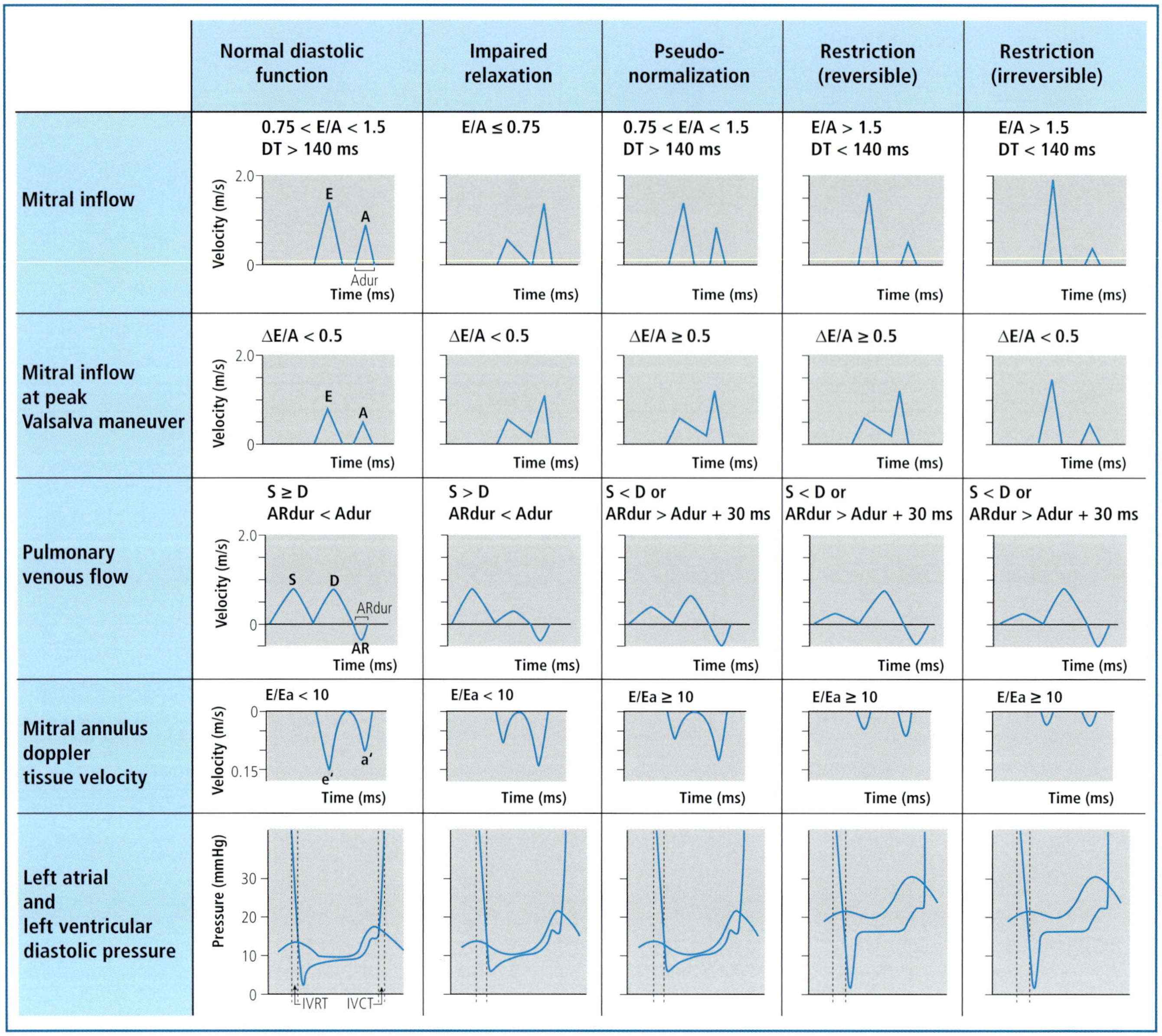

Figure 5-14 Schematic of the mitral inflow at rest and at peak Valsalva maneuver, pulmonary venous flow, and Doppler tissue imaging of the mitral annular motion together with left atrial and left ventricular diastolic pressures in different stages of diastolic dysfunction. E: early diastolic filling phase; A: atrial diastolic filling phase; Δ: delta; Adur: duration of transmitral A-wave; S: systolic antegrade pulmonary venous flow; D: diastolic antegrade pulmonary venous flow; AR: pulmonary venous atrial reversal flow; ARdur: duration of atrial reversal flow; IVRT: isovolumetric relaxation time; IVCT: isovolumetric contraction time; a': tissue velocity with atrial contraction; e': early diastolic filling velocity (modified from Redfield et al. 2003).

Karwatowski et al. (1996) compared LV diastolic myocardial velocities in PC-CMR with color Doppler echocardiography and showed that the onset of diastolic long-axis velocity preceded flow across the MV by a mean of 46 ms. The maximal myocardial long-axis velocity correlated significantly with the peak early filling velocity, and the mean myocardial long-axis velocity correlated significantly with mitral inflow parameters. In a recent study Paelinck et al. (2005) demonstrated the feasibility of using PC-CMR for estimating pulmonary capillary wedge pressure (PCWP) by normalizing MV inflow E velocity with mitral annular septal tissue velocity E'. 18 patients referred for cardiac catheterization including pulmonary capillary wedge pressure (PCWP) measurements were studied with PC-CMR and Doppler for mitral flow and tissue velocities and compared with PCWP. A strong relation between PC-CMR assessed E/E' (11.6 ± 4.3) and Doppler E/E' (12.1 ± 3.5) was found ($r = 0.89$, $p < 0.001$), and also a close relation of mitral A-wave velocities with both techniques but an underestimation by PC-CMR measurements. For both techniques, correlations between invasive PCWP and E/E' were strong (PC-CMR: $r = 0.80$, $p < 0.001$, Doppler: $r = 0.85$, $p < 0.001$), and an E/E' less than 8 had 100% positive predictive value (PPV) for PCWP less than 15 mmHg, and E/E' greater than 15 had a 100% PPV for PCWP greater than 15 mmHg. Thus, similar to Doppler echocardiography assessment of E/E' by PC-CMR is an easily obtainable parameter for non-invasive estimation of PCWP.

5.7.4 Myocardial Tissue Tagging

In contrast to ventricular filling, flow velocity and myocardial velocity as indirect parameters of diastolic function, diastolic relaxation mechanics such as LV torsion recovery or strain rate recovery, reflect directly diastolic function. After application of the tagging pulses during cardiac contraction and relaxation, distortions of the grid permit direct measurements of myocardial deformation, described as units of strain (% S) or torsion (degrees). Clockwise diastolic recoil or untwisting due to release of systolic compressive forces leads to diastolic suction with consecutive enhancement of MV opening, which occurs primarily in the isovolumic relaxation time (IVRT) before opening of the MV. LV recoil or untwisting rate is an intrinsic property of the myocardium, and is correlated to the time constant τ (tau) of ventricular relaxation (30–40 ms in normal humans, "completion" after 3 times τ = 90–120 ms), and has been shown to be independent from left atrial pressure, LV pressure, or dP/dt, as shown in dogs by Dong et al. (2001). In patients with aortic stenosis, it has been shown that diastolic torsion recovery is prolonged until the end of diastole due to pathologic hypertrophy (Stuber 1999, Nagel 2000b), and torsion was reported to be elevated before aortic valve replacement (AVR) and normalized to normal range one year after AVR in concert with regression of LV mass and increase in ejection fraction (Biederman 2005).

Deformation pattern based on circumferential or radial strain may be principally used to evaluate diastolic function or dysfunction. One limitation of the current strategies for diastolic strain analysis is, however, that typical myocardial tag density drops off exponentially as a function of time unless the sampling is specifically adapted to obtain late cardiac cycle data. There are few data on strain analysis regarding diastolic function. In a total of 1,100 patients of the MESA cohort, Fernandes et al. (2007) found direct linear relationships between EF and regional systolic and diastolic functions, as measured by peak regional circumferential strains (E_{cc}), peak systolic strain rate (SRS), and peak early filling strain rate (SRE) in 4 LV segments (anterior, lateral, inferior, and septal). Similar analyses of diastolic strains are actually not available for the right ventricle.

5.8 Measurement of Flow in the Aorta and Pulmonary Artery

PC-Mapping proved to be the gold standard for exact non-invasive in vivo measurement of blood flow in the heart and great arteries. To measure aortic blood flow, a scout image is placed at the level of pulmonary bifurcation in a coronal section, using a VENC value slightly higher than the expected regular aortic flow profile (1.5 m/s at normal conditions, higher in patients with aortic stenosis). Using a set of modulus images to measure cross-sectional area of the aorta and a set of velocity-encoded images, the instantaneous velocity values are determined by integrating the velocity values of each voxel along the aortic axis over the cross-sectional area of the vessel. By multiplying cross-sectional area with the mean blood flow velocity, the volume of blood per time unit can be measured. Pulmonary blood flow is determined in a similar way. The flow measurements are presented either by a time-flow-volume diagram or a time-flow-velocity diagram that can be quantitatively evaluated by a computer program.

> Comparison of aortic and pulmonary flow is extremely useful for a series of clinical situations with the following **main aspects**:
> - concordance or discordance in timing of peak flow within the aorta or pulmonary artery,
> - absolute differences in the amount of right and left ventricular stroke volume,
> - assessment of intracardiac left-to-right or right-to-left shunts by comparing pulmonary with aortic flow volume per time (l/min),
> - quantitative measurements of valvular incompentences.

Therefore assessment of aortic and pulmonary flow is always performed as a routine part of our clinical CMR studies.

5.9 Assessment of Biophysical Mechanical Properties of the Aortic Wall

Arterial and aortic walls consist of three distinct layers, the intima, media, and adventitia. To compensate for the high pressure, wall thickness of the aorta is 2.5 mm and radius 12.5 mm. The media of the aorta contains collagen, smooth muscles and elastic fibers. The passive stretch of a vessel depends on the difference of intra- and extravasal pressure (P_i and P_e), called transmural pressure (Pt_m): $Pt_m = P_i - P_e$

Transmural pressure induces a tangential wall stretch S_t directly poroportional to the inner radius r_i and negatively proportional to wall thickness w: $S_t = (P_i - P_e) \times r_i / w$

Due to the continuous decrease of elastin content in the aortic wall from the proximal part into the periphery, the local compliance of the aorta and arterial vessels decreases continuously. Compliance of the aorta is extremely important for the aortic "Windkessel" function. Arterial compliance (C) is defined as the change in volume (ΔV) per unit change in pressure (ΔP), its reciprocal value is the volume elasticity modulus (E'): $C = 1 / E' = \Delta V / \Delta P \, t_m$

Mean arterial compliance of a distinct vessel can be determined by pulse wave velocity or by the velocity of flow wave. In the aorta the LV derived pressure wave runs along the aortic wall with a speed of 3–5 m/s, and of 5–10 m/s in greater arteries, but with only 1–2 m/s via the vein walls. These pressure waves are significantly faster than flow velocity within the vessel lumen, whereas flow waves have a similar high speed. The speed of both the pressure and flow waves depends significantly on the elasticity of the aortic and arterial walls.

Arterial stiffness describes the resistance of arterial wall to deformation; it is very difficult to measure stiffness in vivo due to the complex mechanical behavior of arterial wall. In vitro arterial compliance has been measured from pressure-volume curves in post-mortem arteries. In vivo estimation of arterial wall compliance is more difficult; it has been performed by pulse wave velocity measurements in animals and humans, pressure-radius relationship, X-ray contrast angiography in humans, and sonography. CMR is a particularly useful tool to measure aortic compliance, since using high-resolution cine imaging with SSFP sequences or by ECG-triggered spin echo imaging, the cross-sectional area of the ascending and descending aorta (A) can be measured simultaneously with high precision during systole and diastole, and segmental volume (V) be determined using slice thickness: $\Delta V = \Delta A \times$ slice thickness

Aortic pulse pressure (ΔP) is measured non-invasively by sphygmomanometry, and regional aortic compliance (C) can be measured: $C\ (\mu l / mmHg / m^2 / N) = \Delta V / \Delta P$

Further biophysical parameters of the aorta can be calculated, e.g. the elasticity modulus (E_P), i.e. the fractional distensibility ΔV/V of the arterial lumen per unit pressure pulse: ΔP: $E_P = 2\ \Delta P / (\Delta V/V)$, or the stiffness index (β), using systolic (BP_s) and diastolic (BP_d) blood pressure: $\beta = BP_s / BP_d$ /area strain

Despite the limitations of measuring blood pressure at the radial artery (i.e. remote from aorta), there is a good correlation between measurement of regional aortic compliance and measurement of global compliance from the speed of propagation of the flow wave within the vessel (Mohiaddin 1993).

Another technique to measure aortic compliance or stiffness is the measurement of aortic flow wave velocity, using high-resolution 2D cine PC-velocity mapping in a plane perpendicular to the ascending and descending aorta to take the time for the flow wave to travel between the two points. The instantaneous flow (l/s) in the ascending and descending aorta can be calculated from cross-sectional area and the mean flow velocity in this area. Pulse wave velocity (PWV in m/s) can then be calculated from the transit time (T) of the foot of flow wave and from the distance (D) between the two points obtained from an oblique sagittal spin echo image. The distance between the two points is determined manually by drawing a line in the center of the aorta joining the two points, and the foot of the flow wave defined by extraopolation of the rapid upstroke of the flow wave to baseline (Mohiaddin 1993), and PWD is then calculated by: $PWV = D / T$

It should be noted that pulse wave velocity is faster the higher arterial stiffness is, and vice versa.

Aortic compliance as measured by CMR may be altered in different situations. Mohiaddin et al. (1989) demonstrated that it falls with age and is abnormally low in patients with CAD, in contrast to high performance athletes with a high compliance. Patients with aortic coarctation and those with Marfan's syndrome have an abnormally low aortic compliance (Rees 1989, Manzara 1990). Recently Robinson et al. (2008) reported that obesity is associated with reduced aortic compliance and distensibility and a higher stiffness index compared with controls, and in multiple regression analysis fat mass, leptin, and body mass index were independent predictors of aortic function. Van der Meer et al. (2007) found a higher pulse wave velocity (PWV) in patients with type 2 diabetes mellitus compared with healthy subjects independent from blood pressure, and PWV correlated significantly with fasting plasma glucose and insulin levels. Aortic distensibility was lower in patients compared with healthy controls and was correlated negatively with PWV and positively with LV diastolic function. Further studies have to show whether these aortic biophysical parameters measured by CMR imaging may be helpful in the early recognition of patients at high risk and for follow-up of dedicated treatments.

References

Biederman RW, Doyle M, Yamrozik J et al. Physiologic compensation is supranormal in compensated aortic stenosis: Does it return to normal after aortic valve replacement or is it blunted by coexistent coronary artery disease? An intramyocardial magnetic resonance imaging study. Circulation 2005; 112 (Suppl): I429–36.

Bloomer TN, Plein S, Radjenovic A et al. Cine-MRI using steady-state free precession in the radial long-axis orientation is a fast accurate method of obtaining volumetric data of the left ventricle. J Magn Reson Imaging 2002; 14: 685–92.

Bloomgarden DC, Fayad ZA, Ferrari VA et al. Global cardiac function using breath-hold MRI: validation of new acquisition and analysis techniques. Magn Reson Med 1997; 37: 683–92.

Bogaert J, Dymarkowski S, Taylor AM. Clinical Cardiac MRI. Berlin, Heidelberg, New York: Springer Publishers 2005.

Bottini PB, Carr AA, Prisant M et al. Magnetic resonance imaging compared to echocardiography to assess left ventricular mass in hypertensive patients. Am J Hypertens 1995; 8: 221–8.

Castillo E, Osman NF, Rosen BD et al. Quantitative assessment of regional myocardial function with MR-tagging in a multi-center study: interobserver and intraobeserver agreement of fast strain analysis with Harmonic Phase (HARP) MRI. J Cardiovasc Magn Reson 2005; 7: 783–91.

Cerqueira MD, Weissman NJ, Dilsizian V et al. Standardized myocardial segmentation and nomenclature for tomographic imaging of the heart. A statement for healthcare professionals from the Cardiac Imaging Committee of the Council on Clinical Cardiology of the American Heart Association. Circulation 2002; 105: 539–42.

Chatzimavroudis GP, Oshinski JN, Franch RH et al. Evaluation of the precision of magnetic resonance phase velocity imaging for blood flow measurements. J Cardiovasc Magn Reson 2001; 3: 11–9.

Constable RT, Rath KM, Sinusas AJ, Gorec JC. Development and evaluation of tracking algorithms for cardiac wall motion analysis using phase velocity MR imaging. Magn Reson Med 1994; 32: 33–42.

Corsi CF, Veronesi F, Lamberti C et al. Automated frame-by-frame endocardial border detection from cardiac magnetic resonance images for quantitative assessment of left ventricular function: validation and clinical feasibility. J Magn Reson Imag 2009; 29: 560–8.

Dong SJ, Hees PS, Siu CO et al. CMR assessment of LV relaxation by untwisting rate: a new isovolumic phase measure of tau. Am J Physiol Heart Circ Physiol 2001; 281: H2002–9.

Fernandes VRS, Edvardsen T, Rosen BD et al. The influence of left ventricular size and global function on regional myocardial contraction and relaxation in an adult population free of cardiovascular disease: a tagged CMR study of the MESA cohort. J Cardiovasc Magn Reson 2007; 9: 921–30.

Firmin DN, Nayler GL, Klipstein RH et al. In vivo validation of magnetic resonance velocity imaging. J Comput Assist Tomogr 1987; 11: 751–6.

Grothues F, Moon JCC, Bellenger NG et al. Interstudy reproducibility of right ventricular volumes, function and mass with cardiovascular magnetic resonance. Am Heart J 2004; 147: 218–23.

Grothues F, Smith GC, Moon JCC et al. Comparison of interstudy reproducibility of cardiovascular magnetic resonance with two-dimensional echocardiography in normal subjects and in patients with heart failure or left ventricular hypertrophy. Am J Cardiol 2002; 90: 29–34.

Helbeing WA, Rebergen SA, Maliepard C et al. Quantification of right ventricular function with magnetic resonance imaging in children with normal hearts and with congenital heart disease. Am Heart J 1995; 130: 828–37.

Hess AT, Zhong X, Spottiswoode B et al. Myocardial 3D strain calculation by combining cine displacement encoding with stimulated echoes (DENSE) and cine strain encoding (SENC) imaging. Magn Reson Med 2009; 62: 77–84.

Jauhainen T, Jarvinen VM, Hekali PE et al. MR gradient echo volumetric analysis of human cardiac casts: focus on the right ventricle. J Comput Assist Tomogr 1998; 22: 899–903.

Karwatowski SP, Brecker SJ, Yang GZ et al. A comparison of left ventricular myocardial velocity in diastole measured by magnetic resonance and left ventricular filling measured by Doppler echocardiography. Eur Heart J 1996; 17: 795–802.

Karwatowski SP, Mohiaddin RH, Yang GZ et al. Regional myocardial velocity imaged by magnetic resonance in patients with ischemic heart disease. Br Heart J 1994; 72: 332–8.

Katz J, Milliken MC, Boxt LM et al. Estimation of human myocardial mass with MR imaging. Radiology 1988; 169: 495–9.

Katz J, Wang J, Boxt LM et al. Estimation of right ventricular mass in normal subjects and in patients with primary pulmonary hypertension by nuclear magnetic resonance imaging. J Am Coll Cardiol 1993; 21: 1475–81.

Keenan NG, Pennell DJ. CMR of ventricular function. Echocardiography 2007; 24: 185–93.

Kondo C, Caputo GR, Semelka R et al. Right and left ventricular volume measurements with velocity-encoded cine-MR imaging: in vitro and in vivo validation. Am J Roentgenol 1991; 157: 9–16.

Korosoglu G, Futterer S, Humpert PM et al. Strain-encoded cardiac MR during high-dose dobutamine stress testing: comparison to cine imaging and to myocardial tagging. J Magn Reson Imaging 2009; 29: 1053–61.

Kramer CM, Barkhausen J, Flamm SD et al. Standardized cardiovascular magnetic resonance imaging (CMR) protocols, society for cardiovascular magnetic resonance: board of trustees task force on standardized protocols. J Cardiovasc Magn Reson 2008; 10 (1): 35.

KühneT, Yilmaz S, Steendijk P et al. Magnetic resonance imaging analysis of right ventricular pressure-volume loops: in vivo validation and clinical application in patients with pulmonary hypertension. Circulation 2004; 110: 2010–6.

Longmore DB, Klipstein RH, Underwood SR et al. Dimensional accuracy of magnetic resonance in studies of the heart. Lancet 1985; 1: 1360–2.

Maceira AM, Prasad SK, Khan M et al. Normalized left ventricular systolic and diastolic function by steady-state free precession cardiovascular magnetic resonance. J Cardiovasc Magn Reson 2006; 8: 417–26.

Manzara CC, Mohiaddin RH, Pennell DJ et al. Magnetic resonance assessment of thoracic aorta in Marfan's syndrome (abstr). Circulation 1990; 82 (Suppl III): 497.

Mohiaddin RH, Firmin DN, Longmore DB. Age-related changes of human aortic flow wave velocity measured non-invasively by magnetic resonance imaging. J Applied Physiol 1993; 74: 492–9.

Mohiaddin RH, Underwood SR, Bogren HG et al. Regional aortic compliance studied by magnetic resonance imaging: the effects of age, training, and coronary artery disease. Br Heart J 1989; 62: 90–7.

Mooij CF, de Wit CJ, Graham DA et al. Reproducibility of MRI measurements of right ventricular size and function in patients with normal and dilated ventricles. J Magn Reson Imaging 2008; 28: 67–73.

Moon JCC, Lorenz CH, Francis JM et al. Breath-hold FLASH and FISP cardiovascular MR imaging: left ventricular volume differences and reproducibility. Radiology 2002; 223: 789–97.
Myerson SG, Bellenger NG, Pennell DJ. Assessment of left ventricular mass by cardiovascular magnetic resonance. Hypertension 2002; 39: 750–5.
Nagel E, Schneider U, Schalla S. Magnetic resonance real-time imaging fort he evaluation of left ventricular function. J Cardiovasc Magn Reson 2000a; 2: 7–14.
Nagel E, Stuber M, Burkhard B et al. Cardiac rotation and relaxation in patients with aortic valve stenosis. Eur Heart J 2000b; 21: 582–9.
Osman NF, Kerwin WS, McVeigh ER, Prince JL. Cardiac motion tracking using CINE harmonic phase (HARP) magnetic resonance imaging. Magn Reson Med 1999; 42: 1048–60.
Paelinck BP, de Roos A, Bax JJ et al. Feasibility of tissue magnetic resonance imaging: a pilot study in comparison with tissue Doppler imaging and invasive measurement. J Am Coll Cardiol 2005; 45: 1109–16.
Rathi VK, Biederman RWW. Expanding role of cardiovascular magnetic resonance in left and right ventricular diastolic function. Heart Fail Clin 2009; 5: 421–35.
Rathi VK, Doyle M, Yamrozik J et al. Routine evaluation of left ventricular diastolic function by cardiovascular magnetic resonance: A practical approach. J Cardiovasc Magn Reson 2008; 10 (1): 36.
Redfield MM et al. Burden of systolic and diastolic ventricular dysfunction in the community-appreciating the scope of the Heart Failure Epidemic. JAMA 2003; 289: 194–202.
Rees RSO, Somerville J, Ward C et al. Magnetic resonance imaging in late post-operative assessment of coarctation of the aorta. Radiology 1989; 173: 499–504.
Rehr RB, Malloy CR, Filipchuk NG et al. Left ventricular volumes measured by MR imaging. Radiology 1985; 156: 717–9.
Robinson MR, Scheuermann-Freestone M, Leeson P et al. Uncomplicated obesity is associated with abnormal aortic function assessed by cardiovascular magnetic resonance. J Cardiovasc Magn Reson 2008; 10 (1): 10.
Rutz AK, Ryf S, Plein S et al. Accelerated whole-heart 3D CSPAMM for myocardial motion quantification. Magn Reson Med 2008; 59: 755–63.
Rüssel IK, Götte MJ, Kuijer JP, Marcus T. Regional assessment of left ventricular torsion by CMR tagging. J Cardiovasc Magn Reson 2008; 10 (1): 26.
Salm LP, Schuijf JD, DeRoos A et al. Global and regional left ventricular function assessment with 16-detector row CT: comparison with echocardiography and cardiovascular magnetic resonance. Eur J Echocardiogr 2006; 7: 308–14.
Sechtem U, Pflugfelder PW, Gould RG et al. Measurement of right and left ventricular volumes in healthy individuals with cine-CMR imaging. Radiology 1987; 163: 697–702.
Sechtem U, Tscholakoff D, Higgins CB. MRI of the normal pericardium. Am J Roentgenol 1986; 147: 239–44.
Semelka RC, Tomei E, Wagner S et al. Interstudy reproducibility of dimensional and functional measurements between cine magnetic resonance imaging studies in the morphologically abnormal left ventricle. Am Heart J 1990; 119: 1367–73.
Shapiro EP, Rogers WJ, Beyar R et al. Determination of left ventricular mass by MRI in hearts deformed by acute infarction. Circulation 1989; 79: 706–11.
Stuber M, Scheidegger MB, Fischer SE et al. Alterations in the local myocardial motion pattern in patients suffering from pressure overload due to aortic stenosis. Circulation 1999; 100: 361–8.
Thiele H, Paetsch I, Schnackenburg B et al. Improved accuracy of quantitative assessment of left ventricular volume and ejection fraction by geometric models with steady-state free precession. J Cardiovasc Magn Reson 2002; 4: 327–39.
Van der Meer RW, Diamant M, Westenberg JJM et al. Magnetic resonance assessment of aortic pulse wave velocity, aortic distensibility, and cardiac function in uncomplicated type 2 diabetes mellitus. J Cardiovasc Magn Reson 2007; 9: 645–51.
Youssef A, Ibrahim ESH, Korosoglou G et al. Strain-encoding cardiovascular magnetic resonance for assessment of right-ventricular regional function. J Cardiovasc Magn Reson 2008; 10 (1): 33.
Zhong X, Spottiswoode B, Meyer CH et al. Imaging three-dimensional myocardial mechanics using navigator-gated volumetric spiral cine-DENSE MRI. Magn Reson Med 2010; 64: 1089–97.

6 Coronary Artery Disease – Stable Angina

Nico Merkle

6.1 Definition

Coronary artery disease (CAD) represents the clinical manifestation of atherosclerotic coronary lesions (stenoses or occlusions) onto the target organ, the heart. Primary manifestation of CAD may vary to include angina pectoris, acute myocardial infarction, ventricular tachyarrhythmias, chronic heart failure from unrecognized myocardial infarctions, or sudden cardiac death.

Coronary artery disease (CAD) or ischemic heart disease (IHD) is the primary cause of morbidity and mortality not only in industrialized, but also in developing countries. In Europe, cardiovascular diseases were the direct cause of more than 4 Mio deaths in the year 2000, accounting for

43% of all deaths in men and for 55% in women (Graham 2007). Cardiovascular diseases are also the major cause of hospital discharges, with an average rate of 2,557 per 100,000 of population in 2002; out of these 695 per 100,000 were caused by CAD and 375 per 100,000 by stroke. In the US it is estimated that 13.2 Mio Americans have CAD, 6.5 Mio of whom have angina pectoris and 7.2 Mio have myocardial infarction. In 2003, CAD accounted for 53% of all deaths caused by cardiovascular disease, resulting in 1 in 5 deaths in the US. Thus, CAD is the major cause of death worldwide.

6.2 Physiology of Coronary Circulation

6.2.1 Myocardial Oxygen Supply and Consumption and Coronary Blood Flow (CBF)

The heart as an anaerobic organ is totally dependent on the oxidation of substrates for the production of energy. The heart cannot undergo a significant oxygen deficit such as e.g. the skeletal muscle. Myocardial perfusion amounts to 70–80 ml/min per 100 g tissue, and the total oxygen consumption of the heart distributes to 20% of basal maintenance of structure, to 1% of the electrical energy, 15% of volume load, and 64% of pressure load. The main determinants of myocardial oxygen consumption are systolic wall stress, diastolic wall stress, heart rate and contractility. Myocardial oxygen supply depends on coronary blood flow and oxygen binding capacity of the blood, diastolic coronary perfusion, and alterations of coronary resistance determine total coronary blood flow. The heart receives approximately 5% of the resting cardiac output, although it represents less than 0.5% of total body weight.

The entire blood supply to the myocardium derives from the right and left coronary arteries, which originate at the root of the aorta behind the cusps of the aortic valves. Coronary blood flow depends on the pressure difference between the aorta and the left and right ventricular end-diastolic pressure, on the diastolic interval and on coronary vascular resistance. Conditions that shorten diastole or lower the driving pressure between the aorta and end-diastolic pressure reduce coronary perfusion, should coronary flow resistance fail to decrease. Coronary vascular resistance is controlled by a host of mechanisms such as metabolic factors, endothelial function, autoregulation, extravascular compression as well as by neuronal influences. In patients with CAD, the effect of coronary stenoses and of collateral circulation adds to the effect of reducing coronary perfusion.

Alterations of myocardial oxygen balance are regulated very quickly, when occluding a coronary artery. In less than 1 s, coronary blood flow increases by reactive hyperemia that reaches its maximum after 15–20 s. The main vasodilatory substances for acute metabolic regulation are adenosine, NO and prostanoids. Adenosine exerts the greatest influence on increase of coronary flood flow during reactive hyperemia, under conditions of hypoxia, and following inotropic stimulation with isoproterenol and dobutamine, as well as during mental stress. The relative vasodilatory impact of adenosine and NO during reactive hyperemia after 10–20 s of occlusion may be estimated by the fact that after administration of an adenosine blocking agent, the hyperemic reaction is reduced by 30% and by concomitant administration of an NO-blocker by 60% (Yanabe 1992).

A second component for regulation of coronary flow is coronary vascular endothelium, which produces strong vasodilator substances such as the endothelial-derived relaxing factor (EDRF), which was identified as NO, prostacyclin and the endothelial-derived hyper polarizing factor (EDHF). NO production may be stimulated by acetylcholine, aggregating platelets via the release of ADP and serotonin, by thrombin, the mast cell product histamine, and by an increased shear stress from increased blood flow in the vessel. A continued release of NO is the most important determinant for regulating vascular flow resistance under resting conditions. Coronary atherosclerosis and hypercholesterolemia may significantly reduce the reactivity of the resistance vessels to endothelial-derived vasodilator substances. Blunted reactivity of the resistance vessels due to endothelial dysfunction may be an important factor for a reduced flow reserve in the coronary microcirculation under conditions of increased oxygen consumption. By this means myocardial ischemia with typical angina pectoris may occur, and this mechanism is considered the pathophysiological cause of microvascular angina (syndrome X) in patients without stenoses in the large epicardial coronary arteries. The endothelium also produces a very potent vasoconstrictor substance, endothelin 1 (ET-1) that may be involved in the regulation of the vascular tone by continuous vasotonic vasoconstrictor effects.

Coronary autoregulation is an intrinsic mechanism of myocardial perfusion. Regional coronary blood flow remains constant as coronary artery pressure is reduced below aortic pressure over a wide range when the determinants of myocardial oxygen consumption are kept constant. When perfusion pressure falls to the lower limit of autoregulation, coronary resistance vessels are maximally dilated due to intrinsic stimuli, and flow becomes pressure-dependent, resulting in the onset of subendocardial ischemia. Under normal hemodynamic conditions blood flow in the coronary arteries averages 0.7–1.0 ml/min/gm and can increase between 4-

and 5-fold during vasodilatation; the ability of flow to increase above resting values in response to pharmacological vasodilatation is termed coronary reserve. Coronary reserve is reduced when diastolic time available for subendocardial perfusion is decreased, or the compressive determinants of diastolic perfusion are increased by an enlarged pre-load. The lower pressure limit of autoregulation in men is about 70 mmHg, in conscious dogs coronary flow can be autoregulated to a mean coronary pressure of 40 mmHg and diastolic pressures of 30 mmHg.

There are important transmural variations in the lower autoregulatory pressure limit, which result in increased susceptibility of the subendocardium to ischemia. Subepicardial flow occurs throughout the cardiac cycle and is maintained until coronary pressure falls below 25 mmHg. In contrast, subendocardial flow primarily occurs in diastole and begins to decrease below a mean coronary pressure of 40 mmHg. This difference is primarily related to the increased oxygen consumption in the subendocardium requiring a higher resting flow level, and to the more pronounced effects of systolic contraction on subendocardial vasodilator reserve. This transmural difference in the lower autoregulatory pressure limit determines the vulnerability of the subendocardium to ischemia at a reduced pressure distal to a coronary stenosis. In contrast to normal individuals without detectable autoregulation, in patients with high grade stenoses in the epicardial arteries, autoregulation plays a significant role. Pressure drops distal to a stenosis may be compensated by autoregulation for up to 80% diameter stenoses, but following a significant decrease of aortic pressure with simultaneous increase of endiastolic pressure in response to myocardial ischemia, distal perfusion pressure may drop to critical values of autoregulation, which results in myocardial ischemia of the subendocardium. Similar effects may be seen in patients with left ventricular hypertrophy due to arterial hypertension or severe aortic stenosis, where autoregulation in the subendocardium is much more limited than in the subepicardium. Pharmacologiacal substances with a dilatory effect on coronary resistance vessels, such as adenosine or dipyridamole, can decrease the perfusion pressure distal to a stenosis, and thus may increase subepicardial flow relative to the subendocardial flow and may blunt subendocardial autoregulation. These phenomena are the main factor underlying the so-called steal-effect after administration of adenosine or dipyridamole. Coronary collateral vessels don't develop autoregulation, which explains the effect that patients with extensive collateral-dependent myocardial perfusion do not tolerate arterial hypotension very well (Canty Jr. 2012).

During cardiac contraction, intramyocardial tissue pressure increases around compliant arterioles and venules, which results in a concealed arterial backflow with reduction of systolic inflow in the epicardial arteries. Compression of venules accelerates venous outflow. During diastole, compressive effects are related to tissue pressures that decrease from the subendocardium to the subepicardium, and at diastolic LV-pressures greater than 20 mmHg pre-load determines the effective back pressure to coronary diastolic perfusion. The effect of compression or wash-out is considerably strong when the intraventricular pressure is higher than the coronary perfusion pressure, e.g. in patients with aortic stenosis or aortic valve incompetence or subvalvular aortic stenosis. Limitation of CBF reserve by extravascular compression during systole is exaggerated by lowering coronary vascular resistance after administration of arterial vasodilators, or by metabolic dilatation from physical activity. Diastolic perfusion pressure also significantly influences coronary perfusion at least in special pathophysiological conditions. The extravascular compressive forces exert their most prominent effects on the subendocardium, since this is supplied by long transversal blood vessels, which are particularly exposed to the transmural and intraventricular pressure. The relatively larger shortening of the subendocardial layers together with a 20% higher oxygen consumption necessitate a 20% higher subendocardial blood flow compared to the subepicardial layers. In the presence of a critical stenosis of the epicardial coronary artery with consecutive reduction of coronary blood flow below 40%, the normal ratio of subendocardial to subepicardial blood flow of 1–1.16 diminishes to 1–0.37 (Bache 1977). Such an imbalance of subendocardial to subepicardial flow may be furthermore exaggerated by physical activity, arterial stimulation, or by the administration of adenosine or dipyridamole. Similar effects may also be observed with pressure-induced left ventricular hypertrophy (e.g. arterial hypertension, aortic stenosis, or aortic incompetence), as well as by chronic heart failure with increased endiastolic pressures.

Coronary backflow may also be influenced by neuronal influences, by baroreceptor activity, and by tonic coronary vasoconstriction. Sympathetic and parasympathetic nerves innervate coronary conduit arteries and segments of the resistance vessels. Neural stimulation affects vascular tone through mechanisms that alter vascular smooth muscle, as well as by stimulating the release of NO from the endothelium. When risk factors impairing endothelium-dependent vasodilatation are present, diametrically opposite effects on coronary tone may occur. Coronary endothelial activation with release of acetylcholine normally increases coronary flow by dilatation of resistance arteries. In conduit arteries, acetylcholine normally induces mild coronary vasodilatation, which reflects the net action of a direct muscarinic constriction of vascular smooth muscle counterbalanced by an endothelium-dependent vasodilatation caused by direct stimulation of NOS with release of NO and an increased flow-mediated dilatation from concomitant resistance vessel vasodilatation. In human coronary arteries with atherosclerosis, the dilatation of resistance vessels to acetylcholine is attenuated or blunted and the reduction in flow-mediated NO production leads to net epicardial conduit artery vasoconstriction. This phenomenon is particularly prominent in stenotic coronary artery segments. With respect to sympathetic innervation under basal conditions, there is no resting sympathetic tone in the heart, and no effect of denervation on resting myocardial perfusion. During sympathetic activation in conduit arteries, α_1-mediated constriction and β_2-mediated vasodilatation occurs, the net effect is dilatation of epicardial coronary arteries. This effect may be potentiated by concomitant flow-mediated vasodilatation from metabolic regulation of coronary resistance vessels. When NO mediated vasodilatation is impaired α_1-mediated constriction predominates and may dynamically increase the severity of stenosis in asymmetrical lesions (so-called dynamic coronary artery stenosis). For further details see Canty Jr. 2012.

6.2.2 Endothelial Dysfunction

In normal coronary arteries, activation of the sympathetic nervous system due to physical activity, cold pressure test or heart rate increase results in a flow and catecholamine mediated increase and endothelium dependent vasodilatation, and thereby an increased blood flow. In the case of dysfunctional endothelium the arterial vessels react with vasoconstriction under these circumstances, and this effect may be detected by an injection of acetylcholine into the coronary arteries. This paradoxical effect of endothelial dependent vasoconstriction by acetylcholine was observed under provocative testing of vascular tone by physical stress, cold pressure test or during increases of heart rate.

Serotonin released from platelets induces a dilatation of coronary arteries under normal conditions; however, in patients with coronary heart disease and dysfunctional endothelium, serotonin may produce coronary constriction. This mechanism plays an important role in case of plaque ruptures with consecutive activation of circulatory platelets that results in thrombus formation.

> In patients with syndrome X with stress induced angina pectoris and normal coronary arteries, a diminished endothelium dependent dilatation of the coronary resistance vessels was observed. Increases of serum cholesterol, cigarette smoking and arterial hypertension as well as advanced age are also correlated with endothelial dysfunction in a significant number of individuals.

6.3 Pathophysiology of Myocardial Ischemia

Myocardial ischemia occurs with an imbalance of oxygen supply and oxygen consumption of the myocardium. Oxygen supply may be impaired by thrombus formation or vascular spasm, as well as chronic underperfusion in the great epicardial vessels that are most frequently induced by atherosclerosis of the coronary arteries. In addition, special disease states with reduced oxygen supply with adequate perfusion are cyanotic congenital heart diseases, cor pulmonale, severe anemia, asphyxia and CO-intoxication.

With commencing myocardial ischemia, a cascade of biological, functional and electrocardiographic events such as decrease of energy rich phosphates in the myocardium, impaired relaxation, regional myocardial dysfunction, increase of filling pressure, ST segment depression within the ECG and angina pectoris ensues (Figure 6-1). The primary event of reduced perfusion may be detected by SPECT or PET flow measurements, as well as by first-pass perfusion assessment with MRI. In patients with coronary stenoses, myocardial ischemia is induced by increased oxygen consumption due to e.g. physical activity, tachycardia or psychosocial stress. This type of demand-ischemia is responsible for most episodes in patients with chronic stable CAD. On the other hand an increased coronary vascular tone, platelet aggregation, or thrombus formation may lead to a reduced oxygen supply (supply-ischemia) that is responsible for most clinical episodes of unstable angina or myocardial infarction. In many cases of myocardial ischemia, both factors of increased myocardial oxygen consumption and reduced oxygen supply play a significant role.

6.3.1 Effects of Coronary Stenoses on Coronary Blood Flow

According to fluid dynamics, blood looses pressure or energy from flow through a stenotic segment, mainly due to viscous friction of fluid segments within a stenotic arterial segment, due to an increase of blood flow with higher kinetic energy and through turbulences at the distal end of the stenosis (separation losses). Fluid resistance through a stenosis shows an exponential correlation to the severity of the stenosis. Increasing blood flow through the stenotic segment produces a higher pressure gradient and a stronger decrease of the post-stenotic perfusion pressure. In the case of distensible stenotic segments that are mostly present in eccentric stenoses, the stenotic segment collapses to a certain degree by increased blood flow due to dilatation of the arterial vessels distal to the stenosis.

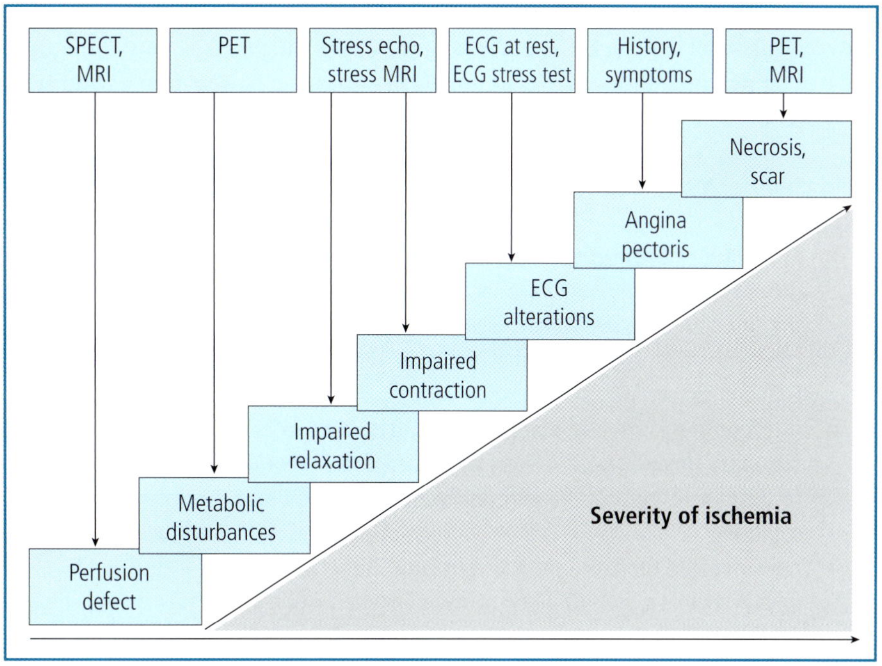

Figure 6-1 Sequence of time-dependent ischemia-induced functional and morphological alterations (stepwise increasing cascade), beginning with a perfusion defect and ending with myocardial necrosis or scar; corresponding diagnostic tests **(upper row)** for adequate assessment of the myocardial alteration in question.

Flow dependent pressure gradient and pressure drop with increased flow play a significant role in the pathogenesis of myocardial ischemia during physical exercise and significant coronary stenosis, at pharmacological dilatation of the coronary resistance vessels, and of myocardial ischemia due to anemia during physical exercise. During physical exercise, myocardial oxygen demand increases together with an increased flow through the stenotic segment with a resultant increase of pressure gradient over, and pressure drop distal to the stenosis. These hemodynamic alterations may redistribute driving pressure and perfusion from the subendocardial to subepicardial layers, together with a pressure drop dependent collapse of the vessel, and may induce myocardial ischemia and angina pectoris.

A similar hemodynamic condition may be induced when vasodilatory drugs such as Adenosine or Dipyridamole are administered: the trans-stenotic flow and pressure gradient over the stenosis are increased, and with maximal dilatation the perfusion of resistance vessels directly depends on the pressure gradient; with increased flow through the stenosis and decreased pressure distal to the stenosis, a redistribution of blood flow from subendocardium to subepicardium is induced (transmural "steal effect"). If aortic pressure falls simultaneously the driving pressure difference is reduced and thereby the steal effect will be further exaggerated.

The shape and length of the stenosis play a significant role in myocardial ischemia, as well, since separation loss from turbulences is mainly dependent on the degree of laminar flow. Since most coronary stenoses begin and end abruptly, a significant turbulent flow at the distal end of the stenosis will occur. Turbulent flow may also arise in very long stenotic segments, whereby the energy loss at the transition of laminar flow to turbulence will be released into the vessel wall. This is the reason why long stenotic segments in a coronary artery create a limited blood flow during physical activity.

Gold and Lipscomp (1974) were able to show that under resting conditions, resting myocardial blood flow will not be limited until there is a degree of coronary stenosis of up to 80%, whereas the maximal coronary blood flow steadily decreased beginning with a stenosis degree of more than 50%. A stenotic segment of more than 90% will exhaust the capacity of further flow increase in the coronary circulation to compensate an increased oxygen consumption during physical activity. It should be stressed that the hemodynamic effect of stenoses within the coronary angiogram cannot be exactly assessed by mere measurements of diameter or cross-sectional obstruction, since important geometric characteristics such as the absolute diameter, length, exit angle and the eccentricity cannot be clearly assessed with three-dimensional imaging. This has been confirmed by White et al. (1984) who were able to show that there is a wide range of hemodynamic compromise with nearly normal coronary reactive hyperemia due to 80% stenosis and impaired coronary vascular flow reserve from 40–50% stenoses. Therefore, measuring coronary flow reserve on drug induced hyperemia will provide better information on the flow limiting degree of a coronary obstruction than morphological feature of the stenosis within the angiogram.

Coronary flow reserve is defined as the difference between the basal and maximal coronary blood flow during reactive hyperemia induced by a short lasting coronary occlusion (e.g. PTCA balloon) or due to vasodilatory drugs.

In principle, **three methods** to assess coronary flow reserve may be used:

- **thermodilution method** with assessing the flow in the great cardiac vein that drains the perfusion territory of the left anterior descendent artery (LAD), or within the coronary sinus that drains the perfusion territory of the LAD and circumflex artery (LCx),
- **intracoronary measurement of phasic and mean coronary flow** via Doppler-wire, or intracoronary pressure measurement by pressure-wire (pressure drop distal to a stenosis),
- **non-invasive measurement of regional flow** by SPECT flow techniques, by PET flow, or by magnetic resonance PC-flow mapping in coronary arteries or coronary sinus, or by first-pass perfusion of left ventricular myocardium.

6.3.2 Role of Coronary Collateral Circulation

Coronary collateral circulation plays a significant role to compensate an acute or chronic occlusion of a coronary artery. Pre-existent collateral vessels are thin walled vessel structures with a diameter of 20–200 µm. The existence of collaterals is extremely species-dependent, in men the density of pre-existent collateral vessels seems to be similar to those in the canine heart. Pre-existent collateral vessels are normally closed and functionally inactive since no pressure gradient exists between a connecting epicardial coronary artery. Following coronary artery occlusion, the distal pressure falls abruptly and the collateral channels immediately open. Transformation of pre-existent collaterals into mature collaterals follows three steps: passive dilatation, cell proliferation and inflammation and finally, arterialisation. Collateral growth is directed by pressure gradients, shear stress, ischemia, hypoxia and the influence of growth factors. The degree of coronary obstruction that must be at least 80 % to induce collateral growth and the dynamicity and developmental speed of the stenoses significantly influence the degree of collateral growth. In contrast regular physical activity may not have a significant influence on collateral growth. In general collaterals can proliferate to a degree where they are sufficient to maintain resting perfusion, and sometimes prevent stress induced ischemia at submaximal cardiac work loads. It should be stressed that there is tremendous individual variability in the function of coronary collaterals among patients with chronic coronary artery stenoses or occlusions. Therefore, in an individual patient it is very difficult to predict the immediate course in the case of an abrupt occlusion of a large epicardial coronary artery, which may remain clinically silent without any visible myocardial infarction on the one hand, or may end up with a large transmural myocardial infarction.

From a clinical point of view it is important that coronary collateral vessels can be dilated by Nitrates and β-agonist drugs, whereas calcium blockers or β-receptor blockers, as well as α-adrenergic agonists, do not have a significant influence on collateral circulation. Vasopressin and serotonin are potent constrictor drugs in collateral vessels. Following platelet aggregation or arterial thrombosis, platelets may release serotonin within the flow territory of collaterals leading to constriction and myocardial ischemia within the collateral perfusion area. The naturally occurring endogenous vasodilator NO and prostacyclin keep collateral vessel in a dilated state, while an inhibition of NO synthase e.g. with L-NAME, causes a significant reduction of collateral flow (for further details see Canty Jr. 2012).

6.3.3 Metabolic and Functional Consequences of Myocardial Ischemia

Because of the close coupling of oxygen supply to coronary blood flow, a sudden cessation of regional perfusion quickly leads to the cessation of aerobic metabolism, depletion of creatine phosphate, and the onset of anarerobic glycolysis, followed by the accumulation of tissue lactate, progressive reduction of ATP levels, and accumulation of catabolytes. With continued ischemia, tissue acidosis develops and an efflux of potassium into the extracellular space ensues. Finally, ATP levels fall below those required to maintain critical membrane and cellular function with consecutive onset of myocyte death.

The temporal evolution and extent of irreversible tissue injury following coronary occlusion is variable and depends on residual coronary blood flow, transmural location, and the hemodynamic determinants of oxygen consumption. In the absence of significant coronary collaterals, irreversible myocardial damage begins after 20 min of coronary occlusion, whereby injury begins in the subendocardium and progresses as a wave front over time to the subepicardium. Transmural progression of infarction is largely completed within 4–6 h after coronary occlusion, whereby factors that increase myocardial oxygen consumption or reduce oxygen delivery accelerate the progression of irreversible injury. The magnitude of residual coronary flow through collateral vessels or through a subtotal coronary occlusion is the most important determinant factor of the actual time course of irreversible injury in patients with chronic CAD. The relationship between infarct size and the area at risk of ischemia during a total occlusion is inversely related to collateral flow.

Myocardial infarction will be prevented after ischemia periods longer than 1 h, when subendocardial collateral flow remains more than approximately 30% of resting flow values. If a subtotal occlusion is present with subsequent more moderate subendocardial ischemia, no significant irreversible injury may occur over a period of at least 5 h (Kloner 2001). This fact is clinically relevant in that signs and symptoms of ischemia may be present for long periods of time without producing significant myocardial necrosis, and may also explain the observation that late coronary perfusion beyond 6 h of ongoing ischemia can salvage myocardium.

With long-term myocardial ischemia, cell-death arises from myocyte necrosis and membrane disruption with a further amplification of injury by the re-entry of leucocytes into the area of damage. The second mechanism may be that cells undergo programmed cell death (so-called apoptosis) with further contribution to delayed myocardial damage (for further details see Canty Jr. 2012).

6.4 Etiology and Pathogenesis of Coronary Atherosclerosis

Atherosclerosis may begin early in the adsolescent ages beyond 10 yrs with extracellular lipid accumulation and leukocyte recruitment within the vessel wall (so-called fatty streaks), and may develop over decades with growing of atheromas between the ages of 40–50 yrs; stenotic atherosclerotic lesions may lead to ischemia in the perfusion dependent area, e.g. with coronary stenoses in myocardial ischemia, and rupture of a thin-capped atheroma may result in a rapid occlusion of a coronary artery followed by myocardial infarction. According to Stary (2000), a continuous development of characteristic stages of atheromata may be diagnosed based on patho-anatomic studies, *starting* with **Stary I lesions** (fatty streaks) and *ending* with **Stary VI atheromas** (end-stage complicated atheroma). Smoking, hypertension, hyperlipidemia and diabetes mellitus, including the metabolic syndrome, are classic risk factors for the initiation and propagation of atherosclerosis. Novel atherosclerostic risk factors include elevated levels of high-sensitivity-C-reactive protein and other markers of inflammation such as homocysteine, fibrinogen, and lipoprotein (a). Genetic factors may also play a significant role in the genesis of coronary atherosclerosis, particularly in individuals who have few or none of the known risk factors.

6.5 Clinical Presentation and Therapy

Patients with stable flow-limiting coronary stenoses and stable angina pectoris experience chest discomfort on exercise or stress induced emotion that disappears after cessation of the initiating stimulus. Typical angina pectoris is described as viselike, constricting, suffocating, crushing, or squeezing retrosternal chest discomfort with frequent radiation down the ulnar surface of the left arm, the neck or jaw or into the epigastrium; typical angina is relieved within minutes by rest or the use of nitroglycerine. A system of grading the severity of angina pectoris proposed by the Canadian Cardiovascular Society (CCS Class I through IV) is widely accepted.

Diagnosis of chronic stable angina is made by taking the history (precipitating risk factors, family history of cardiovascular disease, typical angina), clinical examination, exercise testing (ST segment deviations), and in unclear situations by stress echocardiography, stress magnetic resonance imaging (CMR), or by myocardial perfusion imaging using nuclear techniques (SPECT, PET) or CMR first-pass perfusion imaging.

Medical therapy in low- to medium risk patients includes β-blocking drugs, long-term nitrates, and/or calcium channel blockers and aspirin as well as treatment of risk factors (statins for hyperlipedimia, antihypertensive drugs for hypertension, and drug treatment of diabetes mellitus). In high-risk or drug-resistant angina pectoris patients, interventional (PTCA without/with stenting) or surgical bypass grafting will be considered according to the results of invasive coronary angiography.

6.6 CMR Protocols

6.6.1 CMR-Based Diagnosis of Structure and Function/Dysfunction of the Heart

Global and regional function is typically assessed on a cine data set in true short-axis covering the heart in 10–14 consecutive two-dimensional slices. In addition, long-axis scans can be aquired in every possible geometry.

In addition, regional contractile function can be assessed either by visual interpretation of cine loops or by measuring wall motion, thickening, and strain using myocardial tagging methods. Myocardial tagging during low dose dobutamine stress has been used to measure parameters of diastolic dysfunction such as the time to peak untwist, which may identify coronary stenosis.

6.6.2 Detection of Myocardial Ischemia and Diagnostic Performance of the Tests

Dobutamine Stress MR

Dobutamine is a synthetic catecholamine derivate with a predominantly β_1-adrenergic effect. At low doses (< 10 µg/kg/min) it exerts a predominant positive inotropic effect. In addition dobutamine has a positive chronotropic effect (at doses > 20 µg/kg/min). The rationale of using dobutamine as a stress agent is its comparability with physical exercise. Dobutamine induced increase of myocardial contractility and heart rate result in an increase of myocardial oxygen consumption. The main advantage of dobutamine is its rapid onset of action and short half-life. This allows an operator-controlled level of stress by drug titration. According to the guidelines of the American Heart Association (AHA) and the Society of Cardiovascular Magnetic Resonance (SCMR), high-dose protocols with step-wise infusion rates of 10–40 µg/kg/min were adopted for dobutamine stress MRI. If only submaximal heart rates are achieved, additional fractionated atropine doses (0.25 mg i.v. every 60 s up to a maximal dose of 2 mg) are administered (Ling 1996, Nagel 2001).

Safety, Side Effects and Contraindications for Dobutamine Stress

Side effects and complications of high dose dobutamine testing are well-known from its widespread use in stress echocardiography. Potential side effects of dobutamine are due to its sympathomimetic activity. Most frequent sensations are anxiety, agitation, palpitations and tachypnea. Normally, those effects do not affect the course of the examination, and can be minimized by accurate patient education. In addition, single ventricular premature beats may occur, they do not fulfill criteria for termination of dobutamine stress, but rather may reduce image quality due to trigger problems. Atrial fibrillation occurs in approximately 1 % of examinations and is usually reversible after termination of the stress test. Malignant cardiac arrhythmias, including sustained ventricular tachycardia and ventricular fibrillation, are rare (incidence 0.15 %). Myocardial infarction from severe myocardial ischemia can be observed in 0.1 % of all high-dose dobutamine examinations. In contrast to a regular increase of blood pressure hypotensive dysregulation may sometimes occur.

Possible reasons for hypotensive dysregulation are:

- inotropic obstruction of the left ventricular outflow tract,
- β_2-dobutamine-induced peripheral vasodilatation, or
- left ventricular failure due to extensive myocardial ischemia.

Termination of the examination is required if blood pressure drops > 40 mmHg.

Although serious complications are rare, special safety measures are required when scanning cardiovascular patients. Regarding cardiac stress tests, it is recommended that medication for emergency treatment be readily available. A defibrillator should be placed nearby outside the scan room. In case of malignant arrhythmias, patients must be immediately removed from the scanner room. Another problem is that the ECG can only be used for monitoring the patient's heart rhythm. Magnetic field effects may alter ST segments and T-waves in the ECG rendering the detection of ischemia impossible. Therefore it is necessary that a physician supervises the procedure to ensure online assessment of global and regional myocardial performance during drug infusion. After finishing stress testing, dobutamine side effects can be reversed by β-blocker administration (e.g., esmolol 0.5 mg/kg slowly i.v.).

In addition to the general contraindications for CMR, there are a number of **specific safety concerns** to use sympathomimetic agents for stress testing:

- unstable angina,
- acute coronary syndromes,
- severe arterial hypertension (> 220 mmHg),
- severe aortic stenosis (gradient > 50 mmHg, valve opening area < 1.0 cm^2),
- obstruction of the left ventricular outflow tract,
- high grade ventricular arrhythmia,
- acute inflammatory myocardial and pericardial diseases.

Patient Preparation

Essentials of patient preparation include:

- to ensure maximal effect of the drug and increase sensitivity of the test, patients should refrain from medication with β-blockers and nitrates for at least 24 h prior to the examination,
- informed consent must be obtained beforehand,
- intravenous line,
- physiological monitoring (ECG, blood pressure, and pulse oxymetry).

Scan Protocol

The usual scan protocol is summarized as follows:

- scout/survey for determining heart position and optimize coil positioning,
- reference scan if parallel imaging techniques are used,
- functional scans at rest:
  - SSFP sequences in short-axis geometry (at least 3 slices) and long-axis geometry (2-ch, 3-ch and 4-ch view); image geometry should be stored as reference for the functional stress images,
  - infusion of dobutamine in increments of 10 µg/kg/min every 3 mins to a maximum dose of 40 µg/kg/min; if the targeted heart rate ([220 – age] × 0.85) is not achieved, atropine is added in incremental doses of 0.25 mg to a maximum of 2 mg,
- functional scans at stress:
  - after each increase in dosage SSFP sequences are performed in short- and long-axis orientation in identical scan geometry; due to increasing heart rate it might be necessary to adapt scan parameters for optimization of temporal resolution.

Monitoring

Regular monitoring of the patients includes:

- patient monitoring must be compatible with the CMR environment,
- continous monitoring of heart rate, heart rhythm and, if applicable, oxygen saturation,
- blood pressure should be monitored every minute,
- online review of functional scans after each increment of the stress agent.

Termination Criteria for Dobutamine Stress Test

Absolute criteria for terminating a dobutamine stress test are:

- targeted heart rate ([220 – age] × 0.85) achieved,
- severe symptoms, e.g. angina, arrhythmias,
- new wall motion abnormalities in at least two segments,
- decrease in blood pressure (> 40 mmHg decrease of systolic blood pressure),
- increase in blood pressure (> 240 mmHg systolic, > 120 mmHg diastolic).

Image Analysis

Functional rest and stress images of each dosage should be reviewed simultaneously on a designated work station in multi-screen format allowing direct comparison of the scans. Regional wall motion is qualitatively assessed and categorized on a per segment analysis using the 17-segment model adopted by the ACC/AHA guidelines (Cerqueira 2002) for non-invasive testing. Wall motion is described as normokinetic, hyperkinetic, hypokinetic, akinetic, and dyskinetic. Normokinetic wall motion is characterized by normal endocardial inward movement and wall thickening, whereas hypokinetic wall motion is characterized by decreased endocardial inward movement or wall thickening. Akinetic regions show no endocardial inward movement or wall thickening, and dyskinetic regions reveal paradoxical endocardial outward movement (Figure 6-2 and Figure 6-3).

Usually wall motion scores are applied, and the scoring for normokinetic segments includes 1, of hypokinetic segments 2, akinetic segments 3, and dyskinetic segments 4. These numbers are added and divided by the total number of analyzed segments. Values for wall motion scores > 1 represent a pathological stress test and indicate the presence of hemodynamically relevant coronary stenoses. Alternatively, images can also be assessed quantitatively using parameters such as regional wall motion thickening measured between endo- and epicardial borders during contraction. In addition, there are other techniques for quantitative wall motion assessment, e.g. myocardial tagging or strain. However, complex and time consuming algorithms limit their use in clinical practice; they lack standardization, and are most frequently used in research applications.

Diagnostic Performance of the Test

Stress MRI has recently emerged as a promising alternative to nuclear SPECT and stress echocardiography in the non-invasive functional evaluation of CAD. In a meta-analysis by Nandalur et al. published in 2007, 14 datasets on 754 patients were evaluated using stress induced wall motion abnormalities on dobutamine CMR (DSMR) compared with coronary angiography. Detection of wall motion abnormalities by DSMR demonstrated a sensitivity of 0.83 (95% confidence interval [CI] 0.79–0.88) and specificity of 0.86 (95% CI 0.81–0.91) for the detection of a relevant stenosis > 50% on a patient level. Overall disease prevalence was 70.5%. The authors concluded that in studies with high disease prevalence, DSMR demonstrates overall good sensitivity and specificity for the diagnosis of CAD. However, limited data are available regarding the use of this technique in populations with low disease prevalence. In a direct comparison of CMR and echocardiography, Nagel et al. (1999) performed DSMR and dobutamine stress echocardiography (DSE) in 208 patients referred for conventional coronary angiography. DSMR showed better sensitivity (89 vs. 74%) and specificity (86 vs. 70%) than DSE for the detection of ≥ 50% coronary artery stenosis identified on angiography. The superior performance of DSMR was most striking in

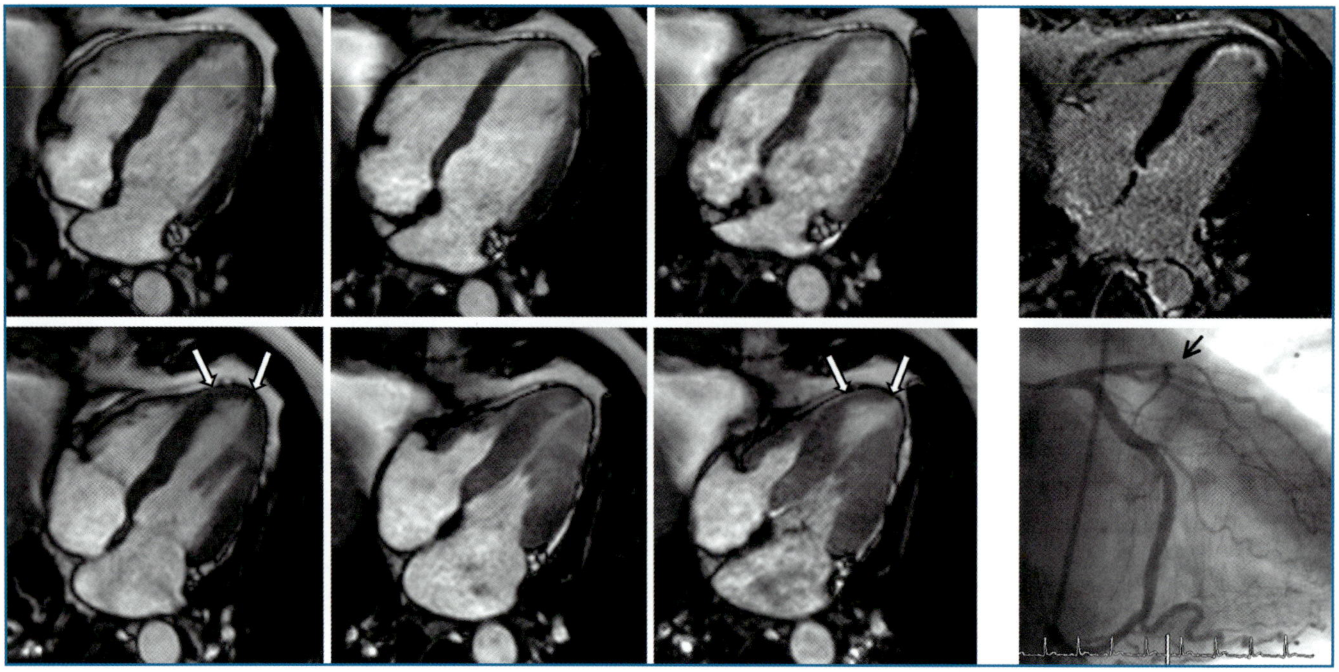

Figure 6-2 Regional contraction analysis in 4-ch view of a dobutamine stress CMR examination in a patient with high grade stenosis of the LAD **(bottom, extreme right**, arrow**)**. Diastolic images top row **(left)** at 3 increasing dobutamine doses, corresponding systolic images bottom row **(left)**. Normokinesis of all segments of the left ventricular wall at rest **(bottom left**, arrows**)**, akinesis and lack of systolic thickening of the apex and apico-inferoseptal segments of the left ventricular (LV) wall at maximum dobutamine administration **(bottom right**, arrows**)**. Delayed enhancement study showed a near 50 % transmural scar in the apical region of the LV wall **(top, extreme right)** (courtesy PD I. Paetsch, University Hospital of Aachen, Germany).

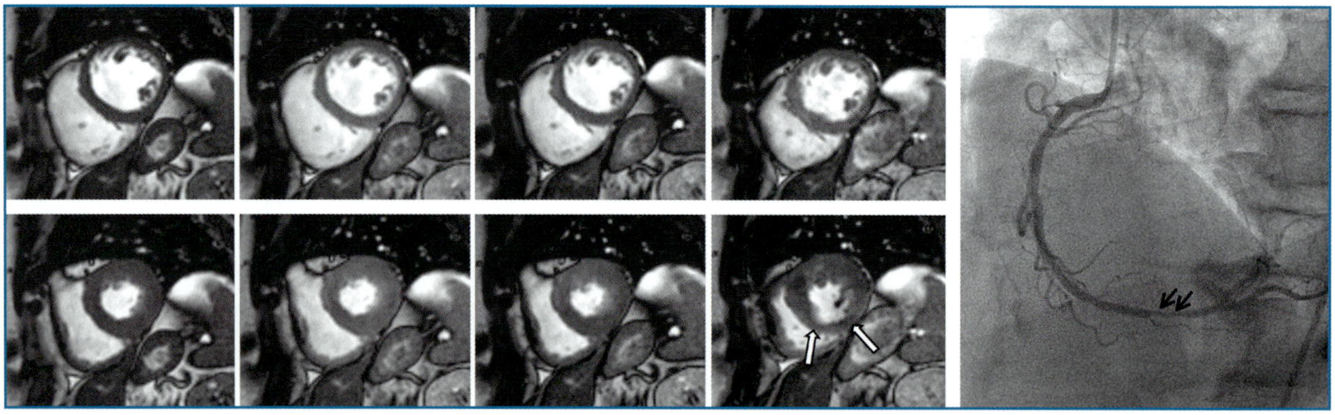

Figure 6-3 Regional contraction analysis in short-axis view of a dobutamine stress CMR examination in a patient with high grade stenosis of the right coronary artery proximal to the crux cordis **(extreme right**, arrows**)**. Diastolic images top row **(left)** at 4 increasing dobutamine doses, corresponding systolic images bottom row **(left)**. Normokinesis of all segments of the left ventricular (LV) wall at rest **(bottom left)**, akinesis and lack of systolic thickening of the inferoseptal and inferior segments of the LV wall at maximum dobutamine administration **(bottom right**, arrows**)** (courtesy PD I. Paetsch, University Hospital of Aachen, Germany).

patients with moderate image quality. It is important to note that only slightly more than half of patients had echocardiographic image quality judged to be good or better, while 40 % were of moderate image quality, and 8 % were non-diagnostic. In patients with moderate image quality, overall accuracy was only marginally better than chance. Conversely, with DSMR, over 80 % of patients had image quality judged as good to very good, while 16 % were of moderate image quality, and only 2 % were non-diagnostic. Furthermore, there was no significant difference in diagnostic accuracy of DSMR between patients with moderate and good to very good image quality. Hundley et al. (1999) performed DSMR in 153 patients with poor acoustic windows that prevented adequate transthoracic echocardiographic imaging. When compared with contrast coronary angiography, the sensitivity and specificity of DSMR were both 83 % for detecting coronary arterial luminal narrowing of ≥ 50 %.

Dobutamine Stress CMR in Patients after Revascularisation

Wahl et al. (2004) studied the diagnostic accuracy of DSMR in 160 patients with resting LV wall motion abnormalities who had a prior MI and/or prior coronary arterial revascularization (bypass surgery or percutaneous intervention). Overall sensitivity and specificity for detecting coronary arterial luminal narrowing of ≥ 50 % were 89 and 84 %, respectively. Diagnostic accuracy was 88 %, and positive and negative predictive values were 94 and 73 %, respectively. The sensitivity for detecting luminal narrowing of ≥ 50 % in one, two, or three epicardial arteries was 87, 91, and 100 % respectively. The authors concluded that high-dose DSMR imaging can be used for follow-up of patients after coronary revascularization procedures. Diagnostic accuracy was similar to stress cardiovascular MR imaging data for patients with suspected CAD, and compares favorably with that of other established non-invasive techniques.

Prognostic Implications

Compared with DSMR in the detection of myocardial ischemia, there is less evidence of its role in clinical decision making and predicting prognosis. In a study by Kelle et al. (2009a), 123 patients were consecutively followed for 24 mths after DSMR testing. Beside the good diagnostic power of positve stress test for detecting CAD, the main finding of this study was an excellent prognosis of patients with a negative DSMR test with an annual event rate of 0.0 %. A larger cohort of patients was published by Jahnke et al. (2007) using a combined CMR protocol with adenosine first-pass perfusion (MRP) and high-dose dobutamine stress protocol in 513 patients with suspected CAD, known CAD and prior CABG or PCI. Patients were followed-up for a median of 2.3 yrs. The 3-yrs event-free survival was 99.2 % for patients with normal MRP and DSMR and 83.5 % for those with abnormal MRP and DSMR. By multivariate analysis, ischemia on magnetic resonance stress testing (MRP or DSMR) was an independent predictor of cardiac events. Futhermore, an abnormal magnetic resonance stress test result had significant incremental value over clinical risk factors and resting wall motion abnormality. To determine the utility of DSMR for assessing peri-operative cardiovascular risk in patients undergoing noncardiac surgery, Rerkpattanapipat et al. (2002) followed 102 patients for the occurrence of cardiac death, MI, or congestive heart failure during or after noncardiac surgery. Among 84 patients with intermediate clinical predictors of MI or cardiac death (as defined by the ACC and AHA criteria), 35 patients with evidence of inducible ischemia had a 20 % rate of perioperative cardiac death, MI, or congestive heart failure compared with a 2 % event rate in those without ischemia. Patients without evidence of ischemia by DCMR, who achieved a heart rate response of ≥ 80 % of the maximal targeted heart rate for age during testing, had no perioperative events.

6.6.3 First-Pass Perfusion

Over the last decade, myocardial perfusion has become a top application of CMR. Several studies have shown high diagnostic accuracy in the detection of coronary stenoses, comparable to alternative standard myocardial perfusion imaging techniques. The advantage of the method is the non-invasivness of the procedure, the lack of radiation, and the high spatial resolution of 2–3 mm. This is by far superior to other imaging modalities, so that even subendocardial ischemia can be more reliably identified. The most commonly used approaches for CMR first-pass perfusion (CMR-FPP) utilize contrast media (CM) to track the first-pass of a contrast bolus through the myocardium. Perfusion defects seen during intravenous vasodilator-stress (most commonly with adenosine) compared with normal scans at rest indicate relatively underperfused regions associated with myocardial ischemia.

Contrast Agents

Most commonly commercially available extravascular contrast agents with different gadolinium chelates are used for FPP studies. Due to their small molecular size they rapidly diffuse from the intravascular to the extravascular space. This results in a high signal intensity in myocardium due to T1 shortening effects at low doses. The optimal dose of extravascular contrast agents ranges from 0.05–0.15 mmol/kg body weight. Signal intensity of left ventricular myocardium not only depends on the concentration of the contrast agent, but also on the tissue blood volume, size of extravascular compartment, and capillary permeability. At higher doses additional T2* and T2 effects may occur resulting in a higher rate of artifacts.

Another approach may be the use of intravascular contrast agents. These gadolinium containing drugs show a prolonged intravascular presence due to higher molecular size or binding to blood proteins. One potential advantage for the use of intravascular agents is that they are not limited to first-pass. Limiting effects may be their smaller distribution volume leading to lower signal intensity within the myocardium. As yet, a widespread experience with the use of intravascular contrast agents has been prevented due to their limited availability. Therefore, existing data on FPP is sparse and predominantely limited to animal studies leaving the potential clinical impact still unclear.

Drug Induced Hyperemia

Adenosine is an endogenous nucleotide and a potent vasodilator. Alternatively, the prodrug dipyridamole with a long half life of 30 min can be used, but this drug is only available in Europe. Adenosine exerts its hemodynamic effect through stimulation of A_1- and A_2-adenosine receptors. As the half-life of adenosine is extremely short, optimal handling of the substance in clinical practice is guaranteed. Comparable to protocols from nuclear medicine/SPECT mainly adenosine is used at a rate of 140 µg/kg/min for at least 3 min ensuring maximal coronary vasodilatation.

Safety, Side effects and Contraindications for Adenosine Stress

Most common side effects of adenosine application are heat sensations, uneasiness, headache and chest pain. These effects are often mild and do not require intervention. It must be noted that patients should be aware of these effects prior to examination. Careful education results in enhanced patient comfort and better image quality. In patients with known obstructive pulmonary disease, bronchospasm may occur. This may lead to abortion of the stress exam. In cases requiring medical intervention aminophylline can be used as an antagonist. Possible hemodynamic side effects of adenosine include a decrease in systolic and diastolic blood pressure, and a reflectory increase in heart rate. This effect is often mild and rarely exeeds 10 mmHg. Moreover, adenosine has a depressive effect on sinus and AV node. However, the incidence of symptomatic bradycardia and high grade AV blocks requiring medical intervention is negligible.

Recently, two studies have shown that adenosine stress perfusion is safe even in patients at high risk with aortic stenosis (Burgstahler 2008) or severe CAD (Karamitsos 2009).

However, there are a number of **contraindications** of using adenosine for FPP stress testing:

- COPD, Asthma bronchiale requiring medication with theophylline,
- high-grade AV blocks (> IIa),
- sinus node dysfunction,
- unstable angina,
- acute coronary syndroms,
- severe arterial hypotension (< 90 mmHg systolic blood pressure).

Patient Preparation

Essentials of patient preparation include:

- informed consent must be obtained,
- patients should refrain from medication with β-blockers or nitrates 24 h before examination,
- patients should refrain from beverages or food containing xanthines, e. g. coffee, black tea, cola, chocolate,
- two separate intravenous lines are required, since the consecutive application of adenosine followed by contrast agent via one line may result in an inadequate bolus of the drug; this increases the risk of higher grade AV blocks,
- physiological monitoring (ECG, blood pressure and pulse oximetry); care should be taken that blood pressure monitoring does not interfere with infusion of stress or contrast agents.

CMR-Perfusion Sequences

There are several requirements for the optimal perfusion sequence. First, high temporal resolution of data with acquisition every one to two heart beats is essential. Second, high spatial resolution is needed to reduce artifacts and differentiate transmural differences in perfusion and third, complete coverage of the heart to assess the extent of disease is needed. The basic contrast-enhanced myocardial perfusion sequence is strong T1-weighted imaging that can be obtained by applying a non-slice selective or slice-selective 90° saturation prepulse with recovery times as short as 100–150 ms. In contrast, with application of inversion recovery (IR), prepulse preparation times range from 300–400 ms. Due to the long acquisition window IR-pulses are no longer recommended.

For contrast-enhanced perfusion imaging T1-weighted turbo gradient echo (T1-TFE, FLASH) or fast gradient echo sequences with echoplanar imaging (hybrid-EPI) sequences can be used. Spoiled T1-TFE or FLASH sequences are hampered by a low signal-to-noise ratio (SNR) and long acquisition times per slice (150–250 ms). Hybrid-EPI sequences have the advantage of shorter acquisition times per slice (< 100 ms). Alternatively, steady-state free precession (SSFP, balanced FFE, true-FISP) sequences can be used. The advantages of SSFP sequences are a higher SNR, and possible acceleration of data acquisition by parallel imaging techniques that allow the implementation of a prepulse before each slice (Wang 2005). Furthermore, shorter acquisition times may reduce motion artifacts and allow for better coverage of the left ventricle. Nowadays, hybrid-EPI and SSFP perfusion techniques are the standard in most imaging centers.

Coverage of the Left Ventricle

There is some argument about the optimal coverage of the left ventricle during first-pass. With standard perfusion sequences and the need of high temporal and spatial resolution, three representative short-axis slices seem to be sufficient (Figure 6-4, Figure 6-5, and Figure 6-6). This approach is supported by data from Nagel et al. (2003), who found 3 slices more reliable than 5 slices. One reason for better performance might be that apical and basal slices are prone to susceptibility artifacts, and basal image data may be mixed with tissue texture of the left ventricular outflow tract. Second, strict apical perfusion defects may occur from stenoses of small diameter vessels not eligible for reasonable revascularisation strategies.

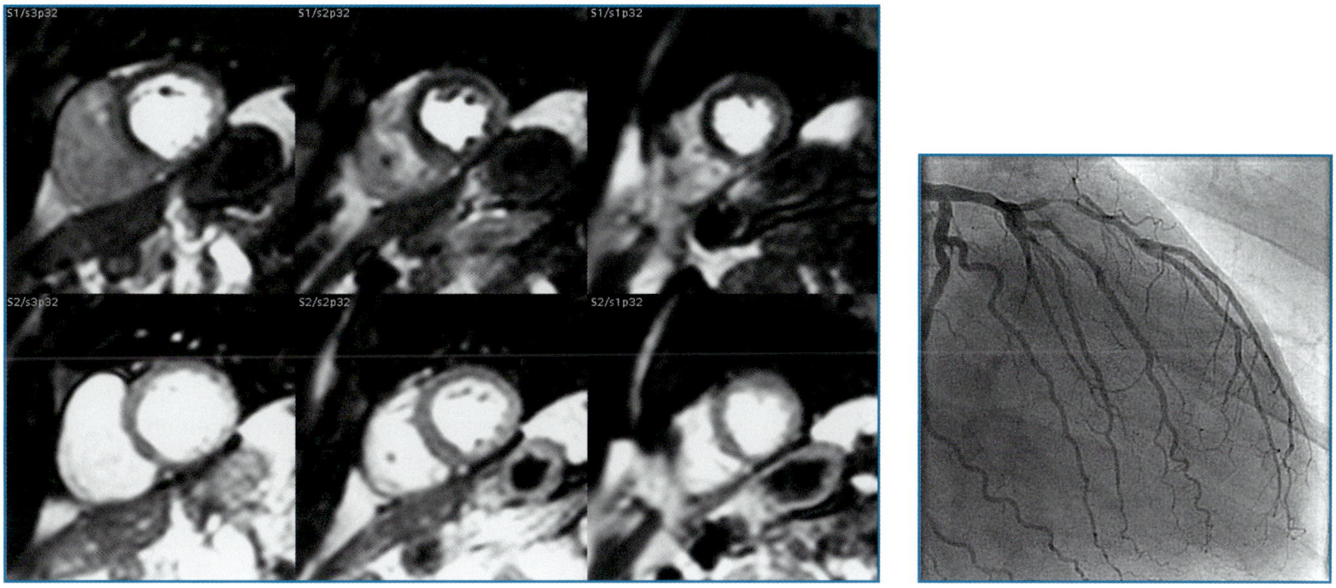

Figure 6-4 Screenshot of an abnormal first-pass perfusion study in a patient with a high grade stenosis of the LAD **(right)**; short-axis basal **(left slice)**, medial **(middle slice)**, and apical **(right slice)** slices with normal even perfusion of all segments at rest **(lower row left)**, and perfusion defect in the anterior and anteroseptal segment particularly in the medial slice **(top row)**.

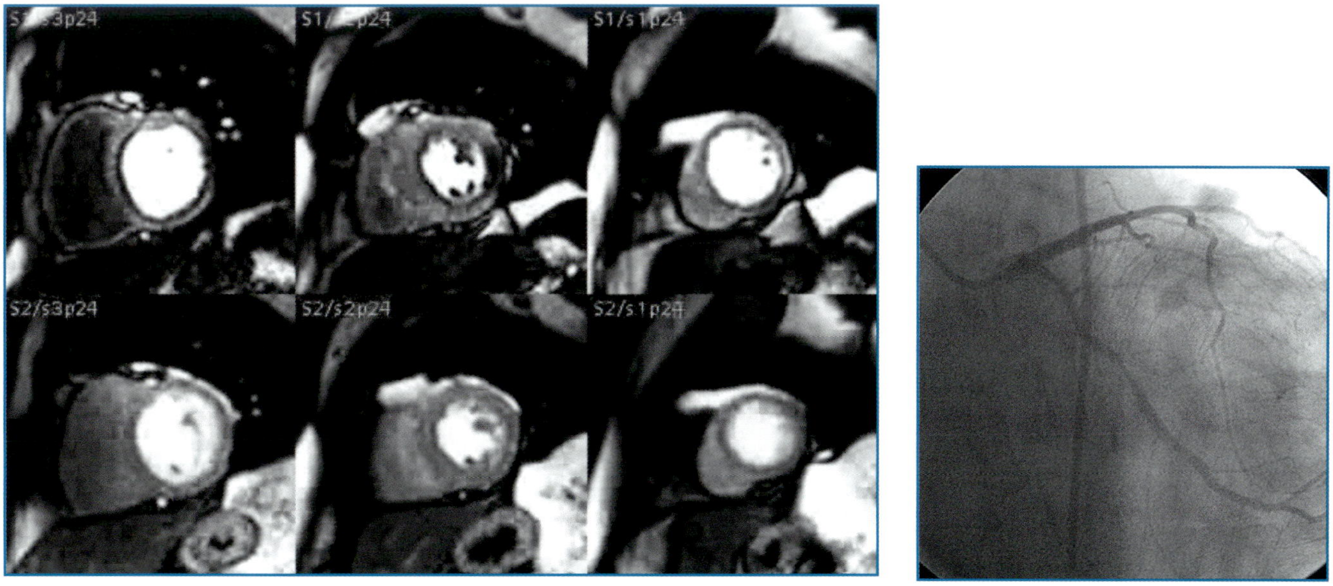

Figure 6-5 Abnormal first-pass perfusion study in a patient with a high grade stenosis of the LCx **(right)**; short-axis basal, medial, and apical slices with normal even perfusion of all segments at rest **(lower row left)**, and perfusion defect in the lateral segment of the left ventricular wall particularly within the medial slice **(top row)**.

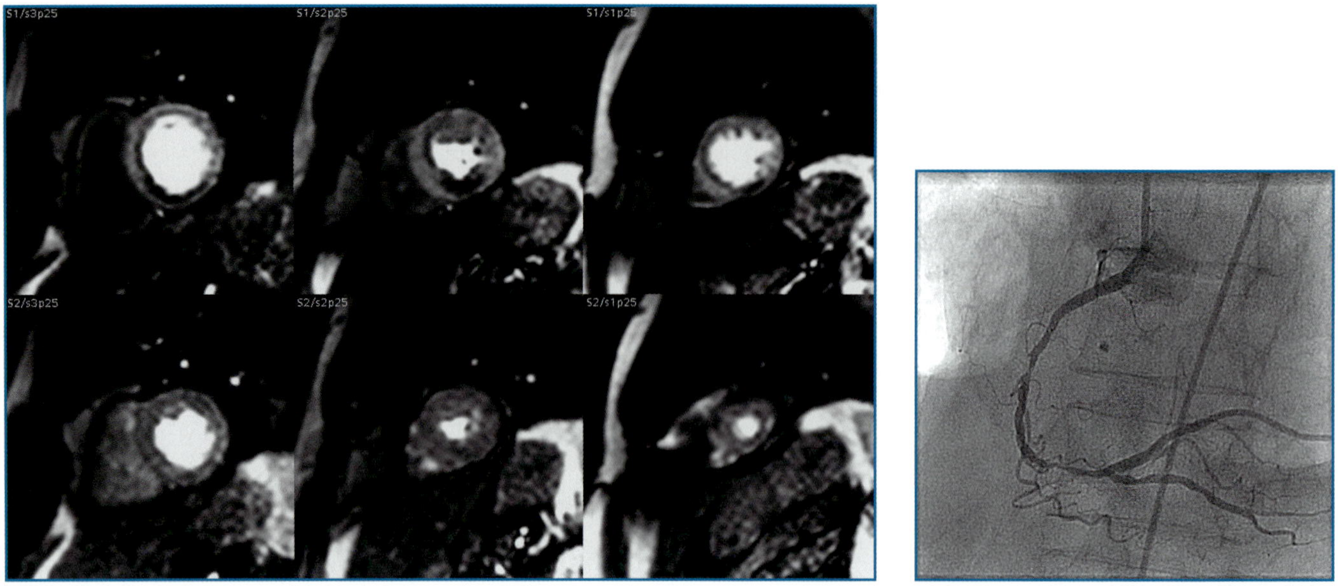

Figure 6-6 Abnormal first-pass perfusion study in a patient with a high grade stenosis of the RCA **(right)**; short-axis basal, medial, and apical slices with normal even perfusion of all segments at rest **(lower row left)**, and perfusion defect in the posterior and posteroseptal segment particularly in the medial but also in the basal slice **(top row)**.

Scan Protocol

The usual scan protocol is summarized as follows:

- scout/survey for determining heart position and optimizing coil positioning,
- reference scan if parallel imaging techniques are used,
- functional scans: SSFP sequences in short-axis and long-axis geometry (2-ch, 3-ch and 4-ch view) for detection of potential wall motion abnormalities,
- first-pass perfusion during adenosine induced hyperemia: adenosine is applied for at least 3 min with an injection rate of 140 µg/kg/min; for first-pass an extracellular contrast agent is applied at a dose of 0.05–0.1 mmol/kg body weight with an injection rate of at least 3 ml/s, flushed with 20 ml NaCl 0.9%; data acquisition should encompass 50–60 heart phases; at the start of data acquisition patients should be advised to hold their breath for native images without breathing motion as baseline data, if semiquantitative analysis is considered; as soon as the contrast is seen in the right ventricle, patients should be advised to hold their breath as long as possible to ensure consistent image geometry and avoid breathing artifacts throughout the contrast agents first-pass through the left ventricular myocardium; adenosine application can be stopped after completion of first pass image acquisition,
- resting period,
- to ensure complete recovery from adenosine effects and allow partial wash out of contrast agent, the resting period should be at least 10 min,
- perfusion scan at rest,
- first-pass perfusion under resting condition is performed using identical scan parameters and geometry and same contrast agent application protocol as with stress scan; direct comparison is advised to differentiate between real perfusion deficits and artifacts,
- late gadolinium enhancement (LGE) imaging,
- at least 10 min after acquisition of resting perfusion data, late gadolinium enhancement images are acquired to differentiate viable from infarcted myocardium.

Monitoring

Regular monitoring of the patients includes:

- continuous: symptoms, heart rate, rhythm, oxygen saturation,
- every minute: blood pressure.

Termination Criteria for Adenosine Stress Test

Absolute criteria for terminating an adenosine stress test are:

- bronchospasm,
- symptomatic hypotension,
- higher grade AV block,
- as an antidote i.v. aminophylline can be used with at a dose of 2–2,5 mg/kg body weight.

Image Analysis

Analysis of perfusion data can be performed visually by segmental assessment of changes in myocardial signal intensity during first-pass using the AHA segment model (a 16-segment model can be used, leaving out the apex). This is still the method of choice in clinical routine, since semiquantitative or quantitative methods remain time consuming. Visual assessment is highly observer dependent and prone to inter-reader variability and reduced reproducibility. Visual reading necessitates high experience with the scans used. Therefore, for better interobserver variability, clear and applicable reading criteria should be pre-defined. In particular, knowledge of possible artifacts is essential. Besides breathing-related motion and trigger artifacts due to premature beats or arrhythmias, dark subendocardial artifacts (i. e. susceptibility artifacts) resulting from rapid changes in magnetization at tissue borders of blood pool and subendocardium are still a challenging problem. The incidence of these artifacts depends on the imaging sequence, the type, and dosage of the contrast agent (CA) used. Dark rim artifacts can be differentiated from real perfusion defects by temporal analysis of first-pass perfusion images. Susceptibilities often diminish during the first few dynamics after CA arrival in the left ventricular cavity due to rapid decline of CA concentration in the blood pool during first-pass. In contrast, perfusion defects usually persist beyond the point of peak myocardial enhancement. A second aspect is that artifacts often appear circular in the subendocardial layer, whereas perfusion defects are restricted to coronary supply regions. It is notable that susceptibilities can also occur in rest perfusion scans. Concomitant appearance of subendocardial hypointensities in stress and rest perfusion images can provide valuable hints regarding the identification of artifacts. For semi-quantitative assessment of ischemia, perfusion-linked parameters such as time to peak signal, maximum signal intensity, signal upslope, and myocardial perfusion reserve index can be used.

Diagnostic Performance in the Detection of Relevant CAD

The diagnostic impact of CMR perfusion for detecting CAD is well-documented. In a recent meta-analysis, Nandalur et al. (2007) reviewed 24 datasets including 1,516 patients using perfusion imaging for the detection of relevant CAD, defined as stenoses of at least > 50 % on coronary angiography. Perfusion imaging demonstrated a sensitivity of 91 % and specificity of 81 % on a patient level with a disease prevalence of 57.4 %. The authors concluded that stress perfusion imaging yields an overall good sensitivity and specificity for the detection of CAD in patients with high disease prevalence. Since in most reports fast gradient echo or hybrid-EPI sequences for first-pass perfusion studies were used, data on the use of SSFP sequences is limited. We examined the largest cohort of 228 patients with suspected CAD or suspected progress of disease by using a SSFP sequence in combination with SENSE, a slice-selective saturation pulse, and a 3-slice coverage of the left ventricle. Sensitivity, specificity, and accuracy for detection of a coronary artery stenosis (> 50 % luminal narrowing) in the total patient group were 93.0, 85.7 and 91.2 %, and for a significant lesion (> 70 % luminal narrowing) 96.1, 72.0, 88.2 %, respectively; disease prevalence was 45 % in the group with suspected CAD and 100 % (i. e. known CAD) in the group with suspected restenosis or progression of CAD (Merkle 2007). We were also able to show that diagnostic accuracy of CMR-FPP is equally high in women compared with men: sensitivity, specificity, and accuracy 90.9, 90.6, and 90.8 % in women compared with 91.4, 74.4, and 87.7 % in men, respectively (Merkle 2010). Similar but slightly lower numbers (84, 88, and 87 %) have been published by Klem et al. (2008).

One challenging problem in interpreting and comparing data is the variety in design of perfusion sequences, contrast protocols and image analysis rendering data hardly comparable. Giang et al. (2004) reported data from three imaging centers. In 94 patients with known or suspected CAD, first-pass-perfusion was performed and was compared with results of invasive coronary angiography. Since the aim of the study was dose finding, patients were randomized to 0.05, 0.10, or 0.15 mmol/kg body weight of an extravascular CA (Gd-DTPA). A multi-slice hybrid-EPI with identical hardware and software in all centers was used during adenosine induced hyperemia, and data were analyzed semi-automatically. For CAD detection (> 50 % stenosis) the area under the receiver operator characteristics (ROC) curve for subendocardial perfusion defects was 0.91 and 0.86 for doses 2 and 3, respectively, with a significantly lower diagnostic performance for the lowest dose. It is notable that protocol violations resulted in 12 % drop outs. Another multi-center dose ranging study published by Wolff et al. (2004) reported different results for visual reading of a segmented EPI perfusion sequence in three imaging centers. In their study, no differences were seen for the three dose groups of 0.05, 0.10, or 0.15 mmol/kg body weight of Gd-DTPA for detection of a > 70 % stenosis.

Data on performance of CMR-FPP in patients with prior coronary bypass graft (CABG) surgery is limited, since these patients were excluded from most of the studies. In a recent study, Klein et al. (2009) found good diagnostic performance of a combined perfusion and late gadolinium enhancement protocol with high specificity. However, sensitivity was reduced compared with published data in patients without CABG. In a study by Bernhardt et al. (2009), diagnostic performance was lower in patients with prior CABG surgery as compared to patients with suspected CAD or patients with prior PCI. Sensitivity and specificity in CABG patients were 79 and 77 %, respectively. A possible reason for the lower sensitivity and specificity might be the complex flow and perfusion kinetics in the myocardium supplied by bypass grafts.

Combination of First-Pass Perfusion with Late Gadolinium Enhancement for the Detection of CAD

In a single center study in 100 consecutive patients scheduled for coronary angiography, Klem et al. (2006) showed a significantly better diagnostic performance of a combined perfusion and late gadolinium enhancement (LGE) protocol compared with stress and rest FPP alone. In this cohort with intermediate disease prevalence (40 % relevant CAD), the combination of perfusion and LGE had a sensitivity, specificity, and accuracy of 89, 87, and 88 %, respectively, for the diagnosis of relevant CAD (> 70 % stenosis), compared with 84, 58, and 68 %, respectively, for stress and rest perfusion alone. This result might be due the extremly high sensitivity and specificity of LGE for detection of even small infarcted myocardial tissue (Wagner 2003). The combination of perfusion and scar information can help to distinguish real perfusion defects from artifacts. This seems to be extremely helpful since image quality of perfusion scans remains still challenging. The combined protocol of FPP and LGE not only provides a better diagnostic performance in the detection of relevant CAD, but also a robust risk stratification for patients presenting with anginal symptoms. Steel et al. (2009) showed that identification of perfusion defects and the presence of LGE have a strong and complementary prognostic implication for cardiac death or acute myocardial infarction.

Comparison with Other Imaging Techniques

To overcome potential limitations of comparing a functional test with morphological data, testing of MRI perfusion against other functional diagnostic modalities is crucial. Watkins et al. (2009) compared CMR-based myocardial perfusion reserve index (MPRI) with invasively measured fractional flow reserve (FFR) in 103 patients. The sensitivity and specificity of MPRI for the detection of functionally significant coronary stenoses were 91 and 94 %, respectively, with positive and negative predictive values of 91 and 94 %. The authors concluded that MPRI can detect functionally significant coronary heart disease with excellent sensitivity, specificity, and positive and negative predictive values compared with FFR. Another study by Rieber et al. (2006) using MPRI reported a sensitivity of 88 % and a specificity of 90 % for detection of hemodynamically relevant stenoses as compared to FFR.

The diagnostic power of CMR stress perfusion imaging appears comparable if not superior to SPECT. In a meta-analysis, Underwood et al. (2004) reviewed 79 studies on 8,964 patients using SPECT in the diagnosis of CAD and found a sensitivity of 86 % and specificity of 74 %. Ishida et al. (2003) compared MR perfusion imaging and SPECT in 69 patients who also underwent conventional coronary angiography and found a significantly greater area under the ROC curve for MR perfusion imaging compared with SPECT. Sakuma et al. (2005) found superior but statistically insignificant diagnostic accuracy for MR perfusion imaging compared with SPECT in 40 patients. In 2008 the results of the largest multi-center trial was published by Schwitter et al. (2008). In a double-blind, multi-vendor study at 18 imaging centers, diagnostic efficiency of MRI first-pass perfusion in the detection of coronary stenoses > 50 % was evaluated against SPECT and coronary angiography. Overall, 234 patients with suspected CAD were randomly dosed with 0.01, 0.025, 0.05, 0.075, or 0.1 mmol/kg Gd-DTPA-BMA. Coronary artery disease (CAD) was defined as diameter stenosis > 50 % on quantitative CA. For first-pass stress and rest perfusion, a fast gradient echo sequence in combination with EPI read out (where available) was used with a 3 short-axis slice coverage of the left ventricle. The main finding of the study was that the highest contrast dose in visual reading of MRI perfusion data performed best. This study was limited by suboptimal SPECT results, which was in part due to a lack of gated SPECT data resulting in a poor specificity of SPECT. ROC analyses suggest CMR perfusion to be a valuable alternative to SPECT for detection of CAD, showing at least an equal performance in head-to-head comparison with gated SPECT techniques.

Microvascular Disease and Syndrome X

Panting et al. (2002) observed subendocardial hypoperfusion in patients with syndrome X following intravenous administration of adenosine that potentially represents an ischemic cause of chest pain. In our own study (Wöhrle 2006) we were able to show that an impaired myocardial MR perfusion reserve index is significantly correlated with a decrease in coronary blood flow reserve for endothelium-dependent (by intracoronary acetylcholine administration) and endothelium-independent (by intracoronary adenosine administration) stimulation. These findings are supported by a study by Yilmaz et al. (2009), which shows that patients with a reversible stress-induced perfusion defect had a pathological coronary epicardial or microvascular vasoreaction during intracoronary acetylcholine testing significantly more often than those without a perfusion defect. These findings suggest that myocardial hypoperfusion on MRI first-pass perfusion in patients without significant CAD may be the result of endothelial dysfunction in epicardial coronary arteries and/or coronary microvascular dysfunction, and may be the reason for a lower specificity of MRI first-pass perfusion in these patients.

Prognostic Implications

In patients with known or suspected CAD, stress myocardial perfusion imaging is important not only for detecting or excluding relevant CAD, but also for assessing prognosis. Jahnke et al. (2007) evaluated the prognostic value of MRI first-pass perfusion in 533 patients with chest pain or dyspnea and suspected coronary artery disease. Over a median follow-up of 2.3 yrs, ischemia by CMR perfusion was found to be the single best predictor of cardiac death or nonfatal myocardial infarction and was superior to ischemia on dobutamine stress CMR. The presence of a normal perfusion test was predictive of 99 % for a 3 yrs event-free survival. Pilz et al. (2008) followed 218 patients with suspected CAD and a negative MR perfusion test. The 12-mths MACE rate was 2/218 with no cardiac death or myocardial infarction, and the negative predictive value of a negative MR first-pass perfusion was 99.1 %. The authors concluded that a negative first-pass perfusion result may reduce the number of redundant coronary angiographies.

6.6.4 Assessment of Myocardial Viability

In the last decade, late gadolinium enhancement (LGE) as a correlate of contrast agent deposition in fibrotic or scarred tissue has been increasingly used for the detection and characterization of myocardial infarction and myocardial fibrosis. Altered contrast kinetics and increased distribution volume from the enlarged interstitium result in a high gadolinium concentration within abnormal myocardium, which appears bright on T1-weighted inversion recovery MR images. Signal intensities in regions with LGE are shown to be 485 % higher than in normal regions. The LGE technique has shown an excellent correlation with histopathological acute and chronic infarctions in animal models (Kim 1999). Due to the high spatial resolution and high contrast to normal myocardium, LGE proved to be superior to radionuclide imaging in the detection of even small subendocardial infarctions. Another advantage is its excellent interobserver and longitudinal reproducibility, allowing the reduction of sample size in dedicated viability studies.

LGE Sequences

LGE MRI is usually acquired by a 2D or 3D segmented k-space gradient echo sequence prepared with an inversion recovery prepulse to null signal intensity of normal myocardium after administration of gadolinium-based contrast media. The conventional 2D gradient-echo approach provides excellent delineation of myocardial scar, but it is time-consuming for adequate SNR and resolution. Repeated breath-holds are required to cover the entire heart, since scan duration ranges from 8–12 s per slice. Another approach may be the use of three-dimensional (3D) IR gradient sequences allowing rapid acquisition of 3D images that cover the LV within one breath-hold (Kuhl 2004). If patients are not able to maintain breath-hold for the necessary length, respiratory navigator-based scans can be combined with LGE imaging sequences.

Image acquisition is performed in breath-hold technique and triggered to mid- or end-diastole to minimize motion artifacts. Acquistion time should be below 200 ms to avoid blurring artifacts due to shorter myocardial resting periods. In the case of tachycardia, scan parameters should be modified for even shorter acquisition times. There are some issues to be kept in mind. Image quality is limited by the optimal balance of SNR and spatial and temporal resolution. In-plane resolution of the LGE images is typically 1.4–1.8 mm × 1.4–1.8 mm, with a slice thickness of 6–8 mm to guarantee optimal assessment of transmurality and to avoid partial volume effects. As contrast agent, gadolinium chelates are used at doses of 0.1–0.2 mmol/kg in most clinical scenarios. In our center a dose of 0.2 mmol/kg gadolinium-DTPA or gadolinium-DOTA is used. LGE images are acquired at least 10 min after intravenous contrast application to allow the wash out of contrast in blood pool, thus ensuring maximum signal differences in blood pool, normal, and infarcted myocardium. When lower doses are used, the delay may be shorter due to faster increase of blood pool signal. If the delay is too short, the high signal intensity of blood may impair the differentiation of small subendocardial infarcts from blood filled cavity. This issue may be negligible in clinical routine but be critical in quantitative LGE studies. It has been shown that LGE imaging is still possible 40 min after contrast application without significant changes in measured infarct size (Marholdt 2002).

The most critical parameter in LGE imaging is accurate adjustment of inversion time. By applying a 180° inversion, pulse magnetization of tissue is reversed. Due to the variable T1 in the blood pool, normal and scarred myocardium relaxation times for each tissue are different. In principle, image acquisition should be done at the point when the net magnetization of relaxing normal myocardium is zero. As a visible result, the signal of normal myocardium is nulled, and differences between signal intensities of scar tissue and intact myocardium are maximal. An inappropriate choice of inversion time leads to decreased signal differences in both tissues. If the inversion time is set too short, the signal of normal myocardium increases while the signal of scar decreases. Ultimately this may lead to equal signal intensities rendering the identification of scar impossible. If the inversion time is set too long, the signal of both tissues is increasing and thus, relative signal difference is decreasing. Both inappropriate inversion times can increase the variation in apparent infarct size. The inversion time is also dependent on the dose of contrast agents and on heart rate. With lower doses of contrast agents, longer inversion times are needed. With normal heart rates, data acquisition is performed every second heart beat to ensure full longitudinal relaxation before applying the next prepulse. In the case of severe bradycardia, imaging every heartbeat is appropriate, whereas with tachycardia, acquisition should be done every second heart beat. The optimal inversion time can be easily determined using a Look-Locker sequence before acquisition of the LGE images (Messroghli 2004). Using this approach, multiple images with different TI times are acquired during a single breath-hold. A phase-sensitive inversion recovery (PSIR) method is another approach that can simplify the choice of correct inversion times. Phase sensitive reconstruction allows imaging across a broad range of inversion times while maintaining good contrast between the infarcted and normal myocardium (Kellman 2002).

Scan Protocol

LGE imaging should be performed in patients with suspected or known CAD, since it may provide additional valuable information regarding the diagnosis and prognosis of CAD.

Essentials of the protocol are:

- for best image quality, the optimal time point of image acquisition is at least 10 min after gadolinium injection; the optimal dose is 0.2 mmol/kg; the delay may be shorter than 10 min if lower doses are used,
- 2D or 3D segmented inversion recovery GRE sequences are used during mid- or end-diastole,
- same views should be applied as for cine imaging (short- and long-axis views),
- slice thickness should be the same as for cine imaging,
- when combining LGE and perfusion scans, LGE image and perfusion geometry should be identical,
- acquisition duration per R-R interval should be lower than 200 ms,
- inversion time is set to null normal myocardium by using a Look-Locker approach; alternatively fixed TI with a phase-sensitive sequence may be used.

Image Analysis

Most commonly, in a clinical setting LGE images are visually assessed using the 17-segment model (Cerqueira 2002). This seems to be appropriate due to the excellent agreement of LGE transmurality judged by visual and quantitative analyses (Schuijf 2004). However, in some instances, e.g. for study purposes, quantification of LGE mass and transmurality may be needed. Most commercial software platforms offer threshold-based LGE quantification tools. After segmentation of endocardial and epicardial myocardial borders, scarring by LGE is defined as image intensities of least > 2 standard deviations (SD) above the mean of image intensities in a remote myocardial region in the same image (Mahrholdt 2002). Alternatively, the "full width half maximum technique" may be used. After measuring the peak LGE signal in the images, scarred myocardium is identified as having signal > 50 % of the peak LGE signal (Amado 2004). However, quantification methods or models have only been validated by post-mortem animal studies. In a recent study in patients before and after coronary revascularisation, different quantification methods were compared to functional outcome in patients with CAD. These various methods showed a strong influence on total and regional infarct size. Best prediction for functional recovery was obtained by applying a > 6 SD threshold, but differences were small and insignificant (Beek 2009). To offer a standardised proceeding, a threshold approach using > 2 SD is favored by the guidelines of the SCMR (Hundley 2009).

Detection of Chronic Myocardial Scar

In numerous animal and in vivo studies, LEG has shown its diagnostic potential and superiority to other imaging techniques to detect even minimal scarring. Kim et al. (1999) in a chronic infarct dog model showed a perfect agreement between the extent of scar tissue on LGE and the histological extent of necrosis using triphenyltetrazolium chloride (TTC) staining. In another animal study CMR imaging using LGE detected 92 % of segments with subendocardial infarction as compared to 28 % with SPECT. This result was transferred into a clinical setting. In 91 patients with CAD, SPECT missed 48 % of subendocardial infarctions as detected by LGE MRI (Wagner 2003). In another study Klein and colleagues (2002) evaluated the diagnostic performance of FDG-PET and CMR-based LGE in a clinical setting. The agreement between both techniques for assessing scar tissue was 91 %. However, 11 % of segments assessed viable on FDG-PET had some extent of scar tissue on contrast-enhanced CMR.

> These data reflect the superior resolution of CMR imaging allowing the discrimination of small subendocardial infarcts in vivo.

Prognostic Implications

Viability and Functional Recovery by LGE

Since the high spatial resolution allows assessment of the transmural extent of infarction, several studies have shown the potential of this technique in prediction of functional recovery in chronic CAD after revascularisation. In a landmark paper, Kim et al. (1999) have shown that the likelihood of segmental functional recovery is paralleled by the transmurality of scarring. In their study, 78% of dysfunctional segments without contrast enhancement improved in function, as compared to 2% of segments with scar tissue extending 75% of the LV wall. Using a cut-off value of 25% transmurality of scar tissue, the sensitivity and specificity were 86% and 61% to predict improvement of function. Changing the cut-off value to 75% transmurality, sensitivity and specificity would be 100 and 15%, respectively. Intermediate extents of infarction (25–50%) showed an intermediate likelihood of recovery. These results were confirmed by another study in a cohort of patients with chronic CAD after surgical revascularisation by Selvanayagam et al. (2004). Furthermore they showed that diagnostic accuracy in predicting functional recovery was best for regions with severe dysfunction.

Low-Dose Dobutamine

In all studies testing transmurality of LGE as a surrogate for functional recovery, the lower values for sensitivity are remarkable. This fact indicates that the presence of viable myocardium will not inevitably predict improved function. A possible reason for this might be the variable functional state of viable myocardium, since the tissue surrounding the scar may be normal, remodeled, or ischemic. Therefore, low-dose dobutamine stress can give valuable information on functional recovery by detecting the contractile reserve (Baer 1998). Dobutamine simulates effects of revascularization by improving contractile function, cellular energetics in hypoperfused myocardium, and perfusion by collaterals or dynamic stenoses. As in echocardiography, CMR assessment of contractile reserve is performed using the infusion of low doses of dobutamine (5–20 µg/kg/min). Several studies have shown that low-dose dobutamine in CMR imaging is superior to LGE in predicting functional recovery. Bove et al. (2006) reported a superior specificity for dobutamine stress CMR in 15 patients undergoing surgical revascularisation. In 29 patients undergoing revascularization, Wellnhofer et al. (2004) demonstrated a higher sensitivity for LGE, but a higher specificity for low-dose dobutamine stress CMR to predict functional recovery. This advantage seems to be largest in segments with an infarction transmurality of 1–74%. Similar results were reported by Kaandorp et al. (2004).

Some controversy exists as to which test performs best for predicting functional recovery among CMR-based techniques. LGE has a high sensitivity in prediction of functional recovery. In contrast, low-dose dobutamine has a significantly higher specifitiy. A complementary use of dobutamine CMR and LGE may prove to be the optimal strategy for predicting post-revascularization functional recovery in patients with intermediate infarct transmurality (LGE 25–75% transmurality), since the information is redundant in small subendocardial infarcts (LGE $<$ 20% transmurality) and transmural infarcts (LGE $>$ 75% transmurality). Nevertheless, a combination of both modalities can provide valuable prognostic information in patients with medically treated CAD. Kelle et al. (2009b) recently showed that overall LGE is a stronger predictor of clinical outcome than contractile reserve. However, in medically treated patients with large myocardial scars, the presence of contractile reserve is more important for the prediction of events than scar tissue. There also seems to be a benefit beyond measurable functional improvement, since clinical outcome may be related to positive effects on adverse remodeling, improved contractile response under stress, prevention of recurrent myocardial ischemia/infarction, and prevention of arrhythmias (Kim 2004).

Prognostic Significance of Unrecognized Myocardial Scarring/Infarction (UMI)

Furthermore, there is some data indicating that LGE imaging can reveal previously unknown myocardial infarction (Meijs 2009) and that presence of LGE has a strong prognostic impact. Unrecognized myocardial scarring is more frequent than expected. In a population-based study in Sweden including 259 randomly selected individuals aged 70-years, LGE indicating scarring was detected in 19.8% of the subjects without a history of myocardial infarction (Barbier 2006). The prevalence of unrecognized myocardial scarring seems to be increased in patients with higher cardiovascular risk. In a study by Kwong et al (2006), LGE was present in 44 of 195 patients with suspected CAD but without known prior myocardial infarction. The authors could show that the presence of even small amounts of LGE indicates a high risk and provides incremental prognostic value for MACE and cardiac mortality beyond common clinical, angiographic, and functional predictors. In another study the same group found similar results in diabetic patients without known prior infarction (Kwong 2008). The presence of LGE as a sign of previous coronary events was the strongest predictor for an adverse cardiac outcome.

In our opinion these findings strongly support the use of LGE imaging in patients with suspected CAD for improving risk assessment.

6.7 Conclusions

Over the last decade, CMR imaging has become an increasingly accepted and valuable tool for the diagnosis and risk assessment of patients with known or suspected CAD. One indication for using CMR imaging is the detection of impaired left ventricular global and regional function. The patient-independent high image quality of CMR and low intra- and interobserver variability are extremely relevant in patients with technically limited echocardiograms, and in the course of clinical studies. To detect functionally relevant coronary stenoses, adenosine perfusion CMR or high-dose dobutamine CMR show excellent diagnostic performance compared with other non-invasive techniques. CMR is of great value as a second test in symptomatic patients with intermediate to high pre-test probability of CAD and ambiguous stress ECG. In our center, stress CMR is performed as a first test in patients without known CAD, who are unable to perform physical exercise, and in patients with uninterpretable stress ECGs. There is no data on the screening of asymptomatic patients. The detection of myocardial ischemia by adenosine CMR has a very high sensitivity, and high negative predictive value for detection of relevant CAD (Merkle 2007, Costa 2007), and some data exists for excellent mid to long term prognosis in patients with a negative adenosine CMR test. One may speculate that adenosine CMR may be used as a first line in patients with suspected CAD. In contrast, in patients with known CAD the use of dobutamine CMR may be preferable because of its higher specificity. In asymptomatic patients with a known history of CAD, indication for stress CMR as a pre-invasive test depends on the severity of CAD. With respect to prognosis, stress CMR may be useful in this scenario in patients with 3-vessel disease, left main and proximal LAD stenoses. Alternatively, stress CMR can be performed to evaluate the functional relevance of borderline stenoses seen on coronary angiograms. In symptomatic patients following coronary revascularization, stress CMR can provide valuable information on the presence and location of ischemia. However, significance and therapeutic implications of CMR stress testing remain critical in patients with large myocardial scarring and multiple coronary bypass grafts.

LGE imaging should be performed in every patient with suspected or known CAD, because its detection is fast, stable and reproducible. Additional imaging of LGE strengthens the pre-interventional diagnostic accuracy of the stress test, provides additional prognostic information, and supports differential diagnosis. Furthermore, analysis of LGE transmurality provides valuable information on potential functional recovery of dysfunctional myocardium after revascularisation. In cases of intermediate LGE transmurality and the need for complex revascularisation strategies adding a low-dose dobutamine protocol for evaluation of functional reserve may be considered. Another rationale for the use of LGE is differentiation between ischemic cardiomyopathy and non-ischemic myocardial disorders, e.g. dilatative cardiomyopathy or myocarditis. However, beneficial use of CMRI in patients with suspected or known CAD strongly depends on the availability of adequate technology and the users experience in image acquisition and analysis.

6.8 Future Perspectives

CMR has been the subject of technological advances during recent years, including ongoing evolution of both hardware (high-field imaging, faster gradients, multi-channel receiver coils) and software (data acquisition and reconstruction), resulting in higher SNR and improved temporal and spatial resolution. In terms of cost effectiveness, scan times for many CMR methods continue to be shortened allowing more patients to be evaluated in a given period of time. With regard to CMR, in stress and viability testing improvement of temporal resolution may be adopted for 4D-whole heart imaging in functional or stress scans (Jahnke 2006, Hamdan 2008). Higher resolution at 3 T-CMR is supposed to reduce imaging artifacts in perfusion scans and has shown a higher diagnostic accuracy compared with 1.5 T-CMR perfusion imaging (Plein 2008). In a further study, similar results were reported, i.e. diagnostic performance of 3 T perfusion imaging was significantly better than at 1.5 T in identifying both single- and multi-vessel disease. The conclusion was that 3 T may become the preferred CMR field strength for myocardial perfusion assessment in clinical practice (Cheng 2007).

Besides the conventional approach of using contrast media for perfusion CMR there are promising new techniques to examine myocardial perfusion and oxygenation. Arterial spin-labeling (ASL) and blood oxygen level-dependent (BOLD) imaging have shown some potential for quantifying myocardial blood flow and myocardial oxygen consumption. ASL utilizes arterial water as an endogenous tracer and can be measured through changes in myocardial and blood T1 (Zhang 2005). ASL imaging is prone to low SNR that impairs image quality. Use of this technique in a 3 T environment may be beneficial due to the higher SNR and the intrinsic longer T1 relaxation times in higher magnetic fields (Northrup 2008). In contrast, BOLD imaging utilizes changes in hemoglobin oxygenation. Whereas oxygenated hemoglobin is slightly diamagnetic, deoxygenated hemoglobin is paramagnetic and causes a signal loss in T2*- or T2-weighted images (Fieno 2004, McCommis 2010, Karamitsos 2010). ASL and BOLD imaging have been applied in both animal and clinical studies, and showed good correlation with positron emission tomography (PET). Yet both techniques are still at an early experimental stage and not ready for routine clinical use.

Improved spatial resolution may result in further improvement in detecting myocardial scarring. Imaging of changes in myocardial microstructure is another promising development. Preliminary results reveal the use of diffusion-tensor CMR and diffusion-spectrum CMR tractography in assessing tissue integrity and fiber architecture in patients with myocardial infarction. These studies demonstrated both microstructural changes in the infarction zone, and microstructural improvement associated with improvement of wall thickening and macrostructure after myocardial infarction. This may be helpful in providing insight into the structural mechanism of infarcted tissue and remodeling of the myocardium after myocardial infarction (Wu 2006, Sosnovik 2009, Wu 2009).

In addition, recent developments focus on molecular CMR imaging. Targeted molecular imaging of the myocardium requires the imaging agent to be small (< 50 nm), sensitive (nanomolar to picomolar levels), and to diffuse into the interstitial space. Novel gadolinium constructs and very small iron-oxide-based magnetic nanoparticles (MNP) seem to meet these requirements, and have shown the potential to assess myocardial alterations on a molecular level. Contrast agent labeled antibodies against antimyosin and annexin and MNP phagocyted by macrophages have shown potential in imaging cardiomyocyte necrosis and apoptosis as well as macrophage infiltration into damaged myocardium in ex vivo and in vivo animal studies. The role of targeted molecular imaging in the myocardium is thus likely to further evolve in both research and clinical settings, and will be translated into patient examinations within the next years (Sosnovik 2008).

References

Amado LC, Gerber BL, Gupta SN et al. Accurate and objective infarct sizing by contrast-enhanced magnetic resonance imaging in a canine myocardial infarction model. J Am Coll Cardiol 2004; 44: 2383–9.

Baer FM, Theissen P, Schneider CA et al. Dobutamine magnetic resonance imaging predicts contractile recovery of chronically dysfunctional myocardium after successful revascularization. J Am Coll Cardiol 1998; 31: 1040–8.

Barbier CE, Bjerner T, Johansson L et al. Myocardial scars more frequent than expected: magnetic resonance imaging detects potential risk group. J Am Coll Cardiol 2006; 48: 765–71.

Beek AM, Bondarenko O, Afsharzada F, van Rossum AC. Quantification of late gadolinium-enhanced CMR in viability assessment in chronic ischemic heart disease: a comparison to functional outcome. J Cardiovasc Magn Reson 2009; 11 (1): 6.

Bernhardt P, Spiess J, Levenson B et al. Combined assessment of myocardial perfusion and late gadolinium enhancement in patients after percutaneous coronary intervention or bypass grafts: a multi-center study of an integrated cardiovascular magnetic resonance protocol. JACC Cardiovasc Imaging 2009; 2: 1292–300.

Bodi V, Sanchis J, Lopez-Lereu MP et al. Prognostic and therapeutic implications of dipyridamole stress cardiovascular magnetic resonance on the basis of the ischemic cascade. Heart 2009; 95 (1): 49–55.

Bodi V, Sanchis J, Lopez-Lereu MP et al. Prognostic value of dipyridamole stress cardiovascular magnetic resonance imaging in patients with known or suspected coronary artery disease. J Am Coll Cardiol 2007; 50 (12): 1174–9.

Bolli R, Marban E. Molecular and cellular mechanisms of myocardial stunning. Physiol Rev 1999; 79: 609–15.

Bove CM, DiMaria JM, Voros S et al. Dobutamine response and myocardial infarct transmurality: Functional improvement after coronary artery bypass grafting – initial experience. Radiology 2006; 240: 835–41.

Burgstahler C, Kunze M, Gawaz M et al. Adenosine stress first-pass perfusion for the detection of coronary artery disease in patients with aortic stenosis: a feasibility study. Int J Cardiovasc Imaging 2008; 24: 195–200.

Canty Jr JM. Coronary Blood Flow and Myocardial Ischemia. In: Braunwald's Heart Disease. A Textbook of Cardiovascular Medicine. Bonow RO, Mann DL, Zipes DP, Libby P (eds). Philadelphia, London, Toronto, Montreal, Sydney, Tokyo: WB Saunders 2012; 1049–75.

Cerqueira MD, Weissman NJ, Dilsizian V et al. Standardized myocardial segmentation and nomenclature for tomographic imaging of the heart: a statement for healthcare professional from the Cardiac Imaging Committee of the Council on Clinical Cardiology of the American Heart Association. Circulation 2002, 105: 539–42.

Cheng AS, Pegg TJ, Karamitsos TD et al. Cardiovascular magnetic resonance perfusion imaging at 3-T for the detection of coronary artery disease: a comparison with 1.5-T. J Am Coll Cardiol 2007; 49 (25): 2440–9.

Cheng AS, Selvanayagam JB, Jerosch-Herold M et al. Percutaneous treatment of chronic total coronary occlusions improves regional hyperemic myocardial blood flow and contractility: insights from quantitative cardiovascular magnetic resonance imaging. JACC Cardiovasc Interv 2008; 1 (1): 44–53.

Costa MA, Shoemaker S, Futamatsu H et al. Quantitative magnetic resonance perfusion imaging detects anatomic and physiologic coronary artery disease as measured by coronary angiography and fractional flow reserve. J Am Coll Cardiol 2007; 50 (6): 514–22.

Doesch C, Seeger A, Doering J et al. Risk stratification by adenosine stress cardiac magnetic resonance in patients with coronary artery stenoses of intermediate angiographic severity. JACC Cardiovasc Imaging 2009; 2 (4): 424–33.

Favallvollita JA, Perry PJ, Canty Jr. JM. 18F-2-deoxyglucose deposition and regional flow in pigs with chronically dysfunctional myocardium: Evidence for transmural variations in chronic hibernating myocardium. Circulation 1997; 95: 1900–7.

Fieno DS, Shea SM, Li Y et al. Myocardial perfusion imaging based on the blood oxygen level-dependent effect using T2-prepared steady-state free precession magnetic resonance imaging. Circulation 2004; 110: 1284–90.

Gerber BL, Raman SV, Nayak K et al. Myocardial first-pass perfusion cardiovascular magnetic resonance: history, theory, and current state of the art. J Cardiovasc Magn Reson 2008; 10 (1): 18.

Giang TH, Nanz D, Coulden R et al. Detection of coronary artery disease by magnetic resonance myocardial perfusion imaging with various contrast medium doses: first European multicentre experience. Eur Heart J 2004; 25 (18): 1657–65.

Gold KL, Lipscomb K. Effects of coronary stenoses on coronary flow reserve. Am J Cardiol 1974; 34: 48–55.

Graham I, Atzar D, Borch-Johnsen K et al. European guidelines on cardiovascular disease prevention in clinical practice: executive summary. Eur J Cardiovasc Prev 2007; 14 (Suppl 2): E1–E40.

Hamdan A, Kelle S, Schnackenburg B et al. Single-breathhold four-dimensional assessment of left ventricular volumes and function using k-t BLAST after application of extracellular contrast agent at 3 T. J Magn Reson Imaging 2008; 27 (5): 1028–36.

Hundley WG, Bluemke D, Bogaert JG et al. Society for Cardiovascular Magnetic Resonance guidelines for reporting cardiovascular magnetic resonance examinations. J Cardiovasc Magn Reson 2009; 11 (1): 5.

Hundley WG, Hamilton CA, Thomas MS et al. Utility of fast cine magnetic resonance imaging and display for the detection of myocardial ischemia in patients not well suited for second harmonic stress echocardiography. Circulation 1999; 100: 1697–702.

Ingkanisorn WP, Kwong RY, Bohme NS et al. Prognosis of negative adenosine stress magnetic resonance in patients presenting to an emergency department with chest pain. J Am Coll Cardiol 2006; 47 (7): 1427–32.

Ishida N, Sakuma H, Motoyasu M et al. Noninfarcted myocardium: correlation between dynamic first-pass contrast-enhanced myocardial MR imaging and quantitative coronary angiography. Radiology 2003; 229: 209–16.

Jahnke C, Nagel E, Gebker R et al. Prognostic value of cardiac magnetic resonance stress tests: adenosine stress perfusion and dobutamine stress wall motion imaging. Circulation 2007; 115 (13): 1769–76.

Jahnke C, Paetsch I, Gebker R et al. Accelerated 4D dobutamine stress MR imaging with k-t BLAST: feasibility and diagnostic performance. Radiology 2006; 3: 718–28.

Kaandorp TA, Bax JJ, Schuijf JD et al. Head-to-head comparison between contrast-enhanced magnetic resonance imaging and dobutamine magnetic resonance imaging in men with ischemic cardiomyopathy. Am J Cardiol 2004; 93 (12): 1461–4.

Kaandorp TA, Lamb HJ, van der Wall EE et al. Cardiovascular MR to assess myocardial viability in chronic ischemic LV dysfunction. Heart 2005; 91 (10): 1359–65.

Karamitsos TD, Arnold JR, Pegg TJ et al. Tolerance and safety of adenosine stress perfusion cardiovascular magnetic resonance imaging in patients with severe coronary artery disease. Int J Cardiovasc Imaging 2009; 25 (3): 277–83.

Karamitsos TD, Leccisotti L, Arnold JR et al. Relationship between regional myocardial oxygenation and perfusion in patients with coronary artery disease: insights from cardiovascular magnetic resonance and positron emission tomography. Circ Cardiovasc Imaging 2010; 3 (1): 32–40.

Kelle S, Egnell C, Vierecke J et al. Prognostic value of negative dobutamine-stress cardiac magnetic resonance imaging. Med Sci Monit 2009a; 15 (10): 131–6.

Kelle S, Roes SD, Klein C et al. Prognostic value of myocardial infarct size and contractile reserve using magnetic resonance imaging. J Am Coll Cardiol 2009b; 54 (19): 1770–7.

Kellman P, Arai AE, McVeigh ER, Aletras AH. Phase-sensitive inversion recovery for detecting myocardial infarction using gadolinium-delayed hyperenhancement. Magn Reson Med 2002; 47: 372–83.

Kim HW, Klem I, Shah DJ et al. Unrecognized non-Q-wave myocardial infarction: prevalence and prognostic significance in patients with suspected coronary disease. PLoS Med 2009; 6 (4): e1000057.

Kim RJ, Fieno DS, Parrish TB et al. Relationship of MRI delayed contrast enhancement to irreversible injury, infarct age, and contractile function. Circulation 1999; 100: 1992–2002.

Kim RJ, Manning WJ. Viability assessment by delayed enhancement cardiovascular magnetic resonance: will low-dose dobutamine dull the shine? Circulation 2004; 109 (21): 2476–9.

Klein C, Nagel E, Gebker R et al. Magnetic resonance adenosine perfusion imaging in patients after coronary artery bypass graft surgery. JACC Cardiovasc Imaging 2009; 2: 437–45.

Klein C, Nakolla SG, Bengel FM et al. Assessment of myocardial viability with contrast-enhanced magnetic resonance imaging: comparison with positron emission tomography. Circulation 2002; 105: 162–7.

Klem I, Greulich S, Heitner JF et al. Value of cardiovascular magnetic resonance stress perfusion testing for the detection of coronary artery disease in women. JACC Cardiovasc Imaging 2008; 1: 436–45.

Klem I, Heitner JF, Shah DJ et al. Improved detection of coronary artery disease by stress perfusion cardiovascular magnetic resonance with the use of delayed enhancement infarction imaging. J Am Coll Cardiol 2006; 47: 1630–8.

Kloner RA, Jennings RB. Consequences of brief ischemia: Stunning, preconditioning, and their clinical implications. Part 2. Circulation 2001; 104: 3158–64.

Kuhl HP, Papavasiliu TS, Beek AM et al. Myocardial viability: Rapid assessment with delayed contrast-enhanced MR imaging with three-dimensional inversion recovery prepared pulse sequence. Radiology 2004; 230: 576–82.

Kwon DH, Halley CM, Carrigan TP et al. Extent of left ventricular scar predicts outcomes in ischemic cardiomyopathy patients with significantly reduced systolic function: a delayed hyperenhancement cardiac magnetic resonance study. JACC Cardiovasc Imaging 2009; 2 (1): 34–44.

Kwong RY, Chan AK, Brown KA et al. Impact of unrecognized myocardial scar detected by cardiac magnetic resonance imaging on event-free survival in patients presenting with signs or symptoms of coronary artery disease. Circulation 2006; 113 (23): 2733–43.

Kwong RY, Sattar H, Wu H et al. Incidence and prognostic implication of unrecognized myocardial scar characterized by cardiac magnetic resonance in diabetic patients without clinical evidence of myocardial infarction. Circulation 2008; 118 (10): 1011–20.

Ling LH et al. Atropine augmentation in dobutamine stress echocardiography: role and incremental value in a clinical practice setting. J Am Coll Cardiol 1996; 28 (3): 551–7.

Mahrholdt H, Wagner A, Holly TA et al. Reproducibility of chronic infarct size measurement by contrast-enhanced magnetic resonance imaging. Circulation 2002; 106: 2322–7.

Marcu CB, Versteeg KS, Beek AM, Van Rossum AC. Prognostic value of delayed gadolinium enhancement MRI in patients with ischemic cardiomyopathy. Conn Med 2009; 73 (4): 197–203.

McCommis KS, Goldstein TA, Abendschein DR et al. Quantification of regional myocardial oxygenation by magnetic resonance imaging: validation with positron emission tomography. Circ Cardiovasc Imaging 2010; 3 (1): 41–6.

Meijs MF, Bots ML, Cramer MJ et al. for the SMART Study group. Unrecognised myocardial infarction in subjects at high vascular risk: prevalence and determinants. Heart 2009; 95 (9): 728–32.

Merkle N, Wöhrle J, Grebe O et al. Assessment of myocardial perfusion for detection of coronary artery stenoses by steady-state, free precession magnetic resonance first-pass imaging. Heart 2007; 93: 1381–5.

Merkle N, Wöhrle J, Nusser T et al. Diagnostic performance of magnetic resonance first-pass perfusion imaging is equally potent in female compared with male patients with coronary artery disease. Clin Res Cardiol 2010; 99: 21–8.

Messroghli DR, Radjenovic A, Kozerke S et al. Modified Look-Locker inversion recovery (MOLLI) for high-resolution T1 mapping of the heart. Magn Reson Med 2004; 52: 141–6.

Nagel E, Lorenz C, Baer F et al. Stress cardiovascular magnetic resonance: consensus panel report. J Cardiovasc Magn Reson 2001; 3 (3): 267–81.

Nagel E, Klein C, Paetsch I et al. Magnetic resonance perfusion measurements for the non-invasive detection of coronary artery disease. Circulation 2003; 108: 432–7.

Nagel E, Lehmkuhl HB, Boksch W et al. Non-invasive diagnosis of ischemia-induced wall motion abnormalities with the use of high-dose dobutamine stress MRI: comparison with dobutamine stress echocardiography. Circulation 1999; 99: 763–70.

Nandalur KR, Dwamena BA, Choudh AF et al. Diagnostic performance of stress cardiac magnetic resonance imaging in the detection of coronary artery disease: a meta-analysis. J Am Coll Cardiol 2007; 50: 1343–53.

Northrup BE, McCommis KS, Zhang H et al. Resting myocardial perfusion quantification with CMR arterial spin labeling at 1.5 T and 3.0 T. J Cardiovasc Magn Reson 2008; 10 (1): 53.

Panting JR, Gatehouse PD, Yang GZ et al. Abnormal subendocardial perfusion in cardiac syndrome X detected by cardiovascular magnetic resonance imaging. N Engl J Med 2002; 346: 1948–53.

Pilz G, Jeske A, Klos M et al. Prognostic value of normal adenosine-stress cardiac magnetic resonance imaging. Am J Cardiol 2008; 101 (10): 1408–12.

Plein S, Schwitter J, Suerder D et al. K-Space and time sensitivity encoding-accelerated myocardial perfusion MR imaging at 3.0 T: comparison with 1.5 T. Radiology 2008; 249 (2): 493–500.

Rerkpattanapipat P, Morgan TM, Neagle CM et al. Assessment of pre-operative cardiac risk with magnetic resonance imaging. Am J Cardiol 2002; 90: 416–9.

Rieber J, Huber A, Erhard I et al. Cardiac magnetic resonance perfusion imaging for the functional assessment of coronary artery disease: a comparison with coronary angiography and fractional flow reserve. Eur Heart J 2006; 27 (12): 1465–71.

Sakuma H, Suzawa N, Ichikawa Y et al. Diagnostic accuracy of stress first-pass contrast-enhanced myocardial perfusion MRI compared with stress myocardial perfusion scintigraphy. Am J Roentgenol 2005; 185: 95–102.

Schuijf JD, Kaandorp TA, Lamb HJ et al. Quantification of myocardial infarct size and transmurality by contrast-enhanced magnetic resonance imaging in men. Am J Cardiol 2004; 94 (3): 284–8.

Schwitter J, Wacker CM, van Rossum AC et al. MR-IMPACT: comparison of perfusion-cardiac magnetic resonance with single-photon emission computed tomography for the detection of coronary artery disease in a multi-centre, multi-vendor, randomized trial. Eur Heart J 2008; 29: 480–9.

Selvanayagam JB, Kardos A, Francis JM et al. Value of delayed-enhancement cardiovascular magnetic resonance imaging in predicting myocardial viability after surgical revascularization. Circulation 2004; 110 (12): 1535–41.

Soriano CJ, Ridocci F, Estornell J et al. Late gadolinium-enhanced cardiovascular magnetic resonance identifies patients with standardized definition of ischemic cardiomyopathy: a single centre experience. Int J Cardiol 2007; 116 (2): 167–73.

Sosnovik DE, Nahrendorf M, Weissleder R. Targeted imaging of myocardial damage. Nat Clin Pract Cardiovasc Med 2008; 5 (Suppl 2): S63–70.

Sosnovik DE, Wang R, Dai G et al. Diffusion spectrum MRI tractography reveals the presence of a complex network of residual myofibers in infarcted myocardium. Circ Cardiovasc Imaging 2009; 2 (3): 206–12.

Stary HC. Natural history and histological classification of atherosclerotic lesions: an update. Arterioscler Thromb Vasc Biol 2000; 20: 1177–8.

Steel K, Broderick R, Gandla V et al. Complementary prognostic values of stress myocardial perfusion and late gadolinium enhancement imaging by cardiac magnetic resonance in patients with known or suspected coronary artery disease. Circulation 2009; 120 (14): 1390–400.

Syed MA, Paterson DI, Ingkanisorn WP et al. Reproducibility and inter-observer variability of dobutamine stress CMR in patients with severe coronary disease: implications for clinical research. J Cardiovasc Magn Reson 2005; 7 (5): 763–8.

Tsukiji M, Nguyen P, Narayan G et al. Peri-infarct ischemia determined by cardiovascular magnetic resonance evaluation of myocardial viability and stress perfusion predicts future cardiovascular events in patients with severe ischemic cardiomyopathy. J Cardiovasc Magn Reson 2006; 8 (6): 773–9.

Underwood SR, Anagnostopoulos C, Cerqueira M et al. Myocardial perfusion scintigraphy: the evidence. Eur J Nucl Med Mol Imaging 2004; 31: 261–91.

Wagner A, Mahrholdt H, Holly TA et al. Contrast-enhanced MRI and routine single photon emission computed tomography (SPECT) perfusion imaging for detection of subendocardial myocardial infarcts: An imaging study. Lancet 2003; 361: 374–9.

Wahl A, Paetsch I, Roethemeyer S et al. High-dose dobutamine-atropine stress cardiovascular MR imaging after coronary revascularization in patients with wall motion abnormalities at rest. Radiology 2004; 233: 210–6.

Wang Y, Moin K, Akinboboye O, Reichek N. Myocardial first-pass perfusion: steady-state free precession versus spoiled gradient echo and segmented echo planar imaging. Magn Reson Med 2005; 54: 1123–9.

Watkins S, McGeoch R, Lyne J et al. Validation of magnetic resonance myocardial perfusion imaging with fractional flow reserve for the detection of significant coronary heart disease. Circulation 2009; 120 (22): 2207–13.

Wellnhofer E, Olariu A, Klein C et al. Magnetic resonance low-dose dobutamine test is superior to scar quantification for the prediction of functional recovery. Circulation 2004; 109: 2172–4.

White CW, Wright CB, Doty DB et al. Does visual interpretation of the coronary arteriogram predict the physiological importance of a coronary stenosis? New Engl J Med 1984; 310: 819–25.

Wöhrle J, Nusser T, Merkle N et al. Myocardial perfusion reserve in cardiovascular magnetic resonance: Correlation to coronary microvascular dysfunction. J Cardiovasc Magn Reson 2006; 8: 781–7.

Wolff SD, Schwitter J, Coulden R et al. Myocardial first-pass perfusion magnetic resonance imaging: a multi-center dose-ranging study. Circulation 2004; 110: 732–7.

Wu MT, Su MY, Huang YL et al. Sequential changes of myocardial microstructure in patients post-myocardial infarction by diffusion-tensor cardiac MR: correlation with left ventricular structure and function. Circ Cardiovasc Imaging 2009; 2 (1): 32–40.

Wu MT, Tseng WY, Su MY et al. Diffusion tensor magnetic resonance imaging mapping the fiber architecture remodeling in human myocardium after infarction: correlation with viability and wall motion. Circulation 2006; 114 (10): 1036–45.

Yanabe H, Okimura K, Ishikaza H et al. Role of endothelium-derived nitric oxide in myocardial reactive hyperemia. Am J Physiol 1992; 263: H8–14.

Yilmaz A, Athanasiadis A, Mahrholdt H et al. Diagnostic value of perfusion-CMR in patients with angina pectoris but normal coronary angiograms assessed by intracoronary acetylcholine-testing. Heart 2009; 96: 372–9.

Yokota H, Heidary S, Katikireddy CK et al. Quantitative characterization of myocardial infarction by cardiovascular magnetic resonance predicts future cardiovascular events in patients with ischemic cardiomyopathy. J Cardiovasc Magn Reson 2008; 10 (1): 17.

Zhang H, Shea SM, Park V et al. Accurate myocardial T1 measurements: toward quantification of myocardial blood flow with arterial spin labeling. Magn Reson Med 2005; 53 (5): 1135–42.

7 Coronary Artery Disease – Acute Coronary Syndromes

Loren Budge, Christopher M. Kramer and Peter Bernhardt

7.1 Definition and Spectrum

The term "acute coronary syndromes" (ACS) refers to any group of clinical symptoms compatible with acute myocardial ischemia and covers the spectrum of clinical conditions ranging from unstable angina (UA) to non-ST segment elevation myocardial infarction (NSTEMI or NSTE-ACS) and to ST segment elevation myocardial infarction (STEMI or STE-ACS). UA and NSTEMI are closely related conditions, but though their pathophysiological origin and clinical presentations are similar, they differ in severity. STEMI refers to prolonged myocardial ischemia resulting in myocyte cell death that may be diagnosed by biochemical, electrocardiographic, and imaging modalities. The differentiation between these three types of ACS depends on clinical presentation, electrocardiographic changes and biochemical cardiac markers (Figure 7-1).

Serum concentration of cardiac enzymes and markers of necrosis define the diagnostic categories of acute coronary syndrome, unstable angina and myocardial infarction (Thygesen 2007). Troponin T (cTnT) and troponin I (cTnI) are cardiac markers, which are extremely sensitive to myocardial injury and damage. Minimal myocardial damage can be detected by elevation in troponin concentration without significant rise in creatine kinase or other cardiac enzymes. The guidelines of the European Society of Cardiology and American College of Cardiology state that any elevation of troponin or creatine kinase MB (muscle, brain) isoenzyme is evidence of myocardial necrosis and should be classified as myocardial infarction (Van de Werf 2003, Antman 2004).

The **three types** of ACS include:

- **myocardial infarction (MI) with ST segment elevation** = STEMI = STE-ACS: severe refractory chest pain, persistent > 20 min of ≥ 0.2 mV ST elevation in at least two contiguous leads in men or ≥ 0.15 mV in women in leads V2–3 and/or ≥ 0.1 mV in other leads (Thygesen 2007) and elevated markers of myocardial necrosis;

- **myocardial infarction (MI) with no ST segment elevation** = NSTEMI = NSTE-ACS: severe chest pain, ST segment and/or T-wave alterations without ST-elevation, elevated markers of myocardial necrosis; and
- **unstable angina** = UA: intermittend chest pain, varying ECG alterations except ST segment elevations, e. g. ST segment depression and/or T-wave alterations, normal serum concentrations of markers of myocardial necrosis.

The differentiation between UA, NSTEMI and STEMI is made by ECG changes and biomarkers of myocardial necrosis (Figure 7-1).

7.2 Etiology and Pathophysiology

It is well established that ACS in their different clinical presentations share a widely common pathophysiological substrate. Pathological, biological, and angioscopic observations have demonstrated that atherosclerotic plaque erosion or rupture with differing degrees of superimposed thrombosis and distal embolization with consecutive regional myocardial ischemia represent the basic mechanism in most ACSs. After fissuring or rupture of these plaques the core constituents such as collagen, lipids, and smooth muscle and foam cells are exposed to flowing blood resulting in platelet aggregation and adhesion and the formation of intracoronary thrombus by concomitant generation of thrombin and deposition of fibrin. Such fresh thrombus – if persistent –

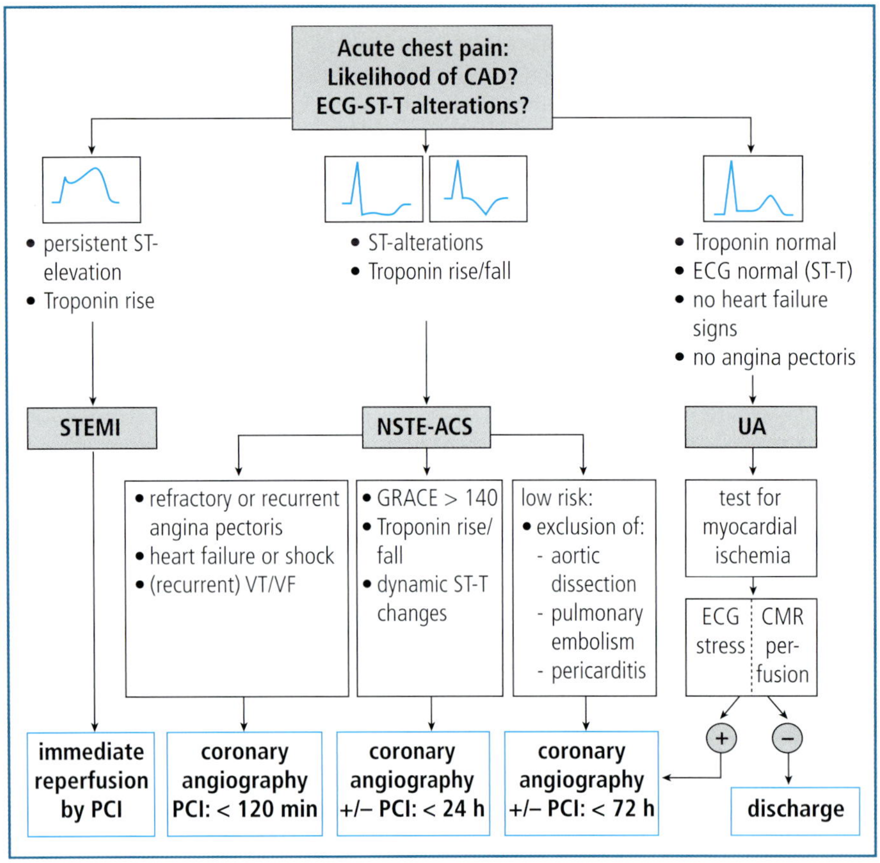

Figure 7-1 Stepwise diagnostic approach, risk stratification, and treatment in patients with acute coronary syndromes (ACS) (adapted and modified from the current Guidelines of the European Society of Cardiology; Hamm et al. 2011). Patients with obvious STEMI should immediately undergo reperfusion. Patients with NSTEMI and high risk (refractory angina, heart failure or shock, VT) should have coronary angiography within 12 h, those with intermediate risk (GRACE score > 140, troponin rise/fall, dynamic ST-T changes) within 24 h, and those with low risk within 72 h. Patients with unstable angina (UA) (no or insignificant ECG changes, troponin normal, no heart failure or angina pectoris) should undergo a stress test (treadmill stress test, stress echo, stress CMR) to detect myocardial ischemia. If the stress test is negative, patients can be treated medically and followed without any further intervention; in case of a positive test with demonstrable myocardial ischemia patients should undergo coronary angiography and revascularization, if appropriate and necessary. Note that using CMR imaging (for stress perfusion or stress regional function to detect myocardial ischemia with high accuracy, exact measurement of infarct size, and detection of microvascular obstruction) independent prognostic parameters can be obtained that may influence further diagnostic and therapeutic work-up of the patients.

may occlude the respective vessel resulting in STEMI or STE-ACS, or cause luminal narrowing resulting in NSTEMI or NSTE-ACS with subsequent myocardial ischemia of the corresponding myocardial perfusion territory. Plaque rupture and thrombus formation may also induce local vasoconstriction that may further reduce regional myocardial perfusion and exacerbate ischemia. Prolonged myocardial ischemia, e.g. in thrombotic occlusion, causes myocyte cell death within 2–4 h or longer, depending on the presence of collateral circulation, persistent or intermittent coronary artery occlusion, the sensitivity of myocytes to ischemia, and individual myocardial oxygen demand. In case of an acute myocardial infarction myocardial edema occurs prior to myocardial necrosis (Willerson 1977).

7.3 Clinical Presentation and Therapy

7.3.1 Relevance of Clinical Signs of Acute Coronary Syndromes (ACS)

A systematic review of 21 studies examined the usefulness of sixteen different clinical signs and symptoms for the diagnosis of acute coronary syndromes and found that no single sign or symptom taken in isolation was discriminatory (Mant 2004).

The guidelines of the American Heart Association/American College of Cardiology (AHA/ACC) recommend that **five factors should be considered together** when assessing the likelihood of myocardial ischemia related to ACSs (Antman 2004). These are:

- the nature of the symptoms,
- the history of ischemic heart disease,
- gender,
- increasing age, and
- the number of traditional cardiovascular risk factors present.

High risk features include worsening angina, prolonged pain, pulmonary edema, hypotension and arrhythmias.

7.3.2 ST-Elevation Myocardial Infarction (STEMI or STE-ACS)

Patients present with severe chest pain lasting for 10–20 min or more not responding fully to nitroglycerine. Often located in the substernal region the pain or pressure frequently radiates to the neck, jaw, left shoulder, or left arm. Other primary locations of pain my be epigastric or interscapular. Though there are no individual physical signs diagnostic of STEMI, many patients have evidence of autonomic nervous system activation (pallor, sweating) and either hypotension or narrow pulse pressure, as well as irregularities of the pulse including bradycardia or tachycardia. The 12-channel ECG shows persistent (> 20 min) ST segment elevation or presumed new left bundle branch block (LBBB). Blood sampling in the early hours for cardiac markers of necrosis (troponins, creatinine kinase) should be done, but immediate reperfusion therapy should not be deferred for getting the results of laboratory tests. Echocardiography may detect regional wall motion abnormalities that occur within seconds after coronary artery occlusion well before myocardial necrosis. After establishing the working diagnosis of STEMI patients should be treated for pain relief (i.v. opiods), oral O_2 (2–4 l/min), and anxiety (tranquilizer), if necessary. In addition, a β-blocker (i.v. low dose, contraindicated in patients presenting with hypotension) and a loading dose of a platelet aggregation inhibitor (clopidogrel, aspirin) has to be given in the acute setting, as well as anticoagulant agents (heparin). The patients should immediately undergo a reperfusion therapy, preferably catheter-based mechanical coronary reperfusion (PCI), because of the wavefront evolution of infarct size over time ("time is muscle"). In cases without PCI facility (PCI not manageable within 90 min from symptom onset) systemic thrombolysis should be performed followed later on by PCI ("facilitated PCI"). Longterm routine treatment includes oral platelet inhibitor, β-blocker, ACE-inhibitor, and a statin. Post-interventional follow-up includes regular clinical and echocardiographic examinations and – if available – serial CMR studies for early detection of infarct complications, adverse ventricular remodeling, and for determining prognosis.

7.3.3 Non-ST-Elevation Myocardial Infarction (NSTEMI or NSTE-ACS) and Unstable Angina (UA)

Patients present with chest or left arm pain or discomfort of varying duration that reproduces previously documented angina. A high likelihood of an ACS (NSTEMI or UA) exists, if patients with chest pain have a known history of CAD, including MI, have transient mitral regurgitation murmur, hypotension, diaphoresis, pulmonary edema, or rales on clinical examination, show new or presumably new transient ST segment deviation (≥ 1 mm) or T-wave inversion in multiple precordial leads of the ECG, and have elevated cTnT, cTnI, or CK-MB levels (Kumar and Cannon 2009). Patients with unstable angina (UA) present with chest pain of varying duration, ST segment depression and/or T-wave alterations, but normal levels of biomarkers of necrosis (cTnT, cTnI, CK-MB). Diagnosis is established by clinical examination, serial ECG recordings (ST-T-abnormalities, often dynamic changing ECG patterns), blood sampling (cTnT, cTnI, CK-MB), and echocardiography (regional wall motion abnormalities). CMR imaging may be extremely helpful in clinically stable patients for detecting old infarcts (scars by LGE), assessing global or regional wall motion abnormalities or involvement of the right ventricle, and to detect and quantify the severity of myocardial ischemia on stress testing (dobutamine stress CMR or adenosine stress first-pass CMR).

The goal of immediate treatment of patients with NSTEMI/UA is to provide relief of ischemia and to prevent the recurrence of adverse ischemic events. Therefore, treatment with anti-ischemic (nitroglycerine, morphine, β-blocker, calcium channel blocker, ACE-inhibitor), antiplatelet (aspirin, clopidogrel, newer P2Y12 ADP inhibitors like Prasugrel, Ticagrelor), and anticoagulant agents (unfractionated heparin, low-molecular heparin, direct thrombin inhibitors, factor Xa inhibitors) is fundamental (ACC/AHA 2007 guidelines).

In addition to aggressive medical therapy, **two treatment pathways** have emerged for treating NSTEMI/UA patients:

- an **early invasive strategy**, i.e. routine cardiac catheterization within 4–12 h after admission followed by PCI or bypass grafting, and
- an **initial conservative strategy**, i.e. initial medical management, followed by catheterization and revascularization only if ischemia recurs despite vigorous medical therapy, according to a risk stratification protocol (Figure 7-1).

High risk patients with the need of immediate invasive strategy are those with recurrent angina or ischemia at rest or low level activities despite intensive medical therapy, elevated biomarkers (cTnT, cTnI), new or presumably new ST segment depression, signs or symptoms of heart failure or new or worsening mitral regurgitation, hemodynamic instability, high-risk findings from non-invasive testing, PCI within 6 mths or prior CABG, high risk score (TIMI, GRACE), and reduced LV ejection fraction. Low risk patients with initial conservative therapy are those with a low risk score (TIMI, GRACE), and patient or physicians preference in the absence of high risk features (Kumar and Cannon 2009). Long-term follow-up includes regular clinical examinations, echocardiographic controls, and stress tests, and CMR imaging may play a significant role in the long-term surveillance of patients with NSTEMI/UA.

7.4 CMR Sequences and Protocols

CMR is regarded the gold standard in the measurement of left ventricular volumes and mass, because it relies on the acquisition of a 3D stack of contiguous short-axis cines covering the entire left and right ventricles without any geometric assumptions. Left and right ventricular end-diastolic and end-systolic volumes are assessed by planimetry for each slice and consecutive summation. CMR offers higher diagnostic accuracy and reproducibility in comparison to other imaging techniques and may be used in longitudinal studies over time and for reducing sample size for drug studies. Steady-state free precession (SSFP) cine images in short-axis orientation with complete biventricular coverage, from the atrioventricular valve plane to the apex are recommended for functional analysis (Kramer 2008). For further details see Chapter 5.

In acute coronary syndromes (ACS) early myocardial edema occurs in many forms of acute myocardial injury. CMR can visualize myocardial areas of edema by T2-weighted sequences (Aletras 2006, Friedrich 2008). In ACS edematous regions represent areas of myocardium at risk. First-pass myocardial perfusion CMR visualizes myocardial passage of a bolus of contrast agent and may detect regional perfusion abnormalities in stable angina as well as in ACS (Schwitter 2001). CMR is superior to most other imaging

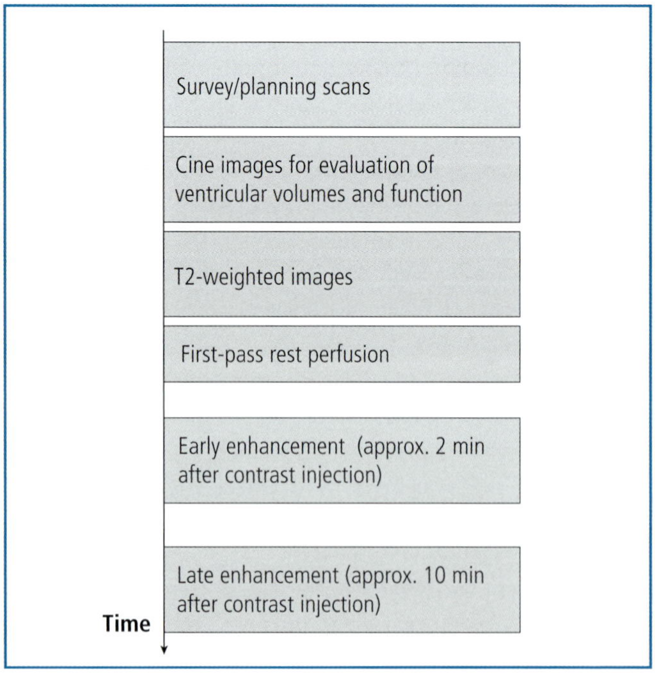

Figure 7-2 CMR protocol to investigate patients with an acute coronary syndrome (ACS).

modalities regarding spatial resolution. Thus, subendocardial ischemia could be identified more reliably compared with nuclear imaging techniques. Imaging at 3 T promises improved signal-to-noise ratio (SNR) and diagnostic accuracy, and acceleration techniques, such as e. g. k-t sense, promise even higher spatial resolution (Plein 2007). Areas of ischemia and microvascular obstruction could be seen in the early stage of MI by contrast-enhanced first-pass perfusion. The area of infarction as well as myocardial necrosis could be visualized by T1-based inversion recovery sequences (LGE) after contrast injection. Thus, in patients with ACS the CMR imaging protocol may be used as outlined in Figure 7-2.

7.5 CMR Examinations in Patients with UA

7.5.1 CMR-Based Diagnosis of Structure and Function/ Dysfunction of the Heart

CMR assessment of left and right ventricular structure and function is usually based on a short-axis cine data set in multiple consecutive slices covering both ventricles entirely. Due to different acceleration techniques 3D cine data sets covering both ventricles could be acquired in a single breath-hold (Jahnke 2007). For the assessment of regional kinetics visual analysis is usually performed in clinical routine (Hoffmann 2006). Alternatively, wall motion, thickening and strain may be measured using myocardial tagging methods (Garot 2002). Low-dose dobutamine cine-CMR can be used after acute myocardial infarction to predict functional recovery and viability (Kramer 2002). However, systematic CMR studies on structure and function of patients with unstable angina have not been performed as yet.

7.5.2 Assessment of Myocardial Viability – Pathophysiology of LGE

Early and late gadolinium enhancement is based on the different myocardial distribution of gadolinium-based contrast agents, i. e. the distribution volume is increased in acute MI due to myocyte necrosis, cell debris, capillary loss etc., as well as in chronic myocardial fibrotic tissue (scar) resulting in differences of contrast distribution between normal and necrotic/scarred myocardium. Early enhancing myocardium can be visualized by a T1-weighted inversion-recovery sequence, as well as late gadolinium enhancement with a dark central zone of the infarcted area, the socalled microvascular obstruction, sometimes emerging from the endocardium. In acutely injured or chronic infarcted myocardium a delayed wash-out of the contrast agents causes a high T1 signal and the respective tissue appears bright (Kim 2000). Imaging time for late gadolinium enhancement (LGE) sequences should be between 10 and 20 min after contrast agent administration. At that time signal differences between necrotic tissue, normal myocardium, and blood pool are maximal. This method has become the reference standard for assessment of myocardial viability in vivo due to its high spatial resolution and high contrast between injured and normal myocardium. The technique has been validated in animal models, showing excellent agreement with histology, and has been applied in many human studies, as well (Kim 1996, Wu 1998a, Kim 2000, Hombach 2005).

7.6 CMR Examinations in Patients with NSTEMI and STEMI

7.6.1 Assessment of Infarct Size and Myocardial Area at Risk in the Acute Setting

Evolution of Myocardial Infarction

A complex cascade of events occurs with the onset of myocardial ischemia. On a cellular level, myocardial ischemia initially causes depletion of energy stores, and an accumulation of osmotically active substances in the intra- and extracellular space. This, in turn, results in cellular and interstitial edema, an event which is further potentiated by reperfusion with iso-osmotic blood into the ischemic myocardium. If the ischemic process continues, there is gradual loss of cellular structure (Steenbergen 1985) and eventual irreversible cell death. Necrosis within ischemic myocardium occurs in a predictable pattern, beginning at the subendocardial surface and gradually extending in a "wavefront" to the epicardium as it becomes a transmural infarct (Reimer 1977). The area of ischemic myocardium is termed the "area at risk" of infarction. It corresponds to the perfusion bed of an occluded coronary artery, and represents the myocardium potentially salvageable with appropriate and timely intervention.

> Cardiac magnetic resonance (CMR) is ideally suited to evaluate ischemic events within the myocardium because of its excellent tissue characterization and spatial resolution. CMR is currently the gold-standard for assessing the presence, location and size of non-viable, infarcted myocardium using delayed contrast-enhanced imaging, and has recently become an invaluable tool for visualizing viable, but acutely ischemic myocardium using T2-weighted imaging.

Measurement of Infarct Size

CMR is able to measure infarct size and location with histological accuracy. This was established in a landmark study by Kim et al. (1999), who demonstrated that the spatial extent of infarction in a canine model assessed by *ex vivo* late gadolinium-enhanced (LGE) CMR was indistinguishable from histology in both acute and chronic infarcts. This was corroborated in a study by Fieno et al. (2000), who confirmed that the spatial extent of LGE was nearly superimposable with triphenyltetrazolim chloride staining for infarction at multiple time points in acute, subacute and chronic infarct stages. It has been shown clinically that infarct size on LGE is highly reproducible and compares favourably with single photon emission computed tomography (SPECT) and positron emission tomography (PET) (Klein 2002). Additionally, the increased spatial resolution of CMR allows visualization of much smaller infarcts than can be seen with SPECT or PET (Klein 2002, Wagner 2003). As discussed in detail in Chapter 6, the importance of this is highlighted by the marked adverse prognostic implications of even small, otherwise unrecognized infarcts seen on CMR (Kwong 2006).

It should be noted that infarct size is dynamic. Measurement of infarct size histologically or with late gadolinium-enhanced CMR demonstrates a peak in infarct size within the first few days after MI, followed by a gradual decline until 4–6 wks after the event, after which infarct size is generally stable. Infarct size in a representative canine MI study was 41 % of LV size at 4 d, but only 11 % of LV size at 28 d. Histological examination revealed a 25 % increase in water content within the acute infarct at 4 d, with dense scarring and decreased water content after 28 d (Reimer 1979). In humans, infarct size has been shown to decrease by 25–30 % over the first 8–12 wks post-MI as evidenced by the decline in size of late gadolinium enhancement (Choi 2004). Early on after MI, the increase in infarct size is likely due to an increase in interstitial edema and necrotic cellular debris, whereas chronic infarcts are characterized by dense scarring with an increase in collagen deposition and loss of cellular structure and edema. In both acute and chronic infarcts there is an increase in extracellular space, which causes an increased volume of distribution for gadolinium, and thus increased signal intensity. Regions of microvascular obstruction, which are characterized by hypoenhanced necrotic and infarcted tissue in the infarct core, should be included with hyperenhanced LGE when assessing infarct size.

T2 is the tissue-specific time constant of the rate of decay of transverse magnetization after a radiofrequency pulse. Tissues with higher water content have longer T2 relaxation times, leading to a brighter signal on T2-weighted images. Free water is the single most important contributor to T2 relaxation time. T2-weighted signal intensity correlates well in a linear manner with directly measured myocardial water content, and has been extensively validated in animal studies. In a landmark study using a porcine model of myocardial infarction, Garcia-Dorado et al. (1993) elegantly showed that the area at risk as measured by T2-weighted CMR correlated very well to the area at risk determined histologically with fluorescein staining ($r = 0.92$) when measured *ex vivo* 78 min after coronary occlusion. Similarly, Aletras et al. (2006) used a canine myocardial infarction model to demonstrate that T2-weighted *in vivo* CMR measurement of the area at risk 2 d following MI showed excellent correlation to the area at risk determined by fluorescent microspheres at the time of coronary occlusion. When compared to SPECT, which has been the clinical gold-standard for measurement of the area at risk, there was no difference in the location or size of the area at risk assessed with T2-weighted CMR (Carlsson 2009). SPECT has several disadvantages compared to CMR in estimation of myocardium at risk. For example SPECT requires injection of a radioactive tracer prior to any coronary intervention, coupled with the need to undergo scanning with a gamma camera within hours of injection, and the need for a second radiolabelled injection and scan to measure the area of infarction. CMR is able to accurately assess all of these measures in one scan, which can be performed days after the event without radiation, while also giving detailed information regarding cardiac structure and function.

Area at Risk and Myocardial Salvage Index

Accurate assessment of infarct size and the area at risk allows non-invasive measurement of a potentially clinically important parameter: the amount of myocardial salvage. The myocardial salvage index is defined as follows: (area at risk – infarct size)/area at risk.

This index is a measure of the myocardium that has been spared infarction, presumably due to a given procedure or treatment, and might be a better surrogate endpoint in studies evaluating therapies for MI than the extent of late gadolinium enhancement. The prognostic significance of myocardial edema is just beginning to be elucidated. CMR trials of STEMI patients undergoing PCI have repeatedly shown that an increase in the time from symptom onset to PCI leads to a significant incremental increase in infarct size and microvascular obstruction, with a corresponding decrease in myocardial salvage, while the extent of myocardial edema, or area at risk remains unchanged (Francone 2009, Eitel 2010). Several animal models have demonstrated that increased myocardial edema adversely affects both systolic and diastolic left ventricular function in the acute setting, as well as chronically, through inducement of myocardial fibrosis. Clinical studies are also beginning to paint a picture of myocardial edema as a predictor of worse outcomes. A trial of 208 ST elevation MI patients who underwent percutaneous coronary interventions (PCI) within 12 h of symptom onset demonstrated that patients with a myocardial salvage index (MSI) above the study median experienced significantly fewer death, reinfarction, or heart failure events at 6 mths when compared with those with an MSI below the median (2.9 % vs. 22.1 %, $p < 0.001$) (Eitel 2010). They also found that MSI was a better predictor of outcome on multivariate regression than infarct size, microvascular obstruction, left ventricular ejection fraction, TIMI flow grade after PCI, or ST segment resolution. Because of this, CMR may become an extremely valuable surrogate measure of outcome in studies of reperfusion therapy. An observational study of 88 patients with non-ST elevation acute coronary syndromes found that CMR-assessed edema was modestly predictive of the need for intervention (Raman 2010a), although it is still unclear whether CMR will be able to accurately and cost-effectively guide intervention in clinical practice.

Time Course of Myocardial Edema

A correct understanding of the time course of edema after cardiac injury is a major key to the accurate interpretation of T2-weighted imaging. In a canine model of myocardial infarction, Abdel-Aty et al. (2009) noted that the onset of edema on CMR first became apparent 28 ± 4 min after experimental coronary artery occlusion, and well before delayed contrast enhancement or troponin elevation, signifying that CMR can visualize edema before the onset of irreversible myocardial injury. This was corroborated in another canine MI study (Dibona 1980). A human trial evaluated eight patients with CMR who were undergoing septal coronary artery embolization for relief of hypertrophic obstructive cardiomyopathy (Schulz-Menger 2003). Each patient received repeat CMR at serial time points, from 1 h to 180 d. They found that increased T2-weighted signal was frequently,

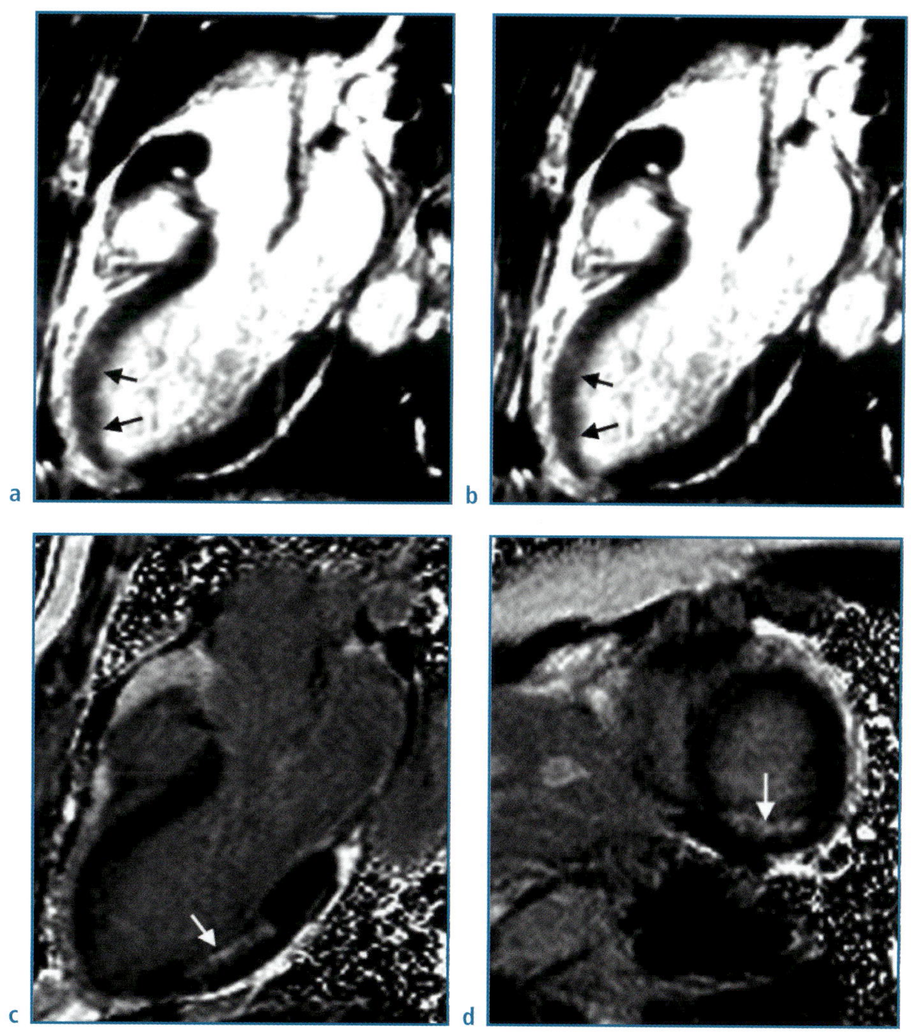

Figure 7-3 T2-weighted images in the 3-ch long-axis (a), and short-axis (b) views of a patient presenting with chest pain and transient anterior ST elevation, showing bright signal (edema) in the anterior wall of the left ventricle (arrows). Late gadolinium delayed images of the same patient and same image orientations are shown in (c) and (d), demonstrating a > 50 % transmural infarct in the inferior wall (arrows), but no infarct in the anterior wall. T2-weighted edema imaging is able to differentiate the acute episode (anterior wall) from the patient's old infarct (inferior wall).

although not always present in the infarct area at the initial time point of 1 h, and was consistently observed from day 1 through 28, after which it tended to resolve by day 90. Another small study evaluating 10 patients with transmural ST-elevation MI found that myocardial T2 signal persisted a median of 6 mths after the event, with 3 of the 10 cases persisting out to one year, although even in these cases, the extent and intensity of the T2 signal intensity diminished over time (Nilsson 2001). Larger clinical studies have shown that increased myocardial T2 signal after an ischemic event gradually dissipates over 1–3 mths (Abdel-Aty 2004). In the first 2–4 wks after myocardial infarction, the edematous area at risk of patients or experimental animals, as determined by T2-weighted CMR or histology, is nearly always transmural (Friedrich 2008), however, multiple studies have noted that T2 signal resolves early on in the epicardium, whereas persistent T2 signal, if present, is often limited to the endocardial surface (Nilsson 2001, Abdel-Aty 2004). When used in conjunction with late gadolinium-enhanced CMR, T2-weighted imaging thus confers the ability to differentiate acute from chronic infarcts (Figure 7-3). This was nicely demonstrated in a study by Abdel-Aty et al. (2004), who used LGE and T2-weighted CMR to evaluate 58 patients with either acute or chronic infarcts. Blinded observers were able to differentiate acute from chronic infarction with a specificity between 92–100 %, and a sensitivity between 91–94 %, depending on the observer.

Myocardial edema is also an important feature of non-ischemic acute cardiac injury including Tako-Tsubo cardiomyopathy, myocarditis, cardiac sarcoid, pulmonary hypertension, acute transplant rejection, and recent cardiac surgery. The pattern of late gadolinium enhancement in these patients is often helpful in differentiating the cause of injury, and is discussed in greater detail in Chapter 10.

Limitations of T2-Weighted Imaging

There are several potential limitations of traditional T2-weighted imaging (Giri 2009). First, the T2-weighted signal intensity is dependent on proximity to the phased array coil. This leads to a propensity to overestimate edema in myocardium close to the chest wall due to its brighter signal, and to under appreciate the T2-weighted signal from more distant structures. Another potential shortcoming with currently employed dark blood T2-weighted sequences is that slow-flowing blood appears bright, making it difficult at times to discern between a true increase in sub-endocardial T2 signal and blood pool artifact. Finally, T2-weighted imaging tends to be sensitive to motion. Experimental protocols have used T2 mapping to overcome these limitations (Giri 2009), but are not yet available for clinical use.

Another potential confounder of quantitative assessment of myocardial edema using T2-weighted imaging is intramyocardial hemorrhage. Interstitial hemorrhage occurs primarily in infarcted regions with microvascular obstruction and causes a change in the T2 signal, which may affect measurement of the area at risk. Hemorrhage can have variable effects on the MR signal depending upon the acuity of the event, but within the first week following infarction, the paramagnetic effects of iron in deoxyhemoglobin usually predominate. This causes a decrease in T2 and T2*, resulting in signal loss and potential underestimation of the area at risk, depending on the method of assessment. A recent CMR study using T2* mapping of 15 acute STEMI patients undergoing PCI found that significant intramyocardial hemorrhage was seen in 40 % of STEMI patients, was frequently found in the infarct core within areas of microvascular obstruction, and that using a boundary detection tool more accurately delineated the area at risk than thresholding, due to signal dropout in the infarct core (O'Regan 2009). A larger CMR study of 70 STEMI patients demonstrated that significant T2-weighted signal dropout within the infarct core was sufficient to impair threshold-based assessment of the area at risk in 11 % of STEMI patients (Francone 2009). Thus boundary detection methods for quantitative assessment of edema are probably more accurate than thresholding methods.

7.6.2 Detection of Infarct Complications

Due to CMR's high spatial resolution and unique tissue characterization abilities, it is an ideal imaging modality for assessing complications arising after MI. CMR is widely considered the gold-standard for analyzing both regional and global ventricular function after MI, and can comprehensively evaluate both systolic and diastolic function. CMR can also readily detect ventricular wall pathology such as ventricular septal defects, or free wall aneurysms, and can differentiate aneurysms from pseudoaneurysms, with its accompanying treatment implications (Figure 7-4 and Figure 7-5).

Visualization of LGE within the papillary muscles is indicative of infarction, and has been reported in post-MI CMR studies to occur in 26–53 % of patients (Hombach 2005, Okayama 2010). In a study of 60 patients with old MI, bilateral papillary muscle infarction was seen by LGE in 17 % of cases, and was associated with a higher incidence of severe mitral regurgitation and LV remodeling than in those with unilateral or no papillary muscle infarction (Okayama 2010). Inflammatory pericarditis is visualized by LGE of the pericardium with high sensitivity and specificity after MI (Taylor 2006), and has been reported to occur in as many as 40 %

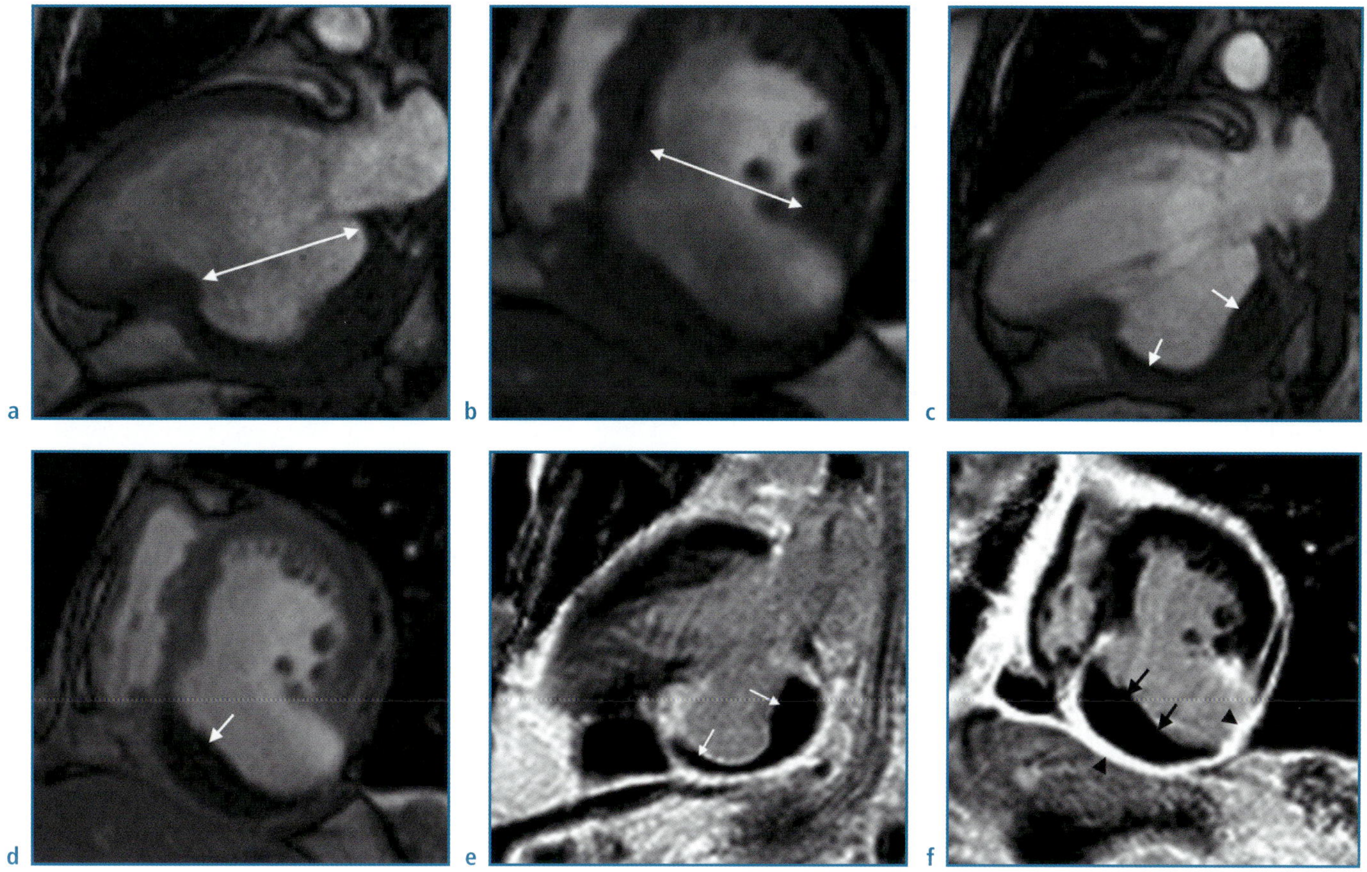

Figure 7-4 Steady-state free precession (SSFP) images in the 2-ch long-axis (a), and short-axis (b) views before contrast was given showing a pseudoaneurysm of the inferior left ventricular wall. Note the relatively narrow neck of the outpouching (double-sided arrow), differentiating this as a pseudoaneurysm, as opposed to the relatively wide neck seen in an inferior aneurysm shown in Figure 7-5. SSFP images in the same image positions shortly after contrast was given are shown in (c) and (d), demonstrating thrombus (arrows) partially filling the pseudoaneurysm. Late gadolinium-enhanced images seen in (e) and (f) further show a large thrombus (arrows) contained within a thin layer of fibrinous tissue (arrowheads).

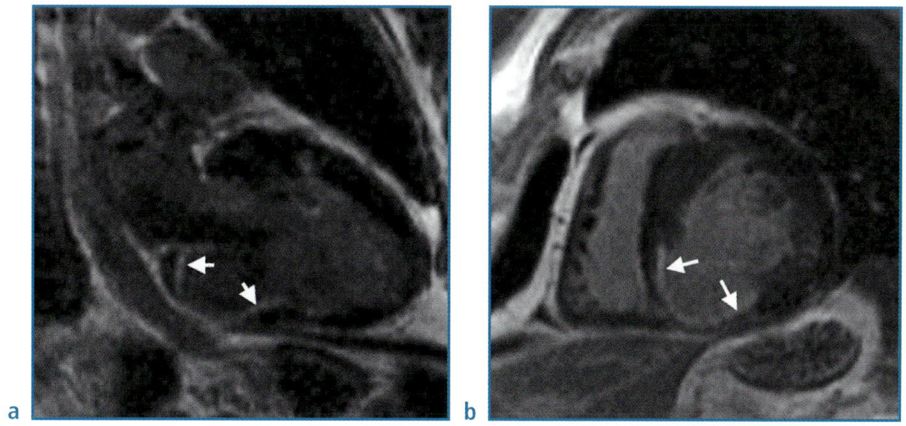

Figure 7-5 Late gadolinium-enhanced images in the 2-ch (a), and short-axis (b) views demonstrating a basal inferior aneurysm. Notice the relatively wide neck (double-sided arrow) of the aneurysm when compared to the pseudoaneurysm shown in Figure 7-4.

of STEMI patients (Hombach 2005). High T2-weighted signal can be visualized in inflammatory pericarditis, although this has not been studied specifically in post-MI patients. Right ventricular infarction is very well-visualized by CMR and is discussed later in this chapter. CMR can also be beneficial in the evaluation of intraventricular thrombi (Figure 7-6). The presence of intraventricular thrombi has been reported in 7–29 % of patients with decreased ejection fraction, depending on the population studied (Srichai 2006, Weinsaft 2008), and is associated with a higher risk of thromboembolic events, including stroke (Srichai 2006). The most prominent risk factors for the development of LV thrombus include anterior infarction, infarct size, LV aneurysm, and decreased ejection fraction (≤ 40%) (Weinsaft 2008). Contrast-enhanced (LGE) CMR has been shown to more accurately diagnose thrombi within the ventricle than transthoracic echocardiography (TTE) or transesophageal echocardiography (TEE). In a multi-modality imaging study of 361 patients with ischemic cardiomyopathy undergoing cardiac surgery, the presence of LV thrombus by LGE CMR, TTE, and TEE were compared to pathology and were found to have sensitivities and specificities of 88 and 99% for LGE, 23 and 96% for TTE, and 40 and 96% for TEE, respectively (Srichai 2006). While contrast echocardiography nearly doubles the sensitivity of non-contrast echo, mural and small apical LV thrombi are still frequently missed (Weinsaft 2009). Recently, the use of prolonged inversion times (600 ms) during LGE imaging has been shown to increase the sensitivity of LGE for detecting thrombus even further (Weinsaft 2008).

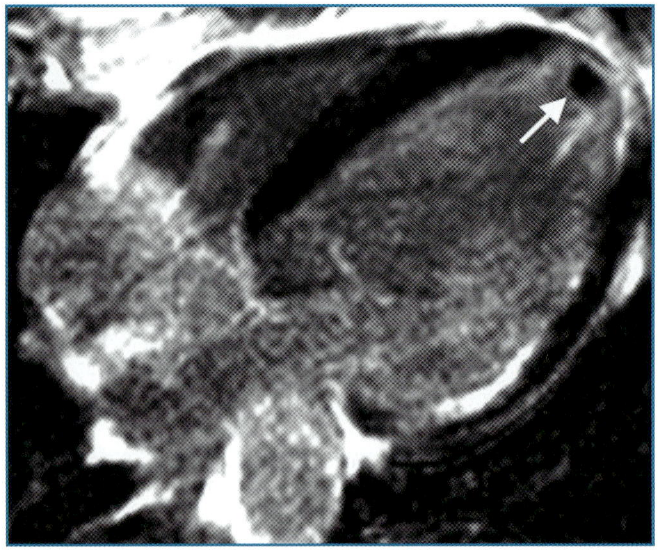

Figure 7-6 Late gadolinium-enhanced image in the 4-ch long-axis view, demonstrating a small apical thrombus (arrow).

7.6.3 Prediction of Left Ventricular Remodeling

In the aftermath of myocardial infarction, the left ventricle undergoes a series of adaptive and maladaptive changes, proportional to the size and transmurality of the infarct, which extend well beyond the infarcted segment. Remodeling in the early post-MI period is characterized by infarct expansion and thinning, with subsequent cavity dilatation in the infarcted area due to weakening of the infarct from myocyte slippage and loss. Over time, the necrotic, infarcted myocardium is replaced by fibrous scar, while adjacent viable segments undergo eccentric hypertrophy and fibrous deposition, causing global increases in ventricular volumes and worsened mechanical function. Although these changes restore stroke volume and cardiac output, they are associated with worsened mortality (Moss 1983, White 1987). Therapies which successfully attenuate post-MI remodeling (e. g. ACE-inhibitors, β-blockers, and aldosterone receptor antagonists) have been shown to improve outcomes after MI.

Because of its marked prognostic significance after MI, there is substantial interest in finding accurate predictors of remodeling which can be assessed at the time of MI. Baseline measurements of left ventricular function and volumes are a tempting target, and baseline ejection fraction and LV volumes have been shown to be modestly predictive of remodeling on follow-up (Larose 2010). However, due to the remodeling process and the frequent presence of stunned, but viable myocardium in the peri-infarct area, measurements of systolic performance immediately post-MI are inherently unreliable. Clinical parameters, such as ST segment resolution and the time from symptom-onset to reperfusion have also been shown to be associated with poor LV function at follow-up, but are also relatively poor and indirect markers of follow-up function. Multiple studies have demonstrated that several CMR-based parameters are much better predictors of long-term LV remodeling. In a study of 73 STEMI patients in whom CMR was performed within 1 wk and again 3 mths after MI, infarct size, as measured by LGE, was shown to be a better determinate of follow-up EF than was the baseline EF (Rubenstein 2008). Larose et al. (2010) confirmed this finding in a study of 103 STEMI patients, demonstrating that infarct size was the most powerful predictor of 6 mths LV dysfunction, with an area under the receiver-operator characteristic curve of 0.92 for infarct size, compared to 0.84, 0.79, and 0.71 for baseline ejection fraction, peak enzyme elevation, and time from symptom onset to revascularization, respectively. Infarct transmurality was shown to be predictive of late LV function after MI in a study by Taylor et al. (2004), who studied 20 MI patients and found that greater than 75% infarct transmurality was predictive of 3 mths LV dysfunction. They also found that poor microvascular perfusion, visualized as a delay (> 2 s) of contrast wash-in in the infarcted segment compared to remote myocardium, was a potent determinant of worsened follow-up LV function. Microvascular obstruction (MO) as a marker for subsequent remodeling was first demonstrated angiographically (Morishima 2000), and CMR-based assessment of MO has since been shown to be a powerful predictor of poor LV function, as discussed later in this chapter. Myocardial salvage index is a relatively recent measure for post-

MI prognosis, but initial studies are very promising. In a study of 137 reperfused acute STEMI patients, MSI was shown to be more predictive of adverse LV remodeling at 4 mths than infarct size, MO, or traditional measures of prognosis (Masci 2010).

7.6.4 Assessment of Post-Myocardial Infarction Prognosis

Left and Right Ventricular Function, Infarct Size and Border Zone

Left Ventricular Volumes and Ejection Fraction

In a landmark study of 866 medically-managed MI patients, a resting left ventricular (LV) ejection fraction (EF) less than 0.40 independently predicted an increase in mortality at 1 yr (Moss 1983). Peak exercise ejection fraction, or the change in EF from rest to peak exercise, has not been shown to add to the prognostic value of resting EF. The CASS study registry of 20,088 patients who were medically-managed after MI similarly demonstrated that a decreased resting EF was predictive of 4-yrs mortality, and was a more powerful predictor of poor outcome than was the number of diseased vessels. The prognostic value of a resting LVEF less than 0.40 after MI is maintained in patients receiving thrombolytic therapy or percutaneous coronary intervention (PCI). In a study of 605 male patients under the age of 60 who were evaluated by left ventriculography 4–8 wks after MI and followed for an average of 6.5 yrs, it was found that LV end-systolic volume (ESV) was a more powerful predictor of death than ejection fraction or end-diastolic volume (EDV) (White 1987).

> In contemporary CMR studies of post-MI patients, LVEF and LVESV are consistently predictive of outcomes; however, multiple studies have shown that other CMR-based parameters of infarction, such as infarct size, microvascular obstruction, and myocardial edema are more powerful predictors of outcomes than simple LV function or volume assessments (Wu 1998, Hombach 2005, Yokota 2008, Eitel 2010).

Myocardial Infarct Size

Early estimation of infarct size using radionuclide imaging demonstrated a clear association of infarct size with long-term clinical outcomes. When measured in 274 MI patients using quantitative tomographic Tc-99M sestamibi imaging, infarct size was strongly predictive of 1-yr mortality (Miller 1995). CMR-based assessment of infarct size using late gadolinium enhancement (LGE) is well-validated and has been shown to be highly predictive of cardiac events at follow-up. In a study by Yokota et al. (2008), 86 patients with prior MI were evaluated by CMR and followed for an average of 20 mths. They found that infarct size by LGE was a better predictor of cardiac events than LV ejection fraction, LVESV or LVEDV. Cheong et al. (2009) followed a cohort of 857 patients with and without coronary artery disease for a median of 4.4 yrs, and demonstrated that LGE, LVEF and heart failure were independent predictors of mortality. Interestingly, patients with LGE and an ejection fraction more than 0.50 had the same outcomes as those with an LVEF less than 0.50 without LGE. A recent study by Larose et al. (2010) investigated 103 acute ST elevation MI (STEMI) patients by CMR within 12 h of PCI, after which they received a 6-mths CMR and were followed for clinical events for an average of 2.4 yrs. It was demonstrated that LGE measured immediately after revascularization strongly and independently predicted 6 mths LVEF and long-term major cardiac events better than LVEF or clinical parameters. This was corroborated in a study of 122 STEMI patients who received CMR after revascularization and were followed for 2 yrs. Infarct size was again a stronger indicator of worsened LV function and clinical outcomes at follow-up than were baseline measurements of LV systolic performance (Wu 2008). It has been shown that the ratio of infarct size (by LGE) to the amount of ischemia (visualized by adenosine stress first-pass perfusion) was significantly higher in patients with Q-wave STEMI than in those with non Q-wave STEMI or non-STEMI (Plein 2008). Conversely, the amount of ischemia present was higher in NSTEMI patients than in STEMI patients, while the total area of ischemia and infarction was not different between the 3 groups. This may explain some of the prognostic discrepancy between these categories of MI.

Peri-Infarct Zone and Ventricular Arrhythmias

Ventricular arrhythmia and sudden cardiac death are a major cause of morbidity and mortality in the post-MI period. The border zone of an infarct is often composed of areas of viable myocardium interspersed with infarcted tissue or scar, which can become a substrate for re-entrant circuits and impaired conduction, leading to malignant arrhythmia. It has been postulated that this peri-infarct zone can be visualized by CMR on LGE images as areas along the infarct border of intermediate signal intensity. A study of 40 patients undergoing an electrophysiology study (EPS) prior to ICD placement for primary prevention confirmed that the size of the infarct border zone by CMR predicted inducibility of monomorphic ventricular tachycardia on EPS (Schmidt 2007). Yan et al. (2006) demonstrated that the size of the peri-infarct zone as measured by CMR was predictive of all cause and cardiac mortality over 2.4 yrs of follow-up. A CMR study of 91 post-MI patients scheduled for ICD implantation for either primary or secondary prevention of

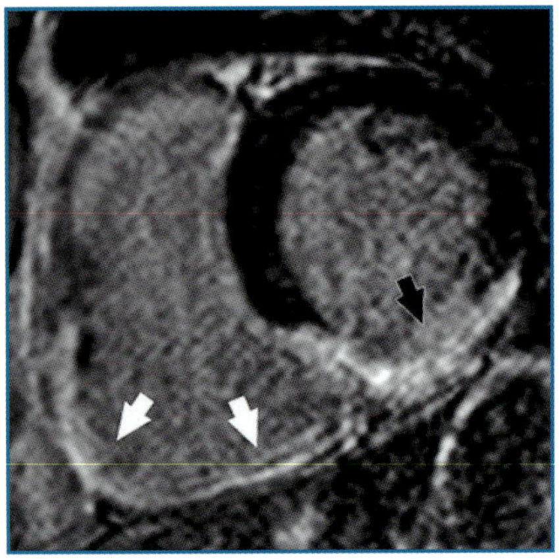

Figure 7-7 Late gadolinium-enhanced image in the short-axis view, demonstrating hyperenhancement of the inferior and inferoseptal LV wall (black arrow), with extension to the right ventricular wall (white arrows) (from Hombach V, Grebe O, Merkle N et al. Sequelae of acute myocardial infarction regarding cardiac structure and function and their prognostic significance as assessed by magnetic resonance imaging. Eur Heart J 2005; 26: 549–57; with permission of Oxford University Press, Oxford, UK).

sudden cardiac death found that the size of the peri-infarct zone was a stronger predictor of appropriate ICD therapy (a surrogate measure of sudden cardiac death), than LVEF or total infarct size (Roes 2009). This was corroborated in a study of 70 patients with a history of MI and ischemic cardiomyopathy being evaluated for ICD placement and followed for 18 mths (Heidary 2010), which revealed that the size of the peri-infarct zone as well as total infarct size were predictive of cardiac events. More work is needed to standardize the methodology used to measure the peri-infarct zone between centers and between studies.

Right Ventricular Infarction

The incidence of right ventricular (RV) infarction in autopsy studies in conjunction with LV infarction varies widely, and depends on the population studied, with isolated RV infarction occurring relatively rarely. Small portions of the anterior and apical RV are frequently involved in anterior LV infarcts seen at autopsy, although these are not often diagnosed clinically. Clinically recognized RV infarction classically occurs along with inferior LV infarction due to proximal occlusion of the right coronary artery (Figure 7-7). RV infarction is usually diagnosed by physical exam, ST elevation on right-sided electrocardiogram leads or by echocardiographic evidence of RV dysfunction; however, CMR has been demonstrated to be much more sensitive for detecting small or medium RV infarcts than physical exam, ECG or echocardiography (Jensen 2010). Before the current era of prompt, effective revascularization after MI, RV infarction was associated with high in-hospital mortality; however, there are conflicting reports regarding its prognostic significance in the current era. Bueno et al. (1997) studied 198 elderly patients with inferior MI, 75% of whom did not receive revascularization. RV infarction in this cohort occurred in 41%, with a mortality of 47%, compared to 10% mortality in those without RV infarction. The incidence of cardiogenic shock, atrioventricular conduction block, and rupture of the interventricular septum was also markedly higher in those with RV involvement. In a study of 200 inferior MI patients, 36% of whom received thrombolytic therapy, Zehender et al. (1993) similarly found that RV infarction occurred in 54%, and was strongly predictive of in-hospital mortality and events, but among survivors, did not predict long term outcomes. In a more recent study of 88 inferior MI patients, 87 of whom underwent PCI, RV infarction was present in 31% and no longer had significant short-term prognostic implications (Giannitsis 2000). This was corroborated in a CMR study of 110 MI patients followed for 7.5 mths, 85% of whom were revascularized (Hombach 2005). Late gadolinium enhancement of the RV was seen in 17% of these patients, with RV wall motion abnormalities in 43%. RV infarction in this study was not associated with worse outcomes. On the other hand, RV infarction on LGE after MI was shown to be predictive of RV dilatation at 6 mths follow-up (Kaandorp 2007). Furthermore, a recent CMR study of 50 MI patients undergoing successful PCI and followed for an average of 32 mths reported RV involvement by LGE in 47 and 65% of inferior and anterior MIs, respectively, and found that RV infarction was a significant independent predictor of cardiac events (odds ratio: 15.8; 95% CI: 4–63), even after controlling for LV infarct size and location (Jensen 2010).

Presence of Microvascular Obstruction (MO)

Pathophysiology

The concept of microvascular obstruction (MO) was first reported in the 1960's, after which it was conclusively demonstrated in the coronary arteries in 1974 in a canine model of MI and reperfusion (Kloner 1974). In this latter study, Kloner et al. demonstrated that reperfusion of a coronary artery after 40 min of ischemia led to homogenous blood flow within the infarcted tissue; however, reperfusion after 90 min led to areas within the infarcted tissue core of no-reflow. Electron microscopy of these areas revealed severe capillary and endothelial cell damage, as well as occasional intraluminal thrombi. This and other studies suggest that endothelial cells have a somewhat higher tolerance to ischemia than myocytes, but once this threshold is reached there is significant disruption of the microvasculature within the core of infarcted myocardium. Disruption of the endothelial layer due to ischemia and necrosis is also likely

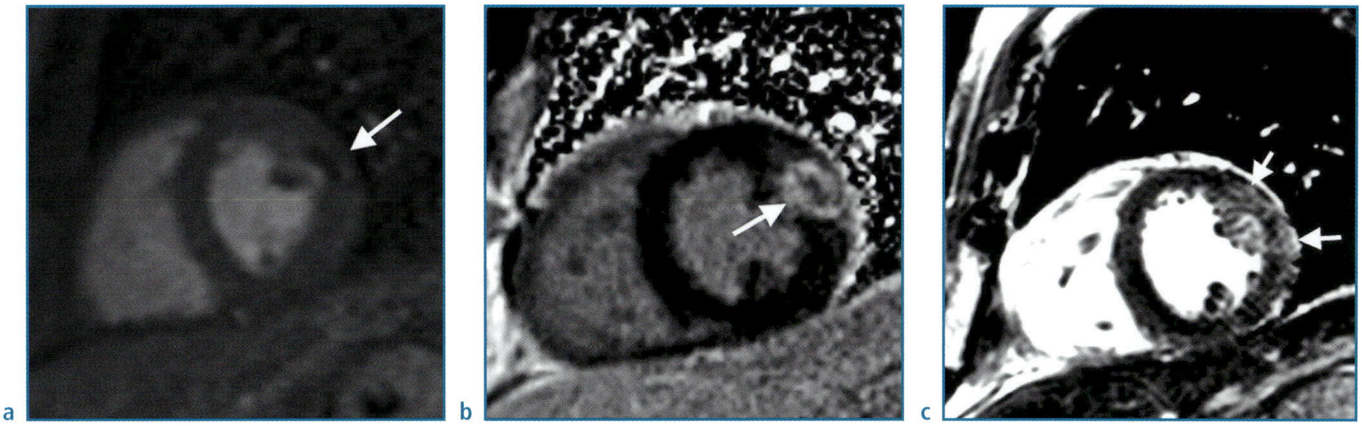

Figure 7-8 Microvascular obstruction, as seen by a perfusion defect in the anterolateral wall (arrow) persisting for 2 min after contrast injection in (a). Late microvascular obstruction is seen in the same patient and location as an area of hypoenhancement surrounded by hyperenhanced (infarcted) tissue on late gadolinium-enhanced imaging in (b). T2-weighted imaging (c) in the same location reveals anterolateral edema (arrows), consistent with an acute event.

responsible for intramyocardial hemorrhage, a phenomenon occurring almost exclusively in areas of no reflow. Other proposed mechanisms for microvascular obstruction include compression on the capillary bed due to marked edema of endothelial cells, myocytes and the interstitium, as well as microemboli of thrombus or necrotic tissue originating in the infarcted area or from the site of coronary occlusion. Reperfusion injury has also been shown to potentiate MO.

Methods to Assess Microvascular Obstruction

Several methods have been developed to assess microvascular perfusion after MI. Early methods used angiographically derived markers such as the thrombolysis in myocardial infarction (TIMI) flow grade, corrected TIMI frame count (cTFC), or myocardial blush grade. An angiographic study of 120 MI patients undergoing PCI and followed for almost 6 yrs showed that no reflow (TIMI flow grade ≤ 2) independently predicted worse outcomes in terms of cardiac death, MI, and LV remodeling (Morishima 2000). Subsequent studies found that cTFC and myocardial blush grade lend additional prognostic information to TIMI flow. Myocardial contrast echocardiography (MCE) involves intracoronary or intravenous infusion of microbubbles, usually at the time of catheterization, and is able to quantitate MO immediately after intervention with modest spatial resolution. MCE-based measurements of MO correlate well with histology (Wu 1998a), and have been found to more accurately predict functional recovery than any of the angiographically-based measures (Greaves 2003). MCE, however, requires patient stability, adequate acoustic windows, and the capability to inject microbubbles and perform measurements in the acute setting, which can be challenging after hours.

The time course of MO is an important factor in the selection of an ideal imaging modality for MO assessment. Several studies have shown that the extent of MO usually peaks from 2 h to 2 d after reperfusion occurs, after which it tends to be stable in size until at least day 9 (Wu 1998a). Thereafter areas of MO involute and regress and are rarely seen on follow-up CMR beyond 1–2 mths after MI. Because of the timing of MO, techniques performed at the time of intervention are likely to underestimate the final extent of MO. CMR thus offers a potential advantage in that it can measure MO up to 7–10 d after infarction with good spatial resolution and without dependence on acoustic windows.

CMR Assessment of Microvascular Obstruction and its Prognostic Significance

Microvascular obstruction can be assessed by CMR using two separate techniques. Early MO is visualized early after first-pass perfusion. Typical protocols using this method define MO as hypoenhancement persisting longer than 1–2 min after contrast injection. The second technique incorporates late gadolinium-enhanced (LGE) CMR images 10–15 min after contrast injection, and appears as an area or areas of hypoenhancement encompassed within the core of hyperenhanced infarcted myocardium, often extending from the subendocardium (Figure 7-8). This latter method in the literature is sometimes termed persistent or late MO (Hombach 2005). There is still no definite consensus on whether early or late MO should be the preferred technique for evaluating MO; however, recent trials have shed considerable light on this issue. The spatial extent of early MO correlates well with histology and myocardial contrast echo (Wu 1998a). It has been shown to be predictive of LV function and remodeling at 1 yr follow-up, and was a better marker of 1 yr infarct size than late MO (Orn 2009). Wu et al. (1998b) found that early MO predicts infarct transmurality, LV function and remodeling after 16 mths, and is also a powerful independent prognostic indicator of hard cardiac events even after controlling for infarct size. In a study of 60 MI patients undergoing CMR at 5 d and 4 mths, it was found that both early and late MO correlated with poor ST segment resolution, and that neither method correlated well with angiographic parameters of TIMI flow grade or angiographic blush grade (Nijveldt 2008). Late MO does, however, correlate with invasive coronary flow velocity measures of microvascular obstruction (Hirsch 2008). It has been demonstrated that late MO better predicted follow-up LV function and remodeling than did early MO, and lent additional prognostic information beyond that of infarct size or transmurality. In another study by Nijveldt et al. (2009), 63 acute MI patients who received PCI and optimal medical management were followed by CMR with assessment of early, mid, and late MO 4–7 d after MI and follow-up CMR at 4 mths. They found that late MO was a better predictor of follow-up LV ejection fraction, LV end-diastolic volume and LV end-systolic volume than early MO. In a study of 110 MI patients, Hombach et al. (2005) found that late MO independently portended an increase in cardiac events at 8 mths follow-up and gave additional prognostic information than infarct size alone. This was corroborated in a CMR study of 67 STEMI patients followed for 14 mths (Bruder 2008). In this study, Bruder et al. similarly reported that late MO was a better predictor of adverse cardiac events than infarct size or baseline ejection fraction. The timing of the CMR examination after MI is also important when assessing MO using first-pass perfusion. Studies demonstrate that early MO is more often seen when CMR is performed 2 d after MI than on days 7 or 9, but is not predictive of long term functional or clinical outcomes until the later time points (Wu 1998b, Orn 2009).

Intramyocardial hemorrhage (IMH) occurs frequently within areas of microvascular obstruction, and is visualized by an area of hypoenhancement within the edematous area on T2-weighted imaging. The presence of IMH correlates highly with the presence of MO, and there are conflicting reports as to whether it lends any additional prognostic significance beyond that of MO (Ganame 2009, Beek 2010).

7.6.5 Assessment of Therapeutic Interventions

Because of ongoing improvements in evidence-based medical therapy and revascularization for MI, the prognosis after MI has steadily improved. While this is obviously desirable, it presents a challenge when assessing new therapies for MI. In order to detect significant differences in those outcomes which are meaningful to the patient, such as mortality or major adverse events, large sample sizes with long-term follow-up are required, which can be prohibitively expensive and time consuming, posing a barrier to the evaluation of emerging therapies. Validated surrogate endpoints allow clinical studies to be performed with fewer patients, shorter follow-up and decreased cost, thus facilitating the investigation of promising new treatments. As discussed by Kim et al. (2009), the required sample size of a study is proportional to the variance (square of the standard deviation) of the measured endpoint in the study population, and inversely proportional to the square of the expected difference in outcome affected by the therapy being tested. Because of this, even small improvements in measurement reproducibility and accuracy can potentially lead to large decreases in required sample size. CMR has been shown to be gold-standard for the reproducible and accurate assessment of parameters such as LV function and infarct size (Kim 1999, Grothues 2002), leading to a decrease in required study size and cost. As such, CMR is an attractive imaging modality for studying new revascularization therapies or treatments aimed at improving remodeling after MI. For example, several recent trials have used CMR to evaluate the efficacy of an intracoronary administration of bone marrow-derived autologous progenitor cells after acute MI, using either LVEF or infarct size as surrogate endpoints (Lunde 2006, Wollert 2004). Wollert et al. (2004) randomized 60 STEMI patients to receive either intracoronary injection of bone marrow cells 5 d after PCI or standard care, and followed them with baseline and 6-mths CMR. They demonstrated a significant improvement in LVEF in the treatment group, while no change in EF was observed in the control group. Another study used CMR to assess infarct size, LVEF and end-diastolic volume in 100 acute MI patients randomized to intracoronary bone marrow cell injection (Lunde 2006), and failed to see any difference between groups in the measured endpoints. Although studies of intracoronary stem cell injection for improvement in post-MI healing have shown conflicting results, CMR provides a relatively rapid and cost-efficient modality to assess emerging therapies.

As mentioned earlier in this chapter, the myocardial salvage index (MSI) has been shown in initial studies to be a more potent prognostic indicator than infarct size or other clinical and CMR-based measures (Eitel 2010). In addition, the MSI effectually controls for some of the variation in infarct size within a study population by indexing infarct size to the area at risk, thus allowing a potentially greater decrease in the sample size required. If this is validated in further studies, the MSI could become a more powerful surrogate endpoint than infarct size in the evaluation of emerging revascularization therapies.

7.7 Non-Invasive Triage of Patients with Acute Chest Pain

Among patients presenting to the emergency department (ED), chest pain or other symptoms suggestive of acute coronary syndrome (ACS) are common complaints, and present a significant challenge to the emergency department physician. In addition to the history and physical examination, the tools available for diagnosis, including the electrocardiogram (ECG) and serum cardiac biomarkers (troponin I or T, myocardial fraction of creatine kinase), are usually helpful in diagnosing the highest risk patients, such as those with ST elevation MI. However, for the majority of patients who do not have obvious evidence of MI on arrival to the emergency department, these tests lack the sensitivity required to make a rapid diagnosis. Due to the high prevalence and mortality associated with coronary artery disease, low and intermediate risk patients with possible acute coronary syndrome typically require lengthy observation periods or hospital admission. Once patients have "ruled out" for MI, further functional or anatomic testing is often performed for better risk stratification. Even so, less than a third of patients admitted to the hospital with suspicion for ACS will eventually be given the diagnosis and importantly, about 2% of patients are discharged from the emergency department with unrecognized MI, a mistake which can have dire consequences.

CMR has been found to improve the diagnostic accuracy of ACS in the emergency department setting. Kwong et al. (2003) performed CMR within 12 h of presentation on 161 patients presenting to the ED with symptoms consistent with ACS, but without ST elevation on ECG. The CMR exam in this study included cine-MRI for LV function, resting first-pass perfusion and LGE. Total CMR scan time was 38 min, and patients were gone from the ED for less than 1 h. The sensitivity for CMR was found to be 84 and 85%, respectively, and added independent diagnostic value to clinical parameters. The main limitation of CMR in this study was its inability to differentiate acute from chronic MI. This problem was addressed by Cury et al. (2008), who added T2-weighted imaging and quantitation of LV wall thickness to distinguish acute events. 62 patients with chest pain, normal ECG, and negative initial cardiac biomarkers, who were being admitted to the hospital to rule out MI, received CMR with an average scan time of 32 min. The new CMR protocol accurately identified all acute MI cases, often before cardiac biomarkers became elevated. Compared with conventional CMR, the addition of edema imaging and wall thickness quantitation increased the specificity from 84 to 96%, the positive predictive value from 55 to 85%, and the overall accuracy from 84 to 93%, respectively. Plein et al. (2004) studied 72 high risk patients diagnosed with non-ST elevation ACS and scheduled to undergo catheterization with a CMR protocol consisting of adenosine stress perfusion, coronary imaging, and LGE. Despite 53% of these patients having elevated troponin levels, there were no complications from vasodilator stress imaging. CMR in this setting was superior to clinical parameters, with a sensitivity and specificity of 96 and 83%, respectively for significant coronary stenosis. In a low risk population of 103 patients with chest pain, negative ECG and negative serial cardiac biomarkers, CMR was performed which included adenosine stress and rest CMR, LV function, and LGE (Lerakis 2009). None of the patients with a normal CMR study had any clinical events at 9 mths follow-up. This was corroborated in a similar study of 135 low risk patients presenting to the ED with chest pain who received adenosine stress CMR after excluding the diagnosis of MI with serial troponin I measurements (Ingkanisorn 2006). At 1 yr follow-up, no patients with a normal stress CMR were found to have a significant coronary stenosis or cardiac event, yielding a sensitivity and specificity of 100 and 93%, respectively.

The cost-effectiveness of using stress CMR to evaluate intermediate and high risk patients in the ED setting was evaluated in a study of 110 patients with chest pain, negative ECG, and negative initial biomarkers, being admitted to the hospital to rule out MI (Miller 2010). These patients were randomized to obtain adenosine stress CMR while in the ED or usual inpatient care. All health care costs relating to their hospitalization and cardiac care over 30 d were included. There was no difference in 30 d clinical outcomes between the groups. A diagnostic protocol which included stress CMR was found to reduce inpatient admissions and produced a cost savings of over 20% in this study. Further cost-effectiveness studies are still needed to address the financial implications of utilizing stress CMR in lower risk populations.

7.8 Summary and Conclusions

CMR has emerged as a robust diagnostic imaging modality capable of providing a comprehensive cardiac evaluation for patients with acute coronary syndromes. CMR is widely regarded as the reference standard for assessment of cardiac structure and function. In patients with acute myocardial infarction, CMR provides powerful diagnostic and prognostic information, allowing evaluation of cardiac function, infarct size and location, infarct complications, the extent of edema or the area at risk, the amount of myocardial salvage, and the status of the microvasculature – all in a single scan.

The prognostic information garnered from a single CMR study in the acute aftermath of MI cannot be rivalled by any other imaging modality. This has been a driving force in making CMR the modality of choice for evaluating new reperfusion therapies. CMR has been shown to be safe, even immediately after PCI in STEMI patients (Larose 2009), and a comprehensive exam can typically be performed in less than 45 min without exposing the patient to radiation. For those with normal coronary arteries in the setting of MI, CMR provides clues to the underlying diagnosis in the majority of cases. In patients with acute or chronic ischemic cardiomyopathy, viability assessment by CMR correctly predicts recovery of function after intervention, which can directly affect patient management decisions. For patients presenting to the emergency department with symptoms and risk factors concerning for acute coronary syndrome, but without evidence of MI, a comprehensive CMR study can also include stress perfusion imaging, allowing accurate functional assessment of the coronary circulation, which has been validated in both low and high risk study populations. T2-weighted imaging of edema and late gadolinium enhancement have the ability to detect infarction and severe ischemia early in the course of MI, even before cardiac biomarkers become elevated, and can differentiate acute from chronic infarction. Importantly, adding CMR to the emergency physician's toolbelt has been shown to improve diagnostic accuracy compared to current standards of care and to be cost effective in certain populations. Taken together, CMR provides a wealth of meaningful diagnostic and prognostic data for a wide range of patient populations with suspected or confirmed acute coronary syndrome.

7.9 Future Perspectives

CMR has a bright future in the evaluation of patients with acute coronary syndrome. Relatively recent improvements in CMR technology have made a comprehensive CMR exam in the acute setting much more practical because of shortened acquisition times, better image quality, and improved CMR protocols yielding higher diagnostic accuracy. New data confirming the efficacy and prognostic importance of existing CMR protocols are accumulating rapidly, and will continue to do so. Of special importance will be emerging data regarding the ability of CMR to improve patient outcomes and to be cost effective for increasing numbers of indications and patient populations. Advancements on the CMR horizon include marked improvements in image acquisition times and image quality with techniques such as compressed sensing and model-based image reconstruction. Another achievement may include exercise stress CMR. One major impediment to the widespread use of pharmacologic stress CMR is that an exercise stress test yields valuable prognostic information for patients who are able to exercise. With pharmacologic stress, regardless of the imaging modality used, much of this prognostic information is lost. This has given imaging modalities more compatible with exercise stress, such as SPECT and echocardiography, an edge in the patient population able to exercise. A recent study demonstrated the feasibility of exercise stress CMR, in which an MR compatible treadmill was placed in the scan room, and a specialized mattress on the MR table ensured proper patient repositioning. Both peak stress perfusion and LV function were assessed within 90 s of exercise termination, and yielded favourable accuracy for prediction of events when compared with SPECT in the same patients (Raman 2010b). If this is validated and becomes clinically practical, the appropriate patient population for stress CMR would increase significantly.

Another area of development within CMR is coronary magnetic resonance angiography (MRA). The ability of MRI to perform plaque characterization in larger peripheral vessels has been well-documented. Current coronary MRA protocols are hampered by inadequate spatial resolution for robust analysis of distal coronary vessels. Further development of coronary MR angiography at higher field strengths will likely produce a truly comprehensive CMR exam capable of anatomic and functional evaluation of coronary artery disease in one exam, without exposing the patient to radiation.

Finally, there is ongoing development of molecular imaging agents targeting high risk (vulnerable) coronary plaque. This is based on the finding that at least half of all coronary events, including myocardial infarction, probably originate with plaques which are less than 50% stenosed immediately prior to the event. Because of this, there is a need to assess plaque risk, rather than just plaque stenosis. Current pre-clinical research efforts in this area include development of probes to a wide range of molecular targets including the oxidized low-density lipoprotein receptor (LOX-1), macrophages, matrix metalloproteinases and other proteinases involved in atherogenesis, annexin (a marker of apoptosis), lipoproteins, $\alpha_v\beta_3$ (a marker of angiogenesis), and thrombus formation. A clinically useful molecular imaging probe able to non-invasively target vulnerable plaque could change the stenosis-based cardiology paradigm, and allow vastly improved risk assessment in patients presenting with suspected ACS.

References

Abdel-Aty H, Cocker M, Meek C et al. Edema as a very early marker for acute myocardial ischemia. A cardiovascular magnetic resonance study. J Am Coll Cardiol 2009; 53 (14): 1194–201.

Abdel-Aty H, Zagrosek A, Schulz-Menger J et al. Delayed enhancement and T2-weighted cardiovascular magnetic resonance imaging differentiate acute from chronic myocardial infarction. Circulation 2004; 109 (20): 2411–6.

ACC/AHA 2007 guidelines for the management of patients with unstable angina/non-ST elevation myocardial infarction: executive summary: a report of the American College of Cardiology/ American Heart Association Task Force on Practice Guidelines: developed in collaboration with the American College of Emergency Physicians, the Society for Cardiovascular Angiography and Interventions, and the Society of Thoracic Surgeons: endorsed by the American Association of Cardiovascular and Pulmonary Rehabilitation and the Society for Academic Emergency Medicine. Circulation 2007; 116: 809–77.

Aletras AH, Tilak GS, Natanzon A et al. Retrospective determination of the area at risk for reperfused acute myocardial infarction with T2-weighted cardiac magnetic resonance imaging: histopathological and displacement encoding with stimulated echoes (DENSE) functional validations. Circulation 2006; 113: 1865–70.

Antman EM, Armstrong PW, Bates ER et al. ACC/AHA guidelines for the management of patients with ST-elevation myocardial infarction: a report of the American College of Cardiology/ American Heart Association Task Force on Practice Guidelines. J Am Coll Cardiol 2004; 44: E1–E211.

Beek AM, Nijveldt R, van Rossum AC. Intramyocardial hemorrhage and microvascular obstruction after primary percutaneous coronary intervention. Int J Cardiovasc Imaging 2010; 26: 49–55.

Bruder O, Breuckmann F, Jensen C et al. Prognostic impact of contrast-enhanced CMR early after acute ST segment elevation myocardial infarction (STEMI) in a regional STEMI network. Herz 2008; 33 (2): 136–42.

Bueno H, Lopez-Palop R, Bermejo J et al. In-hospital outcome of elderly patients with acute inferior myocardial infarction and right ventricular involvement. Circulation 1997; 96 (2): 436–41.

Carlsson M, Ubachs JF, Hedstrom E et al. Myocardium at risk after acute infarction in humans on cardiac magnetic resonance: quantitative assessment during follow-up and validation with single-photon emission computed tomography. JACC Cardiovasc Imaging 2009; 2 (5): 569–76.

Cheong BYC, Muthupillai R, Wilson JM et al. Prognostic significance of delayed-enhancement magnetic resonance imaging survival of 857 patients with and without left ventricular dysfunction. Circulation 2009; 120 (21): 2069–76.

Choi CJ, Haji-Momenian S, DiMaria JM et al. Infarct involution and improved function during healing of acute myocardial infarction: The role of microvascular obstruction. J Cardiovasc Magn Reson 2004; 6 (4): 917–25.

Cury RC, Shash K, Nagurney JT et al. Cardiac magnetic resonance with T2-weighted imaging improves detection of patients with acute coronary syndrome in the emergency department. Circulation 2008; 118 (8): 837–44.

Dibona DR, Powell WJ. Quantitative correlation between cell swelling and necrosis in myocardial ischemia in dogs. Circ Res 1980; 47 (5): 653–65.

Eitel I, Desch S, Fuernau G et al. Prognostic significance and determinants of myocardial salvage assessed by cardiovascular magnetic resonance in acute reperfused myocardial infarction. J Am Coll Cardiol 2010; 55 (22): 2470–9.

Fieno DS, Kim RJ, Chen EL et al. Contrast-enhanced magnetic resonance imaging of myocardium at risk – distinction between reversible and irreversible injury throughout infarct healing. J Am Coll Cardiol 2000; 36 (6): 1985–91.

Francone M, Bucciarelli-Ducci C, Carbone I et al. Impact of primary coronary angioplasty delay on myocardial salvage, infarct size, and microvascular damage in patients with ST-segment elevation myocardial infarction insight from cardiovascular magnetic resonance. J Am Coll Cardiol 2009; 54 (23): 2145–53.

Friedrich MG, Abdel-Aty H, Taylor A et al. The salvaged area at risk in reperfused acute myocardial infarction as visualized by cardiovascular magnetic resonance. J Am Coll Cardiol 2008; 51: 1581–7.

Ganame J, Messalli G, Dymarkowski S et al. Impact of myocardial hemorrhage on left ventricular function and remodeling in patients with reperfused acute myocardial infarction. Eur Heart J 2009; 30 (12): 1440–9.

Garcia-Dorado D, Oliveras J, Gili J et al. Analysis of myocardial edema by magnetic resonance imaging early after coronary-artery occlusion with or without reperfusion. Cardiovasc Res 1993; 27 (8): 1462–9.

Garot J, Pascal O, Diebold B et al. Alterations of systolic left ventricular twist after acute myocardial infarction. Am J Physiol Heart Circ Physiol 2002; 282: H357–H362.

Giannitsis E, Hartmann F, Wiegand U et al. Clinical and angiographic outcome of patients with acute inferior myocardial infarction and right ventricular involvement treated with direct PTCA. Z Kardiol 2000; 89 (1): 28–35.

Giri S, Chung YC, Merchant A et al. T2 quantification for improved detection of myocardial edema. J Cardiovasc Magn Reson 2009; 11: 56.

Greaves K, Dixon SR, Fejka M et al. Myocardial contrast echocardiography is superior to other known modalities for assessing myocardial reperfusion after acute myocardial infarction. Heart 2003; 89 (2): 139–44.

Grothues F, Smith GC, Moon JCC et al. Comparison of interstudy reproducibility of cardiovascular magnetic resonance with two-dimensional echocardiography in normal subjects and in patients with heart failure or left ventricular hypertrophy. Am J Cardiol 2002; 90 (1): 29–34.

Hamm CW, Bassand JP, Agewall S et al. ESC Guidelines for the management of acute coronary syndromes in patients presenting without persistent ST-segment elevation: The Task Force for the management of acute coronary syndromes (ACS) in patients presenting without persistent ST-segment elevation of the European Society of Cardiology (ESC). Eur Heart J 2011; 32 (23): 2999–3054.

Heidary S, Patel H, Chung J et al. Quantitative tissue characterization of infarct core and border zone in patients with ischemic cardiomyopathy by magnetic resonance is associated with future cardiovascular events. J Am Coll Cardiol 2010; 55 (24): 2762–8.

Hirsch A, Nijveldt R, Haeck JDE et al. Relation between the assessment of microvascular injury by cardiovascular magnetic resonance and coronary Doppler flow velocity measurements in patients with acute anterior wall myocardial infarction. J Am Coll Cardiol 2008; 51 (23): 2230–8.

Hoffmann R, von Bardeleben S, Kasprzak JD et al. Analysis of regional left ventricular function by cineventriculography, cardiac magnetic resonance imaging, and unenhanced and contrast-enhanced echocardiography: a multi-center comparison of methods. J Am Coll Cardiol 2006; 47: 121–8.

Hombach V, Grebe O, Merkle N et al. Sequelae of acute myocardial infarction regarding cardiac structure and function and their prognostic significance as assessed by magnetic resonance imaging. Eur Heart J 2005; 26: 549–57.

Ingkanisorn WP, Kwong RY, Bohme NS et al. Prognosis of negative adenosine stress magnetic resonance in patients presenting to an emergency department with chest pain. J Am Coll Cardiol 2006; 47 (7): 1427–32.

Jahnke C, Nagel E, Gebker R et al. Four-dimensional single breath-hold magnetic resonance imaging using kt-BLAST enables reliable assessment of left and right-ventricular volumes and mass. J Magn Reson Imaging 2007; 25: 737–42.

Jensen CJ, Jochims M, Hunold P et al. Right ventricular involvement in acute left ventricular myocardial infarction: prognostic implications of MRI findings. Am J Roentgenol 2010; 194 (3): 592–8.

Kaandorp TAM, Lamb HJ, Poldermans D et al. Assessment of right ventricular infarction with contrast-enhanced magnetic resonance imaging. Coronary Artery Dis 2007; 18 (1): 39–43.

Kim HW, Farzaneh-Far A, Kim RJ. Cardiovascular magnetic resonance in patients with myocardial infarction. J Am Coll Cardiol 2009; 55 (1): 1–16.

Kim RJ, Chen AL, Lima JA, Judd RM. Myocardial Gd-DTPA kinetics determine MRI contrast enhancement and reflect the extent and severity of myocardial injury after acute reperfused infarction. Circulation 1996; 94: 3318–26.

Kim RJ, Fieno DS, Parrish TB et al. Relationship of MRI delayed contrast enhancement to irreversible injury, infarct age, and contractile function. Circulation 1999; 100 (19): 1992–2002.

Kim RJ, Wu E, Rafael A et al. The use of contrast-enhanced magnetic resonance imaging to identify reversible myocardial dysfunction. N Engl J Med 2000; 343: 1445–53.

Klein C, Nekolla SG, Bengel FM et al. Assessment of myocardial viability with contrast-enhanced magnetic resonance imaging – comparison with positron emission tomography. Circulation 2002; 105 (2): 162–7.

Kloner RA, Ganote CE, Jennings RB. No-reflow phenomenon after temporary coronary-occlusion in dog. J Clin Invest 1974; 54 (6): 1496–508.

Kramer CK, Barkhausen J, Flamm SD et al. Standardized cardiovascular magnetic resonance imaging (CMR) protocols, society for cardiovascular magnetic resonance: board of trustees task force on standardized protocols. J Cardiovasc Magn Reson 2008; 10: 35.

Kramer CM, Malkowski MJ, Mankad S et al. Magnetic resonance tagging and echocardiographic response to dobutamine and functional improvement after reperfused myocardial infarction. Am Heart J 2002; 143: 1046–51.

Kumar A, Cannon CP. Symposion on cardiovascular disease: acute coronary syndromes: diagnosis and management, Part I. Mayo Clin Proc 2009; 84: 917–38.

Kwong RY, Chan AK, Brown KA et al. Impact of unrecognized myocardial scar detected by cardiac magnetic resonance imaging on event-free survival in patients presenting with signs or symptoms of coronary artery disease. Circulation 2006; 113 (23): 2733–43.

Kwong RY, Schussheim AE, Rekhraj S et al. Detecting acute coronary syndrome in the emergency department with cardiac magnetic resonance imaging. Circulation 2003; 107 (4): 531–7.

Larose E, Cote J, Rodes-Cabau J et al. Contrast-enhanced cardiovascular magnetic resonance in the hyperacute phase of ST-elevation myocardial infarction. Int J Cardiovasc Imaging 2009; 25 (5): 519–27.

Larose E, Rodes-Cabau J, Pibarot P et al. Predicting late myocardial recovery and outcomes in the early hours of ST-segment elevation myocardial infarction traditional measures compared with microvascular obstruction, salvaged myocardium, and necrosis characteristics by cardiovascular magnetic resonance. J Am Coll Cardiol 2010; 55 (22): 2459–69.

Lerakis S, Mclean DS, Anadiotis AV et al. Prognostic value of adenosine stress cardiovascular magnetic resonance in patients with low-risk chest pain. J Cardiovasc Magn Reson 2009; 11: 37.

Lunde K, Solheim S, Aakhus S et al. Intracoronary injection of mononuclear bone marrow cells in acute myocardial infarction. N Engl J Med 2006; 355 (12): 1199–209.

Mant J, McManus RJ, Oakes RAL et al. Systematic review and modeling of the investigation of acute and chronic chest pain presenting in primary care. Health Technol Assess 2004; 8 (2): 1–158.

Masci PG, Ganame J, Strata E et al. Myocardial salvage by CMR correlates with LV remodeling and early ST-segment resolution in acute myocardial infarction. JACC Cardiovasc Imaging 2010; 3 (1): 45–51.

Miller CD, Hwang W, Hoekstra JW et al. Stress cardiac magnetic resonance imaging with observation unit care reduces cost for patients with emergent chest pain: a randomized trial. Ann Emerg Med 2010; 56: 209–19.

Miller TD, Christian TF, Hopfenspirger MR et al. Infarct size after acute myocardial-infarction measured by quantitative tomographic Tc-99M sestamibi imaging predicts subsequent mortality. Circulation 1995; 92 (3): 334–41.

Morishima I, Sone T, Okumura K et al. Angiographic no-reflow phenomenon as a predictor of adverse long-term outcome in patients treated with percutaneous transluminal coronary angioplasty for first acute myocardial infarction. J Am Coll Cardiol 2000; 36 (4): 1202–9.

Moss AJ. Risk stratification and survival after myocardial-infarction. N Engl J Med 1983; 309 (6): 331–6.

Nijveldt R, Beek AM, Hirsch A et al. Functional recovery after acute myocardial infarction. J Am Coll Cardiol 2008; 52 (3): 181–9.

Nijveldt R, Hofman MBM, Hirsch A et al. Assessment of microvascular obstruction and prediction of short-term remodeling after acute myocardial infarction: cardiac MR imaging study. Radiology 2009; 250 (2): 363–70.

Nilsson JC, Nielsen G, Groenning BA et al. Sustained post-infarction myocardial oedema in humans visualised by magnetic resonance imaging. Heart 2001; 85 (6): 639–42.

Okayama S, Uemura S, Soeda T et al. Clinical significance of papillary muscle late enhancement detected via cardiac magnetic resonance imaging in patients with single old myocardial infarction. Int J Cardiol 2011; 146: 73–9.

O'Regan DP, Ahmed R, Karunanithy N et al. Reperfusion hemorrhage following acute myocardial infarction: assessment with T2*mapping and effect on measuring the area at risk. Radiology 2009; 250 (3): 916–22.

Orn S, Manhenke C, Greve OJ et al. Microvascular obstruction is a major determinant of infarct healing and subsequent left ventricular remodeling following primary percutaneous coronary intervention. Eur Heart J 2009; 30 (16): 1978–85.

Plein S, Greenwood JP, Ridgway JP et al. Assessment of non-ST-segment elevation acute coronary syndromes with cardiac magnetic resonance imaging. J Am Coll Cardiol 2004; 44 (11): 2173–81.

Plein S, Ryf S, Schwitter J et al. Dynamic contrast-enhanced myocardial perfusion MRI accelerated with k-t sense. Magn Reson Med 2007; 58: 777–85.

Plein S, Younger JF, Sparrow P et al. Cardiovascular magnetic resonance of scar and ischemia burden early after acute ST elevation and non-ST elevation myocardial infarction. J Cardiovasc Magn Reson 2008; 10: 47.

Raman SV, Dickerson JA, Jekic M et al. Real-time cine and myocardial perfusion with treadmill exercise stress cardiovascular magnetic resonance in patients referred for stress SPECT. J Cardiovasc Magn Reson 2010b; 12 (1): 41.

Raman SV, Simonetti OP, Winner MW et al. Cardiac magnetic resonance with edema imaging identifies myocardium at risk and predicts worse outcome in patients with non-ST-segment elevation acute coronary syndrome. J Am Coll Cardiol 2010a; 55 (22): 2480–8.

Reimer KA, Jennings RB. Changing anatomic reference base of evolving myocardial-infarction – underestimation of myocardial collateral blood-flow and over-estimation of experimental anatomic infarct size due to tissue edema, hemorrhage and acute inflammation. Circulation 1979; 60 (4): 866–76.

Reimer KA, Lowe JE, Rasmussen MM, Jennings RB. Wavefront phenomenon of ischemic cell-death 1. Myocardial infarct size vs duration of coronary-occlusion in dogs. Circulation 1977; 56 (5): 786–94.

Roes SD, Borleffs CJW, van der Geest RJ et al. Infarct tissue heterogeneity assessed with contrast-enhanced MRI predicts spontaneous ventricular arrhythmia in patients with ischemic cardiomyopathy and implantable cardioverter-defibrillator. Circ Cardiovascular Imaging 2009; 2 (3): 183–90.

Rubenstein JC, Ortiz JT, Wu E et al. Imaging and diagnostic testing – the use of periinfarct contrast-enhanced cardiac magnetic resonance imaging for the prediction of late post-myocardial infarction ventricular dysfunction. Am Heart J 2008; 156 (3): 498–505.

Schmidt A, Azevedo CF, Cheng A et al. Infarct tissue heterogeneity by magnetic resonance imaging identifies enhanced cardiac arrhythmia susceptibility in patients with left ventricular dysfunction. Circulation 2007; 115 (15): 2006–14.

Schulz-Menger J, Gross M, Messroghli D et al. Cardiovascular magnetic resonance of acute myocardial infarction at a very early stage. J Am Coll Cardiol 2003; 42 (3): 513–8.

Schwitter J, Nanz D, Kneifel S et al. Assessment of myocardial perfusion in coronary artery disease by magnetic resonance: a comparison with positron emission tomography and coronary angiography. Circulation 2001; 103: 2230–5.

Srichai MB, Junor C, Rodriguez LL et al. Clinical, imaging, and pathological characteristics of left ventricular thrombus: A comparison of contrast-enhanced magnetic resonance imaging, transthoracic echocardiography, and transesophageal echocardiography with surgical or pathological validation. Am Heart J 2006; 152 (1): 75–84.

Steenbergen C, Hill ML, Jennings RB. Volume regulation and plasma membrane injury in aerobic, anaerobic, and ischemic myocardium in vitro. Effects of osmotic cell swelling on plasma membrane integrity. Circ Res 1985; 57 (6): 864–75.

Taylor AJ, Saadi NA, Al Saadi N et al. Detection of acutely impaired microvascular reperfusion after infarct angioplasty with magnetic resonance imaging. Circulation 2004; 109 (17): 2080–5.

Taylor AM, Dymarkowski S, Verbeken EK, Bogaert J. Detection of pericardial inflammation with late-enhancement cardiac magnetic resonance imaging: initial results. Eur Radiology 2006; 16 (3): 569–74.

Thygesen K, Alpert JS, White HD; Joint ESC/ACCF/AHA/WHF Task Force for the Redefinition of Myocardial Infarction. Universal definition of myocardial infarction. Circulation 2007; 116 (22): 2634–53.

Van de Werf F, Ardissino D, Betriu A et al. Management of acute myocardial infarction in patients presenting with ST-segment elevation. The Task Force on the Management of Acute Myocardial Infarction of the European Society of Cardiology. Eur Heart J 2003; 24: 28–66.

Wagner A, Mahrholdt H, Holly TA et al. Contrast-enhanced MRI and routine single photon emission computed tomography (SPECT) perfusion imaging for detection of subendocardial myocardial infarcts: an imaging study. Lancet 2003; 361 (9355): 374–9.

Weinsaft JW, Kim HW, Shah DJ et al. Detection of left ventricular thrombus by delayed-enhancement cardiovascular magnetic resonance – prevalence and markers in patients with systolic dysfunction. J Am Coll Cardiol 2008; 52 (2): 148–57.

Weinsaft JW, Kim RJ, Ross M et al. Contrast-enhanced anatomic imaging as compared to contrast-enhanced tissue characterization for detection of left ventricular thrombus. JACC Cardiovasc Imaging 2009; 2 (8): 969–79.

White HD, Norris RM, Brown MA et al. Left-ventricular end-systolic volume as the major determinant of survival after recovery from myocardial-infarction. Circulation 1987; 76 (1): 44–51.

Willerson JT, Scales F, Mukherjee A et al. Abnormal myocardial fluid retention as an early manifestation of ischemic injury. Am J Pathol 1977; 87: 159–88.

Wollert KC, Meyer GP, Lotz J et al. Intracoronary autologous bone-marrow cell transfer after myocardial infarction: the BOOST randomised controlled clinical trial. Lancet 2004; 364 (9429): 141–8.

Wu E, Ortiz JT, Tejedor P et al. Infarct size by contrast-enhanced cardiac magnetic resonance is a stronger predictor of outcomes than left ventricular ejection fraction or end-systolic volume index: prospective cohort study. Heart 2008; 94 (6): 730–6.

Wu KC, Kim RJ, Bluemke DA et al. Quantification and time course of microvascular obstruction by contrast-enhanced echocardiography and magnetic resonance imaging following acute myocardial infarction and reperfusion. J Am Coll Cardiol 1998a; 32 (6): 1756–64.

Wu KC, Zerhouni EA, Judd RM et al. Prognostic significance of microvascular obstruction by magnetic resonance imaging in patients with acute myocardial infarction. Circulation 1998b; 97 (8): 765–72.

Yan AT, Shayne AJ, Brown KA al. Characterization of the peri-infarct zone by contrast-enhanced cardiac magnetic resonance imaging is a powerful predictor of post-myocardial infarction mortality. Circulation 2006; 114 (1): 32–9.

Yokota H, Heidary S, Katikireddy CK et al. Quantitative characterization of myocardial infarction by cardiovascular magnetic resonance predicts future cardiovascular events in patients with ischemic cardiomyopathy. J Cardiovasc Magn Reson 2008; 10: 17.

Zehender M, Kasper W, Kauder E et al. Right ventricular infarction as an independent predictor of prognosis after acute inferior myocardial-infarction. N Engl J Med 1993; 328 (14): 981–8.

8 Magnetic Resonance Coronary Angiography and Vessel Wall Imaging

Won Yong Kim, René Botnar and Volker Rasche

8.1 Introduction

Despite progress in prevention and treatment, coronary artery disease (CAD) remains the number one cause of death in the developed countries. The current gold standard for the diagnosis and treatment of CAD is cardiac catheterization. Currently, about 1,000,000 US citizens undergo cardiac catheterization each year. In up to 40% of the examined patients, there is no need for further interventional treatment. Due to the risk of invasive catheterization and the related high costs, alternative non-invasive tests are required to exclude significant CAD. Cardiovascular magnetic resonance (CMR) provides a comprehensive evaluation on myocardial perfusion, function and morphology in CAD. Magnetic resonance angiography (MRA) can be applied for direct visualization of the coronary artery lumen (Kim 2001a) and the vessel wall (Spuentrup 2006), thus making CMR a unique tool providing all required diagnostic information in a single examination.

However, up to now coronary MRA for the assessment of the native coronary arteries has not yet become clinical routine and its application is limited to the assessment of anomalies (class I indication) and aortocoronary bypass grafts (class II indication). Thus, coronary MRA remains challenging mainly due to the pronounced cardiac and respiratory motion combined with the need for high spatial resolution due to the small caliber of the coronary arteries (2–3 mm) and their often very tortuous course.

Continued progress in scanner technology is likely to further facilitate imaging of the coronary arteries as well as the coronary veins. Imaging of coronary vein anatomy has become of interest, especially for optimal placement of pacemaker leads in cardiac resynchronization therapy.

The following chapter will provide an update on current improvements in coronary MRA methodology as well as provide an overview of its current clinical use.

8.2 Motion Compensation

The rapid intrinsic cardiac motion and the respiratory motion pose a major challenge to coronary MRA and vessel wall imaging. A variety of techniques has been introduced to reduce motion related artifacts.

8.2.1 Cardiac Motion

To freeze the cardiac motion, data acquisition has to be synchronized with the heart beat. Since high spatial resolution is required for adequate visualization of the small caliber coronary vessels, the data acquisition must be restricted to periods with minimal cardiac motion (Wang 2000, Kim 2001b). Resting periods with relative diastasis occurs during end-systole (~ 50 ms) and mid-diastole (~ 100 ms) (Hofman 1998, Sodickson 1997a, Wang 1999, Mao 2000). Due to the higher blood flow, usually the end-diastolic rest period is preferred. End-systolic imaging is used in patients with high heart rates since they tend to have shortened mid-diastolic rest periods or in cases of highly varying heart rates, causing a temporal shift of the mid-diastolic rest period over the data acquisition period. Furthermore, end-systolic imaging appears favorable for the assessment of the coronary veins, since the veins usually show larger diameters in end-systole (Nezafat 2007). It is important to note that the optimal trigger delay (time between the R-peak of the ECG and the actual start of the data acquisition) and the length of the acquisition window depends on the patient's heart rate. Therefore, the optimal trigger delay with minimal cardiac motion should preferably be identified shortly before the coronary scan from a cine scan in the 4-chamber view.

The use of a vector ECG (Fischer 1999) or acoustic ECG (Becker 2010) recording in combination with optical transmit lines is recommended since the ECG signal is deteriorated by the main magnetic field caused by the magnetohydrodynamic effect (T-wave enhancement) and often becomes disturbed by the rapidly switching gradient waveforms.

8.2.2 Respiratory Motion

The motion of the heart due to respiratory motion can easily exceed 1–2 cm causing a displacement of the coronary vessels during the respiratory cycle. Thus, synchronization of the image acquisition with the respiratory position of the heart is required. Current approaches to coronary artery imaging utilize navigator techniques (Ehman 1989, Nehrke 1999) to avoid long breath-holds and since high-resolution 3D data acquisition is required to cover the entire coronary vasculature. As described in Chapter 1, the principle of a navigator is to monitor the position of the diaphragm prior to the actual data acquisition (Sachs 1994, Wang 1995, Li 1996, Oshinski 1997, Müller 1997, McConnell 1997, Stuber 1999a, Jahnke 2007). This is achieved by performing a one-dimensional MRI acquisition with e.g. a pencil-beam shaped volume, which is usually located at the dome of the right hemisphere of the diaphragm. The navigator technique can be applied for measuring the diaphragmatic position prior to the actual data acquisition. Depending on the identified respiratory position, the data is either accepted when the position is within a certain acceptance window, or rejected. In the latter case, the data has to be remeasured. The rejection percentage depends on the user-defined acceptance window (normally 5–6 mm). A narrow acceptance window reduces the motion artifacts but increases the overall acquisition time since more data is rejected. To enable larger acceptance windows, the position of the imaging slice can be prospectively adapted to the measured respiratory position and thereby follow the respiratory motion. Normally the movement of the heart due to breathing is less pronounced than the motion of the diaphragm and a scale factor of 0.4–0.6 has been used for optimal slice tracking.

The respiratory induced motion of the heart cannot be completely modeled by a simple translation along the feet-to-head direction. Jahnke et al. (2007) showed that in up to 30 % of the patients an affine transformation models the respiratory induced motion more accurately.

8.3 Imaging Techniques

The imaging of the coronary vasculature demands dedicated techniques to optimize image contrast and ensure a high signal-to-noise ratio (SNR) yielding a clear delineation of the blood-filled structures or the vessel walls with high spatial resolution.

The **standard coronary MRA protocol** comprises:

- ECG triggering for synchronization of the heart motion with the data acquisition,
- respiratory navigation for synchronization/compensation of the respiratory motion,
- spin preparation for ensuring sufficient image contrast, and
- the imaging sequence.

Depending on the application, the spin preparation and the imaging sequence and, to a lesser extent, the trigger and navigator component have to be adapted.

8.3.1 Coronary Artery Imaging

The first approaches to coronary angiography by Edelman et al. (1991) and Manning et al. (1993a) applied two-dimensional (2D) gradient-echo techniques. Epicardial fat was suppressed by application of a spectral selective fat suppression pulse. Data acquisition was synchronized with the heart beat and data acquisition restricted to a mid-diastolic window of roughly 100 ms length. Acquisition of a single slice took about 16 heart beats and was performed in a single breath-hold.

Three-dimensional (3D) imaging was initially not possible due to the inherent long acquisition times. With the introduction of the navigator techniques, data acquisition could be performed during free breathing and 3D acquisitions became feasible, which resulted in significantly improved SNR's and enabled higher spatial resolution. However, in 3D acquisitions a reduced contrast between blood and myocardium is observed since inflow effects are less prominent. Therefore, contrast enhancing spin preparation

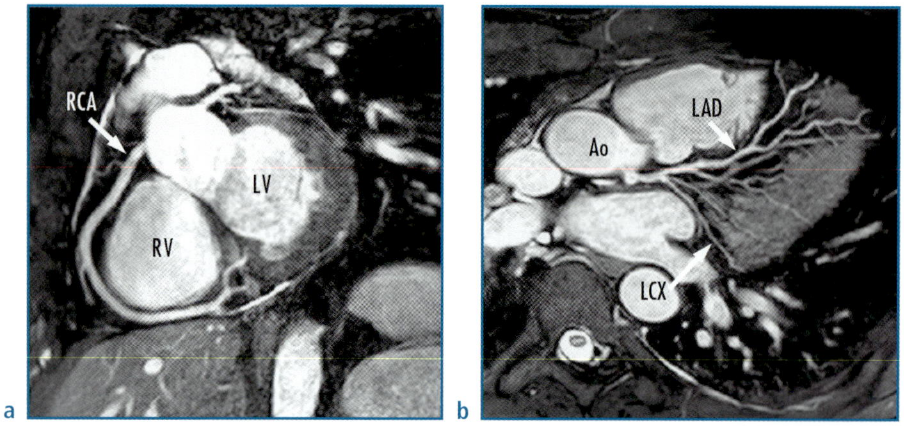

Figure 8-1 Visualization of the right **(a)** and left **(b)** coronary artery tree. Data were acquired by a navigator gated, fat suppressed, T2-prepared steady-state free precession gradient echo sequence. Ao: aorta; LAD: left anterior descendent artery; LCX: left circumflex artery; LV: left ventricle; RCA: right coronary artery; RV: right ventricle.

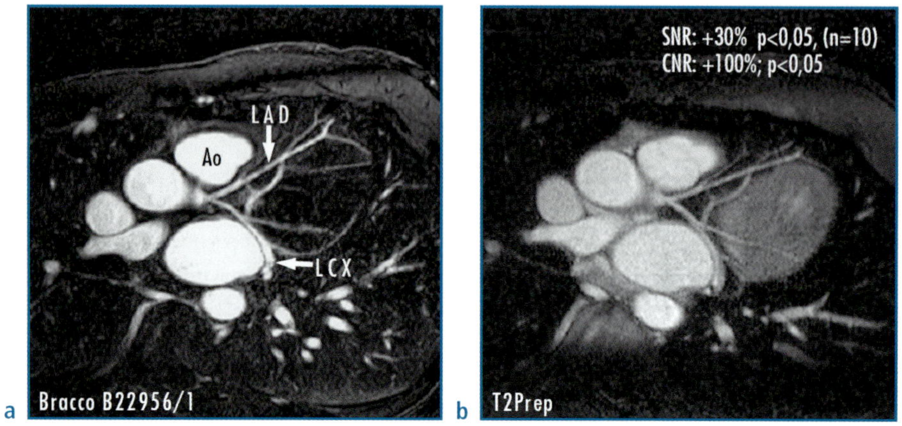

Figure 8-2 Comparison of the conspicuity of the coronary artery with **(a)** and without **(b)** contrast agent (intravascular CA Bracco-B22956) enhancement. The contrast between blood and myocardium and the signal-to-noise ratio appear significantly improved for the CA-enhanced acquisition. Ao: aorta; LAD: left anterior descendent artery; LCX: left circumflex artery.

techniques (Li 1993, Brittain 1995, Botnar 1999) in combination with steady-state free precession (SSFP) techniques have been developed to provide sufficient contrast for delineation of the coronary arteries (Deshpande 2001).

Although a clinical standard has not yet been established, usually a three-dimensional steady-state free precession gradient-echo technique is used (Deshpande 2001, Giorgi 2002, Spuentrup 2002; Figure 8-1). SSFP sequences are normally preferred over T1-weighted gradient echo techniques to benefit from the intrinsic higher SNR and better blood-myocardium contrast. However, due to the off-resonance sensitivity of the SSFP sequence, short repetition times have to be ensured to avoid black-band artifacts caused by the susceptibility differences between lung and myocardium. Furthermore, excellent blood-myocardium contrast needs large flip angles with related high SAR values. This limits the application of the SSFP techniques to 1.5 T systems. At 3 T and higher field strengths (Kaul 2004) T1-weighted gradient echo techniques appear as promising alternative to SSFP techniques.

Further improvement of the contrast between blood and the surrounding tissues can be achieved by application of contrast agents (CA) (Figure 8-2). Contrast agents currently available include extracellular CA (Regenfus 2000), blood-pool CA (Li 1998, Huber 2003, Tang 2009), and slightly albumin binding CA (Nassenstein 2009, Liu 2008, Yang 2009). Ideally, the coronary artery imaging protocol should become part of a routine ischemia/CAD diagnostic imaging protocol. Besides improving vessel conspicuity, the applied CA should also provide late enhancement imaging of scar. The application of the extracellular CAs is limited for vessel enhancement because of the rapid extravasation into the interstitial space. Blood-pool agents may face limitations for late enhancement imaging. Hence, slightly albumin binding CAs appear promising for vessel enhancement due to the prolonged retention time of the CA in the blood pool and its high relaxivities (Laurent 2006), while maintaining late enhancement properties (Krombach 2009).

For faster acquisitions and for reduction of the motion sensitivity of the sequence, alternative encoding of k-space on EPI (Bhat 2010, Slavin 1998), spiral- (Bornert 2001) or radial trajectories (Priest 2007) have been introduced. But due to high off-resonance sensitivity (EPI, spiral) and inefficient k-space sampling (radial), these techniques have not yet been established standards in coronary artery imaging. Parallel imaging techniques such as SMASH (Sodickson

1997b) and SENSE (Pruessmann 1999) are often applied to reduce the overall acquisition time. For the three-dimensional approaches in combination with two-dimensional coil arrays, acceleration along the phase- and slice-encoding direction can be applied. However, acceleration factors above four can hardly be realized due to SNR limitations (Sodickson 1999, Yu 2009).

For non-CA-enhanced imaging, the spin preparation normally includes fat suppression and T2-preparation. Other techniques for improving the blood-myocardium contrast such as spin-locking (Dixon 1996) or magnetization transfer techniques (Li 1993) have been suggested but are not widely applied. In CA-enhanced imaging, the T2-preparation is usually replaced by a saturation (Goldfarb 1998) or an inversion (Stuber 1999b) prepulse. The rapid recovery of the CA filled blood (T1 of blood = 1,200 ms without CA, T1 = 50–100 ms with CA, T1 of the myocardium = 850 ms) ensures excellent contrast between blood and myocardium. The improved contrast and higher magnetization of the blood using CA can either be traded for improving the spatial resolution or for reduction of the image acquisition time.

One major limitation in coronary artery imaging remains to be a limited spatial resolution even at higher field strength. High-resolution imaging with decent SNR is often not possible, since the related very long acquisition times raise severe problems with arrhythmias and drift of the diaphragmatic position.

8.3.2 Coronary Vein Imaging

Assessment of the course of the coronary veins (CV) (Figure 8-3) has recently gained interest for pre-interventional identification of the optimal left ventricular lead placement with biventricular pacemaker devices. A major limitation in CV imaging stems from the low oxygen saturation of venous blood, which causes a strong reduction of the blood T2 value. Contrast enhancement approaches such as the T2-preparation (T2-prep), well-known from coronary artery angiography, cannot be applied to the CV. Current approaches to CV imaging include non-contrast agent approaches (Nezafat 2007, Stoeck 2009), in which optimized magnetization transfer (MTC) preparation is applied for improving blood-myocardial contrast. The usage of contrast agents has recently been published, including the application of blood-pool (Rasche 2007, Chiribiri 2008), extracellular (Yonger 2009), and slightly albumin binding contrast agents (Duckett 2010).

The optimal acquisition window for coronary veins is at end-systole according to a study in healthy subjects. In end-systole, the diameter of the coronary sinus and its major tributaries appeared significantly larger than in the respective mid-diastolic resting phase (Nezafat 2007). In case of heart failure patients, however, the identification of a systolic rest period may become challenging due to the asynchronous contraction and data acquisition during the mid-diastolic rest period may be more promising.

8.3.3 Coronary Arterial Wall Imaging

The first in vivo images of the coronary vessel wall were obtained applying a two-dimensional fat saturated fast spin echo (FSE) technique (Fayad 2000, Botnar 2000). For improved contrast between the blood and the vessel wall, black-blood contrast was established with a double inversion recovery (DIR) prepulse (Edelman 1991). Images were obtained with breath-hold technique as well as during free

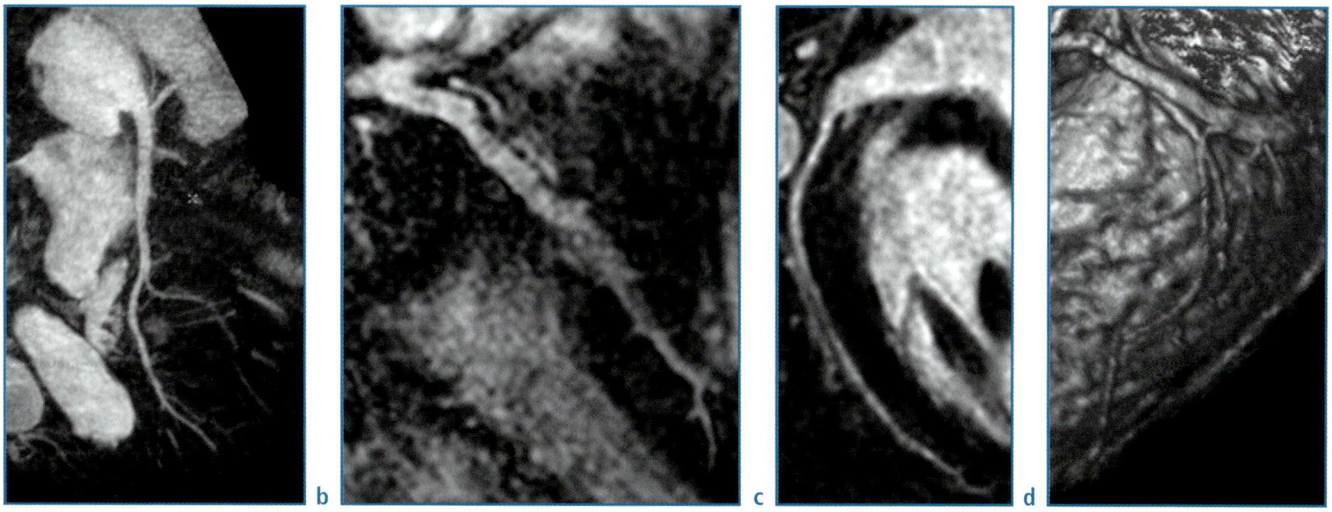

a b c d

Figure 8-3 Volumetric visualization of the coronary veins. Multi-planar reformat (MPR) of the great cardiac vein (a), MPR of the mid cardiac vein (b), MPR of the lateral vein (c), and volume rendered visualization of the coronary sinus and a major lateral vein (d).

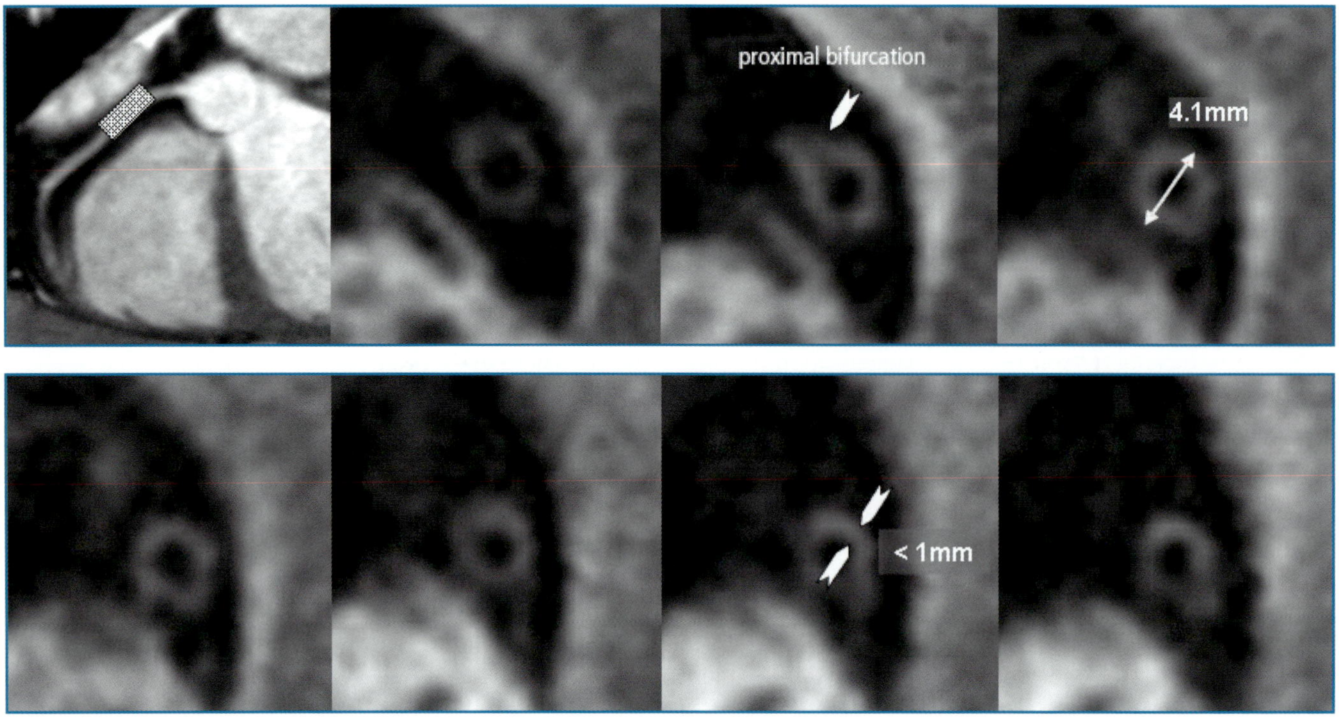

Figure 8-4 High-resolution visualization of the proximal right coronary artery wall. Images were acquired at $250 \times 250\ \mu m^2$ in-plane resolution with 1 mm slice thickness.

breathing. The initial studies demonstrated the applicability of CMR for the assessment of the coronary artery vessel wall in healthy volunteers and in patients with CAD (Figure 8-4). Further approaches include the combination of the DIR techniques with fast gradient echo-based readout schemes (Botnar 2003). For further improvements of the image acquisition, combination with spiral acquisition trajectories (Botnar 2001) and radial acquisition schemes (Katoh 2006) were introduced.

For the specific imaging of atherosclerosis, the application of conventional and specific contrast agents (CA) has been published (Kerwin 2009). In vivo, clinically approved extracellular gadolinium-based CA has been proposed. The uptake of extracellular gadolinium CA in atherosclerotic plaques appears to be non-specific but accumulates in soft plaques both in patients with stable angina pectoris (Yeon 2007) and in patients with acute coronary syndromes (Ibrahim 2009) and conventional late-enhancement techniques can therefore be applied for soft plaque analysis.

Further work has been obtained in experimental animal models. Accumulation of blood-pool CA indicates an increased vascularization and permeability of the vessel wall (Lobbes 2009). The accumulation of iron-oxide particles (USPIO) in the vessel wall indicates inflammation. This is most likely caused by phagocytosis of the USPIOs by macrophages, which more frequently occur in inflamed segments of the vessel wall. A new class of CA is defined by specific CA, which specifically binds to a target molecule. This enables the selective labeling of e.g. inflammatory markers (intercellular adhesion molecule-1 [ICAM-1], vascular cell adhesion molecule-1 [VCAM-1], or matrix metalloproteinase [MMP]). Recent work includes the specific labeling of thrombi by fibrin-specific CA. The specific CAs might open new opportunities for molecular MRI for characterization of early atherosclerotic lesions as well as for the assessment of plaque vulnerability.

8.4 Planning of a Coronary MRI Examination

Due to the anatomical variation of the coronary arteries, an individual planning procedure of the scan geometry is required.

Two **different approaches** are currently used:

- **whole heart imaging**: In the whole-heart approach, an axially oriented volume is acquired. For the coronary arteries, the individual planning of the location of the volume is best done from coronal scout images showing the root of the aorta. To ensure coverage of the entire left and right coronary artery system, the 3D volume should include 2 cm cranial of the aortic root to about 1 cm caudal

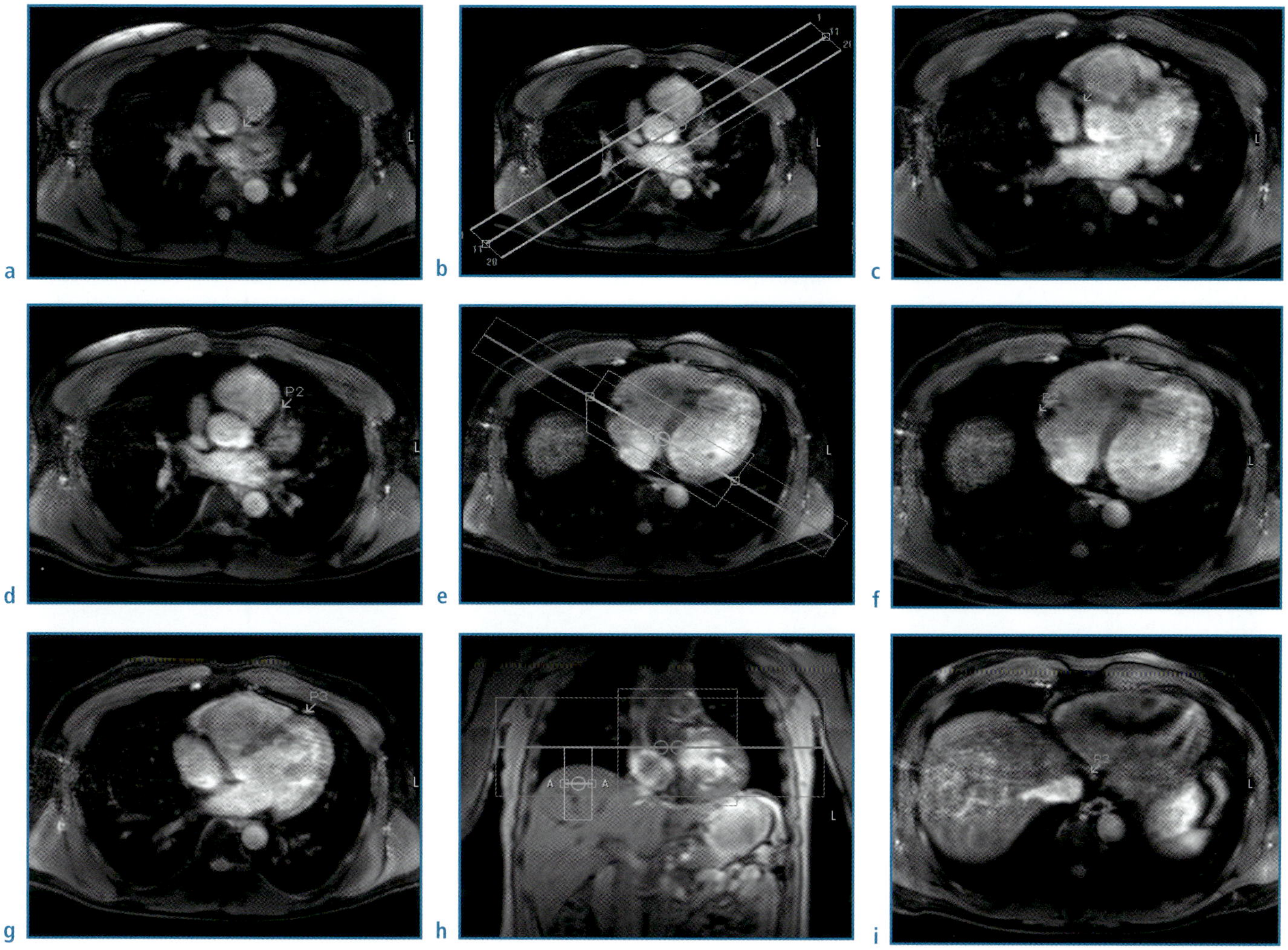

Figure 8-5 Planning and resulting location of the field of view (FOV) for targeted coronary artery imaging of the right **(a, d, g, b)** and the left **(c, f, i, e)** tree, and for whole-heart imaging **(h)**.

to the heart-diaphragm boundary (Figure 8-5h). The volume should preferably be with isotropic spatial resolution to enable reformatting along the entire course of the coronary arteries. The major disadvantages of the whole-heart approach are the inherent longer acquisition time required for the acquisition of the large volume with sufficient spatial resolution and the reduced inflow effects causing less contrast.

- **targeted imaging**: In the targeted approach, the left and right coronary systems are acquired subsequently in two individually planned volumes. The location of the central slice is defined by manual identification of three-points located along the major coronary arteries (Figure 8-5).

For coronary vein imaging, whole heart techniques have been suggested (Nezafat 2007, Rasche 2007). Since the main interest in coronary vein imaging is the identification of tributaries to the coronary sinus and the great cardiac vein, an efficient approach appears to be the alignment of the volume of interest with the mitral valve annulus. This can be planned based on 2- and 4-chamber views. For identification of the off-spring location and angle of the tributaries, the acquisition can be restricted to a small volume of about 5 cm. Further identification of the course of a specific tributary can then be done in a subsequent scan aligned with the lateral wall of the left ventricle located at the respective branch location.

The small caliber of the coronary vasculature demands imaging with sufficiently high spatial resolution. Accurate identification of small changes in the coronary artery diameter or vessel wall thickness demands spatial resolutions in the order of 100 μm. With current MRI systems, this demand cannot be met and compromises have to be made. In whole heart approaches, the required isotropic spatial resolution normally restricts the achievable resolution to about $1.3 \times 1.3 \times 1.3\ mm^3$. For targeted approaches, non-isotropic resolutions yielding high in-plane resolution in the order of 0.5 × 0.5 mm^2 with substantially thicker slices between 2–5 mm are used.

For the identification of the location and off-spring angle of the tributaries, isotropic spatial resolution in the order of 1.3 × 1.3 × 1.3 mm^3 appears necessary. Non-isotropic spatial resolution may be used for scanning the course of a specific lateral vein.

8.5 Clinical Application

8.5.1 Coronary Angiography

Proximal and medial segments of the main branches of the coronary arteries can routinely be well-visualized by free breathing fast gradient echo techniques (Figure 8-6 and Figure 8-7). Especially the proximal segments could be

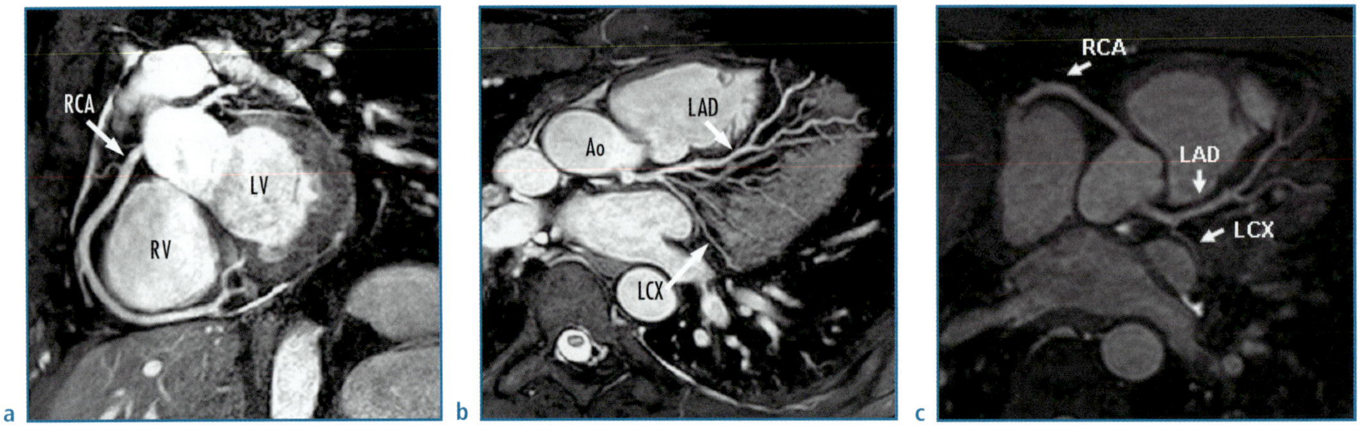

Figure 8-6 Visualization of the coronary arteries by the targeted **(a, b)** and the whole-heart imaging technique **(c)**. Ao: aorta; LAD: left arterior descentend artery; LCX: left circumflex artery; LV: left ventricle; RCA: right coronary artery; RV: right ventricle.

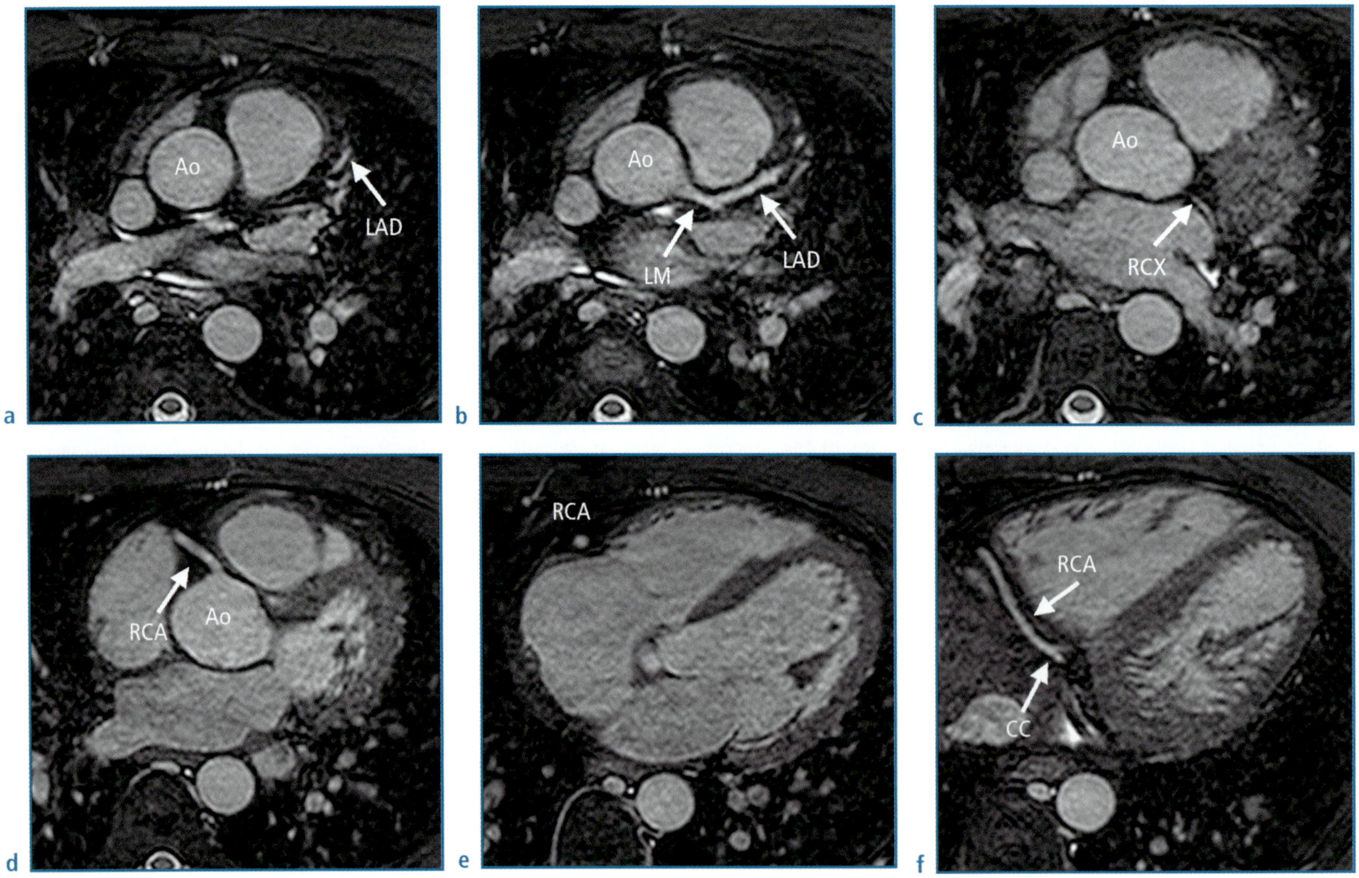

Figure 8-7 Whole-heart imaging of the coronary arteries. Ao: aorta; LAD: left ascending; LM: left main; RCA: right coronary artery; RCX: left circumflex.

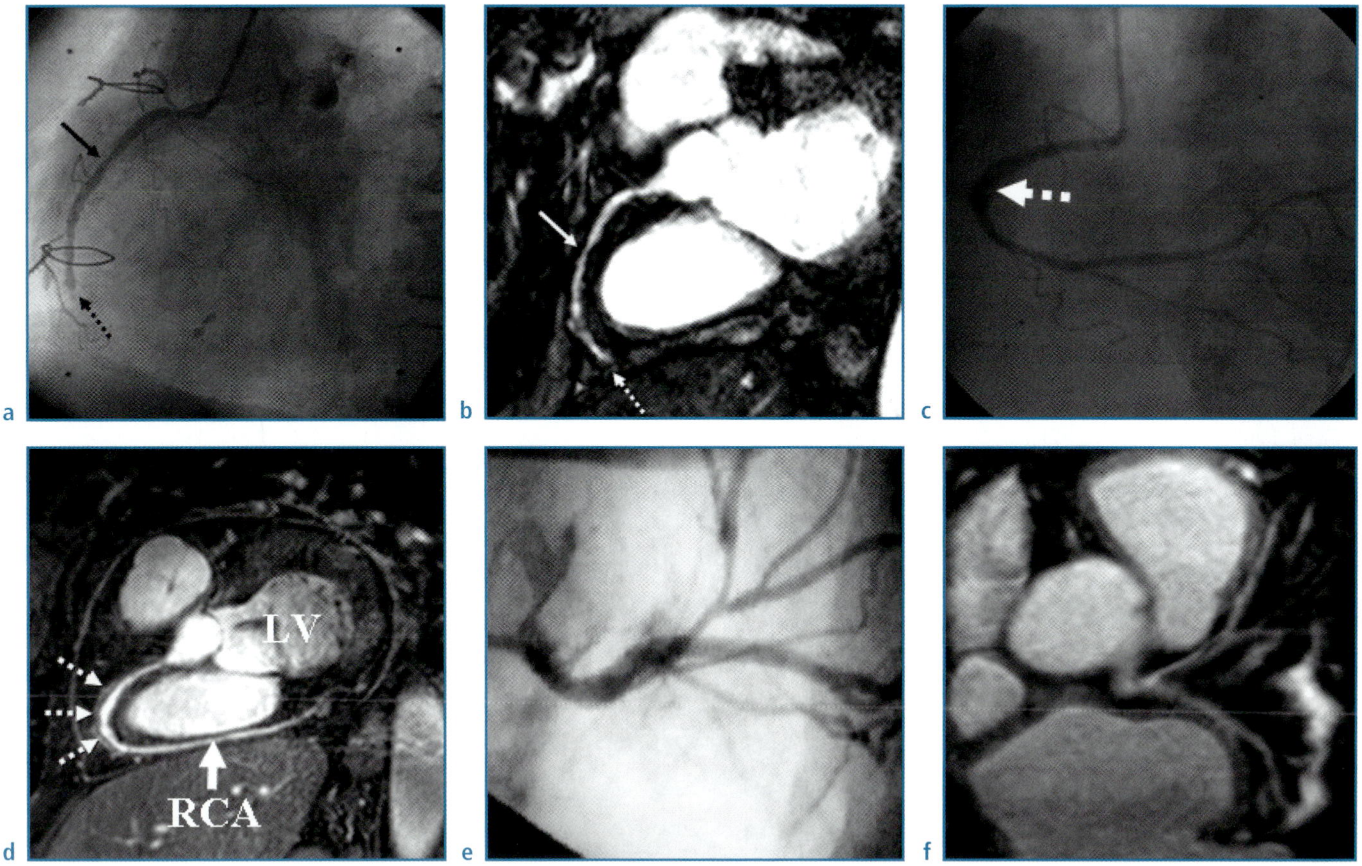

Figure 8-8 Angiographic (a, c, e) and MRI (b, d, f) visualization. Low-grade stenoses of the RCA (a, b); low-grade stenoses with clearly visible plaque in the MRI (dashed arrows) (c, d); high-grade stenoses of the LAD (e, f).

assessed in almost 100 % of the investigated volunteers. Due to the shorter distance to the receive coil and the surrounding epicardial fat, visualization of the LAD and RCA is less demanding than imaging of the LCX, which runs in the direct vicinity of the myocardium at a larger distance to the coil elements. The mean visualized length of the the coronary arteries was 50 mm (LAD), 80 mm (RCA), and 40 mm (LCX) (Paschal 1993, Manning 1993b, Hofman 1995, Oshinski 1996, Post 1996, Botnar 1999, Stuber 1999c, Lobbes 2009). An excellent agreement between the proximal diameter of the vessels was found between coronary MR angiography (MRA) and conventional angiography (Scheidegger 1994).

Although over the past years, a steady improvement in the quality of MR coronary angiography could be achieved, the spatial resolution is still significantly lower than for cardiac catheterization. Despite these limitations, coronary stenoses can often be identified in MRA. On "bright blood" (gradient echo technique) MR coronary angiograms, stenoses appear as a dark signal void in the otherwise bright vessel (Figure 8-8). In addition to a luminal narrowing, the signal loss is attributed to the dephasing of the spins within and distal to the stenosis due to the locally accelerated and often turbulent blood flow, which may cause overestimation of the stenosis in MRA (Pennell 1996).

The initial comparison between coronary MRA and conventional angiography in a selected patient group (Manning 1993) revealed a high sensitivity (90 %) and specificity (92 %) for significant stenoses (> 50 %) in the proximal segments. Later studies using free-breathing, navigator-gated and 3D-segmented gradient echo techniques showed encouraging results for the proximal coronary segments, but a large proportion of segments were not adequately visualized (Bogaert 2003, Botnar 1999, Dewey 2006, Jahnke 2004, Jahnke 2005, Kim 2001a, Maintz 2004, Ozgun 2005, Sakuma 2005, Sakuma 2006, Sommer 2002). An international multicenter study (Kim 2001a) revealed high sensitivity (92 %), but only moderate specificity (59 %). Excellent performance was observed for the exclusion of left main and three-vessel disease (sensitivity: 100 %, negative predictive value: 100 %). Accordingly, coronary MRA may be useful in combination with the late gadolinium enhancement technique in determining the underlying etiology (ischemic vs. non-ischemic) in patients presenting with dilated cardiomyopathy without clinical symptoms of myocardial infarction (Hundley 2010). A recent meta-analysis compared the diagnostic accuracy of

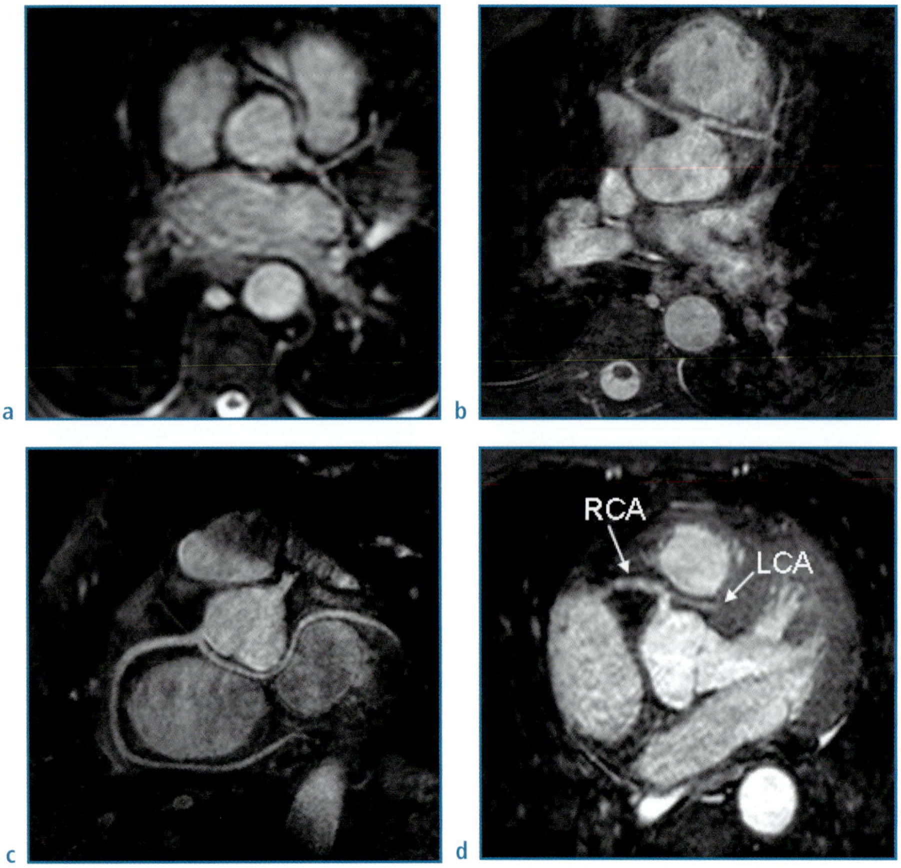

Figure 8-9 Assessment of coronary anomalies. Anterior dislocation of the sinus of the RCA with malign course of the proximal RCA (a); common origin of the right and left coronary artery tree (b, d); atypical offspring of the left circumflex artery (c). LCA: left coronary artery; RCA: right coronary artery.

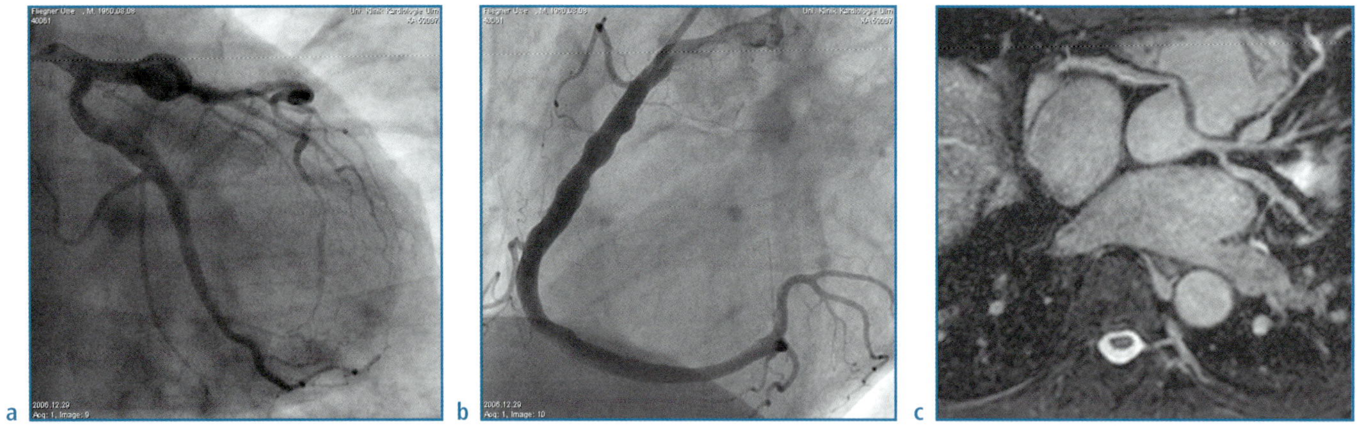

Figure 8-10 MRI of a 46-yrs-old patient (c) showed multiple coronary aneurysms, which could be confirmed angiographically (left coronary artery (a), right coronary artery (b)).

coronary MRA and multi-slice computed tomography (CT) for ruling out significant CAD in adults (Schuetz 2010). The conclusion was that CT is more accurate than CMR for ruling out CAD. Therefore, coronary CT is currently the preferred non-invasive alternative to invasive catherization for the exclusion of significant CAD.

8.5.2 Coronary Anomalies and Aneurysm

Coronary anomalies and aneurysms are usually well-visualized by coronary MRA (Figure 8-9 and Figure 8-10). The major advantage of CMR is the possibility for non-invasive assessment of the origin and course of the proximal coronary arteries. The derived information is usually sufficient

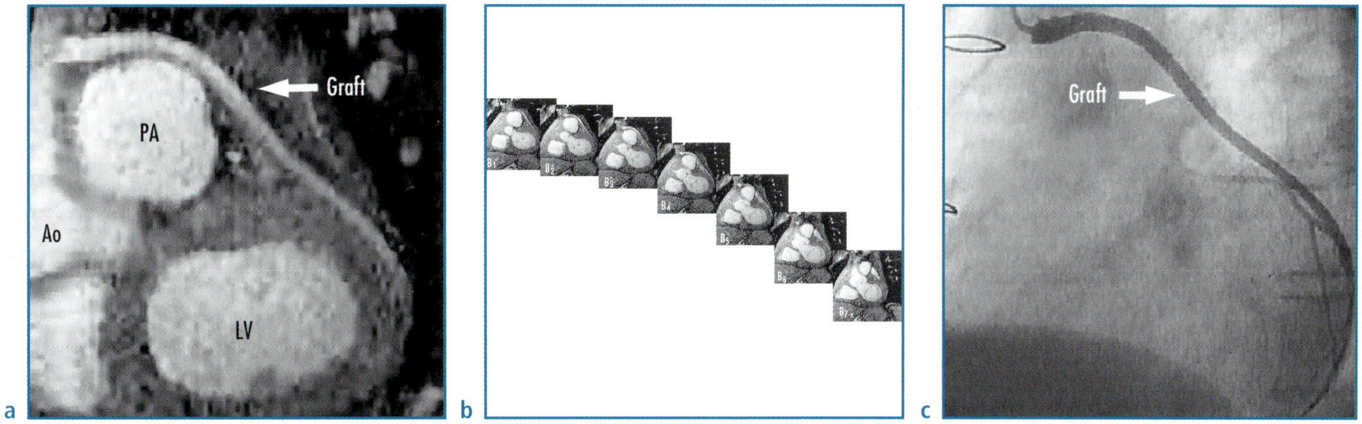

Figure 8-11 Multi-planar reformat (a), single slices (b), and the respective angiographic depiction (c) of an aortocoronary bypass. The images reveal a good agreement between MRI and angiography. Ao: aorta; LV: left ventricle; PA: pulmonary artery.

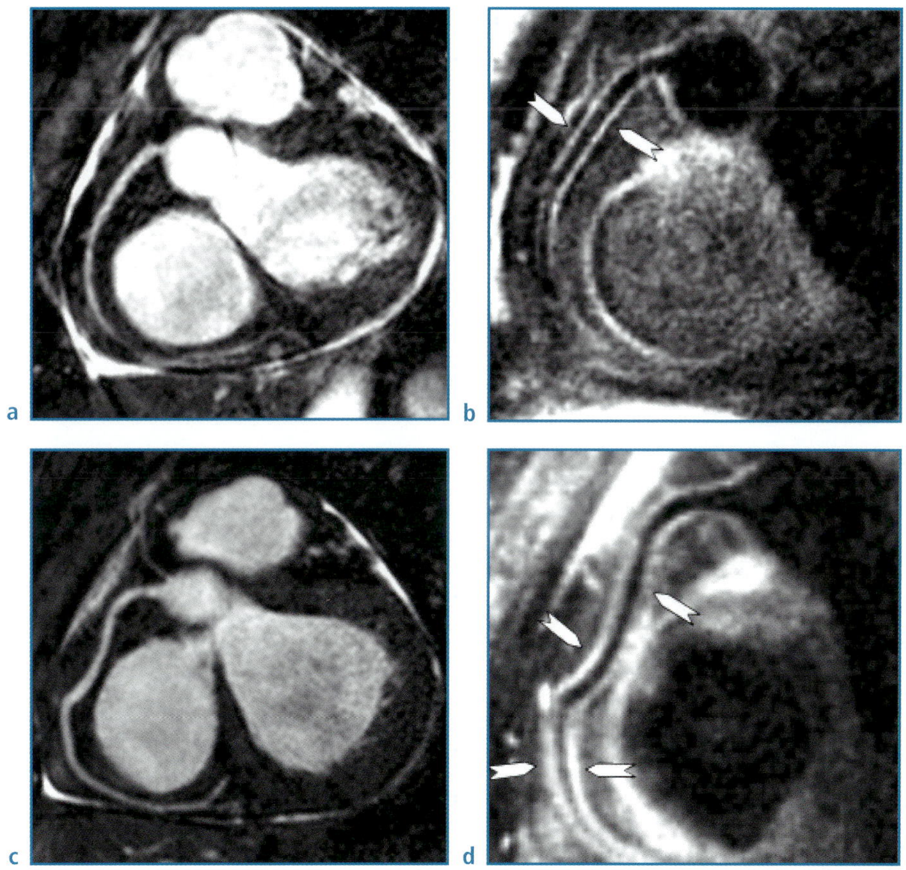

Figure 8-12 Patients with type 1 diabetes without (a, b) and with (c, d) nephropathy. In case of nephropathy, a clear thickening of the vessel wall (arrows) can be appreciated.

for identification of malignant anomalies (course of the vessel between the aorta and pulmonary artery).

Coronary aneurysm can be identified with bright-blood gradient echo techniques (Figure 8-10c).

The recommendation for the use of coronary MRA in clinical practice includes identifying coronary anomalies and aneurysms. This may be especially relevant for children and younger women because of the lack of exposure to ionizing radiation (Hundley 2010).

8.5.3 Coronary Bypass Grafts

The visualization of bypass grafts benefits from their rather stationary position, straight and known course, and large diameter as compared to the native coronary arteries (Figure 8-11). Spin echo techniques (White 1987, Rubinstein 1987, Jenkins 1988, Galjee 1996) as well as gradient echo techniques have been used. Flow can be assessed by signal voids (spin echo) or signal enhancement (bright-blood gradient echo). Contrast agents has been applied for enhancement of the blood signal (Wintersperger 1997, Vrachliotis 1997, Wintersperger 1998), which resulted in reported sensitivities between 95 and 100%.

A major limitation in bypass imaging results from the presence of metallic clips, which cause signal voids due to introduced susceptibility artifacts. Since clips are often located in the proximity of the bypass grafts and coronary arteries, the related signal voids may often not allow the assessment of the respective anatomy.

At specialized centers, coronary MRA may be used to identify coronary arterial stenoses in arterial bypass grafts (Hundley 2010).

8.5.4 Coronary Vessel Wall

The excellent soft tissue contrast of MRI enables the visualization of the vessel wall. By means of black-blood techniques, recent clinical MRI scanners can provide a detailed visualization of the coronary artery wall (Figure 8-4, Figure 8-12, Figure 8-13, and Figure 8-14). Major limitations rise from the need for very high spatial resolution and the related long acquisition times.

The vessel wall can either be visualized in a cross-sectional view (Figure 8-4) or along the long-axis of the

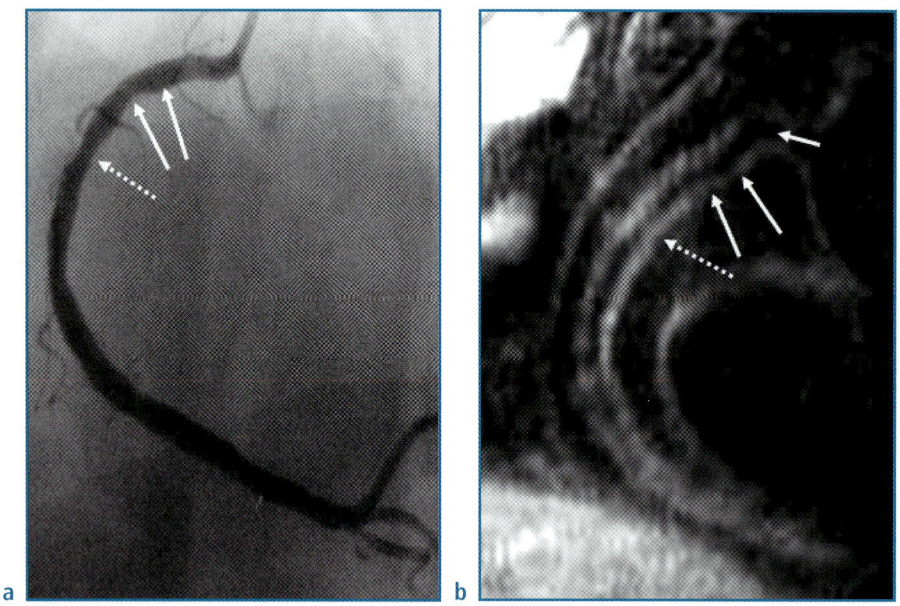

Figure 8-13 Patient with low-grade (< 40%) stenoses of the right coronary artery (a). The respective MRI (b) reveals a pronounced thickening of the vessel wall (arrows in (b)).

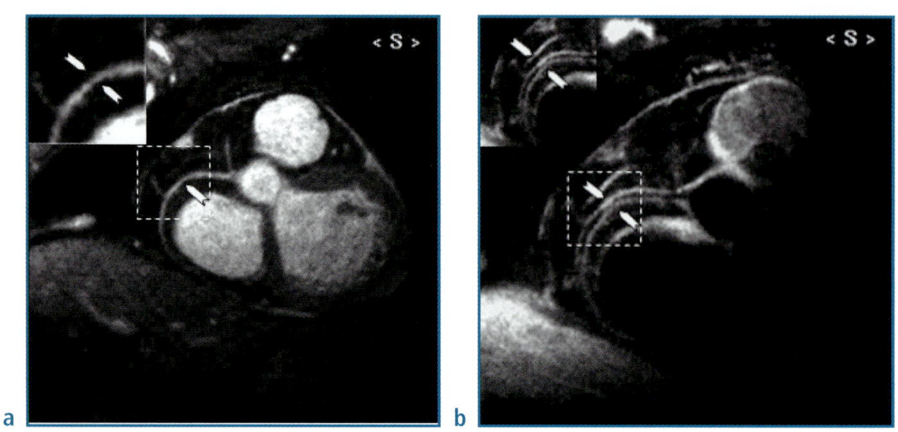

Figure 8-14 Patient with low-grade stenoses in the RCA, clearly visible in the MR angiography (a). A clear thickening of the vessel wall at the location of the lesion is visible in the respective black-blood image (arrows in (b)).

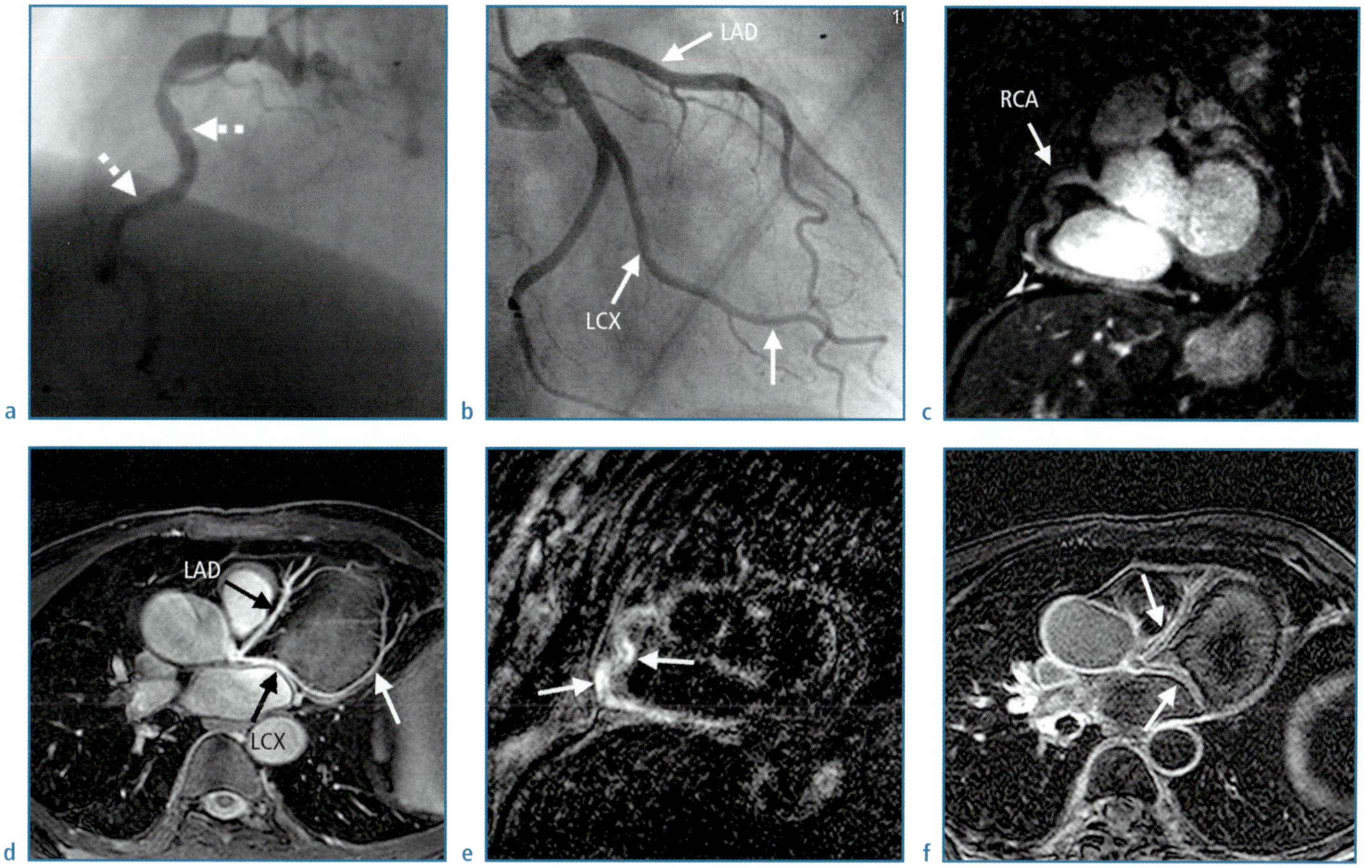

Figure 8-15 Angiography (a, b), MRI angiography (c, d), and late enhancement MRI (e, f) images of a patient with multiple atherosclerotic lesions (a, c, e) and a patient with Mediterranean fever (b, d, f). LAD: left anterior descendent artery; LCX: left circumflex artery; RCA: right coronary artery.

vessel (Figure 8-12, Figure 8-13, and Figure 8-14). Due to reduced partial volume effects, the cross-sectional orientation is supposed to provide more accurate quantification of the vessel wall thickness. Alignment along the long-axis of the vessel allows a quick qualitative assessment of the vessel wall properties along the entire proximal vessel.

Visualization of physiological processes in the coronary vessel wall may benefit from contrast agent-enhanced imaging. After injection of e.g. extracellular CA, the delayed enhancement images show diffuse uptake of CA in the diseased atherosclerotic coronary vessel wall (Figure 8-15c, e, f) and in acute lesions suggestive of coronary vessel wall inflammation (Figure 8-15b, d, f). The current application of atherosclerosis imaging is for research purposes. However, it is very likely that future applications may include CAD risk assessment and monitoring of response to specific therapy of atherosclerosis.

8.5.5 Coronary Vein Imaging

Imaging of the coronary veins may help to guide the left ventricular lead implantation to achieve optimal cardiac resynchronization therapy. Early studies imply that contrast agent-enhanced MRI can be used for the assessment of the course of the coronary sinus, the great cardiac vein, and the respective tributaries. A major limitation in heart failure patients may rise from the asynchronous contraction pattern, causing constant systolic motion of the heart. This may disqualify the suggested usage of an end-systolic trigger window, and the use of a mid-diastolic triggering window may be more effective.

8.6 Future Perspectives

Coronary MRA, coronary vessel wall imaging and coronary vein imaging continuously evolve and CMR holds great promise as a non-invasive imaging modality capable of a comprehensive evaluation of patients with CAD. Further improvements in image quality are expected with higher field strengths (Huber 2004, Gharib 2007, Snyder 2009) and dedicated acquisition and motion compensation strategies. Future developments in target-specific contrast agents will likely make molecular MRI a clinical tool that may facilitate the identification of vulnerable atherosclerotic plaques. Non-invasive atherosclerosis imaging is also expected to advance our knowledge on the natural history of the atherothrombotic process in order to prevent myocardial infarction and ischemic stroke.

References

Becker M, Frauenrath T, Hezel F et al. Comparison of left ventricular function assessment using phonocardiogram- and electrocardiogram-triggered 2D SSFP CINE MR imaging at 1.5 T and 3.0 T. Eur Radiol 2010; 20 (6): 1344–55.

Bhat H, Yang Q, Zuehlsdorff S et al. Contrast-enhanced whole-heart coronary magnetic resonance angiography at 3 T using interleaved echo planar imaging. Invest Radiol 2010; 45: 458–64.

Bogaert J, Kuzo R, Dymarkowski S et al. Coronary artery imaging with real-time navigator three-dimensional turbo-field-echo MR coronary angiography: initial experience. Radiology 2003; 226: 707–16.

Börnert P, Stuber M, Botnar RM et al. Direct comparison of 3D spiral vs. Cartesian gradient-echo coronary magnetic resonance angiography. Magn Reson Med 2001; 46 (4): 789–94.

Botnar RM, Kim WY, Börnert P et al. 3D coronary vessel wall imaging utilizing a local inversion technique with spiral image acquisition. Magn Reson Med 2001; 46 (5): 848–54.

Botnar RM, Stuber M, Danias PG et al. Improved coronary artery definition with T2-weighted, free-breathing, three-dimensional coronary MRA. Circulation 1999; 99: 3139–48.

Botnar RM, Stuber M, Kissinger KV et al. Non-invasive coronary vessel wall and plaque imaging with magnetic resonance imaging. Circulation 2000; 102 (21): 2582–7.

Botnar RM, Stuber M, Lamerichs R et al. Initial experiences with in vivo right coronary artery human MR vessel wall imaging at 3 T. J Cardiovasc Magn Reson 2003; 5 (4): 589–94.

Brittain JH, Hu BS, Wright GA et al. Coronary angiography with magnetization-prepared T2 contrast. Magn Reson Med 1995; 33 (5): 689–96.

Chiribiri A, Kelle S, Köhler U et al. Magnetic resonance cardiac vein imaging: relation to mitral valve annulus and left circumflex coronary artery. JACC Cardiovasc Imaging 2008; 1 (6): 729–38.

Deshpande VS, Shea SM, Laub G et al. 3D magnetization-prepared true-FISP: a new technique for imaging coronary arteries. Magn Reson Med 2001; 46 (3): 494–502.

Dewey M, Teige F, Schnapauff D et al. Combination of free-breathing and breathhold steady-state free precession magnetic resonance angiography for detection of coronary artery stenoses. J Magn Reson Imaging 2006; 23: 674–81.

Dixon WT, Oshinski JN, Trudeau JD et al. Myocardial suppression in vivo by spin locking with composite pulses. Magn Reson Med 1996; 36 (1): 90–4.

Duckett SG, Ginks M, Knowles BR et al. Whole-heart magnetic resonance imaging for visualization of venous anatomy and myocardial scar using slow infusion of Gd-BOPTA in single exam. J Cardiovasc Magn Reson 2010; 12 (Suppl 1): O21.

Edelman RR, Chien D, Kim D. Fast selective black-blood MR imaging. Radiology 1991; 181 (3): 655–60.

Edelman RR, Manning WJ, Burstein D, Paulin S. Coronary arteries: breath-hold MR angiography. Radiology 1991; 181 (3): 641–3.

Ehman RL, Felmlee JP. Adaptive technique for high-definition MR imaging of moving structures. Radiology 1989; 173 (1): 255–63.

Fayad ZA, Fuster V, Fallon JT et al. Non-invasive in vivo human coronary artery lumen and wall imaging using black-blood magnetic resonance imaging. Circulation 2000; 102 (5): 506–10.

Fischer SE, Wickline SA, Lorenz CH. Novel real-time R-wave detection algorithm based on the vectorcardiogram. Magn Reson Med 1999; 42: 361–70.

Galjee MA, van Rossum AC, Doesburg T et al. Value of magnetic resonance imaging in assessing patency and function of coronary artery bypass grafts. An angiographically controlled study. Circulation 1996; 93 (4): 660–6.

Gharib AM, Herzka DA, Ustun AO et al. Coronary MR angiography at 3 T during diastole and systole. J Magn Reson Imaging 2007; 26 (4): 921–6.

Giorgi B, Dymarkowski S, Maes F et al. Improved visualization of coronary arteries using a new three-dimensional submillimeter MR coronary angiography sequence with balanced gradients. Am J Roentgenol 2002; 179 (4): 901–10.

Goldfarb JW, Edelman RR. Coronary arteries: breath-hold, gadolinium-enhanced, three-dimensional MR angiography. Radiology 1998; 206 (3): 830–4.

Hofman MB, Paschal CB, Li D et al. MRI of coronary arteries: 2D breath-hold vs. 3D respiratory-gated acquisition. J Comput Assist Tomogr 1995; 19 (1): 56–62.

Hofman MBM, Wickline SA, Lorenz CH. Quantification of in-plane motion of the coronary arteries during the cardiac cycle: implications for acquisition window duration for MR flow quantification. J Magn Reson Imaging 1998; 8 (3): 568–76.

Huber ME, Kozerke S, Pruessmann KP et al. Sensitivity-encoded coronary MRA at 3 T. Magn Reson Med 2004; 52 (2): 221–7.

Huber ME, Paetsch I, Schnackenburg B et al. Performance of a new gadolinium-based intravascular contrast agent in free-breathing inversion-recovery 3D coronary MRA. Magn Reson Med 2003; 49 (1): 115–21.

Hundley WG, Bluemke DA, Finn JP et al. for the ACC Foundation Task Force on Expert Consensus Documents, ACCF/ACR/AHA/NASCI/SCMR 2010 expert consensus document on cardiovascular magnetic resonance. Circulation 2010; 121 (22): 2462–508.

Ibrahim T, Makowski MR, Jankauskas A et al. Serial contrast-enhanced cardiac magnetic resonance imaging demonstrates regression of hyperenhancement within the coronary artery wall in patients after acute myocardial infarction. JACC Cardiovasc Imaging 2009; 2 (5): 580–8.

Jahnke C, Nehrke K, Paetsch I et al. Improved bulk myocardial motion suppression for navigator-gated coronary magnetic resonance imaging. J Magn Reson Imaging 2007; 26 (3): 780–6.

Jahnke C, Paetsch I, Nehrke K et al. Rapid and complete coronary arterial tree visualization with magnetic resonance imaging: feasibility and diagnostic performance. Eur Heart J 2005; 26: 2313–9.

Jahnke C, Paetsch I, Schnackenburg B et al. Coronary MR angiography with steady-state free precession: individually adapted breath-hold technique vs. free-breathing technique. Radiology 2004; 232: 669–76.

Jenkins JP, Love HG, Foster CJ et al. Detection of coronary artery bypass graft patency as assessed by magnetic resonance imaging. Br J Radiol 1988; 61 (721): 2–4.

Katoh M, Spuentrup E, Buecker A et al. MRI of coronary vessel walls using radial k-space sampling and steady-state free precession imaging. Am J Roentgenol 2006; 186 (Suppl. 2): 401–6.

Kaul MG, Stork A, Bansmann PM et al. Evaluation of balanced steady-state free precession (TrueFISP) and K-space segmented gradient echo sequences for 3D coronary MR angiography with navigator gating at 3 T. Rofo 2004; 176 (11): 1560–5.

Kerwin WS, Zhao X, Yuan C et al. Contrast-enhanced MRI of carotid atherosclerosis: dependence on contrast agent. J Magn Reson Imaging 2009; 30 (1): 35–40.

Kim WY, Danias PG, Stuber M et al. Coronary magnetic resonance angiography for the detection of coronary stenoses. N Engl J Med 2001a; 345: 1863–9.

Kim WY, Stuber M, Kissinger KV et al. Impact of bulk cardiac motion on right coronary MR angiography and vessel wall imaging. J Magn Reson Imaging 2001b; 14 (4): 383–90.

Krombach GA, Hahnen C, Lodemann KP et al. Gd-BOPTA for assessment of myocardial viability on MRI: changes of T1 value and their impact on delayed enhancement. Eur Radiol 2009; 19 (9): 2136–46.

Laurent S, Elst LV, Muller RN. Comparative study of the physicochemical properties of six clinical low molecular weight gadolinium contrast agents. Contrast Media Mol Imaging 2006; 1 (3): 128–37.

Li D, Dolan RP, Walovitch RC, Lauffer RB. Three-Dimensional MRI of coronary arteries using an intravascular contrast agent. Magn Reson Med 1998; 39: 1014–8.

Li D, Kaushikkar S, Haacke EM et al. Coronary arteries: three-dimensional MR imaging with retrospective respiratory gating. Radiology 1996; 201 (3): 857–63.

Li D, Paschal CB, Haacke EM, Adler LP. Coronary arteries: three-dimensional MR imaging with fat saturation and magnetization transfer contrast. Radiology 1993; 187 (2): 401–6.

Liu X, Bi X, Huang J et al. Contrast-enhanced whole-heart coronary magnetic resonance angiography at 3.0 T: comparison with steady-state free precession technique at 1.5 T. Invest Radiol 2008; 43 (9): 663–8.

Lobbes MB, Miserus RJ, Heeneman S et al. Atherosclerosis: contrast-enhanced MR imaging of vessel wall in rabbit model – comparison of gadofosveset and gadopentetate dimeglumine. Radiology 2009; 250 (3): 682–91.

Maintz D, Aepfelbacher FC, Kissinger KV et al. Coronary MR angiography: comparison of quantitative and qualitative data from four techniques. Am J Roentgenol 2004; 182: 515–21.

Manning WJ, Li W, Boyle NG, Edelman RR. Fat-suppressed breath-hold magnetic resonance coronary angiography. Circulation 1993a; 87 (1): 94–104.

Manning WJ, Li W, Edelman RR. A preliminary report comparing magnetic resonance coronary angiography with conventional angiography. N Engl J Med 1993b; 328 (12): 828–32.

Mao S, Lu B, Oudiz RJ, Bakhsheshi H et al. Coronary artery motion in electron beam tomography. J Comput Assist Tomogr 2000; 24 (2): 253–8.

McConnell MV, Khasgiwala VC, Savord BJ et al. Comparison of respiratory suppression methods and navigator locations for MR coronary angiography. Am J Roentgenol 1997; 168 (5): 1369–75.

Müller MF, Fleisch M, Kroeker R et al. Proximal coronary artery stenosis: three-dimensional MRI with fat saturation and navigator echo. J Magn Reson Imaging 1997; 7 (4): 644–51.

Nassenstein K, Breuckmann F, Hunold P et al. Magnetic resonance coronary angiography: comparison between a Gd-BOPTA- and a Gd-DTPA-enhanced spoiled gradient-echo sequence and a non-contrast-enhanced steady-state free precession sequence. Acta Radiol 2009; 50 (4): 406–11.

Nehrke K, Bornert P, Groen J et al. On the performance and accuracy of 2D navigator pulses. Magn Reson Imaging 1999; 17 (8): 1173–81.

Nezafat R, Han Y, Peters DC et al. Coronary magnetic resonance vein imaging: imaging contrast, sequence, and timing. Magn Reson Med 2007; 58 (6): 1196–206.

Oshinski JN, Hofland L, Mukundan Jr. S et al. Two-dimensional coronary MR angiography without breath holding. Radiology 1996; 201 (3): 737–43.

Ozgun M, Hoffmeier A, Kouwenhoven M et al. Comparison of 3D segmented gradient-echo and steady-state free precession coronary MRI sequences in patients with coronary artery disease. Am J Roentgenol 2005; 185: 103–9.

Paschal CB, Haacke EM, Adler LP. Three-dimensional MR imaging of the coronary arteries: preliminary clinical experience. J Magn Reson Imaging 1993; 3 (3): 491–500.

Pennell DJ, Bogren HG, Keegan J et al. Assessment of coronary artery stenosis by magnetic resonance imaging. Heart 1996; 75 (2): 127–33.

Pennell DJ, Keegan J, Firmin DN et al. Magnetic resonance imaging of coronary arteries: technique and preliminary results. Br Heart J 1993; 70 (4): 315–26.

Post JC, van Rossum AC, Hofman MB et al. Three-dimensional respiratory-gated MR angiography of coronary arteries: comparison with conventional coronary angiography. Am J Roentgenol 1996; 166 (6): 1399–404.

Priest AN, Bansmann PM, Müllerleile K, Adam G. Coronary vessel-wall and lumen imaging using radial k-space acquisition with MRI at 3 T. Eur Radiol 2007; 17 (2): 339–46.

Pruessmann KP, Weiger M, Scheidegger MB, Boesiger P. SENSE: sensitivity encoding for fast MRI. Magn Reson Med 1999; 42 (5): 952–62.

Rasche V, Binner L, Cavagna F et al. Whole-heart coronary vein imaging: a comparison between non-contrast-agent- and contrast-agent-enhanced visualization of the coronary venous system. Magn Reson Med 2007; 57 (6): 1019–26.

Regenfus M, Ropers D, Achenbach S et al. Non-invasive detection of coronary artery stenosis using contrast-enhanced three-dimensional breath-hold magnetic resonance coronary angiography. J Am Coll Cardiol 2000; 36 (1): 44–50.

Rubinstein RI, Askenase AD, Thickman D et al. Magnetic resonance imaging to evaluate patency of aortocoronary bypass grafts. Circulation 1987; 76 (4): 786–91.

Sachs TS, Meyer CH, Hu BS et al. Real-time motion detection in spiral MRI using navigators. Magn Reson Med 1994; 32 (5): 639–45.

Sakuma H, Ichikawa Y, Chino S et al. Detection of coronary artery stenosis with whole-heart coronary magnetic resonance angiography. J Am Coll Cardiol 2006; 48: 1946–50.

Sakuma H, Ichikawa Y, Suzawa N et al. Assessment of coronary arteries with total study time of less than 30 min by using whole-heart coronary MR angiography. Radiology 2005; 237: 316–21.

Scheidegger MB, Muller R, Boesiger P. Magnetic resonance angiography: methods and its applications to the coronary arteries. Technol Health Care 1994; 2 (4): 255–65.

Schuetz GM, Zacharopoulou NM, Schlattmann P, Dewey M. Meta-analysis: noninvasive coronary angiography using computed tomography versus magnetic resonance imaging. Ann Intern Med 2010; 152 (3): 167–77.

Slavin GS, Riederer SJ, Ehman RL. Two-dimensional multi-shot echo-planar coronary MR angiography. Magn Reson Med 1998; 40 (6): 883–9.

Snyder CJ, DelaBarre L, Metzger GJ et al. Initial results of cardiac imaging at 7 T. Magn Reson Med 2009; 61 (3): 517–24.

Sodickson DK, Chuang ML, Khasgiwala VC, Manning WJ. In-plane motion of the left and right coronary arteries during the cardiac cycle. In: ISMRM, 5th Annual Meeting 1997; Vancouver: International Society for Magnetic Resonance in Medicine, Berkeley, California, USA 1997a; 910.

Sodickson DK, Manning WJ. Simultaneous acquisition of spatial harmonics (SMASH): fast imaging with radiofrequency coil arrays. Magn Reson Med 1997b; 38 (4): 591–603.

Sodickson DK, Stuber M, Botnar R et al. Accelerated coronary MR angiography in volunteers and patients using double-oblique 3D acquisitions combined with SMASH. J Cardiovasc Magn Reson 1999; 1: 260–1.

Sommer T, Hofer U, Meyer C et al. Submillimeter 3D coronary MR angiography with real-time navigator correction in 107 patients with suspected coronary artery disease. Rofo 2002; 174: 459–66.

Spuentrup E, Bornert P, Botnar RM et al. Navigator-gated free-breathing three-dimensional balanced fast field echo (TrueFISP) coronary magnetic resonance angiography. Invest Radiol 2002; 37 (11): 637–42.

Spuentrup E, Botnar RM. Coronary magnetic resonance imaging: visualization of the vessel lumen and the vessel wall and molecular imaging of arteriothrombosis. Eur Radiol 2006; 16: 1–14.

Stoeck CT, Han Y, Peters DC et al. Whole heart magnetization-prepared steady-state free precession coronary vein MRI. J Magn Reson Imaging 2009; 29 (6): 1293–9.

Stuber M, Botnar RM, Danias PG et al. Submillimeter three-dimensional coronary MR angiography with real-time navigator correction: comparison of navigator locations. Radiology 1999a; 212 (2): 579–87.

Stuber M, Botnar RM, Danias PG et al. Contrast agent-enhanced, free-breathing, three-dimensional coronary magnetic resonance angiography. J Magn Reson Imaging 1999b; 10 (5): 790–9.

Stuber M, Botnar RM, Danias PG et al. Double-oblique free-breathing high resolution three-dimensional coronary magnetic resonance angiography. J Am Coll Cardiol 1999c; 34 (2): 524–31.

Tang L, Merkle N, Schär M et al. Volume-targeted and whole-heart coronary magnetic resonance angiography using an intravascular contrast agent. J Magn Reson Imaging 2009; 30 (5): 1191–6.

Vrachliotis TG, Bis KG, Aliabadi D et al. Contrast-enhanced breath-hold MR angiography for evaluating patency of coronary artery bypass grafts. Am J Roentgenol 1997; 168 (4): 1073–80.

Wang Y, Grimm RC, Rossman PJ et al. 3D coronary MR angiography in multiple breath-holds using a respiratory feedback monitor. Magn Reson Med 1995; 34 (1): 11–6.

Wang Y, Vidan E, Bergman GW. Cardiac motion of coronary arteries: variability in the rest period and implications for coronary MR angiography. Radiology 1999; 213 (3): 751–8.

Wang Y, Watts R, Bezenson J et al. Selecting the optimal period of diastole for eliminating cardiac motion in coronary MRA by the use of an ECG-triggered navigator echo technique. In: ISMRM, 8th Annual Meeting 2000; Denver: International Society for Magnetic Resonance in Medicine, Berkeley, California, USA 2000; 1625.

White RD, Caputo GR, Mark AS et al. Coronary artery bypass graft patency: non-invasive evaluation with MR imaging. Radiology 1987; 164 (3): 681–6.

Wintersperger BJ, Engelmann MG, von Smekal A et al. Patency of coronary bypass grafts: assessment with breath-hold contrast-enhanced MR angiography – value of a non-electrocardiographically triggered technique. Radiology 1998; 208 (2): 345–51.

Wintersperger BJ, von Smekal A, Engelmann MG et al. Contrast media-enhanced magnetic resonance angiography for determining patency of a coronary bypass. A comparison with coronary angiography. Rofo Fortschr Geb Rontgenstr Neu Bildgeb Verfahr 1997; 167 (6): 572–8.

Yang Q, Li K, Liu X et al. Contrast-enhanced whole-heart coronary magnetic resonance angiography at 3.0 T: a comparative study with X-ray angiography in a single center. J Am Coll Cardiol 2009; 54 (1): 69–76.

Yeon SB, Sabir A, Clouse M et al. Delayed-enhancement cardiovascular magnetic resonance coronary artery wall imaging: comparison with multi-slice computed tomography and quantitative coronary angiography. J Am Coll Cardiol 2007; 50 (5): 441–7.

Yonger JF, Plein S, Crean A et al. Visualization of coronary venous anatomy by cardiovascular magnetic resonance. J Cardiovasc Magn Reson 2009; 11 (1): 26.

Yu J, Schär M, Vonken EJ et al. Improved SNR efficiency in gradient echo coronary MRA with high temporal resolution using parallel imaging. Magn Reson Med 2009; 62 (5): 1211–20.

9 Assessment of Myocardial Blood Flow and Oxygenation

Vinzenz Hombach and Volker Rasche

9.1 Physiology of Coronary Circulation and Myocardial Oxygen Consumption

The heart as an anaerobic organ is totally dependent on the oxidation of substrates for the production of energy. The heart cannot undergo a significant oxygen deficit such as e.g. the skeletal muscle. Myocardial perfusion amounts to 70–80 ml/min/100 g tissue, and the total oxygen consumption of the heart splits up in 20% of basal maintenance of structure, 1% of the electrical energy, 15% of volume load, and 64% of pressure load, heart rate, and contractility. The main determinants of myocardial oxygen consumption are systolic wall stress, diastolic wall stress, heart rate, and contractility. Myocardial oxygen supply depends on coronary blood flow and oxygen binding capacity of the blood, diastolic coronary perfusion, and alterations of coronary resistance determine total coronary blood flow. The heart receives approximately 5% of the resting cardiac output, although it represents less than 0.5% of total body weight. During cardiac contraction, intramyocardial tissue pressure increases around compliant arterioles and venules, which results in a concealed arterial backflow with reduction of systolic inflow in the epicardial arteries (Figure 9-1). Compression of venules accelerates venous outflow. During diastole compressive effects are related to tissue pressures that decrease from the subendocardium to subepicardium, and at diastolic LV-pressures greater than 20 mmHg pre-load determines the effective back pressure to coronary diastolic perfusion.

Myocardial oxygen consumption under resting conditions is approximately 7–10 ml O_2/min/100 g myocardial tissue. Myocardial O_2 extraction rate of 140 ml O_2/l blood is very high, i.e. with one passage 140 ml of O_2 are extracted from 1 l of blood. Myocardial oxygen consumption (MVO_2) can be quantified from arteriovenous difference ($AVDO_2$) and coronary blood flow (CBF): $MVO_2 = AVDO_2 \times CBF$.

During physical exercise myocardial oxygen consumption can increase up to 4–5 times the resting values, and this increase is mainly achieved by a significant increase of CBF up to 4–5 times the resting value. Coronary flow reserve is defined as the difference between the basal and maximal coronary blood flow during reactive hyperemia induced by a short lasting coronary occlusion (e.g. PTCA balloon) or due to vasodilatory drugs.

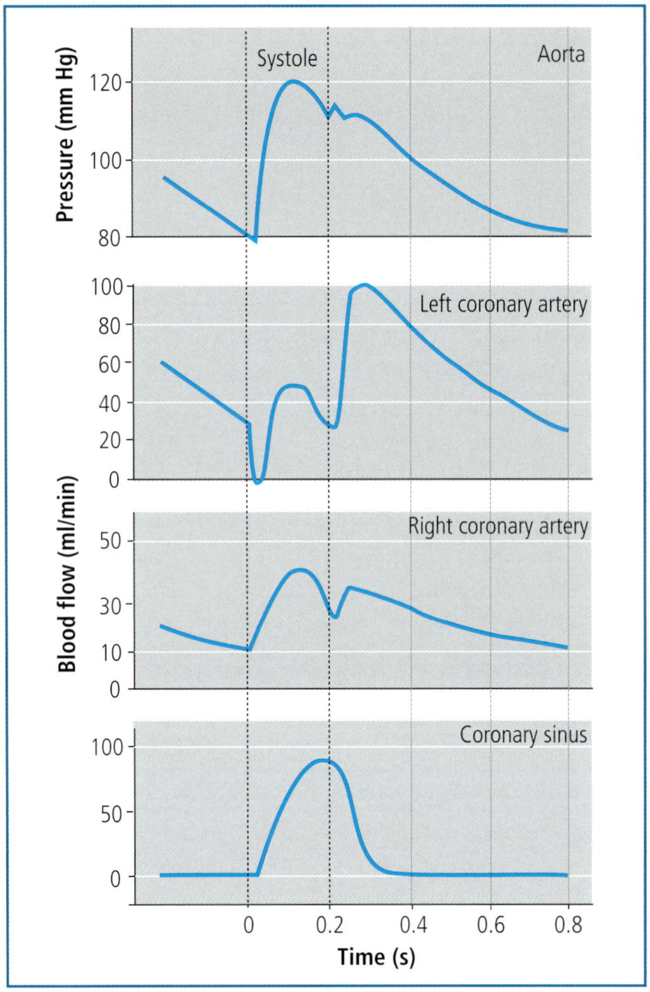

Figure 9-1 Schematic diagram of the flow patterns in the left and right coronary artery and in the coronary sinus.

In principle, **three methods to assess coronary or myocardial flow** may be used:

- **thermodilution method** with assessing the flow in the great cardiac vein that drains the perfusion territory of the left anterior descendent artery (LAD) or within the coronary sinus that drains the perfusion territory of the LAD and circumflex artery (LCFx);
- **intracoronary measurement of phasic and mean coronary flow** via Doppler-wire or intracoronary pressure measurement by pressure-wire (pressure drop distal to a stenosis);
- **non-invasive measurement of regional flow** by SPECT flow techniques, by PET flow, or by magnetic resonance PC-flow mapping in coronary arteries or coronary sinus, or by first-pass perfusion of left ventricular myocardium.

9.2 CMR Protocol for Myocardial Blood Flow and BOLD Imaging

The **CMR protocol** includes sequences for assessing cardiac morphology and function as well as angiography of and PC flow mapping in the respective coronary vessels (coronary artery, coronary bypass graft, coronary sinus):

- scout/survey,
- cine-SSFP sequence with complete short- and long-axis planes, eventually combined with parallel imaging (SENSE) for assessing morphology and function including the coronary sinus,
- transversal MR coronary angiography – scout (ROI for PC flow mapping),
- bright-blood coronary angiography of the coronary vessel to be investigated (coronary artery, or bypass graft),
- optionally: black-blood sequences orthogonal to the coronary vessel segment to be examined,
- high-resolution phase contrast flow mapping within the same coronary vessel segment (orthogonally to the longitudinal axis of the vessel) with motion correction,
- stress testing with adenosine or dipyridamole for detection of myocardial ischemia (suspected coronary artery or bypass graft stenosis) and repeat high-resolution PC-flow mapping in the same vessel segment,
- optional (experimental): T2w- or T2*w-spoiled gradient-echo or steady-state free precession BOLD imaging of myocardium before and after adenosine stress (to detect myocardial ischemia).

9.3 Coronary and Myocardial Blood Flow and Flow Reserve

9.3.1 Native Coronary Arteries

Technical Considerations

Phase contrast (PC) cine-MRI can provide non-invasive assessment of blood flow and flow reserve in human coronary arteries at multiple temporal phases in cardiac cycle. MR measurement of coronary blood flow is challenging because the coronary arteries are small (2–4 mm in diameter) and subject to both cardiac and respiratory motion. Therefore, exact imaging of the vessel segment along its longitudinal direction and positioning of the slab exactly orthogonal to the vessel segment is crucial. This is less problematic for the right coronary artery (RCA), the coronary sinus (CS), and for bypass grafts (CABG) than for the left coronary artery (LAD) and left circumflex artery (LCx). The major limitations of breath-hold MR measurement of coronary blood flow (CBF) are suboptimal spatial and temporal resolution. And if spatial resolution is compromised in relation to vessel size, partial volume averaging of bright signal from flowing blood and attenuated signal from static tissue around the vessel lumen result in overestimation of blood flow volume on phase-difference images. Moreover, peak flow velocity measured by PC-MRI is substantially lower than the peak velocity by intracoronary Doppler flow wire, because the highest velocity at the center and lower velocities at the periphery of the vessel lumen are averaged within MRI voxels (Shibata 1999). Another problem may be the insufficient temporal resolution, when the data acquisition window in the cardiac cycle is to long, blurring of the vessel by in-plane motion results in inaccurate measurement of blood velocity and flow volume. It has been estimated that the duration of acquisition should be < 25 ms for the RCA and 120 ms for the LCA (Hofman 1998). Such optimal conditions (spatial resolution 0.8 mm^2, temporal resolution 23 ms) can be achieved using turbo-field echoplanar MRI to measure blood flow in bypass grafts (Langerak 2001), or using free-breathing spiral sequences (reduction of MRI time by a factor of 10) or breath-hold spiral sequence (temporal resolution 30 ms), as described by Keegan et al. (2004). It should be kept in mind that breath-holding at inspiration causes an increase of intrathoracic pressure with consecutive reduction of venous return, that may significantly influence (reduce) cardiac output and CBF. Therefore PC-sequences that allow shallow breathing should be preferred when measuring CBF.

Evaluation of Coronary Artery Stenosis

In the literature, different values for coronary flow velocity using PC mapping have been reported: in 19 LADs mean 12.5 ± 4.9 cm/s (Shibata et al. 1999), in 13 LADs mean systolic flow velocity 25.0 ± 13.5 mm/s and mean diastolic flow velocity 130.9 ± 32.7 mm/s using a combined water excitation/fat excitation acquisition for through-plane motion correction, and in 10 RCAs 75.3 ± 15.4 mm/s and 96.8 ± 19.8 mm/s, respectively (Keegan 2004); flow velocity in the LAD 6.8 ± 4.3 cm/s, 8.0 ± 3.8 cm/s in the LCx, and 6.0 ± 1.6 cm/s in the RCA, measured in 9 volunteers using PC-mapping at 3 T after validating the technique with a phantom (Johnson 2008). Coronary arterial blood flow values in the LAD were reported by Dall'Armellina et al. (2006) in 11 post-menopausal women with 53 ± 17 ml/min at rest and 74 ±20 after submaximal exercise. Normal coronary flow reserve with volumetric MR flow measurement was 3.14 ± 0.59 according to Sakuma et al. (1996), 4.2 ± 1.8 according to Grist et al. (1997), and 5.0 ± 2.6 according to Davies et al. (1997).

Coronary flow reserve (**CFR**) has also been used to assess the severity of **primary coronary stenoses.** Hundley et al. (1999) reported in 30 subjects that a MRI coronary flow reserve value of < 1.7 identified all subjects with a > 70 % stenosis by QCA within the LAD, the sensitivity and specificity to detect a significant stenosis by MRI flow reserve was 100 and 83 %, respectively. In a similar study Bedaux et al. (2002) compared CFR by MRI with Doppler wire, and found mean CFR values by MRI of 1.5 ± 0.7 in 11 angiographically significantly stenosed arteries vs. 2.7 ± 1.0 in 15 normal coronary arteries ($p = 0.003$); the corresponding values by Doppler flow wire were 1.9 ± 0.7 in stenosed vs. 3.1 ± 0.5 ($p = 0.001$) in normal arteries. To detect a **restenosis after PCI** in 17 patients with recurrent chest pain Hundley et al. (2000) described a CFR value of ≤ 2.0 to be 100 % sensitive and 82 % specific for detecting a ≥ 70 % diameter restenosis, and 82 % sensitive and 100 % specific for a ≥ 50 % diameter restenosis, respectively. Similar results were reported by Saito et al. (2001), who found a significant reduction of CFR in 3 patients with restenosis after PCI from 2.26 ± 0.49 at 1 mth to 1.52 ± 0.09 at 6 mths ($p < 0.05$), compared with 7 patients without restenosis and CFR values of 2.31 ± 0.30 at 1 mth and 2.52 ± 0.25 (ns). In another study, Nagel et al. (2005) reported on 29 successful CFR measurements out of 38 patients after PCI, and found a CFR threshold of 1.2 to be 83 % sensitive and 94 % specific for the detection of a ≥ 70 % restenosis.

9.3.2 Coronary Artery Bypass Grafts (CABG)

Blood Flow at Rest

MR flow measurements may be an effective method of functionally assessing CABGs, and of noninvasively detecting stenoses or occlusions in a graft. Hoogendoorn et al. (1995) reported an average blood flow of 71 ± 17 ml/min in normal saphenous vein grafts vs. 9 ± 8 ml/min in occluded grafts. Several studies reported mean flow values in saphenous vein or arterial (mammary) grafts between 74 ± 17 ml/min and 136 ± 106 ml/min (the latter in sequential grafts), and flow velocities between 7 ± 5 cm/s and 23 ± 12 cm/s (review by Langerak 1999). Using a fast Turbo-Field EPI sequence for flow quantification in CABGs (20 bypass grafts in 15 patients including 18 venous and 2 arterial without stenoses) Langerak et al. (2001) reported peak systolic flow rates of 5.44 ± 2.70 ml/s in internal mammary grafts, and total flow in single vein grafts of 25.35 ± 8.97 ml/min and 40.89 ± 15.33 ml/min in sequential grafts at rest; the corresponding values on adenosine infusion were 65.15 ± 32.64 ml/min and 98.17 ± 35.56 ml/min, respectively.

Flow Reserve on Vasodilatation

Adenosine or dipyridamole stress testing to assess flow reserve may be used to identify stenoses in bypass grafts. Langerak et al. (2003) examined 69 patients with recurrent chest pain with 166 grafts (81 single vein, 44 sequential vein, and 41 arterial grafts) using MR flow mapping at rest and after adenosine stress compared with coronary angiography, dividing the grafts into groups with stenosis ≥ 50% (n = 72) and ≥ 70% (n = 48) in the graft or recipient vessel. For single vein grafts the flow velocity reserve was able to differentiate accurately between those with and without ≥ 70% stenosis (ROC area: 0.89, optimal cut-off value: 1.43). Multivariable analysis using all baseline and stress MR variables resulted in sensitivity/specificity of 94/63% (ROC area: 0.90) and sensitivity/specificity of 96/92% (ROC area: 0.96) for detecting single vein grafts or recipient vessels with stenoses ≥ 50 and ≥ 70%, respectively. Sensitivity/specificity for detecting sequential vein grafts or recipient vessels with luminal stenoses ≥ 50% were 91/82% (ROC area: 0.87) and 94/71% (ROC area: 0.88) for ≥ 70% stenoses, respectively. The conclusion was that MR flow mapping at rest and on adenosine stress is useful for identifying grafts and recipient vessels with flow-limiting stenoses.

Salm et al. (2004) compared the diagnostic accuracy of MR flow velocity and flow volume reserve on MR velocity maps in 49 patients with **single-vein bypass grafts**. Bland-Altman analysis showed close agreement between the two types of analysis. The mean difference between the coronary flow volume reserve and flow velocity reserve was not significantly different for detecting stenoses of 70% or more, and the diagnostic accuracy for volume flow and velocity parameters was 92 and 93%, respectively. The conclusion was that velocity analysis appears to be the preferred method, because it is less time-consuming and has a similar diagnostic accuracy to volume flow analysis. The detection of stenoses in **mammary bypass grafts** is another diagnostic challenge. Ishida et al. (2001) measured blood flow in internal mammary artery bypass grafts in 26 patients (24 successful MR studies, 17 patients without significant stenoses, and 7 patients with > 70% diameter stenosis), and found a ratio of diastolic to systolic peak velocity of 0.61 ± 0.44 in stenosed grafts being significantly lower than a ratio of 1.88 ± 0.96 in patients with fully open grafts (p < 0.01). The average blood flow volume in stenotic grafts (16.9 ± 5.5 ml/min) was significantly lower than that in normal grafts (79.8 ± 38.2 ml/min, p < 0.01). The sensitivity and specificity of MR blood flow measurements in predicting significant stenoses were 86 and 94%, respectively. MR flow mapping may also be used to assess the effect of **PCI in bypass grafts**. Langerak et al. (2003) measured average peak velocity (APV) at rest and stress in 15 patients before and 7.3 ± 1.5 wks after PCI of significant bypass stenoses. After PCI significant improvements were observed in baseline APV (before PCI: 9.2 cm/s ± 6.6; after PCI: 12.9 cm/s ± 7.9, p = 0.008) and stress APV (before PCI: 12.9 cm/s ± 6.3; after PCI: 27.1 cm/s ± 13.9, p < 0.001), while no improvement in velocity reserve was observed in 39 nonstenotic single (2.4 ± 0.8) and in 20 nonstenotic sequential grafts (2.3 ± 0.7). The conclusion was that graft function showed significant improvement after PCI as shown by near to complete restoration of resting and stress flow.

9.3.3 Coronary Sinus (CS)

Technical Considerations

Blood flow through the distal coronary sinus (CS) is a good measure of global LV perfusion, because approximately 96% of LV venous blood drains into the right atrium via the CS. By measuring CS flow (CSF) using cine-MR PC flow mapping, and measuring LV mass with cine-MRI, both total and average coronary blood flow per gram of myocardial mass can be calculated (Figure 9-2). Several investigators validated MR measurements of CSF with different reference techniques. Van Rossum et al. (1992) used phantom studies to assess the accuracy of this technique with good correlations. Lund et al. (2000) used Doppler flow probes in the CS of dogs and found good correlations between total CSF between both techniques (r = 0.98, p < 0.001) with a mean flow per gram muscle mass of 0.40 ± 0.09 ml/g/min by MRI and 0.44 ± 0.08 ml/g/min by Doppler wire. Kosvenkou et al. (2001a) found comparable results between MR flow mapping (VEC-MRI) and PET in 12 male volunteers: with VEC-MRI, MBF was 0.64 ± 0.09 ml/min/g at baseline and 1.59 ± 0.79 ml/min/g at hyperemia (average flow reserve: 2.51 ± 1.29); with PET myocardial blood flow was 0.65 ± 0.20 ml/min/g at baseline and 1.78 ± 0.72 ml/min/g at hyperemia (average flow reserve: 2.79 ± 0.97). In a further study, Kosvenkou et al. (2001b) reported good correlation of CSF at baseline and at hyperemia between VEC-MRI and PET in 20 patients with coronary artery disease (r = 0.80, p < 0.001 for MBF, r = 0.50, p < 0.05 for flow reserve, respectively). Schwitter et al. (2000) examined 16 healthy volunteers at rest and after dipyridamole stress, and found CSF divided by LV mass to correlate highly with the ^{13}N-PET flow data (0.77 ± 0.19 ml/min/g by MRI and 0.73 ± 0.15 ml/min/g by PET; r = 0.95).

VEC-MRI measurements of global CSF are also feasible with 3 T scanners, as has been shown by Bloch et al. (2009) in 12 healthy volunteers. Global CSF was determined at 88 ± 33 ml/min and MBF at 0.60 ± 0.22 ml/min/g, with good

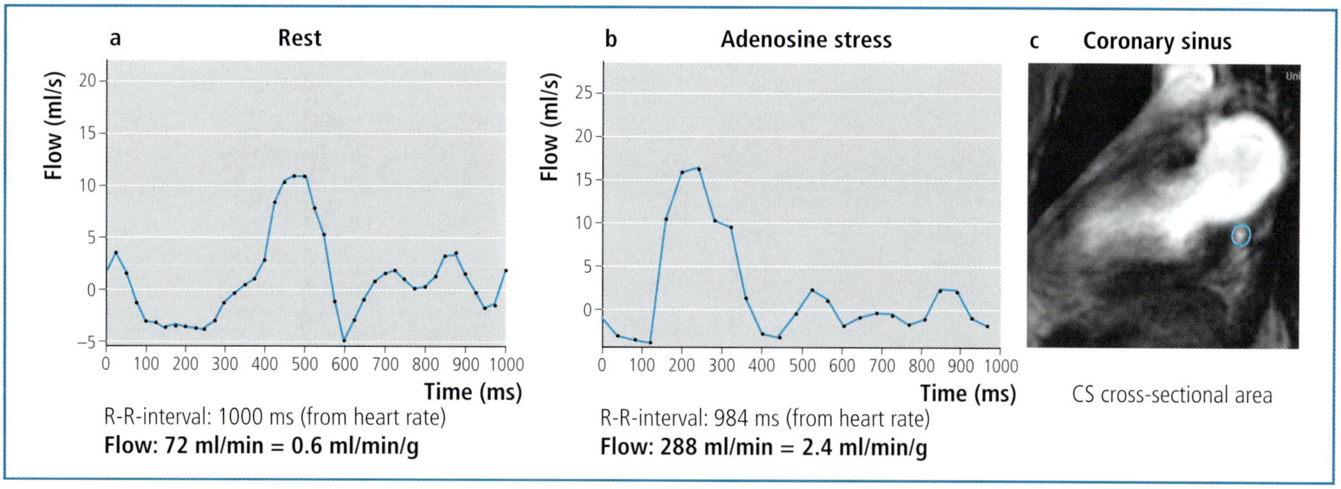

Figure 9-2 Flow measured in the coronary sinus (CS) by PC flow mapping (PC-CMR) in a normal individual at rest (a) and during adenosine infusion (b). Flow is calculated according to the formula: flow (ml/min) = mean flow velocity (cm/s) × cross-sectional area of CS (cm^2); flow rate at rest was 72 ml/min and 288 ml/min on adenosine infusion, coronary flow reserve was 4.0. ROI within the CS for flow measurement by PC-CMR (circle) (c).

repeatability by measuring flow three times. Maroules et al. (2010) examined 14 asymptomatic women with cardiovascular risk factors at baseline and after cold pressure test (CPT), using spiral VEC-MRI at 3 T. A significant increase of CS volume flow was observed after CPT (baseline: 116 ± 26 ml/min, peak stress: 152 ± 34 ml/min, $p = 0.01$, flow reserve was 1.31 ± 0.20). Test-retest variability was 5% at baseline and 6% during peak stress. The conclusion was that spiral VEC-MRI at 3 T is feasible and a reproducible technique for measuring global CSF and changes on CPT, and may be useful in examining asymptomatic women at risk of cardiovascular disease.

Evaluation of Patients with Diffuse Myocardial Diseases

This integrated approach of measuring CSF at baseline and after vasodilator stress with or without measurement of myocardial mass has been used to evaluate patients with diffuse myocardial disease. Lund et al. (2003) studied 10 patients with ischemic cardiomyopathy (iCMP) and 10 healthy controls. LV perfusion was not significantly different at rest (iCMP: 0.46 ± 0.19 ml/min/g vs. normals: 0.52 ± 0.21 ml/min/g, $p = 0.54$), after administration of dipyridamole LV perfusion was significantly lower (iCMP: 1.07 ± 0.64 ml/min/g vs. normals: 2.19 ± 0.98 ml/min/g, $p = 0.03$), and coronary flow reserve (CFR) was also severely reduced (iCMP: 2.3 ± 0.9 vs. normals: 4.2 ± 1.5, $p = 0.01$). Similar results were reported by Aras et al. (2007) in 20 patients with iCMP compared with 11 healthy controls. At rest, global LV perfusion was not significantly different between both groups, but after administration of dipyridamole global LV perfusion and flow reserve were significantly lower in patients with iCMP compared with the control group ($p < 0.001$). An inverse correlation was observed between CFR and the number of infarcted and/or ischemic segments ($p = 0.083$, $p = 0.037$). It was concluded that this MRI-CSF and LVMM assessment protocol may have potential in the monitoring of patients with iCMP, and impaired CFR may contribute to progressive decline in LV function in these patients.

In 29 patients with hypertrophic cardiomyopathy (HCM), Kawada et al. (1999) found different values for global CSF and CFR compared with 9 healthy volunteers. CSF at rest was 0.62 ± 0.27 ml/min/g in HCM patients vs. 0.74 ± 0.23 ml/min/g for healthy subjects, after administration of dipyridamole CSF and CFR were significantly lower (CSF: 1.03 ± 0.49 ml/min/g in HCM patients vs. 2.14 ± 0.51 ml/min/g, $p < 0.01$; CFR: 1.72 ± 0.49 in HCM vs. 3.01 ± 0.75, $p < 0.01$). Similar findings were reported by Watzinger at al. (2005) in 7 patients with idiopathic dilated cardiomyopathy (IDCM) compared with 12 healthy controls. CSF was not significantly different between both groups, but after dipyridamole administration both CSF and CFR were significantly lower in patients with IDCM compared with controls (CSF: 1.05 ± 0.35 ml/min/g vs. 1.99 ± 1.05 ml/min/g, $p < 0.05$; CFR: 2.19 ± 0.77 ml/min/g vs. 3.51 ± 1.29, $p < 0.05$). The conclusion was that measurement of global CSF has the potential to demonstrate an impaired microcirculatory flow in patients with IDCM, and to study the effects of pharmacological interventions on myocardial perfusion. Schwitter et al. (2000) evaluated CSF and CFR in 9 orthotopic heart transplant recipients and found a significantly reduced CFR compared with controls (2.0 ± 0.4 vs. 3.9 ± 1.4, $p < 0.005$), a moderate but significantly negative correlation ($r = 0.56$, $p < 0.005$) was noted between CSF and LV mass.

9.4 Myocardial Oxygenation by BOLD Imaging

9.4.1 Theoretical Background

Hemoglobin in its circulating form alternates between the oxy- and deoxygenated forms as oxygen is exchanged in lungs and capillaries. Deoxygenated hemoglobin has unpaired electrons and is paramagnetic (i. e. shows positive magnetic susceptibility), while oxygenated hemoglobin contains no unpaired electrons and is diamagnetic (i. e. has slightly negative magnetic susceptibility). Because proteins and water are diamagnetic, local magnetic field inhomogeneities will occur surrounding deoxygenated hemoglobin that causes signal loss to blood and the tissue containing blood in T2w- and T2*w-imaging. This effect is referred to the blood oxygen dependent (BOLD) effect.

9.4.2 Animal Studies

High-field experimental studies have shown a significant signal loss in T2w/T2*-images in the LV chamber and myocardium during apnea in rats (Wendland et al. 1993), or on the other hand a significant increase of myocardial signal intensity after administration of dipyridamole in the canine heart, presumably because of increased MBF in the absence of increased oxygen demand (Balaban 1994). These results could be reproduced in healthy volunteers, in whom infusion of dipyridamole (increase of flow without increase of metabolism) caused a near 40% T2* change from baseline, while infusion of dobutamine (increase of both metabolism and flow) did not significantly influence myocardial T2* signal intensity (Li 1999). Foltz et al. (2002) in an instrumented pig model ($n = 7$) were able to show that during intracoronary adenosine infusion, myocardial T2 elevations of mean $17 \pm 8\%$ within the LAD perfusion territory were related to increased perfusion reserve of 3.2 ± 0.4 and coronary venous (sampling in LAD coronary vein) % O_2 of $56 \pm 11\%$ without changes in blood volume and cardiac metabolic rate. The conclusion was that changes in microcirculation oxygen levels of approximately 40% O_2 should be detectable by T2 mapping. Using a newer T2-prepared SSFP BOLD imaging sequence in 13 dogs, Fieno et al. (2004) reported a $33 \pm 4\%$ increase of signal intensity ratio between the LAD (no topic vasodilatation) and LCx region (selective intracoronary adenosine infusion), compared with baseline, corresponding to a 3.8 ± 0.3-fold increase in relative perfusion ($p < 0.01$). At progressive levels of vasodilatation, MR intensity demonstrated a good agreement with microsphere flow ($r = 0.80$, $p < 0.01$). In another study using a canine model of coronary artery stenosis ($n = 21$), McCommis et al. (2010) compared BOLD imaging with PET imaging for myocardial blood flow and oxygenation. MRI data correlated nicely with PET values for myocardial blood flow ($r = 0.79$, $p < 0.01$), myocardial oxygen consumption ($r = 0.74$, $p < 0.001$), and oxygen extraction fraction ($r = 0.66$, $p < 0.01$). The conclusion was that the newly developed MRI oxygenation imaging technique may be a valuable non-invasive tool to directly evaluate myocardial energetics and efficiency.

9.4.3 Human Studies

BOLD imaging in humans may be used for quantitative assessment of myocardial blood flow (MBF) and oxygen consumption (MVO_2), or for qualitative detection of regional ischemia without the need of contrast media. In a basic paper Yang et al. (2009) examined 13 healthy males in MRI studies including measurements of MVO_2 ($n = 11$), whole-body oxygen consumption (VO_2) ($n = 8$), and both MVO_2 and VO_2 ($n = 6$). The protocol included in vitro blood sample T2-% O_2 calibration, coronary sinus and main pulmonary artery (PA) T2- and PC flow measurement, and LV mass (LVMM) calculation. The MVO_2 values were 11 ± 3 ml/min/100 g LVMM, the individual component measurements included CSF of 114 ± 27 ml/min, a CS-T2 of 114 ± 14 ms, a CS-% O_2 of $46 \pm 12\%$, and an LVMM of 108 ± 13 g, the measured VO_2 values were 3.8 ± 0.8 ml/min/g, the main PA flow was 6.5 ± 1.3 l/min. The conclusion was that these MRI techniques that combine coronary sinus and main pulmonary artery T2, flow, and LVMM measurements, appear feasible for quantifying MVO_2 and whole-body VO_2 non-invasively.

To detect myocardial ischemia for clinical purposes, BOLD imaging is used to examine regional tissue oxygenation directly. Friedrich et al. (2003) performed BOLD imaging in 25 patients with stress induced angina before and after adenosine infusion and compared these results with quantitative coronary angiography. During adenosine a mean signal intensity decrease was observed for myocardial segments related to coronary stenoses > 70%, while on average a non-significant increase was observed in the other segments; using a BOLD signal intensity increase cut-off value of 1.2%, BOLD-MRI had a sensitivity and specificity of 88 and 47%, respectively, to correctly classify severe stenoses. However, previously reported MRI approaches using GRE sequences suffered from low signal-to-noise ratio (SNR) and motion-related artifacts with impaired image quality and a limited diagnostic value to detect myocardial ischemia. More recently, BOLD SSFP sequences at 1.5 T

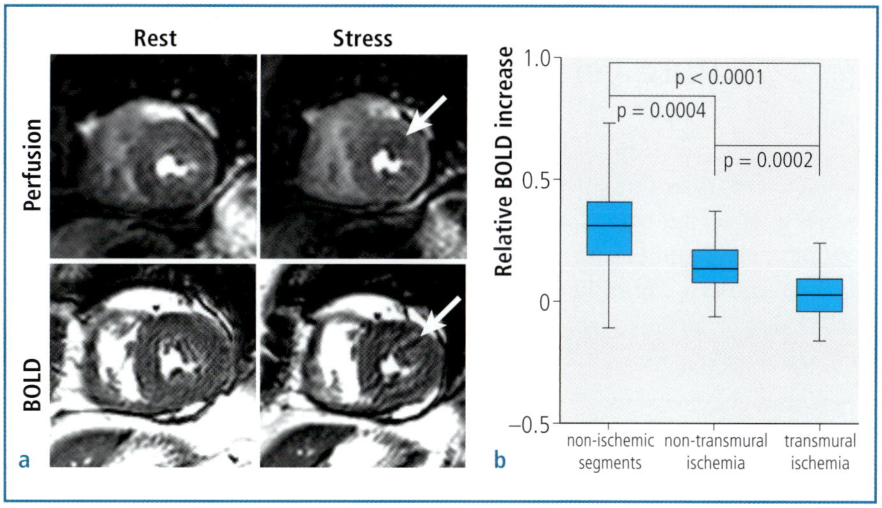

Figure 9-3 Assessment of regional myocardial perfusion on first-pass perfusion MR imaging (MR-FPP) at rest and peak adenosine stress **(top left)** and BOLD perfusion imaging at rest and peak adenosine stress **(bottom left)**; note the perfusion defect in the anterolateral myocardial area of the mid-ventricular slice on MR-FPP, corresponding with stress BOLD imaging **(a)**. Box plots of relative BOLD signal increase on T2-prepared SSFP imaging, showing significant differences of signal intensities for non-ischemic, non-transmural, and transmural ischemic myocardial segments **(b)** (preliminary results on 46 patients) (courtesy PD Bernhardt, University Hospital of Ulm, Department of Cardiology).

(Bernhardt 2011) or at 3 T (Jahnke 2010, Karamitsos 2010) have been examined.

In the study of Bernhardt et al. (2011) in 46 patients with suspected CAD SSFP, BOLD-sensitive images were compared with SSFP first-pass sequences before and after adenosine infusion for detecting myocardial ischemia. Relative BOLD signal increase was significantly lower in patients with perfusion defects compared with patients without perfusion defects ($p < 0.0001$). Patients with non-transmural and transmural first-pass perfusion defects also differed significantly for BOLD signal increase ($p < 0.0001$). ROC analysis showed an AUC of 0.83 for the T2-prepared SSFP sequence regarding the detection of an inducible perfusion deficit.

> The conclusion was that T2-prepared BOLD imaging allows for visualization of myocardial perfusion deficits in a clinical setting without additional use of contrast agents (Figure 9-3).

Jahnke et al. (2010) studied 50 patients with suspected or known CAD using 3D-BOLD imaging at rest and under adenosine stress, followed by stress and rest first-pass perfusion and delayed enhancement, compared with QCA as the reference for assessing coronary stenoses. Semiquantitative evaluation was performed for BOLD imaging using DeltaSI (signal intensity difference between stress and rest) and for myocardial perfusion by MPRI (myocardial perfusion reserve index). DeltaSI differed significantly between normal myocardium, ischemic myocardium, and infarcted myocardium ($p < 0.001$). ROC analysis identified a cut-off value of DeltaSI = 2.7 % for the detection of coronary stenosis, resulting in a sensitivity and specificity of 85.0 and 80.5 %, respectively. The DeltaSI correlated significantly with the degree of coronary stenosis ($r = 0.65$, $p < 0.001$), and DeltaSI and MPRI showed substantial agreement (kappa value: 0.66).

> The conclusion was that navigator-gated 3D-BOLD imaging at 3 T reliably detects stress-induced myocardial ischemia and may be considered a valid alternative to first-pass exogenous contrast-enhancement studies.

Karamitsos et al. (2010) examined 22 patients with CAD (at least 1 stenosis ≥ 50 % on QCA) and 10 normal volunteers by 3 T-BOLD CMR with calculation of mean signal intensities in 6 slices, and by PET with oxygen-15-labeled water to measure myocardial blood flow at rest and during adenosine infusion. Taking ≥ 50 % stenosis on QCA as the gold standard, cut-off values for stress myocardial flow (< 2.45 ml/min/g, AUC 0.83) and BOLD signal intensity change (< 3.47 %, AUC 0.78) were determined to define ischemic segments. BOLD CMR and PET agreed on the presence or absence of ischemia in 18 of the 22 patients (82 %) and in all normal subjects. On a per-segment analysis, 40 % of myocardial segments with stress myocardial blood flow below the cut-off value of 2.45 ml/min/g did not show deoxygenation, whereas 88 % of segments with normal perfusion also had normal oxygenation.

> The conclusion was that regional myocardial perfusion and oxygenation may be dissociated, indicating that in patients with CAD reduced perfusion does not always lead to deoxygenation.

9.5 Conclusions and Future Perspectives

PC-cine-MRI assessment of blood flow and flow reserve in human coronary arteries, bypass grafts, or in the coronary sinus is feasible, but complicated and challenging. In recent years only a few studies have been published using this technique indicating a diminishing interest in this topic. In contrast to measuring flow in the restricted area of a small coronary artery or bypass graft, quantification of blood flow at rest and after vasodilatation within larger segments of left ventricular myocardium seems to be more adequate and accurate. Using sophisticated models and calculations, myocardial flow reserve by CMR imaging can be assessed quantitatively both in healthy subjects and in patients with coronary artery disease in order to detect myocardial ischemia more accurately, as has been recently shown by Ibrahim et al. (2002) and Kurita et al. (2009). Thus, quantitative assessment of regional myocardial perfusion to determine perfusion reserve seems to be the technique of choice for the diagnosis of myocardial ischemia resulting from stenoses in native coronary arteries (primary stenosis, restenosis after PCI) or in coronary bypass grafts (vein grafts, mammaria grafts). Moreover, BOLD imaging using modern 3D-SSFP sequences appears to be a real and valid alternative to exogenous contrast-enhanced first-pass studies to reliably detect myocardial ischemia in patients with suspected or known CAD. But further studies have to be performed to confirm this view. Finally, measurement of global coronary sinus flow and flow reserve may become clinically relevant, since patients with potentially decreased global flow reserve and metabolism, e.g. in coronary artery disease, syndrome X, myocardial hypertrophy, cardiomyopathies, or cardiac transplants, may be functionally characterized and the pathophysiologic severity of these diseases better assessed.

References

Aras A, Anik Y, Balci NC et al. Magnetic resonance imaging measurement of left ventricular blood flow and coronary flow reserve in patients with chronic heart failure due to coronary artery disease. Acta Radiol 2007; 23: 1–9.

Balaban RS, Taylor JF, Turner R. Effect of cardiac flow on gradient recalled echo images of the canine heart. NMR Biomed 1994; 7: 89–94.

Bedaux WLF, Hofman MBM, de Cock CC et al. Magnetic resonance imaging vs. Doppler guide wire in the assessment of coronary flow reserve in patients with coronary artery disease. Coronary Artery Dis 2002; 13: 365–82.

Bernhardt P, Manzke R, Bornstedt A et al. Blood oxygen level-dependent magnetic resonance imaging using T2-prepared steady-state free precession imaging in comparison to contrast-enhanced myocardial perfusion imaging. Int J Cardiol 2011; 147: 416–9.

Bloch KM, Carlsson M, Arheden H, Ståhlberg F. Quantifying coronary sinus flow and global LV perfusion at 3 T. BMC Med Imaging 2009; 9: 9–13.

Dall'Armellina E, Baugh MB, Morgan TM et al. Cardiovascular magnetic resonance measurement of coronary arterial blood flow at rest and after submaximal exercise. J Comput Assist Tomogr 2006; 30: 421–5.

Davis CP, Liu P, Hauser M et al. Coronary flow and coronary flow reserve measurements in humans with breath-hold magnetic resonance phase contrast velocity mapping. Magn Reson Med 1997; 37: 537–44.

Fieno DS, Shea SM, Li Y et al. Myocardial perfusion imaging based on the blood oxygen level-dependent effect using T2-prepared steady-state free precession magnetic resonance imaging. Circulation 2004; 110: 1284–90.

Foltz WD, Huang H, Fort S, Wright GA. Vasodilator response assessment in porcine myocardium with magnetic resonance relaxometry. Circulation 2002; 106: 2714–9.

Friedrich MG, Niendorf T, Schulz-Menger J et al. Blood oxygen level-dependent magnetic resonance imaging in patients with stress-induced angina. Circulation 2003; 108: 2219–23.

Grist TM, Polzin JA, Bianco JA et al. Measurement of coronary blood flow and flow reserve using magnetic resonance imaging. Cardiology 1997; 88: 80–89.

Hofman MB, Wickline SA, Lorenz CH. Quantification of inplane motion of the coronary arteries during the cardiac cycle: implication for acquisition window duration for MR flow quantification. J Magn Reson Imaging 1998; 8: 568–76.

Hundley WG, Hamilton CA, Clarke GD et al. Visualization and functional assessment of proximal and middle left anterior descending coronary stenoses in humans with magnetic resonance imaging. Circulation 1999; 99: 3248–54.

Hundley WG, Hillis LD, Hamilton CA et al. Assessment of coronary arterial restenosis with phase contrast magnetic resonance imaging measurements of coronary flow reserve. Circulation 2000; 101: 2375–81.

Ibrahim T, Nekolla SG, Schreiber K et al. Assessment of coronary flow reserve: comparison between contrast-enhanced magnetic resonance imaging and positron emission tomography. J Am Coll Cardiol 2002; 39: 864–70.

Ishida N, Sakuma H, Cruz BP et al. MR flow measurement in the internal mammary artery-to-coronary artery bypass graft: comparison with graft stenosis at radiographic angiography. Radiology 2001; 220: 441–7.

Jahnke C, Gebker R, Manka R et al. Navigator-gated 3D blood oxygen level-dependent CMR at 3.0 T for detection of stress-induced myocardial ischemic reactions. JACC Cardiovasc Imaging 2010; 3: 375–84.

Johnson K, Sharma P, Oshinski J. Coronary artery flow measurement using navigator echo gated phase contrast magnetic resonance velocity mapping at 3.0 T. J Biomechanics 2008; 41: 595–602.

Karamitsos TD, Leccisotti L, Arnold JR et al. Relationship between regional myocardial oxygenation and perfusion in patients with coronary artery disease. Insights from cardiovascular magnetic resonance and positron emission tomography. Circ Cardiovasc Imaging 2010; 3: 32–40.

Kawada N, Sakuma H, Yamakado T et al. Hypertrophic cardiomyopathy: MR measurement of coronary blood flow and vasodilator flow reserve in patients and healthy subjects. Radiology 1999; 211 (1): 129–35.

Keegan J, Gatehouse PD, Mohiaddin RH et al. Comparison of spiral and FLASH phase velocity mapping with and without breath-holding for the assessment of left and right coronary artery blood flow velocity. J Magn Reson Imaging 2004a; 19: 40–9.

Keegan J, Gatehouse PD, Yang GZ, Firmin DN. Spiral phase velocity mapping of left and right coronary artery blood flow: correction for through-plane motion using selective fat-only excitation. J Magn Reson Imag 2004b; 20: 953–60.

Kosvenkuo JW, Hartiala JJ, Knuuti J et al. Assessing coronary sinus blood flow in patients with coronary artery disease: a comparison of phase contrast MR imaging with positron emission tomography. AJR 2001b; 177: 1161–6.

Kosvenkuo JW, Sakuma H, Niemi P et al. Global myocardial blood flow and global flow reserve measurements by MRI and PET are comparable. J Magn Reson Imaging 2001a; 13: 361–6.

Kurita T, Sakuma H, Onishi K et al. Regional myocardial perfusion reserve determined using myocardial perfusion magnetic resonance imaging showed a direct correlation with coronary flow velocity resreve by Doppler flow wire. Eur Heart J 2009; 30: 444–52.

Langerak SE, Kunz P, de Roos A et al. Evaluation of coronary artery bypass grafts by magnetic resonance imaging. J Magn Reson Imag 1999; 10: 434–41.

Langerak SE, Kunz P, Vliegen HW et al. Improved MR flow mapping in coronary artery bypass grafts during adenosine induced stress. Radiology 2001; 218: 540–7.

Langerak SE, Vliegen HW, Jukema JW et al. Vein graft function improvement after percutaneous intervention: evaluation with MR flow mapping. Radiology 2003; 228: 834–41.

Li D, Oellerich WF, Beck G, Gropler RJ. Assessment of myocardial response to pharmacologic interventions using an improved MR imaging technique to estimate T2* values. AJR 1999; 172: 141–6.

Lund GK, Watzinger N, Saeed M et al. Chronic heart failure: global left ventricular perfusion and coronary flow reserve with velocity-encoded cine-MR imaging: initial results. Radiology 2003; 227: 209–15.

Lund GK, Wendlandt MF, Shimakawa A et al. Coronary sinus flow measurement by means of velocity-encoded cine-MR imaging: validation by using flow probes in dogs. Radiology 2000; 217: 487–93.

Maroules CD, Chang AY, Kontak A et al. Measurement of coronary flow response to cold pressure stress in asymptomatic women with cardiovascular risk factors using spiral velocity-encoded cine-MRI at 3 T. Acta Radiol 2010; 51: 420–6.

McCommis KS, Goldstein TA, Abendschein DR et al. Quantification of regional myocardial oxygenation by magnetic resonance imaging: validation with positron emission tomography. Circ Cardiovasc Imaging 2010; 3: 41–6.

Nagel E, Thouet T, Klein C et al. Non-invasive determination of coronary blood flow velocity with cardiovascular magnetic resonance in patients after stent deployment. Circulation 2003; 107: 1738–43.

Saito Y, Sakuma H, Shibata M et al. Assessment of coronary flow velocity reserve using fast velocity-encoded cine-MRI for non-invasive detection of restenosis after coronary stent implantation. J Cardiovasc Magn Reson 2001; 3: 209–14.

Sakuma H, Blake LM, Amidon TM et al. Non-invasive measurement of coronary flow reserve in humans using breath-hold velocity-encoded cine-MR imaging. Radiology 1996; 198: 745–50.

Salm LP, Langerak SE, Vliegen HW et al. Blood flow in coronary artery bypass vein grafts: volume vs. velocity at cardiovascular imaging. Radiology 2004; 232: 915–20.

Schwitter J, DeMarco T, Kneifel S et al. Magnetic resonance-based assessment of global coronary flow and flow reserve and its relation to left ventricular functional parameters. A comparison with Positron Emission Tomography. Circulation 2000; 101: 2696–702.

Shibata M, Sakuma H, Isaka N et al. Assessment of coronary flow reserve with fast cine phase contrast magnetic resonance imaging: comparison with the measurement by Doppler guide wire. J Magn Reson Imaging 1999; 10: 563–8.

Van Rossum AC, Visser FC, Hofman MBM et al. Global left ventricular perfusion: non-invasive measurement with cine-MR imaging and phase velocity mapping of coronary venous outflow. Radiology 1992; 182: 685–91.

Watzinger N, Lund GK, Saeed M et al. Myocardial blood flow in patients with dilated cardiomyopathy: quantitative assessment with velocity-encoded cine magnetic resonance imaging of the coronary sinus. J Magn Reson Imaging 2005; 21 (4): 347–53.

Wendland MF, Saeed M, Lauerma K et al. Endogenous susceptibility contrast in myocardium during apnea measured using gradient recalled echo planar imaging. Magn Reson Med 1993; 29: 273–7.

Yang Y, Foltz WD, Merchant N et al. Non-invasive quantitative measurement of myocardial and whole-body oxygen consumption using MRIK: initial results. Magn Reson Imaging 2009; 27: 147–54.

10 Cardiomyopathies

Vinzenz Hombach and Markus Kunze

10.1 Definition

Cardiomyopathies are diseases of heart muscle that result from different conditions such as genetic defects, cardiac myocyte injury, or infiltration of myocardial tissue; they are – by classical definition – not induced by coronary artery disease (CAD), valvular heart disease, hypertension, pericardial disease, or congenital heart disease.

According to the WHO/ISFC definition (Konstam 2000), **cardiomyopathies are divided** into:

- **primary cardiomyopathies** (dilated = DCM, hypertrophic = HCM, restrictive = RCM, arrhythmogenic right ventricular = ARVC, and unclassified) with genetic, mixed, or acquired background and, related to the final common pathway phenomenon,
- **specific cardiomyopathies** (ischemic, valvular, hypertensive, inflammatory, metabolic, induced by general systemic diseases, muscular dystrophies, neuromuscular diseases, sensitivity and toxic reactions, and peri-partum cardiomyopathy).

The Working Group of the European Society of Cardiology (ESC) produced a new more clinically oriented classification of cardiomyopathies into the known clinical forms of DCM, HCM, RCM, ARVC and unclassified, and subdividing these forms into familial-genetic and non-familial-non-genetic, and further subdividing the familial-genetic forms into known mutations and unidentified gene defects, and the non-familial-non-genetic into idiopathic and those with known etiology (e.g. myocarditis, Kawasaki, drugs etc.) (Elliott 2008).

10.2 CMR Protocols

CMR imaging should include morphological analysis of the myocardium and the atrial and ventricular cavities, assessment of the hemodynamic impact of myocardial disorder on ventricular systolic and diastolic and on valvular function, and detection and characterization of abnormal myocardial tissue.

To obtain all necessary information for diagnosis and treatment of patients with cardiomyopathies, the following **routine CMR imaging protocol** should be used:

- cine-SSFP sequence, eventually combined with parallel imaging (SENSE) for assessing morphology and function (atria, ventricles, heart valves, regional and global systolic function, wall thickening, myocardial mass, intracardiac abnormal flow pattern),
- T1-, T2- and PD-weighted black-blood sequences in the standard planes for anatomic and morphologic imaging of cardiac structures (atrial and ventricular size, myocardium, great vessels),
- velocity-encoded cine-CMR (valvular dysfunction, intraventricular gradient, shunt calculation, diastolic function by transvalvular flow pattern),
- optional: first-pass perfusion studies of the myocardium (to rule out significant CAD),
- contrast-enhanced imaging in the long (2-ch, 4-ch) and short axes for LGE (myocardial damage, distribution pattern, extent, pericardial enhancement),
- optional: coronary MR angiography and CMR of thoracic vessels (exclusion of concomitant pathology).

The current arsenal of CMR techniques can be used to define most aspects of such complex diseases that provide the clinician with a complete picture of the patient's myocardial disorder. Of course, the huge variety of myocardial disorders requires a CMR study tailored towards the clinical question. CMR imaging should also be considered the preferred tool for following patients for disease progression and/or response to treatment.

10.3 Idiopathic Dilated Cardiomyopathy (IDCM)

Prevalence, Etiology and Pathology

Among the primary cardiomyopathies, dilated cardiomypathy (DCM) is the most common myocardial disorder, with a prevalence of 1:2,500 and an incidence of 5:100,000 per year. In 25–30% of patients a genetic background is present (familial form), 30–50% are caused by a previous viral infection (chronic inflammatory cardiomyopathy), and the remaining are secondary to toxic substances, most commonly alcohol abuse, drugs, cocaine, or further rare or unknown causes. DCM accounts for 25% of cases with congestive heart failure in the US.

At autopsy, examination of the heart of a DCM patient demonstrates four chamber (or in cases of predominant left sided DCM two chamber) enlargement with increased or normal wall thickness and normal valvular structures, eventually combined with dilatation of the valvular orifice. Intracavitary thrombi are often found, and are preferentially located in the ventricular apices. Histological evaluation of the myocardium reveals varying degrees of myocyte hypertrophy and atrophy and interstitial fibrosis. Myocardial hypertrophy consists of myocyte elongation and increase of myocyte diameter with an in-series addition of newly formed sarcomeres that is responsible for the increase in chamber size in DCM. Myocardial fibrosis may be mild and diffuse, severe and diffuse, or segmental, and fibrosis most often affects the left ventricular subendocardium or the entire ventricular myocardium in an interstitial or perivascular pattern. A finding of an island of fibrosis signifying a small area of tissue necrosis suggests an ischemic etiology.

Clinical Presentation, Diagnosis and Therapy

The clinical presentation of DCM is variable. Some patients may be asymptomatic or have minimal **symptoms**, and their prognosis is unclear. Other patients develop dyspnea on exertion, and later on dyspnea at rest and orthopnea, and most of them show cardiac arrhythmias. Right-sided heart failure is rather uncommon and presents only in the most severe cases, particularly those with biventricular dysfunction. **Diagnosis** is made by chest X-ray, and particularly by echocardiography (size, systolic dysfunction, relative valvular insufficiencies). **Treatment** consists of quadruple medical therapy with β-blockers, ACE-inhibitors, diuretics, and aldosterone antagonists. Anticoagulation is necessary in patients with severely depressed LV function and/or atrial fibrillation. Patients with resuscitated SCD or unstable ventricular tachyarrhythmias are candidates for an ICD (secondary prevention), in cases with low ejection fraction (EF below 30%) an ICD is also indicated (primary prevention of SCD). Newer biopsy-based treatments of virus persistence in the myocardium to eradicate the viruses using interferon may be initiated, as well as immunemodulatory agents to suppress chronic myocardial inflammation. However, these treatment strategies are not generally accepted and substantiated by large randomized trials. Prognosis of patients with idiopathic DCM (IDCM) is limited; the median survival rate after 10 yrs is approximately 60% (Felker 2000).

CMR Findings

Morphology and Function

CMR imaging shows enlarged atria and ventricles with increased end-diastolic volume (EDV), end-systolic volume (ESV), and reduced ejection fraction (EF) (Figure 10-1), with individual differences depending on the severity of right vs. left ventricular involvement. Segmental wall motion abnormalities may be present, but are a more characteristic feature of ischemic DCM (ICM). In the right ventricles of

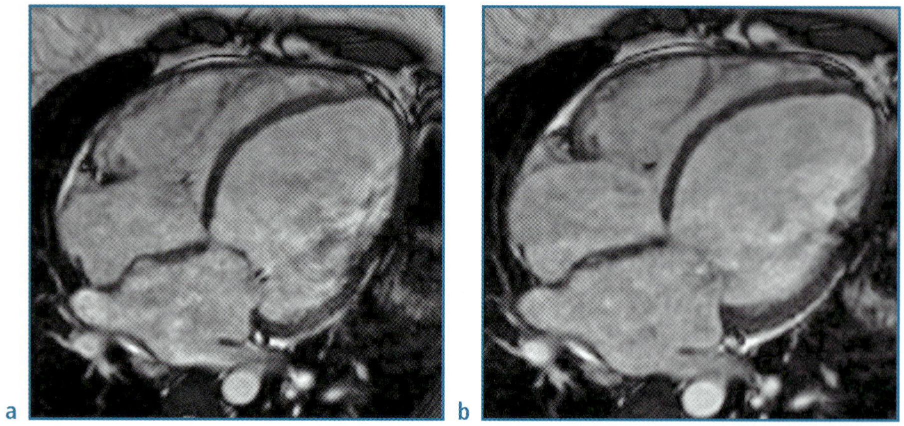

Figure 10-1 26-yrs-old male patient with severe biventricular idiopathic dilated cardiomyopathy in a 4-ch view in diastole (a) and systole (b) on cine-CMR. Note the dilated atria and particularly ventricles with severe global ventricular hypokinesis and relative mitral regurgitation (signal void over mitral valve in systole); right ventricular ejection fraction was 23 %, left ventricular ejection fraction was 11 %.

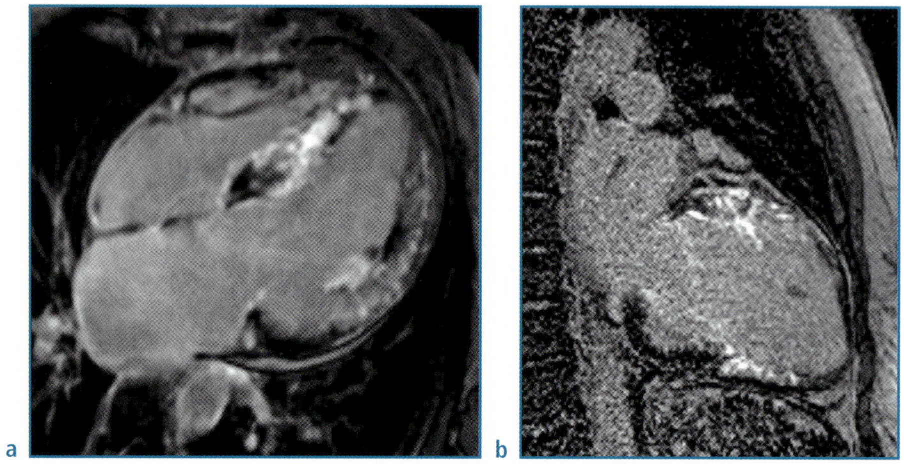

Figure 10-2 Late enhancement phenomenon in a 42-yrs-old male patient with idiopathic dilated cardiomyopathy in a 4-ch (a) and 2-ch view (b). Note the atypical (non-CAD like) bright fibrosis/necrosis zones midwall of the interventricular septum and subepicardially in the lateral left ventricular (LV) wall (a), as well as diffuse patchy enhancement in the basal-anterior and subendocardially in the mid-inferior LV wall (b).

IDCM patients with normal volumes and function diastolic abnormalities, i.e. an increase in time-to-peak filling rate and impaired filling fraction, may be found (Suzuki 1991), indicating that changes in LV morphology and function in IDCM patients influence the behavior even of a healthy looking right ventricle. Left ventricular trabeculae may be enlarged in IDCM patients compared with healthy subjects, and intracardiac thrombi may be detected in the case of severe LV dysfunction and/or atrial fibrillation. Presence and severity of mitral or tricuspid incompetence relative to dilatation of the valvular orifices can be quantitatively assessed by CMR volumetry. Contrast-enhanced imaging may detect presence, type, location, and size of myocardial fibrosis and damage, and LGE has been found to be able to differentiate ischemic from non-ischemic DCM by special scar features, and to provide prognostic information. The increased portion of fibrosis relative to normal myocardium in IDCM patients has been elegantly demonstrated by Jerosch-Herold et al. (2008) by an increased extracellular volume fraction, using the partition coefficient of gadolinium contrast, and this expansion of the extracellular space correlated with reduced myocardial blood flow and ventricular dilatation.

Myocardial Damage by LGE

In several studies, nearly all patients with ischemic DCM (i.e. CAD and prior myocardial infarction) showed subendocardial and/or transmural myocardial hyperenhancement (LGE), whereas patients with IDCM may present LGE in 12–26 % of cases (McCrohon 2003, Soriano 2007, Wu 2008, Hombach 2009). In the study by McCrohon et al., 13 % of patients who had IDCM had CAD-type hyperenhancement, whereas 28 % had non-CAD-type LGE. These rates are nearly identical to the rate of chronic infarcts found at autopsy in patients who had IDCM in a study by Roberts et al. (1987) and in the ATLAS substudy by Uretzky et al. (2000) (14 and 12 %, respectively). Whether the CAD-type of LGE in patients with IDCM is due to coronary embolisation and subsequent recanalisation, remains unclear. The patchy or linear striae of LGE limited to the mid myocardium, as found in McCrohon's study, is not specific for IDCM, according to our own experiences non-CAD-type of

LGE may be found within midwall or subepicardium in any region of the ventricular myocardium (Hombach 2009) (Figure 10-2).

Arrhythmogenicity of Scars and Prognosis

Nazarian et al. (2005) reported that in 26 patients with non-ischemic DCM, scar distribution involving 26–75 % of wall thickness was significantly predictive of inducible VTs on programmed stimulation (EPS), and remained predictive after adjustment for LVEF (OR 9.125, $p = 0.020$). Thus, scar distribution may identify the substrate for inducible VT and may identify high-risk patients with non-ischemic DCM. Similar results were reported by Yokokawa et al. (2008) in 47 patients with IDCM and advanced heart failure (HF). In a total of 101 consecutive patients with non-ischemic DCM and HF, Asomull et al. (2006) found midwall fibrosis by delayed enhancement (DE-CMR) in 35 %, which was associated with a higher rate of predefined combined end-point of all-cause mortality and hospitalization for a cardio-vascular event (HR 3.4, $p = 0.01$) and for prediction of secondary endpoint SCD/VT (HR 5.2, $p = 0.03$). In a series of 65 Patients with non-ICM and EF ≤ 35 % planned for an ICD implantation, Wu et al. (2008) found LGE in 27 (42 %) patients, and 12 of LGE positive patients (44 %) had an index composite outcome event (cardiac death, appropriate ICD firing, and hospitalization for decompensated HF) vs. only 8 % of LGE negative patients ($p < 0.001$). After adjustment for LV volume index and functional class, patients with LGE had an 8-fold higher risk of experiencing the primary outcome (HR 8.2, 95 % CI 2.2–30.9, $p = 0.002$). Hombach et al. (2009) studied 141 consecutive IDCM patients by clinical, conventional ECG, CMR functional parameters, and DE-CMR. Multi-variate analysis revealed cardiac index (CI) ($p < 0.001$) and increased RVEDVI ($p = 0.006$) derived from CMR, the presence of diabetes mellitus ($p = 0.006$), and QRS > 110 ms ($p = 0.0045$) to be significant predictors of the primary endpoint (cardiac death and SCD). In conclusion, it was stressed that prognostically relevant hemodynamic (CI, RVEDVI) and ECG parameters (QRS duration) can be derived from two non-invasive techniques with high precision and without the need for complicated analysis techniques.

10.4 Hypertrophic Cardiomyopathy (HCM)

Prevalence, Etiology and Pathology

HCM is characterized by a thickened non-dilated left ventricle in the absence of any other cardiac condition leading to hypertrophy such as systemic hypertension, aortic valve disease, or athlete's heart. The pathological hallmark of this condition is a triad of myocyte hypertrophy, disarray, and interstitial fibrosis. The prevalence of HCM is about 0.2 % in the general population. The majority of patients have a background of familial disease with mutations in genes that encode the proteins of the contractile apparatus. Approximately 10 % will present with new mutations.

Clinical Presentation, Diagnosis and Therapy

The most common **presentation** of patients with HCM, also in de novo cases, is dyspnea on exertion and dizziness. Chest pain, presyncope, syncope, and arrhythmias (palpitations) are also seen. SCD can be a feature in the familial type of HCM and can occur even if LV hypertrophy is not marked, especially in some mutant carriers of cardiac troponin T. Risk factors for SCD include a LV wall thickness greater than 30 mm, and a significant LVOT obstruction, defined as a pressure gradient of more than 30 mmHg at rest, or with provocation (Maron 2003). **Diagnosis** is usually made by history (dyspnea, palpitations, presyncope), ECG (LV hypertrophy and inverted/negative T-waves in the precordial leads), and echocardiography (LV septal or wall hypertrophy, pressure gradient in the LVOT and SAM-phenomenon in HOCM patients). For full evaluation, CMR is the imaging technique of choice. Patients may be **treated** by drugs (β-blockers, calcium channel blockers), by alcohol septal ablation (TASH), or surgical myectomy (in HOCM patients), and/or by implantation of an ICD in high risk patients (aborted SCD, syncope from VT/VF, episodes of unstable VTs). CMR imaging is particularly useful for following patients on medical maintenance therapy or following TASH or surgical myectomy.

CMR Findings

CMR imaging can meet a number of challenges in the non-invasive evaluation of HCM patients, and provide extremely important information regarding accurate diagnosis by exact phenotypic characterization, regional and global systolic and diastolic function, flow mapping of the LVOT, detection and quantification of fibrosis/necrosis, and follow-up after treatment. CMR is also useful for screening of subjects with suspected HCM and first-degree relatives.

Left Ventricular Hypertrophy (LVH)

Different morphological types of HCM and distribution of LVH are found. HCM typically produces marked asymmetrical LV hypertrophy with an end-diastolic LV wall thickness greater than 15 mm (Figure 10-3). In 70 % of patients the ventricular septum and anterior wall are involved, and significant hypertrophy in the subaortal region results in LVOT obstruction (subaortal type in HOCM: about 25 % of all HCM patients), while mid-ventricular,

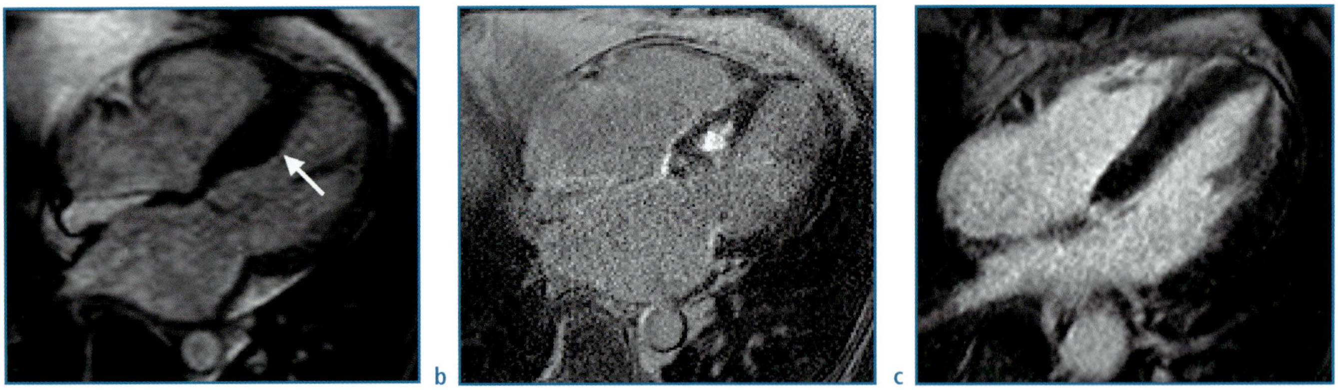

a b c

Figure 10-3 56-yrs-old male patient with atrial flutter and septal hypertrophy (arrow) in a 4-ch view on cine-CMR **(a)** and scar in the center of the hypertrophied region (bright signal) **(b)** using late enhancement technique. 64-yrs-old patient with hypertrophic cardiomyopathy **(c)** without LVOT obstruction in a 4-ch view on cine-CMR showing generalized myocardial hypertrophy (in diastole).

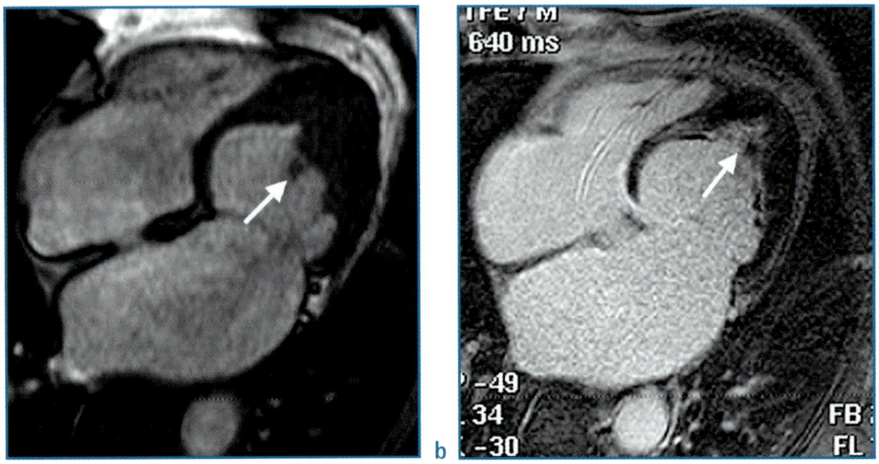

a b

Figure 10-4 Patient with dyspnea on exertion with apical ("spade-like") type of hypertrophy (arrow) in cine-CMR and 4-ch view **(a)**; scar (arrow) in the center of apical hypertrophied area **(b)** using the late enhancement technique (courtesy Dr. J. Schwab, Nuremberg).

apical (Yamaguchi type; Figure 10-4), and RV hypertrophy are less frequent forms of HCM. The left atrium (LA) may be enlarged in patients with HCM, and atrial fibrillation (AF) is commonly encountered in these patients. In the study of Papavassiliu et al. (2009), LA size was superior to late gadolinium enhancement (LGE) for predicting the prevalence of AF; HCM patients with AF showed more LGE, and LA dilatation was related to the extent of LGE irrespective of LV mass, and was a stronger determinant of AF than LGE. The distribution of LV hypertrophy has shown little relation to clinical outcome, but the magnitude of LV wall thickness reveals a direct relationship to SCD risk (Spirito 2000). In contrast to transthoracic echocardiography (TTE) with its limited acoustic window and poor lateral resolution for accurate imaging of the anterolateral free wall of the LV, CMR has the capability of acquiring tomographic images of the hypertrophied LV with tissue contrast and segmental border definition that is superior to TTE. In the study of Rickers et al. (2005) on 48 patients with suspected or confirmed diagnosis of HCM, the degree of LV wall thickness was underestimated by TTE in the anterolateral wall, and the underestimation was significant in 10% of patients with severe LVH (i.e. > 30 mm). In addition, 6% of patients had HCM confirmed by CMR that was missed by TTE. The apical variant of HCM is difficult to diagnose with TTE due to signal dropout, and apical hypertrophy may be missed in 9% of patients with normal TTE but positive CMR for apical hypertrophy, as reported by Eriksson et al. (2002) in a retrospective series of 105 patients. CMR should therefore be considered as the new gold standard imaging modality and diagnostic test of choice in all patients with suspected HCM.

Left Ventricular and Mitral Valve Function

Systolic function and myocardial mass in HCM can be precisely assessed by cine-SSFP imaging and volumetry, and diastolic dysfunction, which is present in about 80% of patients with HCM, can be measured by diastolic mitral

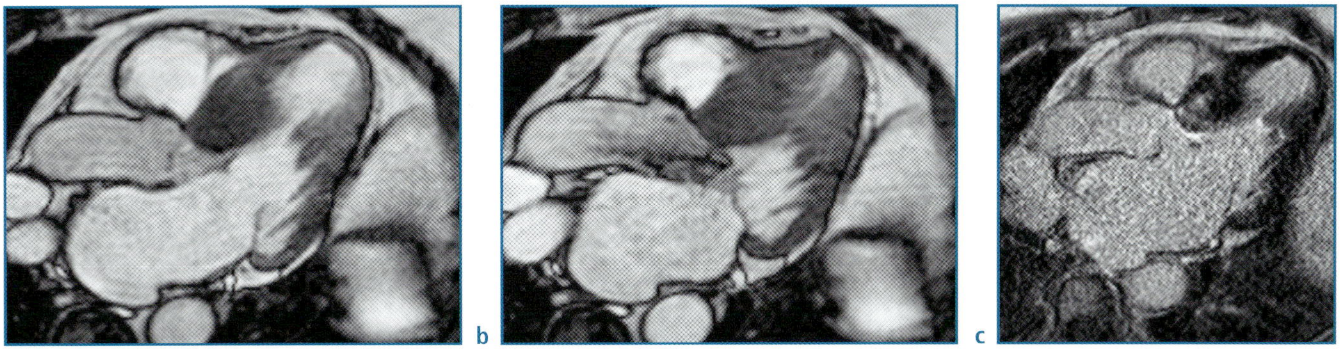

a b c

Figure 10-5 Young patient with hypertrophic obstructive cardiomyopathy: 3-ch view on cine-CMR at diastole (a) and systole (b) showing an enlarged left atrium, subaortal septal hypertrophy, and systolic anterior movement (SAM) of the anterior mitral leaflet (b) with outflow tract obstruction (signal void over LVOT and aortic valve); typical scar in the center of hypertrophied septal muscle after gadolinium administration (c).

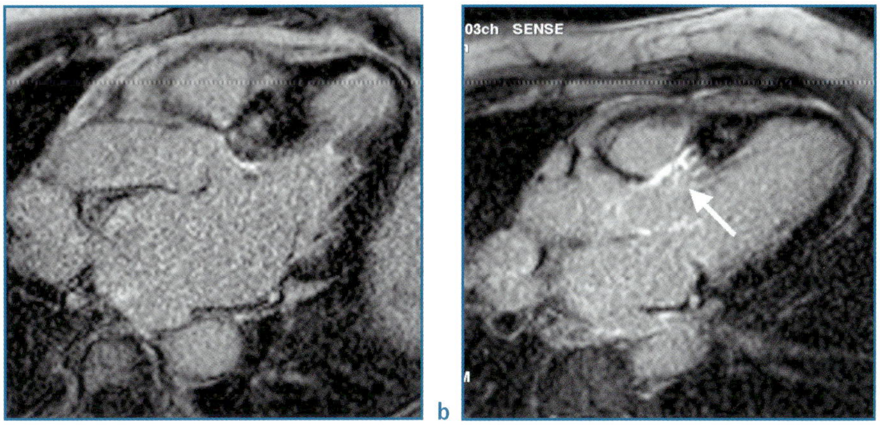

a b

Figure 10-6 Scar sequences in a patient with hypertrophic obstructive cardiomyopathy before (a) and after alcohol septal ablation (= TASH) (b). Note the small scar in the center of hypertrophied septum before, and massive scar with destruction of basal septal muscle after TASH (arrow in (b)).

inflow pattern, using PC flow mapping, and by determining the peak filling rates in time-volume curves. In HOCM patients with significant LVOT obstruction either at rest, or after provocative measures (Valsalva maneuver, administration of amyl nitrite), systolic anterior movement of the mitral leaflet (SAM) can be accurately visualized by CMR, together with the secondary mitral valve incompetence occurring in mid-late systole (Figure 10-5). Regional assessments of segmental wall motion in systole and diastole with measurements of radial and circumferential strain patterns can be performed using CMR tagging techniques. Regarding regional systolic function, several reports have shown that a reduced myocardial contractility (Ghio 2009) or impaired circumferential shortening (Kim 2008) was associated with the extent of late gadolinium enhancement (LGE). Choi et al. (2008) also demonstrated a correlation between the extent of LGE and left atrial volume index, a surrogate marker of chronic diastolic burden in a series of 47 patients with HCM.

LVOT Obstruction in Hypertrophic Obstructive Cardiomyopathy (HOCM)

In patients with HOCM, the severity of LVOT obstruction, which is a second marker of an increased risk of SCD, may be detected visually by flow void and quantitatively assessed by TTE- or CMR-based flow mapping to determine the pressure gradient by a modified Bernoulli formula, or by CMR derived planimetry to measure LVOT cross-sectional area. In 37 patients with HCM, compared with 14 healthy controls, Schulz-Menger et al. (2006) showed that a cut-off value of 2.7 cm^2 cross-sectional area identified the obstruction as defined by TTE with 100% accuracy. Arrtive et al. (1994) reported a correlation between the degree of LVOT obstruction and end-diastolic thickness of the interventricular septum, the systolic anterior movement of the mitral leaflet (SAM), and the zone of signal void within the LVOT. CMR imaging can also be used as a control in alcohol septal ablation (TASH) therapy. Schulz-Menger et al. (2000) reported in 10 patients that the enlargement of cross-sectional

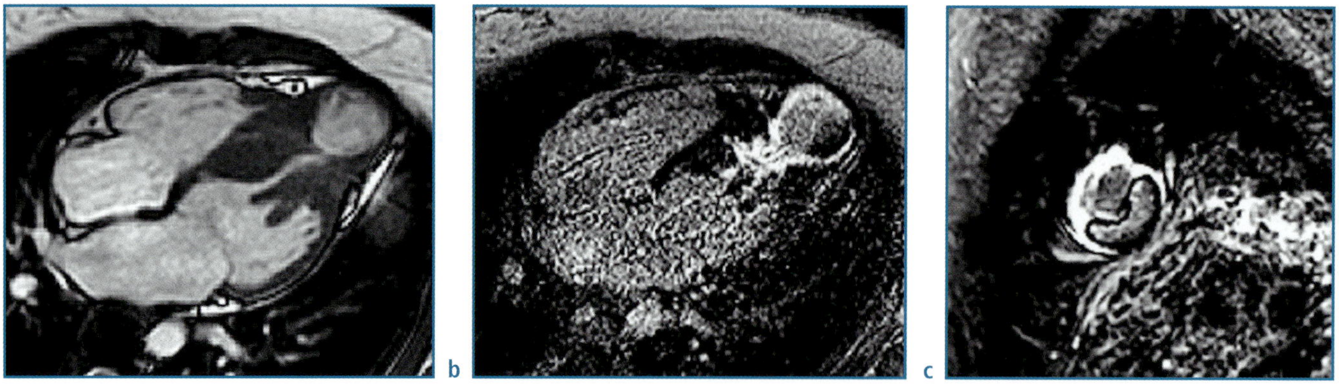
a b c

Figure 10-7 39-yrs-old female patient with unexpected stroke from embolization of an apical thrombus, found in an apical aneurysm in severe hypertrophic obstructive cardiomyopathy in a 4-ch view using cine-CMR imaging (a). Scar sequences revealed a complete necrotic part of the apical left ventricular (LV) musculature together with a visible thrombus in the LV apex (4-ch view) (b). Almost 60 % of the circumference of apical LV musculature were necrotic in a short-axis view (bright signal in (c)). Patient received an ICD because of concomitant near-syncope from sustained ventricular tachycardia and was treated with an ACE-inhibitor, β-blocker, and anticoagulant (phenprocumone).

area by TASH correlated well with improvement of symptoms (r = 0.86). In addition, using the LGE technique, anatomic localization, shape, and size of the TASH-induced septal infarction could be well-documented by CMR (Figure 10-6). The same result with enlargement of the LVOT and reduction of SAM of the mitral valve cusp was reported by White et al. (1996) in 4 patients following surgical myectomy. In a further study using CMR tissue tagging and 3D strain analysis to assess regional myocardial function, van Dockum et al. (2006) reported that septal ablation in 9 patients improved intramural systolic function of the lateral (remote) wall, indicating reversed remodeling.

Left Ventricular Apical Aneurysm

Patients with HCM and LV apical aneurysms represent an underappreciated subset in the heterogenous HCM disease spectrum. Maron et al. (2008) identified LV aneurysms in 28 of 1,299 HCM patients (2 %) between ages of 26–83 yrs. Apical aneurysms varied significantly in size, were dyskinetic/akinetic with thin rims, were associated with transmural myocardial scarring identified by DE-CMR, and 19 patients (68 %) showed an "hourglass" contour with midventricular hypertrophy producing muscular narrowing and intracavitary gradients in 9 patients (example in Figure 10-7). 24 out of 28 patients were treated by β-blockers, calcium channel blockers, or both, 2 patients received an ICD for secondary prevention, and 15 for primary prevention, though the 5 traditional risk factors for HCM were absent in 8 of 15 ICD patients. After a follow-up of 4.1 ± 3.7 yrs, 12 patients (43 %) with LV aneurysms experienced adverse disease complications (event rate 10.5 % per year) including sudden death (2 patients), appropriate ICD discharges (3 patients), nonfatal thromboembolic stroke (2 patients), and progressive heart failure and death (5 patients). The conclusion from this large cohort of HCM patients with LV apical aneurysms was that these patients require a high index of suspicion and CMR imaging for identification, and apical aneurysms in HCM are associated with substantial cardiovascular morbidity and mortality and raise novel treatment considerations.

Myocardial Perfusion and Tissue Characteristics

Myocardial perfusion in hypertrophied regions as well as global myocardial perfusion reserve may be diminished in patients with HCM. Rickers et al. (2002) performed CMR first-pass studies in 40 HCM patients and 40 matched controls, and found a significant reduction of resting blood flow (0.36 ± 0.16 ml/min/g) in patients with HCM compared with normal controls (1.02 ± 0.27 ml/min/g) and in non-hypertrophied regions. The same diminished regional blood flow was measured on stress perfusion, and the ratio of stress to rest perfusion was significantly lower in hypertrophied (2.6 ± 0.72) and non-hypertrophied regions (3.1 ± 0.8) in HCM patients compared with healthy patients (3.7 ± 1.5). It was concluded that abnormal perfusion at rest and on stress in hypertrophied myocardium may induce fibrosis, and may be associated with disease or symptom progression and/or SCD. A similar severe depression of flow reserve ratio in patients with HCM was reported by Kawada et al. (1999), using PC flow measurements in the coronary sinus.

A further strength of CMR in HCM patients is the ability to determine myocardial tissue characteristics by the LGE technique. Typically, HCM patients display a patchy, multifocal, midwall hyperenhancement, occurring only within hypertrophied regions in areas with replacement fibrosis containing a collagenous matrix (Moon 2004). The junction of right ventricular free wall with the interventricular septum is frequently affected in HCM patients, while in

HOCM patients LGE is most commonly located in the center of the hypertrophied septum. To identify high-risk individuals for SCD who are candidates for an ICD, risk factors including family history of SCD, syncope, nonsustained VT, abnormal blood pressure response to exercise, and severe LV hypertrophy have been proposed (Maron 2003). The presence of LGE seems to add new prognostic information, since it has been reported to be associated with progressive ventricular dilatation and markers of SCD (Moon 2003), with higher NYHA classes and prevalence of VT, impaired global LV function and asymmetrical hypertrophy, abnormal Q-waves, and giant negative T-waves (Satoh 2009). It has also been associated with greater likelihood and increased frequency of ventricular tachyarrhythmias, including nonsustained VT on ambulatory Holter ECG (Adabag 2008), and a specially designed LGE score proved to be a significant multi-variable predictor of both clinical VT/VF and of maximal LV wall thickness as markers of high-risk HCM patients (Leonardi 2009). In a mathematical model the 5-yrs probability of SCD in HCM has been calculated to be 0.11 in patients compared with 0.07 in patients without LGE, i.e. the approximate 5-yrs probability of SCD is 1.6-fold higher if scarring is noted on CMR of a patient with HCM (Nazarian and Lima 2008). A recent study (Bruder 2010) showed that in a cohort of 243 patients with largely low or asymptomatic HCM the presence of LGE indicating myocardial scar is a good independent predictor of all-cause and cardiac mortality.

CMR for Screening and Differential Diagnosis

Since first-degree relatives of affected HCM individuals have a 50% chance of being a gene carrier (Maron 2002), determining the presence of HCM in family members is essential and may be achieved most accurately by CMR. Disease expression in HCM patients with certain gene mutations may be very heterogenous, therefore precise phenotyping by CMR with demonstration of LVH is mandatory, providing incremental information to conventional ECG and echocardiographic screening. Particularly in young patients, repeat CMR examinations may be needed every 2–5 yrs for the early observation of disease progression with development of further LVH, ECG abnormalities, and later focal fibrosis (LGE). CMR is also important for differential diagnosis in patients with dyspnea on exertion and abnormal ECG, in whom, apart from HCM, LVH may be induced by underlying arterial hypertension, aortic stenosis, athlete's heart, amyloidosis, or metabolic abnormalities such as Fabry's disease. CMR criteria such as type, extent, and location of LVH, systolic and diastolic function, valvular function, and type, size, and location of LGE may aid differential diagnosis.

10.5 Restrictive Cardiomyopathy

Prevalence, Etiology and Pathology

The hallmark of restrictive cardiomyopathies is abnormal diastolic function due to increased stiffness of the ventricular walls, leading to heart failure. Idiopathic RCM strictly defined to include normal ventricular wall motion, normal wall thickness, and ventricular chamber dimension proved to be relatively rare, and has been observed in single families with sarcomere gene mutations. Approximately 50% of cases with RCM result from specific clinical disorders such as infiltrative (amyloidosis, sarcoidosis, Gaucher disease, Hurler disease, fatty infiltration), storage diseases (hemochromatosis, Fabry's disease, glycogen storage disease), and endomyocardial disorders (endomyocardial fibrosis, hypereosinophilic syndrome, carcinoid heart disease, metastatic cancers, and drugs causing fibrous endocarditis like serotonine, methysergide, ergotamine, mercurial agents, and busulfan). The remaining 50% of patients present with idiopathic RCM.

Clinical Presentation, Diagnosis and Therapy

In early stages of idiopathic RCM (IRC), systolic function may be normal together with impaired filling characteristics, although deterioration in systolic function is usually observed as the disease progresses. Clinically the patients frequently present with exercise intolerance that results from impaired ability to increase cardiac output during increasing heart rate due to the restriction of diastolic filling. Further common **symptoms** are dyspnea and/or chest pain on exertion, weakness, and edema. With advanced disease, profound peripheral edema with hepatomegaly, ascites, and later on anasarca may occur. Many patients report palpitations that are produced by atrial fibrillation. **Diagnosis** is made by history, clinical examination (positive Kussmaul sign, rales, S3–S4 gallop), chest X-ray, and echocardiography, including tissue Doppler (normal systolic function combined with diastolic dysfunction: myocardial relaxation with increased early left ventricular filling velocity, and decreased isovolumetric relaxation time). CMR imaging is a very valuable tool for determining structure, systolic and diastolic function, and tissue characteristics, and to aid in differentiating idiopathic from secondary forms of RCM. The most important differential diagnosis of IRC is constrictive pericarditis, which is also characterized by normal or nearly normal systolic function, but abnormal ventricular filling. Points frequently helpful in favoring constrictive pericarditis over restrictive cardiomyopathy are active pericarditis from history, paradoxical pulse on clinical examination, absence of intraventricular conduction defect within the ECG, calcification on chest X-ray, thickened pericardium on CT/MR imaging, septal notch in the echocardiogram, respiratory variations indicating increased ventricular interdependence on Doppler, close equilibration of diastolic pressures, and absence of amyloid or other infiltrative disease on endomyocardial biopsy (Hanckock 2001). **Treatment** refers to classical drug therapy of heart failure.

CMR Findings

CMR imaging allows precise assessment of atrial and ventricular volumes, systolic and diastolic function, as well as of associated valvular insufficiencies, and provides parameters to differentiate RCM from constrictive pericarditis (CP). In CP a leftward inversion or flattening of the interventricular septum during early ventricular filling is seen, which is not present in patients with RCM. The amount of ventricular coupling can be further evaluated by quantifying the difference in the maximal interventricular septal excursion between inspiration and expiration. This parameter normalized to the end-diastolic biventricular dimension has been shown to be significantly greater with CP (about 20%) than with RCM, where a cut-off value of 11.8% enables such a differentiation (Francone 2006). CMR imaging also provides a detailed description of the morphology of the pericardium in CP vs. RCM (in CP irregular thickening, signal void due to calcifications), an assessment of pericardial motion patterns with cine-SSFP sequences (in CP abolished motion), as well as the impact on ventricular filling by PC flow analysis, i.e. mitral and pulmonary vein inflow patterns.

10.6 Arrhythmogenic Right Ventricular Cardiomyopathy or Dysplasia (ARVD)

Prevalence, Etiology and Pathology

ARVD is a progressive cardiomyopathy primarily affecting the right ventricle (RV) and is characterized by fibro-fatty replacement with myocyte loss, right heart failure, and ventricular (tachy-) arrhythmias with left bundle branch block (LBBB) pattern. Increasing evidence suggests that ARVD is a disease of desmosomal dysfunction. Its prevalence is estimated to be 1:5,000 in the US and 1:10,000 in Europe up to 1:1,000 in the region of Venezia, and it can exist in both sporadic and familial form with a predominantly autosomal dominant inheritance pattern with variable penetrance. ARVD accounts for 5–20% of SCD in young individuals less than 35 yrs, and most SCDs occur during strenuous exercise. There is a 6-fold male predominance over females. The estimated death rate per year is 2.5% (Jain 2008). Morphological features include myocyte loss with fibro-fatty replacement of the ventricular myocardium, focal thinning of the RV wall in diastole, RVOT enlargement, RV dilatation, RV aneurysms and trabecular disarray, and hypertophy. Functionally global or regional contraction abnormalities and RV systolic and/or diastolic dysfunction may be found at least in later stages of the disease.

ARVD is considered a disease of desmosomal dysfunction due to mutations affecting components of the cardiac desmosome, with consecutive disruption of cell-cell adhesion, provoking detachment of myocytes particularly under conditions of mechanical stress, leading in turn to apoptosis and cell necrosis, secondary inflammation, and repair by fatty substitution.

Clinical Presentation, Diagnosis and Therapy

This generally considered progressive disease may present with **four different clinical phases**:

- a concealed phase (subtle RV structural changes, minor ventricular arrhythmias, rarely sudden cardiac death during intense sports or physical exercise in very young individuals),
- an overt clinical disorder (symptomatic RV arrhythmias including VTs associated with overt RV structural and functional abnormalities),
- RV failure due to disease progression, and finally
- biventricular pump failure from significant LV involvement.

Patients most commonly present with ventricular tachycardias (VTs) with LBBB configuration at stage two. **Symptoms** of right-sided heart failure are rare at least in the early stages of disease. **Diagnosis** is confirmed by a set of six major and minor criteria (McKenna 1994) including global and/or regional RV dysfunction and structural abnormalities, tissue characterization of the RV wall, repolarization and depolarization/conduction abnormalities, arrhythmias, and family history (Table 10-1). Patients must have either two major criteria, one major and two minor criteria, or four minor criteria to be labeled as affected with ARVD (Jain 2008). Patients should be **treated** with ACE-inhibitors and β-blockers, and those with high risk or proven ventricular tachyarrhythmias should receive an ICD in order to reduce the major cause of mortality in affected individuals. In patients progressing to overt heart failure, management involves the same principles for the treatment of other forms of cardiomyopathy e.g. DCM. Prognosis of patients with ARVD is moderate, Hulot et al. (2004) reported 21 deaths with an annual death rate of 2.3% in a cohort of 130 patients with ARVD over a follow-up period of 8.1 ± 7.8 yrs, and death from heart failure occurred in 59% of patients compared with 29% SCDs. In a cohort of 61 patients with ARVD, in multivariate analysis Lemola et al.

Table 10-1 Major and minor criteria for the diagnosis of ARVD (modified from Mc Kenna et al. 1994; the CMR criteria have been added to the original concept).

Criterion	Major	Minor
global/regional dysfunction, structural abnormalities of RV	severe RV dilatation, reduced RV-EF, minimal involvement of LV, severe segmental RV dilatation, regional RV aneurysms	mild global RV dilatation, mildly reduced RV-EF, mild segmental RV dilatation, regional RV hypokinesis
tissue characteristics of ventricular myocardium	fibro-fatty degeneration at endocardial biopsy	none
CMR criteria	severe global or segmental RV dilatation, global systolic and diastolic RV dysfunction, severe trabecular disarray of RV, localized RV aneurysms or excavations, presence of LGE in RV wall	intramyocardial fatty infiltration, focal wall thinning of RV, regional wall hypertrophy of RV, moderator band hypertrophy, RVOT enlargement
abnormalities in depolarization and AV conduction	epsilon-wave of the QRS complex in V1 to V3, localized QRS prolongation ≥ 110 ms in V1 to V3	ventricular late potentials in the signal averaged surface ECG
abnormalities in repolarization	none	inverted T-waves in V2 and V3 in patients older than 12 yrs, absent RBBB
cardiac arrhythmias	none	LBBB type of ventricular tachycardias (non-sustained or sustained), frequent ventricular ectopic beats (≥ 1,000/24 h)
family history	familial disease of ARVD confirmed by autopsy or surgery	sudden death victims in the family (victims < 35 yrs) due to suspected ARVD, positive family history by the appropriate criteria of ARVD

(2004) found a history of congestive heart failure and presence of LV involvement as independent predictors of an adverse outcome during a follow-up period of 55 ± 47 mths, with a total death rate of 10 patients (16%).

CMR Findings

CMR abnormalities in ARVD may be divided into structural abnormalities (intramyocardial fatty infiltration, focal wall thinning, regional wall hypertrophy, trabecular disarray and hypertrophy, moderator band hypertrophy, RVOT enlargement), and into functional abnormalities (regional wall motion abnormalities, focal aneurysms and microaneurysms or excavations, RV dilatation, RV diastolic and systolic dysfunction) (Figure 10-8). Of these severe global or segmental dilatation of the RV, global systolic and diastolic dysfunction, and localized aneurysms are considered major CMR criteria, while mild global or regional dilatation of the RV, regional contraction abnormalities, and global diastolic dysfunction are considered minor criteria according to the Task Force (McKenna 1994). Lesions in the RV wall such as fibro-fatty replacement or late-stage fibrosis may be detected by gadolinium-enhanced CMR (LGE). Tandri et al. (2005) found 12 of 30 consecutive patients prospectively evaluated for ARVD to meet the criteria of the Task Force, and 8 of these 10 showed LGE compared with none of 18 patients not meeting the Task Force criteria for ARVD. These LGE areas correlated well with histological findings and with inducibility of VT during electrophysiologic testing. Sen-Chowdrhy et al. (2006) performed comprehensive CMR studies in 232 patients undergoing evaluation of suspected ARVD, and CMR studies were positive in all 64 patients who fulfilled the Task Force criteria (100% sensitivity), while specificity was low (29%) for the whole group. In the group of 26 genotyped individuals (gene-positive) sensitivity of CMR was 96%, specificity 78%, PPV 93% and NPV 88%. Among other diagnostic criteria such as LV or RV dilatation, abnormal trabeculation, and severe RV segmental dilatation/wall motion abnormalities/aneurysms, LGE in the LV had a sensitivity of 100% and specificity of 67%, compared with LGE in the RV with a sensitivity of 59% and a specificity of 100%. The conclusion of this large study on 64 ARVD patients was that CMR including LGE is a valuable component of the diagnostic workup for ARVD when performed with a dedicated protocol by specialists in CMR imaging. In summary, according to the literature and our own experiences severe global or segmental dilatation of RV, global systolic and diastolic RV dysfunction, severe RV trabecular disarray, localized aneurysms, and the presence of LGE within the RV wall should be considered major criteria for ARVD, compared with the other features of CMR imaging considered as minor criteria.

LV involvement in ARVD has been described in 16–76% of cases with subnormal LV ejection fraction, regional wall motion abnormalities, and evolution of LV involvement has

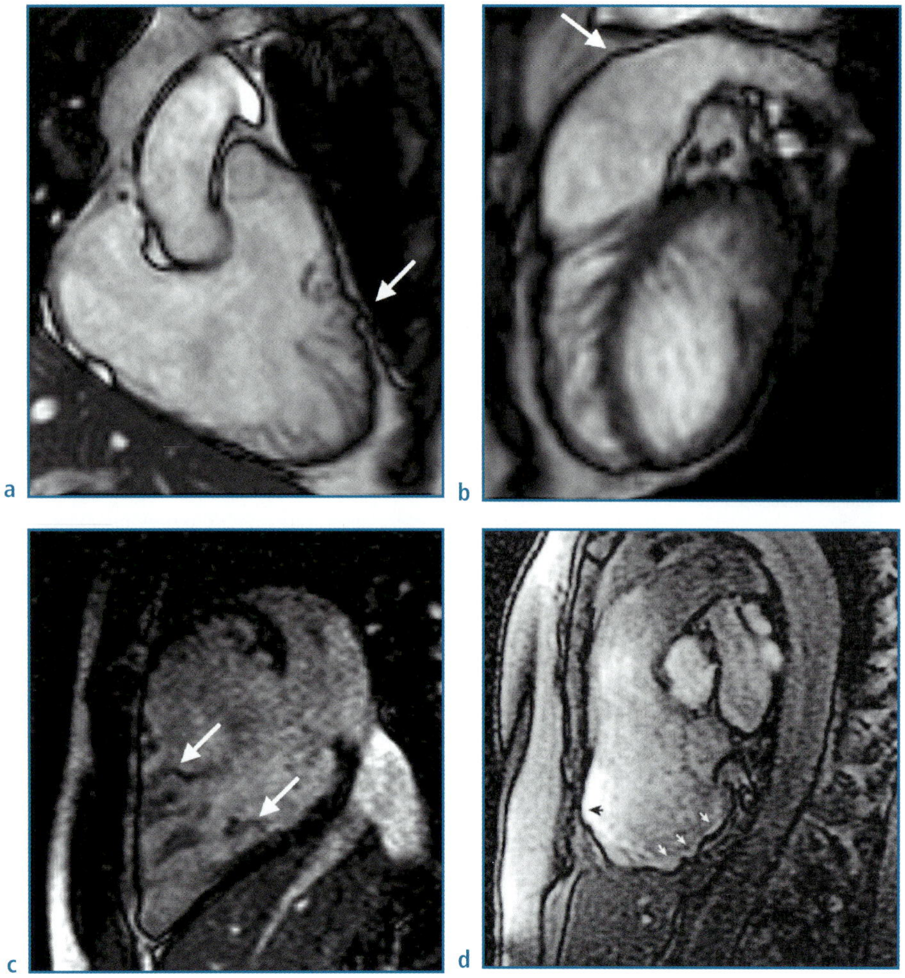

Figure 10-8 Different patients with arrhythmogenic right ventricular dysplasia/cardiomyopathy with circumscribed aneurysm in the anterior right ventricular (RV) wall (arrow) and trabecular disarray **(a)**, circumscribed aneurysm in the RVOT (arrow in **(b)**), severe trabecular disarray (arrows in **(c)**), and multiple small aneurysms/excavations at the basal and anterior part of RV musculature (small arrows in **(d)**) (Figure d by courtesy of Dr. J. Schwab, Nuremberg).

been demonstrated in terms of appearance of new abnormalities or worsening of existing abnormalities or both, with progression of RV disease on long-term follow-up (Jain 2008). The most common variant of ARVD is considered a biventricular form with LV involvement from its early stages, and LV involvement is considered to be part of a larger disease process extending across the entire heart, since ARVD is considered a desmosomal disease and desmosomal genes are expressed in both ventricles. Fibro-fatty changes of the LV located in the subepicardial or mid-ventricular areas can extend across varying thickness of myocardial wall. They can affect both the septum and LV free-wall with a predilection for the posteroseptal and posterolateral areas. CMR imaging provides precise information on LV dilatation and regional wall motion abnormalities including aneurysms, mostly located at the LV apex, by cine-SSFP sequences, and fibro-fatty areas by delayed-enhancement on gadolinium administration. LV involvement is associated with increased myocardial mass, inflammatory infiltrates (i.e. LGE in CMR), clinical arrhythmic events, and more severe RV wall thinning and heart failure, but frank left-sided heart failure is unusual (Jain 2008).

10.7 Tako-Tsubo Cardiomyopathy

Prevalence and Pathogenesis

Tako-Tsubo cardiomyopathy or apical ballooning syndrome (ABS) is a novel acute coronary syndrome that mimics acute myocardial infarction. Its prevalence is very low and was first described by Japanese colleagues, but is now detected worldwide. It is most commonly observed in women secondary to heavy emotional or physiological stress. Its pathogensis is unclear, severe coronary artery spasms are suspected to produce the transient and reversible severe transmural ischemia within the apical region of the left ventricle.

Clinical Presentation, Diagnosis and Therapy

Patients present with the clinical syndrome of acute myocardial infarction with severe acute chest pain, ST segment elevation, and/or elevated cardiac markers (troponin T/I). Typically these patients immediately undergo coronary angiography and show normal coronary arteries together with a typical apical ballooning, i.e. akinesis of the apex up

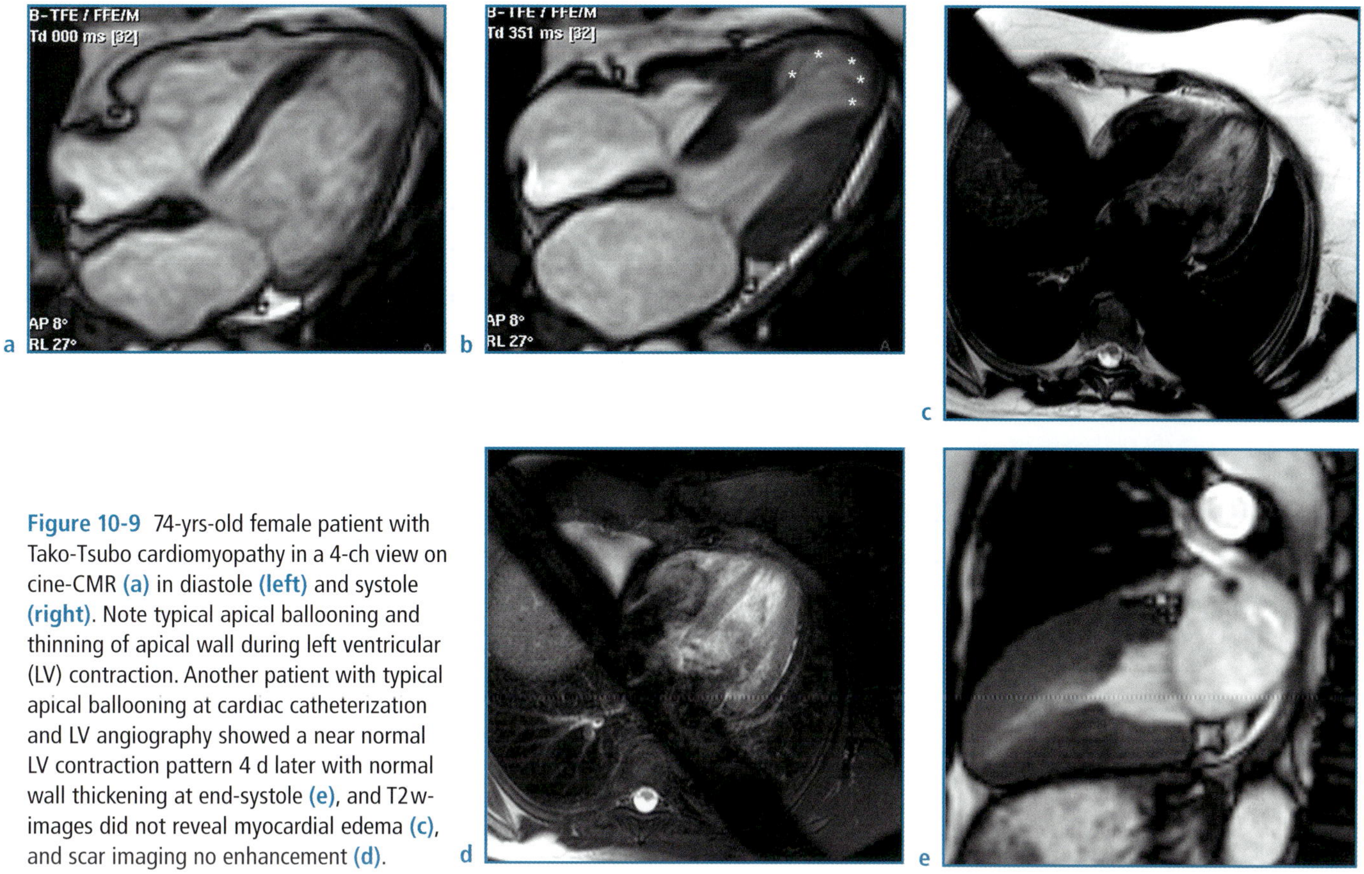

Figure 10-9 74-yrs-old female patient with Tako-Tsubo cardiomyopathy in a 4-ch view on cine-CMR **(a)** in diastole **(left)** and systole **(right)**. Note typical apical ballooning and thinning of apical wall during left ventricular (LV) contraction. Another patient with typical apical ballooning at cardiac catheterization and LV angiography showed a near normal LV contraction pattern 4 d later with normal wall thickening at end-systole **(e)**, and T2w-images did not reveal myocardial edema **(c)**, and scar imaging no enhancement **(d)**.

to the mid-ventricular portion of the left ventricle on left ventricular angiography or echocardiography. Typically wall motion abnormalities disappear within days or weeks on regular treatment with β-blockers and ACE-inhibitors.

CMR Findings

Cine-SSFP imaging shows the typical apical ballooning, and in some patients myocardial edema may be present on T2-weighted imaging (Joshi 2009). In most reports LGE has not been found in ABS (Haghi 2007, Mitchell 2007, Hombach 2008, Koeth 2008, Syed 2008). Myocardial edema disappears and LV dysfunction returns to normal or near normal on follow-up CMR imaging, typically after 3–6 mths a completely normal CMR scan may be present (Figure 10-9).

10.8 Cardiac Non-Compaction (NC)

Prevalence, Etiology and Pathogenesis

This specific (unclassified) cardiomyopathy develops due to a pathological arrest of the compaction process of the loose network of fibers with sinusoids, which are in continuity with the ventricular cavity present during the embryologic period up to the 5th week of intrauterine life. This arrest of compaction leads to the persistence of ventricular hypertrabeculation, which is called spongy myocardium or left ventricular non-compaction (NC). The childhood form of NC was first described in association with other congenital or neuromuscular abnormalities, but NC may be observed in adults without further congenital anomalies. Although NC has generally been regarded as a familial cardiomyopathy, a family history is not always present in adults or children. The prevalence of NC has been estimated at 0.05% in the general population (Ritter 1997). The finding of a ratio of > 2.0 between the thickness of the non-compacted and compacted myocardial layers in systole is considered diagnostic at echocardiographic examination, though using CMR due to its high resolution properties a ratio of > 3.0 has been reported (Fazio 2008).

Clinical Presentation, Natural History and Therapy

Patients may be **asymptomatic** for a longer period, but later on present with dyspnea on exertion, chest pain, palpitations, systemic emboli including stroke, and symptoms of overt heart failure. In a study by Yousef et al. (2009) on 42 patients with non-compaction, the distribution of symptoms was dyspnea in 50%, chest pain in 19%, palpitations in

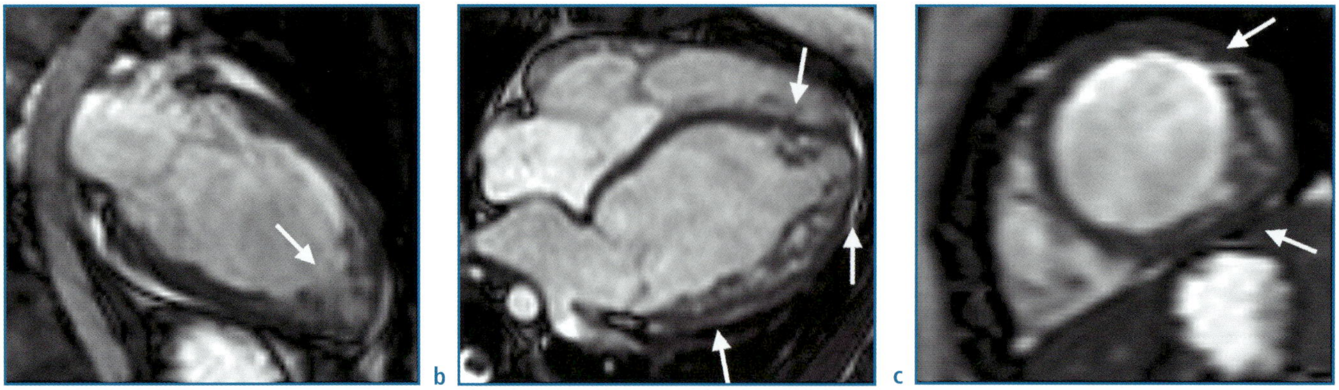

a b c

Figure 10-10 13-yrs-old patient with cardiac non-compaction cardiomyopathy and only slight impairment of physical fitness. Cine-CMR images in the 2-ch (a), 4-ch (b) and short-axis view (c) show the typical spongy myocardium with apical (arrows in (a) and (b)) and lateral wall recessus (arrows in (c)). Left ventricular ejection fraction was 50 % using CMR volumetry.

14 %, and stroke in 5 % of cases. Diagnosis is made by echocardiography, using a ratio of > 2.0 of the non-compacted (NC) and compacted (C) myocardium as diagnostic, though echocardiography poses inherent problems in assessing the LV apex, known to be the most commonly non-compacted area. Therefore, **diagnosis** should be confirmed by CMR imaging using an NC/C ratio of > 2.3 (Petersen 2005) or > 3.0 (Fazio 2008), and by demonstrating the typical non-compacted myocardium at LV apex, anterior and lateral LV wall with open recessus at diastole and obliteration during systole. Patients with overt heart failure are **treated** with ACE-inhibitors, diuretics, and β-blockers. Some patients at high risk of life-threatening ventricular tachyarrhythmias need an ICD implantation, and some may finally undergo heart transplantation. Prognosis of patients with NC is poor. In a study by Oechslin et al. (2000) on 34 patients after a follow-up of 44 ± 40 mths, major complications such as heart failure (18 patients = 53 %), thromboembolic events (8 patients = 24 %), and ventricular tachycardias (14 patients = 41 %) occurred, and 12 patients died (8 suddenly, 4 from end-stage heart failure, and 2 from other causes). 4 patients underwent heart transplantation, and 4 patients received an ICD. Therefore, patients with NC should be carefully observed in shorter time intervals, using CMR imaging as the gold-standard for assessing changes in LV volumes and function over time, and to detect developing thrombi within the non-compacted myocardium prior to systemic embolization.

CMR Findings

In the study by Petersen et al. (2005) on 7 patients, non-compacted myocardial segments were most commonly found at the LV apex (91 % of subjects), followed by mid-cavity levels (78 %), and the basal segments (21 %), and NC was most common in the anterior segment, becoming less frequent in successive segments in a clockwise direction. Yousef et al. (2009) found a slightly different distribution of NC segments with a more or less equal frequency at the apex, apical-inferior, apical-septum, and mid-septal segments between 35 and 40 %. The second CMR criterion to confirm the diagnosis is an NC/C ratio of > 2.3, and the demonstration of open recessus at diastole and obliteration during systole (Figure 10-10). In addition, in NC patients presenting with dyspnea LV volumes may be greater and LV ejection fraction lower than in age-matched healthy controls (Yousef 2009). CMR imaging is the ideal tool to follow NC patients for changes in the myocardial structural and functional status.

10.9 Secondary Types of Restrictive Cardiomyopathy

10.9.1 Amyloidosis

Etiology and Pathogenesis

Infiltrative types of RCM include amyloidosis, sarcoidosis, Gaucher disease, Hurler disease, and fatty infiltration of the myocardium. Amyloidosis results from tissue deposition of special proteins (twisted beta-pleated sheet fibrils) that may be found in almost all organs, but only produce symptoms when tissue infiltration is extensive. **Primary amyloidosis** results from the deposition of portions of immunoglobulin light chain (AL) that result in most cases from a monoclonal expansion of plasma cells in multiple myeloma or Morbus Waldenström. **Secondary amyloidosis** (reactive amyloidosis) results from the excess production of non-immunoglobulin protein known as AA in the setting of rheumatoid arthritis, Morbus Crohn, chronic osteomyelitis, or mucoviscidosis. In rare cases various familial diseases may lead to amyloidosis, most commonly induced by the production of a variant form of prealbumin termed transthyretin. Cardiac amyloidosis is a progressive infiltrative cardiomyopathy that carries a grave prognosis; it shows male predominance, and is rare before age 40. About 25 % of patients with familial (transthyretin-induced) amyloidosis experience clinically significant cardiac involvement, and neurological and renal involvement may also predominate, patients typically present with clinical symptoms after age 35. The amyloid infiltrated heart appears tan and waxy on pathological examination, and is rubbery in consistency. Amyloid deposits may be found within the ventricular and atrial myocardium between the myocytes, atria may be enlarged, and focal thickening of cardiac valves due to amyloid deposition may be present; also amyloid may deposit in the media and adventitia of intramural coronary arteries and may cause impairment of coronary perfusion (Hare 2012).

Clinical Presentation, Diagnosis and Therapy

Most patients with cardiac amyloidosis present with **symptoms** of congestive heart failure, i. e. dyspnea on exertion, reduced exercise capacity, edema etc., blood pressure may be normal or reduced, and pulse pressure may be quite narrow as a result of a low cardiac output. The ECG often reveals low QRS voltage, bundle branch block, atrioventricular blocks of varying degree, and atrial fibrillation with amyloid infiltration of the atria. **Diagnosis** is made by echocardiography revealing increased ventricular wall thickness with small intracavitary chambers, enlarged atria, and a thickened interatrial septum. Systolic function may be normal, but Doppler examination may show a restrictive filling pattern indicating diastolic dysfunction. Diagnosis can be confirmed by endomyocardial biopsy and histologic examination using Sirius red or Congo red staining for amyloid deposition, and immunohistochemistry for identification of specific amyloid proteins. **Therapeutic intervention** includes classic heart failure treatment (digitalis particularly for rate control in atrial fibrillation, diuretics, β-blockers, ACE-inhibitors), pacemaker implantation in AV block, or ICD implantation in severely depressed systolic function, and in AL amyloidosis chemotherapy with alkylating agents alone, or in combination with autologous bone marrow transplantation with a 30–39 % survival rate after 4–5 yrs. The prognosis is rather poor (for details see Hare 2012).

CMR Findings

CMR imaging may reveal the typical homogenous increased thickness of atrial and ventricular walls and the interatrial septum, together with a normal or reduced size (Figure 10-11). Occasionally thickening of papillary muscles or valve leaflets may be seen with CMR. The atria are usually enlarged and pleural and pericardial effusions are commonly observed. Systolic function can be exactly quantified, and diastolic dysfunction can be assessed by PC diastolic mitral and pulmonary vein flow patterns showing a restrictive filling pattern. LGE may also be present and aid in confirming the diagnosis by its type, size and location (Maceira 2005, 2008, Perugini 2005).

T1 and T2 mapping has been tested for confirming amyloid deposition within the myocardium. In the study of Maceira et al. (2005) subendocardial T1 in 30 patients with cardiac amyloidosis was significantly shorter than subepicardial T1, and was correlated with markers of increased myocardial amyloid load such as LV mass, wall thickness, interatrial septal thickness, and diastolic function. In contrast, Sparrow et al. (2009) could not find any difference in T2 relaxation times between the 49 patients with histologically confirmed cardiac amyloidosis and normal controls. LGE has also been found in both studies, in the study of

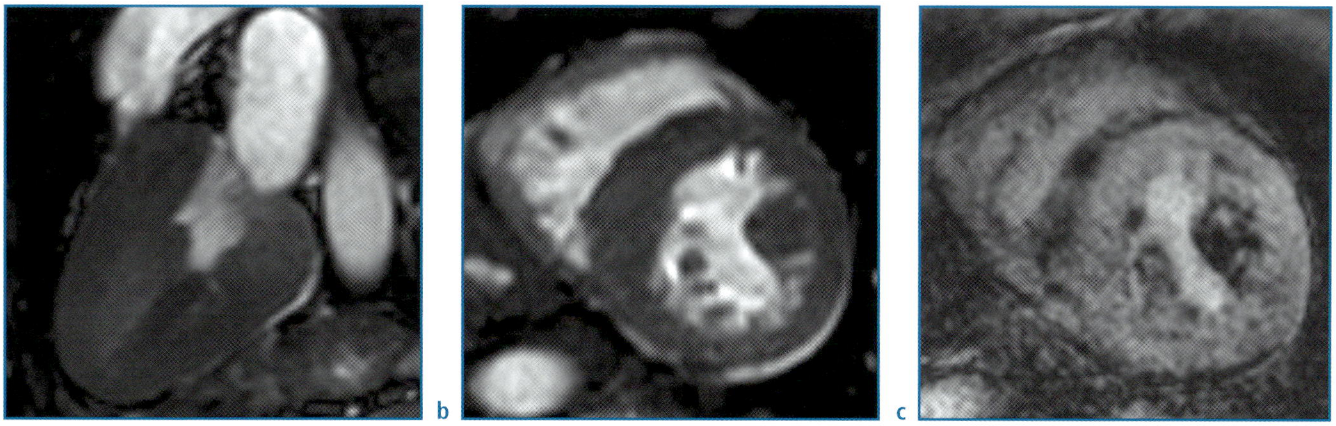
a b c

Figure 10-11 32-yrs-old patient with dyspnea on exertion and NYHA class II–III due to cardiac amyloidosis. Note thickened left ventricular myocardium in a 2-ch (a) and short-axis view (b). After gadolinium administration there was a diffuse patchy myocardial enhancement (short-axis view) (c).

Maceira et al. (2005) in 20/30 patients (69%) with LGE a characteristic pattern of global subendocardial LGE coupled with abnormal myocardial and blood-pool gadolinium kinetics was found. A similar predominant subendocardial location of LGE was described by Sparrow et al. (2009) in 8/12 patients. In addition, Perugini et al. (2006) found LGE in 16/21 patients (66 of 357 myocardial segments = 18%) more often in the mid-ventricular regions. In this study LGE appeared to be associated with impaired segmental and global contractility and a larger atrium (example in Figure 10-11).

CMR imaging may also contribute to assess the prognosis. Maceira et al. (2008) followed 29 patients with cardiac amylodosis for a median of 623 days (IQ range 221, 1,436), and found that the presence of myocardial LGE by itself was not a signidicant predictor of all-cause mortality. However, death was predicted by gadolinium kinetics, with the 2 min post-gadolinium intramyocardial T1 difference between subepicardium and subendocardium predicting mortality with 85% accuracy at a threshold value of 23 ms. Migrino et al. (2009) studied 29 consecutive patients with biopsy-proven amyloidosis and found LGE in 23/29 patients (79%). On follow-up over median 29 mths 14/19 LGE-positive and none of LGE-negative patients died (log rank $p = 0.0061$); presenting NYHA heart failure class was also associated with poor survival ($p = 0.0059$); survival between two LGE groups stratified by heart failure class still showed a significant difference by stratified log-rank test ($p = 0.04$). It was concluded from this study that LGE is common in patients with cardiac light chain amyloidosis and is associated with poor long-term survival even after adjustment for heart failure class presentation. Further prognostic studies on lager patient populations have to be performed to prove the true prognostic potential of CMR in patients with cardiac amyloidosis.

10.9.2 Sarcoidosis

Prevalence, Etiology and Pathogenesis

Sarcoidosis is a systemic inflammatory disease characterized by the formation of noncaseating granulomas in the lungs (most commonly), the reticuloendothelial system, the skin, and in variable frequency in the eyes, heart, and nervous system. Sacoidosis is more commonly seen in young and middle-aged adults, its prevalence ranges from 10 per 100,000 for whites to 35.5 per 100,000 in black, and in Europe, Scandinavians have one of the highest incidence rates of 50–60 cases per 100,000 population. Myocardial involvement occurs in at least 25% of patients and accounts for 12–35% of deaths from sarcoidosis (Silverman 1978). The pathogenesis of sarcoidosis is unclear, infectious or environmental agents are considered the antigens to trigger primarily helper inducer T cells leading to formation of granulomas. At a later stage of lesion evolution there is a shift to the T helper type 2 response during the proliferative phase of granuloma that results in tissue scarring. Pathologic features of cardiac sarcoidosis include granulomas found in every part of the heart, but in decreasing order of frequency in the left ventricular free wall and papillary muscles, the basal aspect of the ventricular septum, the right ventricular free wall, and the atrial walls. Histologically noncaseating granulomas are found with numerous lymphocytes located at their border zone, and a dense band of fibroblasts, collagen fibers, and proteoglycans usually encasing this aggregate of inflammatory cells. The disease process follows three successive histological stages: edema, noncaseating epitheloid granulomatous infiltration, and fibrosis leading to post-inflammatory scarring (for details see Hare 2012).

Clinical Presentation, Diagnosis and Therapy

The clinical manifestations result from infiltration of the conduction system and the myocardium. Patients may be **asymptomatic** in earlier stages, but may present with symptoms of congestive heart failure resulting from direct cardiac involvement or from cor pulmonale due to extensive pulmonary fibrosis, and with cardiac arrhythmias due to AV block 1st to 3rd degree, and atrial as well as ventricular tachyarrhythmias. Ventricular tachycardia (sVT) is the most frequent arrhythmia encountered in cardiac sarcoidosis with an incidence of 23%, and sudden cardiac death as the terminal event in 67% of cases. Supraventricular arrhythmias such as atrial flutter or fibrillation and paroxysmal atrial tachycardias may occur in about 15–17%, and are mostly the result of atrial dilatation rather than the result of atrial granulomas. Other clinical manifestations include chest pain and electrocardiographic changes that may mimic transmural myocardial infarction. In addition, pericardial effusion is encountered in 3–19% of cases and rarely tends to tamponade. **Diagnosis** is made by history, chest X-ray (bilateral hilar lymphadenopathy), echocardiography (global or regional ventricular dysfunction, RV hypertrophy, and pulmonary hypertension by Doppler measurements of systolic pressure gradient via the tricuspid valve), and ECG (T-wave abnormalities, different degrees of AV block), including Holter long-term monitoring (atrial or ventricular arrhymias, non-sTV or sVT). CMR imaging is becoming an extremely valuable tool for confirming cardiac sarcoidosis and assessing both abnormal structure and function of the heart and to characterize myocardial tissue. Therefore this technique is highly important because ante-mortem diagnosis of cardiac sarcoidosis is exceptionally challenging since only 40–50% of patients with cardiac sarcoidosis at necropsy have clinical evidence of myocardial involvement during their lifetime (Silverman 1978). Patients with (cardiac)

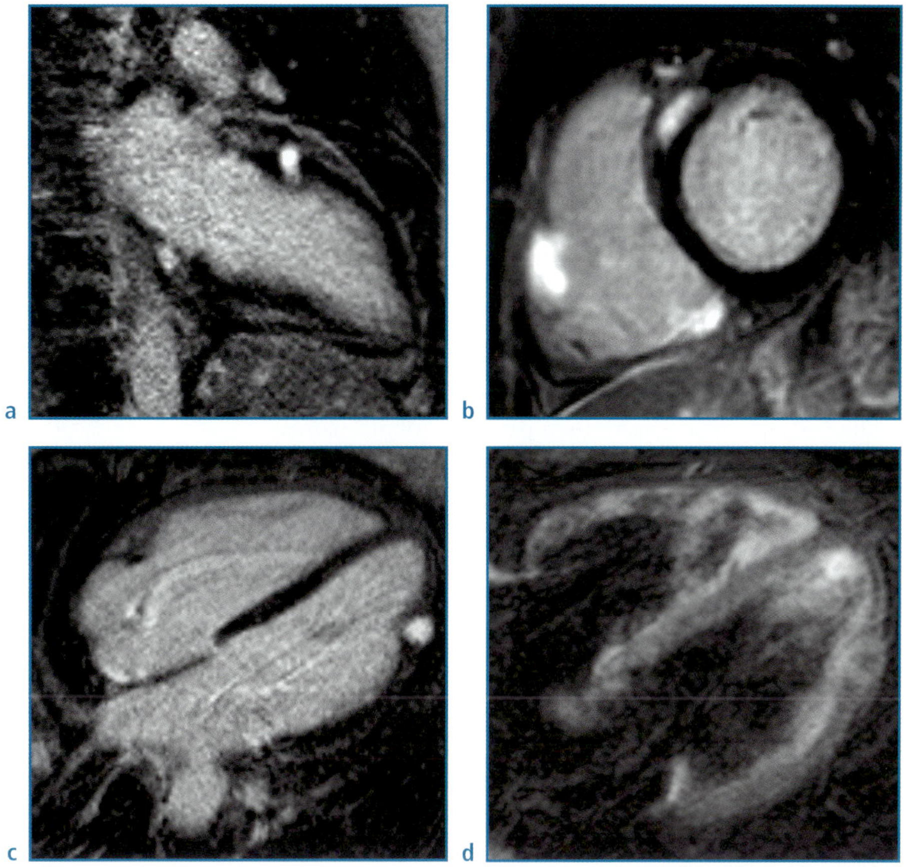

Figure 10-12 36-yrs-old male patient with cardiac sarcoidosis and mild clinical symptoms. Scar imaging showed circumscribed "nodes" within the anterior and posterior left ventricular (LV) wall (2-ch view) (a), the interventricular septum and right ventricular trabeculae (short-axis view) (b), and the apical-lateral LV wall (4-ch view) (c). T2w-images revealed increased signal intensity indicating myocardial edema due to myocardial inflammation (4-ch view) (d).

sarcoidosis are generally **treated** with immunosuppressive agents (corticosteroids, metothrexate, cyclophophamide). Patients with complete AV block should receive a cardiac pacemaker, and those with recurrent ventricular tachyarrhythmias an ICD. Prognosis of patients with cardiac sarcoidosis is not well-defined, recent studies indicate a 5-yrs survival rate of 40–60 % that are better than in older reports, which may be due to earlier diagnosis and treatment of this disease (Doughan and Williams 2006).

CMR Findings

The CMR imaging protocol should include cine-SSFP techniques, T1- and T2-weighted sequences before and after gadolinium administration, and T2-/STIR-weightes images. Wall thickness may be regular, though zones of wall thinning and segmental wall motion abnormalities have been described. Diastolic dysfunction can also be assessed by PC mitral inflow pattern analysis. Myocardial signal intensity may be enhanced in T2w-images because of edema associated with inflammation and granulomatous lesions, and these images can be enhanced by gadolinium injection. The LGE pattern is atypical, i. e. non-CAD specific with intramural or epicardial location (Figure 10-12).

Three CMR patterns of sarcoidosis may be differentiated (Vignaux 2002):

- **a pure nodular pattern** with a peripheral increased and central decreased signal intensity on both T2-weighted and gadolinium-enhanced T1-weighted images, representing hyaline fibrotic tissue,
- **an inflammatory focal or patchy pattern** with increased signal intensity on gadolinium-enhanced T1-weighted images without or with myocardial thickening,
- **a post-inflammatory pattern** with focal increased signal intensity on T2-weighted images, but no gadolinium uptake, and without or with myocardial thinning.

LGE has been tested both as a diagnostic tool for determining cardiac involvement in general sarcoidosis, and for predicting prognosis of patients with proven cardiac sarcoidosis. Smedema et al. (2005) investigated 58 patients with biopsy proven pulmonary sarcoidosis, in 12 patients cardiac sarcoidosis (CS) was found using Japanese guidelines as a gold standard, and in 19 patients LGE was found. In 8 out of 19 patients with patchy LGE scintigraphy was negative, and the overall accuracy of LGE for the diagnosis of CS was 83 %. It was concluded that in patients with sarcoidosis CMR is a useful tool to determine cardiac involvement.

Similar results with a superiority of LGE over the standard Japanese Ministry of Health and Welfare (JMHW) criteria to detect cardiac involvement was described by Manins et al. (2008) in 20 patients with systemic sarcoidosis. Patel et al. (2009) examined 81 consecutive patients with chronic systemic sarcoidosis and normal left ventricular EF. LGE by delayed enhancement-CMR (DE-CMR) identified 21 patients with cardiac involvement (21 %) in contrast to 10 patients (12 %) according to the JMHW criteria. On follow-up of 21 ± 8 mths, patients with myocardial damage on DE-CMR had a 9-fold higher rate of adverse events, i. e. all-cause mortality or symptomatic arrhythmia, and an 11.5-fold higher rate of cardiac death than patients without damage. From this study it was concluded that DE-CMR is more than twice as sensitive for cardiac involvement with sarcoidosis as current consensus criteria, and myocardial damage by DE-CMR appears to be associated with an adverse prognosis; but because of the few events a larger cohort is needed to confirm these prognostic results.

10.9.3 Hemochromatosis

Etiology and Pathology

Hemochromatosis is a storage disease resulting from excessive deposition of iron in a variety of parenchymal tissues including the myocardium. The inherited form results from a mutation in the HFE gene, which codes for a transmembrane protein that is responsible for regulatory iron uptake in the intestine and liver. Hemochromatosis may also arise from ineffective erythropoesis secondary to a defect in hemoglobin synthesis, or from chronic liver disease, or may be aquired as a result of chronic and excessive oral or parenteral intake of iron or blood transfusions for hereditary anemia (e.g. thalassemia or sickle cell anemia). The heart is grossly dilated and ventricular walls are thickened. Iron deposits locate preferentially in the myocyte sarcoplasmic reticulum, more frequently in the ventricular vs. the atrial cardiomyocytes. The conduction system is also frequently involved, and the degree of iron deposition correlates with the extent of myocardial dysfunction. Iron loading of tissues is particularly dangerous, because it leads to tissue damage and fibrosis, and in the heart it will lead to myocardial fibrosis and systolic and diastolic ventricular dysfunction.

Clinical Presentation, Natural History and Therapy

Some patients are asymptomatic at least in the earlier stage of disease. Common **complaints** are exercise intolerance, dyspnea and/or chest pain on exertion, weakness, and peripheral edema in the later stages. ECG changes such as ST segment and T-wave abnormalities and supraventricular arrhythmias may occur. Endomyocardial biopsy may be confirmatory to demonstrate myocardial iron deposition; however a certain sampling error rate should be taken into account. Death results most frequently from cirrhosis and hepatocellular carcinoma, whereas cardiac mortality accounts for an additional 33 % of the mortality with particular importance in the young male patients. **Diagnosis** is usually made by history (anemia, transfusions), and echocardiography including Doppler sonography (thickening of ventricular walls, systolic and diastolic dysfunction with restrictive filling pattern). Continuous subcutaneous **administration of desferrioxamine** or other iron chelators may reduce body iron stores and result in clinical improvement. In rare cases cardiac transplantation may be considered with acceptable 5–10 yrs survival rates (for details see Hare 2012).

CMR Findings

CMR imaging shows a mild increase in LV wall thickness and end-diastolic chamber diameter and sometimes an enlarged left atrium. Diastolic dysfunction with a restrictive filling pattern usually precedes systolic dysfunction. Global systolic dysfunction does not appear until iron concentration within the myocardium reaches a critical level, however subtle wall motion abnormalities may be detected in earlier stages of disease, despite preserved global function. CMR is extremely useful to identify and quantify non-invasively myocardial iron deposition from the image signal intensity (Figure 10-13) or the calculated T2* relaxation time.

The presence of iron disturbs the magnetic field homogeneity and enhances tissue T2 relaxation, and a marked decrease in signal intensity on T2-weighted images will be seen. To determine the T2* value, a single short-axis mid-ventricular slice is acquired at 9–12 separate echo times (ranging from 4.8–163.2 ms, increment 14.4 ms) with ECG gating, using a spoiled gradient echo or a T2*-weighted GRASE sequence, or a black-blood T2* sequence. Myocardial signal intensities are measured in a region of interest (left ventricular septum) and plotted against the echo time to form an exponential decay curve. The intercept of the decay curve with x-axis provides the T2* value of myocardium. Normal values for T2* of myocardium are > 20 ms (33.3 ± 7.8 ms, or 46.4 ± 26.3 ms in the study of He (2008), in patients with iron overload T2* values are typically below 20 ms. He at al. (2008) demonstrated a very good inter- and intra-site reproducibility of T2* measurements, using a breath-hold myocardial T2* technique at four international sites equipped with Siemens MR-scanners and the same software.

Myocardial fibrosis may also be detected by the late enhancement technique (LGE). Pepe et al. (2009) found LGE areas in 28 of 115 patients with thalassemia major, and in 26 patients location of fibrosis was non specific and patchy distribution was present. The LGE group was significantly older than the non-LGE group (31 ± 7.7 yrs vs. 26 ± 7.7 yrs), and no significant relation with heart T2* values and bi-

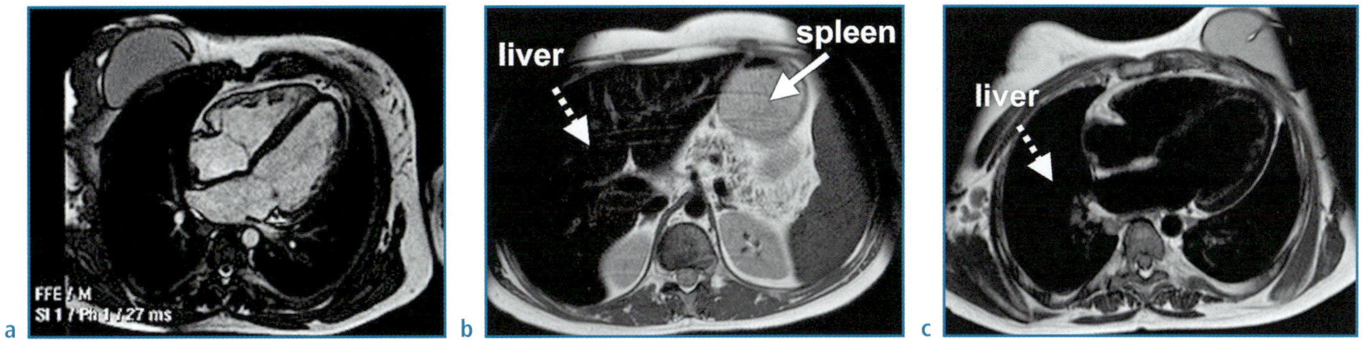

Figure 10-13 Cardiac iron overload in a female patient with primary hemochromatosis. Dark ventricular muscle due to iron deposition within the myocardium, that resulted in slight left ventricular dysfunction (ejection fraction 54 %) in a 4-ch view on cine-CMR (a). Note dark liver (dashed arrows) and relatively bright spleen (arrow) in black-blood sequences (b and c), indicating a primary form of hemochromatosis.

ventricular function was found. The conclusion was that the presence of fibrosis/necrosis seems to be a time-dependent process correlating with cardiovascular risk factors and cardiac complications. Meloni et al. (2009) reported myocardial fibrosis to be present in 31 of 94 patients with thalassemia; the global T2* value in patients with fibrosis was comparable with that of patients without fibrosis ($p = 0.88$), and T2* values in segments with fibrosis were comparable with those in segments without fibrosis ($p = 0.83$). The global T2* value was not correlated with the pO_2. It was concluded that myocardial fibrosis and blood oxygenation did not significantly affect the T2* values supporting the usefulness of taking T2* as an equivalent of iron deposit in the heart in the clinical arena.

10.9.4 Further Storage Diseases

In addition to hemochromatosis by iron overload, further storage diseases such as glycogenosis (type 1 and 2), Fabry's disease (deposition of glycosphingolipids in skin, kidneys and lysosomes of myocytes due to hereditary α-gylcosidase deficiency) (Figure 10-14), Morbus Gaucher (deposition of

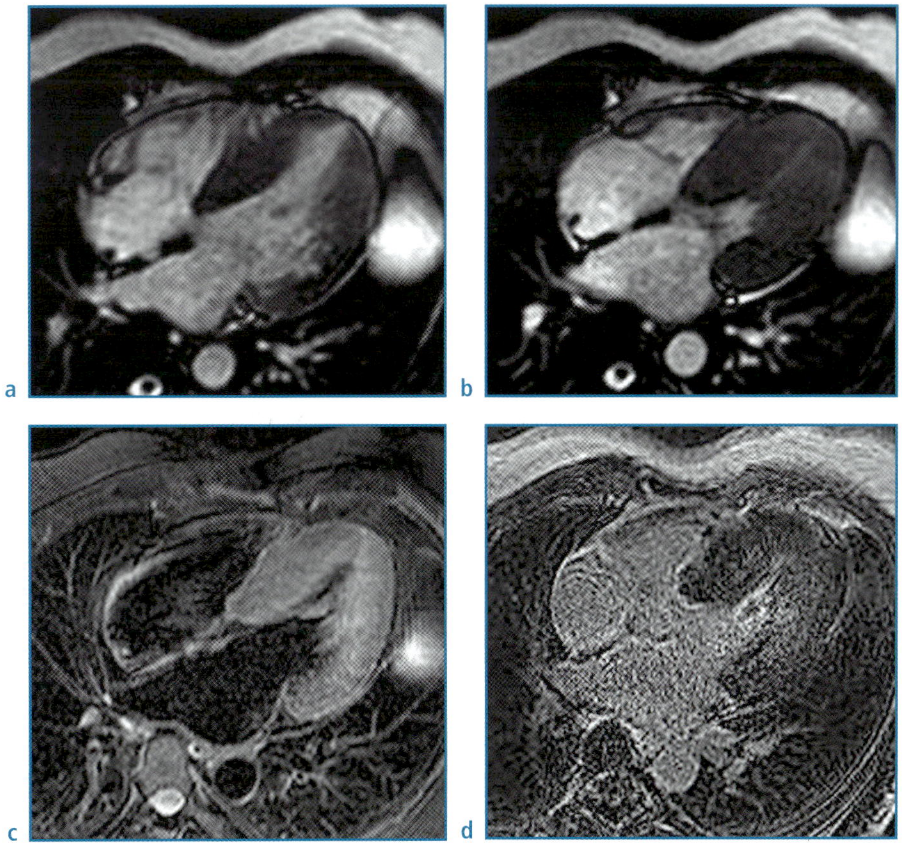

Figure 10-14 Patient with cardiac involvement in Fabry's disease; significant thickening of left ventricular myocardium in diastole (a) and systole (b) on cine-CMR imaging in a 4-ch view. T2w-black-blood imaging with increased signal intensity (4-ch view) (c), and anterolateral gadolinium enhancement (4-ch view) (d) revealed myocardial "damage" from deposition of glykosphingolipids (courtesy Dr. J. Schwab, Nuremberg).

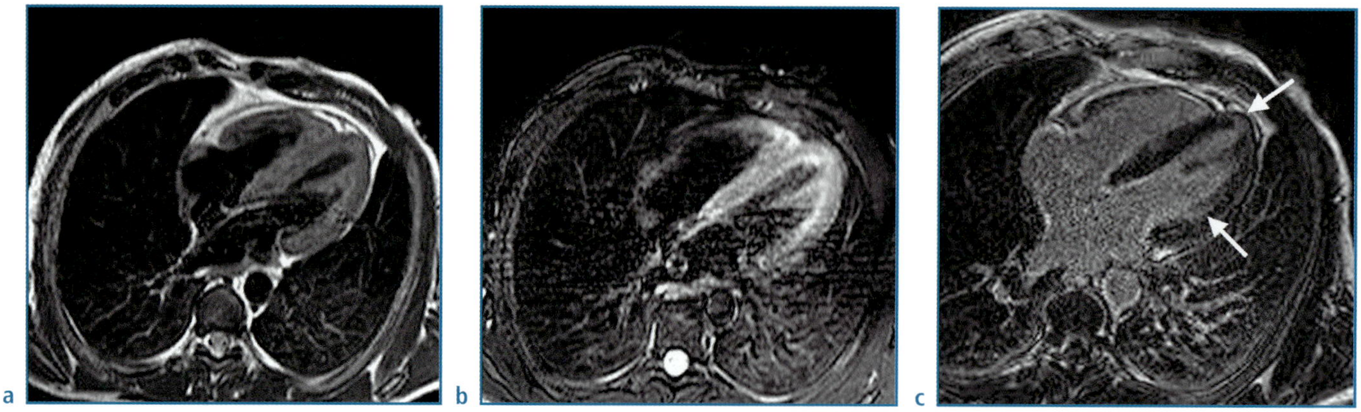

Figure 10-15 Patient with cardiac involvement in Morbus Gaucher in 4-ch views. T2w-images (a) and particularly T2w-black-blood images (b) showed diffuse increased signal intensity, while gadolinium administration revealed only slight enhancement (arrows in (c)) indicating myocardial "damage" from deposition of cerebrosides (courtesy Dr. J. Schwab, Nuremberg).

cerebrosides in spleen, liver, bone marrow, lymph nodes, brain, and interstitum of myocardial tissue due to hereditary β-glucosidase deficiency) (Figure 10-15), and glycogen storage may affect myocardial structure and function. **Clinical presentation** is similar to other storage disease (dyspnea on exercise, arrhythmias, symptoms of heart failure). CMR imaging may show LV wall thickening including the valves, with initially preserved systolic but severely impaired diastolic function, i.e. abnormal mitral and/or pulmonary vein inflow dynamics, and abnormal subepicardial or mid-wall contrast-enhancement. Though systematic studies on these rare diseases have not been reported, CMR imaging may aid significantly to confirm myocardial involvement in addition to other clinical and biochemical finding in these patients, and may also be the ideal tool for following the course of the disease.

10.10 Endomyocardial Diseases

Etiology and Pathogenesis

Endomyocardial diseases with RCM pattern include hypereosinophilic syndrome (Löffler's endocarditis), endomyocardial fibrosis, and carcinoid syndrome, as well as metastatic cancers, toxic effects of anthracyclines, and drugs causing fibrous endocarditis (serotonine, methysergide, ergotamine, mercurial agents, and busulfan). Endomyocardial diseases in the strict sense are Löffler's endocarditis (hypereosinophilic syndrome) and endomyocardial fibrosis (Davies disease), which despite different clinical phenotypes are considered unique disease processes at different stages. The initial hypereosinophilia from different etiologies initializes the **first stage** (necrotic phase due to toxic effects of proteins derived from the granules of eosinophils on myocardial tissue with consecutive myocarditis and arteriitis resulting in Löffler's endocarditis). This first phase occurs during the first months after disease onset, and approximately one year after initial presentation the **second stage** (thrombotic phase) with decreasing inflammation and thickening of the endocardium and variable thrombotic depositions occurs. The putative **third stage** (fibrotic phase) ends up in endocardial fibrosis.

Clinical Presentation, Diagnosis and Therapy

Löffler's Endocarditis

This disease is associated with significant hypereosinophilia, usually characterized by eosonophil counts exceeding 1,500 per mm^3 for at least 6 mths. The eosinophilia may be secondary to leukemia, reactive disorders like parasite infection, allergies, granulomatous syndromes, hypersensitivity, or neoplastic disorders. On **post-mortem examination** both chambers of the heart are involved with endocardial thickening of the inflow regions and ventricular apices, histologically there are varying degrees of eosinophilic myocarditis of the myocardium and subendocardium, thrombosis and inflammation of small intramural coronary vessels, mural thrombosis containing eosinophils, and endocardial thickening of several millimeters. **Clinical presentation** includes fever, cough, rash, weight loss, and heart failure. Early in the disease process patients may be asymptomatic, but more than half of them develop heart failure in the later stages of disease. Systemic emboli are frequently observed. **Diagnosis** is made by chest X-ray (enlarged cardiac silhouette, pulmonary congestion, less frequently pulmonary infiltrates), ECG (ST segment and T-wave abnormalities), and echocardiography (regional thickening of posterobasal LV wall, enlargement of left atrium, impairment of posterior leaflet of mitral valve, occasionally obliteration of LV apex by thrombus, preserved systolic function), and Doppler ultrasound (signs of diastolic dysfunction, atrioventricular regurgitation). Quality and quantity of life may be improved by **medical and surgical therapy**. Corticosteroids or cytotoxic drugs such as hydroxyurea may have important favorable effects on survival, and interferon may offer valuable adjunctive therapy in refractory patients. In addition, supportive therapy includes diuretics, ACE-inhibitors, β-blockers, and anticoagulation. In the fibrotic stage of disease surgical endocardectomy and valve replacement may provide significant symptomatic palliation. **Prognosis** of patients with Löffler's endocarditis is moderate to poor with frequent progression of the disease (Hare 2012).

Endomyocardial Fibrosis (Davies Disease)

This disease is typically found in tropical and subtropical Africa, and is a major cause of morbidity and mortality, accounting for 25% of cases with congestive heart failure and death in these regions. It is also increasingly observed in India, Brazil, Colombia, Sri Lanka, and Saudi Arabia. It affects both sexes equally and is most common in children and young adults, but has also been described in patients aged up to 60 yrs. On **post-mortem examination**, endomyocardial fibrosis affects both ventricles in 50%, only the LV in 40%, and the RV alone in 10% of cases. The heart is normal or slightly enlarged, and right and left atrium may be enlarged, occasionally with atrial thrombi and pericardial effusion. The hallmark feature is fibrotic obliteration of the apex of the ventricles, including fibrosis of papillary muscles and chordae tendineae. Histologically a thick layer of collagen overlaying loosely arranged connective tissues is found with fibrous and granular septations extending into the underlying myocardial tissue. Myocyte hypertrophy and interstitial edema is frequently found, and intramural coronary arteries may show medial degeneration, the deposition of fibrin, and fibrosis. **Clinical presentation** includes symptoms of heart failure (impaired exercise tolerance, dyspnea on exertion, pulmonary congestion in left-sided or peripheral edema in right-sided endomyocardial fibrosis). The disease may be heralded by acute febrile illness or may be insidious. Causes of death include progressive heart failure, infarction, infection, sudden cardiac death, or complications from cardiac surgery, whereby ascites and atrial fibrillation herald a poor prognosis of these patients. **Diagnosis** is made by history, clinical signs of heart failure or AV valve incompetence, laboratory examination, and echocardiography (enlargement of atria, obliteration of ventricular apices, preserved systolic function) including Doppler ultrasound (signs of diastolic dysfunction, atrioventricular regurgitation). **Treatment** includes drugs for heart failure (diuretics, ACE-inhibitors), control of heart rate in atrial fibrillation, anticoagulation, and surgical endocardectomy with atrioventricular valve replacement that usually results in hemodynamic improvement with reduction in ventricular filling pressures, increased cardiac output, and angiographically or echocardiographically normalized cardiac structure. Operative mortality is quite high with death rates of 15–25%, and may be lower if valve replacement is not necessary. **Prognosis** of the patients is usually poor with a 2-yrs mortality of 35–50%, despite single reports on excellent long-term survival in some individuals (for details see Hare 2012).

CMR Findings

CMR imaging is an excellent tool for detecting grossly thickened ventricular walls, narrowing of ventricular cavities, left and right atrial enlargement, and to assess normal or depressed systolic function and impaired diastolic filling characteristics. Ventricular volumes and atrioventricular

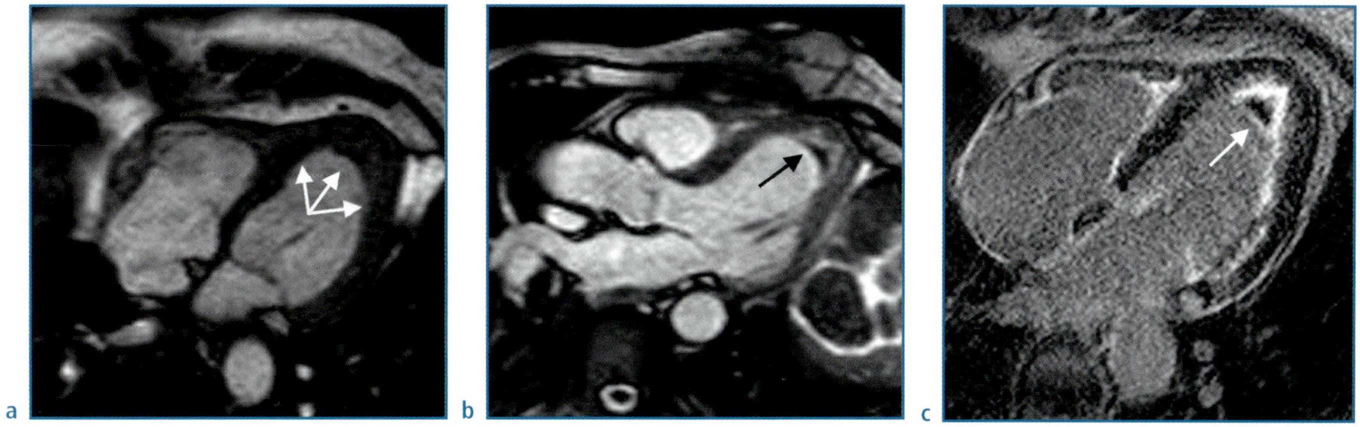

Figure 10-16 Patient with endocarditis fibroplastica (Löffler's endocarditis) with thickened endocardium pronounced in the left ventricular apex on cine-CMR imaging (arrows in (a)). Gadolinium administration revealed apical enhancement in a 3-ch view (b), and 4-ch view (c) indicating endocardial inflammatory activity (courtesy Dr. J. Schwab, Nuremberg).

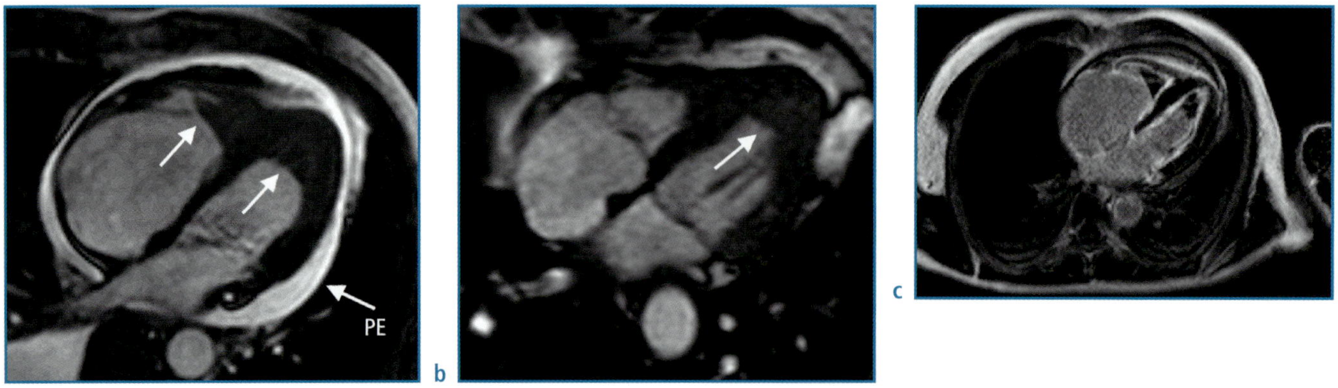

a b c

Figure 10-17 Patient with endomyocardial fibrosis (Davies disease) in 4-ch views with thickened endocardium pronounced in the left (LV) and right ventricular (RV) apex on cine-CMR imaging at diastole (arrows in (a)) and impaired systolic function due to endocardial fibrosis (b). Gadolinium administration revealed moderate enhancement in the apical LV and RV wall regions (c) indicating residual inflammatory activity (courtesy Prof. E. Giannitsis, Heidelberg). PE: pericardial effusion.

regurgitation can be accurately quantified, and contrast-enhanced imaging may be used to differentiate mural thrombus from thickened (inflamed) endomyocardium (Figure 10-16 and Figure 10-17). CMR imaging is the ideal tool to monitor patients with Löffler's endocarditis or endomyocardial fibrosis on drug therapy and after surgical treatment, and to detect progression of the disease.

10.11 Carcinoid Syndrome of the Heart

Etiology and Pathology

The carcinoid syndrome results from the metastasis of carcinoid tumors in the gut, and cardiac involvement usually results from carcinoid of the ileum with regional lymph node and liver metastases that release serotonin and other circulating substances with predominant involvement of the right heart. In only 5–10 % of cases is a left sided involvement observed. The characteristic lesions are fibrous plaques located in areas downstream of the tricuspid and pulmonic valves, the endocardium, and the intima of the venae cavae, pulmonary artery, and coronary sinus. Histologically, plaques appear as a layer of fibrous tissue composed of smooth muscle cells, collagen, and mucopolysaccharides.

Clinical Presentation, Diagnosis and Therapy

Clinical features include marked cutaneous flushing, diarrhea, and bronchoconstriction. A systolic murmur of tricuspid regurgitation is almost always present and systolic or diastolic pulmonic valve murmurs may be found, as well. Chest X-ray may be normal or may show cardiac enlargement and pleural effusion. The ECG may display (unspecific) ST segment and T-wave abnormalities. Echocardiography often reveals enlargement of right atrium and ventricle and tricuspid and pulmonary valve thickening, and sometimes pericardial effusion. These echocardiographic features may be better visualized and quantified by CMR imaging. **Treatment** consists of medical therapy of heart failure using diuretics and ACE-inhibitors. Both somatostatin analogues and chemotherapy may improve symptoms and enhance survival. Balloon valvuloplasty or surgical valve replacement of stenotic valves may relieve symptoms, but operative mortality is high. Prognosis is generally poor, in the series of Pellikka et al. (1993), survival of patients with echocardiographic evidence of carcinoid heart disease in 74 patients was reduced compared with those without cardiac involvement (58 patients, $p = 0.0003$). Thus, cardiac involvement seems to be a significant predictor of a worse outcome in patients with carcinoid syndrome, in addition to disease severity at the time of diagnosis and the presence and extent of myocardial fibrosis.

CMR Findings

The principle features of carcinoid syndrome, such as enlargement of right atrium and ventricle and tricuspid and pulmonary valve thickening, and sometimes pericardial effusion can be precisely visualized, and associated valvular stenoses or incompetences exactly quantified. The effect of therapeutic interventions can also be controlled by CMR imaging, and patient's course safely followed, including the effect of valvuloplasty or surgical intervention. Delayed enhancement imaging may better visualize fibrotic plaques in the typical areas downstream the tricuspid and pulmonary valves and the endocardium. CMR imaging is the ideal tool to monitor patients with carcinoid heart disease on drug therapy and after surgical treatment and to detect regression or progression of the disease.

10.12 Cardiac Involvement in Neuromuscular Diseases (NMD)

Etiology and Pathogenesis

The most relevant neuromuscular diseases with cardiac involvement include Duchenne muscular dystrophy (DMD), Becker-Kiener muscular dystrophy (BKMD), myotonic dystrophies (MD), Emery-Dreifuss muscular dystrophy (EDMD), and Friedreich ataxia. Both Duchenne and Becker muscular dystrophy are X-linked recessive disorders with abnormalities in the dystrophin gene. Myotonic dystrophies are autosomal dominant inherited disorders with two different types 1 and 2. Emery-Dreifuss muscular dystrophy is an X-linked recessive inherited disorder with abnormalities of the STA gene coding for emerin, whose lack is responsible for the phenotype. Friedreich ataxia is an autosomal recessive spinocerebellar degenerative disease with the gene mutation affecting encoding of frataxin leading to mitochondrial dysfunction, poor cellular response to oxidative stress, and apoptosis.

Clinical Presentation, Diagnosis and Therapy

Duchenne Muscular Dystrophy (DMD)

This disease is the most common inherited NMD with an incidence of 30 per 100,000 living male births. Patients typically become **symptomatic** before age 5 with skeletal muscle weakness that progresses rapidly. The majority of DMD patients develop a cardiomyopathy, pre-clinical involvement is present in about 25% of patients by age 6, commonly with clinically apparent cardiomyopathy by age 10. DMD is a progressive disorder with mortality from respiratory or cardiac cause. Clinically patients show **ECG** (tall R-waves and increased R/S amplitude in V1 with deep narrow Q-waves in left precordial leads, persistent sinus tachycardia, atrial arrhythmias including AF or atrial flutter, ventricular ectopic beats) **and echocardiographic abnormalities** (regional wall motion abnormalities in the posterobasal and posterolateral wall, dilated cardiac chambers, systolic and diastolic dysfunction). Steroids and steroid derivatives are effective in delaying skeletal muscle progression, patients with systolic dysfunction should receive classical **heart failure therapy** (ACE-inhibitors, diuretics, β-blockers). Death from cardiac cause is equally distributed to heart failure or sudden death.

Becker Muscular Dystrophy (BKMD)

This disease is less common as DMD with 3 per 100,000 live male births and has a more variable presentation of skeletal muscle weakness. Cardiac involvement is independent of the severity of skeletal muscle involvement, and more than 50% of patients with subclinical or benign skeletal muscle disease may show cardiomyopathy (Figure 10-18) that initially may involve the right ventricle alone. Patients may **present** with dyspnea on exertion, and with mitral regurgitation due to annular dilatation. In the ECG similar alterations are present as in DMD including frequently incomplete right bundle branch block, and occasionally distal conduction system disease with complete heart block and bundle branch re-entrant ventricular tachycardias. Systolic and diastolic dysfunction can be assessed by echocardiography and Doppler ultrasound. **Treatment** of established heart failure includes ACE-inhibitors, diuretics, and β-blockers that may improve LV function. In selected cases heart transplantation may be the ultimate therapeutic option.

Myotonic Dystrophies (MD)

These diseases are the most common inherited neuromuscular disorders in patients presenting as adults. Type 1 with gene mutation on chromosome 19q13.3 is significantly more common (global incidence has been estimated to be 1 in 8,000) than type 2 with gene mutation on chromosome 3q21, and the age of onset of symptoms and diagnosis averages 20–25 yrs. Common early **manifestations** are weakness in the muscles of the face, neck, and distal extremities. Cardiac involvement includes degeneration (fibrosis and fatty infiltration) of the specialized conduction system (sinus node, atrioventricular node, His-Purkinje system), and the working atrial and ventricular myocardium, but the process rarely progresses to symptomatic dilated cardiomyopathy. Patients with type 1 present with ECG abnormalities (1st degree AV block in 42%, right bundle branch block in 3%, left bundle branch block in 4%, and unspecific intraventricular conduction delay in 12%) and a wide variety of arrhythmias (atrial flutter or fibrillation, and bundle branch re-entrant ventricular tachycardias). Echocardiography may reveal left atrial dilatation, mild LV hypertrophy, LV systolic and diastolic dysfunction, regional wall motion abnormalities, and mitral valve prolapse. The incidence of sudden death in MD patients type 1 is primarily considered to be the result of fatal arrhythmias or complete AV block and lack of appropriate escape rhythm. **Treatment** includes pacemaker implantation in case of complete AV block or implantation of an ICD in patients with recurrent ventricular tachycardias. Bundle branch re-entrant tachycardias can be abolished by catheter ablation. The course of patients with MD is variable, death may be the result of respiratory dysfunction or sudden death.

Emery-Dreifuss Muscular Dystrophy (EDMD)

EDMD is a rare familial disorder characterized by the triad of early contractures of the elbow, Achilles tendon and

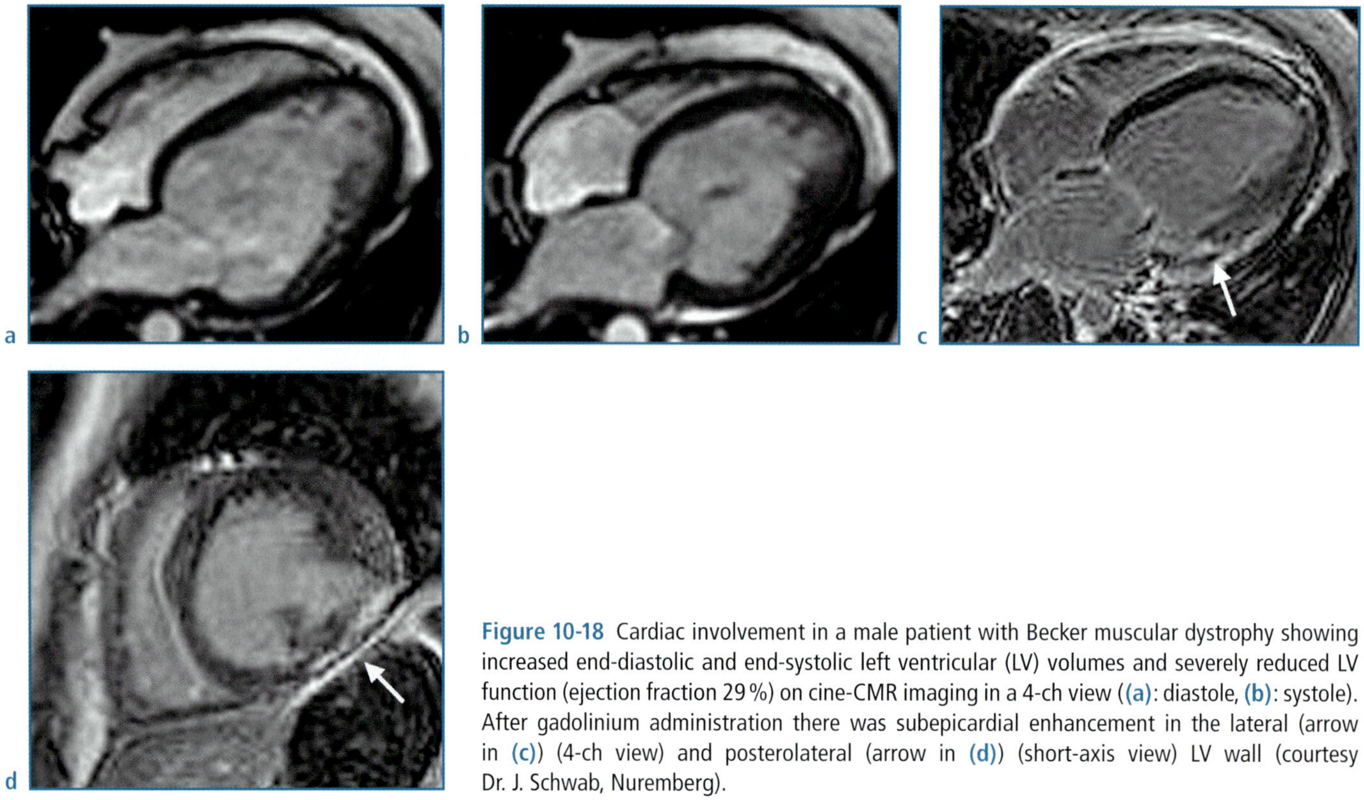

Figure 10-18 Cardiac involvement in a male patient with Becker muscular dystrophy showing increased end-diastolic and end-systolic left ventricular (LV) volumes and severely reduced LV function (ejection fraction 29 %) on cine-CMR imaging in a 4-ch view ((a): diastole, (b): systole). After gadolinium administration there was subepicardial enhancement in the lateral (arrow in (c)) (4-ch view) and posterolateral (arrow in (d)) (short-axis view) LV wall (courtesy Dr. J. Schwab, Nuremberg).

posterior cervical muscles, of slowly progressing muscle weakness and atrophy (primarily in humeroscapular muscles), and of cardiac involvement. Patients present with cardiac impulse formation (permanent atrial standstill, atrial flutter or fibrillation) and conduction disease (atrioventricular and intraventricular block), and dilated cardiomyopathy (Figure 10-19) with dyspnea on exertion and symptoms of heart failure that requires adequate pharmacological therapy. Sudden death in patients with dilated cardiomyopathy is common in those with rapid progression to the extent that heart transplantation is required. Because abnormalities of impulse generation or conduction are present in virtually all patients by age 35–40 yrs, permanent pacing is recommended. Prophylactic implantation of an ICD has been advocated in patients with disorders caused by lamins A and C mutations, once pacing is being considered. In selected cases patients may benefit from heart transplantation. The prognosis is generally poor.

Friedreich Ataxia

Friedreich ataxia usually manifests around puberty with progressive loss of neuromuscular function later on. Its prevalence is 1 : 50,000. It is commonly associated with a concentric hypertrophic cardiomyopathy, sometimes with a LVOT gradient like in HOCM. The dilated cardiomyopathy appears to occur as a progressive transition from HCM in later stages. Up to 90 % of neurologically manifest patients have ECG (signs of LV hypertrophy, T-wave inversion, ventricular arrhythmias) and echocardiographic abnormalities (LV hypertrophy, systolic and diastolic dysfunction). Idebenone, a free-radical scavenger may be a treatment option to reduce myocardial/septal hypertrophy and to improve LV systolic dysfunction. The prognosis is poor with rapid progression to end-stage congestive heart failure.

CMR Findings

CMR imaging is an excellent technique for visualizing cardiac structure, to exactly measure atrial and ventricular volumes and muscle mass, for quantifying the degree of systolic and diastolic as well as valvular dysfunction, and for detecting damage or scar formation within the ventricular myocardium in all types of neuromuscular diseases described above. Myocardial fibrosis has been found by LGE in 7 of 19 patients with Duchenne or Becker muscular dystrophy in the series of Silva et al. (2007), where the lateral wall was the most commonly involved segment. Patients with myocardial fibrosis had lower EF than those without, and correlation between segmental fibrosis and dysfunction was moderate. Yilmaz et al. (2008) investigated 15 male patients with BMD, in whom abnormal echocardiographic results were found in 8 of 15, but CMR imaging revealed abnormal findings in 12 of 15 patients. Myocardial damage assessed by LGE imaging

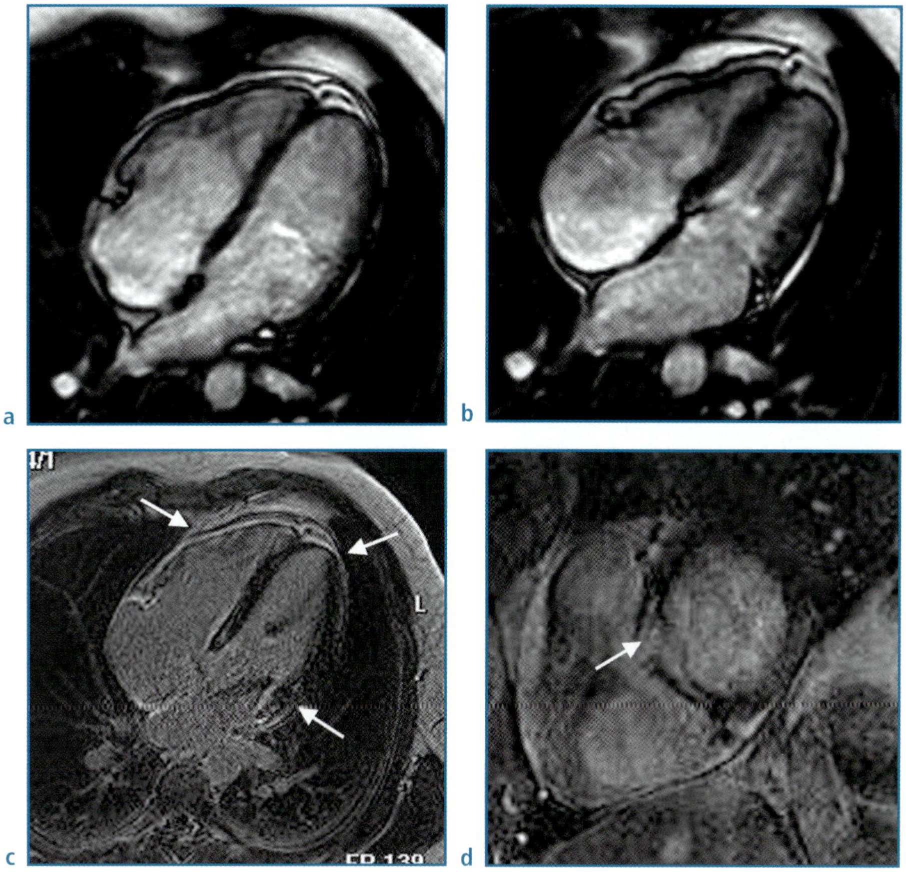

Figure 10-19 Cardiac involvement in a male patient with Emery-Dreifuss muscular dystrophy showing increased end-diastolic and end-systolic left ventricular (LV) volumes and reduced LV function (ejection fraction 38%) on cine-CMR imaging in a 4-ch view ((a): diastole, (b): systole). After gadolinium administration there was subepicardial enhancement in the apical and basal-lateral (arrows in (c)) (4-ch view) and subepicardial to transmural enhancement in the septal wall (arrow in (d)) (short-axis view) (courtesy Dr. J. Schwab, Nuremberg).

was detected in 11 of 15 patients (73%) with a damage volume of 0–38% of LVMM (median 13%), and subepicardial LGE was most commonly found in the inferolateral wall of the left ventricle. Only 4 of 10 patients in need of medical heart failure therapy were in fact treated. The conclusion was that cardiac involvement in BMD is under diagnosed by echocardiography resulting in under treatment of heart failure, and the severity of cardiac involvement is best characterized by state-of-the-art CMR imaging methods.

10.13 Drug Induced Cardiomyopathy

Prevalence and Etiology

Among the drugs that may induce dilated cardiomyopathy and heart failure are **antimitotic drugs** (anthracyclins like adriamycin/doxorubicine, daunorubicin, cyclophosphamide), **antiparasitic drugs** (emetine, dehydroemetine, chloroquine), and **psychotropic drugs** (tricyclic antidepressants, cocaine). The incidence of the different forms of drug-induced cardiomyopathy is unclear. In a large cohort of 19,479 women with anthracycline-containing chemotherapy for breast cancer, the excess cumulative 10-yrs incidence was 4.7% compared to patients without chemotherapy. After adjusting for patients and tumor characteristics patients receiving anthracyclines were 25% more likely to have congestive heart failure than those without chemotherapy (Du 2009). The incidence of cardiac damage by adriamycin occurs acutely with a latency period of several months.

Clinical Presentation

Patients develop a biventricular dilated cardiomyopathy and severe heart failure that often responds poorly to conventional heart failure treatment. The cumulative dose of adriamycin should not exceed 250 mg/m^2. Daunomycin is also cardiotoxic, toxic symptoms occur late, and adults are more vulnerable than children. The antiparasitic drugs emetine and dehydroemetine are used for treatment of amebiasis and schistosomiasis, and they are cardiotoxic with sudden occurrence of global heart failure with a poor prognosis. Chloroquine rarely produces cardiotoxic effects, but may frequently induce ECG alterations. Tricyclic antidepressants (e.g. imipramine, amitryptiline) may also induce tachycardia, orthostatic hypotension, atrioventricular block, and depression of ventricular function. The effect of cocaine

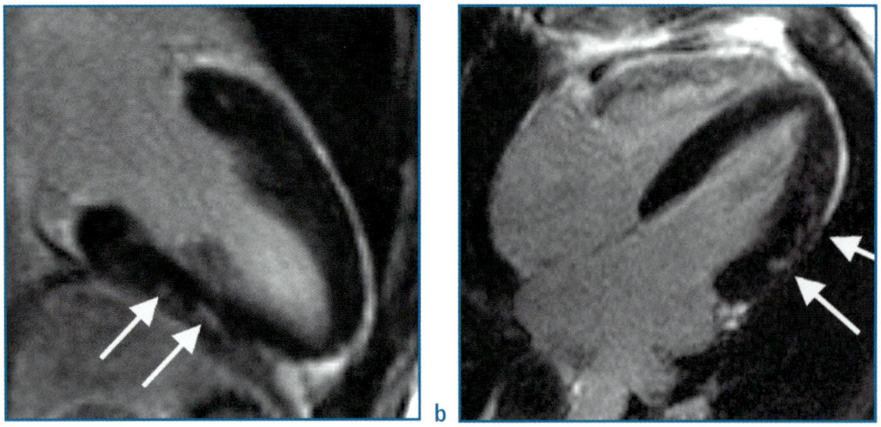

a b

Figure 10-20 41-yrs-old female patient with normal coronary arteries and unremarkable family history. 7 yrs following anthracyclin therapy for breast cancer patient developed the clinical phenotype of dilated cardiomyopathy; in addition to slight left ventricular (LV) dysfunction gadolinium administration revealed intramural enhancement in the inferior (arrows in (a)) (2-ch view) and subepicardial enhancement in the lateral LV wall (arrows in (b)) (4-ch view) (courtesy Prof. J. Schulz-Menger, Berlin).

includes suppression of the fast Na channel with prolongation of both conduction and refractory period, and blockade of the reuptake of catecholamines that results in tachycardia, hypertension, and mydriasis. Coronary vasoconstriction may lead to myocardial infarction, and in chronic abuse an accelerated atherosclerosis may be observed, as well as sudden death, acute myocardial infarction, acute reversible myocarditis, rhabdomyolysis, hypertensive crisis, stroke, aortic dissection, or pneumopericardium.

CMR Findings

There are no specific CMR features in drug induced cardiomyopathies, but dilated ventricles and impaired systolic and diastolic function as well as relative valve insufficiencies can be exactly documented by CMR. In addition, in a variable number of patients LGE with atypical location (midwall, subepicardial) may be found indicating localized damage of the myocardium (Figure 10-20), as described by Fallah-Rad et al. (2008) for all 10 patients with trastuzumab-induced cardiomyopathy out of 160 breast cancer patients. In this series at the time of diagnosis mean LV ejection fraction was 29 ± 4%, and linear subepicardial LGE was found predominantly in the lateral portion of the LV. In individual cases absence of LGE may herald a good prognosis with recovery of myocardial function after termination of the drug, as e.g. described for methamphetamine-induced cardiomyopathy (Lopez 2009). CMR imaging may be extremely useful for earlier detection of slight ongoing alterations of structure and function of the heart that enables early heart failure treatment and timely termination of drug therapy.

10.14 Post-Partum Cardiomyopathy/ Peri-Partum Cardiomyopathy (PPCM)

Prevalence, Etiology and Pathogenesis

Peri-partum cardiomyopathy is defined as a form of dilated cardiomyopathy that presents with signs of heart failure in the last month of pregnancy or within 5 mths of delivery. PPCM is relatively rare and its prevalence is estimated to occur in 1 in every 2,300 live births with a current maternal death rate of 0–9%. The etiology of PPCM is poorly understood, causes and factors discussed include myocarditis, cardiotropic viral infections, chimerism with immune response from fetal cells taken up by the mother, apoptosis of cardiac myocytes, prolonged tocolysis, and an abnormal hemodynamic response of the pregnant mother. In mice lacking the transcription factor STAT3 in cardiac muscle, Hilfiker et al. (2007a) were recently able to show that a lack of antioxidant enzymes, e.g. MnSOD, leads to increased free radical production in the heart with higher oxidative stress and cleavage of prolactin into a proapoptotic and antiangiogenetic 16-kDa subform. This 16-kDa prolactin destroys the endothelium and damages in particular the microcirculation in the myocardium, reducing the metabolic activity of cardiac myocytes with significantly reduced pump function and clinical manifestations of PPCM in the mouse model. There is evidence that this mechanism is also active in human PPCM patients, since increased serum levels of oxLDL (indicator of oxidative stress), of cathepsin D (prolactin cleaving enzyme), and of 16-kDa prolactin have been found in sera of PPCM patients (Hilfiker-Kleiner 2007a). In addition, treatment with bromocriptine that blocks prolactin release has shown favourable results, which further underlines the significance of the prolactin cleavage concept for the development of PPCM.

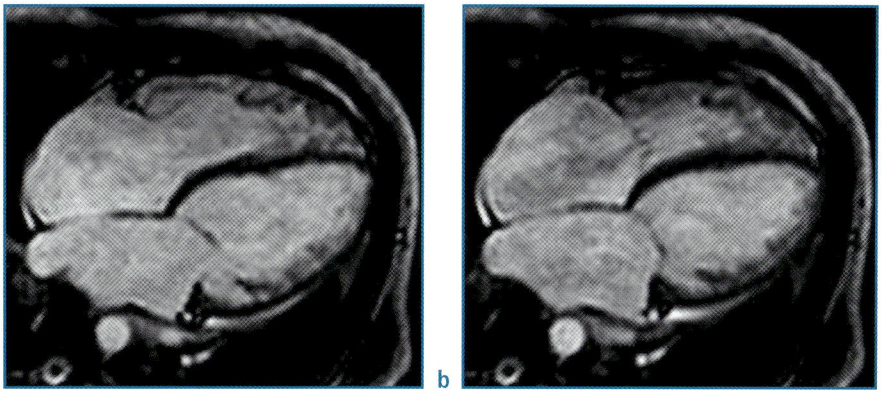

Figure 10-21 39-yrs-old female patient with Caesarian section within the 37th week of pregnancy presenting with heart failure and severely reduced right (RV) and left ventricular (LV) function. Cine-CMR imaging in a 4-ch view revealed increased end-diastolic and end-systolic LV volumes and a severely reduced LV ejection fraction of 26% ((a): diastole, (b): systole). Note the enlarged RV and LV chambers and the severely reduced contractile function of both the right and left ventricle (courtesy Dr. J. Schwab, Nuremberg).

Clinical Presentation, Diagnosis and Therapy

PPCM presents with rapid onset of systolic dysfunction with LV ejection fraction of < 45% and LA and LV enlargement. Apparently healthy women can develop sufficiently severe cardiac failure to require heart transplantation, but approximately 80% of symptomatic patients recover, below 30% of women recover completely with normalization of LV chamber size and function, but in 9–23% terminal heart failure persists. Diagnosis is often made late in the course of disease, since clinical presentation is very variable. The first **symptoms** are dyspnea and cough that may be misinterpreted as pneumonia, and further symptoms or signs like lassitude and exhaustion, cardiac arrhythmias, leg edema, stroke, or peripheral emboli are not always associated with PPCM, but are considered to be consequences of postpartum readjustment. **Diagnosis** is made by careful history, clinical examination (rales, systolic murmur particularly by new-onset of mitral regurgitation), chest X-ray (cardiomegaly, pulmonary congestion), and echocardiography (enlarged atria and ventricles, systolic and sometimes diastolic dysfunction, relative mitral incompetence). CMR imaging may be very helpful in assessing altered structure and ventricular dysfunction, together with the detection of further signs of heart failure such as pleural effusion. **Treatment** consists of classical heart failure medication (ACE-inhibitors, β-blockers, diuretics, aldosterone blockers), and in cases of severe LV dysfunction without/with atrial fibrillation of anticoagulation. Based on recent research results, Hilfiker-Kleiner et al. (2007b) developed a new treatment concept by blocking prolactin release with the dopamine D2 receptor agonist bromocriptine with good clinical results: 6 patients with bromocriptine survived, while 3 of 6 patients without bromocriptine died, and NYHA class 3 mths postpartum was 1 ± 0 in the verum group, but 2.3 ± 0.6 in the control group (Hilfiker-Kleiner 2008). Further prospective randomized studies have to be conducted to confirm this very attractive concept.

CMR Findings

There are no specific CMR features in women with PPVM, but dilated atria and ventricles and impaired systolic and diastolic function as well as relative valve insufficiencies can be exactly documented by CMR (Figure 10-21). In addition, in a variable number of patients LGE with atypical location (midwall, subepicardial) may be found indicating localized damage of the myocardium (Marmursztejn 2009). Whether patients with LGE have a worse prognosis with persistence of LV dysfunction, compared to those without LGE is unknown at present. CMR imaging is also valuable to detect intraventricular or intraatrial (left atrial appendage) thrombi enabling the timely initiation of anticoagulation to prevent arterial emboli. CMR imaging is the ideal tool to follow PPCM patients on heart failure and bromocriptine treatment, and to assess possible improvements of functional status or persistence of cardiac dysfunction.

10.15 Conclusions and Future Perspectives

In patients with suspected cardiomyopathies, taking history and clinical examination together with chest X-ray may often give only hints to the underlying disease, and even echocardiography may fail to exactly assess the type of cardiomyopathy and disease severity because of limited acoustic window, nearfield effect particularly of the LV apex etc. At present CMR imaging is probably the best technique to study patients with cardiomyopathies for demonstrating abnormal structure and function, severity of ventricular systolic and diastolic dysfunction, valvular dysfunction, type and localization of ventricular hypertrophy, and localized damage/fibrosis of ventricular myocardium using the DE-CMR technique. CMR imaging is extremely valuable to assess hypertrophy of the ventricular myocardium that may be the result of a variety of disorders (hypertension, HCM, myocardial storage diseases), and a combination of cine-CMR, SE-MRI, and CE-MRI may be extremely helpful in the differential diagnosis. CMR imaging is also very supportive in the diagnosis of DCM, HCM, RCM, and is the method of choice to confirm the diagnosis of ARVD and non-compaction. The LGE phenomenon is also very useful to demonstrate inflammation in endocardial diseases (Löffler's endocarditis, Davies disease) and myocardial damage in neuromuscular disorders, drug induced cardiomyopathies, and peri-partum cardiomyopthy. In addition, some CMR features seem to be independent prognostic factors, e.g. the degree of hypertrophy or the presence of LGE in the myocardium. In our experience, CMR imaging should be introduced very early in the diagnostic algorithm in patients with suspected cardiomyopathies to save time and to secure the physician and cardiologist in the final diagnosis, which is extremely important for treatment and prognosis of these patients. In the future new concepts of molecular imaging with dedicated contrast molecules that are targeting specific disease mechanisms (e.g. inflammatory targets, fibrosis targets etc.), may further aid in unraveling abnormalities in pathogenesis and to refine the diagnosis of cardiomyopathies.

References

Adabag AS, Maron BJ, Appelbaum E et al. Occurrence and frequency of arrhythmias in hypertrophic cardiomyopathy in relation to delayed enhancement on cardiovascular magnetic resonance. J Am Coll Cardiol 2008; 51: 1369–74.

Asomull RG, Prasad SK, Lyne J et al. Cardiovascular magnetic resonance, fibrosis, and prognosis in dilated cardiomyopathy. J Am Coll Cardiol 2006, 48: 1977.

Bruder O, Wagner A, Jensen CJ et al. Myocardial scar visualized by cardiovascular magnetic resonance imaging predicts major adverse events in patients with hypertrophic cardiomyopathy. J Am Coll Cardiol 2010; 56 (11): 875–87.

Cheung SCW, Chan CWS. Insights of prognostication of Davies disease: what could we learn from serial magnetic resonance imaging studies? Int J Cardiol 2008. doi: 10.1016/j.ijcard.2008.11.181.

Choi DS, Ha YW, Choi B et al. Extent of gadolinium enhancement in cardiovascular magnetic resonance and its relation with left ventricular diastolic function in patients with hypertrophic cardiomyopathy. Circ J 2008; 72: 1449–53.

Doughan AR, Williams BR. Cardiac Sarcoidosis. Heart 2006; 92: 282–8.

Du XL, Xia R, Liu CC et al. Cardiac toxicity associated with anthracycline-containing chemotherapy in older women with breast cancer. Cancer 2009; 115 (24): 5849–51.

Elliott P, Andersson B, Arbustini E et al. Classification of the cardiomyopathies: a position statement from the European Society of Cardiology Working Group on Myocardial and Pericardial Diseases. Eur Heart J 2008; 29: 270–6.

Eriksson MJ, Sonnenberg B, Woo A et al. Long-term outcome in patients with apical hypertrophic cardiomyopathy. J Am Coll Cardiol 2002; 39 (4): 638–45.

Fallah-Rad N, Lytwyn M, Fang T et al. Delayed contrast enhancement cardiac magnetic resonance imaging in trastuzumab induced cardiomyopathy. J Cardiovasc Magn Reson 2008. doi: 10.1186/1532-429X-10-5.

Fazio G, Novo G, Dángelo L et al. Letter to the editor: Magnetic resonance in isolated noncompaction of the ventricular myocardium. Int J Cardiol 2008. doi: 10.1016/j.ijcard.2008.11.080.

Felker GM, Thompson RE, Hare JM et al. Underlying causes and long-term survival in patients with initially unexplained cardiomyopathy. N Engl J Med 2000; 342: 1077–84.

Francone M, Dymarkowski S, Kalantzi M et al. Assessment of ventricular coupling with real-time cine-MRI and its value to differentiate constrictive pericarditis from restrictive cardiomyopathy. Eur Radiol 2006; 16: 944–51.

Ghio S, Revera M, Mori F et al. Regional abnormalities of myocardial deformation in patients with hypertrophic cardiomyopathy: correlation with delayed enhancement in cardiac magnetic resonance. Eur J Heart Fail 2009; 11: 952–7.

Haghi D, Fluechter S, Suselbeck T et al. Cardiovascular magnetic resonance findings in typical versus atypical forms of the acute apical ballooning syndrome (Tako-Tsubo cardiomyopathy). Int J Cardiol 2007; 120: 205–11.

Hanckock EW. Cardiomyopathy: Differential diagnosis of restrictive cardiomyopathy and constrictive pericarditis. Heart 2001; 86: 343–9.

Hare JM. The dilated, restrictive, and infiltrative cardiomyopathies. In: Bonow RO, Mann DL, Zipes DP, Libby P (eds.). Braunwald's Heart Disease. A Textbook of Cardiovascular Medicine. Elsevier Saunders 2012; 1561–81.

He T, Kirk P, Firmin DN et al. Multi-center transferability of a breath-hold T2 technique for myocardial iron assessment. J Cardiovasc Magn Reson 2008. doi: 10.1186/1532-429X-10-11.

Hilfiker-Kleiner D, Kaminski K, Podewski E et al. A cathepsin D-cleaved 16 kDa form of prolactin mediates post-partum cardiomyopathy. Cell 2007a; 128: 589–600.

Hilfiker-Kleiner D, Meyer GP, Schieffer E et al. Recovery from postpartum cardiomyopathy in 2 patients by blocking prolactin release with bromocriptine. J Am Coll Cardiol 2007b; 50: 2354–5.

Hilfiker-Kleiner D, Schieffer E, Meyer GP et al. Review: Postpartum cardiomyopathy. Dtsch Arztebl Int 2008; 105: 751–6.

Hombach V, Merkle N, Kestler HA et al. Characterization of patients with acute chest pain using cardiac magnetic resonance imaging. Clin Res Cardiol 2008; 97: 760–7.

Hombach V, Merkle N, Torzewski J et al. Electrocardiographic and cardiac magnetic resonance imaging parameters as predictors of a worse outcome in patients with idiopathic dilated cardiomyopathy. Eur Heart J 2009; 30: 2011–8.

Hulot JS, Jouven X, Empana JP et al. Natural history and risk stratification of arrhythmogenic right ventricular dysplasia/cardiomyopathy. Circulation 2004; 110: 1879–84.

Ichida F, Tsubata S, Bowles C et al. Novel gene mutations in patients with left ventricular noncompaction or Barth syndrome. Circulation 2001, 103: 1256–63.

Jain A, Tandri H, Calkins H, Bluemke DA. Role of cardiovascular magnetic resonance imaging in arrhythmogenic right ventricular dysplasia. J Cardiovasc Magn Reson 2008; 10: 32.
Jerosch-Herold M, Sheridan DC, Kushner JD et al. Cardiac magnetic resonance imaging of myocardial contrast uptake and blood flow in patients affected with idiopathic or familial dilated cardiomyopathy. Am J Physiol Heart Circ Physiol 2008; 295: H1234–42.
Joshi SB, Chao T, Herzka DA et al. Cardiovascular magnetic resonance T2 signal abnormalities in left ventricular ballooning syndrome. Int J Cardiovasc Imaging 2010; 26: 227–32.
Kawada M, Sakuma H, Yamakado T et al. Hypertropic cardiomyopathy: MR measurement of coronary blood flow and vasodilator flow reserve in patients and healthy subjects. Radiology 1999; 21: 129–35.
Kim YJ, Choi BW, Hur J et al. Delayed enhancement in hypertrophic cardiomyopathy: comparison with myocardial tagging MRI. J Magn Reson Imag 2008; 27: 1054–60.
Koeth O, Mark B, Kilkowski A et al. Clinical, angiographic and cardiovascular magnetic resonance findings in consecutive patients with Tako-Tsubo cardiomyopathy. Clin Res Cardiol 2008; 97: 623–7.
Konstam MA. Progress in heart failure management? Lessons from the real world. Circulation 2000; 102: 1076.
Lemola K, Brunckhorst C, Helfenstein U et al. Predictors of adverse outcome in patients with arrhythmogenic right ventricular dysplasia/cardiomyopathy: long term experience of a tertiary care centre. Heart 2005; 91: 1167–72.
Leonardi S, Raineri C, De Ferrari GM et al. Usefulness of cardiac magnetic resonance in assessing the risk of ventricular arrhythmias and sudden death in patients with hypertrophic cardiomyopathy. Eur Heart J 2009. doi: 10.1093/eurheartj/ehp152.
Lopez JE, Yeao K, Caputo G et al. Recovery of methamphetamine associated cardiomyopathy predicted by late gadolinium-enhanced cardiovascular magnetic resonance. J Cardiovasc Magn Reson 2009; 11: 46.
Maceira AM, Joshi J, Prasad SK et al. Cardiovascular magnetic resonance in cardiac amyloidosis. Circulation 2005; 111: 186–93.
Maceira AM, Prasad SK, Hawkins PN et al. Cardiac magnetic resonance and prognosis in cardiac amyloidosis. J Cardiovasc Magn Reson 2008; 10: 54.
Manins V, Habersberger J, Pfluger H, Taylor AJ. Cardiac magnetic resonance imaging in the evaluation of cardiac sarcoidosis: an Australian single-centre experience. Int Med J 2009; 39: 77–82.
Marmursztejn J, Vignaux O, Goffinet F et al. Delayed-enhanced cardiac magnetic resonance imaging features in paripartum cardiomyopathy. Int J Cardiol 2009; 137: 63–4.
Maron BJ. Hypertrophic cardiomyopathy: a systematic review. JAMA 2002; 287: 1308–20.
Maron BJ, McKenna WJ, Danielson GK at al. ACC/ESC Clinical expert consensus document of hypertrophic cardiomyopathy. A report of the ACC task force on clinical expert consensus documents and the ESC committee for practice guidelines committee to develop as an expert consensus document on hypertrophic cardiomyopathy. J Am Coll Cardiol 2003; 42: 1687–713.
Maron MS, Finley JJ, Bos M et al. Prevalence, clinical significance, and natural history of left ventricular apical aneurysms in hypertrophic cardiomyopathy. Circulation 2008; 118: 1541–9.
Mc Crohon JA, Moon JCC, Prasad SK et al. Differentiation of heart failure related to dilated cardiomyopathy and coronary artery disease using gadolinium-enhanced cardiovascular magnetic resonance. Circulation 2003; 108: 54–9.
Mc Kenna WJ, Thiene G, Nava A et al. Diagnosis of arrhythmogenic right ventricular dysplasia/cardiomyopathy. Br Heart J 1994, 71: 215–8.
Meloni A, Pepe A, Positano V et al. Influence of myocardial fibrosis and blood oxygenation on heart T2* values in thalassemia patients. J Magn Reson Imag 2009; 29: 832–7.
Migrino RQ, Christenson R, Szabo A et al. Prognostic implication of late gadolinium enhancement on cardiac MRI in light chain (AL) amyloidosis on long term follow-up. MBC Medical Physics 2009; 9: 5.
Mitchell JH, Hadden TB, Wilson JM et al. Clinical features and usefulness of cardiac magnetic resonance imaging in assessing myocardial viability and prognosis in Tako-Tsubo cardiomyopathy (transient left ventricular apical ballooning syndrome). Am J Cardiol 2007; 100: 296–301.
Moon JCC, McKenna WJ, McCorhon JA et al. Toward clinical risk assessment in hypertrophic cardiomyopathy with gadolinium cardiocvascular magnetic resonance. J Am Coll Cardiol 2003; 41: 1561–7.
Moon JCC, Reed E, Sheppard MN et al. The histologic basis of late gadolinium enhancement cardiovascular magnetic resonance in hypertrophic cardiomyopathy. J Am Coll Cardiol 2004; 43: 2260–4.
Nazarian S, Bluemke DA, Lardo AC et al. Magnetic resonance assessment of the substrate for inducible ventricular tachycardia in non-ischemic cardiomyopathy. Circulation 2005; 112: 2821–5.
Nazarian S, Lima JAC. Editorial Comment: Cardiovascular magnetic resonance for risk stratification of arrhythmia in hypertrophic cardiomyopathy. J Am Coll Cardiol 2008; 51: 1375–6.
Oechslin EN, Attenhofer Jost CH, Rojas JR et al. Long-term follow-up of 34 adults with isolated left ventricular noncompaction: a distinct cardiomyopathy with poor prognosis. J Am Coll Cardiol 2000; 36: 493–500.
Papavassiliu T, Germans T, Flüchter S et al. CMR findings in patients with hypertrophic cardiomyopathy and atrial fibrillation. J Cardiovasc Magn Reson 2009; 11: 34.
Patel MR, Cawley PJ, Heitner JF et al. Detection of myocardial damage in patients with sarcoidosis. Circulation 2009; 120: 1969–77.
Pellikka PA, Khandheria BK, Seward JB et al. Carcinoid heart disease. Clinical and echocardiographic spectrum in 74 patients. Circulation 1993; 87: 1188–96.
Pepe A, Positano V, Capra M et al. Myocardial scarring by delayed enhancement cardiovascular magnetic resonance in thalassemia major. Heart 2009; 95: 1688–93.
Perugini E, Rapezzi C, Piva T et al. Non-invasive evaluation of the myocardial substrate of cardiac amyloidosis by gadolinium cardiac magnetic resonance. Heart 2005; 92: 343–9.
Petersen SE, Selvanayagam JB, Wiesmann F et al. Left ventricular non-compaction: insights from cardiovascular magnetic resonance imaging. J Am Coll Cardiol 2005; 46: 101–5.
Rickers C, Maron B, Jerosch-Herold M et al. Significance of myocardial ischemia in hypertrophic cardiomyopathy: relation of regional perfusion abnormalities to left ventricular hypertrophy

assessed by magnetic resonance imaging. Circulation 2002; 106: II–652 (abstr.).
Rickers C, Wilke NM, Jerosch-Herold M et al. Utility of cardiac magnetic resonance imaging in the diagnosis of hypertrophic cardiomyopathy. Circulation 2005; 112 (6): 855–61.
Ritter M, Oechslin E, Sutsch G et al. Isolated noncompaction of the myocardium in adults. Mayo Clin Proc 1997; 72: 26–31.
Roberts WC, Siegel RJ, McManus BM. Idiopathic dilated cardiomyopathy: analysis of 152 necropsy patients. Am J Cardiol 1987; 60: 1340–55.
Satoh H, Matoh F, Shiraki K et al. Delayed enhancement on cardiac magnetic resonance and clinical, morphological, and electrocardiographical features in hypertrophic cardiomyopathy. J Cardiac Fail 2009; 15: 419–27.
Schulz-Menger J, Abdel-Aty H, Bujahn A et al. Left ventricular outflow tract planimetry by cardiovascular magnetic resonance differentiates obstructive from non-obstructive hypertrophic cardiomyopathy. J Cardiovasc Magn Reson 2006; 8: 741–6.
Schulz-Menger J, Strohm O, Waigand J et al. The value of magnetic resonance imaging of the left ventricular outflow tract in patients with hypertrophic obstructive cardiomyopathy after septal artery embolization. Circulation 2000; 18: 1764–6.
Sen-Chowdrhy S, Prasad SK, Syrris P et al. Cardiovascular magnetic resonance in arrhythmogenic right ventricular cardiomyopathy revisited. Comparison with task force criteria and genotype. J Am Coll Cardiol 2006; 48: 2132–40.
Silva MC, Meira ZMA, Giannetti JG et al. Myocardial delayed enhancement by magnetic resonance imaging in patients with muscular dystrophy. J Am Coll Cardiol 2007; 49: 1874–9.
Silverman KJ, Hutchins GM, Bulkley BH. Cardiac sarcoid: a clinicopathologic study of 84 unselected patients with systemic sarcoidosis. Circulation 1978; 58: 1204–11.
Smedema JP, Snoep G, van Kroonenburgh MPG et al. Evaluation of the accuracy of gadolinium-enhanced cardiovascular magnetic resonance in the diagnosis of cardiac sarcoidosis. J Am Coll Cardiol 2005; 45: 1683–90.
Soriano CJ, Ridocci F, Estornell J et al. Late gadolinium-enhanced cardiovascular magnetic resonance identifies patients with standardized definition of ischemic cardiomyopathy: A single center experience. Int J Cardiol 2007; 116: 167–73.
Sparrow P, Amirabadi A, Sussman M et al. Quantitative assessment of myocardial T2 relaxation times in cardiac amyloidosis. J Magn Reson Imag 2009; 30: 942–6.
Spirito P, Bellone P, Harris KM et al. Magnitude of left ventricular hypertrophy predicts the risk of sudden death in hypertrophic cardiomyopathy. N Engl J Med 2000; 342: 1778–85.
Sun JP, James KB, Yang XS et al. Comparison of mortality rates and progression of left ventricular dysfunction in patients with idiopathic dilated cardiomyopathy and dilated versus nondilated right ventricular cavities. Am J Cardiol 1997; 80: 1583.
Suzuki J, Caputo GR, Masui T et al. Assessment of right ventricular diastolic and systolic function in patients with dilated cardiomyopathy using cine-magnetic resonance imaging. Am Heart J 1991; 122: 1035–40.
Syed IS, Prasad A, Oh JK et al. Apical ballooning syndrome or aborted acute myocardial infarction? Insights from cardiovascular magnetic resonance imaging. Int J Cardiovasc Imaging 2008; 24: 875–82.
Tandri H, Bomma C, Calkins H, Bluemke DA. Magnetic resonance and computer tomography imaging of arrhythmogenic right ventricular dysplasia. J Magn Reson Imaging 2004; 19: 848–58.
Tandri H, Castillo E, Ferrari VA et al. Magnetic resonance imaging of arrhythmogenic right ventricular dysplasia: sensitivity, specificity, and observer variability of fat detection versus functional analysis of the right ventricle. J Am Coll Cardiol 2006; 48: 2277–84.
Tandri H, Saranathan M, Rodriguez EZ et al. Non-invasive detection of myocardial fibrosis in arrhythmogenic right ventricular cardiomyopathy using delayed-enhancement magnetic resonance imaging. J Am Coll Cardiol 2005; 45: 98–103.
Tsukihashi K, Ueshima K, Uchida T et al. Transient left ventricular apical ballooning without coronary artery stenosis: a novel heart syndrome mimicking acute myocardial infarction. J Am Coll Cardiol 2001; 38: 11–8.
Uretsky BF, Thygessen K, Armstrong PW et al. Acute coronary findings at autopsy in heart failure patients with sudden death: results from the assessment of treatment with lisinopril and survival (ATLAS) trial. Circulation 2000; 102: 611–6.
Van Dockum WG, Kuijer JPA, Götte MJW et al. Septal ablation in hypertrophic obstructive cardiomyopathy improves systolic myocardial function in the lateral (free) wall: a follow-up study using CMR tissue tagging and 3D strain analysis. Eur Heart J 2006; 27: 2833–9.
Vignaux O, Dhote R, Duboc D et al. Detection of myocardial involvement in patients with sarcoidosis applying T2-weighted, contrast-enhanced, and cine-magnetic resonance imaging: initial results of a prospective study. J Comput Assist Tomogr 2002; 26: 762–7.
White RD, Obuchowski NA, Gunawardena S et al. Left ventricular outflow tract obstruction in hypertrophic cardiomyopathy: pre-surgical and post-surgical evaluation by computed tomography magnetic resonance imaging. Am J Card Imaging 1996; 10: 1–13.
Wu KC, Weiss RG, Thiemann DR et al. Late gadolinium enhancement by cardiovascular magnetic resonance heralds an adverse prognosis in non-ischemic cardiomyopathy. J Am Coll Cardiol 2008; 51: 2414–21.
Yilmaz A, Gdynia HJ, Baccouche H et al. Cardiac involvement in patients with Becker muscular dystrophy: new diagnostic and pathophysiolgical insights by a CMR approach. J Cardiovasc Magn Reson 2008; 10: 50.
Yokokawa M, Tada H, Koyama K et al. The characteristics and distribution of the scar tissue predict ventricular tachycardia in patients with advanced heart failure. Pacing Clin Electrophysiol 2009; 32: 314–22.
Yousef ZR, Foley PWX, Khadjooi K et al. Left ventricular noncompaction: clinical features and cardiovascular magnetic resonance imaging. BMC Cardiovasc Dis 2009; 9: 37.

11 Acute Myocarditis and Chronic Inflammatory Cardiomyopathy

Ralf Wassmuth and Jeanette Schulz-Menger

11.1 Definition

In 2006 the American Heart Association defined myocarditis among other acquired cardiomyopathies as an acute or chronic inflammatory process affecting the myocardium produced by a wide variety of toxins and drugs or infectious agents. (Maron 2006). The differentiation of acute and chronic myocarditis was historically based on the Dallas criteria, but they were found to be limited by variability in interpretation, lack of prognostic value and low sensitivity (Baughman 2006). These limitations led to alternative pathologic criteria beyond traditional stained light microscopy that rely on cell-specific immunoperoxidase stains (Maisch 2000, Cooper 2009) or inflammatory cells and cytokines (Kühl 2005).

Lieberman et al. (1991) reported clinicopathologic criteria to differentiate fulminant from acute lymphocytic myocarditis by introducing prognostically useful clinical information. In this classification, fulminant lymphocytic myocarditis, which has a distinct onset within 2 wks, a viral prodrome, hemodynamic compromise, and a good prognosis is distinguished from giant cell myocarditis, which more frequently results in death or heart transplantation (McCarthy 2000, Hare and Baughman 2001). The European classification of cardiomyopathies differentiates dilated cardiomyopathy following cardiac infection and inflammation from active or fulminant myocarditis as an acute inflammatory disorder of the heart, often with preserved ventricular size (Elliott 2008). They defined inflammatory DCM by the presence of chronic inflammatory cells in association with left ventricular dilatation and reduced ejection fraction.

11.2 Etiology and Pathogenesis

Molecular pathogenesis of viral and autoimmune myocarditis has mostly been described in rodent models and isolated cell systems, in particular for coxsackie virus infection. In theory all viruses, non-viral organisms, pharmacologic agents or systemic inflammation may induce a myocardial injury. Most often, however, myocarditis is caused by viral infection (Magnani and Dec 2006). Genetic predisposition, hormonal status, exercise, and other factors might influence the susceptibility for developing disease after viral contact (Yajima and Knowlton 2009). Myocardial damage results either directly from viral damage or develops during immune response (Venteo 2010). Active viral replication, viral persistence, and myocardial remodeling have been described as different phases of myocardial damage after viral infection (Kühl 2005b, Yajima and Knowlton 2009). Autoantibodies (e.g. against myosin heavy chain) are often found in myocarditis (Dennert 2008) and may play an important pathophysiological role in inflammatory heart disease (Rose 2009).

11.3 Clinical Presentation, Natural History and Therapy

Acute myocarditis presents with a wide spectrum of oligosymptomatic disease to fulminant heart failure (Dennert 2008). There is an obvious disparity in gender distribution (Caforio 2007, Kindermann 2008). Young men between 20–35 yrs appear to form a remarkably homogeneous subgroup of infarction-like presentation. After a short episode of acute airway or gastrointestinal infection they present with sudden onset of chest pain. After admission to hospital, typically elevated troponin and CRP, ECG-changes in the inferolateral leads and posterolateral wall motion abnormalities with mildly impaired systolic function are detected. Despite patchy fibrotic lesions on CMR images, their course seems to be rather benign with restored LV function after a few weeks to months (Zagrosek 2009). Typically young people leading a busy life are suddenly no longer active. Their capacity can be impaired for several months even if objective parameters like LVEF, ECG, CRP etc. return to normal after some weeks. In this situation both patient and physician often find it difficult to decide when to return to normal activities. Myocarditis can even result in fulminant heart failure based on a dilated left ventricle with severely reduced systolic function. Some patients show an undulating course of myocarditis with frequent relapses (D'Ambrosio 2001). In this case additional CMR markers beyond late enhancement might help to detect this reactivation.

In acute myocarditis, therapy is limited so far to supportive therapy of heart failure. Certain experimental approaches for inflammatory dilated cardiomyopathy such as interferon therapy (Kühl 2003) or immunoadsorption (Müller 2000) await confirmation in larger trials.

11.4 CMR Protocols

The routine **CMR protocol in patients with suspected myocarditis** includes:

- cine imaging,
- T2-weighted imaging,
- early T1-weighted contrast-enhanced imaging,
- late T1-weighted gadolinium enhancement.

11.4.1 Cine Imaging

Any CMR study of a patient with cardiomyopathy will include cine sequences in long- and short-axis to quantify left ventricular size and systolic function. Steady-state free precession (SSFP) sequences used during breath-hold result in cine loops with a typical temporal resolution of about 40 ms. For further details on LV function, see Chapter 5. We suggest 3 long-axes (4CV, 2CV, 3CV) and at least one short-axis for every patient. A complete stack of short-axis images is added, should the left ventricle appear grossly abnormal. If the right ventricle (RV) is involved, we prefer additional axial slices that allow for measurement of the RV with higher reproducibility (Alfakih 2003).

SSFP sequences will depict acute serous pericardial effusions such as bright rim around the myocardium that might be confirmed in T2-weighted spin echo images. Subacute or organized effusions or effusions rich in protein appear more hypointense than serous effusions. Pleural effusions can be detected on axial scout images either based on spin echo or gradient echo techniques.

11.4.2 T2-Weighted Imaging

Acute myocarditis is characterized by myocardial edema. T2-weighted imaging depicts water accumulation as a bright signal. A short TI inversion recovery sequence (STIR) with additional fat suppression enhances the contrast between bright water and other tissues (Abdel-Aty 2007). In this sequence, three 180° pulses (one non-selective, two slice-selective) precede the readout pulses. The first two ensure blood suppression, the third is for fat suppression.

In fast spin echo imaging, blood is supposed to flow quickly through the image slice to be replaced by blood that has not yet been affected by magnetization, and thereby appears dark. Therefore blood suppression works best in short-axis (perpendicular to the main direction of flow) and in subjects with normal wall motion. In the case of regional or global wall motion abnormality, slow flowing blood stays within the imaging slice, picks up magnetization and appears bright. This bright signal within the cavities close to the endocardial lumen can be difficult to differentiate from bright edematous myocardium. The slice thickness of the blood suppression pulse should be larger than the thickness of the actual imaging slice.

As mentioned above, the STIR sequence consists of three 180° pulses. In cardiac gated imaging an optimal result will only be obtained if all the pulses hit the heart at the same position and at the same time in the cardiac cycle. If the heart has moved during this sequence of pulses, e.g. due to an extrasystole, signal loss will ensue. This can be frequently found in arrhythmia or just higher heart rates above 90 bpm. Unfortunately those patients prone to edema are those acutely ill with higher heart rates. Alternatively SSFP gradient echo imaging (Kellman 2007) or a hybrid of fast spin echo and SSFP gradient echo (Aletras 2008) has been suggested for T2-weighted imaging of edema. While offering more stability even in higher heart rates, these sequences result in less contrast to noise than the fast spin echo sequence.

11.4.3 Early Contrast Enhancement

Acute inflammation results in hyperemia and increased capillary leakage. Edema will result in tissue swelling. All these factors will increase the distribution volume of extracellular contrast agents. Contrast distribution within the extracellular space takes place after the first-pass perfusion within the first 5 min after administration. CMR imaging depicting contrast uptake in this time window should therefore serve as an unspecific marker of acute inflammation, as indicated in an early animal model of soft tissue inflammation (Paajanen 1987). Friedrich et al. introduced double inverted fast spin echo sequences before and after contrast administration for assessment of myocardial inflammation in acute myocarditis (Friedrich 1998). In shallow free breathing, 3–4 short-axis or axial slices are obtained in an interleaved order across the left ventricle. Imaging should cover a time window of 5 min and is repeated instantly after contrast administration. For quantification the relative myocardial signal increase after contrast is divided by skeletal muscle signal increase in the same slice. In normal volunteers, “relative” contrast enhancement should not exceed four.

11.4.4 Late Gadolinium Enhancement

Late gadolinium enhancement (LGE) has been developed to visualize infarction scarring. For myocarditis the images are obtained in the same way (Kim 2003) 15–25 min after a double dose of contrast. We recommend 0.2 mmol/kg gadolininium to ensure visibility of small lesions. Historically, inversion-recovery fast low angle shot (FLASH) gradient echo sequences have been employed. Now, SSFP gradient echo sequences are available as an alternative. Side by side comparisons for the detection of fibrotic lesions are available for large infarction scars (Huber 2005) and a small sample of non-ischemic heart disease (Elgeti 2007). In our experience, the sensitivity for very small lesions might slightly differ between FLASH and FISP gradient echo. Both, FLASH and SSFP, can be obtained as phase-sensitive reconstruction yielding more stable image contrast despite deviation from the optimal inversion time (Kellman 2002). Fibrotic lesions are best seen on long-axis images. However it is crucial to confirm any lesion in a second orthogonal plane. A bright signal originating from subcutaneous fat often results in ghosting artifacts overlaying the myocardium. In this case switching the direction of frequency and phase-encoding gradient will shift the artifacts in a different position and thereby allow them to be differentiated from true lesions. In certain anatomical locations, such as the space between the basal septum and right ventricular trabeculations or the inferior right ventricular insertion point, bright blood between trabecular structures can mimic true lesions. In case of doubt comparison with a cine frame in the same orientation can elucidate the position of myocardium and blood.

11.5 CMR-Based Assessment of Cardiac Structure and Function and Myocardial Tissue Characteristics

11.5.1 Cine Imaging

Cardiac magnetic resonance imaging has been shown to be a precise and reproducible method to quantify left ventricular mass and systolic function (Bellenger 2000, Hoffmann 2005). CMR cine imaging will even detect small changes in LV mass like subtle swelling in acute edema. Zagrosek et al. (2008) demonstrated reversible wall thickening in edema paralled by temporary increase in T2-signal. Puntmann et al. (2010) confirmed increased wall thickness in particular in the posterolateral wall in a series of acute myocarditis patients.

11.5.2 Edema

Myocardial edema is part of any acute myocardial damage and can be found in acute myocardial infarction, but also in acute viral myocarditis, as well as in acute episodes of cardiac sarcoidosis. T2-weighted imaging depicts edematous myocardium as bright. This is easy to detect in the case of focal edema restricted to injured territory as in acute infarction,

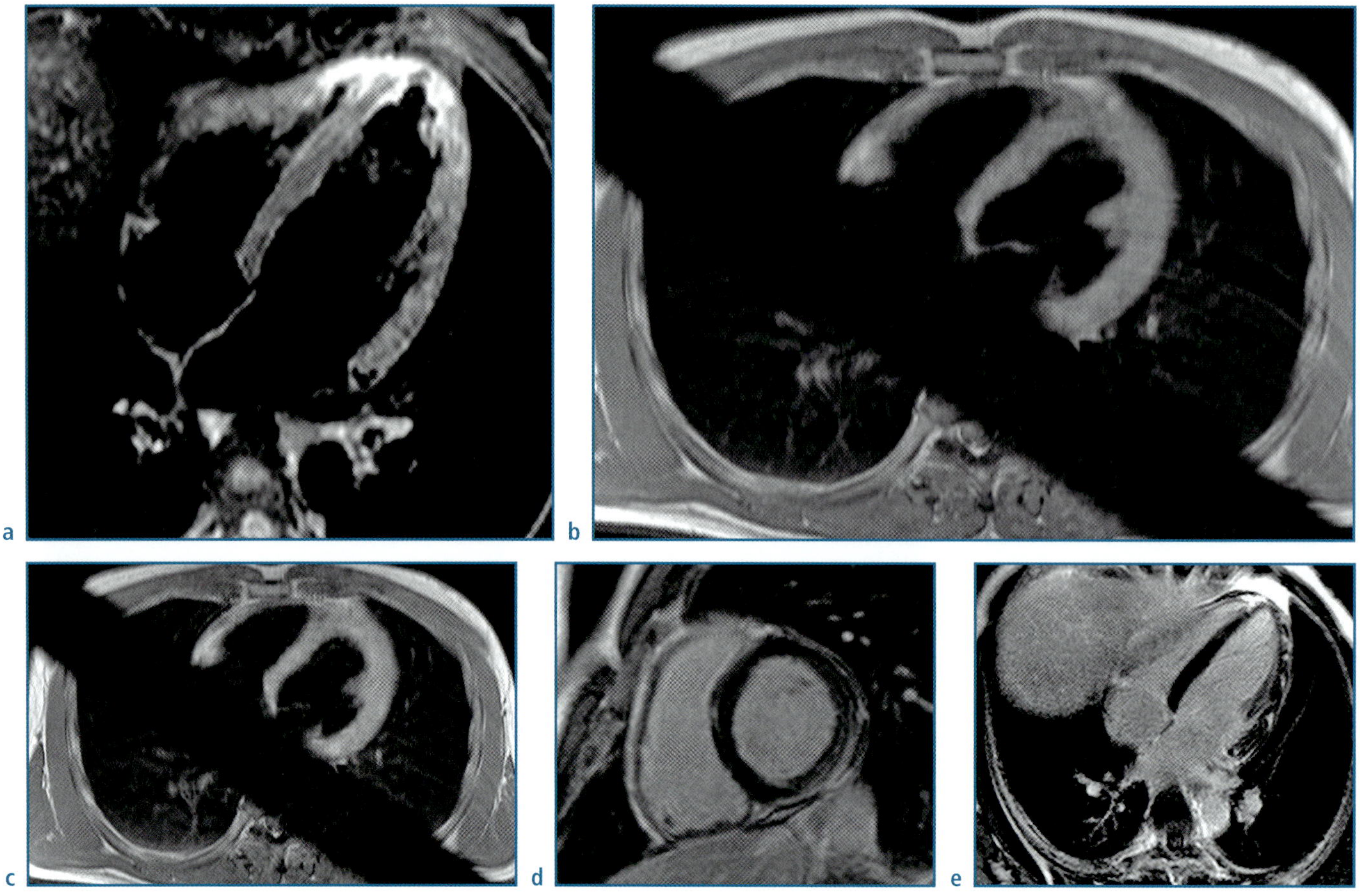

Figure 11-1 A 32-yrs-old male patient was admitted to the emergency room because of sudden onset of chest pain. Troponin was positive, but coronary angiography was normal. CMR depicts typical findings in acute infarction-like viral myocarditis. A triple inverted fast spin echo image in 4-ch orientation displayed hyperintense apical edema **(a)**. Axial T1-weighted fast spin echo images before **(b)** and shortly after **(c)** contrast administration showed global early enhancement. Figure **(d)** indicates posterolateral subepicardial late enhancement in short-axis, while the 4-ch view **(e)** delineates patchy lesions in the lateral wall.

as highlighted in animal models (Aletras 2006, Abdel-Aty 2009) and clinical studies (Abdel-Aty 2004). In very early viral myocarditis, in particular in the "young-male-pattern" that resembles acute inferior infarction, a regional edema can be frequently found as well (Figure 11-1a). The same holds true for acute cardiac sarcoidosis (Figure 11-5b). In subacute viral myocarditis (i.e. 10 d after onset) however, the edema might have expanded over a larger area of myocardium and might therefore be more difficult to delineate. Therefore the contrast between affected and remote tissue might diminish, which makes it more difficult to detect. If one assumes an evenly distributed bright myocardial signal, a reference structure is required to quantify the amount of brightness. In ECG-triggered conventional spin echo imaging, the image contrast depends on the repetition time that is a function of the RR-interval. Therefore direct measurements of myocardial signal intensity are heavily influenced by heart rate. The comparison of myocardial signal intensity and skeletal muscle intensity might allow an abnormal myocardial brightness to be detected regardless of heart rate. Experience in multiple centers suggests that in normal volunteers myocardial signal should not exceed two times the skeletal muscle signal (Friedrich 2009).

11.5.3 Hyperemia and Capillary Leakage

Hyperemia and capillary leakage represent an unspecific marker for acute inflammation not only in viral myocarditis, but also in other forms of acute myocardial inflammation. It often persists for about 4–6 wks, but normalizes afterwards. Therefore measurements of early enhancement may differentiate between active and inactive phases of a chronic disease and may be a useful marker for follow-up studies.

11.5.4 Fibrotic Lesions

Late enhancement lesions are not a mandatory finding in viral myocarditis, but occur in about 50 % of patients depending on the population studied, predominantly in young males. Multiple foci are often located in the subepicardial or midwall layer of the posterolateral myocardium (Figure 11-1d, e), but anteroseptal lesions occur as well. The reason for the posterolateral predominance is unclear, but early pathology reports indicated the same pattern (Shirani 1993). There is no clear relation between the extent of fibrotic lesions and LV function. In fact fulminant myocarditis can occur without any LGE lesions while most of the young men with patchy fibrosis often have only mildly impaired LV function. Late enhancement lesions are not a late complication of myocarditis, but can be found at the very onset of disease. They persist but slightly shrink over time so that very small lesions may disappear on follow-up scans due to partial-volume-effects. So far we have never seen an increase of lesions over time in viral myocarditis. This is different for a chronic inflammation like sarcoidosis. Whether LGE lesions found in a subgroup of dilated cardiomyopathy (Assomull 2006) indicate an inflammatory etiology is unclear.

There is a relation between ventricular arrhythmias and the presence of late enhancement lesions in non-ischemic cardiomyopathy (Nazarian 2005, Bogun 2009). However, there is no evidence yet that the presence or absence of late enhancement lesions influences the prognosis in acute viral myocarditis. In general, the presence of late enhancement lesions was found to be associated with worse outcome, but patients with HCM or inflammatory diseases were excluded from this study (Cheong 2009).

11.6 Characterization

In acute myocarditis with myocardial edema, Zagrosek et al. (2008) demonstrated increased myocardial mass corresponding to hyperintense T2-weighted images compared to follow-up scans. Puntman et al. (2010) confirmed increased wall thickness, in particular in the posterolateral wall, in conjunction with increased signal in T2 in 36 patients with acute myocarditis. Yelgec et al. (2007) described focal edema as a focal bright signal two times more intense than remote areas in half of their acute patients. Jeserich et al. (2009) found an increased ratio of myocardial signal over skeletal muscle of 2.4 ± 0.3 vs. 1.9 ± 0.3 in 36 patients with acute myocarditis compared to controls.

Friedrich et al. (1998), Roditi et al. (2000), and Laissy et al. (2002) reported increased early enhancement based on fast spin echo images in patients with acute myocarditis compared to controls. Wagner et al. (2003) followed patients with acute myocarditis over 30 mths. Early enhancement decreased to values comparable to normal controls after 4 wks and remained normal in most patients. Mahrholdt et al. (2004) were the first to describe late enhancement in acute myocarditis. He proposed a relation between the spatial distribution of lesions and the type of virus (Mahrholdt 2006). Beside focal edema in T2, Yelgec et al. (2007) found LGE lesions in 15 out of 20 of their patients with acute myocarditis. Goitein et al. (2009) found LGE in 21/23 young male patients with acute myocarditis. Danti et al. (2009) confirmed this in a series of 23 young patients (among them 21 young men) with subepicardial LGE after myocarditis.

Abdel-Aty et al. (2005) compared T2-weighting, early and late enhancement in a group of clinically characterized patients with acute myocarditis and found the combination of sequences to be more sensitive than a single technique alone. Zagrosek et al. (2009) followed patients with acute myocarditis over 18 mths. Both T2 and early enhancement decreased over time in parallel to improving systolic LV function, while LGE persisted in all but one patient. In the chronic phase no patient showed both increased signal in T2 and increased early contrast enhancement. Two studies investigated patients beyond the acute phase of myocarditis. De Cobelli et al. (2006) found typical late enhancement lesions in 16/23 patients, but hyperintense signal in T2 in 5/23 only in those patients with chronic myocarditis. Gutberlet et al. (2008) compared T2, early and late T1-weighting in 83 chronic patients with immunohistologic results from biopsy. They found no relation between CMR findings and viral persistence, but a relation between T2, early enhancement and histological evidence of inflammation. In chronic myocarditis, the sensitivity and specificity to detect inflammation was 67 and 69% for T2 and 62 and 86% for early enhancement, respectively. As late enhancement shows little change over time, it appeared less helpful to characterize the degree of inflammation in the chronic setting.

An international group of experts in clinical, pathological and CMR work up of myocarditis issued a consensus paper for CMR in myocarditis, named Lake Louise criteria (Friedrich 2009).

11.7 Special Inflammatory Myocardial Diseases

In systemic inflammatory disease, cardiac involvement often critically influences the prognosis (Knockaert 2007). Even if CMR markers remain unspecific in most instances, they might help to confirm cardiac involvement in a multi-organ disease already known.

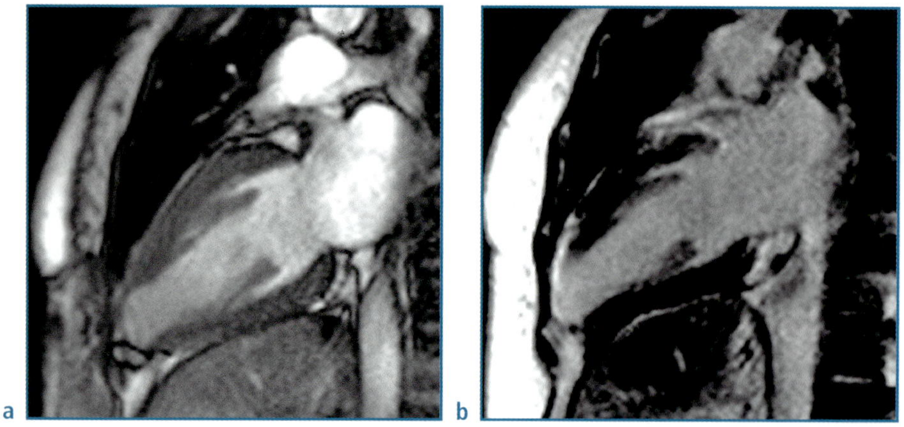

Figure 11-2 Episodes of ventricular arrhythmias in a routine ECG had prompted work-up in an asymptomatic 28-yrs-old female patient from Brazil. CMR revealed apical aneurysm, illustrated in a systolic still frame on a 2-ch view (a), and apical scar (b), indicating Chagas disease.

11.7.1 Chagas Disease

Infection with Trypanosoma cruzi represents a leading cause for heart failure in Latin America (Rassi 2010). About 30% of infected patients present with cardiomyopathy in their forth decade of life. Arrhythmias, chest pain or sudden cardiac death might be other sequelae of Chagas disease (Bestetti and Cardinalli-Neto 2008). Frequently apical aneurysms (Figure 11-2a) and areas of fibrosis (Figure 11-2b) can be found. Rochitte et al. (2005) scanned 51 symptomatic and asymptomatic Chagas patients and found late enhancement lesions in two thirds of them. The frequency of late enhancement corresponded to the clinical status: Only 20% of asymptomatic but seropositive patients had lesions, in contrast to 85% of those with cardiomyopathy and 100% of those with ventricular tachycardia.

11.7.2 Systemic Lupus Erythematosus (SLE)

Systemic lupus erythematosus (SLE) is a multi-system autoimmune connective tissue disorder that often subclinically affects the heart. It can result in pericarditis and pericardial effusions, valvular heart disease (Roldan 2008), but also in premature atherosclerosis (D'Cruz 2007) and myocardial infarction. In a series of 70 consecutive SLE patients Cervera et al. (1992) found echocardiographic abnormalities in 57%. O'Neill et al. (2009) described unexpected infarction scars with late enhancement CMR in a small series of lupus patients.

Autopsy series found evidence of myocarditis in 57% of patients, whereas an in vivo diagnosis was made in 9% only (Wijetunga and Rockson 2002). CMR appears in particular suited to detect subclinical inflammatory tissue changes in lupus. More than 20 years ago Been et al. (1988) reported increased myocardial T1-times in lupus patients. Singh et al. (2005) found increased myocardial T2 relaxation times corresponding to areas of high signal intensity on T2-weighted images in a small group of 6 patients with active myocarditis compared to 5 patients with inactive disease and controls. Using a comprehensive approach including T2-weighted imaging, early and late T1-weighting Abdel-Aty et al. (2008) described abnormalities in a series of 20 lupus patients. LGE lesions appeared intramural in a non-coronary pattern confirming case reports (Edwards 2007, Saremi 2007). Chronic pericardial and even pleural effusions are part of generalized serositis that can be easily visualized with CMR.

11.7.3 Churg-Strauss Syndrome (CSS)

Churg-Strauss syndrome (CSS) belongs to the group of small vessel vasculitis, also including Wegener's granulomatosis and microscopic polyangiitis. In contrast to the other two, CSS frequently affects the heart. CMR can visualize all aspects of acute and persistent myocarditis including edema (Figure 11-3a), early and late contrast enhancement (Wassmuth 2008, Neumann 2009). Interestingly CSS results primarily in subendocardial lesions, whereas most other non-ischemic diseases feature an intramural or subepicardial distribution pattern. Parallel to late enhancement lesions subendocardial perfusion abnormalities at rest have been described in CSS (Hansch 2009). The right ventricle can be affected in particular with fibrous endocardial thickening and thrombus formation. The lesions in CSS are not confined to a single coronary territory (Figure 11-3b) and are most likely related to damaged coronary microvessels. The pattern described for CSS can also be found in cases of other hypereosiniphilic states (Debl 2008). Over time lesions do persist but shrink to a certain extent.

11.7.4 Wegener's Granulomatosis

Compared to Churg-Strauss syndrome, cardiac involvement is less frequent in Wegener's granulomatosis (Hoffman 1992, Reinhold-Keller 2000). Still, myocarditis, pericarditis

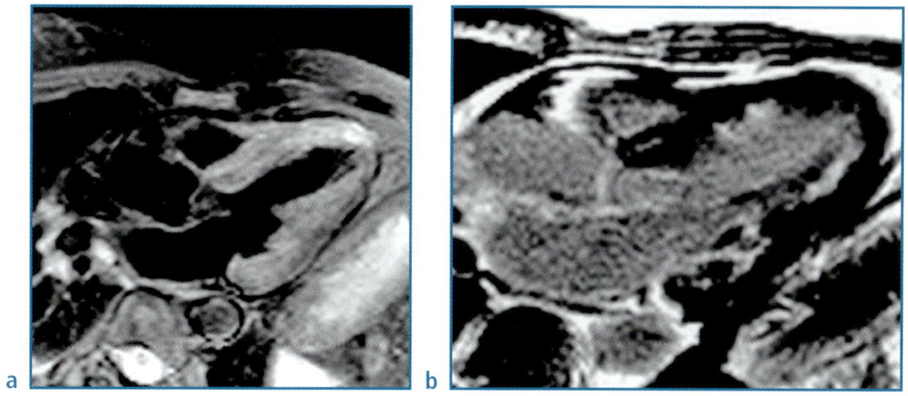

Figure 11-3 A 56-yrs-old woman with unclear pulmonary infiltrates was referred from the Pulmonary to the Cardiology Department because of chest pain and positive troponin. Coronary angiography was normal. CMR was performed in search for any inflammatory change that might explain the increased troponin levels. Figure (a) shows triple inverted T2-weighted fast spin echo in 3-ch view indicating anteroseptal edema. Figure (b) illustrates subendocardial late enhancement not only in the anteroseptal, but also posterolateral area. CMR prompted further workup of vasculitis that finally revealed eosinophilia of 56 %, a history of asthma and sinusitis. The final diagnosis was Churg-Strauss syndrome.

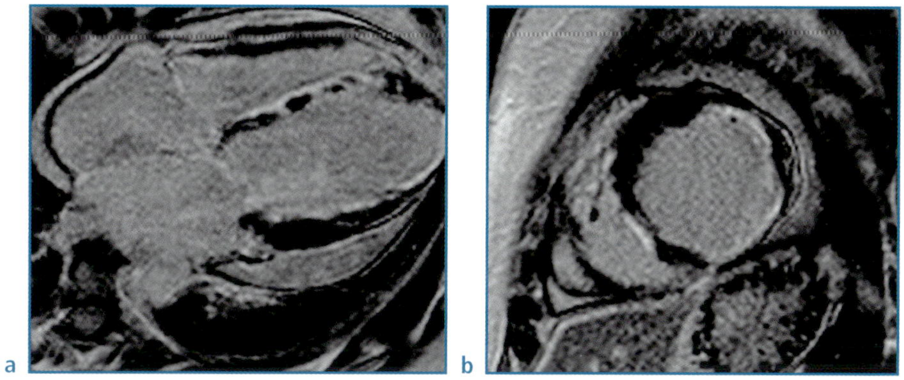

Figure 11-4 Late enhancement imaging in a 52-yrs-old female patient with scleroderma but normal coronary arteries revealed extensive wall thinning, small pericardial effusion and scarring in a 4-ch (a) and short-axis view (b).

and conduction abnormalities have been reported. CMR could delineate temporary edema (Caudron 2009) and persistent either intramural (Brihaye 2008) or subendocardial (To 2007, Mavrogeni 2009) late gadolinium enhancement.

11.7.5 Scleroderma

Systemic sclerosis or scleroderma is a systemic connective tissue disease of unknown etiology that not only results in pulmonary hypertension in about one third of the patients, but might even involve the heart directly (Meune 2010). Frequently chronic pericardial effusions occur. Small but multiple fibrotic lesions in the myocardium have been reported (Figure 11-4) (Nassenstein 2008, Hachulla 2009, Kobayashi 2009).

11.7.6 Sarcoidosis

Sarcoidosis is a systemic granulomatous disease of unknown etiology affecting the heart more often than usually perceived. Autopsy series revealed cardiac infiltration in up to 40 % (Mehta 2008). Myocardial biopsy however has been found to yield a low sensitivity of about 20 % (Silverman 1978). In cases with positive biopsy from extracardiac tissue and CMR evidence of myocardial infiltration one might consider a positive diagnosis of cardiac sarcoidosis. A negative myocardial biopsy cannot exclude myocardial sarcoidosis (Kim 2009).

Multiple reports (Schulz-Menger 2006, Cheong 2009, Patel 2009) found evidence of late gadolinium enhancement in about 25 % of the patients. The presence of fibrotic lesions might represent an advanced state of the disease. Lesions often appear very bright. There is a trend towards subepicardial distribution and large focal spots of late enhancement (Figure 11-5c), matching earlier reports from pathology (Shirani and Roberts 1993). If the patients are

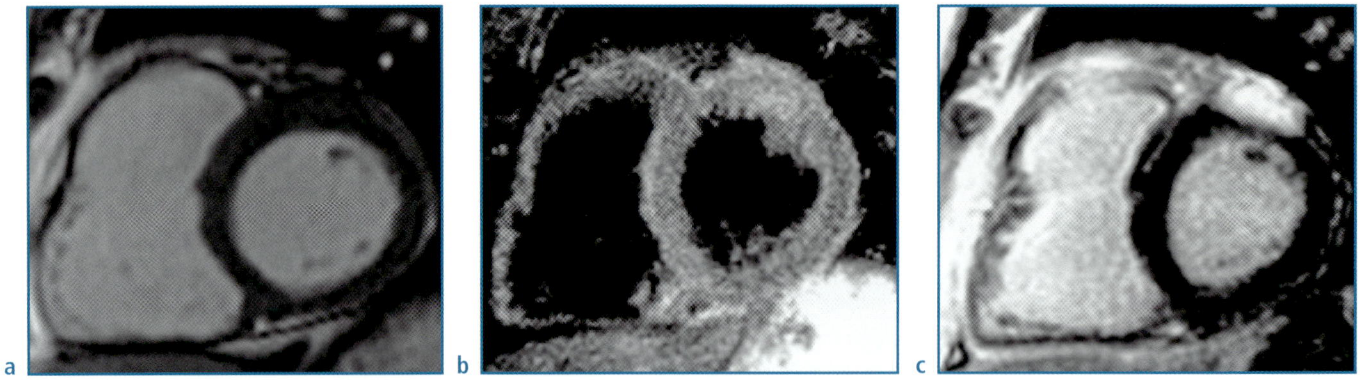

Figure 11-5 A 41-yrs-old patient was admitted to the emergency room with ventricular tachycardia. Instant coronary angiography ruled out coronary artery disease. Figure **(a)** shows a diastolic SSFP cine frame in short-axis. Figure **(b)** illustrates focal anterior edema on triple inverted T2-weighted fast spin echo image, corresponding to very bright, almost transmural, but subepicardial fibrotic lesion on late enhancement images in **(c)**. These findings were suspicious of sarcoidosis that was later confirmed by mediastinal biopsy.

scanned in an active phase of the disease, focal edema (Figure 11-5b) often parallels the LGE lesions (Rieker 2002). Early enhancement might help to detect more subtle forms that have not yet resulted in LGE lesions (Shimada 2001, Schulz-Menger 2006).

11.7.7 Rheumatoid Arthritis

Patients with rheumatoid arthritis suffer from an excess mortality due to premature atherosclerosis that is not explained by traditional risk factors (Roman and Salmon 2007). Small pericardial effusions can be found in up to one out of three patients (Knockaert 2007). Using echocardiography, abnormal diastolic function has been described even in pediatric patients with rheumatoid arthritis (Oguz 2000).

Puntmann et al. (2010) found increased LVEDV with thinner walls and slightly reduced systolic function in 24 patients with rheumatoid arthritis compared to volunteers and patients with acute myocarditis. This is supported by a larger study from Baltimore comparing 75 patients with rheumatoid arthritis to 225 matched controls (Giles 2010). Again myocardial mass, stroke volume and ejection fraction were slightly lower in the diseased group, whereas cardiac volumes were comparable to controls in this study. In a mixed group of patients with inflammatory systemic diseases, including rheumatoid arthritis, Mavrogeni et al. (2009) found increased signal intensity in T2-weighted imaging as well as increased early contrast uptake reflecting myocardial inflammation in these patients.

11.8 Summary and Conclusions

It is important to image patients suspected of acute myocarditis as early as possible, as the sensitivity of CMR decreases over time. Even if a true myocarditis has been present, e.g. 10 wks ago, little imaging evidence will remain in many cases, when the patient still suffers from limited capacity. In young patients with obvious clinical presentation, CMR imaging only needs to confirm a diagnosis already established on clinical grounds. Still, CMR often appears clinically important in the acute setting to exclude other differential diagnoses such as unusual myocardial infarction or Tako-Tsubo cardiomyopathy. Late gadolinium enhancement is widely available, well-standardized, visually impressive and therefore widely accepted as the method of choice for myocarditis. However, not all patients with true myocarditis show LGE. The sensitivity may, depending on the population studied, be as low as 50%. Therefore CMR should not rely on LGE alone in the search for myocarditis. All CMR markers are rather unspecific signs of myocardial damage. Certain patterns of lesions might be found more often in this or that disease, but a CMR finding alone does not allow the diagnosis of a certain type of etiology or even a causative organism.

11.9 Future Perspectives

The stability of T2-weighted imaging needs improvement in higher heart rates and arrhythmias. The quantification of early contrast enhancement appears to be a promising parameter of inflammation that is not yet measured in an optimal way by slow and artifact-prone fast spin echo imaging.

Other sequences have to be tested as an alternative. Instead of measuring signal intensity that often depends on heart rate, it might be more appropriate to measure T1 and T2 relaxation time, which directly reflects tissue properties. Initial experience with T1 quantification is available for myocardial infarction (Messroghli 2003) and amyloidosis (Maceira 2005, Sparrow 2009), but not yet for myocarditis. Pilot studies for T2 quantification have been done in an animal model for acute myocardial infarction (Giri 2009), amyloidosis (Sparrow 2009) and lupus (Singh 2005). Beside technical improvements, clinicians expect data regarding the prognostic impact of CMR findings.

References

Abdel-Aty H, Boye P, Zagrosek A et al. Diagnostic performance of cardiovascular magnetic resonance in patients with suspected acute myocarditis: comparison of different approaches. J Am Coll Cardiol 2005; 45 (11): 1815–22.

Abdel-Aty H, Cocker M, Meek C et al. Edema as a very early marker for acute myocardial ischemia: a cardiovascular magnetic resonance study. J Am Coll Cardiol 2009; 53 (14): 1194–201.

Abdel-Aty H, Siegle N, Natusch A et al. Myocardial tissue characterization in systemic lupus erythematosus: value of a comprehensive cardiovascular magnetic resonance approach. Lupus 2008; 17 (6): 561–7.

Abdel-Aty H, Simonetti O, Friedrich MG. T2-weighted cardiovascular magnetic resonance imaging. J Magn Reson Imaging 2007; 26 (3): 452–9.

Abdel-Aty H, Zagrosek A, Schulz-Menger J et al. Delayed enhancement and T2-weighted cardiovascular magnetic resonance imaging differentiate acute from chronic myocardial infarction. Circulation 2004; 109 (20): 2411–6.

Aletras AH, Kellman P, Derbyshire JA, Arai AE. ACUT2E TSE-SSFP: a hybrid method for T2-weighted imaging of edema in the heart. Magn Reson Med 2008; 59 (2): 229–35.

Aletras AH, Tilak GS, Natanzon A et al. Retrospective determination of the area at risk for reperfused acute myocardial infarction with T2-weighted cardiac magnetic resonance imaging: histopathological and displacement encoding with stimulated echoes (DENSE) functional validations. Circulation 2006; 113 (15): 1865–70.

Alfakih K, Plein S, Bloomer T et al. Comparison of right ventricular volume measurements between axial and short-axis orientation using steady-state free precession magnetic resonance imaging. J Magn Reson Imaging 2003; 18 (1): 25–32.

Assomull RG, Prasad SK, Lyne J et al. Cardiovascular magnetic resonance, fibrosis, and prognosis in dilated cardiomyopathy. J Am Coll Cardiol 2006; 48 (10): 1977–85.

Baughman KL. Diagnosis of myocarditis: death of Dallas criteria. Circulation 2006; 113 (4): 593–5.

Been M, Thomson BJ, Smith MA et al. Myocardial involvement in systemic lupus erythematosus detected by magnetic resonance imaging. Eur Heart J 1988; 9 (11): 1250–6.

Bellenger NG, Davies LC, Francis JM et al. Reduction in sample size for studies of remodeling in heart failure by the use of cardiovascular magnetic resonance. J Cardiovasc Magn Reson 2000; 2 (4): 271–8.

Bestetti RB, Cardinalli-Neto A. Sudden cardiac death in Chagas' heart disease in the contemporary era. Int J Cardiol 2008; 131 (1): 9–17.

Bogun FM, Desjardins B, Good E et al. Delayed-enhanced magnetic resonance imaging in non-ischemic cardiomyopathy: utility for identifying the ventricular arrhythmia substrate. J Am Coll Cardiol 2009; 53 (13): 1138–45.

Brihaye B, Aouba A, Pagnoux C et al. Rituximab reversed cardiac involvement of Wegener's granulomatosis: magnetic resonance imaging assessment. Presse Med 2008; 37 (3 Pt 1): 412–5.

Caforio AL, Calabrese F, Angelini A et al. A prospective study of biopsy-proven myocarditis: prognostic relevance of clinical and etiopathogenetic features at diagnosis. Eur Heart J 2007; 28 (11): 1326–33.

Caudron J, Fares J, Dominique S, Dacher JN. Diagnosis and follow-up of Wegener's granulomatosis by cardiac magnetic resonance. Eur Heart J 2009; 30 (12): 1537.

Cervera R, Font J, Pare C et al. Cardiac disease in systemic lupus erythematosus: prospective study of 70 patients. Ann Rheum Dis 1992; 51 (2): 156–9.

Cheong BY, Muthupillai R, Nemeth M et al. The utility of delayed-enhancement magnetic resonance imaging for identifying non-ischemic myocardial fibrosis in asymptomatic patients with biopsy-proven systemic sarcoidosis. Sarcoidosis Vasc Diffuse Lung Dis 2009; 26 (1): 39–46.

Cheong BY, Muthupillai R, Wilson JM et al. Prognostic significance of delayed-enhancement magnetic resonance imaging: survival of 857 patients with and without left ventricular dysfunction. Circulation 2009; 120 (21): 2069–76.

Cooper Jr LT. Myocarditis. N Engl J Med 2009; 360 (15): 1526–38.

D'Ambrosio A, Patti G, Manzoli A et al. The fate of acute myocarditis between spontaneous improvement and evolution to dilated cardiomyopathy: a review. Heart 2001; 85 (5): 499–504.

Danti M, Sbarbati S, Alsadi N et al. Cardiac magnetic resonance imaging: diagnostic value and utility in the follow-up of patients with acute myocarditis mimicking myocardial infarction. Radiol Med 2009; 114 (2): 229–38.

D'Cruz DP, Khamashta MA, Hughes GR. Systemic lupus erythematosus. Lancet 2007; 369 (9561): 587–96.

Debl K, Djavidani B, Buchner S et al. Time course of eosinophilic myocarditis visualized by CMR. J Cardiovasc Magn Reson 2008; 10 (1): 21.

De Cobelli F, Pieroni M, Esposito A et al. Delayed gadolinium-enhanced cardiac magnetic resonance in patients with chronic myocarditis presenting with heart failure or recurrent arrhythmias. J Am Coll Cardiol 2006; 47 (8): 1649–54.

Dennert R, Crijns HJ, Heymans S. Acute viral myocarditis. Eur Heart J 2008; 29: 2073–82.

Edwards NC, Ferro CJ, Townend JN, Steeds RP. Myocardial disease in systemic vasculitis and autoimmune disease detected by cardiovascular magnetic resonance. Rheumatology (Oxford) 2007; 46 (7): 1208–9.

Elgeti T, Abdel-Aty H, Wagner M et al. Assessment of late gadolinium enhancement in non-ischemic cardiomyopathy: comparison of a fast Phase-Sensitive Inversion Recovery Sequence (PSIR) and a conventional segmented 2D gradient echo recall (GRE) sequence – preliminary findings. Invest Radiol 2007; 42 (10): 671–5.

Elliott P, Andersson B, Arbustini E et al. Classification of the cardiomyopathies: a position statement from the European Society Of Cardiology Working Group on Myocardial and Pericardial Diseases. Eur Heart J 2008; 29 (2): 270–6.

Friedrich MG, Sechtem U, Schulz-Menger J et al. Cardiovascular Magnetic Resonance in Myocarditis: A JACC White Paper. J Am Coll Cardiol 2009; 53 (17): 1475–87.

Friedrich MG, Strohm O, Schulz-Menger J et al. Contrast media-enhanced magnetic resonance imaging visualizes myocardial changes in the course of viral myocarditis. Circulation 1998; 97 (18): 1802–9.

Giles JT, Malayeri AA, Fernandes V et al. Left ventricular structure and function by cardiac magnetic resonance imaging in rheumatoid arthritis. Arthritis Rheum 2010; 62 (4): 940–51.

Giri S, Chung YC, Merchant A et al. T2 quantification for improved detection of myocardial edema. J Cardiovasc Magn Reson 2009; 11 (1): 56.

Goitein O, Matetzky S, Beinart R et al. Acute myocarditis: noninvasive evaluation with cardiac MRI and transthoracic echocardiography. Am J Roentgenol 2009; 192 (1): 254–8.

Gutberlet M, Spors B, Thoma T et al. Suspected chronic myocarditis at cardiac MR: diagnostic accuracy and association with immunohistologically detected inflammation and viral persistence. Radiology 2008; 246 (2): 401–9.

Hachulla AL, Launay D, Gaxotte V et al. Cardiac magnetic resonance imaging in systemic sclerosis: a cross-sectional observational study of 52 patients. Ann Rheum Dis 2009; 68 (12): 1878–84.

Hansch A, Pfeil A, Rzanny R et al. First-pass myocardial perfusion abnormalities in Churg-Strauss syndrome with cardiac involvement. Int J Cardiovasc Imaging 2009; 25: 501–10.

Hare JM, Baughman KL. Fulminant and acute lymphocytic myocarditis: the prognostic value of clinicopathological classification. Eur Heart J 2001; 22 (4): 269–70.

Hoffman GS, Kerr GS, Leavitt RY et al. Wegener's granulomatosis: an analysis of 158 patients. Ann Intern Med 1992; 116 (6): 488–98.

Hoffmann R, von Bardeleben S, ten Cate F et al. Assessment of systolic left ventricular function: a multi-centre comparison of cineventriculography, cardiac magnetic resonance imaging, unenhanced and contrast-enhanced echocardiography. Eur Heart J 2005; 26 (6): 607–16.

Huber AM, Schoenberg SO, Hayes C et al. Phase-sensitive inversion-recovery MR imaging in the detection of myocardial infarction. Radiology 2005; 237 (3): 854–60.

Jeserich M, Olschewski M, Bley T et al. Cardiac involvement after respiratory tract viral infection – detection by cardiac magnetic resonance. J Comput Assist Tomogr 2009; 33 (1): 15–9.

Kellman P, Aletras AH, Mancini C et al. T2-prepared SSFP improves diagnostic confidence in edema imaging in acute myocardial infarction compared to turbo spin echo. Magn Reson Med 2007; 57 (5): 891–7.

Kellman P, Arai AE, McVeigh ER, Aletras AH. Phase-sensitive inversion recovery for detecting myocardial infarction using gadolinium-delayed hyperenhancement. Magn Reson Med 2002; 47 (2): 372–83.

Kim JS, Judson MA, Donnino R et al. Cardiac sarcoidosis. Am Heart J 2009; 157 (1): 9–21.

Kim RJ, Shah DJ, Judd RM. How we perform delayed enhancement imaging. J Cardiovasc Magn Reson 2003; 5 (3): 505–14.

Kindermann I, Kindermann M, Kandolf R et al. Predictors of outcome in patients with suspected myocarditis. Circulation 2008; 118 (6): 639–48.

Knockaert DC. Cardiac involvement in systemic inflammatory diseases. Eur Heart J 2007; 28 (15): 1797–804.

Kobayashi H, Yokoe I, Hirano M et al. Cardiac magnetic resonance imaging with pharmacological stress perfusion and delayed enhancement in asymptomatic patients with systemic sclerosis. J Rheumatol 2009; 36 (1): 106–12.

Kühl U, Pauschinger M, Noutsias M et al. High prevalence of viral genomes and multiple viral infections in the myocardium of adults with "idiopathic" left ventricular dysfunction. Circulation 2005a; 111: 887–92.

Kühl U, Pauschinger M, Schwimmbeck PL et al. Interferon-beta treatment eliminates cardiotropic viruses and improves left ventricular function in patients with myocardial persistence of viral genomes and left ventricular dysfunction. Circulation 2003; 107: 2793–8.

Kühl U, Pauschinger M, Seeberg B et al. Viral persistence in the myocardium is associated with progressive cardiac dysfunction. Circulation 2005b; 112: 1965–19.

Laissy JP, Messin B, Varenne O et al. MRI of acute myocarditis: a comprehensive approach based on various imaging sequences. Chest 2002; 122 (5): 1638–48.

Lieberman EB, Hutchins GM, Herskowitz A et al. Clinicopathologic description of myocarditis. J Am Coll Cardiol 1991; 18 (7): 1617–26.

Maceira AM, Joshi J, Prasad SK et al. Cardiovascular magnetic resonance in cardiac amyloidosis. Circulation 2005; 111 (2): 186–93.

Magnani JW, Dec GW. Myocarditis: current trends in diagnosis and treatment. Circulation 2006; 113 (6): 876–90.

Mahrholdt H, Goedecke C, Wagner A et al. Cardiovascular magnetic resonance assessment of human myocarditis: a comparison to histology and molecular pathology. Circulation 2004; 109 (10): 1250–8.

Mahrholdt H, Wagner A, Deluigi CC et al. Presentation, patterns of myocardial damage, and clinical course of viral myocarditis. Circulation 2006; 114 (15): 1581–90.

Maisch B, Portig I, Ristic A et al. Definition of inflammatory cardiomyopathy (myocarditis): on the way to consensus. A status report. Herz 2000; 25 (3): 200–9.

Maron BJ, Towbin JA, Thiene G et al. Contemporary definitions and classification of the cardiomyopathies: an American Heart Association Scientific Statement from the Council on Clinical Cardiology, Heart Failure and Transplantation Committee; Quality of Care and Outcomes Research and Functional Genomics and Translational Biology Interdisciplinary Working Groups; and Council on Epidemiology and Prevention. Circulation 2006; 113 (14): 1807–16.

Mavrogeni S, Manoussakis MN, Karagiorga TC et al. Detection of coronary artery lesions and myocardial necrosis by magnetic resonance in systemic necrotizing vasculitides. Arthritis Rheum 2009; 61 (8): 1121–9.

Mavrogeni S, Spargias K, Markussis V et al. Myocardial inflammation in autoimmune diseases: investigation by cardiovascular magnetic resonance and endomyocardial biopsy. Inflamm Allergy Drug Targets 2009; 8 (5): 390–7.

McCarthy RE, Boehmer JP, Hruban RH et al. Long-term outcome of fulminant myocarditis as compared with acute (nonfulminant) myocarditis. N Engl J Med 2000; 342 (10): 690–5.

Mehta D, Lubitz SA, Frankel Z et al. Cardiac involvement in patients with sarcoidosis: diagnostic and prognostic value of outpatient testing. Chest 2008; 133 (6): 1426–35.

Messroghli DR, Niendorf T, Schulz-Menger J et al. T1 mapping in patients with acute myocardial infarction. J Cardiovasc Magn Reson 2003; 5 (2): 353–9.

Meune C, Vignaux O, Kahan A, Allanore Y. Heart involvement in systemic sclerosis: evolving concept and diagnostic methodologies. Arch Cardiovasc Dis 2010; 103 (1): 46–52.

Müller J, Wallukat G, Dandel M et al. Immunoglobulin adsorption in patients with idiopathic dilated cardiomyopathy. Circulation 2000; 101: 385–9.

Nassenstein K, Breuckmann F, Huger M et al. Detection of myocardial fibrosis in systemic sclerosis by contrast-enhanced magnetic resonance imaging. Rofo 2008; 180 (12): 1054–60.

Nazarian S, Bluemke DA, Lardo AC et al. Magnetic resonance assessment of the substrate for inducible ventricular tachycardia in non-ischemic cardiomyopathy. Circulation 2005; 112 (18): 2821–5.

Neumann T, Manger B, Schmid M et al. Cardiac involvement in Churg-Strauss syndrome: impact of endomyocarditis. Medicine (Baltimore) 2009; 88 (4): 236–43.

Oguz D, Ocal B, Ertan U et al. Left ventricular diastolic functions in juvenile rheumatoid arthritis. Pediatr Cardiol 2000; 21 (4): 374–7.

O'Neill SG, Woldman S, Bailliard F et al. Cardiac magnetic resonance imaging in patients with systemic lupus erythematosus. Ann Rheum Dis 2009; 68 (9): 1478–81.

Paajanen H, Brasch RC, Schmiedl U, Ogan M. Magnetic resonance imaging of local soft tissue inflammation using gadolinium-DTPA. Acta Radiol 1987; 28 (1): 79–83.

Patel MR, Cawley PJ, Heitner JF et al. Detection of myocardial damage in patients with sarcoidosis. Circulation 2009; 120 (20): 1969–77.

Puntmann VO, Taylor PC, Barr A et al. Towards understanding the phenotypes of myocardial involvement in the presence of self-limiting and sustained systemic inflammation: a magnetic resonance imaging study. Rheumatology (Oxford) 2010; 49 (3): 528–35.

Rassi A, Rassi A, Marin-Neto JA. Chagas disease. Lancet 2010; 375: 1388–402.

Reinhold-Keller E, Beuge N, Latza U et al. An interdisciplinary approach to the care of patients with Wegener's granulomatosis: long-term outcome in 155 patients. Arthritis Rheum 2000; 43 (5): 1021–32.

Rieker O, Mohrs O, Oberholzer K et al. Cardiac MRI in suspected myocarditis. Rofo Fortschr Geb Rontgenstr Neu Bildgeb Verfahr 2002; 174 (12): 1530–6.

Rochitte CE, Oliveira PF, Andrade JM et al. Myocardial delayed enhancement by magnetic resonance imaging in patients with Chagas' disease: a marker of disease severity. J Am Coll Cardiol 2005; 46 (8): 1553–8.

Roditi GH, Hartnell GG, Cohen MC. MRI changes in myocarditis – evaluation with spin echo, cine-MR angiography and contrast-enhanced spin echo imaging. Clin Radiol 2000; 55 (10): 752–8.

Roldan CA. Valvular and coronary heart disease in systemic inflammatory diseases: Systemic disorders in heart disease. Heart 2008; 94 (8): 1089–101.

Roman MJ, Salmon JE. Cardiovascular manifestations of rheumatologic diseases. Circulation 2007; 116 (20): 2346–55.

Rose NR. Myocarditis: infection vs. autoimmunity. J Clin Immunol 2009; 29 (6): 730–7.

Saremi F, Ashikyan O, Saggar R et al. Utility of cardiac MRI for diagnosis and post-treatment follow-up of lupus myocarditis. Int J Cardiovasc Imaging 2007; 23 (3): 347–52.

Schulz-Menger J, Wassmuth R, Abdel-Aty H et al. Patterns of myocardial inflammation and scarring in sarcoidosis as assessed by cardiovascular magnetic resonance. Heart 2006; 92 (3): 399–400.

Shimada T, Shimada K, Sakane T et al. Diagnosis of cardiac sarcoidosis and evaluation of the effects of steroid therapy by gadolinium-DTPA-enhanced magnetic resonance imaging. Am J Med 2001; 110 (7): 520–7.

Shirani J, Freant LJ, Roberts WC. Gross and semiquantitative histologic findings in mononuclear cell myocarditis causing sudden death, and implications for endomyocardial biopsy. Am J Cardiol 1993; 72 (12): 952–7.

Shirani J, Roberts WC. Subepicardial myocardial lesions. Am Heart J 1993; 125 (5 Pt 1): 1346–52.

Silverman KJ, Hutchins GM, Bulkley BH. Cardiac sarcoid: a clinicopathologic study of 84 unselected patients with systemic sarcoidosis. Circulation 1978; 58 (6): 1204–11.

Singh JA, Woodard PK, Davila-Roman VG et al. Cardiac magnetic resonance imaging abnormalities in systemic lupus erythematosus: a preliminary report. Lupus 2005; 14 (2): 137–44.

Sparrow P, Amirabadi A, Sussman MS et al. Quantitative assessment of myocardial T2 relaxation times in cardiac amyloidosis. J Magn Reson Imaging 2009; 30 (5): 942–6.

To A, De Zoysa J, Christiansen JP. Cardiomyopathy associated with Wegener's granulomatosis. Heart 2007; 93 (8): 984.

Venteo L, Bourlet T, Renois F et al. Enterovirus-related activation of the cardiomyocyte mitochondrial apoptotic pathway in patients with acute myocarditis. Eur Heart J 2010; 31 (6): 728–36.

Wagner A, Schulz-Menger J, Dietz R, Friedrich MG. Long-term follow-up of patients with acute myocarditis by magnetic resonance imaging. MAGMA 2003; 16 (1): 17–20.

Wassmuth R, Gobel U, Natusch A et al. Cardiovascular magnetic resonance imaging detects cardiac involvement in Churg-Strauss syndrome. J Card Fail 2008; 14 (10): 856–60.

Wijetunga M, Rockson S. Myocarditis in systemic lupus erythematosus. Am J Med 2002; 113 (5): 419–23.

Yajima T, Knowlton KU. Viral myocarditis: from the perspective of the virus. Circulation 2009; 119 (19): 2615–24.

Yelgec NS, Dymarkowski S, Ganame J, Bogaert J. Value of MRI in patients with a clinical suspicion of acute myocarditis. Eur Radiol 2007; 17 (9): 2211–7.

Zagrosek A, Abdel-Aty H, Boye P et al. Cardiac magnetic resonance monitors reversible and irreversible myocardial injury in myocarditis. JACC Cardiovasc Imaging 2009; 2 (2): 131–8.

Zagrosek A, Wassmuth R, Abdel-Aty H et al. Relation between myocardial edema and myocardial mass during the acute and convalescent phase of myocarditis – a CMR study. J Cardiovasc Magn Reson 2008; 10 (1): 19.

12 Heart Failure and Cardiac Transplantation

Raymond Kim, Igor Klem and Vinzenz Hombach

12.1 Definition and Epidemiology

Heart failure (HF) is a complex clinical syndrome that can result from any structural or functional (inherited or acquired) cardiac disorder that impairs the ability of the ventricle to fill with or eject blood (Hunt 2009). The cardinal manifestations of HF are dyspnea and fatigue, which may limit exercise tolerance, and fluid retention that may lead to pulmonary congestion and peripheral edema. 45–50 % of patients suffer from classical depressed ventricular function (HFrEF), and 50–55 % from diastolic heart failure (HF with normal or preserved ejection fraction of 40–50 % and more = HFpEF).

HF affects worldwide around 23 million people, in the United States 4.7 million people (1.5–2.0 % of total population), with an incidence of 500,000 cases of HF diagnosed annually (Kannel 2000). The prevalence of HF in the European countries is similar to the USA (0.4–2.0 % of total population) and follows an exponential pattern, rising with age and affecting 6–10 % of people older than 65 yrs. The prevalence of systolic HF increases with age and is much higher in men than in women, whereas diastolic HF (HFpEF) increases even more dramatically with age and is much more common in women than in men.

12.2 Etiology and Pathogenesis

The clinical syndrome of HF may result from disorders of the myocardium, endocardium, pericardium, or great vessels, although the majority of patients has symptoms due to an impaired left ventricular myocardial function (systolic or diastolic dysfunction). The most frequent causes of systolic HF are coronary artery disease (CAD), arterial hypertension, valvular disease, and non-ischemic cardiomyopathy. Hypertension has the greatest impact on the development of HF (39% of HF events in men and 59% in women), and myocardial infarction despite its lower incidence (3–10%) has a high attributable risk (34% in men and 13% in women), as well. In 20–30% of patients with HF with a depressed LV ejection fraction (EF) the exact causative basis is unknown; these patients are referred to as suffering from idiopathic dilated cardiomyopathy. Less frequent causes are disorders of heart rhythm, pulmonary heart disease including cor pulmonale and pulmonary vascular disorders, high-output states, metabolic disorders, and excessive blood requirements such as systemic arteriovenous shunting or anemia.

Heart failure may begin after an index event (e.g. an acute myocardial infarction) that produces an initial decline in pumping capacity of the heart. Following this first decline of cardiac pumping capacity, a variety of compensatory mechanisms such as the adrenergic nervous system, the renin-angiotensin-aldosterone system (RAS), and the cytokine systems are activated. The activation of these systems is responsible for maintaining cardiac output through increased retention of salt and water, increased contractility, peripheral arterial vasoconstriction, and activation of inflammatory mediators that are responsible for cardiac repair and remodeling. Thus, in the short term these systems can restore cardiovascular function to a normal homeostatic level and the patients remain asymptomatic. But over time the sustained activation of theses systems can lead to secondary end-organ damage within the ventricle, with worsening of ventricular function, LV remodeling and subsequent cardiac decompensation.

LV remodeling is characterized by an altered biology of cardiac myocytes and nonmyocyte components of the myocardium (extracellular matrix alterations such as degradation and myocardial fibrosis), and alterations of geometry and architecture of the LV chamber (LV dilatation, increased LV sphericity, LV wall thinning, mitral valve incompetence). The pattern of cardiac remodeling in response to hemodynamic overload depends on the nature of the inciting stimulus. When the overload is predominantly due to an increased systolic pressure (e.g. aortic stenosis or hypertension), the increase in systolic stress leads to the parallel addition of sarcomeres and widening of cardiac myocytes, resulting in cardiac concentric hypertrophy. When the overload is predominantly caused by an increase in ventricular volume (e.g. aortic or mitral incompetence), the increase in diastolic wall stress leads to addition of sarcomeres, lengthening of cardiac myocytes, and LV dilatation, which is referred to as eccentric cardiac hypertrophy. As a result of worsening of ventricular function and remodeling of cardiac chambers patients undergo the transition from asymptomatic to symptomatic heart failure. In contrast to the acute event of myocardial infarction other index events may develop gradually over time, e.g. hypertension or valvular heart disease, and may activate the compensatory systems gradually, as well, with a similar transition from asymptomatic to symptomatic HF, when ventricular dysfunction and remodeling are advanced to the level of decompensation (for details see Mann 2012).

12.3 Clinical Presentation and Diagnosis

The cornerstone of clinical assessment of patients with HF remains a detailed history and a careful physical examination. Among the major symptoms of HF cardinal symptoms are dyspnea, exercise intolerance, and fatigue. Additional major HF symptoms are orthopnea, paroxysmal nocturnal dyspnea, pulmonary congestion and edema, and cachexia. Minor symptoms are weight loss, cough, nocturia, palpitations, peripheral cyanosis, and depression. On physical examination major signs are elevated jugular venous pressure, positive hepato-jugular reflux, pulmonary rales, tachypnea, third heart sound, ankle edema, ascites, and pleural effusion. Minor signs are mitral regurgitation, pleural effusion, cardiomegaly, hepatomegaly, splenomegaly, ankle edema, hypotension, pulsus alternans, tachycardia, atrial fibrillation, and ventricular ectopic beats (Ho 1993).

The initial diagnostic algorithm includes a thorough physical examination, routine laboratory testing, an electrocardiogram at rest, an exercise test, chest X-ray, and an echocardiogram. Other non-invasive imaging studies, coronary angiography, and endomyocardial biopsy may be reasonable in specific situations. Initial laboratory evaluation should include complete blood count, urine analysis, serum electrolytes (including calcium and magnesium), blood urea nitrogen, serum creatinine, fasting blood glucose, lipid profile, liver function tests, thyroid stimulating hormone, BNP, CRP, CK, troponin, and possibly screening for HIV, rheumatologic diseases, amyloidosis, and hemochromatosis if there is a clinical suspicion of these diseases. In clinical routine BNP levels have been shown to be useful in distinguishing cardiac from non-cardiac causes of dyspnea in the urgent care setting in whom the clinical diagnosis of HF is uncertain, and to provide prognostic information in patients with chronic HF and/or acute coronary syndromes.

Common ECG abnormalities in HF are pathological Q-waves, LV hypertrophy, left or right bundle branch block (LBBB, RBBB), AV block, or T-wave alterations. Rhythm disorders like atrial fibrillation or ventricular ectopic beats are common in HF patients and of limited prognostic significance, whereas short runs of ventricular tachycardia (VT) may be considered potentially harmful.

While assessment of the patient's ability to perform routine and desired activities of daily living are routinely assessed, maximal exercise testing is of limited value in HF patients. It can be used, however, for functional assessment and prognostic stratification to identify high-risk patients who are candidates for cardiac transplantation or other advanced treatments. The best prognostic parameter is maximal oxygen consumption ($\dot{V}O_2$ max) on a progressively increasing workload, and a $\dot{V}O_2$ of less than 12 ml/kg BW/min heralds a worse prognosis.

In patients with chronic HF chest X-ray can be used to estimate cardiomegaly by a cardiothoracic ratio of more than 0.5 and to detect pulmonary venous hypertension by redistribution of lung perfusion from the base to the upper zone of the lung, and less frequently by the presence of pleural effusion. These alterations are similarly present in both HF patients with preserved (HFpEF) and reduced systolic function (HFrEF). Signs of acute HF in the X-ray are classical lung edema and Kerley-B lines (linear densities representing interlobular interstitial edema).

Two-dimensional echocardiography with Doppler is the most common and convenient method for assessing structure and function of the heart by studying the myocardium and pericardium, evaluating regional and global ventricular function, wall thickness, and detecting the presence and severity of valvular dysfunction (stenosis or incomepetence or both). The most important features in the evaluation of HF patients are assessment of LV ejection fraction (LVEF), severity of LV remodeling, and changes in diastolic inflow properties.

However, there are **general limitations of echocardiography** like unpredictable variation in image quality and patient-related echogenicity, and **specific limitations** regarding:

- the exact quantification of valvular incompetence and ventricular ejection fraction,
- assessment of right ventricular structure and function,
- myocardial tissue characterization,
- measurement of inter- and intraventricular dyssnchrony in left bundle branch block (LBBB) and prediction of cardiac resynchronization therapy (CRT) response, and
- the presence of a limited acoustic window in 10–30 % of patients, in whom transesophageal echocardiography is required.

12.4 Prognosis and Therapy

The overall mortality rate of HF patients is higher than for many cancers despite several recent reports indicating that the prognosis is improving. In the Framingham Study, the median survival was 3.2 yrs for women and 1.7 yrs for men, with only 38 % of women and 25 % of men surviving 5 yrs (Kannel 2000). More recent data from the Framingham Study have examined long-term trends in the survival of HF patients and shown improved survival for both women and men, with an overall decline in mortality of about 12 % per decade from 1950 to 1999 (Lev 2002). Many factors such as demographics, causes of HF, sleep apnea, obesity, clinical symptoms and signs, hemodynamic factors, exercise testing, metabolic factors, ECG parameters, biomarkers, and endomyocardial biopsy have been associated with increased risk. For clinical purposes the Seattle Heart Failure Model provides an accurate estimate of 1-, 2- and 3-yrs survival with the use of easily obtained clinical, pharmacological, device, and laboratory characteristics and is accessible via an interactive web-based program (http://depts.washington.edu/shfm).

Basic pharmacological treatment in HF patients with systolic dysfunction (HFrEF) and ≥ NYHA class II is aimed at reducing HF symptoms and delay progression of the disease and includes quadruple therapy with β-adrenergic blockers, diuretics, ACE-inhibitors and/or angiotensin receptor blockers, and aldosterone antagonists. In patients with severly reduced LV function and intracardiac thrombus or with atrial fibrillation anticoagulation with coumadin is warranted. Patients with tachycardic atrial fibrillation should be treated with cardiac glycosides in order to normalize ventricular rate both at rest and during exercise. Recent ACC/AHA and ESC guidelines recommend to implant an intracardiac defibrillator (ICD) for primary prevention of sudden cardiac death (SCD) in both, non-ischemic cardiomyopathy and ischemic heart disease at least 40 d post-MI, LVEF ≤ 35 %, NYHA functional class II or III symptoms while receiving chronic optimal medical therapy, and life expectancy of > 1 yr (class IA recommendation). And in patients with severe inter-/intraventricular dyssynchrony, who are symptomatic despite optimal medical therapy (NYHA class III or IV), QRS width ≥ 120 ms, and LVEF ≤ 30 %, a cardiac resynchronization (CRT) device (class IA recommendation for sinus rhythm, class IIA for atrial fibrillation or pacemaker-dependent patients), in most cases including an ICD mode (CRT-ICD = biventricular pacer-defibrillator) should be implanted for therapeutic and prognostic reasons.

12.5 CMR Protocols

The CMR examination in HF patients should follow a certain protocol that includes assessment of LV and RV volumes and function as well as evaluation of wall thickness, valve function, atrial dimensions, and the pericardium followed by myocardial tissue characterization. This core exam should include multi-planar (horizontal long-axis, vertical long-axis, 3-chamber, and contiguous short-axis covering of the heart) cine imaging typically using bright-blood cine steady-state free precession techniques (b-SSFP) and delayed-enhancement CMR (DE-CMR) using contrast-enhanced inversion-recovery gradient-echo (IR-GRE) sequences with nulling signal from normal myocardium.

This core exam may be complemented by other pulse-sequences as indicated by clinical history and findings during the exam: black-blood or bright-blood morphological images in anatomic planes may be used to assess the great vessels (systemic and pulmonary veins, aorta, and pulmonary arteries). Single-shot inversion-recovery images with a long inversion time (approx. 600 ms at 1.5 T) may be used to specifically detect thrombus. Phase contrast flow measurements are useful for quantification of left- and right-ventricular cardiac output for quantification of intraventricular shunts and for quantitative assessment of valvular dysfunctions (particularly of valve incompetence). T2-weighted images with increased SI may indicate myocardial edema (e.g. in acute myocardial infarction or acute myocarditis). Given the prevalence of ischemic heart disease, it may be beneficial to include stress with either dobutamine cine imaging or adenosine first-pass perfusion imaging to demonstrate presence and extent of reversible ischemia and the contractile reserve in patients being considered for revascularization. Coronary MR angiography may be used to assess for anomalous coronary arteries if clinically indicated.

12.6 CMR-Based Diagnosis of Structure and Dysfunction of the Heart

For prognostic reasons structure and dysfunction of the heart are the main targets for imaging, and the main parameters for the presence of ventricular dysfunction, following therapy and defining prognosis are the accurate and reproducible measurements of ventricular dimensions, mass and function. For serial studies in large clinical trials echocardiography has been used to assess changes in size, shape and function of the heart. The reasons for using echocardiography are its low-cost, widespread availability and feasibility to perform bedside examination. However, this technique suffers from unpredictable variation in image quality and poor patient-related echogenicity. In contrast, cardiac magnetic resonance imaging (CMR) does not have these limitations and is currently the only imaging technique, which provides a comprehensive study of both structure and function of the heart as well as myocardial perfusion and viability. Moreover CMR examination is independent of slice-orientation or acoustic window, and post-processing does not require any geometric assumptions as in echocardiography to determine ventricular dimensions. This is particularly important when evaluating ventricles of patients with chronic heart failure who have severely altered morphology that may have regional variations in wall thickness and contractility at least in ischemic cardiomyopathy. The highly reproducible results of CMR imaging have turned this technique as a reference for the non-invasive assessment of LV dimensions, mass, and function (Holman 1997), and CMR offers an ideal means of serial assessment of disease progression or response to treatment in an individual patient. Bellenger et al. (2000) were able to show that about 1/10 of sample sizes are needed for CMR imaging in contrast to echocardiography when studying changes of ventricular function with pharmacological treatment.

In recent years it became clear that chronic heart failure occurs at any level of left-ventricular ejection fraction, i.e. patients may present with heart failure with preserved (HFpEF) or reduced ejection fraction (HFrEF). In general, one should keep in mind that LVEF is a mere index of global ventricular pump performance blind to many mechanical ventricular abnormalities in heart failure, such as dysfunctional longitudinal subendocardial muscle fibers, twisting, untwisting, and suction abnormalities, disturbed non-uniformities of strain, or abnormal cross-talk in the pluricellular ventricular tissue pump (De Keulenaer and Brutsaert 2009). At this point CMR imaging offers great advantage over echocardiography, since detailed analysis of twisting and untwisting and suction abnormalities and non-uniformities of strain can be detected by myocardial tissue tagging and special CMR strain analysis. Moreover, diastolic dysfunction can also be assessed by CMR by analysing left ventricular diastolic filling characteristics using PC flow analysis or volume-filling time analysis of cine imaging data (Maceira 2006, Kawaji 2009). Although CMR or other imaging data (echocardiography, radionuclide ventriculography) can contribute to a diagnosis of diastolic dysfunction, no modality is considered sufficiently definite to establish the diagnosis on the basis of isolated measurements. Moreover, the diagnosis of diastolic dysfunction is largely one of exclusion based on the documentation of normal or near-normal systolic function and unequivocal evidence of

HF (e.g. pulmonary edema on chest radiograph plus symptoms of breathlessness or right-sided failure).

12.7 Identification of Etiology and Systematic Diagnostic Approach

Once the diagnosis of HF is established and an abnormality in myocardial function is identified, the next step in patient management is to determine the etiology. As discussed earlier cardiomyopathies, which are myocardial disorders affecting the heart muscle structure and function directly, are frequent causes of heart failure. Though several classification schemes are used to characterize various cardiomyopathies, (Konstam 2000, Maron 2006, Elliott 2008) for clinical purposes, a simple differentiation between patients having ischemic (ICM) or non-ischemic cardiomyopathy (non-ICM) is useful, since this classification can affect patient management directly (e.g. coronary revascularisation in ICM and response to medical therapy; Follath 1998). Moreover, this classification also provides insight into patient prognosis, ICM is associated with reduced survival compared with non-ICM (Felker 2002). As a second step, within the broad category of non-ICM a specific cause must be determined, which affects patient treatment and survival (Felker 2000). In clinical routine stress testing or coronary angiography or both to identify the presence of obstructive epicardial coronary artery disease (CAD) has been the cornerstone in differentiating ischemic from non-ischemic cardiomyopathies. However, this classical approach may have several drawbacks including the moderate accuracy of non-invasive imaging tests for the diagnosis of CAD without coronary angiography, the limited utility of available diagnostic tools for defining the pathology of non-ICM (e.g. reliance on granular sparkling appearance on 2D-echocardiography or sampling error of cardiac biopsies), and finally the finding that correlation between the presence of coronary obstruction to non-ICMs or ICMs is moderate (Felker 2002). These limitations are exemplified by the results of the autopsy study of the ATLAS trial (Uretsky 2000). Of the 171 patients with moderate to severe heart failure who died and had autopsy, 120 patients (70%) were diagnosed in life as having ICM, and 51 patients (30%) were diagnosed as having non-ICM. Autopsy documented that 17% of those diagnosed as having ICM did not have CAD, whereas 31% of those diagnosed as having non-ICM had significant CAD. Overall, 21% had an incorrect clinical diagnosis (Figure 12-1).

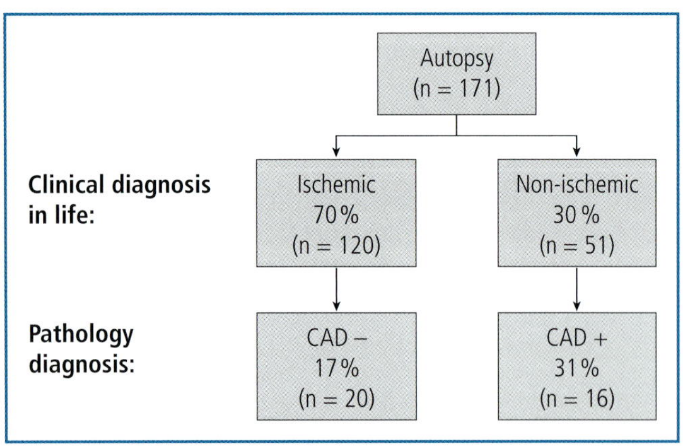

Figure 12-1 The ATLAS study was a multi-center, randomized trial for lisinopril in 3,164 patients with moderate to severe heart failure. Diagram is showing the clinical diagnosis as well post-mortem pathological diagnosis in 171 patients who died during the study and autopsy was obtained (modified from Uretsky et al. 2000). CAD: coronary artery disease.

12.7.1 Detection of Myocardial Damage/Scar by DE-CMR

DE-CMR may provide a non-invasive approach to determining the etiology of cardiomyopathy by allowing direct assessment of the myopathic processes. Comparative histopathologic studies have shown that the presence, extent, and location of late godalinium enhancement (LGE) by DE-CMR is a precise indicator of non-viable myocardium in both ischemic (Kim 1999) and non-ischemic heart disease (Marholdt 2004, Moon 2004). LGE beyond a simple measurement of viability provides additional information by the presence and pattern of hyperenhancement. In acute or chronic myocardial infarction the unifying mechanism for the hyperenhancement of non-viable myocardium may be the absence of viable myocytes rather than any inherent properties that are specific for acutely necrotic tissue, collagenous scar, or other forms of non-viable tissue. Understanding of the "wavefront" expansion of ischemic injury from subendocardium towards the epicardium in the area at risk subtended by a specific coronary artery (Reimer 1977) allows the identification of an "ischemic-type" or "CAD-type" pattern (Figure 12-2). A "CAD-type" of LGE always should involve the subendocardium, i.e. subendocardial or transmural, and should be located in a region that is consistent with a perfusion territory of an epicardial coronary artery. Conversely, a "non-CAD-type" pattern of LGE is one that spares the subendocardium outside a perfusion territory and is secondary to non-ischemic disorders.

In several studies nearly all patients with ICM (CAD and prior myocardial infarction) showed myocardial hyperenhancement, whereas patients with idiopathic dilated

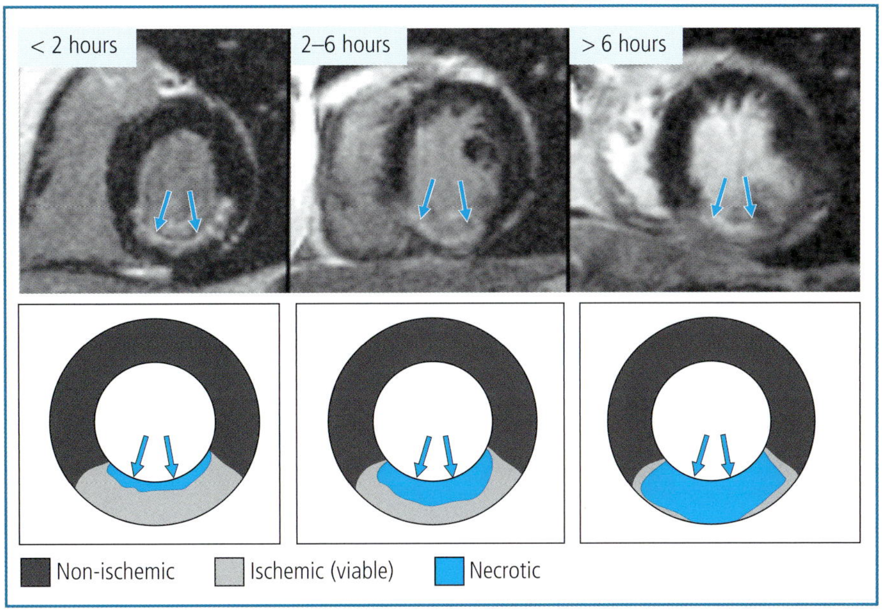

Figure 12-2 The typical enhancement pattern of myocardial infarction can be explained by the pathophysiology of ischemia. Little or no cellular necrosis is found until about 15 min after occlusion. Over the next few hours a wavefront of necrosis begins in the subendocardium and moves progressively towards the epicardium. During this period, the infarcted region (arrows) within the ischemic zone increases continously and ultimately can become transmural (from Mahrholdt H et al. Delayed enhancement cardiovascular magnetic resonance assessment of non-ischemic cardiomyopathies. Eur Heart J 2005; 26: 1461–74; with permission of Oxford University Press, Oxford, UK).

cardiomyopathy (IDCM) may present hyperenhancement in 12–26% of cases (Bello 2003, McCrohon 2003, Soriano 2005, Soriano 2007, Wu 2008, Hombach 2009). In the study of McCrohon et al. (2003) 13% of patients who had IDCM had CAD-type hyperenhancement, whereas 28% had non-CAD-type. These rates are nearly identical to the rate of chronic infarcts found at autopsy in patients who had IDCM in a study of Roberts et al. (1987) and in the ATLAS substudy by Uretzky et al. (2000) (14 and 12%, respectively). Whether the CAD-type of LGE in patients with IDCM is due to coronary embolisation and spontaneous recanalisation after plaque rupture remains unclear. The patchy or linear striae of LGE limited to the mid myocardium as found in the study of McCrohon et al. may be found in patients with longstanding LV dysfunction and in those who have a possible history of myocarditis. According to our own experiences non-CAD-type of LGE may be found within midwall or subepicardium in any region of ventricular myocardium (Hombach 2009).

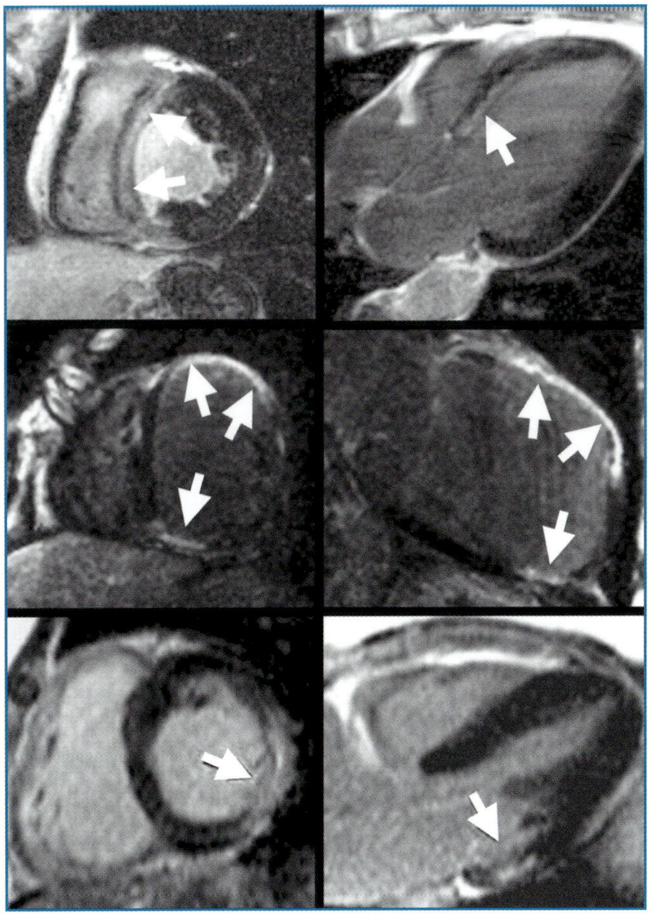

Figure 12-3 Patient example of patterns and locations of LGE typically found in patients with myocarditis, sarcoidosis, and Fabry's disease.

Some recent publications suggest that certain non-ischemic cardiomyopathies have a predilection for specific scar patterns (Figure 12-3). Choudhury et al. (2002) described the presence of mid-wall hyperenhancement in one or both junctions of the interventricular septum and right ventricular free wall in patients with hypertrophic cardiomyopathy (HCM), whereas mid-wall or epicardial hyperenhancement in the inferolateral wall is consistent with Anderson-Fabry disease (Moon 2003). In patients with Chagas disease a relatively disease specific involvement of both the LV basal lateral wall and apex of hyperenhancement was seen (Rochitte 2005). The finding that patients with myocarditis had preferred non-CAD-type of hyperenhancement in the lateral wall of the left ventricle could

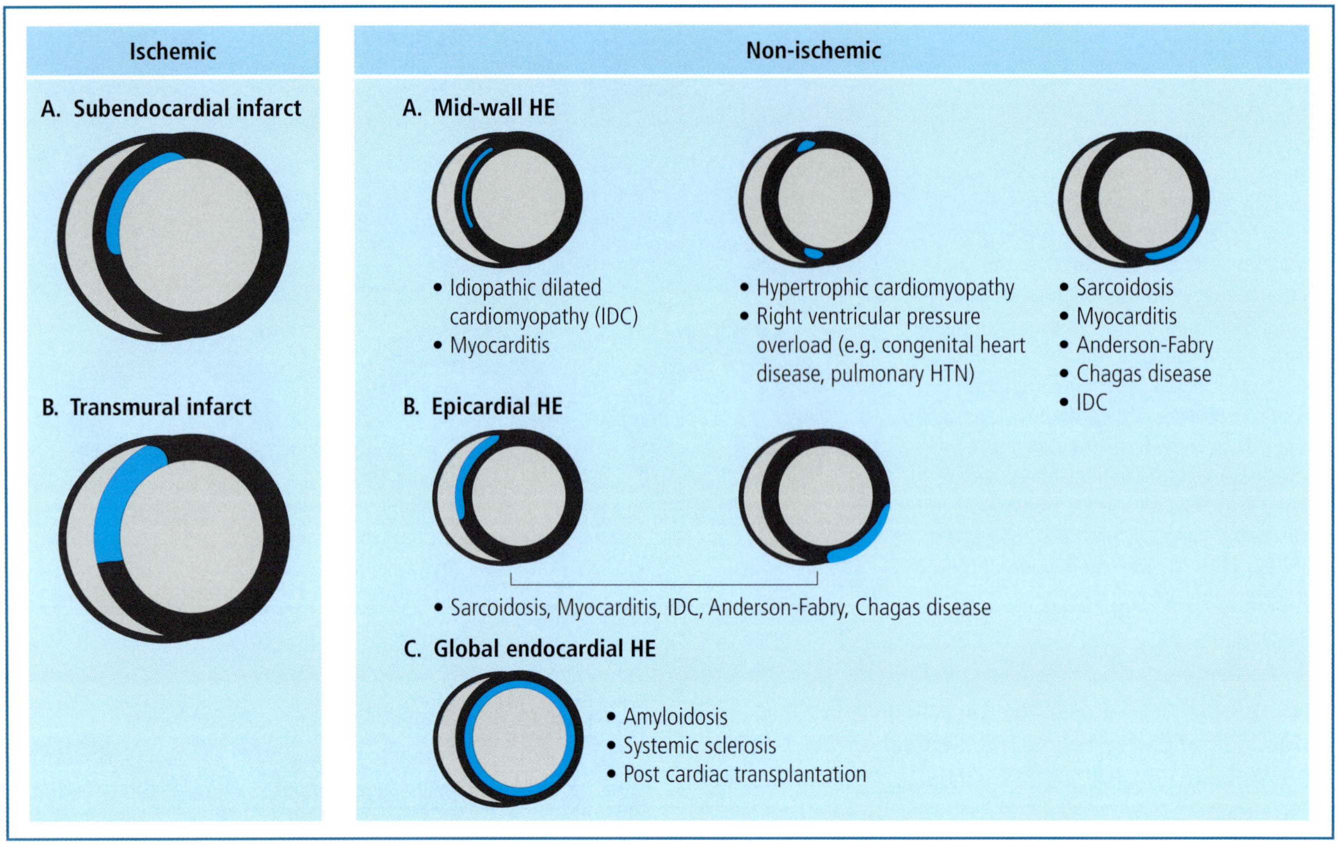

Figure 12-4 Hyperenhancement (HE) patterns encountered in DE-CMR imaging. If hyperenhancement is present, the endocardium should be involved in patients who have ischemic disease. Isolated mid-wall or epicardial hyperenhancement strongly suggests a non-ischemic cause (from Mahrholdt H et al. Delayed enhancement cardiovascular magnetic resonance assessment of non-ischemic cardiomyopathies. Eur Heart J 2005; 26: 1461–74; with permission of Oxford University Press, Oxford, UK).

not be confirmed by our own data, since we found a random distribution of local contraction abnormalities and of LGE in a subgroup of 27 patients with acute myocarditis (Hombach 2008). The locations and patterns of scarring on DE-CMR are often quite distinct, and a pattern-recognition approach based on the visualization of LGE can provide useful diagnostic information about the likely underlying disease process (Figure 12-4). In summary, DE-CMR depicts regions of replacement scarring in vivo that previously could be detected only at autopsy, but DE-CMR currently is unable to identify the presence of diffuse ventricular interstitial fibrosis. Since the voxel resolution of DE-CMR is approximately 1.8 mm × 1.3 mm × 6 mm, a regional hyperenhancement visible on DE-CMR will comprise several voxels, and the pathology analogue would be a macroscopic scar that is visible on gross pathological exam.

12.7.2 Stepwise Diagnostic Approach

Based on the literature a systematic stepwise approach to interpreting DE-CMR images in patients with HF of different origin has been proposed (Shah 2006, Senthilkumar 2009) (Figure 12-5). The **first step** in HF evaluation is to assess the severity and regionality of LV dysfunction, chamber size, wall thickness, and valvular function using cine-CMR. The **second step** will determine the presence or absence of hyperenhancement on DE-CMR. Since almost all patients with longstanding ICM have evidence of prior myocardial infarction (Boucher 1979, Schuster 1980), the diagnosis of non-ICM should be considered strongly in patients who have severe cardiomyopathy without hyperenhancement. Common conditions in which LGE frequently is absent include idiopathic dilated, alcoholic, Tako-Tsubo, and peri-partum cardiomyopathy. The **third step** deals with classification of location and distribution of LGE, if present, as CAD-type or non-CAD-type hyperenhancement. According to the concept of ischemic "wavefront" LGE patterns that spare the subendocardium and are limited to the middle or epicardial portion of the LV wall are clearly non-CAD-type LGE. It should be taken in mind that in a given patient both CAD-type and non-CAD-type LGE may be present. This may represent a mixed CMP, however

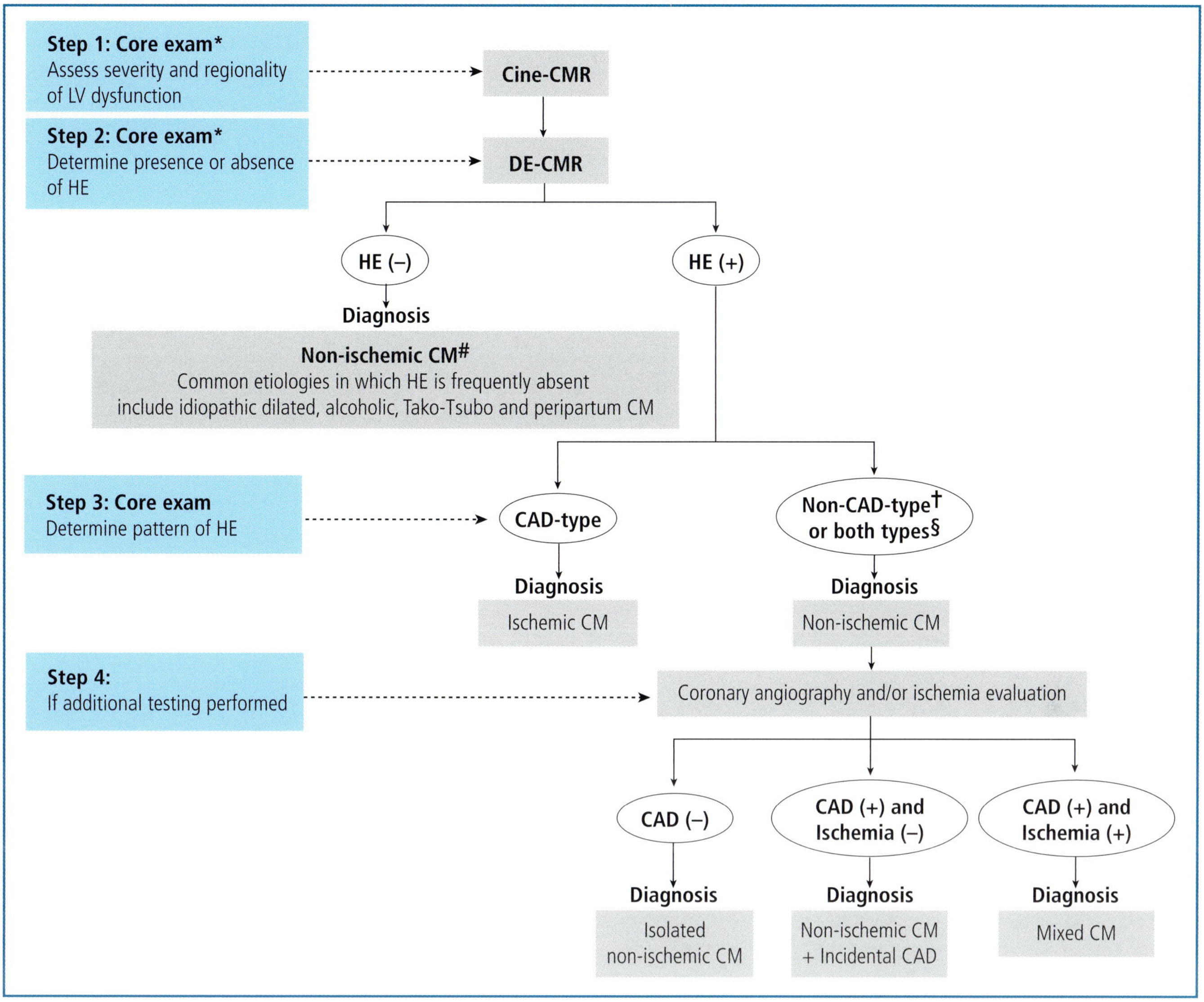

Figure 12-5 A stepwise approach incorporating DE-CMR for evaluation of patients with heart failure. CAD: coronary artery disease; CM: cardiomyopathy; CMR: cardiac magnetic resonance; DE: delayed enhancement; HE: hyperenhancement; LV: left ventricle.

* Core exam typically consists of cine- and delayed-enhancement MRI.

Presumes long-standing, chronic cardiomyopathy and severe ventricular dysfunction.

† See Figure 12-4 for details of non-CAD-type patterns of hyperenhancement in various non-ischemic cardiomyopathies.

§ Patients with non-ischemic cardiomyopathy often can have both CAD and non-CAD-type hyperenhancement (i.e. sarcoidosis).

certain non-ischemic cardiomyopathies (e.g. sarcoidosis) may present with both patterns. Further classification based on specific patterns associated with various non-ischemic disease processes is considered if LGE is present in a non-CAD pattern (Senthilkumar 2009). In some patients additional testing such as coronary angiography and/or stress perfusion CMR as a **forth step** might aid in the interpretation of DE-CMR findings. For example in patients with ICM and CAD-type scarring knowledge of coronary anatomy and/or the presence of ischemia will be useful for decisions regarding treatment, including interventional or surgical revascularisation. In a patient with non-CAD type scarring additional testing may reveal the precise cause or causes of cardiomyopathy. If coronary angiography demonstrates no atherosclerosis, ventricular dysfunction is caused solely by non-ICM. In the presence of coronary atherosclerosis without evidence of ischemia on functional testing the presence of non-ICM with incidental coronary artery disease has to be considered. On the other hand, patients with coronary lesions and inducible ischemia are likely to have a mixed disorder and to have ischemic and non-ischemic cardiomyopathy concomitantly (Senthilkumar 2009).

12.8 Outcome Studies in Heart Failure

Since CMR imaging has proven to be the gold standard for assessing cardiac structure and function several large scale clinical trials are using CMR substudies in the research protocol. In the EARTH study (Lüscher 2001) serial CMR studies were performed to assess changes in LV end-systolic volume (LVESV) over 24 wks from baseline by the endothelin A receptor antagonist darusentan. 642 patients were treated with 10, 25, 50, 100, or 300 mg of darusentan vs. placebo, and the primary endpoint LVESV assessed in 485 patients at baseline and follow-up was not significantly different from placebo with 10 mg (+ 1.28 ml) up to 300 mg (– 4.34 ml) of darusentan (Anand et al. 2004a). Similar adverse results on the dual receptor endothelin antagonist enrasentan were later on reported by Prasad et al. (2006) in asymptomatic individuals with LV dysfunction, who using CMR for LV volume assessment found an increased LVEDVI on enrasentan, in contrast to a decrease with enalapril, together with an increased cardiac index and LV mass index. It was concluded from this study that enrasentan at a dose of 60–90 mg/d over 6 mths causes adverse ventricular remodeling despite an increase in resting cardiac index.

Bello et al. (2003) studied 45 patients with chronic HF with CMR for LV function and viability on β-blocker therapy. Scarring was found in all patients with ICM, but in only 2 of 17 (12%) patients with non-ICM. In the 35 patients who were maintained on β-blockers and had a follow-up study, there was an inverse relationship between the extent of scarring at baseline and the likelihood of contractile improvement 6 mths later ($p < 0.001$). Multi-variate analysis showed that the amount of dysfunctional but viable myocardium by CMR was an independent predictor of the change in EF ($p = 0.01$), mean wall motion score ($p = 0.0007$), LVEDVI ($p = 0.007$), and LVESVI ($p \leq 0.0001$). It was concluded that in patients treated with β-blockers LGE on CMR predicts the response in LV function and remodeling.

Bellenger et al. (2004) reported in 34 patients with chronic HF on LV remodeling in a placebo-controlled trial with carvedilol. LV volumes were assessed before randomisation into carvedilol or placebo. Over the study period of 6 mths there was a significant reduction in ESVI and EDVI between the carvedilol and placebo group (carvedilol -9 ml/m^2 vs. placebo $+3$ ml/m^2, $p = 0.0004$; carvedilol -8 ml/m^2 vs. placebo 0 ml/m^2, $p = 0.05$). The LV ejection fraction increased significantly between the groups (carvedilol +3% vs. placebo −2%, $p = 0.003$). It was concluded that in patients with chronic HF carvedilol results in significant improvement in left ventricular volumes and function that may contribute to the benefits of carvedilol on mortality and morbidity in this patient group.

In a substudy on 69 randomly selected eligible patients out of the 912 patients of the RENAISSANCE Trial CMR was used at entry and 24 wks later to assess LV function, volume and muscular mass index (LVMI) (Anand et al. 2004b). The study revealed that anemia is common in CHF patients and is associated with increasing disease severity, i.e. greater HF severity was found to be associated with lower hemoglobin (Hb) concentrations. An increase in Hb over time was associated with a decrease in LVMI and lower mortality, whereas a decrease in Hb over time was associated with an increase in LVMI and higher mortality. It was concluded that lower Hb is associated with greater disease severity, a greater LVMI, and higher hospitalization and mortality rates.

12.9 Assessment of LV Dyssynchrony

Cardiac resynchronisation therapy (CRT) is a new modality to improve symptoms and prognosis of patients with severe heart failure and interventricular/intraventricular dyssynchrony. Standard CRT criteria are NYHA classification III–IV, left ventricular ejection fraction ≤ 35%, and QRS width ≥ 120 ms. Moreover, several echocardiographic parameter have been developed (e.g. IVMD, SPWMD, LVIVD using tissue Doppler) to assess inter- and intraventricular dyssynchrony. However, in the PROSPECT multi-center study on 498 patients fulfilling standard CRT criteria, 12 echocardiographic parameters of dyssynchrony were tested. Sensitivities for clinical improvement were 6–74%, specificity 35–91%, and for LVESV decrease ≥ 15% sensitivity was 9–77% and specificity 31–93% (Chung 2008). Despite several criticisms of this study alternative imaging methods have to be used in order to quantitate inter- and intraventricular dyssynchrony and to better predict the response to CRT, since 20–30% of patients are non-responders to CRT despite classical CRT entry criteria.

12.9.1 Velocity-Encoded CMR and 3D LV Contraction Analysis

Since CMR provides accurate morphological and functional analysis with excellent temporal and spatial resolution with high accuracy and reproducibility for quantifying LV volumes and function, this technique is increasingly used for assessing dyssynchrony. Westenberg et al. (2006) performed a head to head comparison between tissue Doppler imaging (TDI) and velocity-encoded MR imaging to assess septal-to-lateral delay as a marker of intraventricular dyssynchrony, and found excellent agreement between both techniques for classification according to severity of dyssynchrony. Koos et al. (2008) compared global volumes, ejection fraction and the SDI (standard deviation of the time intervals) of 17 regional systolic volumes to reach a minimum in the volume time curve. In 45 patients including 35 with reduced LV function and wide QRS complex compared to 10 control subjects, SDI differed significantly between patients (14 ± 5%) and controls (5 ± 2%, $p < 0.001$), and an exponential correlation between EF and SDI was observed. Another study by Fornwalt et al. (2008) determined the internal flow fraction defined as the total internal flow as a percentage of stroke volume during systole from LV volume reconstructions within 16 regions; IFF_{whole} (internal flow fraction over whole systole) was significantly increased in 10 patients with dyssynchrony (9.9 ± 5.0% vs. 1.5 ± 0.5% in the controls, $p < 0.001$), and an IFF_{whole} threshold of 4% discriminated between patients and controls with 99% sensitivity and 100% specificity. These three studies were not designed to predict the response to CRT therapy.

Bilchik et al. (2008) used myocardial tagging (MR-MT) to predict response of HF patients to CRT. Two cohorts of patients were studied, a CRT HF cohort (n = 20, LVEF 0.23 ± 0.057) to evaluate the role of MR-MT and DE-CMR prior to CRT and a multi-modality cohort (n = 27, LVEF 0.20 ± 0.066) and 9 healthy controls to compare tagging and tissue Doppler-derived septal-lateral delay for assessment of mechanical dyssynchrony. Short-axis tagged slices were analysed by HARP to assess strain, and regional systolic circumferential strains and time from end-diastole to peak circumferential strain were determined in 24 LV segments. Mechanical dyssynchrony was indexed by the circumferential uniformity ratio estimate (CURE), values for CURE range from 0 (pure dyssynchrony) to 1 (perfectly synchronous). Control subjects had highly synchronous contractions (CURE 0.96 ± 0.01), but TDI indicated dyssynchrony in 44%. Using a cut-off of < 0.75 for CURE 56% of patients tested positive for mechanical dyssynchrony, and the tagging-derived CURE predicted improved function class with 90% accuracy. Adding DE-CMR (% total scar < 15%) data improved accuracy further to 95% (positive and negative predictive values: 93%, 100%). The cohort 2 showed a 30% discordance rate between CURE and TDI septal-lateral delay. It was concluded that MR-MT predicts improvement in function class after CRT and adding scar imaging further improves this predictive value.

12.9.2 Role of Myocardial Scarring

Several investigations have described the role of myocardial scar for CRT response. White et al. (2006) were able to show in 23 patients with HF undergoing CRT that percent total scar was significantly higher in the non-response vs. response group (median and interquartal range of 24.7% [18.1–48.7] vs. 1% [0.0–8.7], $p = 0.0022$). A cut-off value of 15% total scar provided a sensitivity and specificity of 85 and 90%, respectively, for clinical response to CRT. Similarly, septal scar ≤ 40% provided a 100% sensitivity and specificity for response. In contrast Bleeker et al. (2006) examined the role of posterolateral scar tissue on clinical and echocardiographic improvement after CRT. Dyssynchrony was assessed at baseline and immediately after implantation with tissue Doppler imaging. 14 patients (35%) had a transmural (> 50% of LV wall thickness) posterolateral scar, these patients showed a low response rate compared to those without scar (14% vs. 81%, $p < 0.05$) and did not improve in clinical or echocardiographic parameters. In addition, LV dyssynchrony remained unchanged after CRT, whereas patients without posterolateral scar tissue and severe baseline dyssynchrony (≥ 65 ms) showed an excellent response rate of 95% compared with patients with a posterolateral scar and/or absent LV dyssynchrony (11%).

Similar results were reported by Chalil et al. (2007a) who assessed scar size (percentage of LVMM), location, and transmurality prior to CRT using DE-CMR and followed clinical improvement by 6 min walking distance (6 MWD) and quality of life (QoL) before and after CRT. Responders had a higher LVEF ($p = 0.048$), smaller scars (< 33%) ($p = 0.009$), and fewer scars with ≥ 51% transmurality ($p = 0.002$). Scar size correlated negatively with changes in 6 MWD and QoL scores. Among the patients with posterolateral scars, a transmurality value of ≥ 51% was associated with a particularly poor response rate (23%), compared with scars with < 51% transmurality (88%, $p < 0.001$). In multivariate analysis both scar size ($p = 0.022$) and transmurality ($p = 0.004$) emerged as predictors of response in patients with posterolateral scars, pacing outside the scar was associated with a better responder rate than pacing over the scar (86 vs. 33%, $p = 0.004$). It was concluded that in patients with ischemic cardiomyopathy, a scar size ≥ 33%, a transmurality ≥ 51%, and pacing over a posterolateral scar are associated with a suboptimal response to CRT.

12.9.3 Prognostic Impact of CMR Derived Dyssynchrony

Chalil et al. (2007b) could show that the CMR derived tissue synchronisation index (TSI) as a parameter of LV dyssynchrony had prognostic impact in 77 patients with HF undergoing CRT. Kaplan-Meier curves showed that patients with a TSI ≥ 110 ms had worse outcome regarding survival from death from any cause or hospitalisation for MACE, hospitalisation for HF, survival from death from any cause, and survival from cardiovascular death. These results are puzzling because on one hand LV dyssynchrony is a predictor of increased mortality in patients with HF, on the other hand CRT should improve outcome and clinical parameters in patients with HF. This discrepancy may be explained by the study of Leyva et al. (2009), who developed a triple index to predict survival after CRT. Out of 16 prognostic risk factors of HF patients, Cox proportional hazards analyses revealed dyssynchrony, posterolateral scar and elevated creatinine as independent predictors of cardiovascular mortality (DSC index). Compared to patients with a DSC < 3, cardiovascular mortality in patients in the intermediate DSC index (3–5; HR: 11.1 [95% CI 3.00 to 41.1, p = 0.0003]) and high DSC index group (≥ 5; HR: 30.5 [95% CI 9.15 to 101.8, p < 0.0001]) was significantly higher. In this study HR of posterolateral scar location was 12.2 compared to CMR-TSI with a HR 1.01 and creatinine with a HR 1.01, and thus, posterolateral scar was the most significant prognostic parameter within this triple DSC index.

12.9.4 MR Angiography of Coronary Veins

CMR imaging may add another important support for CRT, since non-invasive angiography of the coronary veins can be performed (Rasche 2007, Nezafat 2007, Younger 2009). This offers the opportunity for the implanting cardiologist or surgeon to have a prior look at the venous anatomy (coronary sinus, great cardiac vein, lateral vein), where the left lateral pacing lead has to be implanted. Moreover recent own investigations using multi-modal CMR imaging have shown that a correlation can be made between left lateral local contraction, left lateral myocardial scar, and the location of the lateral vein for lead placement.

In summary, CMR plays an increasing role not only in the evaluation of cardiac dyssynchrony in HF patients, but also for prediction of CRT response and prognosis, and for facilitating and optimizing lead placement for biventricular pacing.

12.10 Prognostic Information

CMR may provide independent prognostic information in HF patients by both LV and RV function and LGE. Nazarian et al. (2005) reported that in 26 patients with non-ICM predominance of scar distribution, assessed by LGE on CMR, involving 26–75% of wall thickness was significantly predictive of inducible VT on EPS and remained predictive after adjustment for LVEF (OR 9.125, p = 0.020). Thus, scar distribution may identify the substrate for inducible VT and may identify high-risk patients with non-ICM. Similar results were reported by Yokokawa et al. (2008) in 47 patients with IDCM and advanced HF.

Yokota et al. (2008) studied 86 patients with ICM with a mean LVEF of 26 ± 12% using DE-CMR with a follow-up of 20 ± 16 mths; patients developing cardiovascular events (CHF 33, VA 9, MI 2, revascularization 5, death 6) had larger scar volume and scar percentage of the myocardium than patients without events (16.8 ± 12.4 cm^3 vs. 11.7 ± 12.6 cm^3, p = 0.023 and 10.2 ± 6.9% vs. 7.2 ± 6.7%, p = 0.037, respectively). Quantification of scar volume was superior to LVEDV, LVESV, and LVEF in prognosticating future cardiovascular events in ICM patients. Similar results were reported by Kwon et al. (2009) in 349 patients with ICM and severely reduced LVEF. Mean scar percentage and transmurality score were higher in patients with events (56 events: 51 deaths, 5 CTx) vs. those without (39 ± 22 vs. 30 ± 20, p = 0.003, and 9.7 ± 5 vs. 7.8 ± 5, p = 0.004). Unrecognized non-Q-wave myocardial infarction was shown in a systematic study in 185 patients with suspected CAD without clinical or ECG evidence of prior infarction to be associated with an 11-fold higher mortality risk independent of LVEF (Kim 2009).

In a total of 101 consecutive patients with non-ICM and HF Asomull et al. (2006) found midwall fibrosis by DE-CMR in 35%, which was associated with a higher rate of pre-defined combined endpoint of all-cause death and hospitalization for a cardiovascular event (HR 3.4, p = 0.01) and for prediction of secondary endpoint SCD/VT (HR 5.2, p = 0.03). In this study RV volumes, CI, and classical ECG parameters were not included in the multivariate model. Wu et al. (2008) in a series of 65 patients with non-ICM and EF ≤ 35% planned for an ICD implantation, found LGE in 27 (42%) patients, and 12 of LGE positive patients (44%) had an index composite outcome event (cardiac death, appropriate ICD firing, and hospitalization for decompensated HF) vs. only 8% of LGE negative patients (p < 0.001). After adjustment for LV volume index and functional class, patients with LGE had an 8-fold higher risk of experiencing the primary outcome (HR 8.2, 95% CI 2.2 to 30.9, p = 0.002). It should be mentioned that this was a small and selected group of the sickest IDCM patients with a depressed LVEF, and ECG and RV volume parameters were not included into the statistical model, as well.

Hombach et al. (2009) studied 141 consecutive IDCM patients by clinical, conventional ECG, CMR functional parameters, and DE-CMR. In 63 patients myocardial biopsy was performed, and chronic inflammation was excluded by molecular analysis. Non-CAD type mid-wall or subepicardial LGE was present in 36 patients (26%). After median follow-up of 1339 d including 483 patient years 25 patients (18%) experienced the primary endpoint (cardiac death 16, sudden death 3 plus 6 with an ICD shock). Kaplan-Meier analysis showed QRS > 110 ms ($p = 0.010$), presence of LGE ($p = 0.037$), and diabetes mellitus ($p < 0.001$) as significant predictors of a worse outcome. Multi-variate analysis revealed CI ($p < 0.001$) and increased RVEDVI ($p = 0.006$) derived from CMR, the presence of diabetes mellitus ($p = 0.006$), and QRS > 110 ms ($p = 0.0045$) as significant predictors of the primary endpoint. In conclusion, it was stressed that prognostically relevant hemodynamic (CI, RVEDVI) and ECG parameters (QRS duration) can be derived from two non-invasive techniques with highest precision and without complicated analysis techniques.

12.11 Cardiac Transplantation

12.11.1 Surgical Technique

Cardiac transplantation continues to be the gold standard for treatment of end stage cardiac diseases refractory to medical therapy. For orthotopic transplantation two techniques are used to replace the recipient heart with the donor heart: the classic Shumway-Lower bi-atrial transplant technique, in which the donor's right atrium is attached directly to the recipient's right atrium, and the bi-caval technique increasingly used, in which the superior and inferior vena cava are attached separately and the left atrial anastomosis is done as a cuff. The standard bi-atrial technique results in disruption of normal atrial geometry, and leads to increased atrial size with abnormal or reduced atrial contribution to ventricular filling, right ventricular dysfunction, tricuspid and mitral insufficiency, and sinus node dysfunction. Although the bi-caval technique results in a slightly longer donor heart ischemia time, it preserves the anatomical integrity of the atria with lower right atrial pressures, a lower incidence of atrial tachyarrhythmias, and less tricuspid valve incompetence. Despite increasing use of the bi-caval technique, tricuspid regurgitation remains a problem early and late after cardiac transplantation.

12.11.2 Pathophysiology, Clinical Course, Complications and Prognosis

The cardiac allograft is functionally and anatomically denervated, and therefore cannot increase heart rate adequately to increase cardiac output acutely during exercise. Therefore, the transplanted heart relies on the Frank Starling mechanism to increase cardiac output in response to an increase in venous return at the onset of acute exercise. Circulating catecholamine levels rise later and provide a delayed chronotropic response to exercise. Within one year after transplantation a partial reinnervation of sympathetic and parasympathetic nerves goes on, these reinnervation phenomena are incomplete and vary from patient to patient. Coronary reserve of the transplanted heart is normal and reduced during periods of acute rejection. The mean 1-yr survival rate of transplanted patients is 85 % or greater, and survival rates of 90–95 % at 1 yr are not uncommon. The biggest impact on survival has been in the early peri-operative phase and in the first few months after transplantation. Beyond this period there has been a consistent slow steady decline in survival with a mortality rate of 4 % per year usually related to the complications of immune suppression or the development of coronary artery vasculopathy. The 10-yrs survival rate is approximately 50 % or even greater.

Acute and subacute complications are allograft rejection, long-term cardiac complications are the development of transplant coronary artery disease (TVP), and the major non-cardiac complications malignancy, infection, hypertension, renal failure, and osteoporosis. Of greatest importance is the timely diagnosis of rejection. The clinical signs are fever, tachycardia, cardiac arrhythmias and peripheral edema. Gold standard for confirming the diagnosis is myocardial biopsy, however, non-invasive techniques such as intramyocardial electrogram, signal-averaged high-resolution surface ECG, serum markers like troponin and others, echocardiography and Doppler echocardiography, and CMR may be used instead of or in combination with endomyocardial biopsy. Recently the CARGO study group was formed in 2001 to investigate the usefulness of molecular testing for gene expression in peripheral blood cells for the diagnosis of cardiac rejection (Al Khaldi and Robbins 2006). This group looked for specific changes in the pattern of gene expression in peripheral blood cells and showed a good correlation and high predictive value for these molecular fingerprinting techniques to predict future acute rejections. Thus, molecular testing for gene expression in peripheral blood cells may ultimately replace routine endomyocardial biopsy for rejection surveillance. In addition, there remains a role for imaging techniques to detect diastolic and systolic dysfunctions, and changes in both myocardial mass, water content, and regional damage.

12.11.3 Detection of Hemodynamic Alterations and Peri-Operative Complications

Following transplantation in case of bi-atrial connection those sections of the recipient and donor atria are intact but do not contract synergistically leading to a decreased atrial input with a consecutive lower net stroke volume than that in the native heart, as shown by Lauerma et al. (1996). In contrast, Walpoth et al. (1995) could show that both right and left-atrial emptying fractions were significantly higher in the bicaval vs. the biatrial patient group, but these parameters were significantly lower in the two transplant groups vs. normal controls. Immediately in the post-operative period a "stiff" heart develops with restrictive hemodynamic patterns resulting in low cardiac output. There are further reasons of low cardiac output such as vasopressor drugs used in the donor, ischemic injury at the time of donor procurement, denervation, high peripheral vascular resistance, myocardial edema, and allograft rejection. There are also possible further complications such as constrictive pericarditis, pleural or pericardial effusion, hemorrhage, and endocardial thrombi. All these altered structural or functional processes can be well-assessed by CMR imaging. Particularly important is thrombus formation most currently in the morphologically abnormal atria and they present as soft tissue mass with heterogenous intensity. On T1- or T2-weighted fast spin echo (TSE) images thrombi appear as intermediate to high signal intensity structures, on CE-MRI images as non-enhancing dark structures, which can be nulled at a specific TI time of about 600 ms at 1.5 T (Weinsaft 2008). Pericardial effusion may also be detected very easily including hemorrhagic contents of fibrotic strains. The abnormal function of the atria and low cardiac output syndrome can also be easily assessed by CMR quantitative LV and RV volumetric measurements including cardiac index.

12.11.4 Allograft Rejection in Animals and Humans

T1 and T2 Relaxation Times

The gold standard for detection of cellular cardiac rejection has been regular transjugular endomyocardial biopsy. However, this technique is uncomfortable for patients and has the potential for rare, but life-threatening complications as well as random biopsy sampling often misses the patchy foci of rejection and there is significant variability in the reporting of histologic specimen. During acute heart transplant rejection the myocardium is inflamed with increased water content (edema), increased myocardial mass and diastolic dysfunction followed by systolic dysfunction. Promising CMR correlates of rejection are assessment of T2- and T1-relaxation times, of diastolic dysfunction, abnormal ventricular twist, late gadolinium enhancement, and paramagnetic iron oxide contrast agents.

Myocardial T2 signal intensity (SI) is influenced by myocardial water content, and T2-SI has been used for CMR-based detection of allograft rejection with mixed results. Therefore T2 quantification by T2 relaxation time has been proposed, which is calculated by plotting the spin echo signal intensity against varying echo times, whereby each CMR laboratory should define its own normal T2 relaxation times from a group of controls and describe abnormal T2 relaxation as more than two standard deviations above the mean (Butler 2009).

In 11 animal trials since 1985 T2 relaxation time and transplant rejection have been evaluated and it has been shown that T2 relaxation times increased with histologic rejection and ex-vivo myocardial water content (Butler 2009). In human cardiac transplants with a total of 302 patients with 521 CMR scans T2 relaxation times were compared to transplant rejection as determined by endomyocardial biopsy, and in four trials a significant correlation between prolonged T2 relaxation times and transplant rejection was reported (Marie 1998, Marie 2001, Lund 1988, Wisenberg 1987). Two trials did not find an association between T2 and rejection, and both gated the image acquisition to ventricular systole that often leads to signal loss and poor image quality. It should be borne in mind that T2 relaxation times are not able to discriminate rejecting and non-rejecting allografts in the early 24 h-peri-operative period due to normal inflammation and edema, induced by cold ischemic time and cardio-protective solution etc. that occurs early after heart transplantation. A prolonged T2 relaxation time appears as a relatively sensitive CMR parameter to predict rejection at grade 2 ESHLT 1990. However, one needs to keep in mind some technical limitations to current T2 imaging, e.g. signal drop-out, motion artifacts, SE vs. TSE sequences, signal gradation, multi-exponential T2 behaviour.

T1-weighted CMR images are influenced by myocardial water content, as well, although to a lesser extent than T2-weighted images. Using myocardial T1 signal intensity only inconsistent correlations with rejections in animal models were reported. In 25 human heart transplant recipients Wisenberg et al. (1987) could show that T1 relaxation times were significantly prolonged for those with rejection compared to non-rejection, and both T1 and T2 relaxation times were only correlated with biopsy proven rejection after 24 d post-transplantation. T1 relaxation times and transplant rejection have been very rarely studied mainly because T2-weighted images have been shown to have superior sensitivity to detect increased water content (Butler 2009). One should note that T1-weighted imaging has been performed primarily using older techniques that are far less sensitive and specific to T1-weighting than DE-CMR techniques.

Gadolinium-Based Contrast Imaging (Early Contrast Enhancement)

T1-weighted images following administration of gadolinium-based contrast agents have also been used to assess myocardial inflammation (concept of early contrast enhancement). In two human trials of transplant rejection, post-contrast signal intensity tended to increase with the degree of rejection although it could not consistently identify the full spectrum of abnormal endomyocardial biopsy diagnostic of rejection (Almenar 2003, Mousseaux 1993). In the study of Alemnar et al. on 40 heart transplant patients no association was found between contrast-enhanced SI with T1 and allograft rejection. Mousseaux et al. examined 39 heart transplant patients and found an increase in myocardial enhancement in rejectors compared with non-rejectors, however, myocardial enhancement was not able to discriminate rejection severity. At present gadolinium-based early enhancement imaging does not seem to be a very strong parameter for allograft rejection.

Morphological and Functional Parameters

Myocardial wall thickness has been shown to increase in animal and human CMR trials of transplant rejection (Butler 2009), and several animal studies showed that increased wall thickness during acute rejection was correlated to total myocardial water content. But wall thickness from CMR imaging was not able to accurately identify the severity of a rejection episode, particularly of the less severe but clinically most important episodes. The same holds true for decreased systolic ventricular function in the phase of acute rejection, and detailed CMR studies on diastolic dysfunction as the earliest sign of acute rejection have not been performed as yet. Another interesting functional parameter is twisting mechanics. Hansen et al. (1987) using radio-opaque intramyocardial markers and biplane fluoroscopy to serially study systolic torsion and diastolic recoil in 12 transplant recipients found a 25% decrease in torsional deformation amplitude and peak systolic torsion during periods of rejection compared to pre-rejection periods. Though CMR-based quantification of myocardial twisting is standardized by myocardial tagging and strain analysis, up to now CMR studies have not been published to prove this non-invasive concept for early non-invasive diagnosis of allograft rejection.

T1 and T2 Contrast Agents (Iron Oxide Particles)

Iron oxide contrast agents (USPIOS) are used for contrast-enhanced angiography and diagnosis of malignant tumors. Moreover, these particles are taken up over time by macrophages, which shortens their T2/T2* relaxation. Thereby, accumulation of iron oxide containing macrophages in inflamed tissues can be visualized as a signal loss on T2-weighted images. Up to now only animal studies with iron oxide particles have been reported. Kanno et al. (2001) showed that T2 signal intensity (SI) decreased 24 h after iron oxide particle injection in rejecting grafts, and after treatment with cyclosporine for 7 d SI returned to baseline. Immunohistochemistry confirmed accumulation of iron oxide containing macrophages in areas of rejection. Johansson et al. (2002) showed that 6 d post-transplant T1-SI increased within the allografts of untreated rat recipients by mean 25% 5 min after injection of iron oxide particles, indicating an increased vascular permeability due to acute rejection-inflammation. Similar results were reported by Penno et al. (2007), who showed that SI in rejecting rat allografts was significantyly elevated compared with immunosuppressed allografts within 4 min post-contrast injection. These preliminary results indicate that CMR with iron oxide particles as a novel and powerful technique to evaluate inflammation of the heart in acute rejection episodes may identify not only increased vascular permeability by T1 imaging early post-iron oxide contrast injection, but also in vivo macrophage accumulation in the inflamed heart by delayed T2 imaging. Whether micrometer-sized iron oxide particles (MIOs) are better suited for detecting acute (Wu 2006) or chronic rejection (Ye 2008), remains to be studied in further animal and later on human studies.

12.11.5 Long-Term Allograft Surveillance

Because the transplanted heart is denervated, heart rate does not vary with respiration and does not respond to Valsalva maneuvers or carotid massage, and altered cardiovascular response to exercise and cardiac electrophysiology is present. Due to the denervation most patients do not experience angina after transplant vasculopathy (TVP) has emerged. In addition, most patients develop concentric myocardial hypertrophy and high ejection fractions in the later stages of transplantation. Due to its excellent tissue contrast and high temporal and spatial resolution CMR imaging may become the ideal tool to perform serial controls on patients with heart transplantation regarding cardiac morphology and function, particularly ventricular volumes and muscle mass. Moreover, CMR imaging may also be used for early detection of TVP, either by performing first-pass perfusion studies (FPP) to detect myocardial ischemia, or by non-invasive MR coronary angiography (MRCA).

TVP is a common phenomenon with an incidence of 5–10% per year and 45–50% of all cardiac transplant patients develop TVP with an incidence of critical coronary stenoses of 5–10% within 5 yrs. Muehling et al. (2003) assessed myocardial perfusion reserve (MPR, CFR) and endo/epi flow ratio in normals and HTx-patients. Patients without LVH or rejection and those with either of this phenotype had CFR ≥ 2.5, patients with Tx-CAD by angiography had a reduced CFR < 2.5 and reduced endo/epi ratio. Tx-CAD could be excluded by a MPR of > 2.3 (sensitivity 100%, specificity 85%) and an endo/epi ratio of > 1.3 (sensitivity 100%, specificity 80%). Further studies are needed to determine the role of FPP for early detection of TVP.

Two studies reported on non-invasive MRCA to diagnose TVP. Mohiaddin et al. (1996) studied 60 patients after heart transplantation compared to conventional invasive coronary angiography about 6 yrs after transplantation. For the right coronary artery sensitivity and specificity for detecting significant stenoses were 100 and 75%, respectively; specificity for detecting stenotic segments in the left main and descending coronary artery was 86%, and combined sensitivity and specificity for left and right coronary arteries were only 56 and 82%, respectively. Davis et al. (1996) studied 18 patients with heart transplantation using MRCA and found normal coronary anatomy of left main in 15 of 15 patients, in 5 of 10 patients 9 discrete 50% diameter stenoses were detected, and MRCA detected 7 of 9 of these stenoses. In a recent study Usta et al. (2009) used multi-slice computer tomography (MSCT), coronary angiography and CMR imaging to assess cardiac allograft vasculopathy in 10 asymptomatic long-term survivors after heart transplantation. MSCT correctly identified lesions in the large epicardial vessel segments in all patients compared to invasive coronary angiography. LGE as a sign of myocardial injury or scarring after prior rejections was found in four patients, a severely reduced LV function in one patient with CAD and two prior acute rejections. The histologically determined degree of rejection in myocardial biopsies correlated positively with the LGE findings confirming fibrosis of the myocardium. None of the examined endomyocardial specimen showed cardiac allograft rejection greater than I R. Whether this combined approach is reliable to detect both chronic rejection and TVP, has to be confirmed by further larger prospective studies.

Another approach towards earlier detection of TVP was reported by Steen et al. (2008), who compared DE-CMR CAD-type of LGE (grade I $\leq$ 25% to IV $\geq$ 75 transmurality) with coronary angiography TVP (mild, moderate 25–75% stenosis, and severe $\geq$ 75% stenosis). CAD-type LGE was already found in TVP grade I and II and increased significantly between groups I (23%), II (33%), and III (84%, $p < 0.05$) and involved only single vessel territories in TVP, but multiple vessels in TVP II and III. Non-CAD-type LGE was equally distributed across all TVP stages and was associated with a significantly higher LV ejection fraction than patients with CAD-type LGE or combined pattern (66 $\pm$ 6% vs. 45 $\pm$ 16% or 60 $\pm$ 13%, $p < 0.05$). It was concluded that DE-CMR allows both identification of silent MIs in apparently event-free HTx patients and disclosure of myocardial fibrosis in patients with absent or mild TVP, and thus, may help to establish an earlier diagnosis of TVP.

12.12 Conclusions and Future Perspectives

CMR imaging has been proven to reliably assess cardiac morphology, function and alterations of myocardial tissue in normals as well as in HF patients, and impaired hemodynamics and reduced response to exercise in HF patients can be accurately measured. In addition, CMR may be useful for unraveling the etiology of HF by a systematic stepwise approach, as well as for serial follow-up of HF patients on maintenance medical therapy, or for identifying HF patients as responders to CRT. In heart transplant patients structural and functional alterations of the allograft may be followed and acute rejection may be diagnosed. Transplant vasculopathy may be detected by first-pass perfusion studies, by detection of CAD-type late gadolinium enhancement, and by MR coronary angiography. In the future larger prospective studies have to be performed to define the ultimate role of CMR imaging in the many different diagnostic and therapeutic tasks in patients with chronic heart failure.

References

Al Khaldi A, Robbins RC. New directions in cardiac transplantation. Annu Rev Med 2006; 57: 455–62.

Almenar L, Igual B, Martínez-Dolz L et al. Utility of cardiac magnetic resonance imaging for the diagnosis of heart transplant rejection. Transplant Proc 2003; 35 (5): 1962–4.

Anand I, McMurray JJ, Cohn JN et al. EARTH investigators. Long-term effects of darusentan on left-ventricular remodeling and clinical outcomes in the endothelin A receptor antagonist trial in heart Failure (EARTH): randomised, double-blind, placebo-controlled trial. Lancet 2004a; 364: 347–54.

Anand I, McMurray JJ, Whitmore J et al. Anemia and its relationship to clinical outcome in heart failure. Circulation 2004b; 110 (2): 149–54.

Assomull RG, Prasad SK, Lyne J et al. Cardiovascular magnetic resonance, fibrosis, and prognosis in dilated cardiomyopathy. J Am Coll Cardiol 2006; 48 (10): 1977–85.

Bellenger NG, Davies LC, Francis JM et al. Reduction in sample size for studies of remodeling in heart failure by the use of cardiovascular magnetic resonance. J Cardiovasc Magn Reson 2000; 2: 271–8.

Bellenger NG, Rajappan K, Rahman SL et al. on behalf of the CHRISTMAS Study Steering Committee and Investigators. Effects of carvedilol on left ventricular remodeling in chronic stable heart failure: a cardiovascular magnetic resonance study. Heart 2004; 90 (7): 760–4.

Bello D, Shah DJ, Farah GM et al. Gadolinium cardiovascular magnetic resonance predicts reversible myocardial dysfunction and remodeling in patients with heart failure undergoing beta-blocker therapy. Circulation 2003; 108 (16): 1945–53.

Bilchick KC, Dimaano V, Wu KC et al. Cardiac magnetic resonance assessment of dyssynchrony and myocardial scar predicts function class improvement following cardiac resynchronization therapy. JACC Cardiovasc Imaging 2008; 1 (5): 561–8.

Bleeker GB, Kaandorp TAM, Lamb HJ et al. Effect of posterolateral scar tissue on clinical and echocardiographic improvment after cardiac resynchronisation therapy. Circulation 2006; 113: 969–76.

Boucher CA, Fallon JT, Johnson RA, Yurchak PM. Cardiomyopathic syndrome caused by coronary artery disease. III: Prospective clinicopathological study of its prevalence among patients with clinically unexplained chronic heart failure. Br Heart J 1979; 41 (5): 613–20.

Butler CR, Thompson R, Haykowsky M et al. Cardiovascular magnetic resonance in the diagnosis of acute heart transplant rejection: a review. J Cardiovasc Magn Reson 2009; 11 (1): 7.

Chalil S, Foley PW, Muyhaldeen SA et al. Late gadolinium enhancement-cardiovascular magnetic resonance as a predictor of response to cardiac resynchronization therapy in patients with ischemic cardiomyopathy. Europace 2007a; 9 (11): 1031–7.

Chalil S, Stegemann B, Muhyaldeen S et al. Intraventricular dyssynchrony predicts mortality and morbidity after cardiac resynchronization therapy: a study using cardiovascular magnetic resonance tissue synchronization imaging. J Am Coll Cardiol 2007b; 50 (3): 243–52.

Choudhury L, Mahrholdt H, Wagner A et al. Myocardial scarring in asymptomatic or mildly symptomatic patients with hypertrophic cardiomyopathy. J Am Coll Cardiol 2002; 40 (12): 2156–64.

Chung ES, Leon AR, Tavazzi L et al. Results of the Predictors of Response to CRT (PROSPECT) trial. Circulation 2008; 117: 2608–16.

Davis SF, Kannam JP, Wielopolski P et al. Magnetic resonance coronary angiography in heart transplantat recipients. J Heart Lung Transplant 1996; 15: 580–6.

De Keulenaer GW, Brutsaert DL. The Heart Failure Spectrum-Time for a phenotype-oriented approach. Editorial. Circulation 2009; 119: 3044–6.

Donofrio MT, Clark BJ, Ramaciotti C et al. Regional wall motion and strain of transplanted hearts in pediatric patients using magnetic resonance tagging. Am J Physiol 1999; 277: R1481–R1487.

Elliott P, Andersson B, Arbustini E et al. Classification of the cardiomyopathies: a position statement from the European Society of Cardiology Working Group on Myocardial and Pericardial Diseases. Eur Heart J 2008, 29: 270–6.

Felker GM, Shaw LK, O'Connor CM. A standardized definition of ischemic cardiomyopathy for use in clinical research. J Am Coll Cardiol 2002; 39: 210–8.

Felker GM, Thompson RE, Hare JM et al. Underlying causes and long-term survival in patients with initially unexplained cardiomyopathy. N Engl J Med 2000; 342: 1077–84.

Follath F, Cleland JG, Klein W, Murphy R. Etiology and response to drug treatment in heart failure. J Am Coll Cardiol 1998; 32: 1167–72.

Fornwalt BK, Gonzales PC, Delfino JG et al. Quantification of left ventricular internal flow from cardiac magnetic resonance images in patients with dyssynchronous heart failure. J Magn Reson Imag 2008; 28: 375–81.

Hansen DE, Daughters GT, Alderman EL et al. Effect of acute human cardiac allograft rejection on left ventricular systolic torsion and diastolic recoil measured by intramyocardial markers. Circulation 1987; 76: 998–1008.

Ho KL, Pinksy JL, Kannel WB et al. The epidemiology of heart failure: The Framingham Study. JACC 1993; 22 (Suppl A): 6A.

Holman ER, Buller VG, Roos A et al. Detection and quantification of dysfunctional myocardium by magnetic resonance imaging. A new three-dimensional method for quantitative wall-thickening analysis. Circulation 1997; 95: 924–31.

Hombach V, Merkle N, Kestler HA et al. Characterization of patients with acute chest pain using cardiac magnetic resonance imaging. Clin Res Cardiol 2008; 97: 760–7.

Hombach V, Merkle N, Torzewski J et al. Electrocardiographic and cardiac magnetic resonance imaging parameters as predictors of a worse outcome in patients with idiopathic dilated cardiomyopathy. Eur Heart J 2009; 30 (16): 2011–8.

Hunt SA et al. for the 2005 Writing Committee Members and Jessup M et al. for the 2009 Focused Update Writing Group Members. 2009 Focused update incorporated into the ACC/AHA 2005 guidelines for the diagnosis and management of heart failure in adults: A report of the American College of Cardiology Foundation/American Heart Association Task Force on Practice Guidelines. Circulation 2009; 119: e391–e479.

Johansson L, Jonsson C, Penno E et al. Acute cardiac transplant rejection: detection and grading with MR imaging with a blood pool contrast agent-experimental study in the rat. Radiology 2002; 225: 97–103.

Kannel WB. Incidence and epidemiology of heart failure. Heart Fail Rev 2000; 5: 167–78.

Kanno S, Wu YJ, Lee PC et al. Macrophage accumulation associated with rat cardiac allograft rejection detected by magnetic resonance imaging with ultrasmall superparamagnetic iron oxide particles. Circulation 2001; 104: 934–8.

Kawaji K, Codella NC, Prince MR et al. Automated segmentation of routine clinical cardiac magnetic resonance imaging for assessment of left ventricular diastolic dysfunction. Circ Cardiovasc Imaging 2009; 2: 476–84.

Kim HW, Klem I, Shah DJ et al. Unrecognized non-Q-wave myocardial infarction: prevalence and prognostic significance in patients with suspected coronary disease. PLoS Med 2009; 6 (4): e1000057.

Kim RJ, Fieno DS, Parrish TB et al. Relationship of MRI delayed contrast enhancement to irreversible injury, infarct age, and contractile function. Circulation 1999; 100: 1992–2002.

Kim RJ, Wu E, Rafael A et al. The use of contrast-enhanced magnetic resonance imaging to identify reversible myocardial dysfunction. N Engl J Med 2000; 343: 1445–53.

Konstam MA. Progress in heart failure management? Lessons from the real world. Circulation 2000, 102: 1076.

Koos R, Neizel M, Schummers G et al. Feasibility and initial experience of assessment of mechanical dyssynchrony using cardiovascular magnetic resonance semi-automatic border detection. J Cardiovasc Magn Res 2008; 10: 49.

Kwon DH, Halley CM, Carrigan TP et al. Extent of left ventricular scar predicts outcomes in ischemic cardiomyopathy patients with significantly reduced systolic function: a delayed hyperenhancement cardiac magnetic resonance study. JACC Cardiovasc Imaging 2009; 2 (1): 34–44.

Lauerma K, Harjula A, Jarvinen V et al. Assessment of right and left atrial function in patients with transplanted hearts with the use of magnetic resonance imaging. J Heart Lung Transplant 1996; 15: 360–9.

Lee DS, Gona P, Vasan RS et al. Relation of disease pathogenesis and risk factors to heart failure with preserved or reduced ejection fraction: insights from the Framingham Heart Study of the National Heart, Lung, and Blood Institute. Circulation 2009; 119: 3070–7.

Lev D, Kenchaiah S, Larson MG et al. Long-term trends in the incidence of and survival with heart failure. N Engl J Med 2002; 347: 1397–406.

Leyva F, Foley PW, Stegemann B et al. Development and validation of a clinical index to predict survival after cardiac resynchronisation therapy. Heart 2009; 95 (19): 1619–25.

Lund G, Morin RL, Olivari MT, Ring WS. Serial myocardial T2 relaxation time measurements in normal subjects and heart transplant recipients. J Heart Transplant 1988; 7: 274–9.

Lüscher TF, Ruschitzka F, Anand I et al. on behalf of the EARTH investigators. EARTH: Endothelin a receptor antagonist trial in heart failure. Heart Drug 2001; 1: 294–8.

Maceira AM, Prasad SK, Khan M, Pennell DJ. Normalized left ventricular systolic and diastolic function by steady-state free precession cardiovascular magnetic resonance. J Cardiovasc Magn Reson 2006; 8: 417–26.

Mahrholdt H, Goedecke C, Wagner A et al. Cardiovascular magnetic resonance assessment of human myocarditis: a comparison to histology and molecular pathology. Circulation 2004; 109: 1250–8.

Mann DL. Pathophysiology of heart failure. In: Bonow RO, Mann DL, Zipes DP, Libby P (eds.). Braunwald's Heart Disease. A Textbook of Cardiovascular Medicine. Elsevier Saunders 2012; 487–504.

Marie PY, Carteaux JP, Angioi M et al. Detection and predicition of acute heart transplant rejection with the myocardial T2 determination provided by a black-blood magnetic resonance imaging sequence. J Am Coll Cardiol 2001; 37: 825–31.

Marie PY, Carteaux JP, Angioi M et al. Detection and prediction of acute heart transplant rejection: preliminary results on the clinical use of a "black-blood" magnetic resonance imaging sequence. Transplant Proc 1998; 30: 1933–5.

Maron BJ, Towbin JA, Thiene G et al. Contemporary definitions and classification of the cardiomyopathies: an AHA scientific statement from the Council on Clinical Cardiology, Heart Failure Research and Transplantation Committee; Quality of care and Outcomes Research and Functional Genomic and Translational Biology Interdisciplinary Working Groups; and Council on Epidemiology and Prevention. Circulation 2006; 113: 1807–16.

McCrohon JA, Moon JCC, Prasad SK et al. Differentiation of heart failure related to dilated cardiomyopathy and coronary artery disease using gadolinium-enhanced cardiovascular magnetic resonance. Circulation 2003; 108: 54–9.

Mohiaddin RH, Bongren HG, Lazim F et al. Magnetic resonance coronary angiography in heart transplant recipients. Coron Artery Dis 1996; 7: 591–7.

Moon JC, Sachdev B, Elkington AG et al. Gadolinium enhanced cardiovascular magnetic resonance in Anderson-Fabry disease. Evidence for a disease specific abnormality of the myocardial interstitium. Eur Heart J 2003; 24 (23): 2151–5.

Moon JCC, Reed E, Sheppard MN et al. The histologic basis of late gadolinium enhancement cardiovascular magnetic resonance in hypertrophic cardiomyopathy. J Am Coll Cardiol 2004; 43: 2260–4.

Mousseaux E, Farge D, Guillemain R et al. Assessing human cardiac allograft rejection using MRI with Gd-DOTA. J Comput Assist Tomogr 1993; 17 (2): 237–44.

Muehling OM, Wilke NM, Panse P et al. Reduced myocardial perfusion reserve and transmural perfusion gradient in heart transplant arteriopathy assessed by magnetic resonance imaging. J Am Coll Cardiol 2003; 42: 1054–60.

Nagel E, Schneider U, Schalla S. Magnetic resonance real-time imaging for the evaluation of left ventricular function. J Cardiovasc Magn Reson 2000; 2: 7–14.

Nazarian S, Bluemke DA, Lardo AC et al. Magnetic resonance assessment of the substrate for inducible ventricular tachycardia in non-ischemic cardiomyopathy. Circulation 2005; 112: 2821–5.

Nezafat R, Han Y, Peters DC et al. Coronary magnetic resonance vein imaging: Imaging contrast, sequence, and timing. Magn Reson Med 2007; 58: 1196–206.

Penno E, Johansson L, Ahlstrom H, Johnsson C. Ultrasmall iron oxide particle contrast agent and MRI can be used to monitor the effect of anti-rejection treatment. Transplantation 2007; 84: 374–9.

Prasad SK, Dargie HJ, Smith GC et al. Comparison of the dual receptor endothelin antagonist enrasentan with enalapril in asymptomatic left ventricular systolic dysfunction: a cardiovascular magnetic resonance study. Heart 2006; 92 (6): 798–803.

Rahimtoola SH, Dilsizian V, Kramer CM et al. Chronic ischemic left ventricular dysfunction: from pathophysiology to imaging and its integration into clinical practice. JACC Cardiovasc Imaging 2008; 1: 536–55.

Rasche V, Binner L, Cavagna F et al. Whole-heart coronary vein imaging: A comparison between non-contrast-agent and contrast-agent-enhanced visualization of the coronary venous system. Magn Reson Med 2007; 57: 1019–26.

Reimer KA, Lowe JE, Rasmussen MM, Jennings RB. The wavefront phenomenon of ischemic cell death. Myocardial infarct size vs. duration of coronary occlusion in dogs. Circulation 1977; 56: 786–94.

Roberts WC, Siegel RJ, McManus BM. Idiopathic dilated cardiomyopathy: analysis of 152 necropsy patients. Am J Cardiol 1987; 60: 1340–55.

Rochitte CE, Oliveira PF, Andrade JM et al. Myocardial delayed enhancement by magnetic resonance imaging in patients with Chagas' disease: a marker of disease severity. J Am Coll Cardiol 2005; 46 (8): 1553–8

Schuster EH, Bulkley BH. Ischemic cardiomyopathy: a clinicopathologic study of fourteen patients. Am Heart J 1980; 100 (4): 506–12.

Senthilkumar A, Majmudar MD, Shenoy C et al. Identifying the etiology: A systematic approach using delayed-enhancement cardiovascular magnetic resonance. Heart Failure Clin 2009; 5: 349–67.

Shah DJ, Judd RM, Kim RJ. Myocardial viability. In: Edelman RR, Hesselinik JR, Zlatkin MB (ed.). Clinical Magnetic Resonance Imaging. 3rd ed. New York: Elsevier 2006.

Soriano CJ, Ridocci F, Estornell J et al. Late gadolinium-enhanced cardiovascular magnetic resonance identifies patients with standardized definition of ischemic cardiomyopathy: A single center experience. Int J Cardiol 2007; 116: 167–73.

Soriano CJ, Ridocci F, Estornell J et al. Non-invasive diagnosis of coronary artery disease in patients with heart failure and systolic dysfunction of uncertain etiology, using late gadolinium-enhanced cardiovascular magnetic resonance. J Am Coll Cardiol 2005; 45: 743–8.

Steen H, Merten C, Refle S et al. Prevalence of different gadolinium enhancement patterns in patients after heart transplantation. J Am Coll Cardiol 2008; 52: 1160–7.

Uretsky BF, Thygessen K, Armstrong PW et al. Acute coronary findings at autopsy in heart failure patients with sudden death: results from the assessment of treatment with lisinopril and survival (ATLAS) trial. Circulation 2000; 102 (6): 611–6.

Usta E, Burgstahler C, Aebert H et al. The challenge to detect heart transplant rejection and transplant vasculopathy non-invasively – a pilot study. J Cardiothorac Surg 2009; 4: 43.

Walpoth BH, Lazeyras F, Tschopp A et al. Assessment of cardiac rejection and immunosupression by magnetic resonance imaging and spectroscopy. Transplant Proc 1995; 27: 2088–93.

Weinsaft JW, Kim HW, Shah DJ et al. Detection of left ventricular thrombus by delayed-enhancement cardiovascular magnetic resonance prevalence and markers in patients with systolic dysfunction. J Am Coll Cardiol 2008; 52: 148–57.

Westenberg JJM, Lamb HJ, van der Geest RJ et al. Assessment of left ventricular dyssynchrony in patients with conduction delay and idiopathic dilated cardiomyopathy. Head-to-head comparison between tissue Doppler imaging and velocity-encoded magnetic resonance imaging. J Am Coll Cardiol 2006; 47: 2042–8.

White JA, Yee R, Yuan X et al. Delayed enhancement magnetic resonance imaging predicts response to cardiac resynchronisation therapy in patients with intraventricular dyssynchrony. J Am Coll Cardiol 2006; 48: 1953–60.

Wisenberg G, Pflugfelder PW, Kostuk WJ et al. Diagnostic applicability of magnetic resonance imaging in assessing human cardiac allograft rejection. Am J Cardiol 1987; 60: 130–6.

Wu KC, Weiss RG, Thiemann DR et al. Late gadolinium enhancement by cardiovascular magnetic resonance heralds an adverse prognosis in non-ischemic cardiomyopathy. J Am Coll Cardiol 2008; 51 (25): 2414–21.

Wu YL, Ye Q, Foley LM et al. In situ labeling of immune cells with iron oxide particles: An approach to detect organ rejection by cellular MRI. Proc Natl Acad Sci U S A 2006; 103 (6): 1852–7.

Ye Q, Wu YL, Foley LM et al. Longitudinal tracking of recipient macrophages in a rat chronic cardiac allograft rejection model with non-invasive magnetic resonance imaging using micrometer-sized paramagnetic iron oxide particles. Circulation 2008; 118: 149–56.

Yokokawa M, Tada H, Koyama K et al. The characteristics and distribution of the scar tissue predict ventricular tachycardia in patients with advanced heart failure. Pacing Clin Electrophysiol 2009; 32 (3): 314–22.

Yokota H, Heidary S, Katikireddy CK et al. Quantitative characterization of myocardial infarction by cardiovascular magnetic resonance predicts future cardiovascular events in patients with ischemic cardiomyopathy. J Cardiovasc Mag Res 2008; 10: 17.

Younger JF, Plein S, Crean A et al. Visualization of coronary venous anatomy by cardiovascular magnetic resonance. J Cardiovasc Magn Reson 2009; 11: 26.

13 Adult Valvular Disease

Bernhard L. Gerber and Jochen Spiess

13.1 Introduction

The recent advances in cardiac MR imaging have allowed this technique to become an important method for the non-invasive evaluation of patients with adult valve disease (Cawley 2009). Indeed, similar to echocardiography, cardiac MR can assess the morphology, severity of stenosis and insufficiency of all four valves in the adult heart. The important strengths of CMR over other techniques are its ability to quantify severity of valve regurgitations, to precisely measure left and right ventricular volumes and function, to evaluate the great thoracic vessels, and finally to assess associated or related pathology of the myocardium such as myocardial fibrosis or necrosis.

13.2 General Principles of Evaluation of Valve Disease by CMR

Similar to echocardiography, the evaluation of patients with valvular heart disease requires a comprehensive approach, appraising the morphology and function all four cardiac valves in terms of opening and closure. For each valve, the degree of opening and closure should be assessed both using anatomical (i.e. respectively valve opening or closing areas) and physiological (i.e. respectively pressure gradients and regurgitant volumes) measurements, since both parameters are complementary. In addition to assessing the severity of valve dysfunction, it is important to evaluate the consequences of valve disease on left and right ventricular size and systolic function. Indeed such functional parameters are usually needed for clinical decision making in patients with valve disease, and in particular for the decision of whether patients should undergo surgery or not. Finally, since it is increasingly feasible to surgically repair valves instead of replacing them by prosthesis, it is important to define precisely the mechanism of dysfunction of valves and to predict surgical reparability. All commonly used cardiac MR techniques are useful for evaluation of patients with valve disease, and readers are referred to Chapter 1 for review of those techniques.

13.3 Identification of Valve Stenosis and Regurgitation by Signal Void

Identification of valve stenosis or valve regurgitation can be performed visually by identifying loss of signal (signal void) due the dephasing of moving protons on cine-imaging SSFP or gradient echo images. Stenosis can be identified when signal void occurs due to flow turbulence upstream of the stenotic valve (Kilner 1993) (Figure 13-1). Valve regurgitation can be identified by signal void due to regurgitant jet downstream of the incompetent valve. Signal void can be identified both for SSFP and gradient echo cine pulse sequences; however SSFP sequences are generally less sensitive for detecting flow disturbances than gradient echo sequences (Krombach 2004). Indeed the sensitivity depends on echo time: the longer the echo time, the larger and more pronounced the regurgitant jet (Suzuki 1990). Similar to color Doppler echocardiography, the size of signal void may allow some semi-quantitative appreciation of the severity of stenosis or regurgitation (Figure 13-2); however the clinical usefulness of this approach is limited by the fact that the size of jet depends on imaging parameters, and may thus vary among patients. By contrast, the direction and location of jets are important to understand the mechanism of dysfunction of the valve disease, in particular to identify valve prolapse (see below).

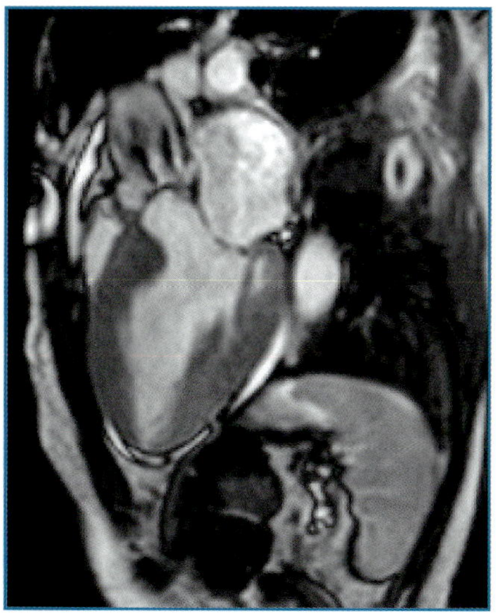

Figure 13-1 Identification of aortic stenosis by dephasing artifacts (signal void) in the ascending aorta beyond the stenotic valve.

13.4 Quantification of Valve Opening and Stenosis

Valve stenosis can be appraised both anatomically and physiologically, i.e.:

- by measuring the surface of opening of the valve, either by direct planimetry of the anatomic valve area or by indirect computation of the effective valve opening using the continuity equation, and
- by evaluating the severity of pressure gradients through the stenotic valve.

Both parameters provide complementary yet independent estimates of severity of stenosis, since pressure gradients are dependent on the amount of flow passing through the stenotic valve.

13.4.1 Direct Planimetry of Anatomical Valve Area

Direct planimetry of **anatomical valve opening area** can be performed by prescribing a stack of serial short-axis cine-SSFP images at different levels through the stenotic valve (Friedrich 2002, John 2003, Kupfahl 2004, Debl 2008). The area of minimal opening at the tips of the valve leaflets is then carefully traced by planimetry on an image where the valve is fully opened, i.e. in mid systole for aortic (Figure 13-3) and pulmonary valves, and in early diastole for mitral and tricuspid valves. High spatial and temporal resolution is required for greatest precision of measurements. The excellent blood-to-myocardium contrast and high signal-to-noise ratio (SNR) provided by SSFP sequences typically allows precise delineation of the valve against the blood, yet potential pitfalls are signal void artifacts resulting from calcifications or turbulent flow.

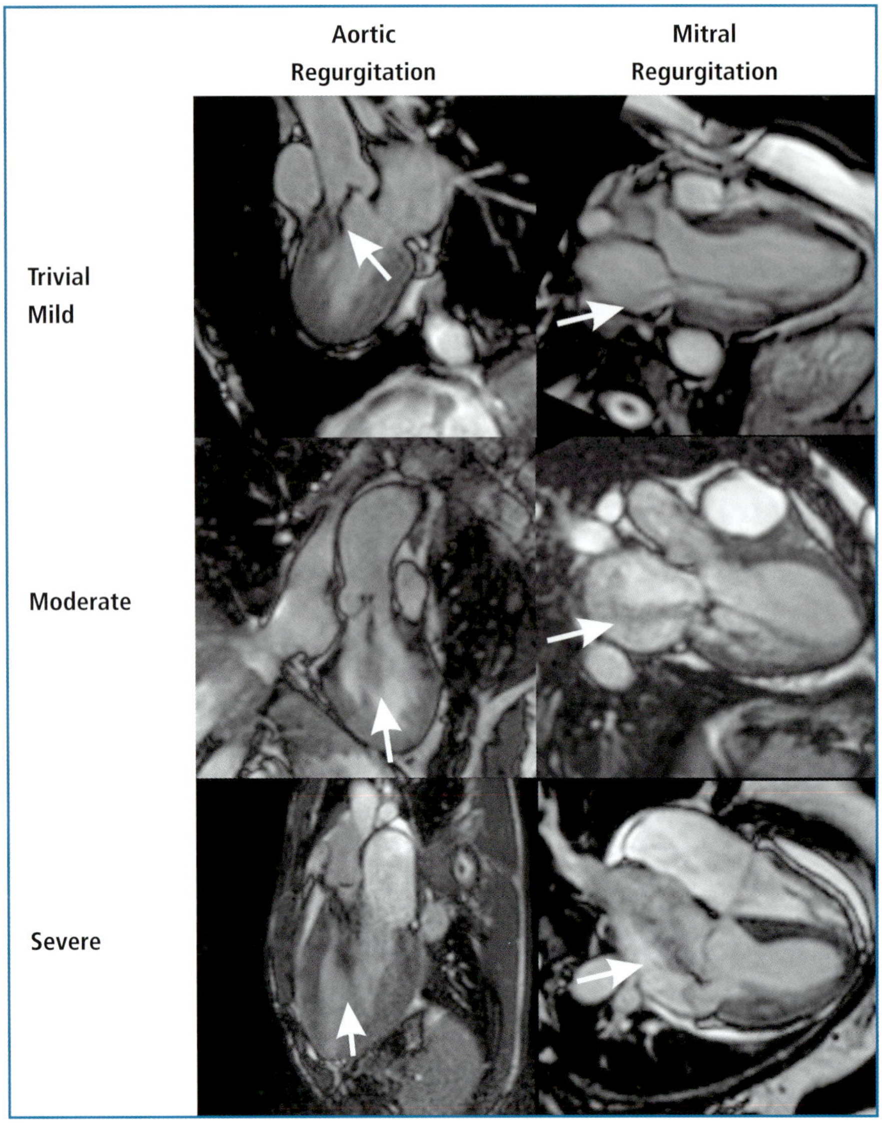

Figure 13-2 Semiquantitave grading of aortic and mitral regurgitation severity based on size and thickness of jet (arrows).

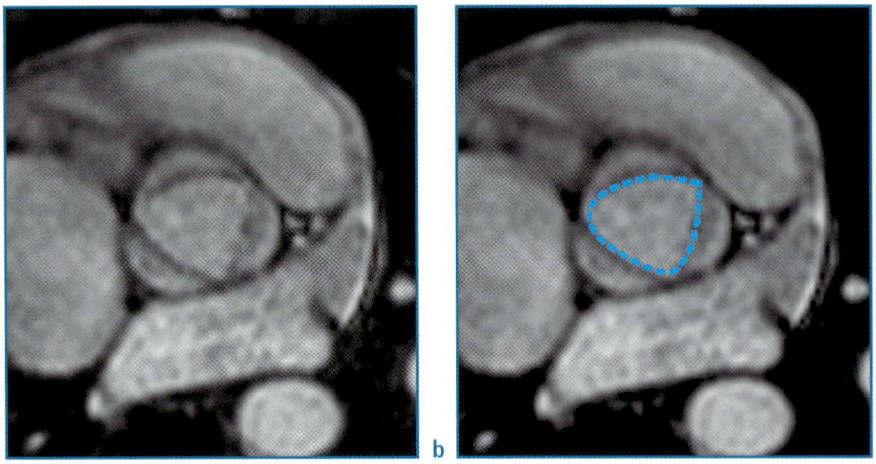

Figure 13-3 Direct planimetry of anatomical aortic valve opening on cine-SSFP images: Maximal opening of aortic valve (a), planimetry of the valve orifice (broken line) (b).

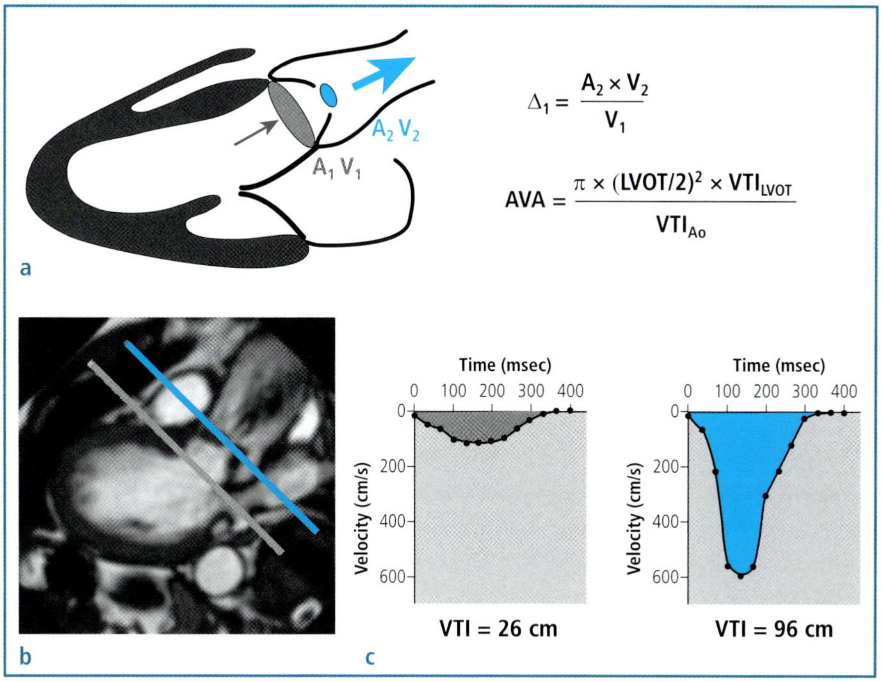

Figure 13-4 Computation of effective aortic valve opening area by means of continuity equation: Schematic diagram of anatomy and parameters (a), imaging plane through the aortic valve region (b), velocity-time integral calculated within the two respective planes (c). A_1 and V_1: area and spatial mean velocity proximal to the obstruction; A_2 and V_2: area and spatial mean velocity at the site of obstruction; Ao: aorta; AVA: aortic valve area (effective aortic valve opening area); LVOT: left ventricular outflow tract; VTI: velocity-time integral.

13.4.2 Indirect Assessment of Effective Valve Opening Using Continuity Equation

Similar to Doppler echocardiography, **effective valve opening area** can also be computed indirectly from phase contrast velocity measurements by means of the continuity equation (Figure 13-4). The continuity equation is based on Newton's second law of thermodynamics, involving the conservation of mass. As it applies to flow velocity imaging, this principle states that the volumetric flow rate through the cardiovascular system is constant, assuming that the blood is incompressible and the conduit is inelastic. Stated differently, the flow rate (or volume of blood passing through any given point in time) is the same at all points along the circuit, and thus the ratio of velocities at two different levels of the cardiac valves is inversely proportional to the ratio of cross-sectional areas, while the product of flow area and flow velocity remains constant. When there is an obstruction in a flow channel, the product of flow area and flow velocity will be constant at the obstructed and the non-obstructed part of the flow channel, according to the continuity equation: $A \times V = A' \times V'$ where V and A are the spatial mean velocity and the area proximal to the obstruction, and V' and A' are the spatial mean velocity and the area at the obstruction. If V, A, and V' are known, the stenotic area can be calculated by rearranging equation 1 as follows: $A' = A \times V/V'$. This equation is valid both in time-steady flow and at each moment during pulsatile flow, provided that the velocity profile does not change from A to A'.

Thus the method requires the assessment of peak velocity using **velocity-encoded phase contrast imaging at 2 levels**:

- at the maximum of the convergence, and
- at another reference level.

It needs also assessment of the area of the reference area, either by planimetry on the magnitude images, or by measuring the diameter of the outflow tract and by computing reference area as $2\pi r^2$. Measurements need thus to be performed at the plane location for accurate location of the maximal flow, which needs to be located beyond the anatomical motion of the valve. Optimally several slices are prescribed to avoid missing the maximal flow velocity. Furthermore the maximal encoding velocity needs to be set higher than the maximal velocity of the turbulent jet to avoid aliasing. Another problem is the through plane motion of the valve during the cardiac cycle. This problem is most important in the tricuspid and mitral valve, therefore the method is more useful for measurement of stenosis of the aortic and pulmonary valves.

Measurements of valve area by continuity equation are usually slightly smaller than those obtained by direct planimetry. This is related to the fact that both methods measure different type of stenotic orifice, the continuity equation estimates *effective valve area*, i.e. a virtual area of flow convergence, situated beyond the true anatomical valve orifice, and which is typically smaller than the true *anatomical valve area* measured by planimetry (Figure 13-4 and Figure 13-5). The ratio of anatomical to effective valve area is often called **coefficient of contraction** and is typically around 0.85 for the aortic valve.

13.4.3 Pressure Gradients

Mean and maximal pressure gradients can also be estimated from the data of velocity-encoded phase contrast imaging employing the simplified Bernouilly equation: $\Delta P = 4 v^2$, with the common assumption that losses of energy due to viscous friction and flow acceleration in pulsatile systems are neglectable, as opposed to the pressure drop resulting from convective acceleration of pressure energy to kinetic energy. This assumption is generally valid for stenoses which are not too severe or last long enough to cause a change from laminar to turbulent flow.

> Similar to what was discussed for the continuity equation, **to avoid errors** in measurements it is important that:
> - flow must be measured at the location of its highest acceleration, i.e. the vena contracta, and
> - velocity encoding setting must be high enough to avoid aliasing.

13.5 Quantitative Measurements of Severity of Valve Regurgitation

Similar to the assessment of stenosis severity, quantitative evaluation of the severity of regurgitation requires both measurement of anatomical and physiological parameters, i.e. the assessment of the anatomical area of the regurgitant orifice by direct planimetry, and the assessment of the regurgitant volume through the incompetent valves using phase contrast imaging.

13.5.1 Evaluation of Anatomical Regurgitant Orifice

Evaluation of the **anatomical regurgitant orifice** is performed in a similar approach as planimetry of valve opening, i.e. by prescribing serial short-axis slices perpendicular to the valve orifice (Figure 13-5), and by planimetring the maximal size of the regurgitant orifice of the incompetent valve (Debl 2008, Buchner 2008, Goffinet 2010) while the

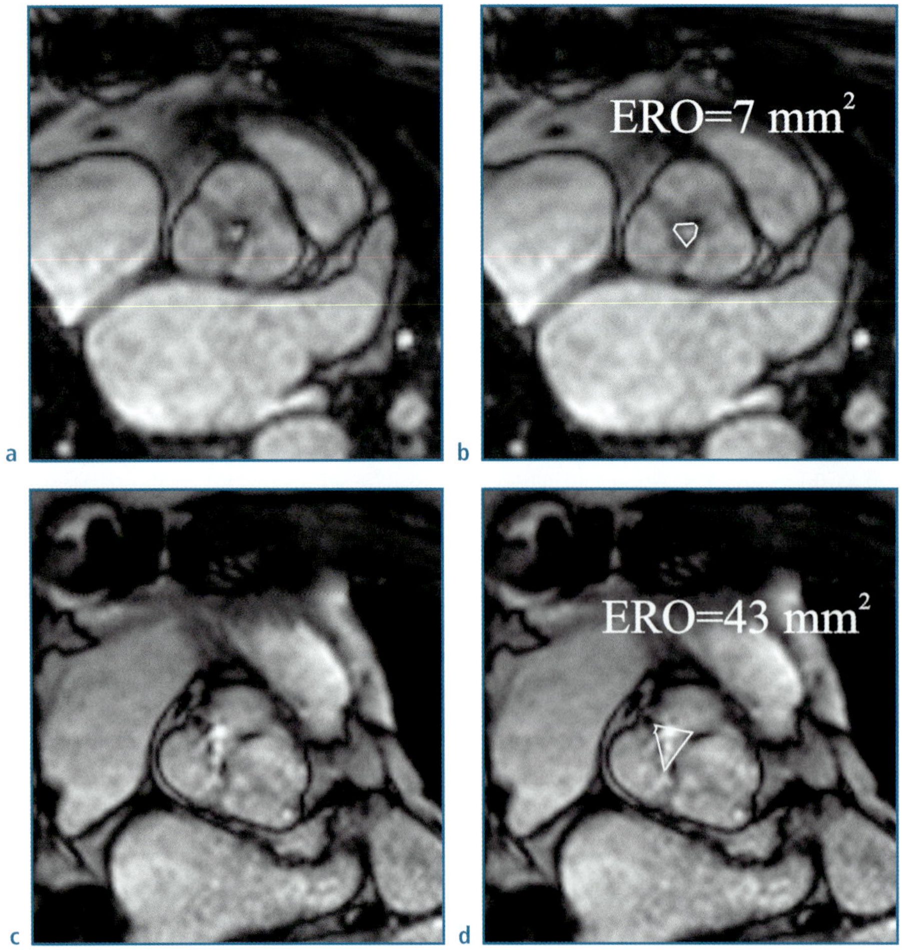

Figure 13-5 Measurement of anatomical regurgitant orifice by direct planimetry on short-axis slices prescribed through the aortic valve. Small anatomical regurgitant orifice in native (a) and planimetry (broken line) (b), larger anatomical regurgitant orifice in native (c) and planimetry (broken line) (d). ERO: effective regurgitant orifice.

valve is closed. The same prescription as for assessment of valve stenosis can be used if regurgitant jets are central. Yet, if regurgitant jets are eccentric, which most often occurs when one or more leaflets present prolapse, care must be taken to prescribe the short-axis slices (Figure 13-5) perpendicular to the direction of the regurgitant jet, in order to avoid overestimation of the regurgitant orifice (Goffinet 2010). Since regurgitant orifices are typically smaller than stenotic valve openings, the magnitude of error in measurements is greater than for assessment of anatomical valve area. It is thus even more important to choose high image resolutions.

13.5.2 Quantification of Regurgitant Volume

Quantification of the regurgitant volume can be performed several ways: in the aortic and pulmonary valve it may be evaluated directly by prescribing a through plane phase contrast image just beyond the incompetent valve (Figure 13-6). By multiplying vessel area times the integral of velocities over time one can compute not only forward volume, but also regurgitant volume through the incompetent valve. The severity of regurgitation can be expressed either in absolute terms, or as a percentage of forward flow (regurgitant fraction). Because the aorta and pulmonary artery have circular shape and relatively less cardiac motion, the direct approach is better suited for assessing regurgitant volumes in the aortic and pulmonary valve than in the mitral and regurgitant valve. For highest precision of measurement, the through phase contrast image should be prescribed as close as possible to the valve. If plane following methods are available, it is also possible to prescribe a plane through the mitral or tricuspid annulus and directly measure the volume of regurgitation of these valves.

In the absence of plane following methods for quantification of mitral and tricuspid valve regurgitant volume, an indirect approach is usually used (Figure 13-7): Indeed mitral or tricuspid regurgitant volume can be computed by comparing right and left ventricular stroke volumes (Sechtem 1988) computed from Simpson's method on serial short-axis slices in the left ventricle (LV) and the right ventricle (RV), if no other valvular regurgitation is present. Another approach which is not affected by regurgitations of

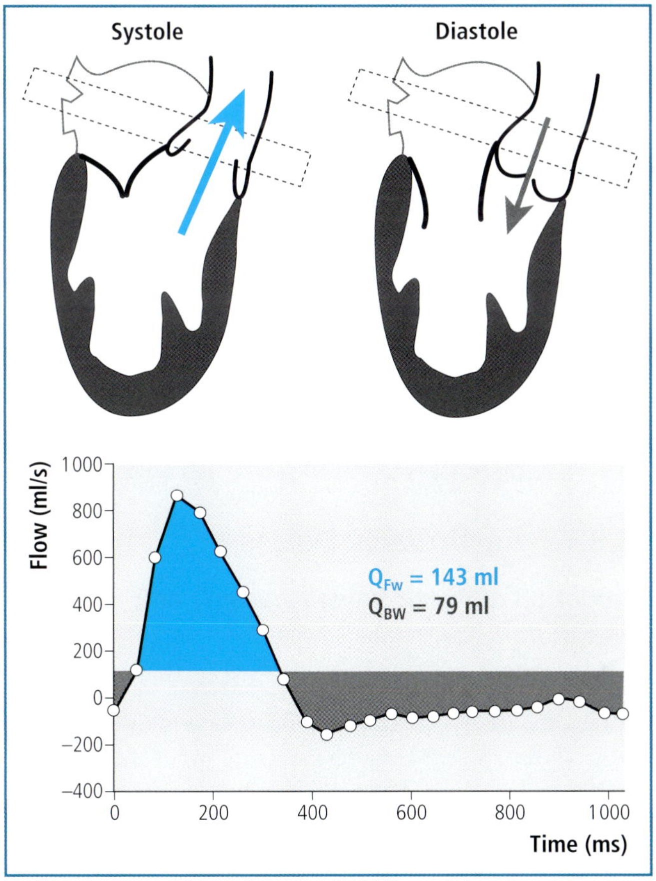

Figure 13-6 Quantification of regurgitant volume in the aortic valve by phase contrast imaging. Q_{BW}: backward flow; Q_{FW}: forward flow.

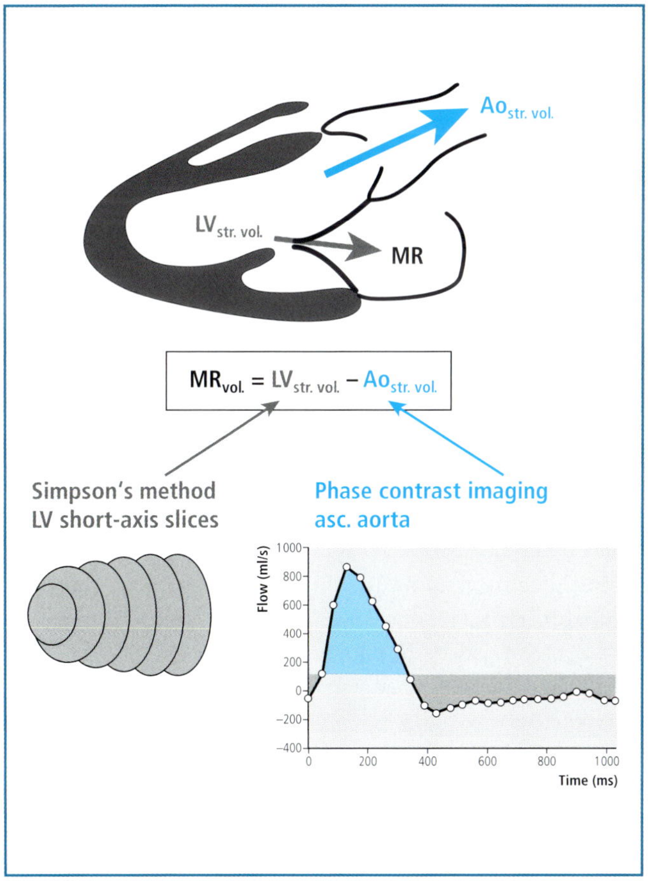

Figure 13-7 Quantification of mitral regurgitant volume (MR_{vol}) by subtraction method. Ao: aorta; asc.: ascending (aorta); LV: left ventricle; str. vol.: stroke volume.

other valves is comparing left and right ventricular stroke volumes from Simpson's method to forward stroke volume in aortic or pulmonary artery using phase contrast imaging. Mitral regurgitant volume, for instance, is then computed as the difference in LV stroke volume (computed using the Simpson's method from serial short-axis slices through the LV) minus aortic stroke volume (computed from phase contrast imaging in the aortic root). Likewise, tricuspid regurgitant volume is computed as the difference in RV stroke volume (from Simpson's method) and pulmonary artery stroke volume (from phase contrast imaging). This approach remains valid even in the presence of aortic and pulmonary regurgitation, however since the method requires two different means for computation of LV/RV and aortic/pulmonary stroke volumes, there is inherently more risk of summation of errors in measurements, resulting of less precision of assessment of regurgitant volumes by this method.

Pitfalls of using phase contrast methods are inaccuracies in stroke volume due to phase offsets due to Eddy or Maxwell currents. To minimize these errors, echo times (TE) should be as short as possible. Furthermore to avoid aliasing, the encoding velocity must be set higher than the maximal velocity encountered in the given vessel.

13.6 Evaluation of Valve Morphology and Mechanism of Dysfunction

Due to the advent of valve repair technique, it has become more and more important to evaluate valve morphology and the functional mechanism of valve dysfunction. This allows the decision of whether and how a dysfunctional valve can be repaired. The main technique for evaluation of valve morphology and reparability remains transesophageal echocardiography (TEE). Due to its 3D imaging capabilities, CMR offers additional information which can not be provided by conventional 2D-TEE: for instance 3D visualization of the mitral annulus, of the aortic cusps and the aortic root. Furthermore using T1-, T2-weighted, fat saturated and post-contrast turbospin echo images, CMR allows alterations in cardiac tissues to be characterized. This may be helpful to differentiate some larger valvular tumors such as myxoma, calcification or lipoma or neighboring structures to the valves. Limitations of CMR for evaluation of valve morphology are lower spatial resolution than TEE and the requirement to image over several cardiac cycles. Therefore very small or highly mobile valvular structures such as vegetations, ruptured chordae, or Lambl's exhissence are generally not as well-visualized by CMR as by TEE.

13.7 Evaluation of Physiological Consequences of Valve Disease

CMR is also capable of precisely measuring left and right ventricular end-diastolic and systolic volumes, mass and ejection fraction, with superior accuracy and interstudy reproducibility compared to 2D echocardiography. It is thus particularly well-suited to evaluate the pathophysiological consequences of valve disease on the left or right ventricle. Since in many types of valve disease, the timing of surgery is determined by the functional repercussions of disease on the ventricles, CMR may thus help to detect the optimal time of intervention in cardiac disease. Because of its high precision, CMR is the method of choice for serially following LV and RV volumes, as well as masses in patients over time. This may be particularly interesting in studies evaluating results of valve surgery on ventricular volumes, mass and function. Indeed because of higher precision sample size of such studies may be reduced in contrast to 2D echocardiography.

Finally CMR has the unique ability to characterize the myocardium by T1 and T2 weighed spin echo sequences, which is, however, done even better by IR gradient echo sequences after injection of contrast (late-enhancement). It may thus detect myocardial fibrosis or necrosis in certain types of valve disease, and also provide valuable information on the viability of tissue in the presence of valve disease. This latter information is particularly important in evaluating operative benefit and risk in patients who have valve disease in the presence of severely depressed cardiac function.

13.8 Place of CMR in the Evaluation of Specific Valvular Diseases

13.8.1 Aortic Valve Disease

Evaluation of Aortic Valve Anatomy and Function by CMR

The aortic valve is a tricuspid semi-lunar valve situated between the left ventricular outflow tract and the ascending aorta. The aortic valve leaflets are supported by the aortic annulus which is part of the fibrous skeleton of the heart. At their level of coaption, which is always situated several mm higher than the annulus, they present a fibrous reinforcement, termed nodule of Arrantius. Distal to the semi-lunar leaflets, the aortic root presents three enlargements termed sinus of Valsalva, into which each of the semi-lunar leaflets

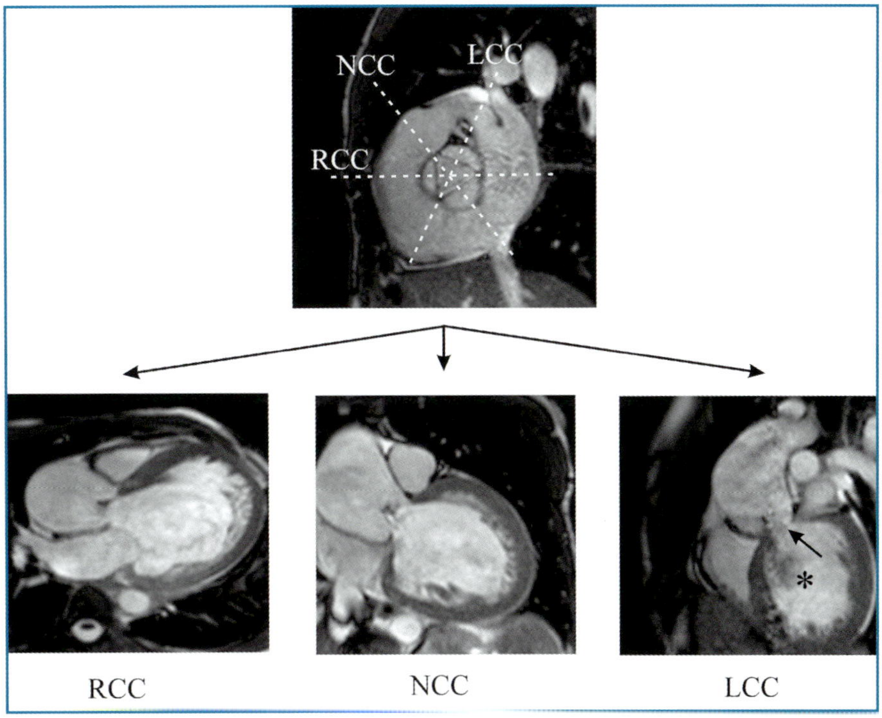

Figure 13-8 Prescription of planes for evaluation of aortic valve morphology and function. LCC: left coronary cusp; NCC: non-coronary cusp; RCC: right coronary cusp.

open during systole. Two of these sinuses give rise to the right and left coronary arteries, and are thus named after their coronary artery, i.e. as right and left coronary leaflets and sinus. The third sinus and leaflet is termed "non-coronary". The aortic sinuses are separated and stabilized by interleaflet triangles of fibrous tissue originating from the aortic annulus, which extends up to the sinotubular junction of the ascending aorta. The entire structure of aortic annulus and interleaflet triangles support the leaflets and contribute to their coaption during closure. Therefore the valve and aortic root are now considered a functional entity, the so-called functional aortic apparatus.

A comprehensive exam of the aortic valve by CMR thus requires not only assessment of aortic valve leaflet anatomy and function, but also appraisal of the anatomy of the functional aortic root. Assessment of aortic valve anatomy and motion is best performed by prescribing serial thin (5 mm) short-axis slices perpendicular to a 3-chamber LV outflow tract view. From these one can prescribe 3 radial long-axis slices separated approximately by 60° angles, which cut through each of the aortic valve leaflets (Figure 13-8). These long-axis slices not only allow the evaluation of the degree of opening of each leaflet in systole, but more importantly also allow the determination of the point of coaptation during valve closure in diastole. They thus allow the detection of prolapse or restriction as mechanism of insufficiency. Furthermore they allow the evaluation of dilatation of the aortic sinuses, the sinotubular junction or ascending aorta. Functional severity of stenosis can be evaluated by prescribing phase contrast images just beyond the level of opening of the aortic valve leaflets. Severity of aortic regurgitation is evaluated by a phase contrast image close to the aortic valve, typically at the level of the sinotubular junction. Because of the coexistence of disease of the ascending aorta, evaluation of aortic valve disease should also be completed by anatomical evaluation of the ascending and descending aorta on contrast-enhanced 3D angiography images.

Aortic Stenosis (AS)

Aortic stenosis (AS) is the most common valve disease in adult patients. The most important cause of AS is calcified degeneration of the valve in elderly patients. The second most common etiology of aortic stenosis is congenital, most often related to bicuspid valve disease. Bicuspid AS presents in younger patients than AS due to degenerative disease. Rheumatic etiology has become rare in the western population.

Aortic stenosis is considered moderate when aortic valve area is < 1.2 cm², and severe when valve area is either < 1.0 cm² or indexed < 0.6 cm²/m² and velocity gradient by continuous Doppler echocardiography exceed 4 m/s. Moderate and even severe aortic stenosis is generally well-tolerated for longer periods, however once symptoms of angina, heart failure or syncope occur, survival becomes rapidly reduced. Outcome of AS is also particularly poor in the setting of low ejection fraction. Therefore current guidelines (Vahanian 2007) recommend surgical valve replace-

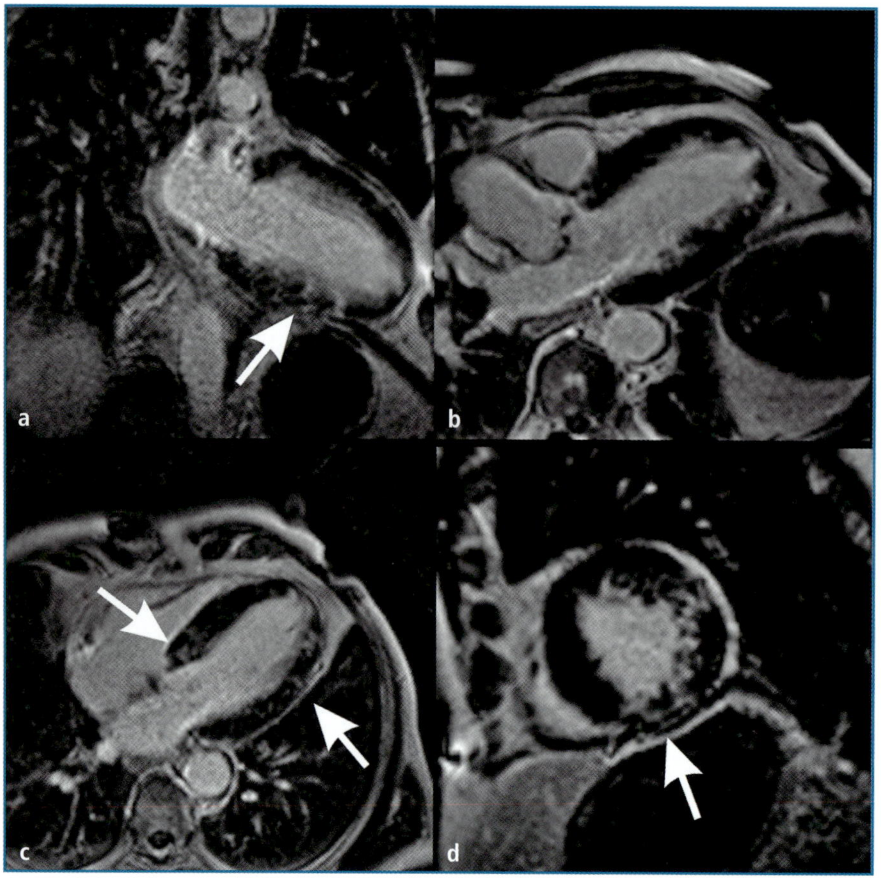

Figure 13-9 Demonstration of fibrosis on delayed Gd contrast-enhanced images (arrows) in a patient with severe aortic stenosis, but without coronary artery disease: 2-ch view (a), 3-ch view (b), 4-ch view (c), and short-axis view (d).

ment when patients with severe aortic stenosis become symptomatic, or in the presence of altered systolic function.

Transthoracic echocardiography (TTE) remains the technique of choice for assessment of the large majority of patients with aortic stenosis. CMR can, however, be an alternative or secondary technique for evaluation of AS if image quality of TTE is poor, for instance in patients with poor echocardiographic image quality, or if results of TTE are inconsistent with the patients symptoms. Assessment of severity of AS by CMR can be performed both by direct planimetry of anatomical valve opening on cine images prescribed at the tips of the aortic valve leaflets (Friedrich 2002, John 2003, Kupfahl 2004) and by computing the effective valve orifice using the continuity equation (Caruthers 2003) in phase contrast encoded velocity images obtained at the aortic valve tips and in the left ventricular outflow tract. Both techniques compare favorably to TTE, however planimetry tends to provide slightly higher aortic valve areas than the continuity equation (Pouleur 2007). This likely reflects that both methods do not exactly measure the same orifice, the effective valve orifice being slightly smaller than the anatomical valve orifice, as discussed earlier.

CMR phase contrast imaging can also estimate the maximal velocity through the stenotic valve, and hence compute maximal pressure gradient using the modified Bernouilly equation. The accuracy of this measurement was found to be high vs. continuous Doppler TTE (Sondergaard 1993a, Caruthers 2003).

Cine-SSFP CMR allows better visualization of the aortic cusps than TTE. Therefore CMR is more accurate in detecting whether valves in AS are bi- or tricuspid. CMR can also more accurately measure LV mass, and thus can better characterize the degree of LV hypertrophy in AS than TTE.

Of greater clinical interest is the recently demonstrated ability of CMR to identify regions of late enhancement in patients with aortic stenosis (Debl 2006) (Figure 13-9). Such delayed enhancement correlates with histological fibrosis (Nigri 2009, Weidemann 2009) and appears to predict functional improvement (Weidemann 2009) and prognosis in aortic stenosis (Azvedo 2010).

Low-flow low gradient stenosis associating apparently severe aortic stenosis with low transvalvular gradients (mean gradient < 30 mmHg), and low ejection fraction is another clinically challenging situation in which CMR could play an important role. Indeed, because of flow dependencies of measurements of AS in the setting of reduced cardiac output, the severity of AS may be overestimated. Therefore it may be difficult to distinguish patients with true aortic stenosis at the stage of LV failure from patients with pseudosevere AS and cardiomyopathy due to other causes. Also in this setting, deciding whether to operate on patients or not is important but often particularly difficult. Indeed, outcome of patients with true severe AS and low ejection fraction under medical treatment is extremely poor. On the other hand, valve replacement in the setting of poor ejection fraction is associated with important peri-operative risk, but may improve long-term outcome. However, patients with pseudosevere AS and cardiomyopathy do not benefit from surgery. Dobutamine echocardiography has been recommended to demonstrate inotropic response and changes in aortic valve area during inotropic stimulation, to decide which patients should undergo surgery (Vahanian 2007). Likewise dobutamine CMR can also be used to demonstrate inotropic response and to separate true from pseudosevere AS. In this setting it may also be interesting to directly image the aortic valve for severity of morphological abnormalities such as calcifications of the aortic valve, which are more severe in true than in pseudosevere AS. Gd-DTPA late enhancement may also be of use in this setting. Indeed presence of myocardial necrosis and fibrosis indicating lack of myocardial viability may be used to predict functional recovery after aortic valve replacement. Although CMR is often used for this purpose, there is still a lack of data demonstrating the value of the technique in this setting, in particular in opposition to dobutamine.

Lastly, similar to CT, CMR has the capability to accurately evaluate the entire ascending aorta. This may be particularly important in the follow-up of patients with bicuspid aortic valve to monitor aortic root dilatation, and determine whether aortic root replacement needs to be associated to AVR. Also such assessment of ascending aorta and of LV outflow tract has become important prior to percutaneous stented aortic valves (TAVI) implantation.

Aortic Regurgitation (AR)

Grading of severity of aortic regurgitation (AR) is illustrated in Table 13-1. Trivial AR is commonly found without clinical significance. Aortic regurgitation may result from a variety of conditions. Calcified degeneration of aortic cusps is the most common cause of aortic regurgitation in older patients. Congenital bicuspid aortic valve is the most common cause of aortic regurgitation in younger patients and is commonly caused by prolapse of the anterior cusp. Functional aortic regurgitation due to aortic root dilatation without structural destruction of aortic cusps is another important cause of aortic regurgitation. Finally aortic regurgitation may also be caused by valve destruction after infective endocarditis of the heart. Once common, rheumatic heart disease has nowadays become an uncommon cause of aortic regurgitation.

Table 13-1 Grading of the severity of aortic regurgitation (Vahanian et al. 2007).

	Mild	Moderate		Severe
regurgitant volume (ml/beat)	< 30	30–44	45–59	> 60
regurgitant fraction (%)	< 30	30–39	40–49	> 50
effective regurgitant orifice (mm^3)	< 10	10–19	20–29	> 30

With the advent of valve sparing AR surgery, a functional classification similar to that of mitral regurgitation has been proposed for description of the mechanism of aortic regurgitation (El Khoury 2005) (Figure 13-10). Type I aortic regurgitation describes AR with normal cusp motion related to dilatation of the sinotubular junction (Ia), sinus of Valsalva (Ib) or annulus (Ic), Type II describes AR due to cusp prolapse, Type III describes aortic regurgitation related to restrictive cusp motion. Type I and II are not mutually exclusive and may often be associated, for instance AR may simultaneously result from cusp prolapse and aortic root dilatation.

Chronic severe aortic regurgitation has typically good prognosis unless patients develop symptoms of heart failure or deteriorate LV function. Therefore symptom onset or deterioration of LV function at rest (resting LVEF < 50 %) in asymptomatic patients constitutes indications for surgery in patients with severe AR. Surgery should also be considered in asymptomatic patients with severe LV dilatation (LV end-diastolic diameter > 70 mm and/or end-systolic diameter > 50 mm or > 25 mm/m^2 BSA by echocardiography) (Vahanian 2007) since the likelihood of heart failure increases beyond these cut-off values. In many other patients with AR, it is the degree of dilatation of the aortic root rather than the severity of aortic regurgitation of LV function that indicates surgery. Indeed because of the associated risk of aortic dissection in severe aortic aneurysms, aortic root dilatation > 55 mm should be surgically repaired, irrespective of the degree of AR. For patients with bicuspid aortic valves or Marfan's syndrome, even lower degrees of root dilatation (< 50 and < 45 mm, respectively) have been proposed as indications for surgery, especially when there is a rapid increase of aortic diameter between serial measurements (5 mm per year) or family history of aortic dissection.

CMR can assess AR by several approaches. Initial work in the 1980's demonstrated the feasibility of semi-quantitatively evaluating aortic regurgitation by the size of signal void in the left ventricle (Cawley 2009). Severity of AR can also be quantified by comparing left to right ventricular stroke volumes (Cawley 2009) in the absence of other valve

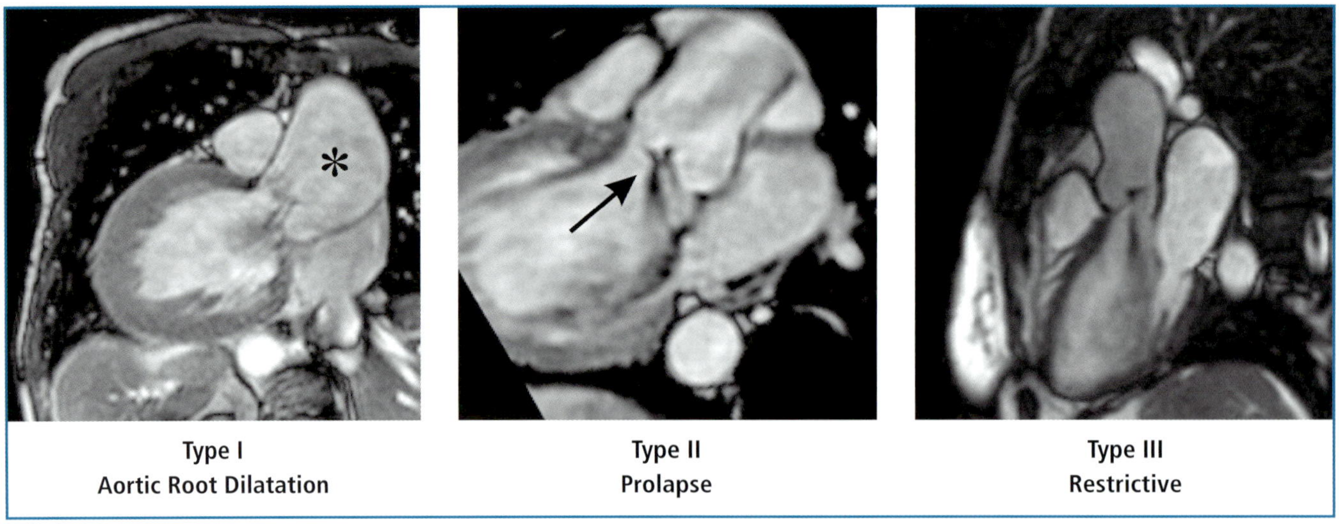

Figure 13-10 Functional classification of mechanism of aortic regurgitation. *: dilated aortic root; arrow: regurgitant jet.

regurgitations. Other parameters of assessing severity of AR are measuring the size of the area of proximal acceleration or the motion of a transverse saturation band in the thoracic aorta to grade severity of aortic regurgitation. A more physiological measure for quantification of severity of AR is direct planimetry of the size of the anatomical regurgitant orifice (Debl 2008, Goffinet 2010). This method was found to be accurate vs. cardiac catheterization (Debl 2008) and vs. estimates of the effective regurgitant orifice by PISA-echocardiography (Goffinet 2010). A limitation of this approach is that because of the smaller size of the regurgitant orifice, this method is less precise in grading anatomical aortic regurgitant than mitral regurgitant orifice. The most accurate measurement of AR is however direct measurement of regurgitant volume from phase contrast imaging slices prescribed through the aortic root (Bogren 1989, van Rossum 1991, Sondergaard 1993b). This method was found to correlate well with estimates of AR from the difference of RV and LV stroke volumes (Sondergaard 1993b) Doppler (Pouleur 2008) and angiographic measurements of AR (Honda 1993) and was demonstrated to have high inter-study reproducibility (Dulce 1992). For highest accuracy measurements should be performed at the level of the coronary ostia, close to the aortic valve (Chatzamavroudis 1997). Because of the ease and accuracy of this method it is currently considered the gold standard for quantification of aortic regurgitation and has been used for assessment of follow-up studies or therapeutic effect in treatment of aortic regurgitation (Globits 1996, Hoffmann 2001). Because the gradient echo sequence is quite robust against field inhomogeneity effects, the technique is also applicable in patients with prosthetic valves (Di Cesare 1995).

While echocardiography remains the primary technique for identification and grading of aortic regurgitation, CMR plays a major role for evaluating patients with AR. This is because quantification of AR by echocardiography is difficult and often relatively imprecise. Although absolute quantification is possible using the proximal isosurface (PISA) method, this method is often challenging, especially in the presence of eccentric regurgitant jets as encountered often in bicuspid valves with prolapse. In this situation, the ability to quantify regurgitant volume by phase contrast CMR helps to better appreciate the severity of AR. Another important role of CMR in the follow-up of patients with aortic regurgitation is the ability to precisely measure the size of the aortic root. Furthermore CMR is more precise than TTE echocardiography for assessment of LV volumes and ejection fraction, which are also major determinants of timing for surgery. Finally because of its 3D imaging ability, which allows the motion of each leaflet to be individually followed, CMR may also clarify the mechanism of AR with precision similar to TEE, making it possible to define whether valve sparing surgery is possible (Goffinet 2010).

13.8.2 Mitral Valve Disease

Evaluation of Mitral Valve Anatomy and Function by CMR

The mitral valve is situated at the junction of the left atrium and left ventricle. It is composed of two leaflets which are orientated obliquely from the anterolateral to the infero-basal part of the base of the heart and perpendicularly to the aortic valve (Figure 13-11). The posterior leaflet is quadrangular and has two well-defined indentations which, divides it into three individual scallops, which are identified as P1 (anteromedial), P2 (middle) and P3 (posterolateral). The anterior leaflet has semi-circular shape and is usually con-

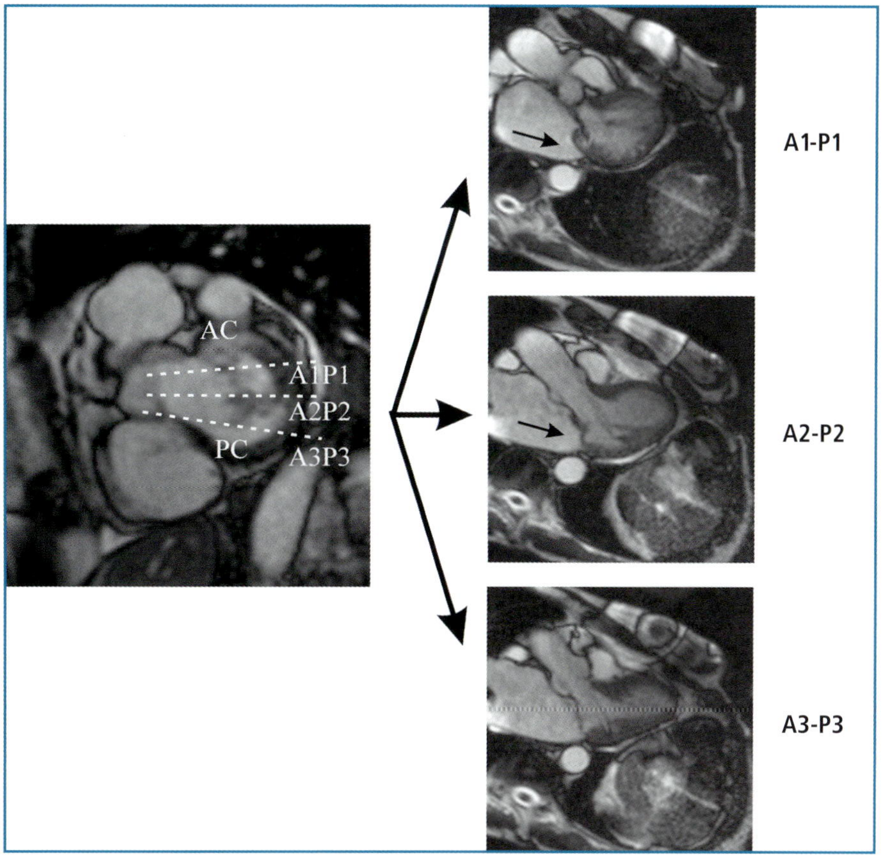

Figure 13-11 Prescription of planes for evaluation of mitral valve morphology and function. AC: anterior leaflet; PC: posterior leaflet; A: anterior mitral valve scallops: segments opposing the posterior scallops are termed A1, A2 and A3; P: posterior mitral valve scallops: P1 (anteromedial), P2 (middle) and P3 (posterolateral).

tinuous without indentations. The segments opposing the posterior scallops are termed A1, A2 and A3. This nomenclature is important to describe specific anatomic segmental anatomy between echocardiographer and surgeon. The commissures define the areas where the anterior and posterior leaflets unite. Both leaflets are attached to both the anterior and posterior papillary muscles by primary and secondary chordae. Primary chordae attach to the free margin of the valve, secondary chordae attach on the ventricular side of the valve. The mitral valve is furthermore attached to the left ventricle by the mitral annulus, a part of fibrous skeleton of the heart. The anterior and posterior leaflets of the mitral valve coapt on the ventricular side below the mitral annulus. The zone and length of coaptation is important for valve competency.

A comprehensive method for evaluation of the mitral valve by CMR has been proposed (Chan 2008, Gabriel 2008). Indeed following a standard imaging of the left ventricle, including cines of 2-, 3- and 4-chamber long-axis views and short-axis slices continuing up to the mitral annulus, a contiguous stack of oblique slices is prescribed on the mitral valve orthogonal to the line of coaptation, approximately parallel to the 3-chamber view (Figure 13-11). This stack of images allows visualization of each of the valves (A1-P1, A2-P2, A3-P3). Another pair of oblique slices acquired orthogonal to the oblique line of leaflet coaptation at each end of the valve allows appreciation of the commissures.

Mitral Stenosis (MS)

Mitral stenosis (MS) is defined as reduced opening of the mitral valve surface. This results in impaired filling of the left ventricle, which is compensated by increased pressure gradients between the left atrium and the left ventricle. Mild mitral stenosis is defined as valve surface between 1.5 and 2.0 cm^2, moderate mitral valve stenosis is defined as valve surface between 1.0 and 1.5 cm^2 and severe mitral stenosis is defined as valve surface < 1.0 cm^2. Mitral valve stenosis is first and foremost the consequence of rheumatic heart disease. With the disappearance of this disease due to antibiotic treatment, mitral valve stenosis has become very uncommon in developed countries. The disease remains however frequent in developing countries. Mitral valve stenosis is typically asymptomatic when mild. Patients with moderate to severe disease require surgery when they remain symptomatic despite medical treatment. Most often valve replacement is performed; however repair may be possible if chor-

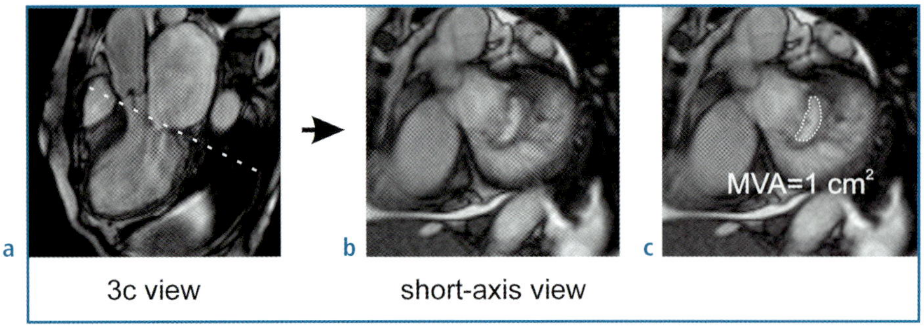

Figure 13-12 Evaluation of mitral stenosis by planimetry of the valve: 3-ch view (a), short-axis view (b), planimetered mitral valve opening area (broken line) (c). MVA: mitral valve area (diastolic mitral orifice).

dae and leaflets are not too severely calcified. Percutaneous balloon valvuloplasty is an alternative treatment in young patients, in particular women to allow pregnancy.

Similar to continuous wave TTE Doppler, CMR can estimate mean pressure gradients through the stenotic valve on phase contrast imaging (Kilner 1993) with good correlation vs. Doppler echocardiography. Also, similar to echocardiography, mitral valve area can be computed indirectly by means of the pressure half-method (Lin 2004), according to the formula: MVA (cm^2) = $220/T_{1/2}$, where MVA is mitral valve area and $T_{1/2}$ is the slope of the rate at which the atrioventricular pressure gradients decays during diastole.

The major limitation of this indirect empirically derived relation between valve area and the rate of transvalvular pressure decay during diastole is that it assumes normal left ventricular compliance (Thomas 1987). Furthermore pressure half-time is also affected when accelerated ventricular filling such as in aortic regurgitation is present. A better means of estimating valve area is probably direct planimetry of the valve area on serial short-axis slices through the mitral valve (Djavidani 2005) (Figure 13-12). This method was found to be accurate, however it slightly overestimated valve area as compared to the Gorlin formula and echocardiography.

Overall TTE and TEE echocardiography remain the preferred method to assess the severity and consequences of MS, as well as the extent of anatomic lesions. Because these techniques are usually sufficient, there is typically no major role for CMR in evaluation of patients with mitral valve stenosis in the clinical setting.

Table 13-2 Grading of the severity of mitral regurgitation (Vahanian et al. 2007).

	Trivial/ Mild	Moderate		Severe
regurgitant volume (ml/beat)	< 30	30–44	45–60	> 60
regurgitant fraction (%)	< 30	30–39	40–49	> 50
effective regurgitant orifice (mm^3)	< 20	20–29	30–39	> 39

Mitral Regurgitation (MR)

Grading of severity of mitral regurgitation (MR) is shown in Table 13-2. Trivial or mild mitral regurgitation can often be seen in healthy individuals and has not significant repercussions. Moderate to severe mitral regurgitation is the second most common form of adult valvular heart disease in Europe. Mitral regurgitation may be due to primary disease of the valve itself, or secondary due to dilatation of the mitral annulus and dysfunction of papillary muscles. Among these, the most common etiology of severe mitral regurgitation is mitral valve prolapse due to myxomatous degeneration of the valve (20–70 % of cases) and ischemic heart disease (13–30 %), followed by rheumatic heart disease (3–40 %), and endocarditis (10–12 %). With the advent of mitral repair techniques, a functional classification for understanding the mechanism of mitral regurgitation has been proposed (Carpentier 1983) (Figure 13-13).

This **functional classification** describes mitral regurgitation as:

- type I (normal valve movement, such as annular dilatation or leaflet perforation),
- type II (excessive movement, i. e. valve prolapse), and
- type III:
  - IIIa (diastolic restriction as in rheumatic disease),
  - IIIb (systolic restriction as in functional disease).

For a comprehensive understanding, mitral regurgitation should be described in terms of severity, functional mechanism (prolapse, restriction etc.) and anatomical location (i. e. A1, P2 etc.).

Surgery is indicated in symptomatic patients with severe MR. In asymptomatic patients with severe MR, surgery is recommended when LV dysfunction (LVEF < 60 % and/or end-systolic dimension > 45 mm), atrial fibrillation or pul-

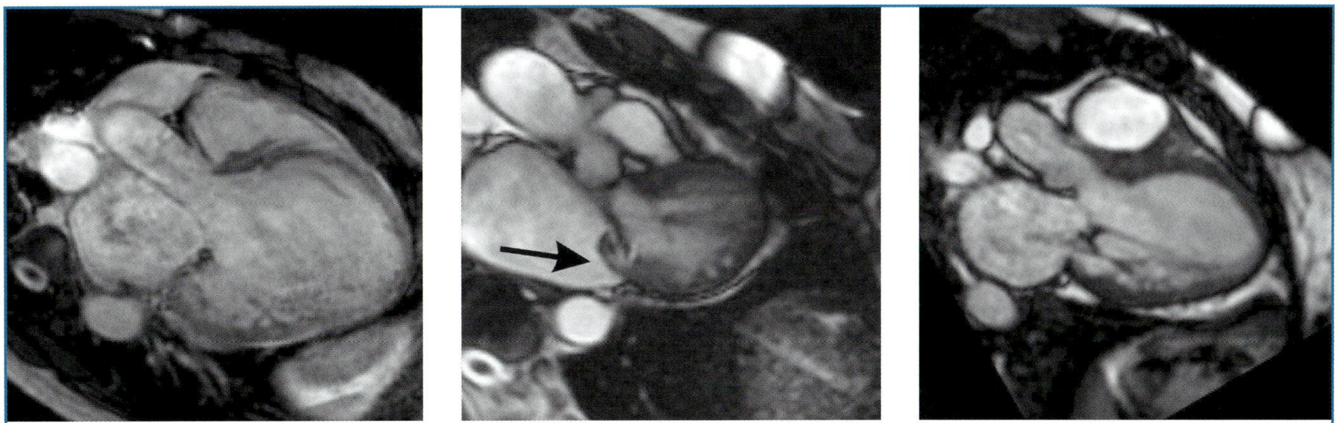

Figure 13-13 Functional classification of the mechanism of mitral regurgitation. arrow: prolapse.

monary hypertension develop. Intervention is debatable in asymptomatic patients with severe MR with neither signs of LV dysfunction, nor AF, nor pulmonary hypertension; however some recent studies suggest benefit of early surgery when the valve can be repaired and operative risk is low. Thus in every case, the indication for surgical intervention is based on grading severity of mitral regurgitation as well as on functional assessment of the left ventricle.

2D Doppler color-TTE is the most commonly used technique for assessment of severity and hemodynamic complications of MR. The proximal isosurface method (PISA) is the preferred technique for quantification of MR and allows computing regurgitant volume and effective regurgitant orifice. TEE and 3D-TTE allow better refinement of mechanism of MR than 2D-TTE. These techniques are typically used in pre-operative evaluation of reparability of MR.

CMR can identify mitral regurgitation by revealing of signal void in the left atrium on cine gradient or SSFP images. It can also semiquantitatively grade the severity of MR-based width and length of the regurgitant jet (Cawley 2009) with good correlation to echocardiographic or angiographic estimation of severity. This semiquantitative assessment is, however, more suited to describe the direction and location of jet, which is important to understand the mechanism of disease (see below). In the presence of moderate to severe mitral regurgitation, true quantification of severity should be performed. Several CMR approaches have been proposed for this purpose. Direct quantification of mitral regurgitant volume by phase contrast imaging through the mitral valve (Fujita 1994) is hampered by the important motion at the mitral annulus through the cardiac cycle. To correct for annual motion, slice following techniques are required (Kozerke 2001, Westenberg 2004). These are however not yet commercially available. Quantification can also be performed by comparing LV and RV stroke volumes (Underwood 1986, Sechtem 1988). The method is accurate, however, only in the absence of other valve regurgitations. The preferred method, which is not affected by such regurgitations of other valves, is computation of mitral regurgitant volume as the difference in LV stroke volume using the Simpson's method from serial short-axis slices through the LV and the aortic stroke volume computed from phase contrast imaging in the aortic root. Despite the risk of summation of errors both from the evaluation of LV and aortic stroke volume, several studies have reported good correlations between this approach and quantitative measurements of severity of mitral regurgitation both vs. phantom studies in vitro (Chatzimavroudis 1998) and in vivo vs. angiography (Hundley 1995) or quantitative Doppler echocardiography (Kizilbash 1998). Also this method was found to be more precise than the comparison of RV and LV volumes (Kon 2004). Another recently proposed approach of grading severity of mitral regurgitation is by direct planimetry of the anatomical regurgitant orifice on serial short-axis slices through the mitral valve (Buchner 2008). This approach was found to correlate well with PISA derived-effective regurgitant orifice (ERO). ERO > 0.4 cm^2 was found to predict severe mitral regurgitation with a sensitivity and specificity of both 94 %, using catheterization as reference standard. Finally phase contrast imaging demonstrating reversed end-systolic flow in the pulmonary veins (Galjee 1995) was also proposed as a characteristic sign of severe mitral regurgitation.

MRI can also be used to unravel the mechanism of mitral regurgitation. For this purpose, serial cine slices are prescribed perpendicular to long-axis 3-chamber LV outflow tract (Figure 13-2). This allows comprehensive evalua-

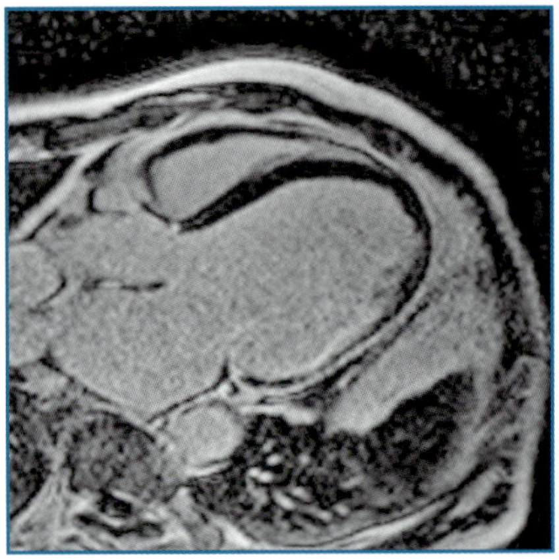

Figure 13-14 Delayed contrast-enhanced viability imaging demonstrating transmural inferior wall necrosis and necrosis of the posterolateral papillary muscle in a patient with ischemic mitral regurgitation (3-ch view).

tion of presence of prolapse or restriction in all parts and scallops of the anterior and posterior mitral leaflet (Stork 2007, Chan 2008, Gabriel 2008). Good agreement for mapping of prolapse between MR and TEE (Gabriel 2008) and surgical inspection (Stork 2007) was found. Another important characteristic of valve prolapse is the presence of an excentric jet. Using a multi-slice prescription through the mitral valve it is also possible to reconstruct the mitral apparatus in 3D and to evaluate geometric alterations (Kaji 2005) such as altered mitral annulus diameter and increased tenting area in functional mitral regurgitation.

Because of the overall good performance of TTE and TEE for quantification and sorting out the mechanism of mitral regurgitation, CMR is rarely required for evaluation of patients with organic mitral regurgitation and preserved LV function. Because of limited temporal and spatial resolution CMR is also not as efficient as TTE and TEE for identifying ruptured chordae. Similarly CMR also performs less well as echocardiography for visualizing vegetations in patients with mitral endocarditis. On the other hand, CMR plays an important role for precise evaluation of LV function, volume and viability in patients with functional or ischemic mitral regurgitation due to ischemic heart disease (Figure 13-14) or dilated cardiomyopathy. Indeed in this setting, CMR is the method of choice to confirm the diagnosis and to evaluate the severity of alterations of the underlying cardiomyopathy.

13.8.3 Tricuspid Valve Disease

The right atrioventricular (tricuspid) valve typically has 3 leaflets which are termed anterior, posterior and septal. The tricuspid annulus is part of the fibrous skeleton of the heart, but is situated slightly more apically than the mitral annulus. The free edges of the leaflets are attached by chordae to several small papillary muscles, which are less well-developed and individualized than in the left ventricle.

Tricuspid stenosis is uncommon, but could be formerly observed in rheumatic heart disease. It is considered clinically significant when valve areas are < 1.5 cm^2.

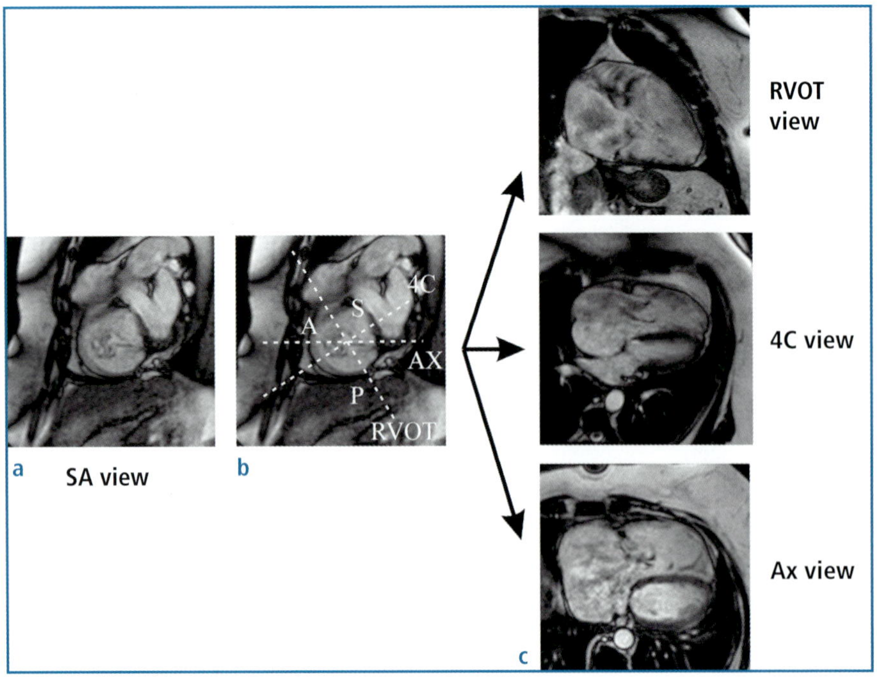

Figure 13-15 Prescription of planes to evaluate morphology and function of the tricuspid valve: Short-axis view with native tricuspid leaflets (a), planned imaging planes through the tricuspid valve (b), prescribed imaging planes for evaluation of morphology and function (c). A: anterior tricuspid leaflet; Ax: axial; 4C: 4-ch; P: posterior tricuspid leaflet; RVOT: right ventricular outflow tract; S: septal tricuspid leaflet; SA: sagittal.

Similar to mitral regurgitation, trivial tricuspid regurgitation is common. Severe tricuspid regurgitation may be primary, resulting from destruction of the valve, but is more commonly secondary (functional). The most common causes of primary tricuspid regurgitation are valve prolapse due to myxomatous degeneration, congenital (Ebstein's anomaly), destruction due to endocarditis, retraction of the valve due to carcinoid syndrome or serotonin blocker abuse, and mechanical destruction, for instance due to abrasions by pacemaker leads. Secondary tricuspid regurgitation most commonly results from severe pulmonary hypertension with secondary annular dilatation of the right ventricle. It may also result from cardiomyopathy of the right ventricle. Similar to the mitral valve, a functional classification is used to describe the mechanism of tricuspid regurgitation. Patients with severe primary tricuspid regurgitation may benefit from surgical repair or valve replacement when they are symptomatic. Tricuspid repair is also suggested as an additional procedure for patients undergoing left sided valve surgery when moderate to severe tricuspid regurgitation coexists. In contrast, surgery should be not proposed for severe tricuspid regurgitation resulting from secondary causes with severe right ventricular heart failure.

CMR can evaluate the tricuspid valve on short-axis slices through the right ventricular base. These may be used to evaluate opening surface, annulus diameter and may also identify leaflet prolapse. Motion of the septal and posterior leaflets can be best evaluated on a 4-chamber view of the heart as well as on axial slices. Motion of the anterior tricuspid leaflet can be best evaluated on a 2-chamber view of the right ventricle (Figure 13-15). The severity of tricuspid regurgitation can be measured as the difference between right ventricular stroke volume computed using Simpson's method and forward stroke volume measured by phase contrast-imaging in the pulmonary artery.

Because quantification of tricuspid regurgitation and visualization of the tricuspid valve are difficult using TTE, CMR has often an important clinical place in the evaluation of the severity and mechanism of tricuspid regurgitation and right ventricular heart disease in general. In particular it may help in understanding whether tricuspid regurgitation is primary or secondary. In this case it has the ability of precisely evaluating right ventricular function and structural abnormalities, such as ischemic necrosis. It may also thereby identify other causes for secondary right ventricular dilatation, such as ARVD, abnormal pulmonary venous return etc.

13.8.4 Pulmonary Valve Disease

Isolated pathology of the pulmonary valve is relatively uncommon in adult patients. Right ventricular outflow tract obstruction may be subvalvular, valvular or supravalvular.

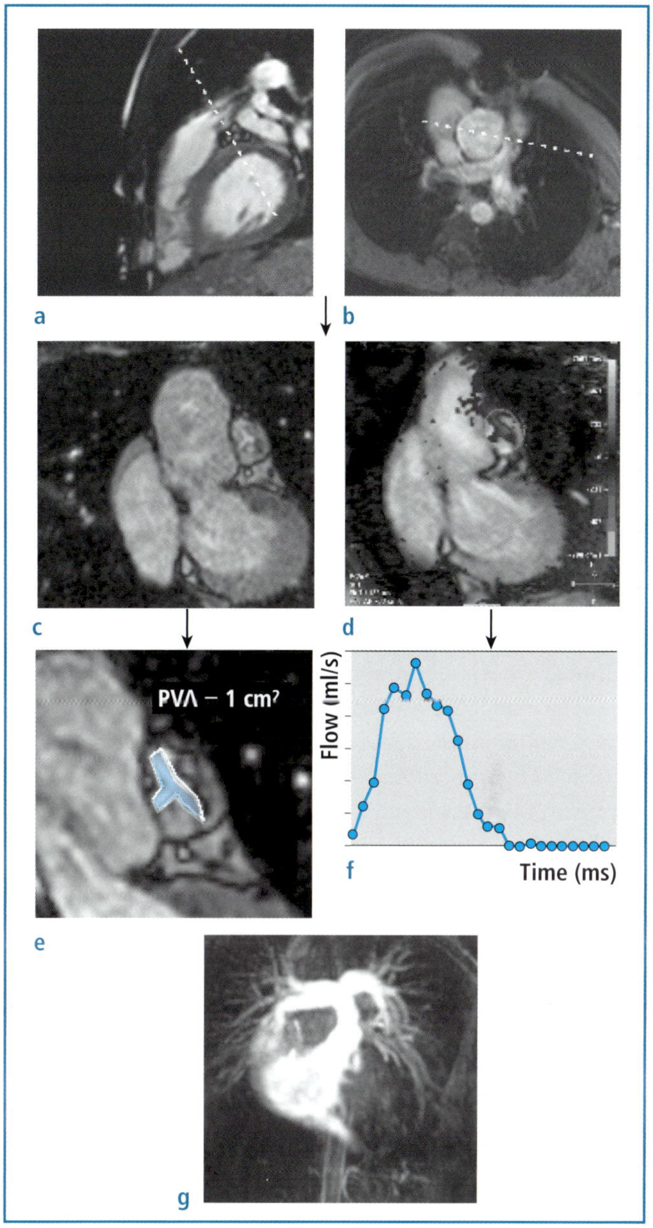

Figure 13-16 Evaluation of a patient with stenosis of the pulmonary homograft following Ross operation. Prescription of a sagittal (a) and horizontal (b) plane through the pulmonary homograft, maximal opening area of the pulmonary homograft valve (c), PC flow mapping through the stenosed pulmonary homograft valve (d), planimetered pulmonary valve area (e), flow curve through the homograft valve (f), pulmonary MR angiography showing the right ventricle, the pulmonary trunk with the homograft, and the peripheral pulmonary arterial tree (g). PVA: pulmonary valve area.

Both sub- and supravalvular stenosis are usually congential and associated with other complex congenital heart disease, such as tetralogy of Fallot. These will be discussed in another section of this book. Also isolated pulmonary stenosis is most often congenital. Only in rare circumstances might it be secondary to rheumatic disease, endocarditis or carcinoid syndrome. Trivial pulmonary regurgitation is frequent. Severe pulmonary regurgitation is often seen in congenital patients after repair of tetralogy of Fallot. It may also occur in carcinoid syndrome or after serotonin drug abuse.

Because both TTE and TEE have limited abilities to visualize the morphology of the pulmonary valve, and the sub- and supravalular parts of the RVOT, and of grading the severity of pulmonary regurgitation, CMR is the method of choice for comprehensive evaluation of the pulmonary valve. With CMR the pulmonary valve is best approached in a stepwise fashion. First a straight axial and a coronal right ventricular outflow tract cine slice may be prescribed. This generally allows visualization of the RV outflow tract and of the pulmonary valve and appreciation of whether RVOT obstruction is subvalvular or valvular. The supravalular part or the pulmonary artery may also be visualized on contrast-enhanced angiographic images (Figure 13-16). From the RVOT outflow tract location, one can then prescribe serial thin (5 mm) perpendicular short-axis slices through the pulmonary valve. These allow the appreciation of the opening surface and the overall morphology of the pulmonary valve. Grading of the severity of pulmonary regurgitation is performed by prescribing a phase contrast imaging plane on a RV outflow tract plane just beyond the pulmonary valve but before the bifurcation of the pulmonary artery. The pulmonary arteries may be evaluated on axial SSFP slices or on a contrast-enhanced angiography.

13.8.5 Evaluation of Valvular Masses and Tumors

CMR is rarely used for evaluation of valvular masses such as endocarditis or valvular tumors such as fibroelastomas. Although it has the possibility to perform tissue characterization, imaging small and highly mobile structures situated on valves is challenging on T1- and T2-weighted turbospin echo images and two-dimensional (2D) TTE and TEE is especially superior for this purpose.

13.8.6 Evaluation of Prosthetic Valves

Evaluation of prosthetic valves by CMR is safe and possible for all type of prosthetic valves (Shellock 2001), however, may be affected by artifacts in variable degrees depending on the amount and type of metal in the prosthesis (Figure 13-17). Mechanical valves yield severe artifacts preventing evaluation of their anatomy and motion on SSFP cine images. Stentless bioprosthetic valves and homo- and autografts have no metallic parts. Therefore leaftlet motion can be imaged without any artifacts. The magnitude of artifacts in stented bioprosthesis depends on the type and quantity of metal used in the stent. For most types of bioprosthesis, artifacts are relatively minor and leaflet morphology and opening surface can be visualized (Knobelsdorf-Brenkenhoff 2009). In contrast the metallic frame surrounding the percutaneously implanted stented bioprosthesis generates severe artifacts, which prevent any visualization of the leaflets. Aortic valve sparing surgery does not require annulus implantation and does not result in artifacts. After mitral and tricuspid valve sparing surgery, the severity of artifacts depends on the type of annulus used.

In general, evaluation of the severity of prosthetic valve incompetence and measurement of peak flow velocity (Botnar 2000) is feasible in all types of prosthetic valves, since phase contrast sequences are less affected by field inhomogeneity artifacts and since measurements can be performed at some distance imaging for evaluation of severity of the regurgitant valve. In contrast, visualization of valve leaflets and evaluation of stenosis is much more arbitrary and CMR should not be recommended as an imaging modality for this purpose.

13.9 Summary and Conclusions

Although transthoracic and transesophageal echocardiography remain today the primary tools for assessment of patients with adult valvular disease, CMR has become an important technique for non-invasive evaluation of patients with adult valvular disease. Indeed CMR is capable of assessing the morphology and function of all four valves of the heart with high precision. The technique has the advantage of providing more consistent image quality than echocardiography, and may thus be used as a secondary method to confirm findings when echocardiography is doubtful or of poor image quality, or when results are inconsistent with clinical findings. More importantly CMR allows better quantification of severity of valve regurgitation, and of left and right ventricular volumes and function than echocardiography. Its three-dimensional abilities also allow individual visualization of the valve leaflets, as well as of the aortic root, thereby allowing characterization of the mechanisms of dysfunction. CMR is therefore the method of choice for quantification of aortic and pulmonary insufficiency and for evaluation of complex valvular disease. Also in assessment of functional mitral regurgitation, CMR plays an important role for precise measurements of LV volumes, function and especially viability. Finally, in all types of valvular disease CMR has the unique ability to assess consequences for myocardial function by allowing computation of regional strains, and for myocardial ultrastructure, demonstrating the presence of fibrosis or necrosis.

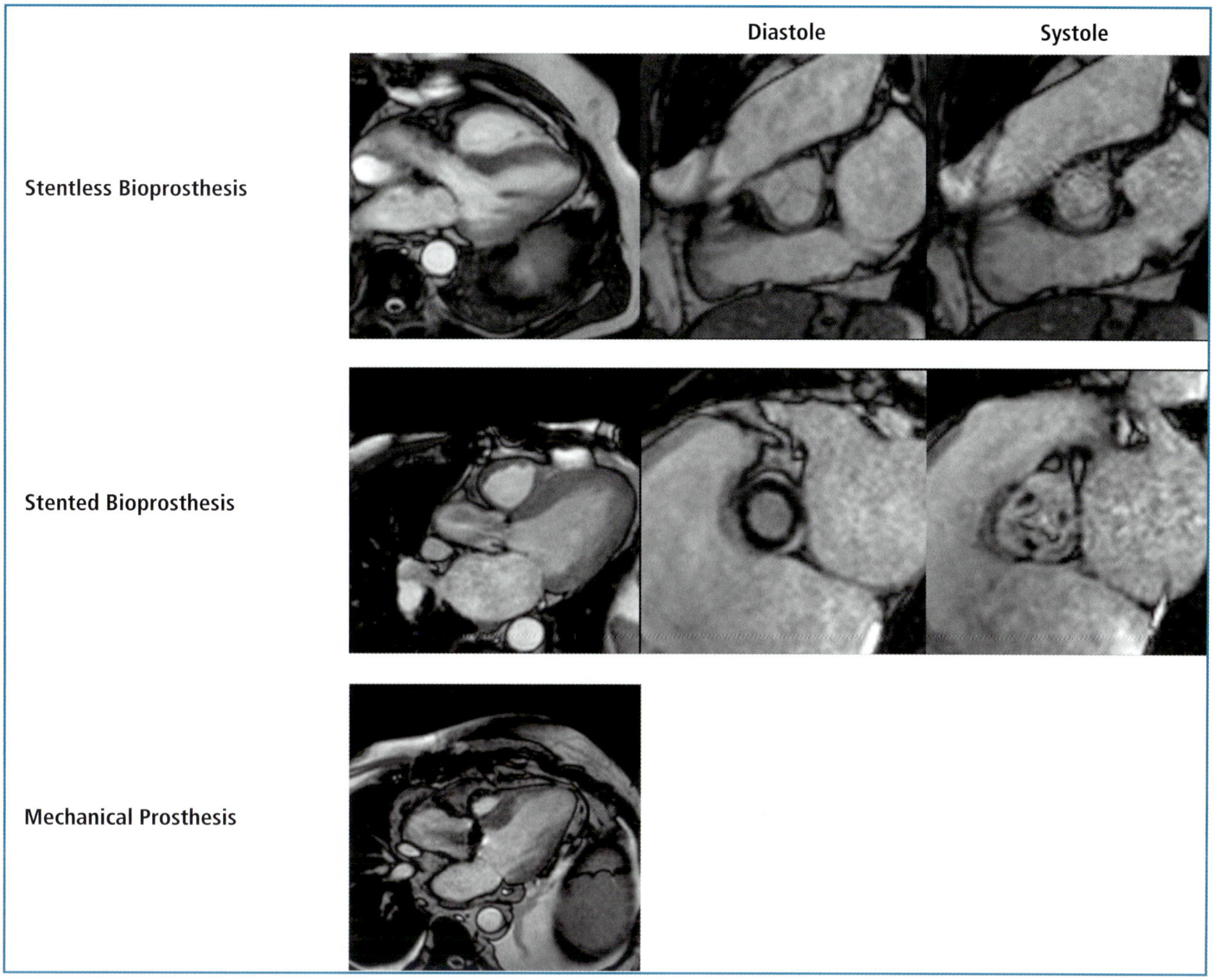

Figure 13-17 Examples of stentless and stented bioprosthesis and mechanical valve in aortic position: 3-ch view showing the different prostheses in situ (left panel), cross-section of the valve leaflets in diastole (middle panel) and systole (right panel).

References

Azevedo C et al. Prognostic significance of myocardial fibrosis quantification by histopathology and magnetic resonance imaging in patients with severe aortic valve disease. J Am Coll Cardiol 2010; 56: 278–87.

Bogren HG, Klipstein RH, Firmin DN et al. Quantitation of antegrade and retrograde blood flow in the human aorta by magnetic resonance velocity mapping. Am Heart J 1989; 117: 1214–22.

Botnar R, Nagel E, Scheidegger MB et al. Assessment of prosthetic aortic valve performance by magnetic resonance velocity imaging. MAGMA 2000; 10: 18–26.

Buchner S, Debl K, Poschenrieder F et al. Cardiovascular magnetic resonance for direct assessment of anatomic regurgitant orifice in mitral regurgitation. Circ Cardiovasc Imaging 2008; 1: 148–55.

Carpentier A. Cardiac valve surgery – the "French correction". J Thorac Cardiovasc Surg 1983; 86: 323–37.

Caruthers SD, Jiuan Lin S, Brown P et al. Practical value of cardiac magnetic resonance imaging for clinical quantification of aortic valve stenosis: comparison with echocardiography. Circulation 2003; 108: 2236–43.

Cawley PJ, Maki JH, Otto CM. Cardiovascular magnetic resonance imaging for valvular heart disease: technique and validation. Circulation 2009; 119: 468–78.

Chan KM, Wage R, Symmonds K et al. Towards comprehensive assessment of mitral regurgitation using cardiovascular magnetic resonance. J Cardiovasc Magn Reson 2008; 10: 61.

Chatzimavroudis GP, Oshinski JN, Pettigrew RI et al. Quantification of mitral regurgitation with MR phase-velocity mapping using a control volume method. J Magn Reson Imaging 1998; 8: 577–82.

Chatzimavroudis GP, Walker PG, Oshinski JN et al. Slice location dependence of aortic regurgitation measurements with MR phase velocity mapping. Magn Reson Med 1997; 37: 545–51.

Debl K, Djavidani B, Buchner C et al. Delayed hyperenhancement in magnetic resonance imaging of left ventricular hypertrophy

caused by aortic stenosis and hypertrophic cardiomyopathy: visualisation of focal fibrosis. Heart 2006; 92: 1447–51.
Debl K, Djavidani B, Buchner S et al. Assessment of the anatomic regurgitant orifice in aortic regurgitation: a clinical magnetic resonance imaging study. Heart 2008; 94: e8.
Di Cesare E, Enrici RM, Paparoni S et al. Low-field magnetic resonance imaging in the evaluation of mechanical and biological heart valve function. Eur J Radiol 1995; 20: 224–8.
Djavidani B, Debl K, Lenhart M et al. Planimetry of mitral valve stenosis by magnetic resonance imaging. J Am Coll Cardiol 2005; 45: 2048–53.
Dulce MC, Mostbeck GH, O'Sullivan M et al. Severity of aortic regurgitation: interstudy reproducibility of measurements with velocity-encoded cine-MR imaging. Radiology 1992; 185: 235–40.
El Khoury G, Glineur D, Rubay J et al. Functional classification of aortic root/valve abnormalities and their correlation with etiologies and surgical procedures. Curr Opin Cardiol 2005; 20: 115–21.
Friedrich MG, Schulz-Menger J, Poetsch T et al. Quantification of valvular aortic stenosis by magnetic resonance imaging. Am Heart J 2002; 144: 329–34.
Fujita N, Chazouilleres AF, Hartiala JJ et al. Quantification of mitral regurgitation by velocity-encoded cine-nuclear magnetic resonance imaging. J Am Coll Cardiol 1994; 23: 951–8.
Gabriel RS, Kerr AJ, Raffel OC et al. Mapping of mitral regurgitant defects by cardiovascular magnetic resonance in moderate or severe mitral regurgitation secondary to mitral valve prolapse. J Cardiovasc Magn Reson 2008; 10: 16.
Galjee MA, van Rossum AC, van Eenige MJ et al. Magnetic resonance imaging of the pulmonary venous flow pattern in mitral regurgitation. Independence of the investigated vein. Eur Heart J 1995; 16: 1675–85.
Globits S, Blake L, Bourns M et al. Assessment of hemodynamic effects of angiotensin-converting enzyme inhibitor therapy in chronic aortic regurgitation by using velocity-encoded cine-magnetic resonance imaging. Am Heart J 1996; 131: 289–93.
Goffinet C, Kersten V, Pouleur AC et al. Comprehensive assessment of the severity and mechanism of aortic regurgitation using multi-detector CT and MR. Eur Radiol 2010; 20: 326–36.
Hoffmann U, Frank H, Stefenelli T et al. Afterload reduction in severe aortic regurgitation. J Magn Reson Imaging 2001; 14: 693–7.
Honda N, Machida K, Hashimoto M et al. Aortic regurgitation: quantitation with MR imaging velocity mapping. Radiology 1993; 186: 189–94.
Hundley WG, Li HF, Willard JE et al. Magnetic resonance imaging assessment of the severity of mitral regurgitation. Comparison with invasive techniques. Circulation 1995; 92: 1151–8.
John AS, Dill T, Brandt RR et al. Magnetic resonance to assess the aortic valve area in aortic stenosis: how does it compare to current diagnostic standards? J Am Coll Cardiol 2003; 42: 519–26.
Kaji S, Nasu M, Yamamuro A et al. Annular geometry in patients with chronic ischemic mitral regurgitation: three-dimensional magnetic resonance imaging study. Circulation 2005; 112: I409–I414.
Kilner PJ, Manzara CC, Mohiaddin RH et al. Magnetic resonance jet velocity mapping in mitral and aortic valve stenosis. Circulation 1993; 87: 1239–48.
Kizilbash AM, Hundley WG, Willett DL et al. Comparison of quantitative Doppler with magnetic resonance imaging for assessment of the severity of mitral regurgitation. Am J Cardiol 1998; 81: 792–5.
Knobelsdorff-Brenkenhoff F, Rudolph A, Wassmuth R et al. Feasibility of cardiovascular magnetic resonance to assess the orifice area of aortic bioprostheses. Circ Cardiovasc Imaging 2009; 2: 397–404.
Kon MW, Myerson SG, Moat NE, Pennell DJ. Quantification of regurgitant fraction in mitral regurgitation by cardiovascular magnetic resonance: comparison of techniques. J Heart Valve Dis 2004; 13: 600–7.
Kozerke S, Schwitter J, Pedersen EM, Boesiger P. Aortic and mitral regurgitation: quantification using moving slice velocity mapping. J Magn Reson Imaging 2001; 14: 106–12.
Krombach GA, Kühl H, Bücker A et al. Cine-MR imaging of heart valve dysfunction with segmented true fast imaging with steady-state free precession. J Magn Reson Imaging 2004; 19: 59–67.
Kupfahl C, Honold MM, Meinhardt G et al. Evaluation of aortic stenosis by cardiovascular magnetic resonance imaging: comparison with established routine clinical techniques. Heart 2004; 90: 893–901.
Lin SJ, Brown PA, Watkins MP et al. Quantification of stenotic mitral valve area with magnetic resonance imaging and comparison with Doppler ultrasound. J Am Coll Cardiol 2004; 44: 133–7.
Nigri M, Azevedo CF, Rochitte CE et al. Contrast-enhanced magnetic resonance imaging identifies focal regions of intramyocardial fibrosis in patients with severe aortic valve disease: Correlation with quantitative histopathology. Am Heart J 2009; 157: 361–8.
Pouleur AC, Le Polain de Waroux JB, Goffinet C et al. Accuracy of the flow convergence method for quantification of aortic regurgitation in patients with central vs. eccentric jets. Am J Cardiol 2008; 102: 475–80.
Pouleur AC, Le Polain de Waroux JB, Pasquet A et al. Planimetric and continuity equation assessment of aortic valve area: Head to head comparison between cardiac magnetic resonance and echocardiography. J Magn Reson Imaging 2007; 26: 1436–43.
Sechtem U, Pflugfelder PW, Cassidy MM et al. Mitral and aortic regurgitation: Quantification of regurgitant volume with cine-MR imaging. Radiology 1988; 167: 425–30.
Shellock FG. Prosthetic heart valves and annuloplasty rings: assessment of magnetic field interactions, heating, and artifacts at 1.5 T. J Cardiovasc Magn Reson 2001; 3: 317–24.
Sondergaard L, Lindvig K, Hildebrandt P et al. Quantification of aortic regurgitation by magnetic resonance velocity mapping. Am Heart J 1993b; 125: 1081–90.
Sondergaard L, Stahlberg F, Thomsen C et al. Accuracy and precision of MR velocity mapping in measurement of stenotic cross-sectional area, flow rate, and pressure gradient. J Magn Reson Imaging 1993a; 3: 433–7.
Stork A, Franzen O, Ruschewski H et al. Assessment of functional anatomy of the mitral valve in patients with mitral regurgitation with cine-magnetic resonance imaging: comparison with transesophageal echocardiography and surgical results. Eur Radiol 2007; 17: 3189–98.
Suzuki J, Caputo GR, Kondo C, Higgins CB. Cine-MR imaging of valvular heart disease: display and imaging parameters affect

the size of the signal void caused by valvular regurgitation. Am J Roentgenol 1990; 155: 723–7.

Thomas JD, Weyman AE. Doppler mitral pressure half-time: a clinical tool in search of theoretical justification. J Am Coll Cardiol 1987; 10: 923–9.

Underwood SR, Klipstein RH, Firmin DN et al. Magnetic resonance assessment of aortic and mitral regurgitation. Br Heart J 1986; 56: 455–62.

Vahanian A, Baumgartner H, Bax J et al. Guidelines on the management of valvular heart disease: The Task Force on the Management of Valvular Heart Disease of the European Society of Cardiology. Eur Heart J 2007; 28: 230–68.

Van Rossum AC, Sprenger M, Visser FC et al. An in vivo validation of quantitative blood flow imaging in arteries and veins using magnetic resonance phase shift techniques. Eur Heart J 1991; 12: 117–26.

Weidemann F, Herrmann S, Störk S et al. Impact of myocardial fibrosis in patients with symptomatic severe aortic stenosis. Circulation 2009; 120: 577–84.

Westenberg JJ, Danilouchkine MG, Doornbos J et al. Accurate and reproducible mitral valvular blood flow measurement with three-directional velocity-encoded magnetic resonance imaging. J Cardiovasc Magn Reson 2004; 6: 767–76.

14 Congenital Heart Disease (CHD)

Philipp Beerbaum, Christoph Galm and Jochen Spiess

14.1 Introduction

Congenital cardiovascular disease (CHD) is defined as an abnormality in cardiocirculatory structure or function that is present at birth, even if it is discovered much later. Congenital cardiovascular malformations usually result from altered embryonic development of a normal structure or failure of such a structure to progress beyond an early stage of embryonic or fetal development. The aberrant flow patterns induced by an anatomical defect may significantly influence the structural and functional development of the remainder of the circulation.

The incidence of CHD is difficult to determine accurately, about 0.8 % of life births are complicated by a cardiovascular malformation, not included are the two most common cardiac abnormalities, the congenital bicuspid aortic valve and prolapse of the mitral valve. Some defects show definite gender preponderance such as patent ductus arteriosus (PDA), Ebstein's anomaly of the tricuspid valve, and atrial septal defect (ASD) for females, and aortic valve stenosis, coarcation of the aorta (CoA), hypoplastic left-heart syndrome (HLHS), pulmonary and tricuspid atresia, and transposition of the great arteries (TGA) to occur more commonly in males.

14.2 General Clinical Signs and Symptoms

There are four cardinal symptoms of complex CHD including congestive heart failure, cyanosis, pulmonary hypertension including Eisenmenger's syndrome, and cardiac arrhythmias. The cardinal findings of fetal **heart failure** are scalp edema, ascites, pericardial effusion, and decreased fetal movements. In pre-time infants of less than 1,500 gm birth weight persistent patency of the ductus arteriosus is the most common cause of cardiac decompensation. In full-term newborns, the main cause of heart failure are hypoplastic left heart and aortic coarctation syndromes, sustained tachyarrhythmia, hepatic or cerebral arteriovenous fistula, and myocarditis. Beyond age 1–2 wks with diminished pulmonary vascular resistance allowing substantial left-to-right shunting are ventricular septal defects (VSD) and atrioventricular septal defects (AVSD), transposition of the great arteries (TGA), truncus arteriosus (TAC), and total anomalous pulmonary venous connection (TAPVC) to induce heart failure. Heart failure in infants mostly occurs secondary to cardiac malformations whilst heart failure in older children is mainly due to acquired disease or a complication of open-heart surgery. The distinction between left and right heart failure is less obvious in infants than in older children or adults. The general aims of treatment are to achieve an increase in cardiac performance, augment peripheral perfusion, and decrease pulmonary and systemic venous congestion.

Central cyanosis refers to arterial oxygen desaturation resulting from the shunting or mixing of systemic venous blood into the arterial circulation. The magnitude of shunting or mixing and the amount of pulmonary blood flow determine the severity of desaturation.

> Most common cardiac defects causing **central cyanosis** are:
> - the **5 Ts** (**t**ransposition of great arteries, **t**etralogy of Fallot, **t**ricuspid atresia, **t**runcus arteriosus, **t**otal anomalous pulmonary venous return),
> - the **2 Es** (**E**bstein's anomaly, **E**isenmenger's physiology) as well as
> - critical pulmonary stenosis or atresia and
> - functional single-ventricle.

The main clinical features of chronic severe central cyanosis include hyperviscosity syndrome, hemostatic abnormalities, neurological complications including cerebral hemorrhage, brain abscess and new neurological symptoms, renal dysfunction, and arthritis including gout, and hypertrophic osteoarthropathy.

Pulmonary hypertension frequently accompanies congenital cardiac disease. In fact, the status of the pulmonary vascular bed is often the principal determinant of the clinical manifestation and impacts on timing and strategy of surgical repair or medical treatment. In contrast to a normal fall of pulmonary vascular resistance after birth, patients with CHD resulting in high pulmonary artery pressure and high pulmonary blood flow due to excessive left-to-right shunting may develop intimal and medial thickening of the pulmonary arteriolar vascular system in early childhood, which may ultimately progress into obliterative changes and irreversible pulmonary hypertension, known as **Eisenmenger's syndrome**. The progressive nature of this condition often results in shunt reversal and central cyanosis once the pulmonary vascular resistance exceeds the systemic vascular resistance. Congenital heart defects that may result in Eisenmenger's syndrome include "simple" defects such as ASD, VSD, and PDA, as well as more "complex" defects such as AVSD, truncus arteriosus, aortopulmonary window, and single-ventricle physiology without pulmonary stenosis to protect the pulmonary vascular bed. Clinical consequences of Eisenmenger's syndrome include palpitations, ventricular tachycardia, hemoptysis, pulmonary thromboembolism, angina, syncope, endocarditis, and congestive heart failure. The diagnosis is made by ECG, chest X-ray, echocardiography and cardiac catheterization. More recently, cardiac MRI has been found to be an excellent tool for non-invasive monitoring of the quantitative ventricular function. Treatment includes oxygen supply or lung-transplantation, as well as pharmacological treatment using calcium channel blockers, ACE-inhibitors, or endothelin receptor antagonists.

In young adults most **arrhythmias** encountered are associated with previously operated CHD. Arrhythmias include atrial arrhythmias (atrial flutter, atrial fibrillation), ventricular tachycardia, atrioventricular block, and sudden cardiac death. Atrial flutter or fibrillation are commonly observed following a Mustard/Senning operation of TGA, following surgical correction of tetralogy of Fallot (TOF), in Ebstein's anomaly, or non-corrected ASD. Ventricular tachyarrhythmias are common following surgically corrected TOF and are primarily induced by right ventricular dilatation and dysfunction. First degree AV block is normally seen in patients with AV septal defects, older ASD patients, Ebstein's anomaly, and complete TGA, as well as following surgical corrective procedures. Sudden death has been reported with arrhythmias, aortic stenosis, hypertrophic obstructive cardiomyopathy, primary pulmonary hypertension, Eisenmenger's syndrome, myocarditis, congenital complete heart block, primary endocardial fibroelastosis, and undiagnosed anomalies of the coronary arteries.

14.3 Systematic Analysis of CHD

The complexity of congenital heart disease requires a systematic sequential segmental analysis of the cardiovascular structures following the blood flow. In sequential order the atrial and visceral situs, the systemic and pulmonary venous connections, the concordance or discordance of atrioventricular (AV) and ventriculoarterial (VA) connections need to be defined. Furthermore, a complete intracardiac morphological diagnosis involves analysis and description of specific features of the right and left atrial anatomy including appendages, atrial septal defects, AV valves, papillary muscles including possible straddling of the valve chordal apparatus, morphological features as well as size and position (d-loop, l-loop) of the ventricles and their outflow tracts. The presence, number and location of ventricular septal defects will need to be assessed as well as their relation to the great arteries. On the arterial level the sequential analysis will include the quality of the semilunar valves, the presence and size of both central and peripheral pulmonary arteries, presence or absence of major aortopulmonary collaterals or a persistent ductus arteriosus (PDA), aortopulmonary windows, as well as the size, patency and position of the aortic arch and its branches. Finally, a detailed description of the proximal coronary anatomy is of vital importance for planning the surgical repair of many CHD, in particular those with conotruncal abnormalities such as transposition of the great arteries, double-outlet right ventricle, truncus arteriosus communis (TAC) and tetralogy of Fallot (TOF).

In terms of extracardiac anatomy, it should be emphasized that a wide variety of cardiovascular malformations (in particular of the aortic arch) may result in compression of the central airways. Moreover, anomalies of the cardiac situs (in particular "isomeric" syndromes) are frequently associated with situs anomalies of the lungs and the abdominal organs. Hence it is important to provide a full systemical cardiovascular diagnosis and relate this to other organ findings as necessary.

14.4 CMR Imaging Techniques

14.4.1 General Aspects

The main goals of cardiovascular magnetic resonance imaging in patients with CHD are the delineation of cardiovascular and extra-cardiac anatomy, assessment of ventricular function by quantifying ventricular volumes without geometric assumptions, and quantifying flow into valves and vessels, as well as cardiac tissue characterisation. As with other cardiac conditions, CMR can also aid in the assessment of myocardial perfusion, ischemia, and viability, as well as assist in the detection of tumor and thrombus. Unlike echocardiography, CMR is not limited by the availability of acoustic windows and provides better 3D spatial information on the relative positions of cardiac and extra-cardiac structures.

> Regarding extra-cardiac anatomy, **contrast-enhanced magnetic resonance angiography** (CE-MRA) is useful for:
> - accurate and reproducible measurement of the **ascending aorta and aortic arch** (bicuspid aortic valves, Marfan's syndrome, Loeys-Dietz syndrome, D-transposition after arterial switch, and coarctation of the aorta),
> - accurate and reproducible measurement of the **pulmonary arteries**, and for
> - delineation of the **pulmonary venous anatomy**:
>   - partial anomalous pulmonary venous return (PAPVR),
>   - complex total anomalous pulmonary venous return (TAPVR), and
>   - pulmonary vein stenosis.

Regarding ventricular volumes this technique is particularly advantageous in right ventricles, systemic right ventricles, and single-ventricles, where no presumptive geometric model exists, and this technique is used to quantify both left and right ventricular volumes and function for nearly all patients undergoing CMR for CHD. Phase contrast (PC) imaging can be used to quantitate aortic, pulmonic and to a lesser extent, tricuspid regurgitant fractions, where through plane motion complicates analysis. By comparing the flow in the main pulmonary artery and the aorta, a Qp/Qs ratio can be calculated in a variety of lesions with intracardiac shunts (ASD, VSD, PDA, and anomalous pulmonary venous return) with good correlation to values obtained invasively by oximetry (Beerbaum 2001). Flow quantification can also be used to measure the proportion of blood flow to each lung in the setting of branch pulmonary artery stenoses.

Tissue characterisation can be obtained using delayed enhancement techniques (DE-CMR), and first-pass perfusion without or with dobutamine or adenosine stress can be used to detect myocardial ischemia or delayed perfusion. A combination of first-pass perfusion, myocardial delayed enhancement imaging, and T1/T2-weighted black-blood imaging can be used to help characterise intracardiac tumor types, myocarditis, arrhythmogenic right ventricular cardiomyopathy, and pericardial disease. Imaging of the coronary arteries by 3D steady-state free precession (SSFP) sequences can be used to detect anomalies or aneurysms of the coronary arteries. Thus, in patients with CHD CMR imaging is a very valuable tool to answer most important questions regarding the abnormal structures and function of the heart, valves and vessels. It has to be emphasised that although standardized protocols may be applicable for routine congenital CMR cases (e.g. assessment of RV size/function and pulmonary regurgitation in post-operative TOF) the examination of the patient with CHD often must be tailored to the clinical indications specified. This means that direct physician involvement in image acquisition is usually required for patients with acyanotic and cyanotic CHD to ensure that all pertinent clinical questions have been addressed.

14.4.2 Performing CMR in Newborns and Children

CMR imaging in children is a technical challenge, and at least 1.5 T scanners should be used to get high temporal and spatial resolution images in a relatively short acquisition time. Cardiac coils for adults may also be used in older children, in children < 5 kg body weight quadratur coils (e.g. head-neck coil) may be appropriate. A key prerequisite is the use of high performance gradient systems for performing contrast-enhanced angiographies and dynamic steady-state free precession (SSFP) sequences for reliable assessment of structural, functional and flow abnormalities.

CMR examinations in **newborns, children** or **teenagers** may be performed under **three different conditions** according to indication of the study, safety aspects, and patient's co-operability:

- in general anesthesia using endotracheal intubation,
- in a sedative state using sedatives,
- spontaneously without any drugs.

Fogel et al. (2008) reported on 660 patients with CHD undergoing deep sedation for CMR studies compared with 161 patients with CHD undergoing general anesthesia. The result was that sedation of appropriately screened pediatric patients with CHD undergoing CMR is safe and well-tolerated and yields high-quality images similar to general anesthesia. General anesthesia should be considered for CHD patients with hemodynamic or airway compromise, in whom sedation has failed. The preparatory protocol may vary considerably according to the condition chosen, and the decision of which preparation scheme is used will be made by the referring pediatric cardiologist, the availability and skills of the anesthetist, and availability of scan time and MR-compatible equipment. As a general rule the indication of general anesthesia should be: the younger and the sicker the child, the more liberal the use of general anesthesia. In this scenario a risk-benefit assessment is important as a CMR examination requires a highly skilled team of intensive care physicians, anesthetists and cardiologists in order to be performed safely in critically ill children or infants. CT angiography may be considered as a viable and much faster alternative, in particular for young infants with cardiovascular airway compression. In children necessitating catecholamine therapy or those with suspected stenoses of the respiratory tract general anesthesia is obligatory. Nevertheless, it should be stressed that in a skilled environment CMR imaging in patients with CHD is safe, as has been shown by Dorfman et al. (2007), who found 22 adverse events among 1,334 CMR studies (1.6%), including 14 minor, 7 moderate, and 1 major adverse event. General anesthesia and examinations of hospitalized patients were independent risk factors for adverse events with the most acutely ill patients at highest risk.

14.4.3 CMR Protocols

The **complete protocol for CMR in CHD** includes scouts and reference scans, sequences for examining intracardiac morphology including vessels and airways, flow assessment, angiography, and function of the cardiac chambers (particularly the ventricles), according to the following scheme:

- scouts and reference scans (SSFP and parallel imaging, e.g. SENSE),
- cine-SSFP sequences, eventually combined with parallel imaging (SENSE) for assessing morphology and function

(atria, ventricles, heart valves, great vessels, regional and global, systolic function, wall thickening, myocardial mass, intracardiac abnormal flow pattern),
- T1-, T2- and PD-weighted black-blood sequences in the standard planes for anatomic and morphologic imaging of cardiac structures (atrial and ventricular size, myocardium, great vessels) and airway structures (tracheal stenoses etc.),
- velocity-encoded cine-CMR for quantitative flow assessment (valvular dysfunction, intraventricular gradient, shunt calculation, diastolic function by transvalvular flow pattern),
- contrast-enhanced angiography or inflow MR angiography for imaging normal and abnormal vessels,
- optional: first-pass perfusion studies of the myocardium (to rule out significant CAD),
- optional: contrast-enhanced imaging in the long- (2-ch, 4-ch) and short-axes for LGE (myocardial damage, distribution pattern, extent, pericardial enhancement),
- optional: coronary MR angiography and CMR of thoracic vessels (exclusion of concomitant pathology).

14.4.4 Quantitative Analysis of Morphology and Function

Quantitative measurements of RV and LV volumes by short-axis volumetry, quantification of flow volumes and maximal flow velocities in areas of stenoses by PC mapping, as well as analysis of myocardial kinetics and wall motion by VENC CMR and tagging are performed according to standard criteria (Simonetti 2006), as described in Chapter 5. Luijnenburg et al. (2010) have shown in 35 patients with CHD (7–62 yrs) that inter-observer (3.9–10.2 %) and intra-observer (2.9–6.8 %) variability of biventricular parameters assessed by CMR imaging is good, i.e. low, with smallest variations for biventricular end-diastolic volumes and highest for biventricular end-systolic volumes. It was concluded that CMR imaging is an accurate and reproducible method and should allow adequate assessment of changes in both ventricular size and global function. However, as shown by Beerbaum et al. in a study of the German Competence Network for Congenital Heart Disease in 2009 it is of vital importance for ventricular volumetric analysis that strict intra-institutional image reading criteria are being consistently applied through observer training; and this is even more important when comparing data from different institutions, or have the same data read by different observers. It is not sufficient to rely on published guidelines but rather necessary to implement on-screen observer training and regular observer variance checks within a given MRI lab to keep observer variances below 10 % (Beerbaum 2009).

14.4.5 Normal Values of Cardiac Volumes/ Function

Normal CMR values for healthy children are sparse. Recently normal gender specific values for CMR measured RV and LV volumes, mass, ejection fraction, and cardiac index have been published by Sarikouch et al. (2010) for 114 healthy children and adolescents at age groups of 5–15 yrs and 16–20 yrs (Table 14-1). Subjects underwent axial volumetry (1.5 T scanner) using standardized 2D SSFP and flow proto-

Table 14-1 Normal pediatric cardiac volumes in CMR imaging according to age and gender.

	LVEDVI (ml/m^2)	LVESVI (ml/m^2)	LVSVI (ml/m^2)	CI ($l/min/m^2$)	RVEDVI (ml/m^2)	RVESVI (ml/m^2)	RVSVI (ml/m^2)	LVEF (%)	RVEF (%)
Total									
girls	77.9 ± 10.8	28.5 ± 6.2	49.3 ± 8.1	3.98 ± 0.7	76.9 ± 12.7	28.6 ± 5.4	48.2 ± 6.8	63.4 ± 6.1	62.8 ± 4.3
boys	85.1 ± 13.8	30.5 ± 7.6	54.6 ± 8.2	4.30 ± 0.85	84.5 ± 12.7	32.5 ± 6.4	52.0 ± 8.4	64.4 ± 4.9	61.6 ± 4.5
8–15 yrs									
girls	78.7 ± 10.7	28.9 ± 6.1	49.7 ± 8.3	3.94 ± 0.62	78.3 ± 9.7	29.2 ± 4.6	49.1 ± 6.8	63.2 ± 6.3	62.6 ± 3.6
boys	81.9 ± 12.9	28.2 ± 6.7	53.7 ± 8.5	4.42 ± 0.85	82.9 ± 12.6	31.3 ± 6.1	51.6 ± 8.4	65.7 ± 4.9	62.3 ± 4.3
16–20 yrs									
girls	80.7 ± 9.5	29.9 ± 7.5	51.7 ± 6.8	3.85 ± 0.86	79.9 ± 10.3	30.4 ± 6.9	49.3 ± 6.3	64.3 ± 7.3	62.1 ± 6.0
boys	93.5 ± 10.9	35.9 ± 7.1	57.6 ± 5.9	4.02 ± 0.79	90.2 ± 10.9	36.1 ± 6.3	54.1 ± 7.3	61.8 ± 4.3	60.0 ± 4.4

Numbers of individuals studied: total group: girls n = 59 and boys n = 55; group of 8–15 yrs: girls n = 35 and boys n = 35; group of 16–20 yrs: girls n = 13 and boys n = 16.

LVEDVI: left ventricular end-diastolic volume index; LVESVI: left ventricular end-systolic volume index; LVSVI: left ventricular stroke volume index; CI: cardiac index; RVEDVI: right ventricular end-diastolic volume index; RVESVI: right ventricular end-systolic volume index; RVSVI: right ventricular stroke volume index; LVEF: left ventricular ejection fraction; RVEF: right ventricular ejection fraction (modified from Sarikouch et al. 2010; with permission of Wolters Kluwer – Lippincott, Williams & Wilkins, Baltimore).

cols. Percentiles were computed for age 8–20 yrs (99 subjects) as breath-holds were more consistent in this group. When indexed for body surface area (BSA) or height, the centile curves of ventricular volumetric parameters showed allometric increase until adolescence, when a plateau was reached, with values comparable to published results, but ventricular mass centiles increased without a plateau. There was a significant gender difference with centiles reflecting larger values in boys than in girls ($p < 0.05$), with ventricular volumes indexed to BSA or height in contrast to no difference when indexing to weight. There was excellent agreement of axial and short-axis volumetry and of volumetric and flow-derived stroke volumes (Sarikouch et al. 2010).

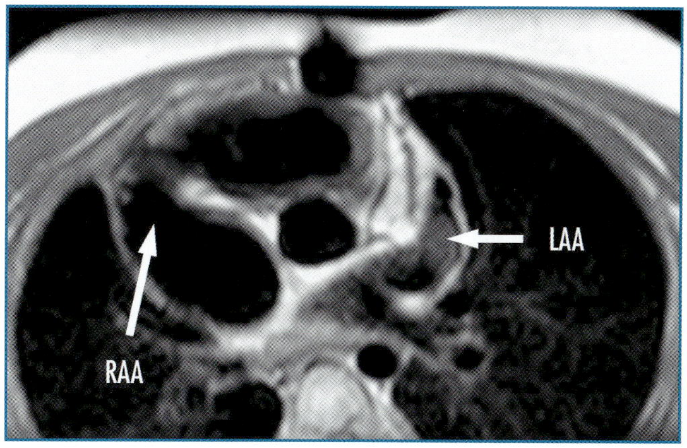

Figure 14-1 Atrial situs solitus with dextroposition of the heart in a SE-EPI sequence showing the position of the left atrial (LAA) and right atrial appendage (RAA).

14.5 Anomalies of the Atrial and Visceral Situs

Pathology

Cardiac **situs solitus** (normal situs) is defined by the position of the morphologically right atrium (RA) at the right-anterior-inferior border to the left atrium (LA), the latter being located posterior-superior in front of the spine (Figure 14-1). Cardiac **situs inversus** shows a mirror image of the relationship of RA to LA (Figure 14-2).

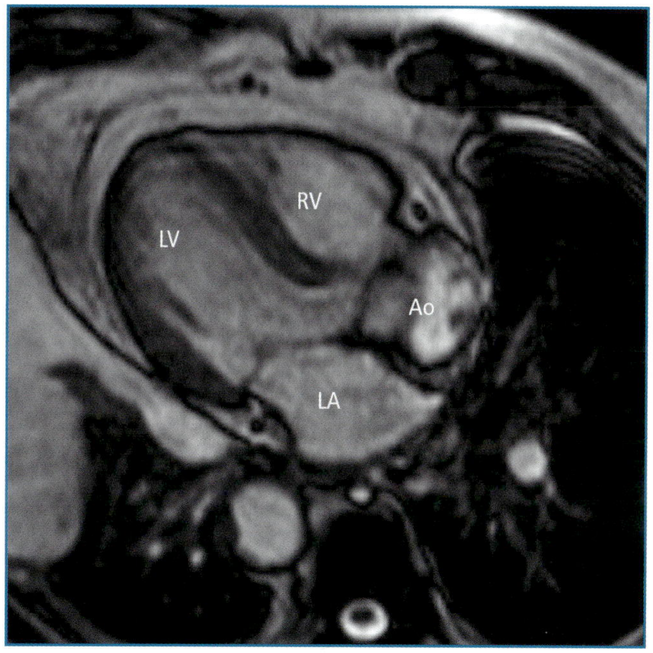

Figure 14-2 Situs inversus in a cine-SSFP image: mirror image of the heart within the thorax – mesoposition with dextrocardia. Ao: aortic root; LA: left atrium; LV: left ventricle; RV: right ventricle.

The **situs ambiguous** may occur in three different forms:
- an indeterminate atrial anatomy,
- "right isomerism" (two morphologically right atria) or
- "left isomerism" (two morphologically left atria).

"Right isomerism" is characterized by right atrial situs, bilateral "right" main bronchi (short with large tracheal angle), both pulmonary artery branches anterior to the upper lobe bronchus, asplenia, central (midway) liver with two lobes, malrotation of the intestine; commonly associated anomalies of the heart include atrium commune, complete AV defect, hypoplastic left ventricle, a double-outlet right ventricle (DORV) with/without ventricular inversion, pulmonary valve stenosis or -atresia with ductus-dependent lung perfusion, and bilateral superior vena cava (SVC) with biatrial orifice and anomalous supracardiac pulmonary vein (PV) drainage.

"Left isomerism" is characterized by left atrial situs with interrupted intrahepatic inferior vena cava (IVC) to morphological LA, continuation of the azygos vein with draining of the blood from the abdominal and retroperitoneal pelvic and leg veins into the SVC, bilateral "left" main bronchi (long with small tracheal angle), both pulmonary artery branches posterior to the upper lobe bronchus, polysplenia, and anomalies of the intestine; commonly associated congenital anomalies of the heart include atrium commune, bilateral draining of PVs into their corresponding atria (RA or LA), separate draining of liver veins into their corresponding atria, partial AV defect, less common unbalanced ventricles, and less common pulmonary valve stenosis or -atresia. As a general rule, the cardiovascular defects tend to be less severe in left atrial isomerism, as compared with right atrial isomerism.

Clinical Presentation

Clinical presentation, diagnosis and therapy depends on associated congenital abnormalities. Most commonly these lesions will have cyanosis in the newborn period as a leading symptom, and in case of pulmonary atresia there is then obviously duct-dependency.

14.6 Anomalies of the Atria, Systemic and Pulmonary Veins

14.6.1 Atrial Septal Defect (ASD)

Pathology and Pathophysiology

ASD is common with a prevalence of 7.5–8.5 % of all CHDs.

> There are **four types of ASDs** or interatrial connections:
> - ostium primum (ASD I, endocardial cushion; Figure 14-6),
> - ostium secundum (ASD II, approximately 80 % of all ASDs; Figure 14-3),
> - sinus venosus (approximately 11 % of all ASDs, associated with anomalous pulmonary vein drainage; Figure 14-5), and
> - coronary sinus defects (very rare).

In any type of ASD left-to-right shunting is present, and its degree depends on the size of the defect and the relative properties (compliance) of the two ventricles and pulmonary vascular resistance.

Clinical Presentation

Most patients with ASD are asymptomatic and develop progressive symptoms by 40 yrs including atrial arrhythmias (atrial fibrillation or flutter), AV block, exertional dyspnea or fatigue, right sided heart failure, and signs of pulmonary hypertension.

Diagnosis and CMR Findings

Diagnosis is made by clinical examination ("left atrialisation" of the jugular venous pressure, widely fixed split of S2, pansystolic murmur of tricuspid regurgitation with RV failure), echocardiography (type and size of defect, direction of shunt, size and function of the right ventricle), and in doubtful cases by CMR imaging (Figure 14-4). CMR provides precise information on the size and function of both atria and ventricles (volume overload of the RV) (Figure 14-7a, b), as well as determining the degree of shunting (PC flow measurement in the pulmonary artery and the aorta) (Beerbaum 2001, 2003a and b). In addition, using inflow-MRA or 3D-CE-MRA the size and location of the defect and PV anomalies can be detected. ASDs should be occluded if the shunt fraction Qp/Qs exceeds 1.5:1 ("significant" ASD) (Figure 14-7c).

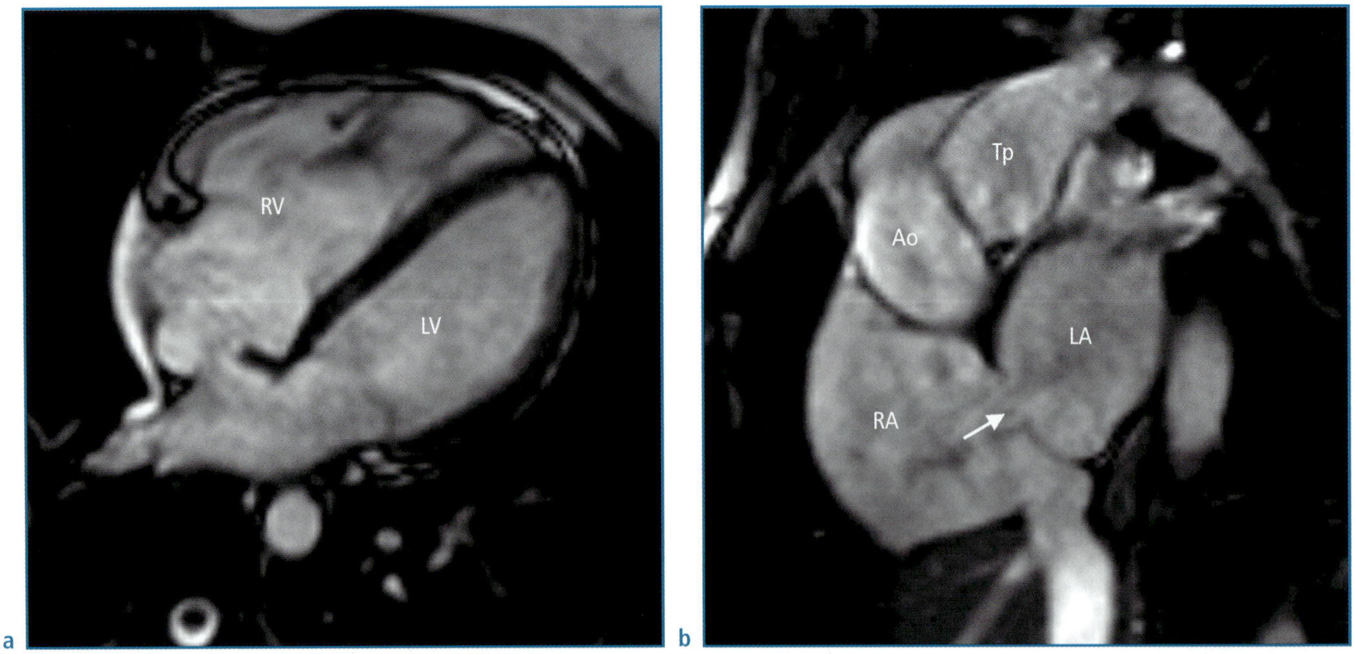

Figure 14-3 Atrial septal defect of secundum type (ASD II) in 4-ch- (a) and short-axis view (b) on a cine-SSFP sequence showing the defect in the membraneous interatrial septum (arrow in (b)), together with a dilated right ventricle due to volume overload (a). Ao: aortic root; LA: left atrium; LV: left ventricle; RA: right atrium; RV: right ventricle; Tp: pulmonary trunk.

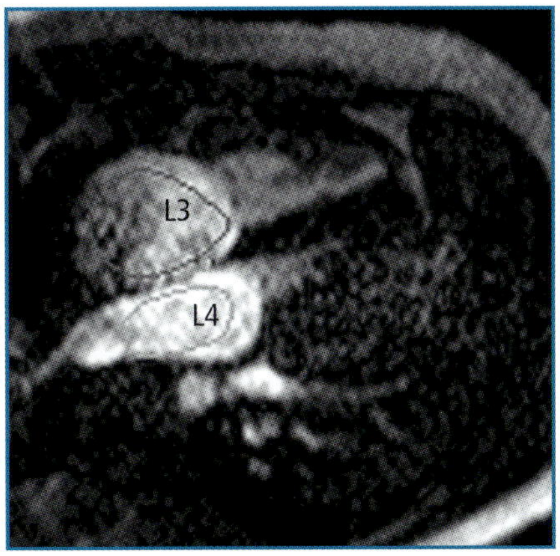

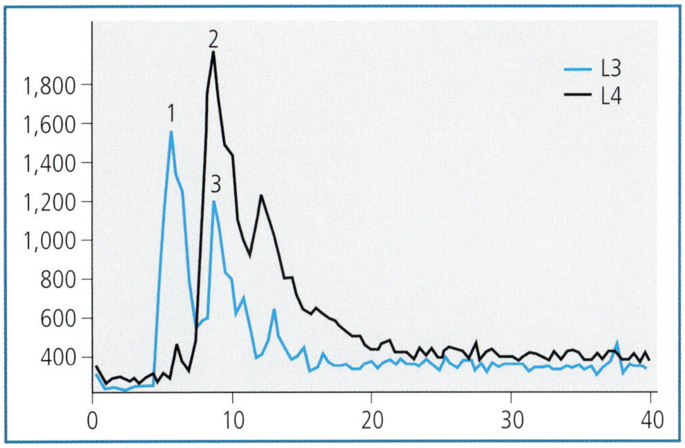

Figure 14-4 Detection of a left-to-right shunt at the atrial level using a single intravenous bolus of 5 ml of gadolinium contrast agent and continuous registration of the time-intensity curves in a dedicated measurement field in the right (L3) and left atrium (L4) in a 4-ch view (a). Initially the contrast bolus passes the right ventricle (blue curve in (b)) with a first peak (1 in (b)); following its passage through the lung the bolus appears in the left atrium (black curve in (b)) with a peak (2 in (b)), while almost simultaneously a second peak in the right atrial signal intensity curve (3 in (b)) occurs due to left-to-right shunting. The amount of the shunt can be calculated by PC flow measurement in the aorta and pulmonary artery.

Therapy

Patients with secundum-type ASD are most commonly treated by catheter-based device closure (occluder). In large secundum ASDs or primum ASD or in sinus venosus defects with concomitant PV anomalies surgical correction is necessary. Long-term outcome of patients with device occluded ASDs or surgical correction is excellent.

Long-Term Effects and CMR Findings

Patients with surgically repaired sinus venosus defect are at risk of developing caval and/or pulmonary vein stenosis and should be kept under regular review. Patients with surgical or device repair as adults, patients with atrial arrhythmias pre- or post-operatively, and those with ventricular dysfunctions should remain under long-term cardiological surveillance. Each of these complications (stenoses or ventricular dysfunction) can be easily detected and quantified by appropriate CMR imaging during follow-up.

14.6.2 Pulmonary Vein Anomalies

Pathology and Pathophysiology

These anomalies are commonly associated with complex CHD, particularly in heterotaxia syndrome. Partial abnormal PV drainage is the rule with **sinus venosus defect** (Figure 14-5), most commonly the veins of the right upper and middle lobe drain into the SVC leading to left-to-right shunting (Figure 14-8a). A special condition is observed with the **Scimitar syndrome**, in which all right-sided PVs drain via a collecting vessel ("Scimitar vessel") into the IVC sometimes with a coexisting PV stenosis with consecutive pulmonary hypertension (Figure 14-8b); in most cases bronchopulmonary sequestration of segments of the lower lobe, abnormal collateral supply to the sequestered segment, and hypoplasia of the right lung exists leading to secondary dextroposition of the heart. Left-sided partial anomalous PVs most commonly drain into the left innominate vein (commonly of the upper lobe), only rarely into the coronary

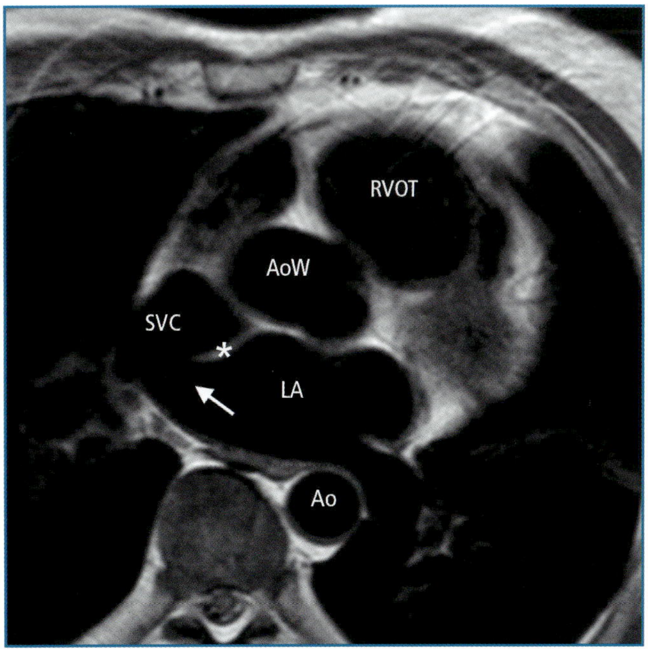

Figure 14-5 Sinus venosus defect in a black-blood sequence in an axial plane at the level of the aortic bulb (AoW). The defect (arrow) is located within the interatrial septum (*) between the left atrium (LA) and the superior caval vein (SVC). Ao: descending aorta; RVOT: right ventricular outflow tract.

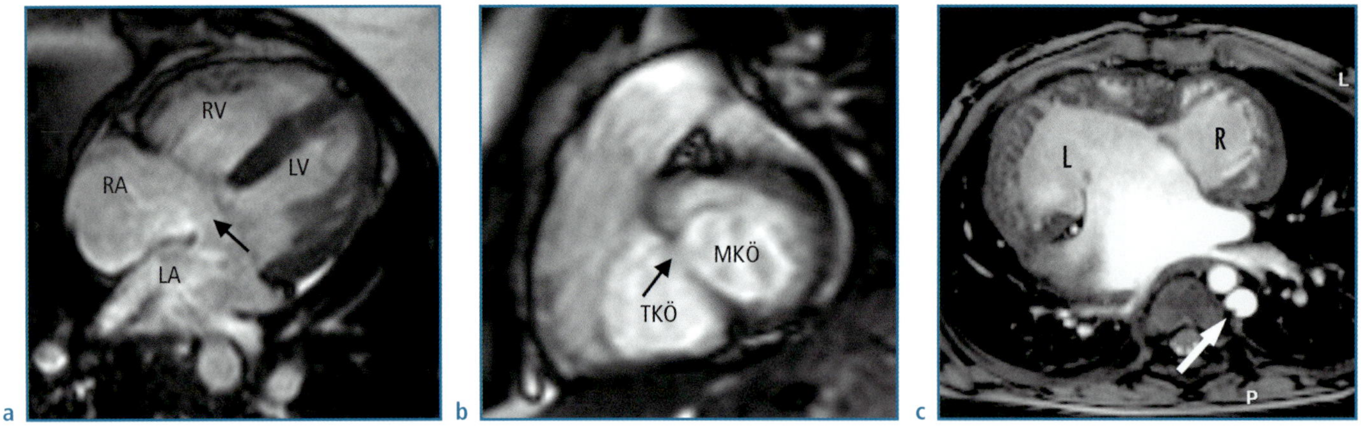

Figure 14-6 Intermediate atrioventricular septal defect (AVSD) with an atrial septal defect of primum type (ASD I), a restrictive ventricular septal defect (VSD) and separate AV valves in a cine-SSFP sequence in 4-ch **(a)** and short-axis view **(b)**. The ASD I is visible at the proximal part of the interatrial septum (arrow in **(a)**) with enlarged right atrium and ventricle; the VSD is seen at the level of the mitral and tricuspid valve (arrow in **(b)**). Complete AV septal defect (AVSD) in a 4-ch view **(c)** through both ventricles with common atrium (atrium commune), dextrocardia and left isomerism. The morphological right ventricle (R) lies on the left and the left ventricle (L) on the right side; the pulmonary veins drain atypically at the dorsal aspect of the common atrium, the inferior caval vein (arrow) lacks an intrahepatic portion, azygos continuation at the left-dorsal aspect of the descending aorta. LA: left atrium; LV: left ventricle; MKÖ: mitral valve orifice; RA: right atrium; RV: right ventricle; TKÖ: tricuspid valve orifice.

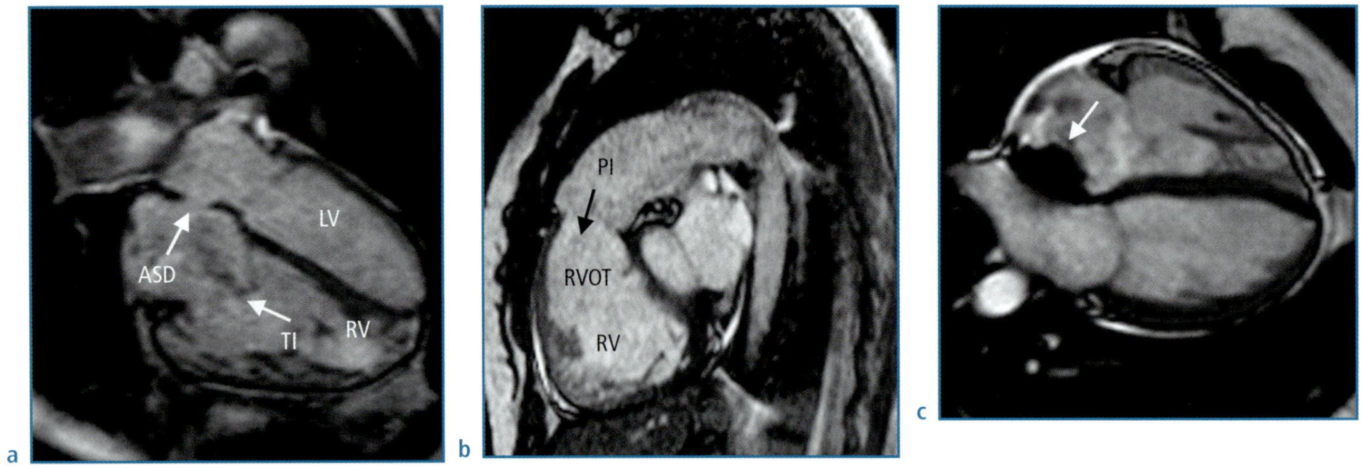

Figure 14-7 Eisenmenger's physiology in a patient with longlasting ASD II in a cine-SSFP sequence in 4-ch view **(a)** and RVOT plane **(b)**. Atrial septal defect (ASD, arrow in **(a)**) with enlarged right ventricle (RV), RV hypertrophy, and secondary tricuspid regurgitation (TI, arrow in **(a)**); enlargement of the RV including the RVOT and pulmonary artery with secondary pulmonary regurgitation (PI, arrow in **(b)**). Interventional treatment of an ASD **(c)** using an atrial septal occluder (arrow in **(c)**). LV: left ventricle; RVOT: right ventricular outflow tract (Figures a and b by courtesy of Dr. J. Schwab, Nuremberg).

sinus or into the right atrium; they are frequently associated with a secundum ASD. **Total anomalous pulmonary vein connection** (TAPVC) describes the situation where all pulmonary veins fail to drain directly into the left atrium (LA), and as a result, all of the systemic and pulmonary venous return eventually drains into the right atrium (RA) (Figure 14-8c). The anomalous connection is most often supradiaphragmatic, connecting via a vertical vein to the left brachiocephalic vein, directly to the RA, to the coronary sinus, or directly to the SVC. In approximately 10–15 % the site of connection is infradiaphragmatic, and the anomalous trunk connects into the portal vein or one of its tributaries, the ductus venosus, or rarely to the hepatic or other abdominal veins. Systemic circulation is only provided by obligatory right-to-left shunting across an open foramen ovale or an ASD to reach the often small-sized left atrium and left ventricle.

Clinical Presentation

In the absence of associated anomalies, the physiological disturbance is determined by the number of anomalous veins and their site of connection, the presence and size of

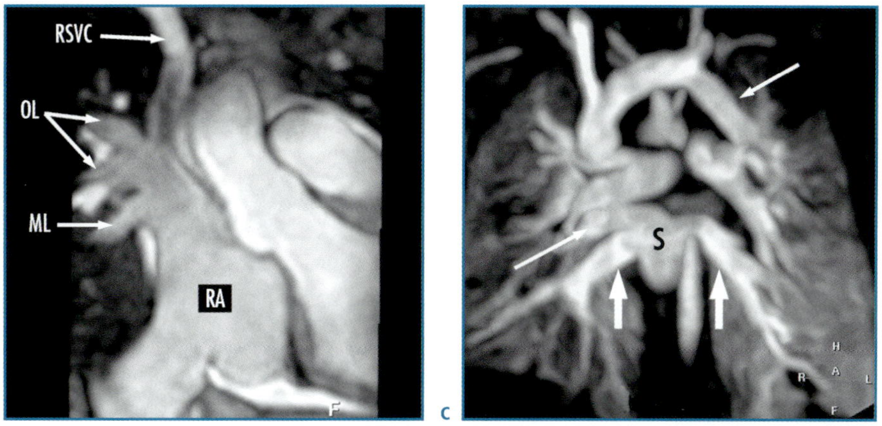

a c

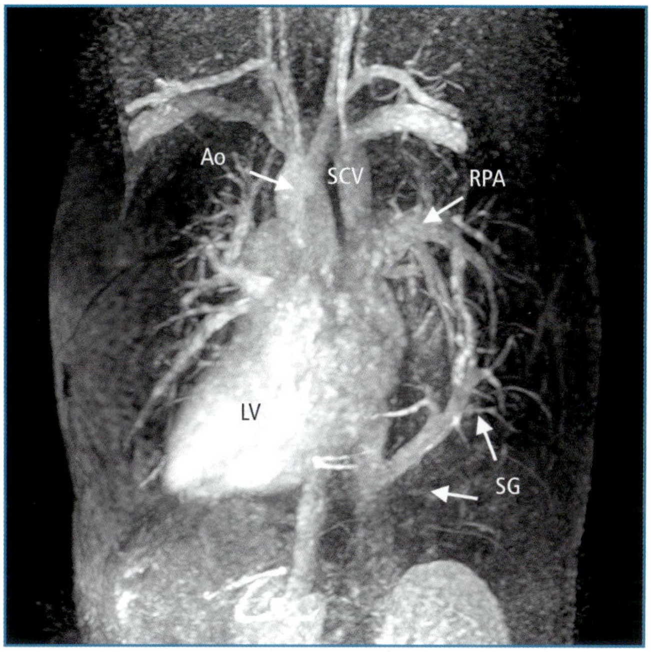

b

Figure 14-8 Anomalous drainage of the right upper (OL) and middle (ML) lobe pulmonary veins into the right superior caval vein (RSVC) just cranial to the orifice of the SCV into the right atrium (RA) (a). Scimitar syndrome from the dorsal aspect showing an anomalous drainage of a right-sided pulmonary vein via a collecting vessel (SG = Scimitar vessel) into the inferior caval vein distal to the orifice of the liver vein (b). Total anomalous pulmonary venous return (TAPVR) in a newborn in a frontal view on CE-MRA (c): the right-sided pulmonary veins and the left lower lobe vein (broad arrows) drain into a common collecting vessel (S) that further drains into the right atrium (not imaged) via the coronary sinus; the left upper pulmonary vein (small arrow) drains directly into the left vena anonyma. Ao: aorta; LV: left ventricle; RPA: right pulmonary artery; SCV and SVC: superior caval vein.

an ASD, and the state of pulmonary vascular bed. In patients with isolated partial pulmonary venous connection, the hemodynamic state, symptoms, and physical findings are similar to those in ASD. Symptomatic infants with TAPVC, usually occurring within the first year of life, present with cyanosis (obligatory right-to-left shunt on atrial level) and signs of heart failure (venous mixing with left-to-right shunt) once the pulmonary vascular resistance falls in the newborn period. Infants with TAPVC and pulmonary venous obstruction present with early onset of severe dyspnea, cyanosis, pulmonary edema, and low-cardiac output state. Without severe venous obstruction symptoms may be minimal and remain undetected in infancy. On auscultation a fixed, widely split second heart sound, galopp rhythm and an accentuated pulmonic component of the second heart sound is present.

Diagnosis and CMR Findings

Diagnosis of single PV connections is made by X-ray (increased pulmonary blood flow), and by echocardiography (RV volume overload, shunt). Anomalous drainage of PVs as well as venous stenoses can be easily detected by inflow MRA or by CE-MRA (Greil 2002). In patients with TAPVC diagnosis is confirmed by ECG (right axis deviation, RA and RV hypertrophy), chest X-ray (cardiomegaly, "figure-of-eight" or "snow-man" heart due to enlargement of heart and presence of dilated right SVC, innominate vein, and left vertical vein), and by echocardiography (marked enlargement of the RV, small LA, entire pathway of anomalous blood flow). Cine-MRI and black-blood CMR can easily detect the abnormal anatomy and blood flow, which can also be assessed by inflow-MRA or CE-MRA. The amount of right-to-left shunt can be quantified by PC mapping of PA and aortic blood flow. In a sick neonate a CT angiogram

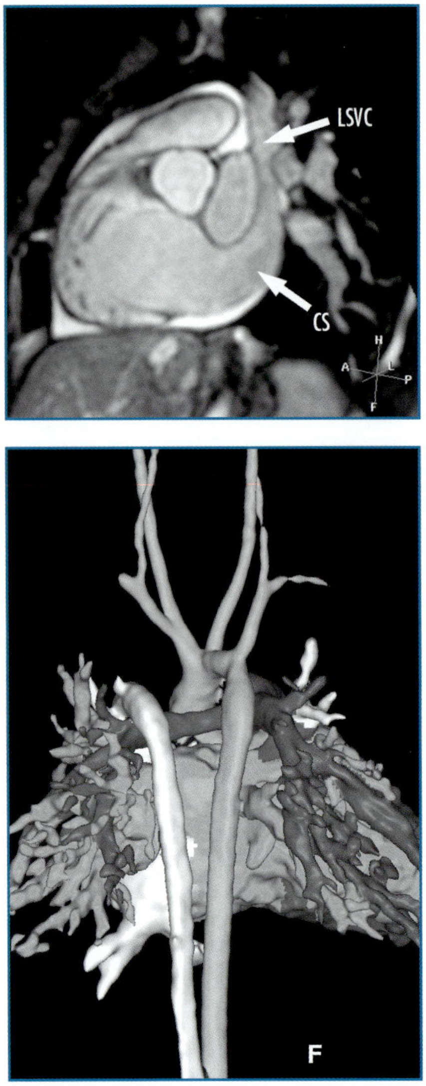

a

b

Figure 14-9 Persistent left superior caval vein (LSVC, arrow) draining into the coronary sinus (CS, arrow) in a sagittal view using a cine-SSFP sequence (a). Complex congenital malformation with an azygos continuity and drainage into the left-sided upper caval vein (vessel with bright signal intensity) (b).

may be a good alternative to MRI should questions remain open after echocardiography.

Therapy

Treatment of isolated abnormal PV connections is surgical correction if Qp/Qs exceeds 1.5 : 1. Obstructed TAPVR is a surgical emergency in newborn/infant age. Urgent transcatheter treatment of the pulmonary venous obstruction by stenting may rarely be required in severe cases to stabilise a patient prior to surgery. Surgical correction is usually performed by connecting the retroatrial collecting sinus with the LA and closing the ASD.

Long-Term Effects and CMR Findings

Historically with the older surgical technique PV stenosis has been a problem on long-term, which can be easily detected and quantified by CMR imaging. With the newer technique stenosis of the PVs or the surgical anastomosis is very rare, and children without stenosis are seen as low- to moderate-risk adults.

14.6.3 Anomalies of the Systemic Veins

Such anomalies are encountered in over 90% of complex CHD with situs ambiguous, they are rare with a lateralized situs (situs solitus or inversus). In more than 90% of cases a persistent left superior caval vein (LSVC) drains into the RA via the coronary sinus (Figure 14-9a). An isolated LSVC has no clinical significance but if associated with congenital malformation the surgeon must be informed for appropriate modification of venous cannulation when connecting the cardiopulmonary bypass. Rarely, a LSVC drains into the LA associated with an "unroofed coronary sinus" and thus, produces a righ-to-left shunt with moderate central cyanosis, combined with a left-to-right shunt via the interatrial cleft.

A LSVC is always present in the very rare cases of absent or atretic right SVC as well as of atresia of the ostium of the coronary sinus. Also very rarely the SVC connects with the LA with resulting cyanosis. In almost 90% of patients with heterotaxia with polysplenia an interrupted IVC with azygos continuation is encountered (Figure 14-9b), whereas bilateral inferior venae cavae are mostly seen in patients with heterotaxia syndrome. All these caval vein anomalies can be simply and reliably detected by inflow MRA or CE-MRA. To differentiate pulmonary venous anomalies from supracardiac PV connections and to delineate systemic venous recirculation at least two dynamic MR studies should be acquired.

14.7 Ventricular Malformations and Ventricular Septal Defects

14.7.1 Ventricular Septal Defects (VSD) and Atrioventricular Septal Defects (AVSD)

Pathology and Pathophysiology

VSDs are classified into defects of the inlet septum, the muscular septum (including apical defects) (Figure 14-10a, b), subaortal "perimembraneous" defects, and subpulmonary VSDs (superior to the crista supraventricularis). VSDs are

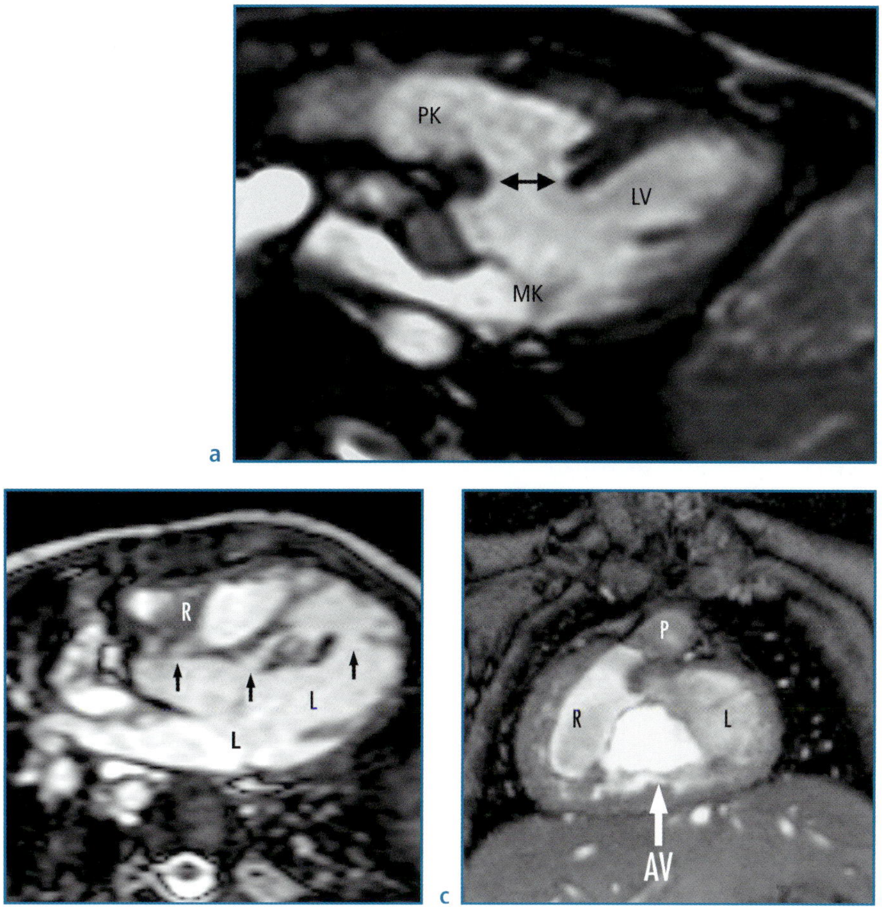

Figure 14-10 Large defect within the muscular interventricular septum (double-sided arrow) (a); LV: left ventricle; MK: mitral valve; PK: pulmonary valve. Multiple ventricular septal defects (arrows) (b); L: left ventricle; R: right ventricle. Complete AV septal defect with a single AV valve (AV, arrow) in a view parallel and inferior to the AV valve plane through the right (R) and left ventricle (L) showing the large defect (c), the pulmonary artery arising from the right ventricle, and the infundibular septum. P: pulmonary artery.

commonly encountered in complex congenital malformations and are always seen in conotruncal defects. In the presence of a normal pulmonary vascular resistance, a restrictive VSD would result in a significant pressure gradient between the LV and RV (pulmonary/aortic systolic pressure ratio < 0.3) and is accompanied by a small shunt (1.4/1.0). A moderately restrictive VSD is accompanied by a moderate shunt (Qp/Qs 1.4–2.2/1.0) with a pulmonary/aortic pressure ratio of < 0.66, whereas a large non-restrictive VSD is accompanied by a large shunt (Qp/Qs > 2.2) and a pulmonary/aortic systolic pressure ratio of ≥ 0.66. A VSD or AVSD is often part of a more complex congenital heart defect, such as with tetralogy of Fallot or double-outlet right ventricle, and the pathophysiology and clinical presentation may then be determined by the additional lesions.

Complete AVSD (as frequently associated with Down's syndrome) is defined as a defect of the septum primum and the inlet or muscular septum, and abnormal configuration of the AV valves (Figure 14–10c). A partitioned orifice has a tongue of tissue that connects the superior and inferior leaflets bridging the interventricular septum with partitioning the AV valve orifice into a separate right and left orifice. A common AV valve orifice lacks such a connecting tongue, resulting in one large orifice that encompasses the left- and right-sided components. The term unbalanced AVSD refers to cases where one ventricle is hypoplastic. Pathophysiology of ASD I (primum ASD) is similar to a large ASD II (secundum ASD) with right-sided RA and RV volume overload. Chronic left AV valve regurgitation may produce left-sided LA and LV volume overload. Complete AVSD has also ventricular-level left-to-right shunting and hence there is both right heart dilatation (ASD component) and left heart dilatation (VSD component). Patients with complete AVSD are at particular high risk for the development of irreversible pulmonary hypertension.

Clinical Presentation

Neonates with a small restrictive VSD may be asymptomatic apart from a pansystolic murmur. On the other side, infants with large non-restrictive VSDs may develop breathlessness, congestive heart failure, and failure to thrive in the 2nd and 3rd month due to progressive increase of pulmonary blood flow with decreasing pulmonary vascular resistance. Patients with moderately restrictive VSD with near-normal pulmonary pressures but excessive left-to-right shunt present with exertional dyspnea, whereas patients with non-restrictive

VSD if left untreated may develop Eisenmenger's physiology with central cyanosis, signs of pulmonary hypertension, and peripheral edema reflecting right-sided heart failure. Symptoms and signs of patients with ASD I are similar to those with ASD II, patients with surgically unrepaired AVSD as adults have a propensity to develop pulmonary hypertension at earlier ages.

Diagnosis and CMR Findings

Diagnosis is made by clinical examination, ECG (notched P-wave, deep Q- and tall R-waves in V5 and V6 in large VSDs), and echocardiography (location, size, and hemodynamic consequences of VSD). CMR imaging can accurately assess location, size and hemodynamic consequences of the VSD (degree of shunting, atrial and ventricular volume and function, pulmonary valve function), particularly in large non-restrictive VSDs (Figure 14-10a). Moreover, CE-MRA can exclude associated cardiovascular malformations. In multiple VSDs CMR imaging is particularly helpful to detect the number and location of each single defect and to quantitate their contributions to shunting (Figure 14-10b). In cases with subaortal and subpulmonary VSDs prolapse of one aortic leaflet into the defect can occur with concomitant aortic regurgitation due to root asymmetry. This situation can be assessed by cine-SSFP with the imaging plane through the aortic root. The degree of shunting can be quantified by volumetry and/or by PC mapping in the aorta and pulmonary artery. In complete AVSD the abnormal anatomy can be assessed by SSFP and black-blood sequences with the imaging plane in parallel to and slightly inferior to the AV valve plane (Figure 14-10c). In complex congenital heart disease including a VSD or AVSD, CMR is particularly useful to fully delineate the anatomy and quantify the hemodynamic consequences.

Therapy

Patients with small restrictive VSDs can be followed without surgical repair. Patients with large VSDs and those with complete AVSD and significant hemodynamic compromise require surgical repair. The results of surgical treatment can be accurately assessed by CMR imaging both after surgery and during follow-up.

14.7.2 Intracavitary Right Ventricular Stenosis

In intracavitary RV stenosis (double-chambered right ventricle) abnormal subinfundibular muscle bundles divide the RV into a proximal high-pressure and distal low-pressure chamber beyond the stenosis. In most cases a VSD exists with connection to the low-pressure area (RVOT) and less common to the high-pressure area (RV sinus portion). Intracavitary RV stenosis progresses and in many cases the VSD occludes over time. Diagnosis is made by echocardiography, while CMR imaging in axial or parasagittal planes may show localisation and expansion of the abnormal muscle bundles. Also the localisation and size of the VSD can be assessed by cine-SSFP and black-blood sequences, and the degree of shunting by PC flow mapping in the aorta and pulmonary artery. In addition, the position of the stenosis relative to the VSD and separation of the stenosis from the infundibulum and the pulmonary valve has to be visualized that can be achieved best using a sagittal plane through the RVOT and the pulmonary valve.

14.7.3 Pulmonary Atresia (PAA) with Intact Interventricular Septum

Pathology and Pathophysiology

This anomaly is rare and represents less than 1 % of all congenital abnormalities. In 80 % of cases a membrane-like occlusion of the pulmonary valve exists, in 20 % an infundibular atresia, whilst valve orifice and pulmonary artery often are hypoplastic but rarely atretic.

> **Three types of RV compartments** may be differentiated:
> - tripartite RV with three RV compartments,
> - bipartite with inlet and outlet portion without trabeculated portion, and
> - monopartite RV with the inlet portion only.

Interatrial connections and an open ductus arteriosus are vital for the survival of patients. The size of the RV varies and determines the prognosis. The high pressure within the RV can be relieved via the coronary arteries and sinusoidal connections to the RV lumen and via a tricuspid incompetence. In cases with proximal coronary artery stenoses the distal coronary vasculature is perfused by desaturated blood. In PAA with VSD pulmonary perfusion is provided by an open ductus arteriosus in 70 % of cases, and via aorto-pulmonary collaterals in 30 % of cases.

Clinical Presentation

Children are symptomatic with central cyanosis after birth and develop right-heart failure with further growth.

Diagnosis and CMR Findings

Diagnosis is made by echocardiography and cardiac catheterization, the latter for visualizing the relationship between the coronary arteries and the RV. CMR imaging is also very useful to visualize the abnormal anatomy and in particular to assess RV size and function, which may be essential for choosing among the variety of surgical and interventional

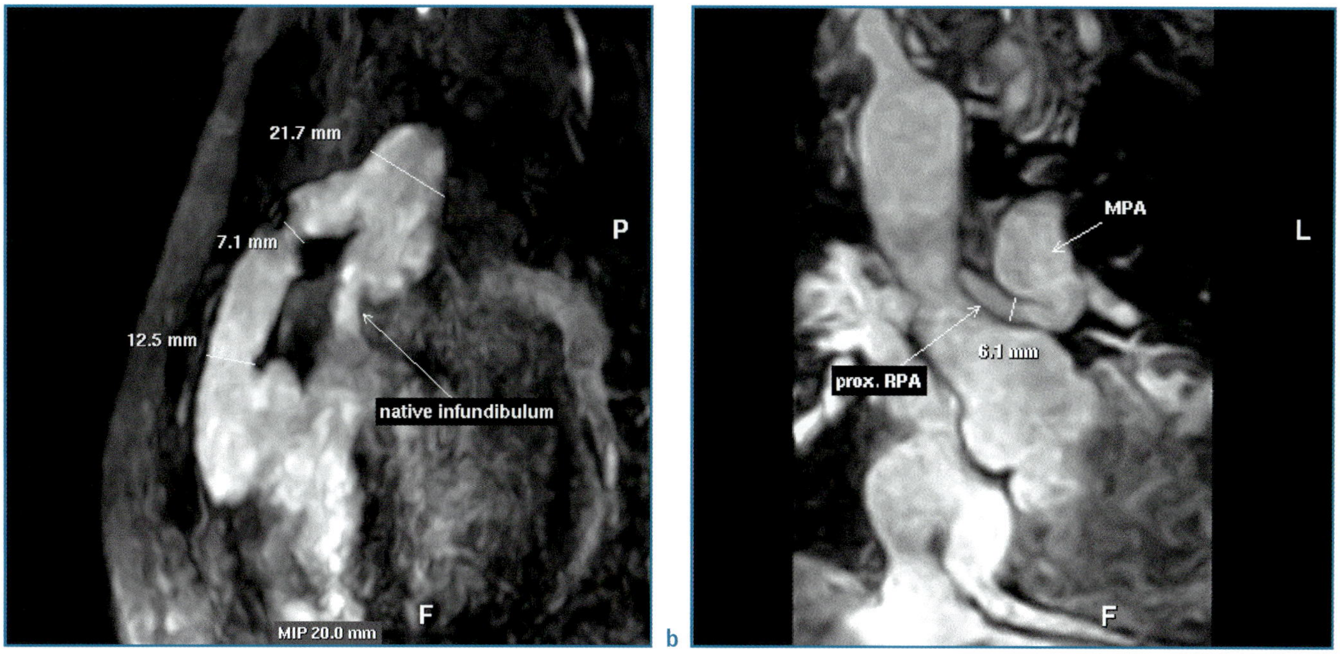

a b

Figure 14-11 Pulmonary atresia with ventricular septal defect after antegrade flow reconstruction and later surgical repair with unifocalizing of the pulmonary artery, right ventricular to pulmonary artery conduit, and patch closure of VSD – stenosis and calcification of the homograft (a), and stenosis of the right pulmonary artery (b). MPA: main pulmonary artery (PA trunk); prox. RPA: proximal right pulmonary artery.

treatment options that ultimately depend on RV size and function. These are often staged procedures, and CMR is very helpful in decision-making.

Therapy

In patients with PAA and intact ventricular septum the decision on repair strategy depends on RV size and function and the quality of the central pulmonary arteries. It is here where CMR has a huge role to play in the clinical decision making through serial follow-up of these variables. In very small RV a Fontan circulation will be established (see below). On the other end of the spectrum, if there is valvular atresia with tripartite RV a surgical or transcatheter perforation of the pulmonary valve may allow biventricular circulation. In combination with the latter, in intermediate cases, an aorto-pulmonary shunt (or stenting of the ductus arteriosus) may be necessary to allow for more time for the RV to growth. Not rarely however a valved conduit needs to be implanted in pulmonary position at some point (Figure 14-11). Some patients are managed best using a "one and a half" approach where the superior vena cava (SVC) is connected to the right pulmonary artery (RPA) and the atrial septum closed. This leaves only the blood from the inferior vena cava to be transported antegradely by the RV.

Long-Term Effects and CMR Findings

Long-term complications include stenoses of the conduit by calcification or neointima proliferation. RV dysfunction can be reliably assed by CMR imaging using cine-SSFP for detection of conduit stenoses and for quantitating RV function or tricuspid regurgitation (Figure 14-11), and PC mapping for assessing the degree of pulmonary incompetence or (conduit) stenosis and of tricuspid regurgitation or residual atrial or surgical shunt communications.

14.7.4 Ebstein's Anomaly

Pathology

This anomaly is rare with a prevalence of 0.5%, and its feature is apical displacement of the septal leaflet in conjunction with leaflet dysplasia and severe tricuspid regurgitation and RV volume overload. The displacement of the tricuspid valve results in "atrialisation" of the RV inflow tract and produces a variably small, functional RV. Associated anomalies include an ASD or patent foramen ovale (about 50% of cases), varying degrees of RVOT obstructions, and accessory pathways with consecutive WPW tachycardias (about 25% of cases).

Clinical Presentation

In mild forms patients are usually asymptomatic. When tricuspid valve deformity and dysfunction is extreme, death in utero from hydrops fetalis is the norm. With severe tricuspid valve deformity, newborns and infants present with right-sided heart failure and failure to thrive. Most adults with moderate to severe forms of Ebstein's anomaly

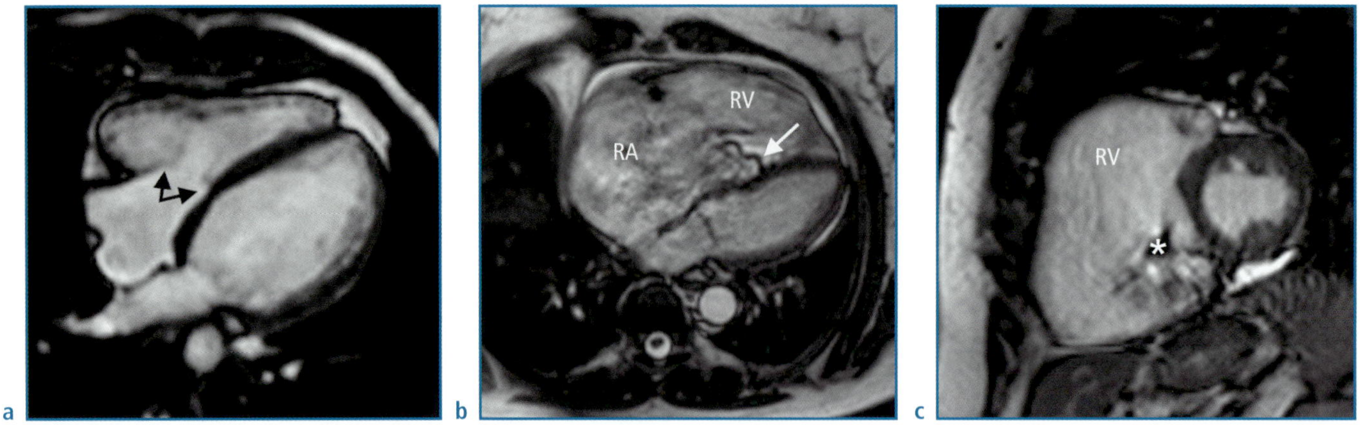

Figure 14-12 Ebstein's anomaly with apical displacement of the septal leaflet of the tricuspid valve in a 4-ch view during early systole (arrows in (a)). Another patient with Ebstein's anomaly in 4-ch (b) and short-axis view (c) showing displacement of the septal leaflet to the RV apex (arrow in (b)) and enlarged right atrium due to atrialization of RV inflow tract (RA); due to severe tricuspid regurgitation severe enlargement of the RV and flow void (* in (c)) representing tricuspid regurgitation. RA: right atrium; RV: right ventricle.

present with exercise intolerance including exertional dyspnea and fatigue, palpitations, or cyanosis from right-to-left shunt at atrial level.

Diagnosis and CMR Findings

Diagnosis is made by clinical examination, chest X-ray ("water bottle" appearance of the heart, cardiomegaly), and echocardiography (apical displacement of the tricuspid valve by 8 mm/m^2 body surface area or more, elongated sail-like appearance of the anterior leaflet, atrialized RV). CMR imaging is very helpful for visualizing the abnormal anatomy and in particular to quantitatively assess RV volume and function in serial follow-up investigations, as well as quantifying the degree of tricuspid regurgitation (Figure 14-12). Moreover, cine-SSFP and inflow-MRA techniques or sometimes CE-MRA are able to detect associated VSDs, pulmonary stenoses or atresia, as well as obstructions of the LVOT.

Therapy

Indications for intervention include substantial cyanosis, deteriorating functional capacity, and right-sided heart failure. The preferable method is surgical tricuspid valve repair if feasible, the closure of an associated ASD, and the division of accessory pathways. If the tricuspid valve is not reparable, valve replacement will be necessary (usually a bioprosthetic valve). In high-risk patients with severe tricuspid regurgitation and inadequate RV function a bidirectional cavopulmonary connection can be added to reduce RV preload if pulmonary pressure is low. Sometimes a Fontan procedure may be indicated in patients with tricuspid stenosis and/or hypoplastic RV.

Long-Term Effects and CMR Findings

Patients should have regular follow-up, particularly those with cyanosis, substantial cardiomegaly, and tricuspid regurgitation following valve repair, and particular attention should be paid to detect degenerating bioprostheses or dysfunctional mechanical valves. These long-term complications can be easily detected by CMR imaging.

14.7.5 Tricuspid Atresia (TA)

Pathology and Pathophysiology

Tricuspid atresia is best described as absence of right AV connection due to agenesis of the tricuspid valve. Its incidence is 1–3% of all congenital anomalies. In concordant ventriculoarterial connection (70–80% of cases) pulmonary circulation is provided by a patent foramen ovale (PFO) or an ASD to the LV and from there to the RV via a VSD; there is often flow restriction towards the pulmonary artery by means of a restrictive VSD and/or a pulmonary valve stenosis, leading to often severe neonatal cyanosis and duct-dependency of the pulmonary circulation. In contrast, in the remaining 20–30% there will be ventricular-arterial discordance such that the aorta is transposed and originates from the right ventricle and the pulmonary artery from the left ventricle (TGA). More often than not the VSD is larger and a pulmonary stenosis is lacking such that heart failure from pulmonary overflow dominates the clinical picture with only mild to moderate cyanosis; also in this group there is often additional aortic arch hypoplasia and coarctation, which may result in duct-dependency of the systemic circulation.

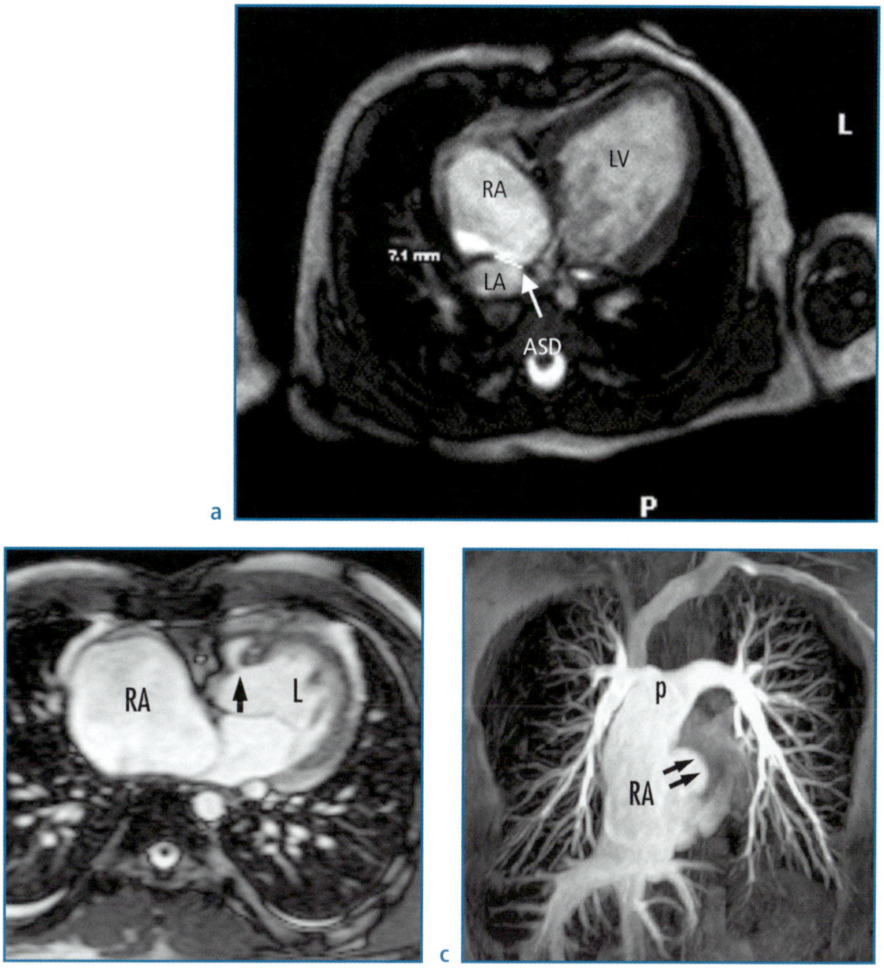

Figure 14-13 Cine-SSFP sequence in a patient with tricuspid atresia (TA) with ASD and dominant LV in an axial view (a). In another patient using cine-SSFP imaging right atrial dilatation in TA after atriopulmonary Fontan anastomosis and ASD closure is present as well as connection via a VSD to the hypoplastic LV (black arrow in (b)), and leftward bulging of the interatrial septum (black arrows in (c)). ASD: atrial septal defect; LA: left atrium; LV and L: left ventricle; p: pulmonary artery; RA: right atrium.

Clinical Presentation

Patients usually present in the neonatal age with different degrees of either pronounced cyanosis or heart failure, according to ventriculoarterial connection as per above. There may be duct-dependency of either pulmonary or systemic circulation as per above.

Diagnosis and CMR Findings

Diagnosis is usually made by ECG (left axis deviation, RA enlargement, LA enlargement with high pulmonary flow), and echocardiography (abnomal anatomy, size of ASD, VSD, and aortic arch). CMR imaging is useful to document abnormal anatomy by cine-SSFP or black-blood sequences (hypoplastic RV and dominant LV, RVOT, size and location of ASD and VSD; Figure 14-13a). CE-MRA may be used to assess morphology and function of RA, RV and LV, and to follow venous flow from the atrial level to the pulmonary artery. Using PC mapping in the aorta and pulmonary artery the amount of shunting can be measured.

Therapy

Acute treatment in cases with restricted atrial communication consists of **balloon atrioseptostomy**. In infants with concordant ventriculoarterial connections and severe cyanosis, a systemic-to-pulmonary shunt is produced (first 6–8 wks of life). In more balanced circulation with better pulmonary antegrade perfusion an elective primary **Glenn procedure** may be performed beyond the third month of life when cyanosis worsenes. In discordant ventriculoarterial connection, early palliation ranges from banding of the pulmonary artery to **Norwood stage I procedure** in cases with severe subaortic stenosis (restrictive VSD!) and hypoplastic aorta and arch. The aim of all early palliation is to prepare for the eventual Fontan procedure which is the most accepted long-term palliation in cases of good ventricular function, unobstructed systemic blood flow, minimal AV valve regurgitation, and low pulmonary vascular resistance. The **original Fontan procedure** in patients with tricuspid atresia included an end-to-end anastomosis of the superior vena cava (SVC) with a proximally cut right pulmonary artery (RPA) as a so-called **Glenn shunt**, connection of the right atrium with the pulmonary artery via a valved homograft (Figure 14-13b, c), and implantation of a bioprosthesis between the inferior vena cava (IVC) and right atrium as well as closure of the ASD. Following the initial procedure total cavopulmonary anastomosis has been introduced using an anastomosis from the SVC to the right pulmonary artery and a patched tunnel baffle from the IVC to the right pulmonary artery. Another technique consists of creating an extra-cardiac tunnel (18–22 mm prosthesis) between IVC and pulmonary artery, eventually with a fenestration to the pulmonary-venous atrium.

Long-Term Effects and CMR Findings

Long-term sequelae of Fontan procedure may be a stenosis of the Fontan anastomosis including the intraatrial or extracardiac tunnel, atrial arrhythmias (AV nodal tachycardias), and systemic ventricular or mitral valve dysfunction. Moreover, right-to-left shunt through (for example) re-opening of veno-venous connections or intraatrial baffle leaks may cause recurrence of cyanosis. In addition to this, aortopulmonary collaterals may produce relevant left-to-right shunt and volume load for the single ventricle. All these changes can be easily detected and quantified by CMR imaging: cine-SSF for baffle and conduit stenosis, and RV and LV volumetry and residual ASD and AV valve regurgitation, black-blood sequences for imaging the intraatrial baffle, and PC flow mapping to assess conduit stenosis, pulmonary blood flow (Rebergen 1993), and residual shunt of the fenestrated baffle. Contrast-enhanced 3D imaging and 3D "whole-heart" imaging is very useful to image the patency of the Fontan connections and pulmonary arteries or diagnose veno-venous and aortopulmonary collaterals.

14.7.6 Subvalvular Aortic Stenosis

In 80 % of cases a membraneous or fibromuscular obstruction, in 10–15 % a tunnel forming obstruction of LVOT is present, in 30–50 % of cases associated with aortic valve regurgitation due to malformations of valve leaflets (20 % of patients). Most patients are asymptomatic, only associated VSD or cleft of the anterior mitral leaflet produce symptoms and clinical signs. Diagnosis is made by echocardiography as a rule, but in addition, CMR imaging may be helpful to demonstrate abnormal anatomy and severity of stenosis (Figure 14-14) including the degree of LV hypertrophy. Treatment can be challenging and usually includes transaortic resection or myocardial incision, but recurrence rates are high. In cases with tunnel forming stenoses and relevant aortic regurgitation an aortoventriculoplasty (**Konno procedure**) including aortic valve replacement is indicated. The post-operative and long-term results of operative repair can be easily controlled by CMR.

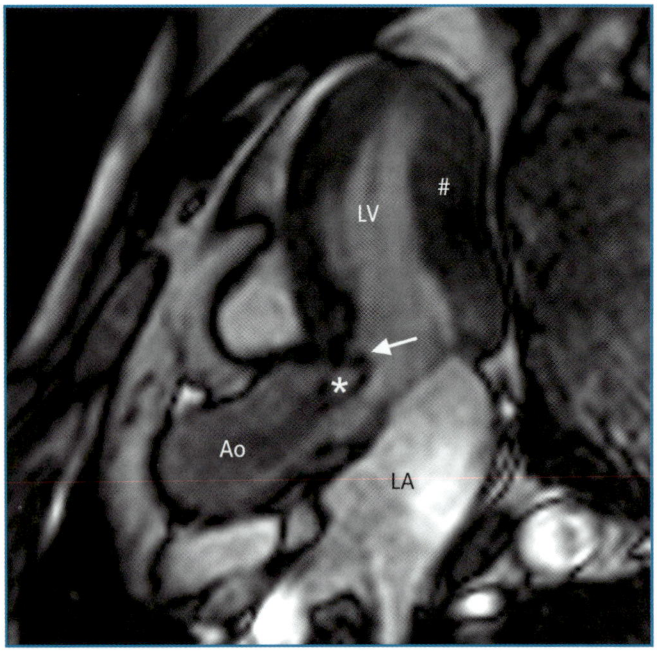

Figure 14-14 Subvalvular aortic stenosis in a 3-ch view on cine-SSFP imaging in early systole with increased flow velocity (*) due to a subvalvular membrane (arrow) extending into the left ventricular outflow tract. Ao: aorta; LA: left atrium; LV: left ventricle; #: descending aorta.

14.7.7 Hypoplastic Left Heart Syndrome (HLHS)

Pathology and Pathophysiology

This term describes a group of closely related cardiac anomalies characterized by underdevelopment of the left cardiac chambers, endocardial fibroelastosis, stenosis or atresia of the aortic and/or mitral orifices, and hypoplasia of the aorta or coarctation. HLHS is rare with a prevalence of about 1 % of all cardiac anomalies, but it is the most common cause of death in newborns.

Clinical Presentation

HLHS is characterized by duct-dependent systemic circulation (Figure 14-15), it tends to present with severe symptoms within the first week of life when ductal constriction occurs. Infants after birth may present with sudden onset of circulatory collapse and severe lactic acidosis resulting from duct-closure related coronary ischemia. More recently, the availability of fetal echocardiography has vastly improved the post-natal management avoiding cardiogenic shock as the first clinical presentation.

Diagnosis

Diagnosis is made by echocardiography (small LV cavity, diminuative mitral valve, thinned or normal myocardium

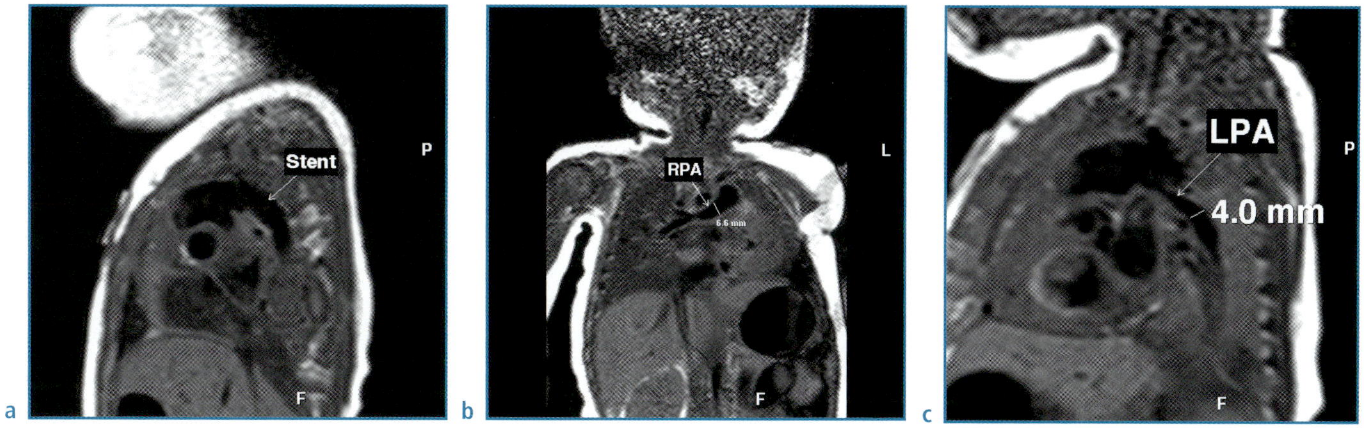

Figure 14-15 Hypoplastic left heart syndrome after initial palliation using a "hybrid" procedure (stenting of the patent ductus arteriosus and bilateral banding of the pulmonary arteries) showing the stent in the ductus arteriosus (a), right pulmonary artery banding (b), and left pulmonary artery banding (c). LPA: left pulmonary artery; RPA: right pulmonary artery.

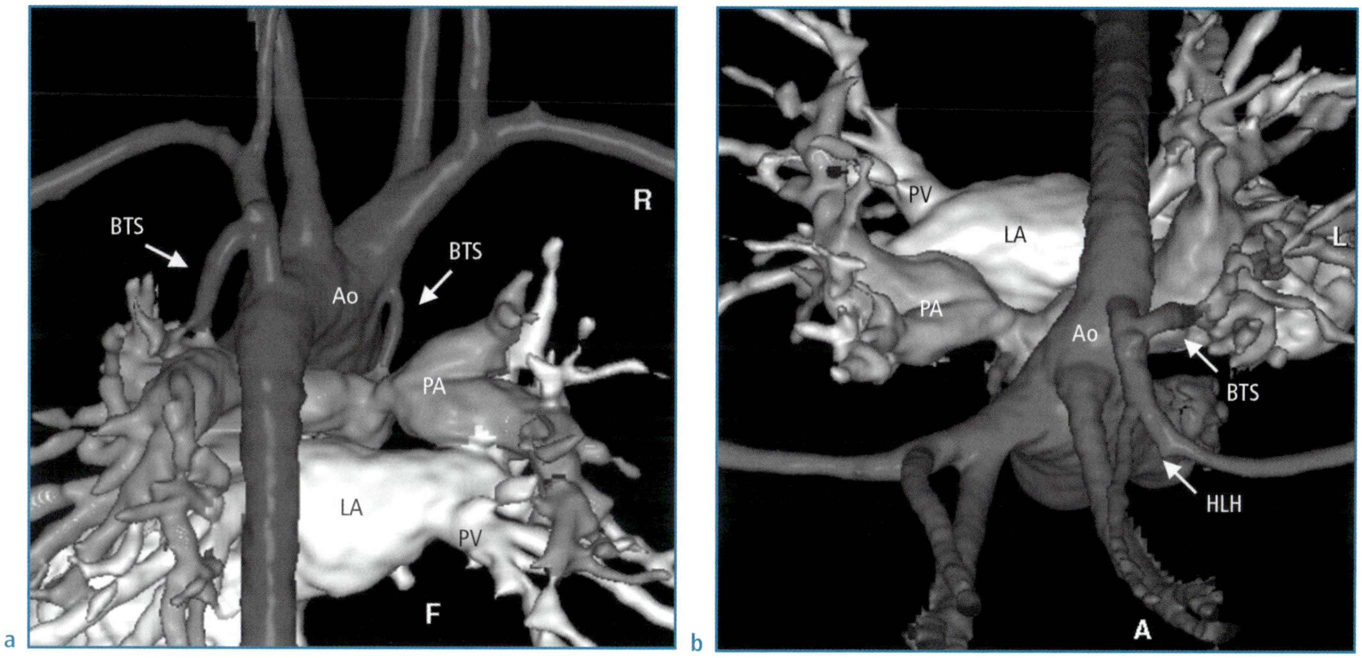

Figure 14-16 Moderate hypoplastic left heart syndrome after initial Norwood palliation. To stimulate LV growth a second left-sided modified Blalock-Taussig shunt (BTS) was installed. Anatomy is shown from dorsal with both shunts (a) and from superior (b). Ao: aorta; BTS: Blalock-Taussig shunt; HLH: hypoplastic left heart; LA: left atrium; PA: pulmonary artery; PV: pulmonary vein.

with thickened endocardium, diminuative aortic root, and juxtaductal coarctation). The duct varies in size according to treatment, and assessment of this and the interatrial communication are crucial to managing the patients.

Therapy

Treatment includes administration of prostaglandins and the *first step* of palliation, the **Norwood procedure**: creation of an unobstructed communication between RV and unobstructed aorta by direct connection between the transsected proximal pulmonary trunk and ascending aorta with a patch extending around the augmented aortic arch, systemic-to-pulmonary shunt or right-ventricle-to-pulmonary artery conduit to establish pulmonary blood flow, and creation of a large interatrial communication (Figure 14-15, Figure 14-16, and Figure 14-17).

Step two consists of an end-to-side SVC-to-pulmonary artery connection (bidirectional **Glenn procedure**) or a **Hemi-Fontan** (incorporating the roof of the atrium into the pulmonary artery anastomosis).

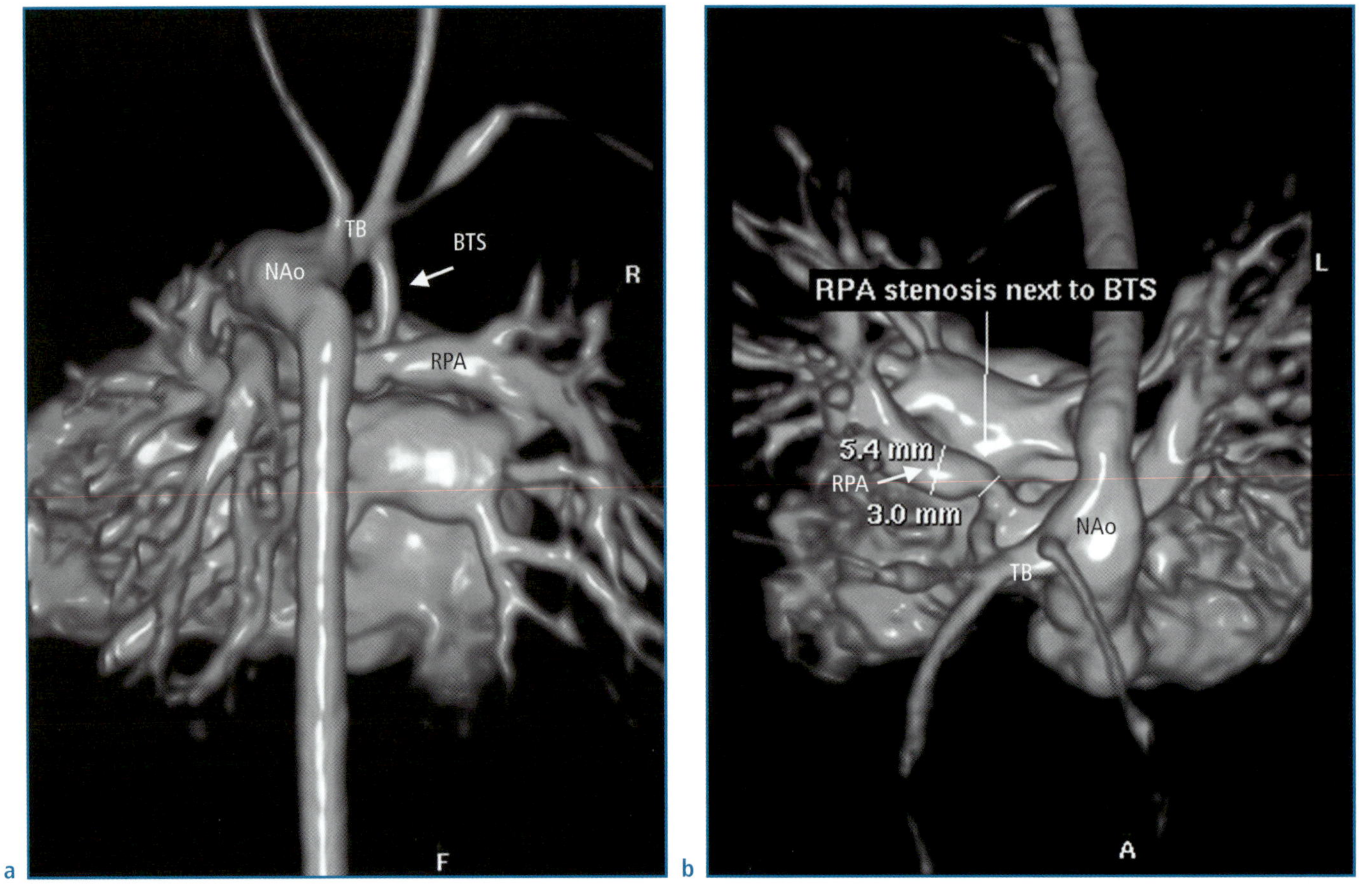

Figure 14-17 Hypoplastic left heart syndrome after initial Norwood palliation showing the reconstructed neo-aorta (NAo) and the modified Blalock-Taussig shunt (BTS) between the brachiocephalic trunk (TB) and the right pulmonary artery **(a)**. Demonstration of the stenosis of the right pulmonary artery (RPA) next to the BTS **(b)**.

Step three is the **Fontan palliation**. The **conduit procedure** (atriopulmonary anastomosis) includes a valved conduit from RA to pulmonary artery, a bioprosthesis from the IVC to the RA, and closure of an ASD, if present. The **De Leval/Jonas procedure** includes total cavopulmonary connection (TCPC) with connecting the SVC bidirectionally with the right pulmonary artery and crossing the blood from IVC via a patch-tunnel to the right pulmonary artery, temporarily with fenestration of the baffle.

Long-Term Effects and CMR Findings

Several long-term sequelae of the staged Norwood and Fontan procedure were discussed under Chapter 14.7.5. As explained there all hemodynamically relevant Fontan complications may be readily assessed by CMR imaging: cine-SSFP for volumetry, function and muscle mass of the systemic ventricle; CE-MRA for systemic and pulmonary flow, and imaging of the TCPC; black-blood sequences for intracardiac thrombi or morphology of the conduit; PC flow mapping for measuring right and left pulmonary blood flow, flow rates within the SVC and IVC, and for cardiac output. In fact, the use of CMR has become the cornerstone in the follow-up of these patients, due to its completeness and non-invasiveness, and the quantitative nature of CMR's functional data on pulmonary flow and single ventricle performance.

14.7.8 Univentricular Atrioventricular Connections

Pathology

This congenital anomaly is rare with a prevalence of about 1% of CHD. Univentricular hearts are defined by having more than 50% of both AV connections connected to a dominant ventricle, i.e. the whole or one and greater than 50% of alternative junction is connected to either a left or right ventricle. Regarding atrioventricular connections a double inlet (two AV valves), a common inlet (one common AV valve), and a singular inlet (one atretic and one normal AV valve) can be differentiated. In about 75–80% of patients the dominant ventricle is a left ventricle separated from the right ventricle by a VSD, in 20 % the dominant ventricle is a right ventricle and the small, incomplete left ventricle is of LV apical morphology. In only 5 % of cases is there a truly single ventricle. In 85 % of cases a transposition of the great arteries is found, and the most common constellation is a "double-inlet left ventricle" (DILV) with origin of the aorta from a left-anterior rudimentary outlet chamber in L-transposition (75 % of cases), and in about 50 % with associated pulmonary stenosis or -atresia.

Clinical Presentation

Infants with critical reduction of systemic outflow may become duct-dependent and present with cardiogenic shock. In contrast, when pulmonary blood flow is critically reduced infants may present with severe cyanosis or with duct-dependent pulmonary blood flow. Other patients may remain asymptomatic and develop heart failure later on because of increased pulmonary blood flow.

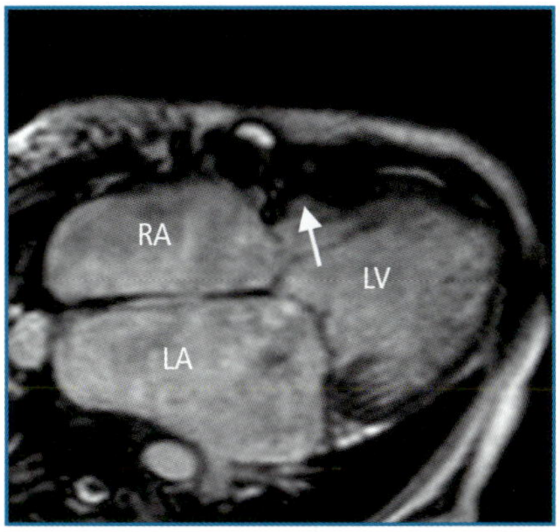

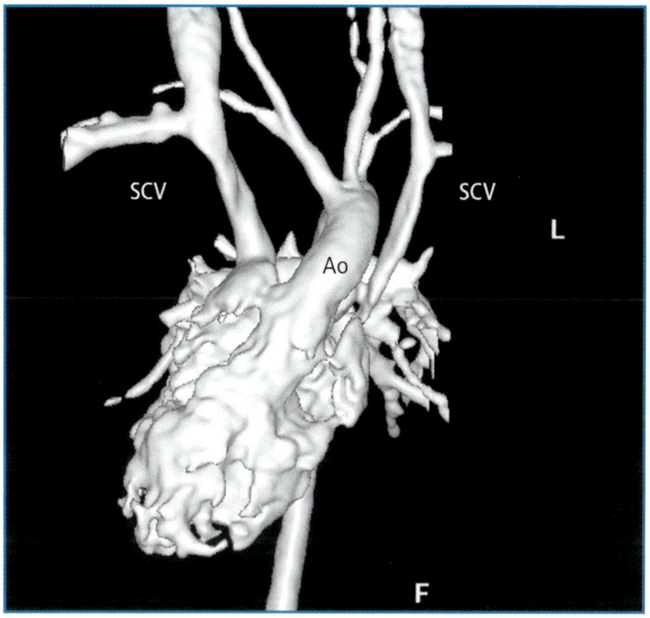

Figure 14-18 LV type single ventricle (double inlet left ventricle) with L-transposition of the great arteries and right-sided Blalock-Taussig anastomosis **(a)**: enlarged left ventricle (LV) with double inlet from right (RA) and left atrium (LA) and two AV valves and a rudimentary right ventricle (arrow) (courtesy Dr. J. Schwab, Nuremberg). Another patient with univentricular heart, dextrocardia, and indeterminate ventricular morphology, bilateral superior caval veins (SCV), L-malposition of the aorta (Ao), and sub-pulmonary stenosis **(b)** (ventral view).

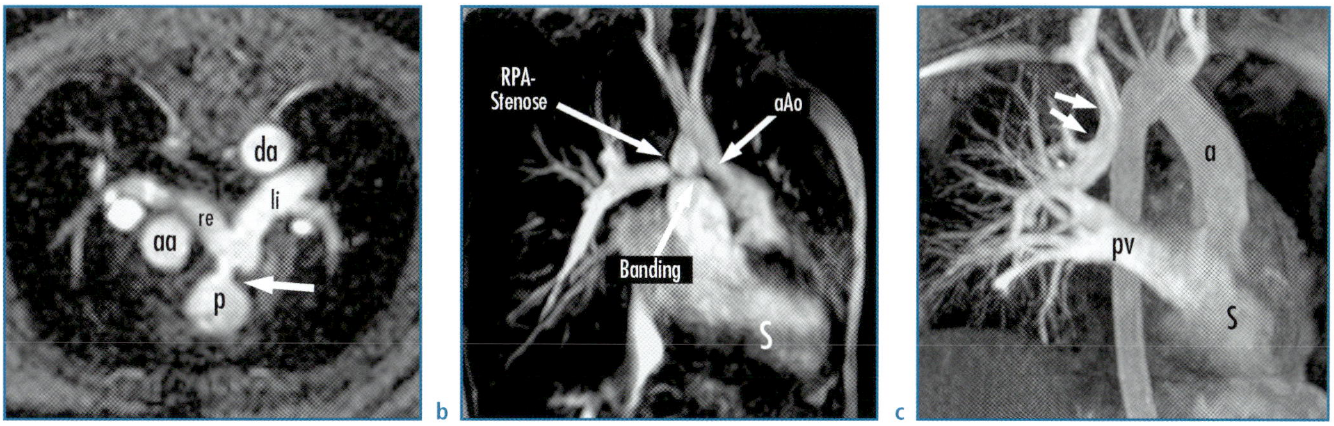

Figure 14-19 Patient with single ventricle with correct pulmonary artery banding (arrow) **(a)**. Another patient with single ventricle of LV type showing a hypoplastic RV outlet chamber to the aorta (aAo, short white arrow), L-transposition of the aorta, and dislocated pulmonary banding with a high-grade stenosis of the right pulmonary artery (RPA, long white arrow) **(b)**. A third patient with single ventricle with a Glenn shunt (white arrows) between the superior caval vein and the right pulmonary artery **(c)**. a: aorta; aa: ascending aorta; aAo: ascending aorta; da: descending aorta; li: left pulmonary artery; p: pulmonary artery trunk; pv: pulmonary vein; re: right pulmonary artery; RPA-Stenose: stenosis; S: single ventricle.

Diagnosis and CMR Findings

Diagnosis is made by echocardiography (AV valve anomalies, presence and anatomy of subaortic obstruction). CMR imaging may be useful to visualize the anatomic abnormalities, and to assess ventricular function, subaortic stenosis, and left- vs. right-sided pulmonary blood flow (Figure 14-18).

Therapy, Long-Term Effects and CMR Findings

Patients follow the same surgical algorithms as those with tricuspid atresia (Figure 14-19), finally undergoing Fontan procedure. Long-term sequelae are similar to those described for tricuspid atresia (see Chapter 14.7.5).

14.8 Conotruncal Defects

14.8.1 Tetralogy of Fallot (TOF) and Pulmonary Atresia with Ventricular Septal Defect and Pulmonary Valve Agenesis

Pathology

Tetralogy of Fallot (TOF) is the most common cyanotic congenital anomaly with a prevalence of ~ 10 %.

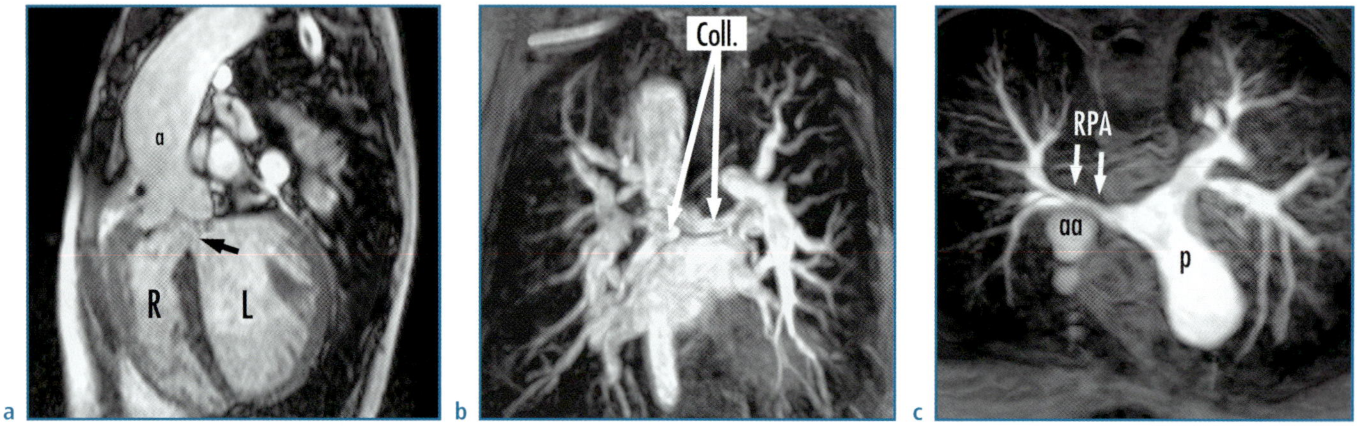

Figure 14-20 Tetralogy of Fallot (TOF) with ventricular septal defect (arrow) with overriding aorta (a). Another patient with TOF and significant aortopulmonary collateral vessels (Coll) from the descending aorta to the right lower lobe and left upper lobe pulmonary arteries (b). A third patient with TOF and long tubular stenosis (arrows) of the right pulmonary artery (RPA) following a former Waterston anastomosis between the ascending aorta (aa) and the right pulmonary artery (RPA) (c). a: ascending aorta; L: left ventricle; R: right ventricle.

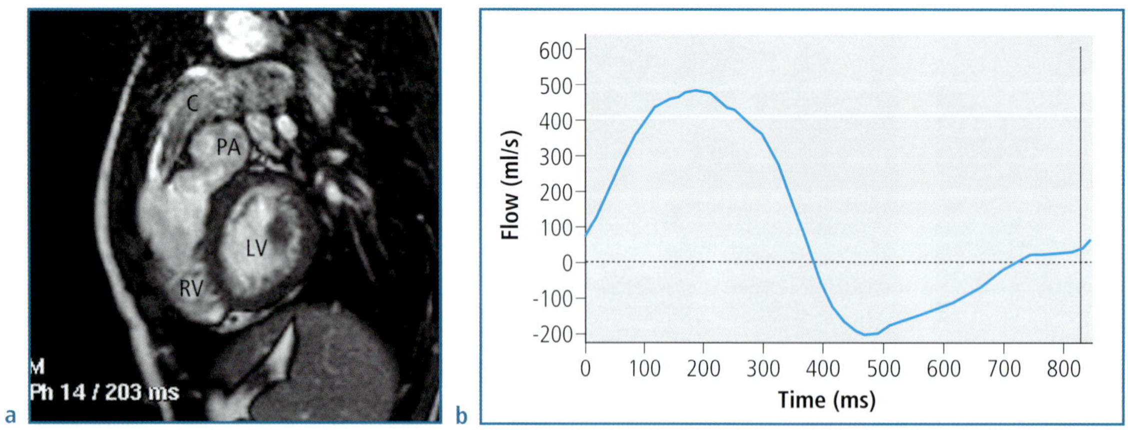

Figure 14-21 Surgical repair of a patient with tetralogy of Fallot (TOF) showing a closed pulmonary trunk (PA), flow void in systole in the conduit and pulmonary artery due to conduit stenosis (a), and significant pulmonary (conduit) regurgitation (not shown). Measurement of regurgitant fraction (RF) over the pulmonary (conduit) valve using PC flow mapping (b): forward flow was 130 ml, backward flow was 40.5 ml, and RF was 31 %. C: conduit; LV: left ventricle; RV: right ventricle.

The **four components** of TOF are:

- obstruction to the right ventricular outflow with infundibular and usually also additional valvular pulmonary stenosis,
- an outlet VSD,
- overriding of the aorta over the VSD, and
- RV hypertrophy.

In "pentalogy" of Fallot an additional ASD is present. In some cases the outflow tract is atretic with major aorto-pulmonary collaterals. Associated anomalies are a right aortic arch (25% of patients), peripheral pulmonary stenoses, and abnormal course of coronary arteries (5% of cases).

Clinical Presentation

Patients present early with cyanosis due to right-to-left shunting via the VSD, and the degree of cyanosis depends on the severity of RVOT obstruction and the level of systemic vascular resistance. Progressive hypoxia and finger clubbing develop with further aging, and patients without timely palliation have a limited prognosis.

Diagnosis and CMR Findings

Diagnosis can be achieved by echocardiography (abnormal structure and stenotic flow in the RVOT, VSD, pulmonary valve function), but CMR imaging may provide additional information on abnormal structure (Figure 14-20a), function, and degree of shunting: cine-SSFF and black-blood sequences for pathomorphology of RVOT, VSD, pulmonary stenosis, and eventually associated stenoses of the trachea; CE-MRA to demonstrate the anatomy of the central and peripheral pulmonary arteries and additional angiography of the aortic arch via the VSD, and to demonstrate anomalies of the veins on blood flow return. PC flow mapping in the aorta and pulmonary artery provides an exact measure of the right-to-left shunt.

Therapy

Surgical repair is usually performed during the first year of life (often during the first 6 mths), and includes infundibulectomy, transatrial closure of the VSD using a patch,

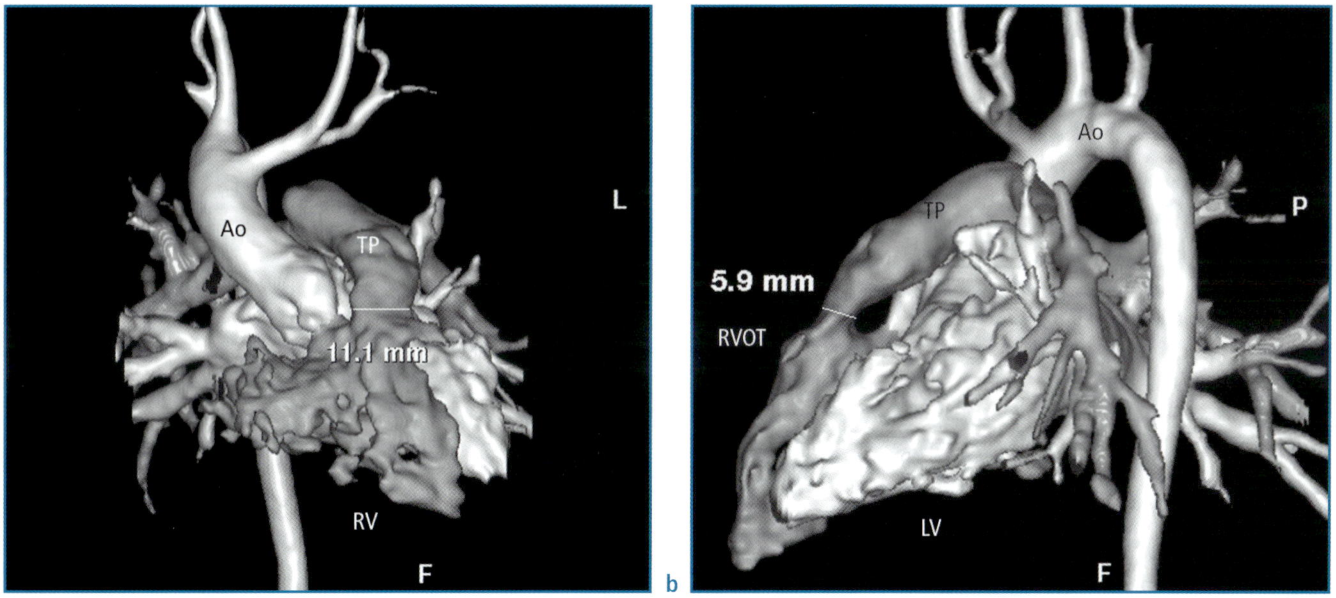

a b

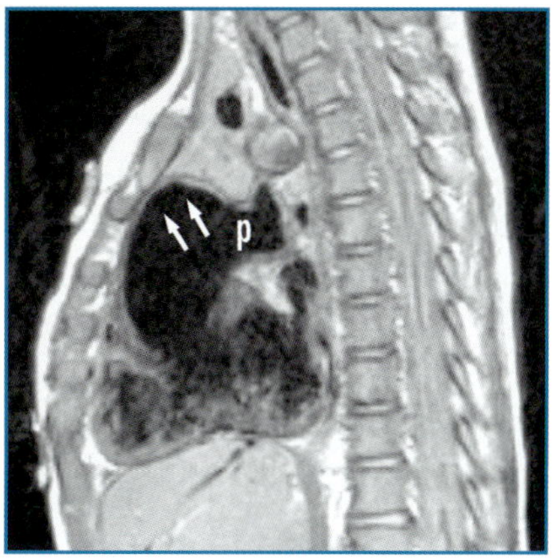

c

Figure 14-22 Surgical repair of a patient with tetralogy of Fallot (TOF) with right-sided aortic arch, malalignment of the aortic root, and residual moderate stenosis of the right ventricular outflow tract (RVOT). Volume rendering reconstruction in a frontal (a) and sagittal plane (b). Another patient with surgical repair of TOF showing a huge aneurysm (arrows) within the right ventricular outflow tract after patch repair (c). Ao: aorta; LV: left ventricle; p: pulmonary artery; RV: right ventricle; TP: pulmonary trunk.

widening of the RVOT by a patch, and pulmonary valvular commisurotomy (Figure 14-21 and Figure 14-22).

Long-Term Effects and CMR Findings

The goal of CMR soon after TOF repair includes quantitative evaluation of RV and LV volumes and function (stroke volume, ejection fraction), imaging of the morphology of the RVOT, the pulmonary arteries, the aorta and aorto-pulmonary collaterals (Figure 14-20b), and quantifying pulmonary, aortic, and tricuspid regurgitation (Dorfman and Geva 2006). Long-term sequelae of surgically repaired TOF include central or peripheral pulmonary stenoses (Figure 14-20c), restenosis or residual stenosis of the pulmonary valve, pulmonary regurgitation (Figure 14-21), and RV dysfunction (dilatation, hypertrophy, diastolic dysfunction, tricuspid regurgitation). The degree of RV dysfunction is an important determinant of clinical status late after TOF repair and is also closely associated with LV dysfunction (ventriculo-ventricular interaction; Fogel 1995). Many studies have shown that the degree of pulmonary regurgitation, measured by PC mapping, is closely associated with RV dilatation (Helbing 1996, Dorfman and Geva 2006). The degree of pulmonary regurgitation and RV and LV dysfunction can be reliably assessed by CMR imaging (Cheung 2008). In cases with severe pulmonary (Figure 14-21 and Figure 14-22c) or aortic regurgitation reoperation may be warranted. Recently percutaneous implantation of pulmonary valves (PPVI) in surgically repaired TOF have been introduced, and this type of treatment can also easily be planned and followed by CMR imaging.

14.8.2 Truncus Arteriosus Communis (TAC)

Pathology and Pathophysiology

This anomaly is rare, its prevalence is 1% of all cyanotic CHDs. One single vessel forms the outlet of both ventricles and gives rise to the systemic, pulmonary, and coronary arteries (Figure 14-23a, b). The anomaly is always accom-

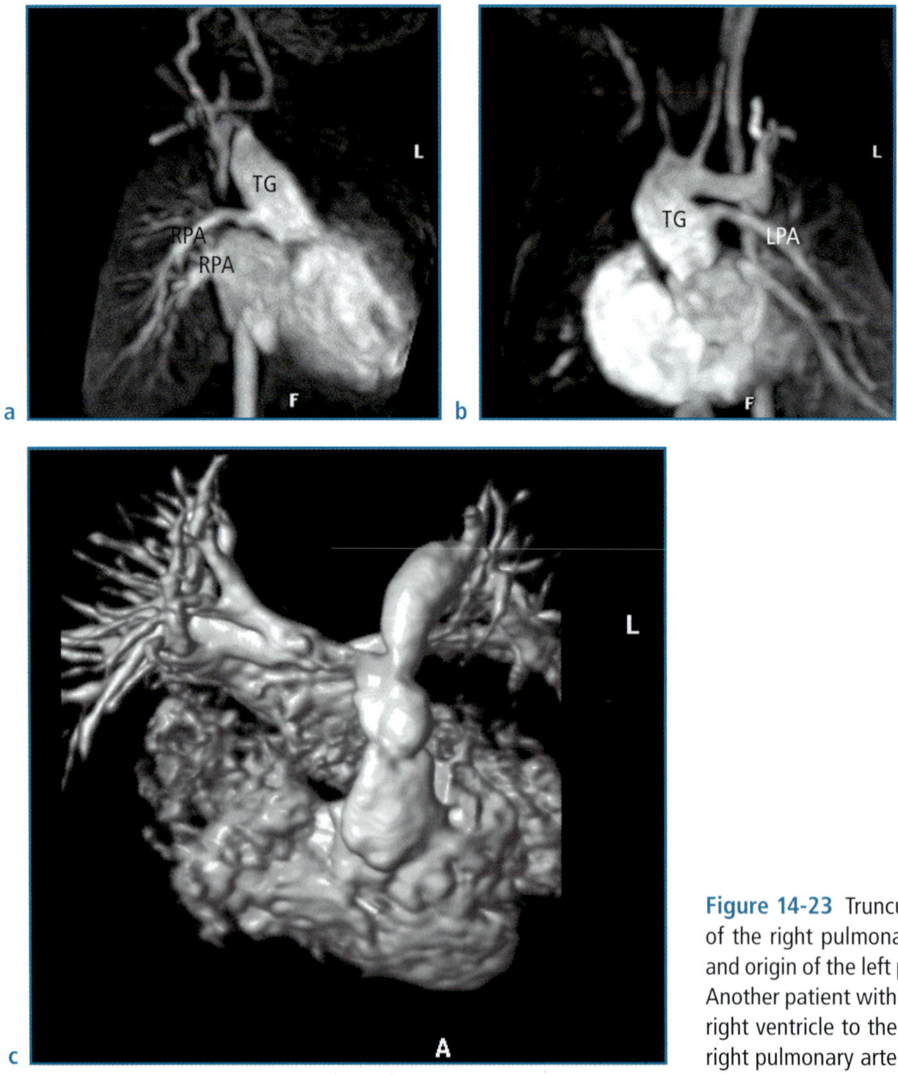

Figure 14-23 Truncus arteriosus communis (TAC) type III with origin of the right pulmonary artery (RPA) from the truncal vessel (TG) (a), and origin of the left pulmonary artery (LPA) from the truncal vessel (b). Another patient with TAC after surgical repair with homograft from the right ventricle to the pulmonary artery and a proximal stenosis of the right pulmonary artery (c) (superior view).

panied by a large VSD (the trunk overrides the VSD), and frequently with a right-sided aortic arch (30% of cases), in 10–15% of cases an interrupted aortic arch is present. The valve is frequently bicuspid or quadruple cuspid with significant regurgitation.

Type I of TAC is defined by a partially separate pulmonary trunk of variable length giving rise to the left and right pulmonary artery (PA); in **Type II** each PA arises separately but close to the other from the posterior aspect of the trunk; in **Type III** each PA arises from the lateral aspect of the trunk. Pulmonary blood flow is governed by the size of the PAs and the pulmonary vascular resistance (PVR). In infants with low PVR pulmonary blood flow is usually excessive and cyanosis minimal, but with aging and constantly increasing PVR pulmonary blood flow decreases at the cost of ventricular volume load and increasing cyanosis. When PVR reaches systemic levels, Eisenmenger's physiology with bidirectional shunting occurs, and significant truncal valve regurgitation produces volume load on both the RV and LV.

Clinical Presentation

Initially infants with TAC present with mild cyanosis, with ageing cyanosis increases. Usually poor physical development and symptoms of heart failure occur. The prevalence of truncal valve regurgitation increases with age causing biventricular heart failure and susceptibility to endocarditis.

Diagnosis and CMR Findings

Diagnosis is achieved by clinical examination (collapsing peripheral pulse, cardiomegaly, loud single 2nd heart sound, a harsh systolic murmur, and low-pitched mid-diastolic rumbling murmur, bounding pulses), chest X-ray (cardiomegaly, prominent PA markings, right aortic arch in 50% of cases), and by echocardiography (overriding truncal root, origin of pulmonary arteries, VSD size, functional status of truncal valve). Differential diagnosis includes PA with VSD and aortopulmonic window. Using CMR imaging a complete diagnosis regarding abnormal anatomy and function of the ventricles and truncal valve, the size of VSD, and the amount of right-to-left shunt can be made, as well.

Therapy

Operative repair consists of closure of the VSD, leaving the aorta arising from the LV, excision of the pulmonary arteries from their trunk, and implantation of a valve-containing prosthetic conduit (e.g., aortic or pulmonary homograft valve) between the RV and the pulmonary arteries to establish biventricular repair (Figure 14-23c). Insufficiency of the truncal valve requires valve replacement or repair.

Long-Term Effects and CMR Findings

Patients operated < 1 yr may outgrow the size of the initial homograft, and conduit change may be indicated later. Children with significant truncal valve stenosis or regurgitation may require valve replacement. Both long-term changes can be easily detected and quantified by CMR imaging.

> The **goals of CMR imaging** after truncal repair are similar to those after Fallot repair and include:
> - quantitative assessment of LV and RV volumes, function, and mass,
> - measurements of pulmonary and neo-aortic valve regurgitations,
> - imaging of the RVOT, the homograft, and the branch pulmonary arteries,
> - assessment of residual shunts, and
> - imaging of the aortic arch and isthmus (Dorfman and Geva 2006).

14.8.3 Double Outlet Right Ventricle (DORV)

Pathology and Pathophysiology

This is a rare complex anomaly with a prevalence of 1% of all CHDs. Both great arteries arise predominantly from the right ventricular chamber, with the only single outlet from the LV being a VSD. The relationship of the great arteries to each other is variable, in most cases the position of the aorta is right-lateral (side-by-side), sometimes right-anterior, right-posterior, or left-anterior to the pulmonary artery. The semilunar valves are at the same level, and the arteries may run in parallel. A conal septum divides the subvalvular region of both vessels. Because both vessels possess a conus (normally the aorta lacks a conus), no fibrous continuity is present between the AV valves and the semilunar valves; this is an important feature that allows differentiation of DORV from TOF and D-TGA.

Clinical Presentation

The hemodynamic situation in DORV is determined by the relative position of the VSD to the aorta and PA, and the presence and localization of a pulmonary stenosis. When a **subaortal VSD** is present (60–70% of cases) with the defect below the crista supraventricularis, oxygenated blood is directed to the aorta and venous blood predominantly to the PA, that results clinically in a mild or no cyanosis. However, in 50% of cases a concomitant pulmonary stenosis, most commonly a subvalvular stenosis, exists resulting in a TOF hemodynamics with significant cyanosis. The **subpulmonary VSD** (10% of cases, Taussig-Bing complex) is located

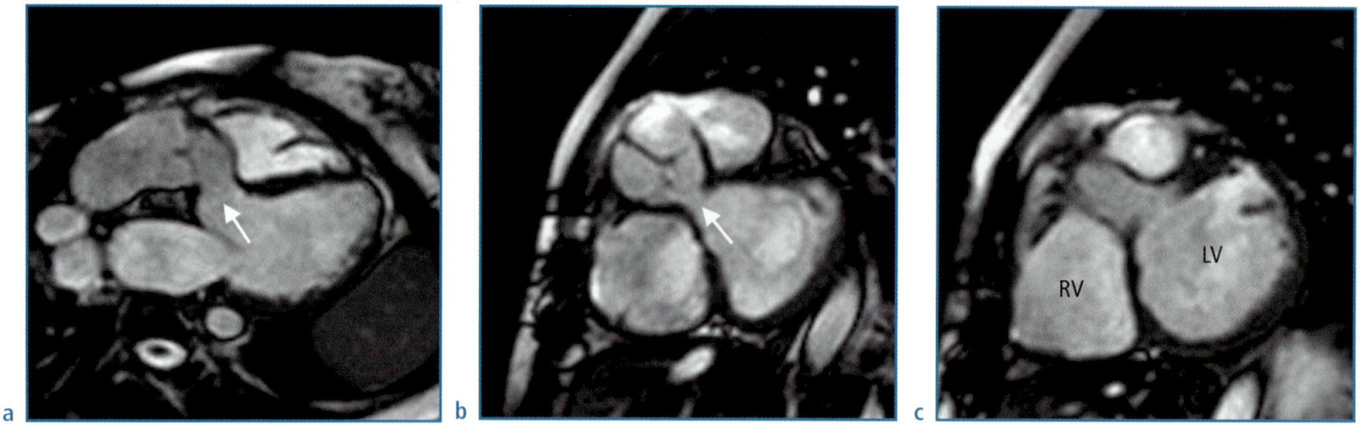

Figure 14-24 Double-outlet right ventricle (DORV) after Rastelli procedure with prolongation of the interventricular septum at closure of the VSD to redirect LV outflow to the aorta (arrow in (a) and (b)). LV: left ventricle; RV: right ventricle (courtesy Dr. J. Schwab, Nuremberg).

superior of the crista supraventricularis, usually without a coexisting pulmonary stenosis, and the oxygenated blood is redirected to the pulmonary artery, the deoxygenated blood to the aorta, and a severe cyanosis is present (hemodynamics similar to D-TGA). In **"double-committed VSD"** the supracristal defect has a narrow distance to the great arteries, in **"remote VSD"** the distance is wide, such as with AVSD or inlet VSD.

Diagnosis and CMR Findings

Diagnosis is usually made by echocardiography (commitment of the semilunar valves, subaortic or subpulmonic stenosis, abnormalities of the aortic arch). CMR imaging using cine-SSFF-, black-blood- and 3D contrast-enhanced angiography sequences as well as flow imaging has been reported to visualize the complex anatomical featues and also associated defects such as aortic arch anomalies, branch pulmonary artery stenoses, aortopulmonary collaterals, and systemic or pulmonary venous anomalies. Several investigators demonstrated the use of CMR to assess the relationship between the great vessels and the VSD (Hoppe 1996) as well as the position of the great vessels in relation to the conal septum (Niezen 1999, Beekman 2000). Imbalanced ventricles, i.e. with hypoplasia of one chamber, can be assessed by volumetry, and structure and dysfunction of concomitant AV valve abnormalities can be documented.

Therapy

Appropriate treatment is surgical repair to establish left ventricle-to-aorta continuity, create adequate right ventricle-to-pulmonary continuity, and repair associated lesions. Complete repair is now performed as a primary procedure in the majority of cases. In subaortic VSD this includes creating an intracardiac baffle that conducts the blood from the LV to the aorta (with coexisting pulmonary stenosis the repair is similar to that of TOF). In subpulmonary VSD without subpulmonary stenosis repair is accomplished by closure of the VSD and arterial switch; in cases with subpulmonary stenosis the aorta is connected to the LV using an intraventricular baffle, and a right-ventricle-to-pulmonary artery conduit is placed to complete the repair (**Rastelli procedure**; Figure 14-24). In cases with remote VSD (and the VSD cannot be baffled to the aorta) a **Mustard** or **Senning atrial redirection procedure**, closure of the VSD, and placement of a conduit between the LV and the pulmonary trunk is required.

Long-Term Effects and CMR Findings

CMR can provide useful information for planning the complex repair, in particular when using 3D "whole-heart" SSFP. More commonly CMR is used for follow-up after repair as late complications in patients with repaired DORV are relatively frequent, depending on the underlying anatomy, pathophysiology, and the applied surgical repair technique. Subaortic stenosis may develop after the LV is baffled, and the complications after DORV repair with pulmonary outflow tract obstruction are similar to those after TOF repair i.e. pulmonary regurgitation, RV dilatation and dysfunction, and arrhythmias. Aortic arch obstruction can be found in patients after coarctation or interrupted aortic arch repair. Using tailored CMR protocols all these long-term postoperative complications can be easily visualized and dysfunctions (stenoses, ventricular dysfunction) be exactly quantified.

14.8.4 D-Transposition of the Great Arteries (TGA)

Pathology and Pathophysiology

Congenital malformations of the great arteries in D-transposition are relatively common (5–7% of all CHDs). The anomaly consists of the origin of the aorta from the morphological RV (about 50% of cases) with a subaortal infundibulum (conus, no continuity between aortic and tricuspid valve), and origin of the pulmonary artery from the morphological LV (Figure 14-25a) without an infundibulum (continuous connection between pulmonary and mitral valve). Thus, the systemic and pulmonary circulations are connected in parallel rather than the normal in-series connection. Almost all patients have an interatrial communication to sustain life, two-thirds have a patent ductus arteriosus (PDA), one-third an associated VSD. **"TGA simplex"** is defined as d-TGA without further significant malformations except a PDA, persistent foramen ovale, and eventually a small VSD. **"Complex TGA"** is defined as TGA associated with a large VSD (about 25–30% of cases) and eventually associated obstructions of the LVOT (about 10% of cases; fibrous or fibromuscular circular obstructions), and rarely, associated AV valve abnormalities or RV hypoplasia. Anomalies of coronary arteries are also common in d-TGA, this fact is very important when planning an arterial switch repair.

Clinical Presentation

After birth neonates present with cyanosis, dyspnea, progressive hypoxemia, and congestive heart failure. The most severe hypoxemia and cyanosis are observed in infants who have only a small patent foramen ovale or ductus arteriosus and an intact ventricular septum, or in those infants with relatively reduced pulmonary blood flow because of LVOT obstruction. On the contrary, with a large PDA or large VSD, cyanosis can be minimal, and heart failure is the dominant problem.

Diagnosis and CMR Findings

Diagnosis is usually achieved in the neonate by clinical examination and echocardiography, that provides all necessary informations for pre-operative assessment. In rare cases CMR imaging may be used to gain additional information on associated malformations.

Therapy

An initial palliative and life-saving procedure is balloon atrial septostomy to improve atrial-level mixing. However, in all cases surgical repair has to be performed, and the two most common surgical procedures are atrial switch or arterial switch operation. **Atrial switch**, either as Mustard or Senning procedure (Figure 14-25b, c), is the most common surgical procedure in patients who are currently adults. Blood is redirected at the atrial level using a baffle made of Dacron or pericardium (**Mustard procedure**) or atrial flaps (**Senning procedure**), achieving physiological correction by diverting systemic venous return through the mitral valve into the subpulmonary LV, and rerouting the pulmonary venous return through the tricuspid valve into the subaortic region. Using **arterial switch** operation the arterial trunks are transsected and reanastomosed to the contralateral root (Figure 14-26a). The coronary arteries must be transposed together with the aorta. If present, a VSD is closed. Infants with TGA plus a VSD and LVOT obstruction may require early systemic-to-pulmonary artery anastomosis and a later

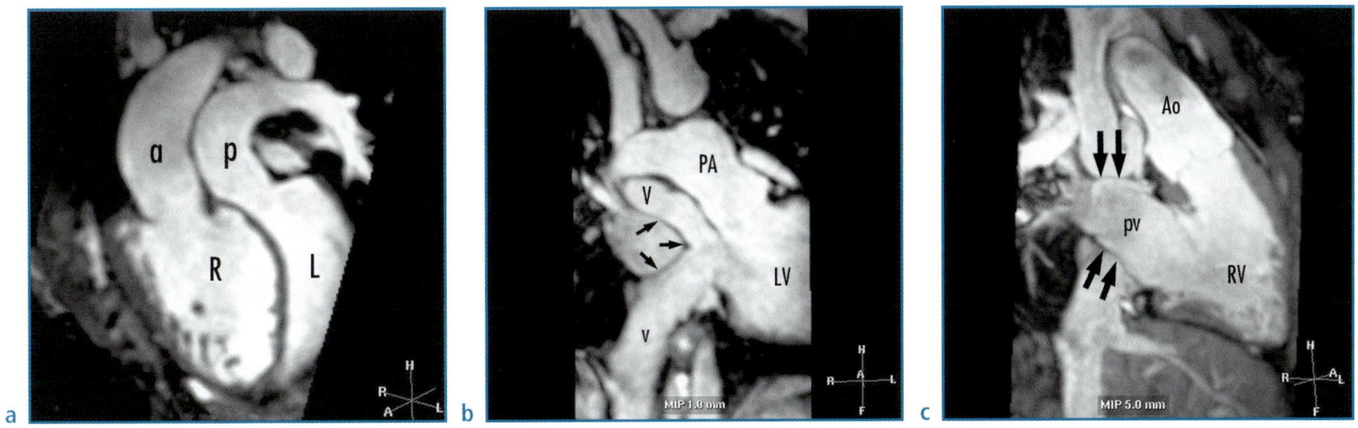

Figure 14-25 D-transposition of the great arteries (TGA) with the aorta (a) right-anterior to the pulmonary artery (p) arising from the right ventricle (R), while the pulmonary artery arises from the left ventricle (L) **(a)**. Another patient with D-TGA after Mustard procedure **(b and c)**: Atrial baffle (small arrows in **(b)**) for redirecting blood flow from caval veins (v, V) subpulmonary to the left ventricle (LV), and to redirect blood flow from the pulmonary veins (pv, broad arrows in **(c)**) to the right ventricle (RV). PA: pulmonary artery; Ao: aorta.

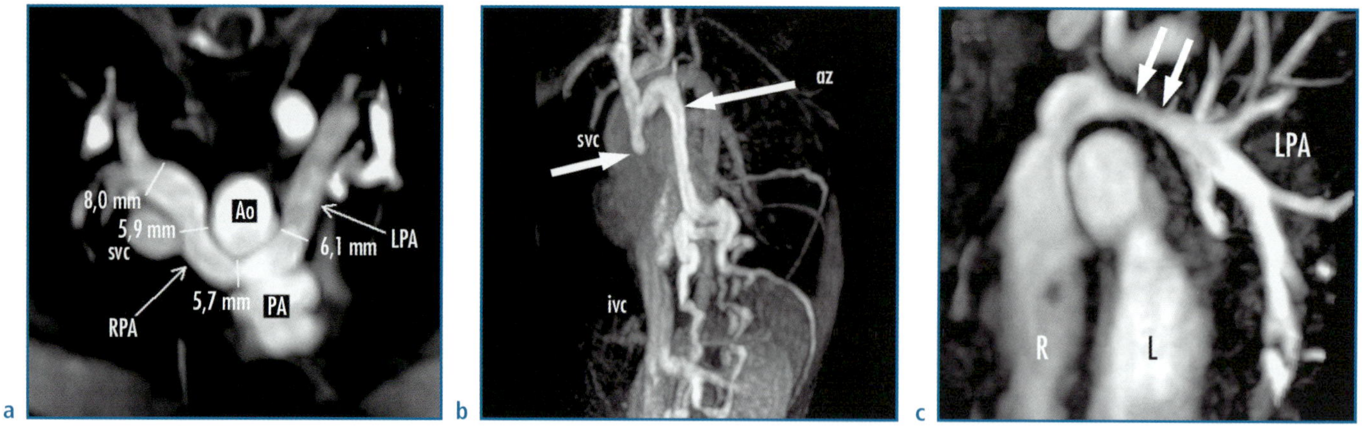

Figure 14-26 D-transposition of the great arteries (TGA) after arterial switch procedure **(a)** – the ascending aorta (Ao) including the coronary arteries was shifted posterior over pulmonary artery bifurcation, and the pulmonary artery (PA) was shifted anterior. The right pulmonary artery (RPA) courses between the ascending aorta and the superior caval vein (svc) to the right hilus. Another patient with TGA with occlusion of the superior caval vein (svc) due to an obstructing baffle after Mustard procedure and collateral circulation via the azygos vein system (az) to the inferior caval vein (ivc) **(b)**. Tubular stenosis (arrows) of the left pulmonary artery (LPA) in a patient with TGA after arterial switch procedure **(c)**. L: left ventricle; R: right ventricle.

corrective procedure according to **Rastelli** (aorta connected to the LV using an intraventricular baffle, and right-ventricle-to-pulmonary artery conduit placed).

Long-Term Effects and CMR Findings

Following **atrial switch** several long-term complications may occur. Among these are moderate to severe RV dysfunction with consecutive tricuspid regurgitation, baffle leak with significant left-to-right shunt and pulmonary vascular disease, SVC or IVC baffle obstruction (Figure 14-26b) or pulmonary venous baffle obstruction with elevated pulmonary artery pressures and RV pressure load. Potential sequelae of **arterial switch operation** include coronary occlusion, supravalvular pulmonary stenosis (Figure 14-26c) that may be treated by balloon angioplasty or reoperation, supravalvular aortic stenosis, usually treated by reoperation, and neoaortic dilatation and regurgitation. Although most of these adverse sequelae may be detected by echocardiography, CMR imaging plays a significant role due to its ability to non-invasively evaluate most clinically relevant issues (Rebergen 1995, Gutberlet 2000).

The **goals of CMR in post-operative atrial switch** include:

- quantitative evaluation of the size and function of the systemic RV,
- imaging of the systemic and pulmonary venous pathways for obstruction and/or baffle leaks,
- assessment of tricuspid valve regurgitation, evaluation of the LVOT and RVOT for obstruction, and
- detection of aortopulmonary collateral vessels and other associated anomalies (Dorfman and Geva 2006).

The **goals of CMR in post-operative arterial switch** include:

- evaluation of the global and regional LV and RV size and function,
- evaluation of the LVOT and RVOT for obstruction,
- qualitative estimation of RV systolic pressure based on the configuration of the interventricular septum,
- imaging of the great vessels with emphasis on evaluation of the pulmonary arteries for stenosis and the aortic root for dilatation, and
- detection of aortopulmonary collaterals and other associated anomalies (Dorfman and Geva 2006).

14.8.5 Congenitally Corrected Transposition of the Great Arteries (ccTGA)

Pathology and Pathophysiology

This rare malformation (prevalence of < 1% of all CHDs) consists of ventricular inversion with concomitant transposition of the great arteries, i.e. discordant AV connections combined with discordant ventriculoarterial (VA) connections ("double discordance"). With the usual atrial arrangement systemic venous blood passes from the RA through a mitral valve to the LV and then to the posteriorly located pulmonary artery, while pulmonary venous blood passes from the LA through a tricuspid valve to a left-sided RV and then to an anterior, left-sided aorta. The circulation is thus "physiologically" corrected, but the morphological RV supports the systemic circulation which may lead to RV failure (Figure 14-27). Associated anomalies (in 95% of

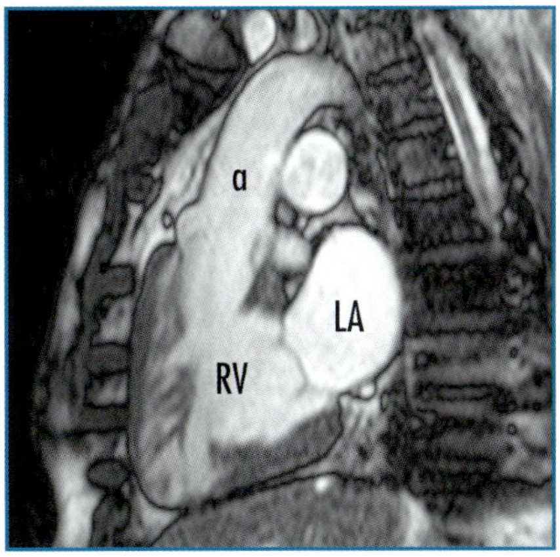

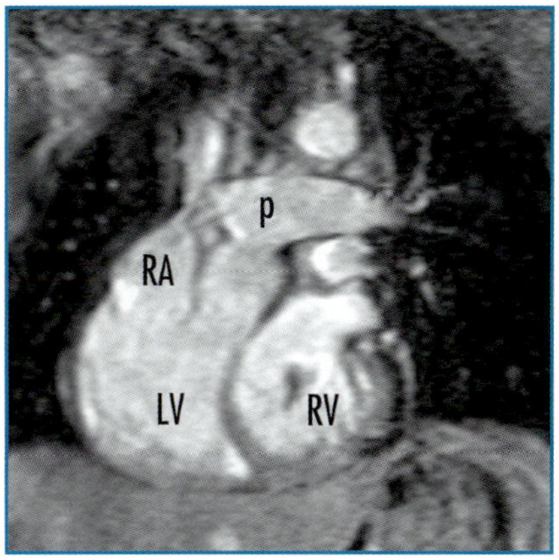

Figure 14-27 Congenitally corrected transposition of the great arteries (ccTGA) with ventricular inversion and concomitant TGA in a sagittal (a) and frontal view (b). The aorta (a) is situated left-anterior and arises from the right ventricle (RV) that receives its blood from the left atrium (LA); the pulmonary artery (p) arises from the left ventricle (LV) that is connected to the right atrium (RA).

patients) include VSD (75%), pulmonary or subpulmonary stenosis (75%) or (rarely) pulmonary atresia with ductus-dependent pulmonary perfusion, and left-sided tricuspid, often "Ebstein-like" valve abnormalities (more than 75%). Dextrocardia or mesocardia is present in about 25% of patients, and situs inversus in 5%.

Clinical Presentation

Patients without associated defects (< 5% of cases) may remain asymptomatic, but particularly those with associated anomalies may develop cyanosis, exercise intolerance, congestive heart failure, and palpitations from supraventricular arrhythmias (symptoms usually arising in the 5th or 6th decade).

Diagnosis and CMR Findings

Diagnosis is generally made by echocardiography, the role of CMR imaging in ccTGA is to evaluate the systemic right ventricular volume and ejection fraction, and to assess associated anomalies.

Therapy

Treatment includes valve replacement in case of moderate to severe AV valve regurgitation, but when tricuspid regurgitation is associated with poor systemic RV function, the double-switch procedure may be considered. Patients with significant VSD and pulmonary stenosis or RVOT obstruction may require surgical repair including VSD closure and LV-to-pulmonary artery conduit.

Long-Term Effects and CMR Findings

Possible long-term problems after operation for ccTGA can be reliably detected and quantified by CMR imaging.

14.9 Aortic Arch Anomalies (including Ring Formation)

CMR imaging is meanwhile the gold standard for evaluating patients with aortic arch anomalies and has substituted classical invasive angiography and simultaneous bronchography. Its main advantage is precise visualization of all vascular territories and their relation to the neighboring structures e.g. the tracheobronchial tree and the esophagus, and when combining CMR with bronchoscopy all anatomic and functional relations and interactions can be assessed. The anatomy of the vascular structures is imaged by cine-SSFP and black-blood sequences in end-expiratory breath-hold. In addition, TSE sequences may be used to examine the morphology of the trachea and the esophagus by using transversal orthogonal planes to the trachea, and additional in coronal plane exactly within and parallel to the course of the trachea. In case of suspected compression of the trachea CMR imaging should be performed in endotracheal anesthesia with end-expiratory breath-hold, but the endotracheal tube should not be advanced through the compressed lumen to avoid splinting of the stenosed area. Moreover, during endotracheal anesthesia and artificial ventilation a positive end-exspiratory airway pressure is present that may alleviate the degree of tracheal stenosis. These issues have to be borne in mind, and in combination with all clinical informations a definite assessment of structure and dysfunction of a compressed trachea should be made; in unclear situations a tracheobronchoscopy should be performed during spontaneous breathing.

14.9.1 Anomalies with Left Aortic Arch

Normal anatomy of aortic arch and its branches includes the first branch of the truncus brachiocephalicus with branching into the right subclavian (rSA) and carotid artery (rCA). The second arch branch is the left common carotid artery (lCCA), and the third branch is the left subclavian artery (lSA). The ligamentum arteriosum originating just distal to the lSA connects the aortic arch with the pulmonary bifurcation in the region of the origin of the left pulmonary artery (lPA). A harmless variant is the origin of the lCCA from the truncus brachiocephalicus, as is the separate origin of the left vertrebral artery from the aortic arch between the lCCA and the lSA. The only situation with four arch vessels is the retroesophageal course of the rSA (**arteria lusoria**; Figure 14-28a, b); all arch vesssels have the same calibre, and the arteria lusoria origins as the last branch from the posteromedial aspect of the aortic arch. This is a frequently encountered anomaly with a prevalence of about 0.5 % of the general population, patients are usually asymptomatic and do not require treatment; surgical repair is only indicated if patients present with significant dysphagia.

A rare anomaly is a **left aortic arch with a right descending aorta** that compresses the esophagus. The rSA arises also as the last arch vessel with a non-retroesophageal course. The clinical symptoms are caused by a ring completed by a right ductal ligament connected with the right PA. This is the only anatomic constellation with left aortic arch where patients present with stridor. Surgical access to correct this anomaly is from the right-thoracic or, rarely, via a transsternal approach, while for all other ring formations access is from left-thoracic region.

14.9.2 Anomalies with Right Aortic Arch

The most common of the five variants is a **right aortic arch with mirror image origin of the arch arteries** – first is the left truncus brachiocephalicus dividing into the lCCA and lSA, second is the rCCA, and third the rSA. This variant is not associated with a vascular ring. The clinical relevance of this anomaly relates to associated malformations such as TOF and other "conotruncal" defects.

In right **aortic arch and retroesophageal Kommerell's diverticulum** a ring is present because the ductal ligament is located between the Kommerell diverticulum and the pulmonary bifurcation, and vessel branching includes the lCCA as the first aortic branch, followed by rCCA and rSA, while the small lSA originates from the large Kommerell diverticulum coursing to the left side (Figure 14-28c). If patients present with significant dysphagia, stridor, or recurrent pneumonia, surgical transsection of the ligament is necessary using a left-thoracic surgical access.

A similar but rarer malformation is a **right aortic arch with retroesophageal lSA without a Kommerell diverticulum**, where a ring is absent. A further rare malformation is a right aortic arch with left descendent aorta, that includes a ring due to a left ductal ligament originating from the retroesophageal leftward coursing aorta at the level of the 4th to 5th thoracic vertrebra to join the left PA. Arch branches are organized in mirror image, or with a lSA as the last arch branch. Another ring is present in **right aortic arch and a retroesophageal truncus brachiocephalicus sinister**, the ring being built by the left ductal ligamentum from the base of the trunk to the left PA.

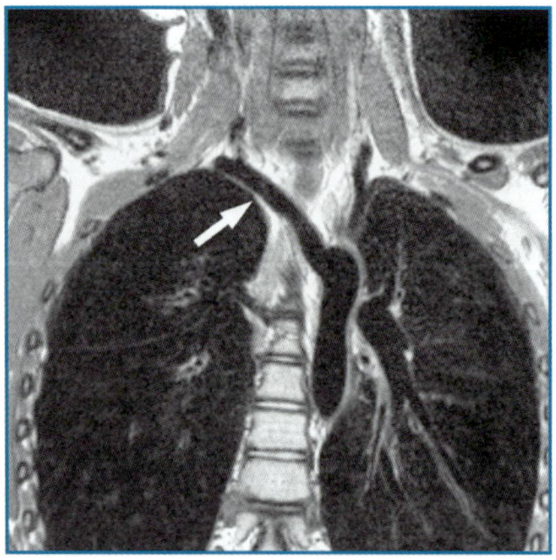
a

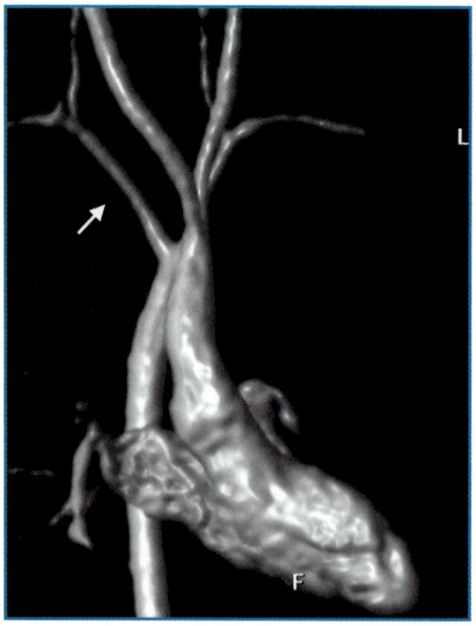

b

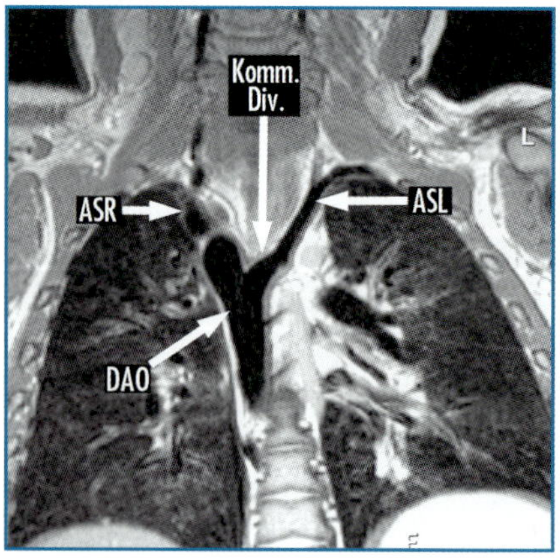

c

Figure 14-28 Right subclavian artery arising from the descending aorta with retroesophageal course ("arteria lusoria", arrow) in a frontal view (a). Arteria lusoria (arrow) in a volume-rendered image in a lateral view (b). Right aortic arch with origin of the left subclavian artery (ASL) from a Kommerell diverticulum (Komm Div.) in a frontal view (c). ASR: right subclavian artery; DAO: descending aorta.

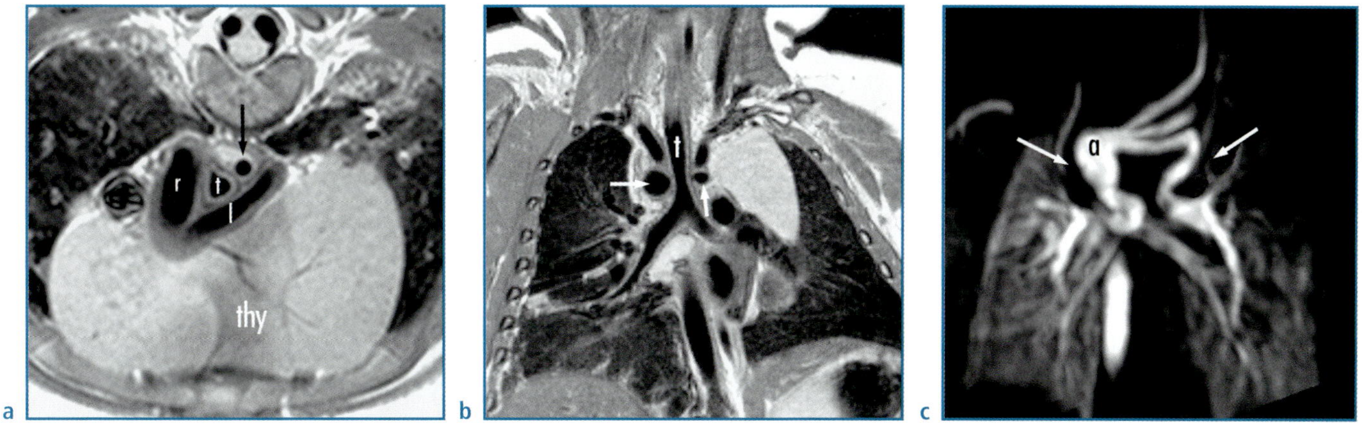

Figure 14-29 Double aortic arch in an axial (a) and frontal view (b) with ring-like course around the trachea (t in (a), small upward arrow in (b)); the right part of the arch (r in (a), horizontal arrow in (b)) shows a larger lumen than the left part (l in (a), broad upward arrow in (b)). Bilateral persistent patent ductus arteriosus (arrows) arising from the aortic arch (a in (c)) in a patient with pulmonary atresia and absence of a confluens of the pulmonary arteries (c).

14.9.3 Double Aortic Arch

A double aortic arch always presents with a ring around the esophagus and the trachea, because both aortic arches course at the left and right side around these structures in dorsal direction, the right aortic arch being situated slightly higher than the left (Figure 14-29a, b). Both arches may be widely open (narrow ring with early symptoms within the first year of life), but most often the left arch is hypoplastic or atretic resulting in less obstruction with symptoms often presenting later in life.

The **branching pattern** of the arch vessels depends on the preponderant patency of the individual arches:

- both arches patent with symmetric origin of their arch branches: lCCA anterior and lSA posterior originating from the left, and rCCA anterior and rSA posterior originating from the right arch,
- left arch atretic distal to the origin of the lSA: the anatomy of branching vessels is a mirror image to the right aortic arch but with the aorta descending on the left,
- double aortic arch with atresia of the left part between the lCCA and lSA: this anomaly is difficult to differentiate from right aorta with the origin of the lSA from a Kommerell diverticulum,
- in the rare case of an atretic right arch variants of the left arch are "simulated".

Associated cardiac malformations are rare (e.g. TOF) as well as further arch anomalies (e.g. coarctation). In addition, a ductal ligament (most commonly left-sided) may be present, that has to be dissected, as well, in case a symptomatic ring is formed, in order to avoid a residual airway stenosis postoperatively.

14.9.4 Persistent Fifth Aortic Arch

This is a very rare anomaly most commonly associated with further congenital cardiac malformations. The aortic arch has a double lumen, whose both parts are located on the same site of the trachea. The upper arch corresponds to the embryologically normal forth arch, while the lower persistent arch develops from the fifth arch coursing from the base of the truncus brachiocephalicus dorsal to shortly distal to the origin of the lSA. Both arches may be patent, or the upper arch is atretic or interrupted, while all branches originate from the ascending aorta.

14.9.5 Interrupted Aortic Arch

In this very severe anomaly the circulation of the lower body depends on the ductus arteriosus that regularly renders newborns symptomatic with the need of an early diagnosis. A steep course of the ascending aorta and a long atretic part is characteristic of this anomaly.

Three types can be differentiated:

- **Type A**: The interruption begins distal to the subclavian artery that is ipsilateral to the second common carotid artery; this correlation is necessary to differentiate from the right subclavian artery that may be isolated or retroesophageal, as well; Type A interrupted aortic arch is frequently associated with an aortopulmonary window or with a transposition of the great arteries (TGA).
- **Type B**: The interruption of the aorta is between the second common carotid artery and the ipsilateral subclavian artery, and this anomaly is always associated with a VSD as part of a conotruncal defect with malalignment of the infundibular septum; most commonly a DiGeorge

syndrome is the cause at least when a right arch persists (the first arch branch represents the carotid artery of the contralateral site; a retroesophageal or isolated subclavian artery always origins from the contralateral site of the arch).

- **Type C**: The atretic part lies between both carotis arteries, the "contralateral" subclavian artery may originate retroesophageally or isolated.

14.9.6 Aortopulmonary Window

This rare anomaly with a prevalence of 0.6% of all CHDs is most commonly associated with further congenital malformations (in about 50% of cases).

There are **three types of the deficient septum between both great arteries**:

- in **Type I** the defect is halfway between the semilunar valves and the pulmonary bifurcation,
- in **Type II** the defect is located in the posterior aortic wall near the pulmonary bifurcation with the right PA originating from the aorta,
- **Type III** is a combination of I and II.

Because of the large non-restrictive communication often a significant left-to-right shunt exists with consecutive pulmonary hypertension. Children present symptomatic within the first weeks after birth. Diagnosis is usually made by echocardiography (assessment of the defect, qualitative evaluation of the shunt). In cases with suspicion of associated congenital anomalies CMR imaging is the technique of choice to assess abnormal anatomy, dysfunctions, pulmonary flow, and amount of left-to-right shunt. Therapy includes surgical repair of the window and, if present, correction of associated anomalies. CMR imaging is also extremely valuable in immediate post-operative and follow-up examinations.

14.9.7 Patent Ductus Arteriosus (PDA) Botalli

The ductus arteriosus derives from the left sixth primitive aortic arch and connects the proximal left PA to the descending aorta. It is widely open in the normal fetus and closes shortly after birth from vasoconstriction, while anatomic closure from intimal proliferation and fibrosis takes place several weeks later to complete. A patent ductus arteriosus (PDA) is relatively frequent with a prevalence of 5–10% of all CHDs and occurs isolated or in combination with a multitude of CHD (Figure 14-29c).

In PDA a left-to-right shunt is present, its amount depends on both the size and length of the duct, and the difference between systemic and pulmonary vascular resistance, and thus, **several degrees of shunts** can be differentiated:

- silent PDA (detected by chance and nonclinical means),
- small PDA (no significant hemodynamic derangement, continuous murmur, Qp/Qs < 1.5 : 1.0),
- moderate PDA (volume load on LA and LV, continuous murmur, dyspnea and palpitations, Qp/Qs = 1.5–2.2 : 1.0),
- large PDA (hypoxemia in the feet more than in the hands, short systolic ejection murmur, Eisenmenger's physiology, Qp/Qs > 2.2 : 1.0), and
- Eisenmenger's syndrome (dyspnea at rest or exertion, continuous murmur absent, differential hypoxemia, differential cyanosis, bidirectional or right-to-left shunt).

Diagnosis is usually made by echocardiography (presence, size and degree of shunting). CMR imaging may be useful in assessing size and location of the defect, volume overload (LA and LV), and to precisely measure the amount of shunt. Treatment includes either interventional closure of the duct with a plug (in ducts smaller than 8 mm), or surgical closure by duct ligation and/or division. Post-operative and long-term control can be made by either echocardiography or CMR imaging.

14.9.8 "Aberrant" Truncus Brachiocephalicus

This anomaly is frequently found in infants with exspiratory stridor and a right-ventrally pulsating obstruction of the trachea without a demonstrable arterial ring. It is unclear whether there is a primary tracheomalacia with close contact to the trunk, or the trunk plays a causal role for tracheal obstruction. Diagnosis can be easily confirmed by CMR imaging to demonstrate the anatomical relation of the trunk to the trachea, and to quantitate the degree of tracheal obstruction (Figure 14-30a). Treatment consists of aorto-ventro-pexia with antefixation of the vessel to the sternum. Pre- and post-operative control (location of the trunk relative to the trachea, deobstruction of the trachea) is best achieved by CMR imaging.

14.9.9 Cervical Aortic Arch

This very rare anomaly consists of an elongated aorta ascendens with an arch that exeeds the clavicula (Figure 14-30b), in almost all cases a right aortic arch is present. The abnormal arch may cause compression of the trachea with consecutive tracheomalacia that in rare cases needs an operative correction with right-sided fixation of the ascending aorta. There are combinations with ring structures, e.g.

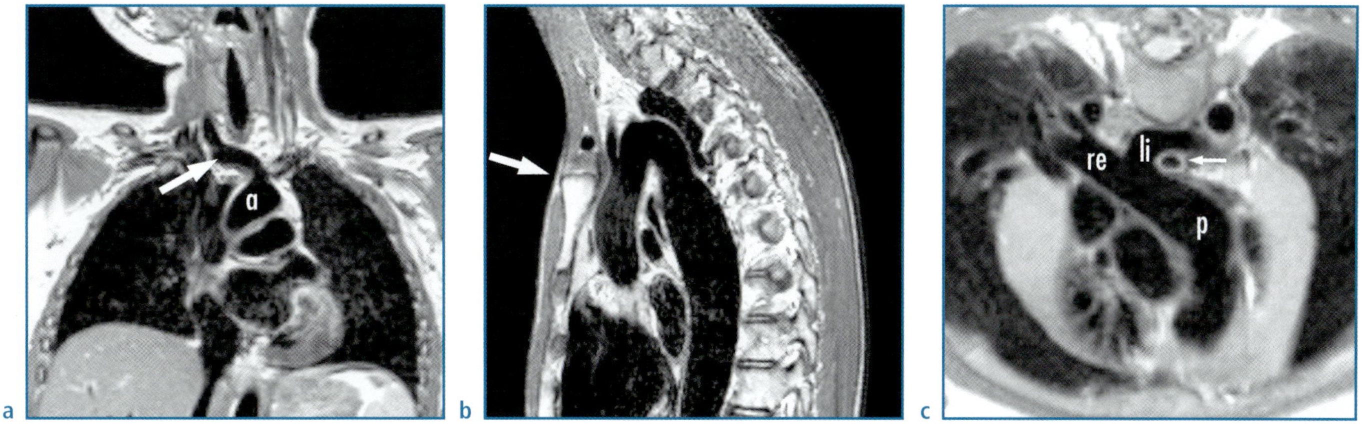

Figure 14-30 Aberrant truncus brachiocephalicus (arrow) with its origin from the aortic arch (a) in a frontal view (a). Cervical aortic arch with its vertex in the fossa jugularis superior to the sternum (arrow) (b). Pulmonary sling with origin of the left pulmonary artery (li) from the right pulmonary artery (re) (c); notice tracheal stenosis by a cricoid cartilage (arrow). p: pulmonary trunc.

by a ductal ligament in left descendent aorta. CMR using black-blood sequences and 3D CE-MRA is the imaging tool of choice to assess abnormal anatomy and (dys)function of the aorta both pre- and post-operatively.

14.10 Anomalies of the Pulmonary Artery

14.10.1 Origin of one Pulmonary Artery from the Ascending Aorta

In this syndrome one pulmonary artery branch with a normal pulmonary trunk originates from the ascending aorta. This configuration is different to the truncus arteriosus communis with only one pulmonary artery branch originating from the ascending aorta ("hemitrunk") and perfusion of the contralateral lung via a ductus arteriosus or aortopulmonary collaterals. In more than 75 % of cases it is the right branch, commonly associated with aortopulmonary window with a left aortic arch. If the left branch is affected, as a rule a right aortic arch is present and/or TOF. CMR imaging is a valuable tool to visualize the abnormal anatomy, but lacks information on pulmonary vascular resistance in elderly patients.

14.10.2 Origin of Left Pulmonary Artery from the Right Pulmonary Artery ("Pulmonary Sling")

In this anomaly the left PA arises from the right PA and courses dorsal to the trachea but ventral to the esophagus (Figure 14-30c). Children present with dyspnea and stridor, the cause may not always be the anomaly itself, but may be associated with ring cartilage of the trachea. Operative repair, if necessary, includes both retransplant of the PA and – if present – correction of the tracheal ring cartilage.

14.11 Anomalies of the Aorta

14.11.1 Coarctation of the Aorta (CoA)

Pathology

Aortic arch obstruction may be divided into localized coarctation in close proximity to a PDA or ligamentum, tubular hypoplasia of some part of the aortic arch system, and aortic arch interruption (Figure 14-31 and Figure 14-32). The lesion consists of a localized shelf in the posterolateral aortic wall opposite to the ductus arteriosus. It is relatively common with a prevalence of 6–8 % of all patients with CHD. Coarctation of the aorta is not a simple anomaly, but is highly associated with Turner syndrome (gonadal dysgenesis) and bicuspid aortic valve.

Clinical Presentation

Severe obstruction in infancy is a prominent cause of left heart failure and systemic hypoperfusion. Also, if infants or children are rapidly presenting with symptoms (about 50 % of cases), associated malformations such as tubular aortic arch hypoplasia, aortic or mitral valve dysfunctions, subaortic stenosis, VSD, or PDA are usually present. Not infrequently CoA is associated with complex CHD, e.g. AVSD, DORV with subpulmonary VSD, or d-TGA with/without tricuspid atresia.

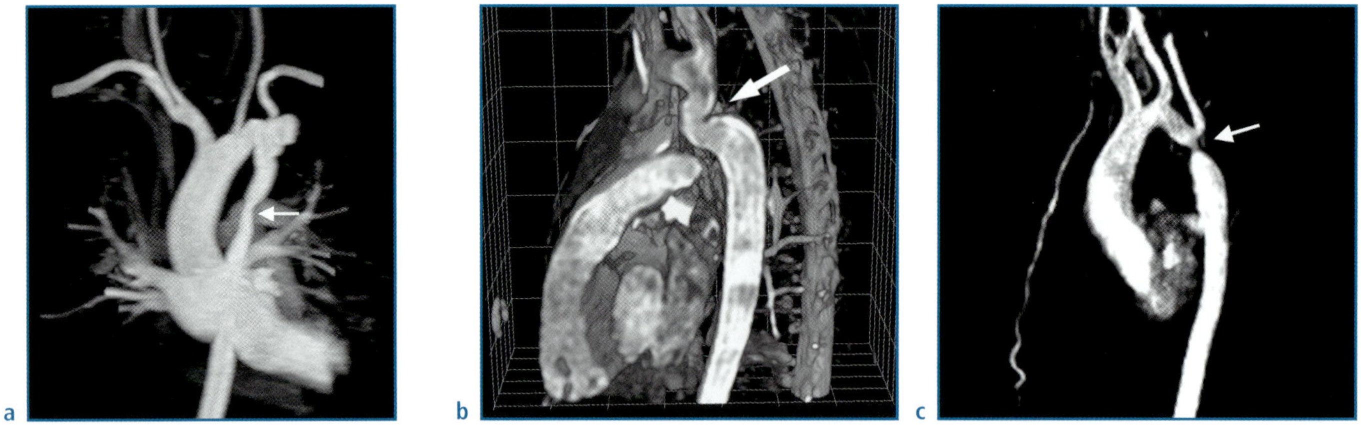

Figure 14-31 Coarctation of the aorta (CoA) with a moderate excentric stenosis in the descending aorta (arrow) (a). Another patient with a special type of CoA with a siphon-like course of the aortic arch (arrow) after the origin of the left subclavian artery (b). A third patient with a ring-like high-grade CoA just after the origin of the left subclavian artery (arrow) (c).

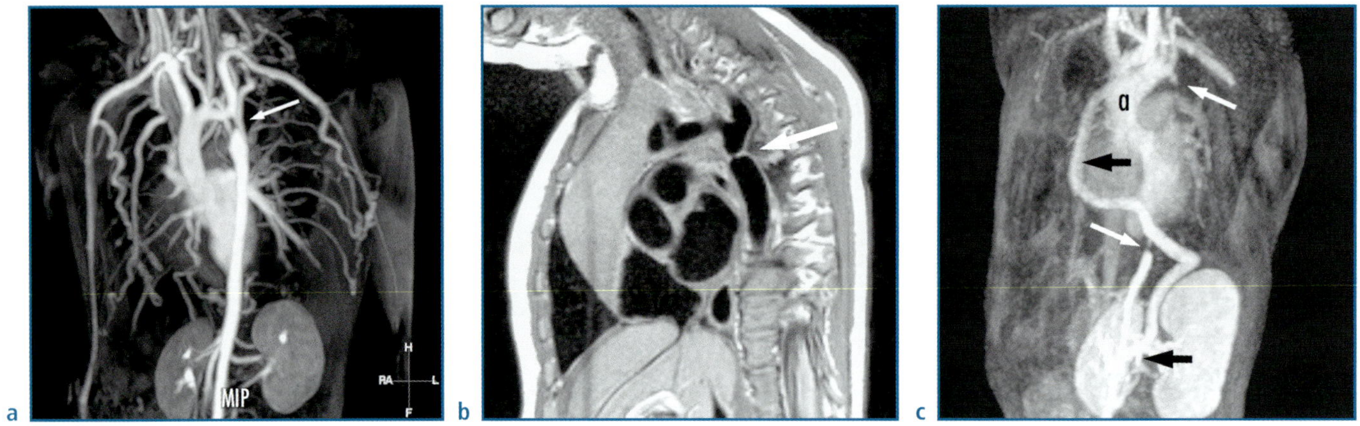

Figure 14-32 Coarctation of the aorta (CoA) in a frontal view (a) with a tubular-stenotic segment in the descending aorta (arrow) and numerous large collateral vessels via intercostal arteries and both subclavian arteries to bypass the stenotic aortic segment. High-grade circumscript CoA in a newborn due to a membrane-like structure ("ductus shelf") in a sagittal view (arrow) (b). Thoracic aorta interrupted between the isthmus and the diaphragmatic level (white arrows) in an 8-yrs-old girl following surgical repair (c): a 10 mm conduit (black arrows) was inserted between the ascending aorta (a) and the abdominal aorta with the distal anastomosis distal to the origin of the renal arteries. MIP: Maximum Intensity Projection (image).

Diagnosis and CMR Findings

Diagnosis is achieved by clinical examination (pulse discrepancies between arms and legs, blood pressure difference between arms and legs or between right arm and left arm, inter-rib pulsations from collaterals) and echocardiography (posterior shelf, degree of hypoplasia, pressure gradient over the obstructed area). CMR imaging may also be very helpful in visualizing the anatomy (Figure 14-32), and to measure blood flow in the upper and lower body region by PC mapping, as well as to demonstrate collateral circulation between the upper trunk and abdomen (Figure 14-32a). This is achieved by black-blood sequences axial through-plane and parasagittal in-plane along the aortic arch to measure the degree of stenosis. Using flow-sensitive cine-GRE or cine-SSFP sequences the origin of stenotic flow turbulences can be detected that may clarify whether a significant stenosis exists within a hypoplastic aortic segment that was not seen within the spin echo image. 3D-contrast-enhanced MRA is able to visualize the whole arch, the stenotic segment, and the descending aorta, and to demonstrate collateral arteries between the upper and lower trunk (Figure 14-32a, c). Using PC mapping the gradient via the stenotic segment can be assessed as well as the flow volume via the collateral arteries (flow volume just downstream the stenotic segment minus the flow volume at the diaphragmatic level; Mohiaddin 1993).

Therapy

Management usually involves prostaglandin E1 infusion, and surgical repair including excision of the area of coarctation and extended end-to-end repair, or end-to-side anastomosis with absorbable sutures to allow remodeling of the aorta with time. Subclavian flap or patch repair employed extensively in the past are now less popular because of long-term problems (late aneurysm development, perfusion problems of the subclavian artery). An alternative approach at least in elderly patients is the implantation of a stent graft after prior balloon dilatation of the coarcted area.

Long-Term Effects and CMR Imaging

CMR imaging is an ideal tool for immediate and late post-operative follow-up of the patients, it is also extremely useful to detect long-term complications, e.g. aneurysms after patch repair.

14.11.2 Supravalvular Aortic Stenosis

Pathology

Three different types of supravalvular aortic stenosis are recognized:

- the **hourglass type** (marked thickening and disorganization of the aortic media producing a constrictive annular ridge at the superior margin of the sinus of Valsalvae),
- the **membraneous type** (fibrous or fibromuscular semicircular diaphragm with small central opening), and
- a **diffuse type** (diffuse hypoplasia of the ascending aorta).

The coronary arteries arise proximal to the site of outflow obstruction and thus, are subjected to elevated pressure that exists within the LV, with premature coronary atherosclerosis in some patients. In some patients the origin of coronary arteries may be included in the stenotic segment, or some or all aortic cusps adhere to the site of supravalvular stenosis leading to compromised coronary inflow.

Clinical Presentation

Supravalvular aortic stenosis may be associated with a special cardiac and multi-system disorder, called **Williams-Beuren syndrome**. Infants with this syndrome may present with feeding difficulties, failure to thrive, gastrointestinal problems with vomiting, constipation and colic, auditory hyperacusis, inguinal hernia, a horse voice, intellectual impairment, "elfin" facies, strabismus, and abnormalities of dental development.

Diagnosis and CMR Findings

Diagnosis of supravalvular aortic stenosis is confirmed by clinical examination (stenotic murmur, clinical signs of Williams-Beuren syndrome), ECG (signs of LV hypertrophy or biventricular hypertrophy), and echocardiography (site of stenosis, dilated sinuses of Valsalva, pressure gradient by Doppler sonography). CMR imaging is an ideal tool to visualize the anatomy of the entire thoracic aorta (Figure 14-33), and to assess both the degree of stenosis and function of both ventricles.

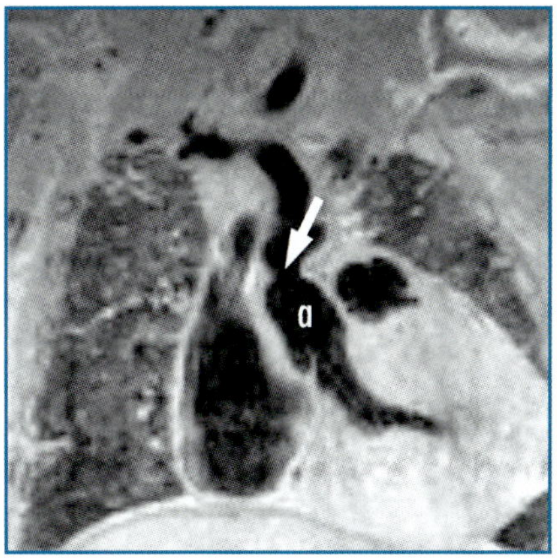

Figure 14-33 Supravalvular aortic stenosis (arrow) in a newborn in a frontal view. a: ascending aorta.

Therapy

Therapy includes surgical resection with end-to-end anastomosis, use of an Y patch, or a **Ross procedure**. Also useful information on the proximal coronary anatomy and possible involvement of coronary origins into the supraaortic stenosis can be obtained by a 3D "whole-heart" SSFP sequence.

Long-Term Effects and CMR Imaging

The immediate and long-term post-operative results including possible complications can be easily controlled by CMR imaging.

14.12 Congenital Valvular Disease

Pathology

Congenital mitral valve abnormalities are rare and include **mitral stenosis** (parachute deformity with shortened chordae tendineae converging and inserting into a single papillary muscle, or thickened leaflets with shortening and fusion of the chordae tendineae, or an anomalous arcade of obstructing papillary muscles, or accessory mitral valve tissue), and **mitral regurgitation** (isolated cleft of the anterior mitral valve leaflet, or leaflet dysplasia). Cardiac defects associated with congenital mitral stenosis are common including LVOT obstruction, PDA, coarctation of the aorta, or endocardial fibroelastosis. Complex mitral regurgitation is more frequently seen in DORV, TGA and VSD, and corrected TGA.

Isolated congenital tricuspid valve stenosis or **regurgitation** is extremely rare, and is diagnosed by echocardiography. **Congenital pulmonary stenosis** (cPS) with intact ventricular septum is more common, with a wide range of isolated valvular stenosis to complete atresia of the pulmonary outflow tract. In isolated cPS the pulmonary valve may vary from well-formed triflet valve with different degrees of commissural fusion to an imperforate membrane. Infants with a high-grade cPS present with central cyanosis due to right-to-left shunting at the atrial level. Children and adults with isolated mild to moderate cPS are usually asymptomatic.

Diagnosis and CMR Findings

Diagnosis of congenital mitral valve abnormalities is achieved by clinical examination, ECG, and echocardiography (abnormal mitral valve structure, degree of stenosis or incompetence, atrial and ventricular dimensions and function). CMR imaging is a useful adjunct at least in cases with incomplete echo studies to visualize the abnormal anatomy, degree of stenosis or regurgitation (measurement of regurgitant fraction), and to precisely assess atrial and ventricular volumes and function.

Diagnosis of congenital pulmonary stenosis is confirmed by clinical examination (systolic murmur with a single or split S_2), ECG (RV hypertrophy), and echocardiography (valve abnormality, degree of stenosis by Doppler sonography).

CMR imaging may be a valuable adjunct for visualizing the abnormal anatomy and to assess both the degree of stenosis and RV function.

Therapy

Therapy in symptomatic mitral stenosis includes surgical repair by removing a supramitral ring if present, and splitting the papillary muscles and fused chordal apparatus in the most common form of mitral stenosis. Ballon dilatation is not a realistic option for congenital mitral valve stenosis. In patients with congenital mitral regurgitation surgical correction should be performed before patients become symptomatic. Surgery involves suture of an isolated cleft, with or without associated commissuroplasties. In cases with a dysplastic mitral valve, leaflet extension and additional annuloplasty and commissuroplasty are used to achieve effective control of regurgitation in the short and medium term. Treatment of congenital pulmonary stenosis includes balloon dilatation (treatment of choice), or rarely, surgical repair in case of failure of balloon dilatation. CMR imaging may be used for post-treatment control.

14.13 MR Imaging after Surgical Palliation

14.13.1 Separation of Circulation at the Atrial Level (Fontan Procedure)

The Fontan procedure is a palliative operation to separate the systemic venous and the pulmonary venous blood flow in patients with only one functioning ventricular chamber. Such congenital anomalies include tricuspid atresia, univentricular atrioventricular connections, the hypoplastic left heart syndrome following Norwood palliation, and DORV with hypoplastic left ventricle. The indication for Fontan procedure is given, if a separation of the circulation at the level of the ventricles by creating a 2-chamber system is impossible or if the risk of ventricular septation is higher than the Fontan palliation. The principle of this procedure is diversion of the systemic venous return directly to the pulmonary arteries without passing through a subpulmonary ventricle, while the oxygenated blood is conducted via the single-chamber to the systemic circulation. The original Fontan procedure in patients with tricuspid atresia included an end-to-end anastomosis of the superior vena cava (SVC) with a proximally cut right pulmonary artery (RPA) as a so-called **Glenn shunt**, connection of the right atrium with the pulmonary artery via a valved homograft, and implantation of a bioprosthesis between the inferior vena cava (IVC) and right atrium as well as closure of the ASD. Following the initial procedure total cavopulmonary anastomosis has been introduced using an anastomosis from the SVC to the right pulmonary artery, and using a patched tunnel baffle from the IVC to the right pulmonary artery. Another technique consists of creating an **extra-cardiac tunnel** (18–22 mm prosthesis) between the IVC and pulmonary artery, eventually with a fenestration to the pulmonary-venous atrium.

CMR imaging has become an extremely important tool for follow-up of these surgically treated patients to assess the post-operative result and incidental post-operative problems. The main objectives of CMR are the assessment of the systemic ventricular function by volumetry, to quantify perfusion of the left vs. the right lung, to assess the flow rate via the caval veins, and to measure cardiac output (see also Chapter 14.7.5).

14.13.2 Surgical Palliation Prior to Correction or Fontan Procedure

Operative palliation often becomes necessary in newborns and younger children when biventricular surgical correction or a Fontan procedure in single-ventricle physiology seems impossible or too risky at the time of diagnosis, on the other hand the natural history would be associated with a high mortality. **Pulmonary artery banding** to reduce lung perfusion used in patients with single ventricle without pulmonary stenoses can be reliably controlled with CMR imaging, including obstructions of the orifices of the pulmonary arterial side branches from this location of the banding. To improve perfusion of the lung in cyanotic congenital anomalies many variant surgical shunt techniques between the aorta and the central part of the pulmonary artery have been introduced. The earliest were the **Waterston-Cooley anastomosis** between the posterior wall of the ascending aorta and the anterior wall of the right pulmonary artery, or **Pott anastomosis** between the descending aorta and the left pulmonary artery. Most techniques often result in volume overload of the ventricles and result in pulmonary hypertension, or stenoses of the involved pulmonary artery with consecutive malperfusion of the contralateral site. These post-operative situations can be easily assessed by CMR imaging including contrast-enhanced MR angiography.

Further techniques are **central aortopulmonary anastomoses** and the *classical* **Blalock-Taussig anastomosis** (shunt between the subclavian artery to the pulmonary artery), and the *modified* **Blalock-Taussig anastomosis** using a goretex tube from the left subclavian artery to the pulmonary artery in left-sided aortic arch (and vice versa). Using phase contrast techniques stenoses of the shunt or occlusions may be easily detected, in unclear cases CE-MRA can be used. In addition, the performance of the volume loaded ventricles and thereafter with increasing cyanosis confronted systemic ventricles can be exactly quantified by CMR-based volumetry.

14.14 Conclusions and Future Perspectives

Present standard CMR sequences allow the assessment of all aspects of morphology, structure, and function at least in children and adolescents with congenital cardiac malformations. Contrast-enhanced CMR imaging of myocardial tissue is used to detect myocardial scars post-operatively, particularly when heart-lung machines were used. Stress testing for evaluating ventricular function is established and increasingly applied in clinical routine. Fast imaging techniques using partial k-space coverage, acquisition of larger k-space elements, or parallel imaging and k-t acceleration techniques have been established to allow high-quality real-time CMR, that obviates the limitations of breath-hold maneuvers or ECG triggering problems. For reasons of radiation protection MR-compatible materials (catheters, devices) are being developed to facilitate non-invasive catheterizations and catheter-based interventions under real-time MR "fluoroscopy" in younger patients with CHD (Rezavi 2006, Kuehne and Ewert 2006).

References

Beekman RP, Roest AA, Helbing WA et al. Spin echo MRI in the evaluation of hearts with a double outlet right ventricle: usefulness and limitations. Magn Reson Imaging 2000; 18: 245–53.

Beerbaum P, Barth P, Kropf S et al. Cardiac function by MRI in congenital heart disease: impact of consensus training on interinstitutional variance. J Magn Reson Imaging 2009; 30: 956–66.

Beerbaum P, Körperich H, Barth P et al. Non-invasive quantification of left-to-right shunt in pediatric patients: phase contrast cine magnetic resonance imaging compared with invasive oximetry. Circulation 2001; 103: 2476–82.

Beerbaum P, Körperich H, Esdorn H et al. Atrial septal defects in pediatric patients: non-invasive sizing with cardiovcascular MR imaging. Radiology 2003b; 228: 361–9.

Beerbaum P, Körperich H, Gieseke J et al. Rapid left-to-right shunt quantification in children by phase contrast MRI combined with sensitivity encoding (SENSE). Circulation 2003a; 108: 1355–61.

Cheung EW, Lam WW, Cheung SC, Cheung YF. Functional implications of the right ventricular myocardial performance index in patients after surgical repair of tetralogy of Fallot. Heart Vessels 2008; 23 (2): 112–7.

Dorfman AL, Geva T. Magnetic resonance imaging evaluation of congenital heart disease: conotruncal anomalies. J Cardiovasc Magn Reson 2006; 8: 645–59.

Dorfman AL, Odegard KC, Powell AJ et al. Risk factors for adverse events during cardiovascular magnetic resonance in congenital heart disease. J Cardiovasc Magn Reson 2007; 9: 793–8.

Fogel MA, Rychik J. Right ventricular function in congenital heart disease: pressure and volume overload lesions. Progr Cardiovasc Dis 1998; 40: 343–56.

Fogel MA, Weinberg PM, Fellows KE et al. A study in ventricular-ventricular interaction. Single right ventricles compared with systemic right ventricles in a dual-chamber circulation. Circulation 1995; 92: 219–30.

Fogel MA, Weinberg PM, Parave E et al. Deep sedation for cardiac magnetic resonance imaging: a comparison with cardiac anesthesia. J Pediatr 2008; 152: 534–9.

Greil GF, Powell AJ, Gildein HP, Geva T. Gadolinium-enhanced three-dimensional magnetic resonance angiography of pulmonary and systemic venous anomalies. J Am Coll Cardiol 2002; 39: 335–41.

Gutberlet M, Boeckel T, Hosten N et al. Arterial switch procedure for D-transposition of the great arteries: quantitative midterm evaluation of hemodynamic changes with cine-MR imaging and phase shift velocity mapping-initial experience. Radiology 2000; 214: 467–75.

Helbing WA, Niezen RA, Le Cessie S et al. Right ventricular diastolic function in children with pulmonary regurgitation after repair of tetralogy of Fallot: volumetric evaluation by magnetic resonance velocity mapping. J Am Coll Cardiol 1996; 28: 1827–35.

Hoppe UC, Dederichs B, Deutsch HJ et al. Congenital heart disease in adults and adolescents: comparative value of transthoracic and transesophageal echocardiography and MR imaging. Radiology 1996; 199 (3): 669–77.

Kuehne T, Ewert P. Endovascular intervention – congenital heart disease. In: Higgins CB, de Roos A (eds.). MRI and CT of the Cardiovascular System. 2nd ed. Lippincott Williams & Wilkins 2006; 593–9.

Luijnenburg SE, Robbers-Visser D, Moelker A et al. Intra-observer and interobserver variability of biventricular function, volumes and mass in patients with congenital heart disease measured by CMR imaging. Int J Cardiovasc Imaging 2010; 26: 57–64.

Mohiaddin RH, Kilner PJ, Rees S, Longmore DB. Magnetic resonance volume flow and jet velocity mapping in coarctation. J Am Coll Cardiol 1993; 22: 1515–21.

Niezen RA, Beekman RP, Helbing RP et al. Double outlet right ventricle assessed with magnetic resonance imaging. Int J Card Imaging 1999; 15: 323–9.

Rebergen SA, Helbing WA, van der Wall EF et al. MR velocity mapping of tricuspid flow in healthy children and in patients who have undergone Mustard or Senning repair. Radiology 1995; 194: 505–12.

Rebergen SA, Ottenkamp J, Doornbos J et al. Post-operative pulmonary flow dynamics after Fontan surgery: assessment with nuclear magnetic resonance velocity mapping. J Am Coll Cardiol 1993; 21: 123–31.

Rezavi R. Magnetic resonance guided cardiac catheterization. In: Higgins CB, de Roos A (eds.). MRI and CT of the Cardiovascular System. 2nd ed. Lippincott Williams & Wilkins 2006; 610–28.

Sarikouch S, Kuehne T, Peters B et al. Gender specific pediatric percentiles for ventricular size and mass as reference values for cardiac magnetic resonance imaging. Circ Cardiovasc Imaging 2010, 3: 65–76.

Simonetti OP, Cook S. Technical aspects of pediatric CMR. J Cardiovasc Magn Reson 2006; 8: 581–93.

15 Pericardial Diseases

Vinzenz Hombach

15.1 Anatomy and Function of the Pericardium

The pericardium is composed of **two layers**:

- the **inner serous membrane** (visceral pericardium) composed of a single layer of mesothelial cells adherent to the epicardial surface of the heart, and
- an **outer fibrocollagenous layer** (parietal pericardium) that is 2 mm thick, largely acellular and contains collagen and elastin fibers.

The visceral pericardium reflects back near the origins of the great vessels, becoming continuous with and forming the inner layer of the parietal pericardium. The pericardium contains two major pericardial sinuses with a transverse recess connecting the two tubes of pericardium to envelop the great vessels (the aorta and pulmonary artery enclosed in one anterosuperior tube, the vena cava and pulmonary veins in a posterior tube), and the oblique sinus behind the left atrium (LA) with the posterior LA wall separated from the pericardial space. The small pericardial cavity contains 10–50 ml of fluid (ultrafiltrate of plasma) produced by the visceral pericardium and drained out of the cavity towards the thoracic duct and right lymphatic duct.

The function of the pericardium is, by exerting a restraining force, to prevent sudden dilatation of the cardiac chambers, especially of the right atrium (RA) and right ventricle (RV), during exercise and with hypervolemia. It also restricts the anatomic position of the heart, minimizes friction between the heart and kinking of the great vessels, and probably retards the spread of infections from the lung and pleural cavities to the heart. The pericardial sac has a relatively small reserve volume and when exceeded, the pressure in the sac located on the surface of the heart increases rapidly and is transmitted into the cardiac chambers according to the exponential pressure-volume relation. On the other hand, chronic pericardial stress, e.g. by slowly accumulating pericardial effusion or left ventricular remodeling and dilatation, may occur without pericardial constriction, when pressure-volume relation shifts to the right. Moreover, the pericardium equalizes the compliance between the right and left ventricle, and produces interdepencence of filling between the ventricles (so-called ventricular coupling). This phenomenon plays an important role in cardiac tamponade with increased intrapericardial pressure, or in fixed pericardial cavity by constrictive pericarditis (for details see Le Winter and Tischler 2012).

15.2 CMR Protocols

Normal pericardium is visible on spin echo CMR as a thin, smooth, hypointense curvilinear structure surrounded by hyperintense mediastinal and epicardial fat with a normal diameter of 1.2 mm in diastole and 1.7 mm in systole. These diameters are larger than found in anatomical studies with values of 0.4–1.0 mm, and this overestimation is due to motion of pericardial layers, lack of sufficient spatial resolution, and chemical shift artifacts at the fat-fluid interface on cine-CMR. Comprehensive CMR imaging aims at assessing the morphology of pericardium and pericardial sac and fluid, at detecting inflammatory involvement of both the pericardium and myocardium, or fibro-calcified pericardium in constrictive pericarditis, and at accurately measuring RV and LV volumes and function as well as ventricular inflow characteristics to detect a restrictive filling pattern.

The **CMR protocol should include** the following sequences:
- scouts (with a small field of view and a saturation block positioned on the frontal chest wall in the following protocol),
- spin echo sequences to visualize pericardial morphology (width, localization, extent, pericardial delineation) and cardiac/ventricular structure,
- cine-SSFP sequences to visualize pericardial morphology and function (motion pattern), to assess size and shape of ventricles, myocardial morphology, and regional and global ventricular function, and to assess caval vein size and detect pleural fluid or ascites,
- real-time cine-CMR for detecting ventricular coupling (ventricular septal shape, septal motion pattern, respiratory-related septal shift),
- black-blood sequences for pericardial and cardiac morphology,
- contrast-enhanced CMR to detect myocardial scars, infiltrations, storage disease, or inflammation and pericardial inflammation, as well as to characterize pericardial layer/fluid,
- phase contrast mapping to assess cardiac filling characteristics (mitral inflow, pulmonary vein flow),
- CMR tagging to detect fusion of pericardial layers.

15.3 Pericarditis and Pericardial Effusion

Etiology and Pathophysiology

Acute pericarditis is the most common pathologic process involving the pericardium.

Etiologic factors are:
- **infections**:
  - viral: coxsackie virus A and B, echovirus, mumps, adenovirus, HIV,
  - bacterial: pneumococcus, streptococcus, staphylococcus, tuberculosis, treponema pallidum,
  - fungal: histoplasmosis, coccidiomycosis, candida, and
  - protozoal, parasitic etc.,
- **non-infectious diseases**: acute myocardial infarction, uremia, neoplasia, myxedema, trauma, aortic dissection, familial pericarditis, Whipple's disease, sarcoidosis, and
- **factors presumably related to hypersensitivity or autoimmunity**: rheumatic fever, collagen vascular diseases like SLE, rheumatoid arthritis, scleroderma, drug-induced e.g. by hydralazine, phenytoin, isoniazide, minoxidil, and post-cardiac injury like Dressler's syndrome/post-myocardial infarction, post-pericardectomy, or post-traumatic.

The clinical classification includes:
- **acute** pericarditis < 6 wks (fibrinous, effusive),
- **subacute** pericarditis: 6 wks to 6 mths (effusive-constrictive, constrictive), and
- **chronic** pericarditis > 6 mths (constrictive, effusive, adhesive-nonconstrictive).

Acute inflammation of the pericardial layers is characterized by formation of fresh, highly vascularized granulation tissue with fibrin deposition, and usually a variable amount of pericardial fluid is present, while the fibrin deposition may lead to fibrous adhesion of the pericardial layers. Chronic inflammation is characterized by a progressive sclerosing pericarditis with collagen, fibroblasts and lesser amount of fibrin deposition. This process may proceed towards an end-stage, i.e. chronic fibrosing pericarditis with collagen and fibroblasts, with consecutive forming of a stiff pericardium with constriction of the heart (constrictive pericarditis). **Pericarditis** without significant effusion does not produce any negative hemodynamic effects, while a significant **effusion** may cause impairment of ventricular filling and reduction of cardiac output. If the quantity of pericardial effusion is sufficient to cause serious obstruction to inflow of blood to the ventricles, this results in **cardiac tamponade**, and this complication may be fatal if it is not recognized and treated promptly. The quantity of fluid necessary to produce the critical stage of tamponade may be as small as 200 ml when the fluid accumulates rapidly, or > 2,000 ml in slowly developing effusion when the pericardium has had the opportunity to stretch and adapt to an increasing volume. In cardiac tamponade the normal inspiratory augmentation of the RV volume causes an exaggerated reciprocal reduction in LV volume together with leftward bulging of the interventricular septum. Further hallmarks of cardiac tamponade are the diastolic inversion or collapse of the RV free wall, right atrial compression during early systole, exaggerated respiration in cardiac inflow, and abnormal flow patterns in the caval veins (Spodick 2003).

Clinical Presentation

Patients present with chest pain particularly in acute pericarditis, a pericardial friction rub on auscultation, and ECG alterations. These include elevation of the ST segment (*stage 1*), often with upward concavity, followed by return to normal (*stage 2*), negative T-waves (*stage 3*), and return to normal (*stage 4*). In acute pericarditis, effusion is usually associated with pain and/or these ECG changes. However, if

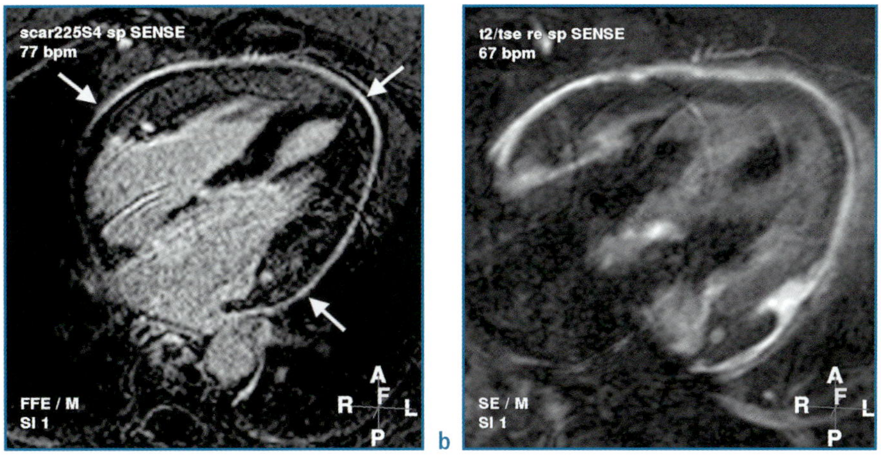

Figure 15-1 Acute pericarditis with a small amount of pericardial effusion and strong pericardial enhancement after gadolinium administration (arrows) (a), and slight myocardial edema on T2w-image (b).

pericardial effusion develops within a relatively short time, it may lead to cardiac tamponade with siginificant hemodynamic consequences. With effusion the heart sounds may be fainter, friction rub may disappear, and apex impulse may vanish. The three clinical features of tamponade are hypotension, soft or absent heart sounds, and a jugular venous distention with prominent x descent but an absent y descent (Beck's triad). In slowly developing tamponade patients may present with dyspnea, orthopnea, and hepatic engorgement. Paradoxical pulse is an important clue to the diagnosis of cardiac tamponade. This sign consists of a greater than normal (10 mmHg) decline in systolic arterial pressure that can be detected by palpating the weakness or disappearance of the arterial pulse during inspiration, or by sphygmomanometrically measured systolic pressure during slow respiration. Paradoxical pulse may not only be observed in cardiac tamponade, but also in about one-third of patients with constrictive pericarditis. It may also be observed in hypovolemic shock, acute or chronic obstructive airways disease, and in pulmonary embolus.

Diagnosis

Clinical diagnosis of pericarditis may be derived from chest pain depending on position of the thorax, by auscultation (pericardial friction rub), and by significant ECG alterations (ST segment elevation). Pericardial effusion may be confirmed clinically by low ECG voltage (with large effusions), and be confirmed by echocardiography (localisation and quantity of pericardial fluid, "swinging heart" in large effusions). Pericardial tamponade may be diagnosed clinically by Beck's triad (hypotension, soft or absent heart sounds, and jugular venous distention), and by paradoxical pulse (pulsus paradoxus: inspiratory decline of systolic arterial pressure greater than 10 mmHg). Diagnosis is confirmed by echocardiography (reduced RV cavity diameter, late diastolic inward motion of RV free wall and of right atrium = collapse), and by Doppler echocardiography (markedly increased tricuspid and pulmonic valve flow velocities during inspiration, in contrast to diminished pulmonic vein, mitral, and aortic flow velocities). These alterations can also be detected with high accuracy using CMR imaging.

CMR Findings

In acute pericarditis (pericardial inflammation) both thickening of pericardial layers, and associated pericardial effusion can be well-detected on T1w-spin echo images or cine-CMR. T2w-STIR-spin echo sequences allow visualization of edema of the inflamed pericardial layers (Figure 15-1). In addition, pericardial inflammation can be easily demonstrated by contrast enhancement after gadolinium injection (Figure 15-1 and Figure 15-2), while addition of a fat suppression prepulse may be helpful to enhance visualization of pericardial inflammation. In cases of more chronic pericarditis delineation of pericardial layers may be most important to demonstrate more irregular contours of thickened pericardium and streaky enhancement of the surrounding fat and enhancement of adjacent myocardial tissue, indicating associated epicarditis and/or myocarditis. Tagging CMR techniques may be used to evaluate fibrotic adhesions of pericardial layers.

Pericardial **transsudate**s typically have a low signal intensity on T1w-spin echo and a high signal intensity on T2w-images (Figure 15-3). **Exudates** with their high protein and cell content show higher signal intensity on T1w- and lower signal intensity on T2w-images. CMR imaging is an excellent method for detection of small pericardial effusions based on the typical signal intensities. Even a small volume of fluid appears as a high signal space between the epicardial layers. However, non-linear motion of pericardial fluid during cardiac motion may falsely cause high signal on T1w-spin echo images within the effusion even in the presence of a simple exudate. Pericardial fluid motion

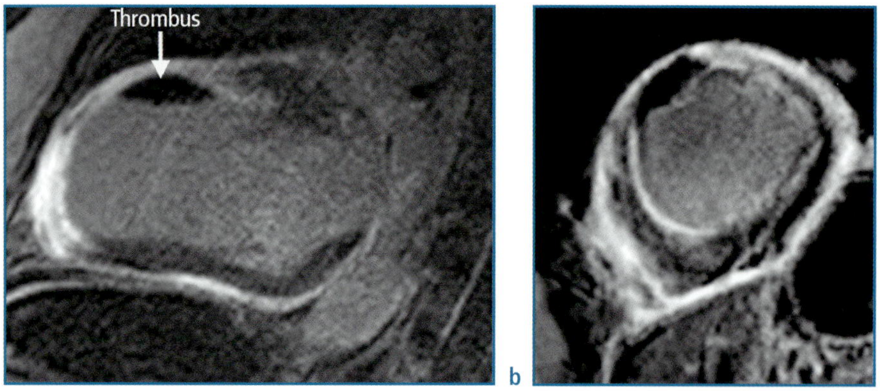

a b

Figure 15-2 Acute pericarditis following an acute anteroseptal myocardial infarction (Dressler's syndrome): strong pericardial enhancement after gadolinium administration in the 2-ch (a) and short-axis view (b). Note myocardial enhancement in the left ventricular apical myocardium due to myocardial infarction, and a thrombus (arrow) at the basal anterior LV wall.

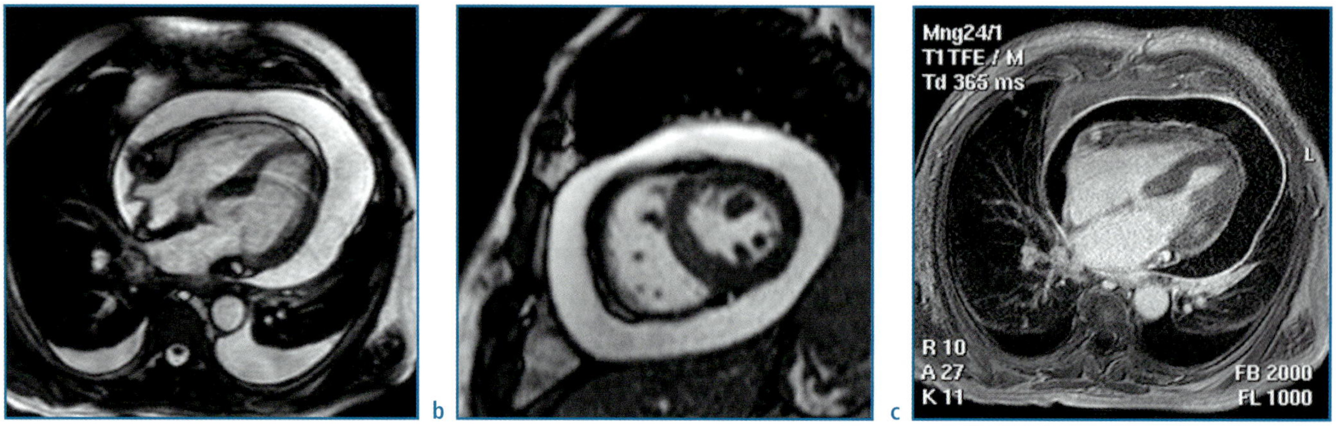

a b c

Figure 15-3 Subacute large pericardial effusion in the 4-ch (a), and short-axis view (b) together with enhancement of the pericardium after gadolinium administration (c) representing pericardial inflammation (courtesy Dr. J. Schwab, Nuremberg).

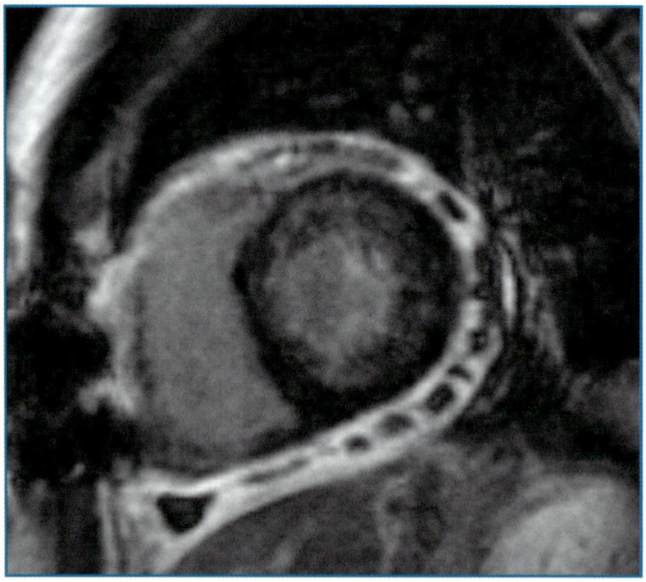

Figure 15-4 Pericardial effusion (bright signal) with blood coagula in the pericardial sac (dark particles) in the short-axis view (= subacute hemorrhagic pericardial effusion) (courtesy Prof. J. Schulz-Menger, Berlin).

during cardiac cycle on cine-GRE sequences may help in differentiating pericardial fluid and pericardial thickening, as well as excluding the presence of adherences in the regions where fluid motion is seen between parietal and visceral pericardium. Typically pericardial effusion shows no increase in signal intensity on T1w-images after administration of gadolinium contrast agent, which aids in distinguishing between pericardial fluid and pericardial or myocardial tumor on T1w-spin echo images. The appearance of **hemorrhagic effusions** depends on the age of pericardial blood. Acute hemopericardium shows high signal intensity on T1w-spin echo images and a low signal intensity on cine-GRE sequences. Subacute and chronic hematomas are usually heterogenous with both high- and low-signal intensity regions on T1w-images, and balanced SSFP sequences often better characterize the pericardial hemorrhagic fluid by visualizing fibrinous strands or presence of coagulated blood (Figure 15-4).

Therapy

Acute pericarditis and small pericardial effusions usually do not require specific treatment, though antiinflammatory drugs may relieve symptoms of pericarditis and prevent the transition to chronic pericarditis. However, patients with acute pericarditis should be observed frequently for the development of an effusion or tamponade. Cardiac tamponade is a life-threatening condition and requires immediate pericardiocentesis with subsequent draining of the pericardial cavity as completely as possible. Follow-up of the patients can be easily performed by echocardiography or CMR.

15.4 Constrictive Pericarditis

Etiology and Pathophysiology

This disease results when the healing of an acute fibrinous or serofibrinous pericarditis or the resorption of a chronic pericardial effusion is followed by obliteration of the pericardial cavity with the formation of granulation tissue. This granulation tissue gradually contracts and forms a firm scar, encasing the heart and interfering with filling of the heart. The basic physiologic abnormality of this condition is the inability of the ventricles to fill because of the limitations imposed by the rigid, thickened pericardium or the tense pericardial fluid. During early diastole ventricular filling is unimpaired, while reduced abruptly when the elastic limit of the pericardium is reached. This is in contrast to cardiac tamponade where ventricular filling is impeded throughout diastole. In both diseases, ventricular end-diastolic and stroke volumes are reduced and the end-diastolic pressures in both ventricles as well as the mean pressures in the atria, pulmonary veins, and systemic veins are all elevated to similar levels (within 5 mmHg of one another). Yet myocardial function may be normal or slightly impaired, but the fibrotic process may extend into the myocardium causing myocardial scarring and atrophy. Ultimately venous congestion may then be due to the combined effect of pericardial and myocardial damage.

The **three main hemodynamic consequences** of encasement of the heart are:

- dissociation between intrathoracic and intracardiac pressure, isolating the heart from normal respiratory changes in intrathoracic pressure,
- increased ventricular coupling, and
- increased cardiac filling pressures with pressure equalization in all four cardiac chambers.

Clinical Presentation

Patients present with weakness, fatigue, weight gain, increased abdominal girth, abdominal discomfort, and edema, in advanced cases with anasarca, cachexia, and skeletal muscle wasting. The cervical veins are distended and venous pressure may fail to decline during inspiration (Kussmaul's sign). Right and left atrial pressure pulses display an M-shaped contour, with prominent x and y descents. The y descent reflecting the early filling period is interrupted by a rapid rise in atrial pressure during early diastole due to impeded filling of the ventricle by the constricting pericardium. These changes are transmitted to the jugular veins and can be assessed by inspection of the patient. Pulse pressure is normal or reduced, and in about 30% of cases a paradoxical pulse can be detected. The apical pulse is reduced and may retract in systole, and an early third heart sound (pericardial knock) may be heard occurring with the rapid cessation of ventricular filling.

Diagnosis

Diagnosis is made by clinical examination, ECG (low voltage, flattened or inverted T-waves), chest X-ray (thickened and calcified pericardium), and echocardiography including Doppler sonography (pericardial thickening, dilatation of the inferior vena cava and hepatic veins, sharp halt in ventricular filling in early diastole, flattening of the posterior wall, and normal ventricular systolic function). Thickened pericardium including calcifications can also be detected by CT or by CMR imaging (Figure 15-5 and Figure 15-6).

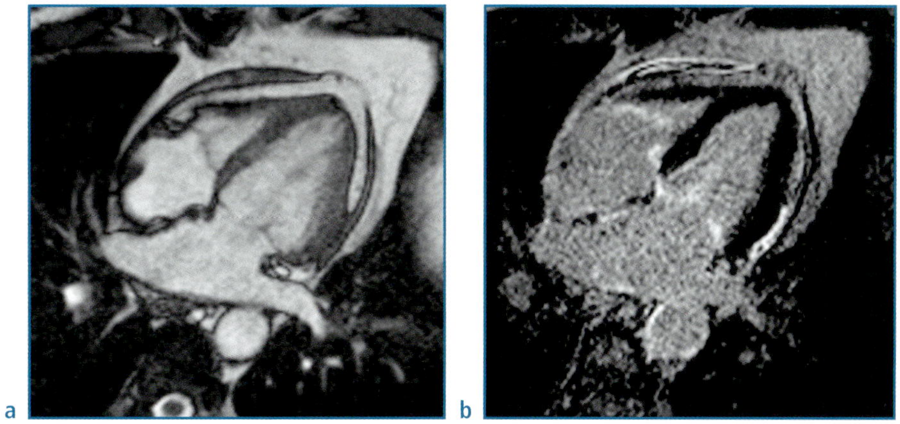

Figure 15-5 Pericardial fibrosis in a SSFP cine-CMR (a) with bright epicardial fat layer and thickened pericardium (7 mm in diameter) over the whole right and left ventricular circumference; localized pericardial enhancement after gadolinium administration (b) representing residual pericardial inflammation.

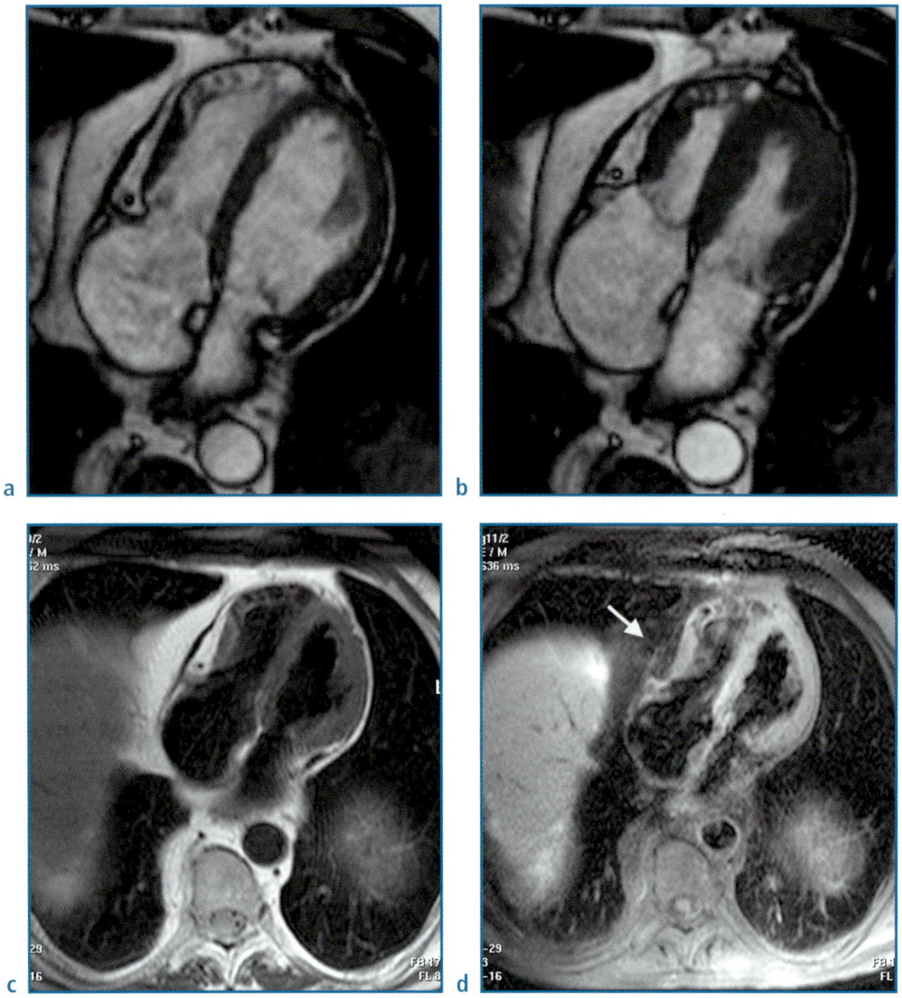

Figure 15-6 Constrictive pericarditis in the 4-ch view: restricted motility of the right and – to a lesser extent – the left ventricular myocardium in diastole (a) and systole (b) in the SSFP cine-CMR. In the black-blood sequence loss of the calcified pericardial structure (c), and in a fat-sat sequence (d) massive impression (arrow) of the right ventricular lateral myocardial wall (courtesy Dr. J. Schwab, Nuremberg).

CMR Findings

Various patterns of distribution of constrictive tissue have been described including global, right-sided, left-sided, or focal types of constriction. The focal type usually involves the atrioventricular groove and thereby may impede right atrial, and less frequently left atrial emptying. In global constriction cine-SSFP images show flattened or tubular-shaped cardiac cavities, and as a result of increased filling pressures unilateral or bilateral atrial enlargment, dilatation of caval and hepatic veins, pleural effusion, and ascites. Pericardial thickness may be defined with a thickness of 2 mm or less as normal, thickness greater than 4 mm in patients with appropriate clinical presentation as suggestive of pericardial constriction, and thickness greater than 5–6 mm as highly specific for pericardial constriction (Soulen 1985, Maisch 2004). The thickened fibrotic and/or calcified pericardium has a low signal intensity in T1w-, T2w-spin echo, as well as in cine imaging, and calcified regions appear with signal void (Figure 15-6). In end-stage chronic fibrosing pericarditis there is no enhancement after gadolinium injection, while pericardial enhancement is suggestive of residual inflammation (Bogaert and Francone 2009).

Velocity-encoded CMR typically shows a restrictive filling pattern with an enhanced early filling, and a decreased or absent late filling, depending on the degree of pericardial constriction and increased filling pressures. A similar restrictive filling pattern can be detected in the pulmonary and caval veins with diminished or absent forward, or even reversed systolic flow, and increased early diastolic forward flow and late backflow. In contrast to restrictive cardiomyopathy, constrictive pericarditis typically shows a strong respiratory-related variation in cardiac filling, i.e. enhanced RV filling on inspiration, and enhanced LV filling on expiration (Talreja 2008, Bogaert and Francone 2009). Increased ventricular coupling is another important sign of cardiac constriction. Under normal loading conditions due to the positive LV to RV pressure gradient the interventricular septum has a right-sided convex shape, which is maintained during the entire cardiac cycle and is minimally influenced by respiration. The lack of pericardial stretch in constrictive pericarditis leads to an increased ventricular coupling with septal flattening or inversion on early diastolic ventricular filling (Nishimura 2001). These septal abnormalities are most pronounced at onset of respiration and rapidly fade away, while at onset of expiration an opposite, i.e. right-sided septal shift occurs. Using real-time CMR these dynamic respiration-dependent changes of the septum can be dynamically visualized, i.e. inspiratory septal inversion (i.e. notable movement toward LV), and expiratory increased right-sided septal motion, leading to an increased respiratory septal shift. Pericardial mobility is also an interesting feature to differentiate normal pericardium, which slightly moves during cardiac cycle often synchronous with the underlying myocardial motion, from constrictive pericarditis with limited or almost no displacement of the pericardium. The restricted expansion of the myocardium during cardiac filling abutting against the stiff pericardium can be well-demonstrated in cine- or real-time CMR.

Therapy

The definitive treatment of constrictive pericarditis is pericardial resection with an operative mortality of 5–10%, depending on the extent of penetration of the myocardium by the calcific process, on the severity of myocardial atrophy, on the extent of secondary impairment of hepatic and/or renal function, and on the patient's general condition. The benefits derived from surgical cardiac decortication are usually progressive over a period of months, and can be easily monitored by CMR imaging for both structural and functional improvement.

15.5 Pericardial Cysts, Defects and Diverticula

Etiology and Pathophysiology

Pericardial cysts are congenital encapsulated cysts implanted on the pericardium with no connection with the pericardial cavity. Their location is typically in the cardiophrenic sulcus (90%), and most often right-sided (70%). **Pericardial defects** are congenital malformations with a wide range of small defects to total absence of pericardium, and may be secondary to abnormalities of vascular supply to the pericardium. **Pericardial diverticulum** is an extremely rare congenital or acquired condition, it corresponds to a herniation through a defect in the parietal pericardium, which communicates with the pericardial cavity. It typically occurs in the cardiophrenic angles and has a tendency to change in size over time. These diverticula result from failure in the fusion of one of the mesenchymal lacunae that normally concur to form the pericardial sac.

Clinical Presentation

Pericardial cysts are usually asymptomatic, only in some rare cases they become symptomatic by compressing other cardiac structures. Pericardial cysts should be differentiated from other cysts like bronchogenic cysts and thymic cysts, and from encapsulated pericardial effusion. Clinical presentation of **pericardial defects** is variable, patients are often asymptomatic, but symptoms occur when cardiac structures are transiently entrapped or incarcerated in the defect. Left atrial appendage may herniate into the defect, resulting in infarction of the appendage, or the left coronary artery may be compressed with consecutive myocardial ischemia and chest pain particularly during exercise. Patients with **pericardial diverticulum** are usually asymptomatic.

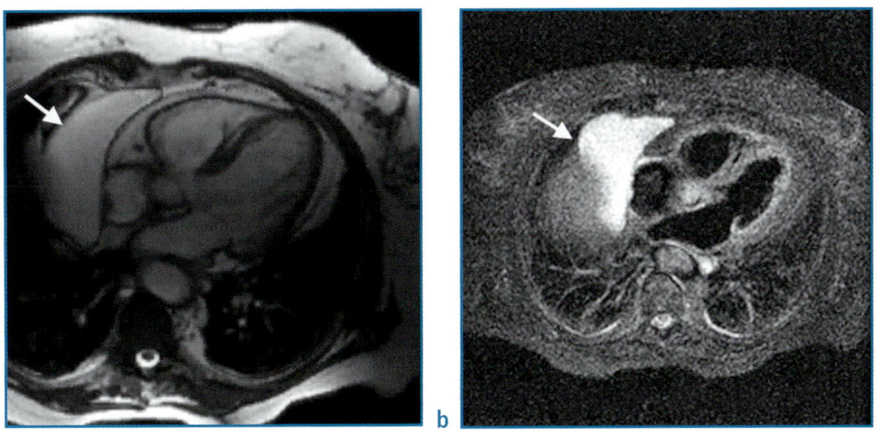

a b

Figure 15-7 Pleuro-pericardial cyst in the right-atrial-right-ventricular angle (arrows) in a cine-SSFP sequence (a) and a T2w-triple inversion recovery sequence (b) with high signal intensity.

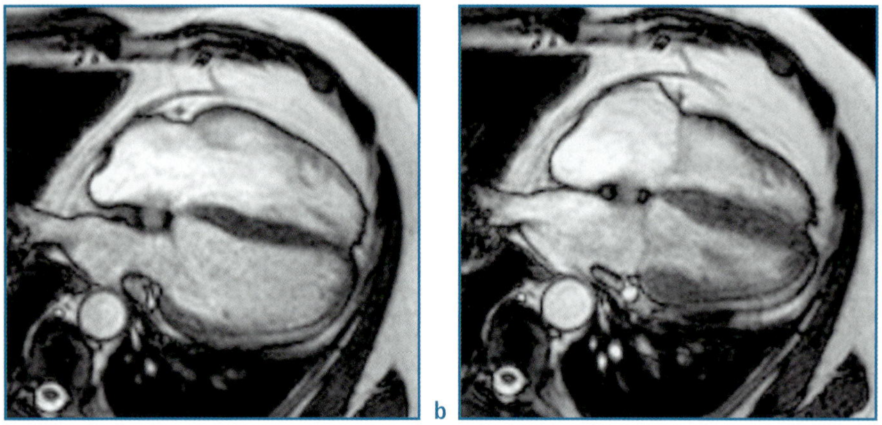

Figure 15-8 Partial congenital aplasia of the pericardium in front of the entire lateral wall of the right ventricle in diastole (a) and systole (b) using a SSFP sequence in a 4-ch view. Note cardiac long-axis deviated to a left-dorsal direction. Patient was asymptomatic.

Diagnosis and CMR Findings

Pericardial cysts may be detected by chest X-ray as a well-defined outpouching on the lateral border of the heart. On CMR they appear as a well-defined homogenous paracardiac structure with signal characteristics of water (low signal intensity on T1w- and high signal intensity in T2w-spin echo images) (Figure 15-7). Occasionally a highly proteinaceous content causes a moderate to high signal intensity on T1w-images. **Pericardial defects** are characterized by a discontinuation of the pericardial line (partial defects more commonly located on the left side, but rarely at the right side at the diaphragmatic surface), together with paucity of surrounding fat (Figure 15-8). The most reliable sign of complete absence of pericardium is interposition of lung between the aorta and main pulmonary artery in the aorto-pulmonary window, and a rotation of the cardiac axis to the left side. In addition, in contrast to the relative stationarity of normal cardiac apex during cardiac contraction and relaxation, excessive mobility of cardiac apex may be indicative of a pericardial defect. In case of herniation of the heart this can be detected at cine-CMR by positional changes such as positioning the patient in the left lateral decubitus. CMR imaging may also be helpful in the diagnosis of a **pericardial diverticulum** for visualizing the abnormal structure that may resemble a pericardial cyst. However, if a complete cardiac wall cannot be identified in all parts of the lesion, a diverticulum may be suspected. Moreover, on cine-CMR the diverticulum shows a changing size with changing body positioning.

Therapy

Pericardial cysts usually do not require any treatment. **Pericardial defects** may need surgical correction, if excessive mobility or herniation of the heart is present. The same holds true for **pericardial diverticulum**. Surgical results and follow-up of surgically treated patients can be accurately controlled by CMR imaging.

15.6 Tumors of the Pericardium

15.6.1 Mesothelioma

Prevalence and Pathology

Pericardial mesothelioma is the most common primary pericardial malignant tumor, followed by fibrosarcoma, angiosarcoma, and teratocarcinoma. Pericardial mesothelioma represents less than 1% of all malignant mesotheliomas, but accounts for 50% of all primary pericardial tumors. Pericardial mesotheliomas arise from the mesothelial cells of the pericardium. Their manifestation is in the ages from 2–78 yrs with a 2:1 male predominance. Microscopically the tumor is typically biphasic composed of epithelial areas resembling a carcinoma, and spindled areas similar to a sarcoma (Grebenc 2000).

Clinical Presentation

Clinical symptoms include chest pain, dyspnea, cough, and palpitations. Patients with diffuse pericardial involvement may have symptoms and signs mimicking pericarditis or cardiac tamponade. Patients with advanced disease often present with widespread metastases.

Diagnosis

Preliminary diagnosis is made by clinical examination, ECG, and echocardiography for detecting the tumor and its localization, and chest radiography demonstrating cardiac enlargement and/or irregular cardiac contour or diffuse mediastinal enlargement. The diagnosis can be confirmed by cardiac CT or most efficiently by CMR imaging.

CMR Findings

CMR imaging will show cardiac encasement by a soft-tissue pericardial mass with irregular and diffuse pericardial thickening, as well as an associated pericardial effusion. The amount and hemodynamic significance of pericardial fluid

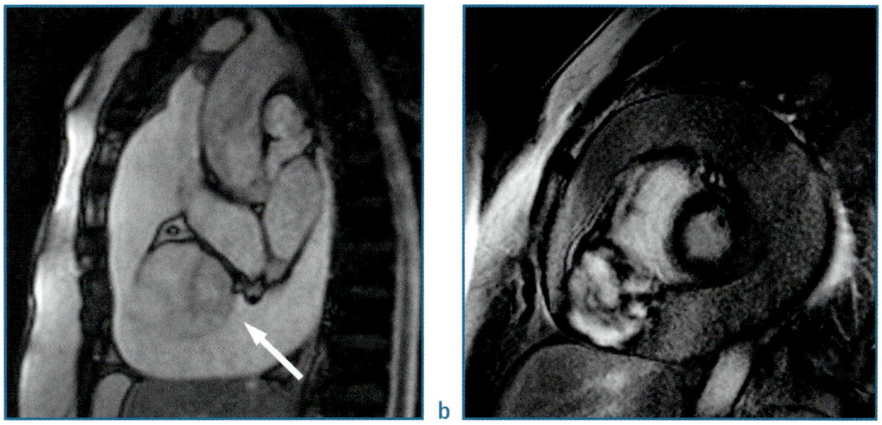

Figure 15-9 Large circular pericardial effusion secondary to a malignant tumor in the right-atrial-right-ventricular angle (arrow) (a) with irregular late contrast enhancement after gadolinium administration (b).

can be accurately assessed by CMR. On T1w-TSE-images the tumor shows low-signal intensity, whereas T2w-TSE images typically demonstrate increased signal intensity. Following gadolinium administration the lesion shows slight enhancement.

Therapy

Surgery combined with radiation therapy may be palliative. However, the prognosis of all patients even those who are treated is extremely poor with a survival rate of 6 mths to 1 yr after diagnosis and/or treatment.

15.6.2 Extracardiac (Secondary) Tumors

Prevalence and Pathology

Extracardiac tumors like bronchogenic carcinoma, breast cancer, lymphoma, leukemia, Hodgkin disease, and melanoma may either directly invade the pericardium, or may deliver metastases to the pericardium. Pericardial metastases occur late in the course of a neoplasm, usually as recurrent disease, while malignant pericardial effusion as the first sign of a neoplasm is rare. Lung cancer, the most frequent source of neoplastic pericardial disease, accounts for about one-third of cases. In addition, autopsies have shown that about one-third of patients with lung cancer also had metastatic involvement of the pericardium (Chiles 2001). Breast cancer is the second most common cause of malignant pericardial effusion (25% of patients with breast cancer have pericardial involvement at autopsy). The third largest group are patients with hematologic malignancies such as leukemia, non-Hodgkin- and Hodgkin lymphoma (altogether about 15% of cases).

Clinical Presentation

Patients with metastatic pericardial involvement most frequently present with pericardial effusion of variable amounts of fluid and/or ill-defined chest pain and fatigue.

Diagnosis

The diagnosis of effusion is made by chest X-ray and by echocardiography, the diagnosis of malignant pericardial effusion is achieved by means of pericardiocentesis, pericardioscopy, or both (Millaire 1992).

CMR Findings

In most malignant tumors invading the pericardium or those with metastatic pericardial disease pericardial effusion and thickening of the pericardium with irregular nodular linings are seen with CT or CMR imaging. Pericardial effusion can be easily detected and quantified using CMR (Figure 15-9). If CT or CMR imaging demonstrate obliteration of the superior pulmonary vein, intrapericardial extension of tumor and invasion of the left atrium should be suspected. Enhancement of the pericardium after gadolinium or pericardial nodularity suggests malignant involvement, but pericardiocentesis is required for definitive diagnosis.

Therapy

Therapy refers to the treatment of the primary malignant tumor disease, only in the rare cases of hemodynamic compromise from pleural effusion pericardiocentesis is required.

15.7 Summary and Conclusions

CMR imaging has become a particularly valuable technique in the workup of patients with all types of pericardial diseases. In particular, when pericardial tumors are suspected optimal tumor characterization may be achieved due to the different imaging sequences in combination with contrast enhancement studies, as well as due to the unrestricted field of view and superior soft tissue characterization without ionizing radiation. The different imaging sequences allow optimum evaluation of anatomy and tissue features of pericardial tissue and the adjacent myocardium, thus enabling accurate assessment of functional and hemodynamic impact of pericardial involvement. Therefore, CMR imaging should be used early in the diagnostic process of suspected or known pericardial disease, as well as for follow-up of patients after treatment, and to timely detect recurrence of the disease.

References

Bogaert J, Francone M. Cardiovascular magnetic resonance in pericardial diseases. J Cardiovasc Magn Reson 2009; 11 (1): 14.

Chiles C, Woodward PK, Gutierrez FR, Link KM. Metastatic involvement of the heart and pericardium: CT and MR imaging. RadioGraphics 2001; 21: 439–49.

Grebenc ML, Rosado de Christenson ML, Burke AP et al. Primary cardiac and pericardial neoplasms: radiologic-pathologic correlation. RadioGraphics 2000; 20: 1073–103.

Le Winter MM, Tischler MD. Pericardial diseases. In: Bonow RO, Mann DL, Zipes DP, Libby P (eds.). Braunwald's Heart Disease. A Textbook of Cardiovascular Medicine. Elsevier Saunders 2012; 1651–71.

Maisch B, Seferovic PM, Ristic AD et al. for the Task Force on the Diagnosis and Management of Pericardial Diseases of the European Society of Cardiology. Guidelines on the diagnosis and management of pericardial diseases: executive summary. Eur Heart J 2004; 25: 587–610.

Millaire A, Wurtz A, De Groote P et al. Malignant pericardial effusions: usefulness of pericardioscopy. Am Heart J 1992; 124: 1030–4.

Nishimura RA. Constrictive pericarditis in the modern era: a diagnostic dilemma. Heart 2001; 86: 619–23.

Soulen RL, Strak DD, Higgins CB. Magnetic resonance imaging of constrictive pericardial disease. Am J Cardiol 1985; 55: 480–4.

Spodick DH. Acute cardiac tamponade. N Engl J Med 2003; 349: 684–90.

Talreja DP, Nishimura RA, Oh JK, Holmes DR. Constrictive pericarditis in the modern era: novel criteria for diagnosis in the cardiac catheterization laboratory. J Am Coll Cardiol 2008; 51: 315–9.

16 Cardiac Magnetic Resonance Control of Cardiovascular Interventions

Vinzenz Hombach

16.1 Introduction

Since the introduction of atrioseptostomy by Rashkind in the 1960 years, the first interventional closure of an open Ductus of Botalli by Porstmann by an Ivalon plug in 1967, the first percutaneous balloon angioplasty of coronary stenoses by Grüntzig in 1977, and percutaneous aortic valve implantation by Cribier in 1992, a host of different interventional procedures for non-operative treatments of cardiovascular diseases have been developed and introduced into clinical routine. Simultaneously cardiovascular surgical techniques have been further developed and refined, so that in addition to reducing operative mortality, long-term surgical results have also been significantly improved. Further, the spectrum of surgical interventions in relation to age and severity of diseased patients has been significantly extended.

Systematic follow-up of interventionally and surgically treated patients includes clinical, electrocardiographical and echocardiographical techniques, and occasionally cardiac catheterisation and coronary angiography to control the success of an intervention and to diagnose early progression of disease. In principle, CMR imaging has the potential for a comprehensive non-invasive survey of patients after invasive interventional or surgical treatment, as important information on myocardial structure and function, the effect of revascularising techniques and myocardial perfusion, myocardial viability, and function of implanted devices can be assessed with high precision. In the following the theoretical advantages and practical applications of CMR imaging for control and follow-up of patients with treated cardiovascular diseases shall be described.

16.2 Medical Treatments

16.2.1 Heart Failure (HF)

CMR imaging has proven to be the gold standard for assessing cardiac structure and function in different disease cohorts. Regarding **medical treatment of heart failure** in the EARTH study (Lüscher 2001), serial CMR studies were performed to assess changes in LV end-systolic volume (LVESV) from baseline by the endothelin A receptor antagonist darusentan in 642 patients over 24 wks. The primary endpoint LVESV assessed in 485 patients at baseline and follow-up did not significantly differ from placebo with doses ranging from 10 mg (+ 1.28 ml) to 300 mg (– 4.34 ml) of darusentan (Anand 2004a). Similar adverse results from the dual receptor endothelin antagonist enrasentan were later on reported by Prasad et al. (2006) in asymptomatic individuals with LV dysfunction. Using CMR for LV volume assessment, an increased LV end-diastolic volume index (LVEDVI) for patients on enrasentan was found, in contrast to a decreased LVEDVI as well as an increased cardiac index and LV mass index on enalapril. It was concluded from this study that enrasentan at a dose of 60–90 mg/d over 6 mths causes adverse ventricular remodeling despite an increase in resting cardiac index. Bello et al. (2003) studied 45 patients with chronic HF with CMR for LV function and viability on β-blocker therapy. Scarring was found in all patients with ischemic cardiomyopathy (ICM), but in only 2 of 17 (12%) patients with non-ICM. The main finding was that in patients treated with β-blockers, late gadolinium enhancement (LGE) on CMR predicts the response in LV function and remodeling. Bellenger et al. (2004) reported in 34 patients with chronic HF on LV remodeling in a placebo-controlled trial with carvedilol. They found that in patients with chronic HF carvedilol results in significant improvement in left ventricular volumes and function, which may contribute to the benefits of carvedilol on mortality and morbidity in this patient group. In a substudy on 69 randomly selected eligible patients, taken from a group of 912 patients in the RENAISSANCE Trial, CMR was used at entry and 24 wks later to assess LV function, volume, and muscular mass index (LVMMI) (Anand 2004b). The study revealed that anemia is common in CHF patients and is associated with increasing disease severity, i.e. greater HF severity was found to be associated with lower Hb concentrations. An increase in Hb over time was associated with a decrease in LVMMI and lower mortality, whereas a decrease in Hb over time was associated with an increase in LVMMI and higher mortality. It was concluded that lower Hb is associated with greater disease severity, a greater LVMMI, and higher hospitalization and mortality rates.

16.2.2 Chelation Therapy in Thalassemia Major

T2*-weighted imaging is not only valuable to confirm the diagnosis of myocardial iron overload, e.g. in thalassemia major, but also to control medical therapy. Tanner et al. (2008) reported on the effect of subcutaneous desferoxamine monotherapy in 167 patients with thalassemia major, 22 of whom had severe myocardial siderosis (T2* < 8 ms) with impaired LV function. 15 patients received combination therapy with subcutaneous deferoxamine and oral deferiprone and had CMR follow-up. After 12 mths myocardial T2* improved (from 5.7 ± 0.98 ms to 7.9 ± 2.47 ms, $p = 0.010$), with concomitant improvement in LV ejection fraction (from 51.2 ± 10.9% to 65.6 ± 6.7%, $p < 0.001$) and no deaths or occurrence of new cardiovascular complications. T2* CMR has also been shown to be one of the main factors for decreasing death rates in thalassemia major, mainly driven by the reduction in the rate of deaths from iron overload, whereby T2* imaging identifies patients at highest risk who require intensified iron chelation treatment (Modell 2008). Similar improved survival has been reported from Italy, where T2* CMR has been available since 2002 to identify individuals at highest risk, and establish the definite link to deferiprone use (Piga 2003, Borgna-Pignatti 2006). Comparable results were reported from Cyprus (Telfer 2006). Thus, T2* CMR should be the first-line diagnostic technique to detect and quantify myocardial iron overload. Repeated T2* myocardial scans should be used to monitor clearance of myocardial iron and improved LV function, and to guide adjustments of chelation therapy.

16.3 Catheter Ablation of Cardiac Arrhythmias

16.3.1 Electro-Anatomic Mapping

CMR imaging may be used for electro-anatomic mapping, control of RF-induced lesions around the pulmonary veins, detection of left atrial (LA) scar, assessment of the LA after catheter ablation, and prediction of recurrence of atrial fibrillation (Kolandaivelu 2009). CMR has been used most extensively to assist planning and guidance of atrial fibrillation (AF) ablation procedures. To improve procedural success and reduce complications, 3D-CMR angiography has been used to assist in the planning of radiofrequency (RF) ablation. Pulmonary vein (PV) anatomic variants may be found in 38% of patients. Identification of these variants is important because AF triggering foci can be located within additional veins. To improve electro-anatomic mapping

3D reconstruction of the left atrium may be helpful (Dong 2006). In their study the segmented 3D MR/CT LA reconstruction was accurately registered to the real-time mapping space, with a combination of landmark registration and surface registration. The registered anatomic reconstructions were successfully used to guide deployment of RF applications for encircling the pulmonary veins (PV). The distance between the surface of the registered 3D MR/CT LA reconstruction and the multiple electro-anatomic map points was 3.05 ± 0.41 mm. The authors concluded that this type of 3D reconstruction provided detailed and accurate anatomic information during the procedure and enabled tailored RF ablation to individual PV and LA anatomy.

16.3.2 Assessment and Implications of Radiofrequency-Induced Scars

The DE-CMR technique has been used to detect pulmonary vein and left atrial scars after catheter ablation. In the study on 23 patients by Peters et al. (2007), post-ablation LGE was identified in all, but only 62% of patients demonstrated more than 90% circumferential delayed enhancement of PVs, using high spatial resolution MR imaging. Wylie et al. (2008) assessed LA and RA systolic function in 33 consecutive patients before and after RF ablation. After ablation LA size decreased and left atrial systolic function was reduced by 14%. This change strongly correlated with the volume of LA scar, and this finding might have implications for post-procedural thromboembolic risk and for procedures involving more extensive RF ablations. Taclas et al. (2009) compared the sites of RF application with the sites of post-procedural scar formation in the LA. The distance between each Carto point and the nearest scar was measured and the gaps inside of LGE and in Carto ablation assessed qualitatively. The main results of this study were that the custom registration method provided a mean integration error between Carto and CMR of 2.7 ± 0.7 mm with an average distance between Carto and LGE scar of 3.6 ± 1.3 mm, and that 20% of sectors with sites of Carto ablation showed no evidence of LGE. The conclusion was that there was a visual and quantitative correspondence between Carto ablation site and LGE scar, however, for 20% of Carto ablation sites there was no visible corresponding LGE scar.

McGann et al. (2008) measured the amount of LA scarring by 3D LA reconstruction and correlated this with arrhythmia recurrence at 3 mths. Patient rhythm correlated with the degree of wall enhancement, with > 13% injury predicting freedom from AF (odds ratio: 18.5, 95% confidence interval 1.7–268, $p = 0.032$). The conclusion was that detection and quantification of LA wall scaring is feasible and that there seems to be a correlation between the extent of LA wall injuries and short-term procedural outcome. Similar findings were reported by Peters et al. (2009) who found that in 35 patients with AF after RF ablation, those without recurrence had a greater amount of completely circumferentially scarred veins (55 vs. 35% of veins, p = ns), and patients without recurrence had more frequent scarring in the inferior portion of the right inferior pulmonary vein (82 vs. 31%, $p = 0.025$). Moreover the volume of scarring in the right inferior PV was quantitatively greater in patients without AF recurrence ($p \leq 0.05$). The conclusion was that AF recurrence during the first year after AF ablation was associated with a lesser degree of PV and LA scarring on 3D-LGE CMR. In this context the results of Oakes et al. (2009) are interesting, who reported on the use of DE-CMR before RFA for detection of LA remodeling in patients with AF undergoing pulmonary vein isolation (PVI) and on the correlation with AF recurrence after RF treatment. In 81 of the 118 patients, 3D-CMR-LGE imaging was successfully performed, and varying degrees of LGE in LA walls were found: patients with mild LGE (< 15%, n = 43) had a 14% AF recurrence rate during follow-up (mean 9.6 mths), compared to 43% in patients with moderate LGE (15–35%, n = 30) and 75% in those with severe LGE (> 35%, n = 8). The extent of LGE correlated well with the number of low-voltage regions identified by EPS mapping, and multivariate analysis revealed that the extent of LA wall enhancement was a stronger predictor of patient response to drug and pulmonary vein antrum isolation (PVI) therapies for AF than LA volume. If these results are confirmed by larger studies, CMR quantification of LA scarring could become clinically useful for the identification of patients with AF who would benefit from PVI as opposed to those who might be better treated by rate control and anticoagulation.

Another valuable contribution of DE-CMR imaging was that the esophagus is frequently involved in post-AF ablation damage, as shown by Meng et al. (2010). In their study the prevalence of esophageal late enhancement on DE-CMR was investigated prior to and following PVI in 74 patients. The pre- and post-PVI esophageal position was measured relative to the vertebral body. The result was that prior to PVI, 3% of patients had esophageal LGE, and 23 of 74 patients (30%) demonstrated new esophageal LGE adjacent to an ablation site. The presence of post-procedural esophageal LGE was not associated with longer ablation time, use of irrigated catheters, or the timing of the LGE-CMR study after PVI. The conclusion was that new esophageal LGE is seen in almost one third of patients after pulmonary vein isolation. The clinical implications of this finding remain to be explored.

16.3.3 Future Role of CMR Imaging in Radiofrequency Ablation

In the future CMR imaging may play a significant role not only in providing more anatomic information on the geometry of the left atrium and the pulmonary veins before RF ablation, but also and particularly important for immediate control of the RF lesions' completeness by T2-weighted imaging (Kolandaivelu 2009). Another possible application will be the use of DE-CMR imaging for planning VT ablation procedures, and using real-time CMR combined with intraprocedural lesion imaging to allow physicians to accurately guide devices and establish completeness of ablation lines without concern for radiation exposure.

16.4 Myocardial Revascularisation

16.4.1 Percutaneous Coronary Interventions (PCI)

CMR imaging has been used to improve or control myocardial revascularization procedures. In a landmark study Syed et al. (2006) were able to show that in 119 patients with acute MI and emergency bare metal stent implantation, CMR imaging on a 1.5 T scanner was safe when performed 2.7 ± 3.1 d after PCI. The imaging procedure was not associated with an increased risk of adverse clinical outcomes. Taylor et al. (2006) investigated 15 patients with stable CAD undergoing PCI and compared them to 10 control subjects. Using CMR imaging, microvascular perfusion and regional wall motion was assessed. PCI resulted in a regional contrast delay and a reduction of the relative upslope of the signal-intensity curve compared to pre-PCI values, consistent with reduced microvascular perfusion, and unaccompanied by any change in regional systolic thickening. It was concluded that these data show PCI-induced impairment of resting microvascular perfusion in the area of myocardium subtended by the treated artery after PCI, a likely consequence of iatrogenic atherosclerotic plaque rupture.

16.4.2 Functional Outcome after Revascularization

As already found in patients with suspected CAD or progression of CAD after PCI, CMR first-pass perfusion (FPP) analysis together with DE-imaging is also able to detect myocardial ischemia after coronary artery bypass grafting (CABG) with high sensitivities, specificities, and accuracies, as reported from our institution by Bernhardt et al. (2009) and by Klein et al. (2009). Thus, CMR-based diagnosis of myocardial ischemia is a reliable technique used to detect progression of coronary artery disease after successful myocardial revascularisation using the CMR FPP technique.

The functional outcome after myocardial revascularization using CMR imaging and LGE technique was studied in 45 patients with chronic ischemic LV dysfunction by Bondarenko et al. (2007), who tested the predictive accuracy of the extent of LGE (transmural), the amount of residual non-enhanced viable myocardium, and procedure related necrosis. 60 % of segments without LGE showed functional improvement, but no improvement was seen in segments with > 75 % segmental extent of LGE. Procedure related necrosis was found in 27 % of patients, and its presence was the only negative predictor of changes in LV volumes and ejection fraction. The conclusion was that functional outcome after revascularization was influenced by both transmural extent of LGE and procedure related necrosis, but no additional value was found with the presence of a residual, viable myocardial rim. Similar results were reported by Krittayaphong et al. (2008) in 50 patients scheduled for CABG. Abnormal wall motion and the LGE area were detected in 1,226 segments (71.6 %) and in 1,196 segments (59.2 %), respectively. Wall motion improvement was demonstrated in 481 of 1,227 segments (39.2 %) with initial wall motion abnormalities at baseline. Statistical analysis proved LGE and end-diastolic wall thickness (EDWT) to be independent predictors for functional recovery after revascularisation, but LGE appeared to be a more important factor and independent from EDWT.

In another study by Cheng et al. (2008) the effect of recanalisation by PCI of chronic total occlusions (CTO) on regional hyperemic myocardial blood flow (MBF) and contractility was investigated. 17 patients scheduled for PCI of CTO, 17 scheduled for PCI of a stenosed but not occluded coronary artery (non-CTO), and 6 control patients with CTO not scheduled for revascularization were recruited. In both interventional groups hyperemic MBF increased 24 h after PCI compared to baseline: CTO group, 2.1 ± 0.2 ml/min/g vs. 1.4 ± 0.2 ml/min/g ($p < 0.01$); non-CTO group, 2.5 ± 0.2 ml/min/g vs. 1.6 ± 0.2 ml/min/g ($p < 0.01$). This improvement persisted 6 mths after PCI for both groups. Contractility in treated segments was improved at 24 h and 6 mths after PCI of CTO, but only 6 mths after non-CTO PCI. It was concluded that PCI of CTO increases hyperemic MBF as early as 24 h after the procedure, with a greater and earlier improvement in regional contractility, than after non-CTO PCI, despite a greater likelihood of irreversible injury in CTO segments.

Rahimi et al. (2009) investigated the prognostic impact of procedural myocardial injury during PCI or CABG in 152 consecutive patients, in whom myocardial necrosis was quantified by DE-CMR imaging shortly before and after PCI or CABG. The primary endpoint was defined as death, non-fatal myocardial infarction, sustained ventricular arrhythmia, unstable angina or heart failure. During a median follow-up of 2.9 yrs, 27 patients (18 %) reached the primary endpoint, and 49 patients (32 %) had evidence of new procedure-related myocardial LGE with a median mass of 5.0 g. After adjustment for age and sex, these patients had a 3.1-fold (95 % confidence interval 1.4–6.8, $p = 0.004$) higher risk of adverse outcome than patients without new LGE. It was concluded that myocardial injury during PCI or CABG identified by LGE adversely affects clinical outcome. This suggests the benefits from revascularisation could partially be offset by new myocardial injury caused by the intervention itself.

16.5 Catheter-Based Closure of Atrial Septal Defects and of Patent Foramen Ovale

There are only few reports regarding the role of CMR imaging for assessing post-procedural success (Figure 16-1) and changes of atrial and ventricular volumes. Nusser et al. (2006) performed contrast-enhanced CMR and transesophageal echocardiography (TEE) in 75 patients before and 12 mths after catheter-based PFO occlusion to assess completeness of closure. High-resolution cine-CMR was used to detect atrial septal aneurysms (ASA). Before PFO closure, ASA was seen in 28 of 75 patients (37 %) using CMR, compared to 47 of 75 cases (63 %) using TEE. A total of 211 CMR studies with corresponding TEE were performed in 75 pa-

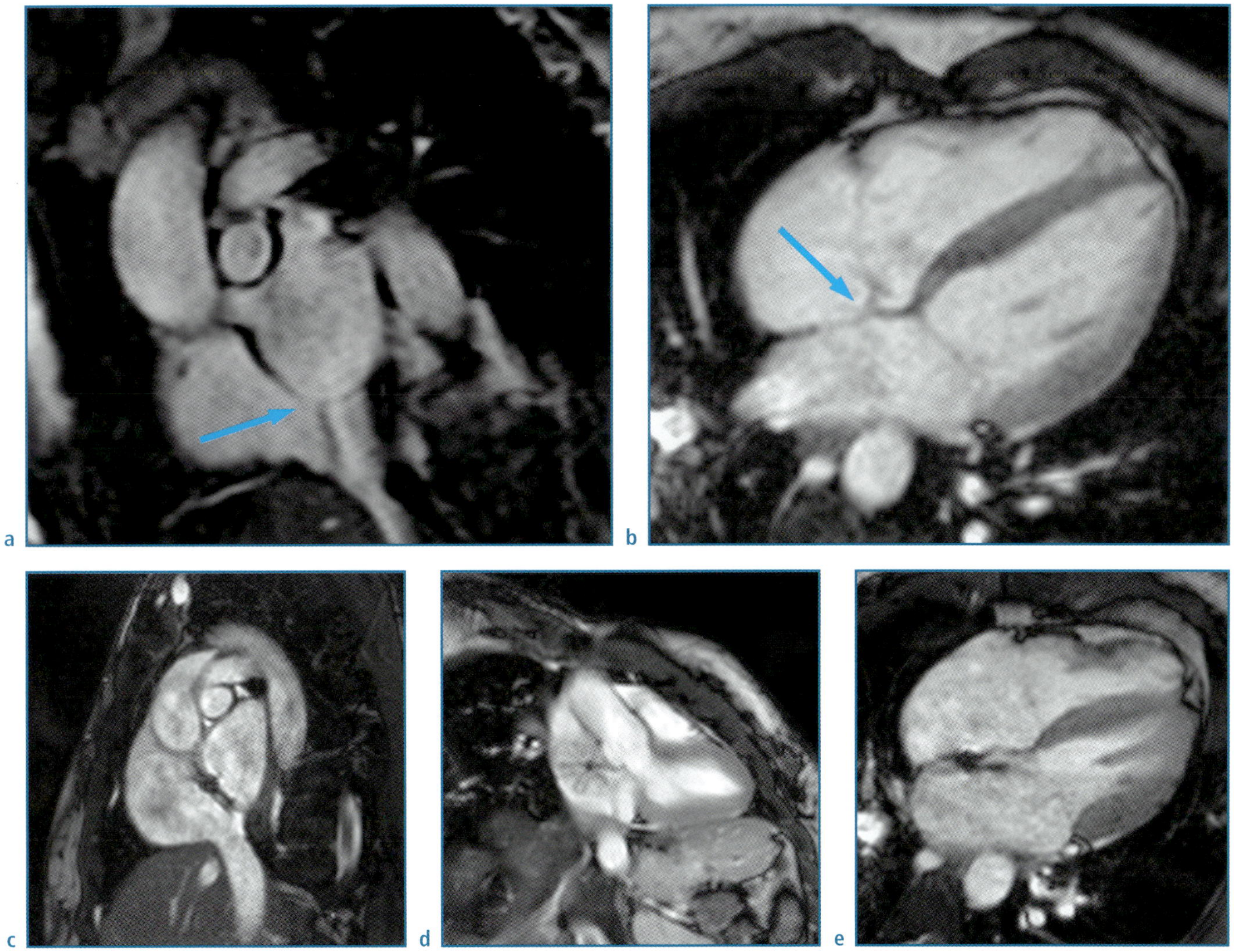

Figure 16-1 Patent foramen ovale (PFO) in a female patient with left-to-right shunting and cryptogenic stroke **(a and b)**: Small jet from the left to the right atrium in cine-SSFP images in short-axis (arrow in **(a)**) and 4-ch view (arrow in **(b)**). Control after interventional closure using an occluder-device "CardiaStarASD®" **(c–e)**: Occluder in situ without residual shunt in short-axis **(c)**, long-axis along the atrial septum **(d)**, and 4-ch view **(e)**.

tients. No shunt was present in 107 of the 211 studies with both techniques. Contrast-enhanced right-to-left shunting on Valsalva maneuver was detected by CMR in 48 of 72 (67%) cases with moderate or severe shunts seen with TEE as the reference technique, but in only 6 of 32 (19%) studies with mild shunts. Anomalous venous returns were excluded in all patients, and coronary anomalies were seen in 2 patients with CMR but not with TEE. The conclusion was that at present the CMR technique is inferior to TEE in detecting contrast-enhanced right-to-left shunting and identifying ASA, but provides reliable information on the anatomic location of the occluding device.

Burgstahler et al. (2007) performed CMR planimetry of left and right atria (LA and RA) and volumetry of ventricles (RV and LV) in 14 patients before and 24 h after catheter-based ASD closure. They were able to show that RA decreased significantly from 27.6 ± 6.4 cm^2 before to 24.4 ± 5.6 cm^2 after closure ($p = 0.0018$), whereas LA area did not change. RV volumes, volume index, and ejection fraction decreased significantly from 229 ± 64 ml to 181 ± 43 ml ($p < 0.001$, average reduction = 19 ± 15%), from 126.0 ± 25 ml/m^2 to 96.6 ± 28.6 ml/m^2 ($p < 0.0001$), and from 64 ± 5% to 58 ± 7% ($p = 0.01$), respectively. LV volumes and volume indexes remained unchanged. Left-to-right shunting decreased from 40 ± 15% to 9 ± 15% ($p < 0.001$). The conclusion was that CMR is able to detect acute changes in RA and RV parameters within 24 h after transcatheter implantation of an ASD closure device with significant reductions in RA size and RV volumes and EF, whereas LA and LV parameters remain unchanged.

Similar results were reported by Teo et al. (2008) before and 6 mths after percutaneous ASD closure in 23 patients. During follow-up RA volumes significantly decreased together with a significant decrease in right ventricular volumes. However, in contrast to the results of Burgstahler et al. (2007), left ventricular volumes significantly increased without a significant difference in LV ejection fraction or LV mass post-ASD closure. The conclusion was that ASD closure leads to normalisation of ventricular volumes and also to a reduction in right atrial volume. Further follow-up is required to assess how this predicts outcomes e.g. the risk of atrial arrhythmias after such procedures.

16.6 Interventional and Surgical Septal Ablation in HOCM

CMR imaging is a reliable tool to control the effect of alcohol septal ablation (TASH) on both septal remodeling (scar) and improvement of LV function (Figure 16-2). One of the first studies to assess the effect of TASH using CMR imaging was published by Schulz-Menger et al. (2000), who measured the circumference of the left ventricular outflow tract (LVOT) before and after TASH in 10 patients with HOCM. During 12 mths of follow-up a continuous but not linear improvement of LVOT was found over time (increase of LVOT area from 1.3 ± 0.1 cm^2 to 3.5 ± 0.6 cm^2). The increase in LVOT area correlated well with the decrease in septal wall thickness ($r = 0.93$; $p < 0.018$; $r^2 = 0.86$) and with the amelioration of symptoms ($r^2 = 0.86$). Van Dockum et al. (2005) found that at 1 and 6 mths not only septal muscle mass decreased significantly after TASH compared with baseline, but also remote non-septal muscle mass in 29 patients with HOCM. Remote mass reduction was associated with transmural or left-sided septal infarct location at 6 mths ($p < 0.01$), and percentage remote mass reduction correlated significantly ($p = 0.03$) with LVOT gradient reduction at 6 mths follow-up. This finding was explained to be in part the result of afterload reduction following TASH with concomitant reduction in remote muscle mass. In another paper van Dockum et al. (2006) were able to show using CMR tissue tagging in 9 patients that in addition to a reduction in remote muscle mass after TASH, improvement of intramural systolic function in the lateral (remote) wall occurred at 6 mths follow-up, indicating reversed LV remodeling. The same group (van Dockum 2009) measured LAD coronary blood flow (CBF) in 7 patients with HOCM by MR phase contrast velocity mapping (background CMR flow mapping). Changes in MBF compared to baseline were correlated to LV mass reduction, enzyme release, volume of ethanol administered, LVOT gradient reduction, and LV rate pressure product (LVRPP) at 1 and 6 mths after TASH. A significant correlation was only found between the change in LVRPP and LAD blood flow. It was concluded that the reduction of blood flow in the LAD is primarily associated with diminished LV loading conditions, whereas the induction of metabolically inactive myocardial scar tissue by TASH did not significantly influence the changes in coronary blood flow.

One paper by Valeti et al. (2007) reported on the effects of surgical septal myectomy in 24 patients and TASH (24 patients), using cine- and contrast-enhanced CMR images, to compare location of septal reduction, extent of myocardial necrosis, and conduction system abnormalities with each technique. With septal myectomy, there was a discrete area of resected tissue consistently localized to the anterior septum, while TASH resulted in a more variable effect. TASH caused a transmural region of tissue necrosis, located more inferiorly in the basal septum than myectomy, and usually extending into the right ventricular side of the septum at the midventricular level. There were 6 patients after TASH in whom there was no injury to the basal septum with residual gradients at follow-up. After the procedure, left bundle branch block developed in 46% of septal myectomy

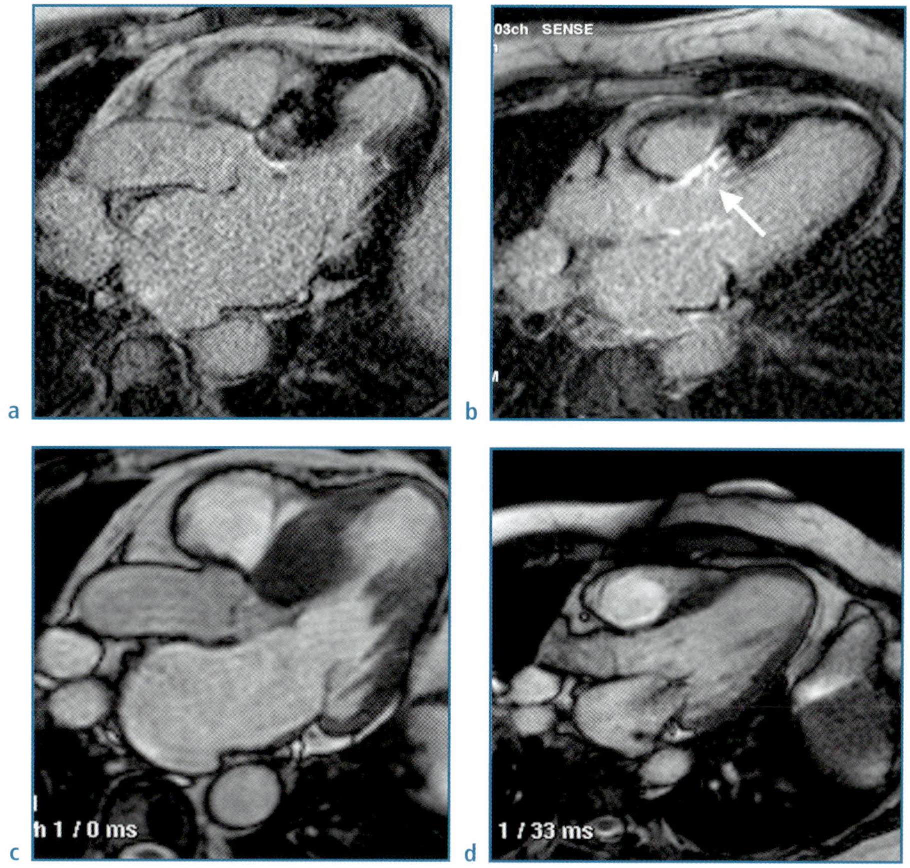

Figure 16-2 Effect of alcohol septal ablation (TASH) in a young patient with severe hypertrophic obstructive cardiomyopathy using scar imaging in the 4-ch view: Small scar in the center of hypertrophied basal septum (before TASH) (a), and large scar with abolished basal septal muscle substituted by scar (after TASH) (b). Effect of TASH on functional parameters in cine-CMR imaging in a 3-ch view: Before TASH severe left ventricular outflow tract (LVOT) obstruction with systolic anterior movement (SAM) of the anterior mitral leaflet and flow void in the LVOT and ascending aorta (c), while LVOT obstruction, SAM and flow void are no longer observed after TASH (d).

patients, and right bundle branch block was evident in 58 % of TASH treatments. It was concluded that these different effects of septal myectomy vs. alcohol septal ablation may have important implications for patient selection and management as well as long-term outcome of patients with HOCM.

16.7 Transcutaneous Aortic Valve Implantation (TAVI)

In principle, CMR imaging may be used to select patients for TAVI and to control procedural success (Figure 16-3). However, there are no systematic studies on the significance of CMR imaging in patients with high-grade aortic stenosis undergoing TAVI, though important informations may be gained both before and after the transcutaneous procedure. LV and RV function/dysfunction, presence of myocardial scars, anatomy of the LVOT, the aortic root and ascending aorta as well as the abnormal structure of the stenotic valve and aortic valve area can reliably be imaged in 3D with multiple planes. There is one paper (Koos 2011) that compared CMR with dual-source CT (DSCT) for analysis of aortic root dimensions and showed a good correlation of CMR measurements with DSCT. Aortic annulus measurements using TEE, CMR and DSCT were close but not identical and, as concluded by the authors, the method used has important implications on TAVI strategy.

Patients may be monitored after the procedure by CMR for function of the implanted prosthesis, degree of concomitant aortic regurgitation, possible LV functional remodeling, and early detection of complications or malfunctions of the prosthesis. Sherif et al. (2011) compared quantitative assessment of post-TAVI aortic regurgitation (AR) by CMR with qualitative angiography in 16 patients and found a better correlation of CMR with angiography than of echocardiography. It was concluded that echocardiography may underestimate the degree of AR and CMR has great potential in reliably measuring the severity of AR in a quantitative manner. Historically, multi-detector CT is used routinely to provide all necessary informations on structure and dimensions of aortic valve, aortic root and ascending aorta pre-implantation, as well as for post-procedural control of the prosthesis and vessel anatomy. However, CMR may be used alternatively to assess these parameters both pre- and post-operatively, yet in addition functional parameters, e.g. the degree of AR post-TAVI or longterm-LV function and

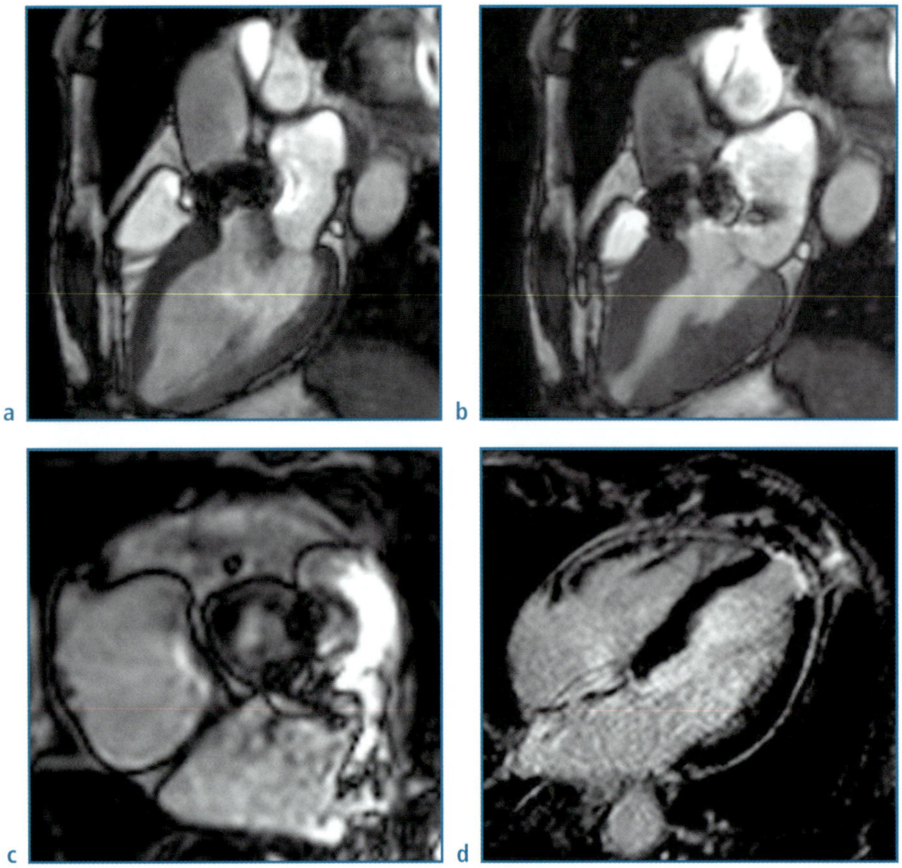

Figure 16-3 Percutaneous implantation of an aortic valve (TAVI) in a patient with severe calcified aortic stenosis on cine-SSFP imaging showing prosthesis in situ at diastole (a) and systole (b) in 2-ch view; normal opening function of the prosthesis leaflets on axial plane (c), and small subendocardial infarct at the LV apex on scar imaging in 4-ch view (d), probably due to a small coronary embolus at TAVI.

muscle mass can be precisely measured and frequently followed by CMR without exposing patients to radiation.

Recently first attempts have been made at real-time MR-guided TAVI using deployment of the valve devices in a phantom model (Kahlert 2010). The two commercially available delivery devices and the stainless steel-based Edwards SAPIEN™ prosthesis proved to be not suitable for the implantation procedure because of severe susceptibility artefacts exceeding the valve's dimensions and hindering an exact placement. In contrast, the Medtronic CoreValve® was excellently visualized with delineation of even small details and thus, was regarded as suitable for implantation under CMR control. Reliable flow measurements could be performed for both stent-valves after deployment using phase-contrast sequences. Whether this fascinating new technique may be used in patients remains to be investigated in detail in the future.

16.8 Interventional Treatment or Operative Repair of Aortic Dissection or Aneurysm

16.8.1 Stenting

CMR imaging may be principally used to follow patients after surgical repair of type A aortic dissection or aortic aneurysm (Figure 16-4), as well as for interventional stent placement for aortic type B dissection (Figure 16-5). There are only few systematic studies on the usefulness of CMR imaging in patients with such aortic diseases. Mosquera et al. (2009) used either 64-slice CT or CMR imaging to follow 20 surgical high risk patients (8 type B dissections, 5 atherosclerotic aneurysms, 4 penetrating ulcers, 3 traumatic aortic ruptures) undergoing thoracic endovascular aortic repair (TEVAR) for assessing mean (reduced) diameter of the descending aorta and reduction of diameter of the previous aneurysm. Attia et al. (2008) analyzed 75 patients undergoing endovascular stent grafting (EVAR) of lesions involving the descendent thoracic aorta (31 aneurysms, 8 chronic and 6 complicated type B dissections, 4 penetrating ulcers, and 26 aortic ruptures). CMR imaging was

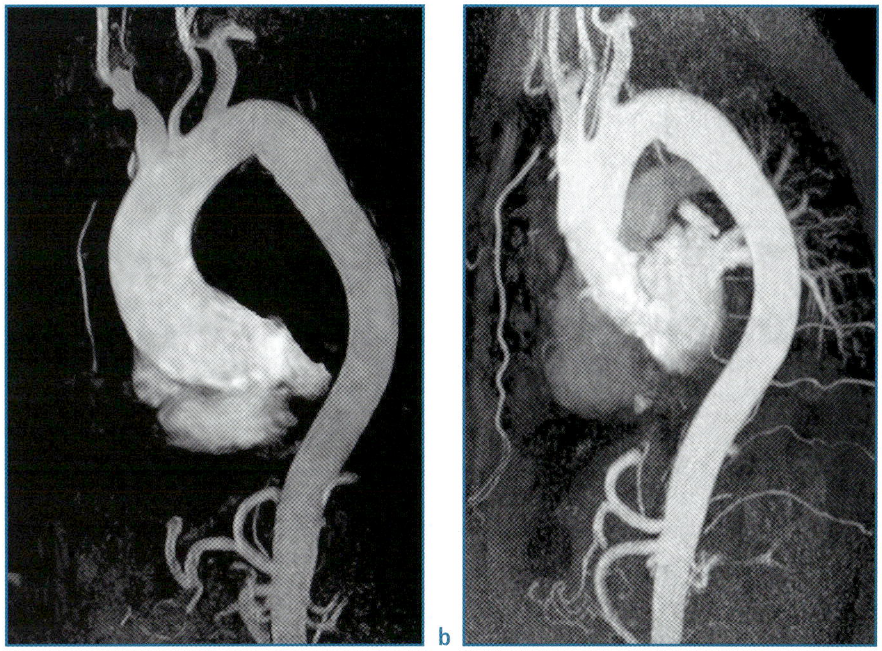

Figure 16-4 Aneurysm of the ascending aorta on contrast-enhanced MRA before (a), and after prosthetic operative repair (b). Note the significant reduction of aortic diameter and the insertion site of the prosthesis in the native aortic wall, as well as the appropriate closure of the artificial aortic valve incorporated in the prosthesis. a b

generally used to detect secondary endoleaks and changes in aneurysmal dimension. Total mortality was 14 patients (18.6%) after a follow-up of 31.5 mths (3–60 mths). Late endoleaks occurred in 12 (16%) patients, in 9 with aneurysms, and in 3 with type B dissection: de novo type I endoleak due to enlargement of the distal neck in 3 patients, proximal endoleaks in 6, endoleaks type II (reperfusion of the aneurysmal sac from an intercostal artery) in one, and type III endoleaks due to stent-graft migration distally in 2 patients. Aneurysm dimensions showed a significant regression of > 5 mm in 23 of 54 patients, significant progression of > 5 mm in 3 patients, and stability of the aneurysmal sac in 28 patients. These limited reports suggest that CMR imaging may be a reliable technique to assess complications after stenting and to reveal changes in the morphology and dimensions of aortic diseases treated with endovascular stenting. In clinical routine, however, angiography and particularly multi-detector CT are the most frequently used methods for providing all necessary information on structure and dysfunction of the diseased aortic wall, both before and after interventional treatment.

Regarding post-stenting control of abdominal aortic aneurysms (AAA) four studies are available. Engellau et al. (1998) using MR angiography (MRA) and CT aimed at assessing changes in the stent graft itself for AAA, of aneurysmal neck, endoleaks or thrombi, and found MRA superior to CT in detecting thrombi within the aneurysm and infarction of a vertebral body. Haulon et al. (2001) looked for endoleaks type II in 64 patients after stent-graft implantation using abdominal X-ray, CT, and MRA and found MRA superior to X-ray and CT in detecting such endoleaks. Similar superiority of MRA over CT in detecting endoleaks after EVAR was reported by van der Laan et al. (2006) in 28 aneurysm patients treated with 2 different stent-grafts.

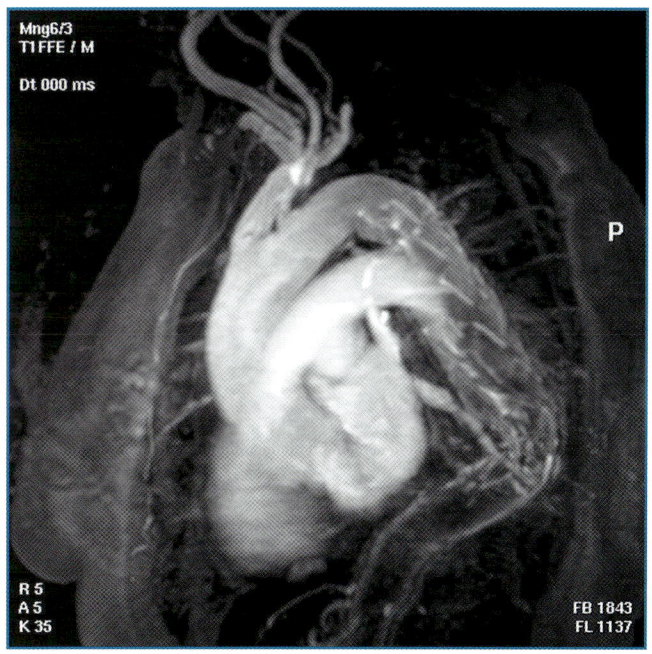

Figure 16-5 Stentgraft in the descending thoracic aorta in a patient with type B aortic dissection using contrast-enhanced MRA. Note the exact fit of the stent with the aortic wall without a residual dissection membrane (courtesy Dr. J. Schwab, Nuremberg).

Dynamic MRA imaging may also offer biomechanical information, as shown by van Herwaarden et al. (2006), who measured aortic stiffness (β) and elastic modulus (Ep) in the region of an AAA before and after stent-graft treatment (EVAR) in 11 consecutive male patients. Pre-operatively, Ep and β were significantly higher ($p < 0.05$) at the level of the aneurysmal sac compared to all other levels (3 cm above renal arteries, between, and 1 cm below renal arteries, and at the level of maximum aneurysm sac diameter). Following EVAR, stiffness increased at this level ($p < 0.05$). After implantation, patients with an Excluder endograft demonstrated Ep and β at the aneurysm neck to be 94 and 60% higher, respectively, compared to those with a Talent endograft ($p < 0.05$). The presence of an endoleak had no effect on Ep or β. The conclusion was that patients with AAA demonstrate an increased aortic elastic modulus and stiffness at the level of the aneurysmal sac, and stent-graft design seems to alter Ep and β within the aneurysmal neck, which may have consequences for endograft durability.

16.8.2 Operative Repair

There are some reports related to CMR imaging in the evaluation of patients before and after surgical repair of aortic aneurysms. Lepore et al. (1996) investigated 27 patients, 9 with aortic dissection, and 18 with aortic aneurysm, 0–167 d after surgical reconstruction of the aortic root. In all patients LVOT, mechanical function of the implanted valve prosthesis, the proximal coronary arteries after being anastomosed to the graft, and the remaining aorta could be successfully imaged. In none of the patients' aortic regurgitation, ectasia of the proximal coronary arteries or pseudoaneurysms were found. Similar results were reported by Moore et al. (1996) studying 28 patients after surgical repair of type A dissection with excellent imaging of the postoperative anatomy, in whom a distal perfused false lumen was detected for 22 of 28 patients (78%). Todd et al. (1998) investigated 115 patients with surgical repair, 6 patients with interventional stent graft repair, and another 10 patients with combined interventional-surgical repair of aortic aneurysms. At post-operative CMR control the authors concluded that smaller proximal parts of the aneurysms remained patent and were not detectable by MR or CT imaging. Before patient discharge angiography should be chosen to document a complete thrombotic occlusion of the proximal part of an aneurysm. In a series of 114 patients, 45 with type A dissection (group 1), and 69 patients with other types of aneurysms of the ascending aorta (group 2), Mesana et al. (2000) used CMR imaging for post-operative control of periprosthetic hematoma (in 26 patients of group 1, and in 52 patients of group 2), false aneurysms as an indication for reoperation (in 15 in group 1, and in 8 in group 2), and persistent dissection in all 45 patients in group 1. The conclusion was that periprosthetic hematomas may occur in both types of surgically repaired aneurysms, and may be a pre-existing cause of false periprosthetic aneurysms; the authors suggested performing a CMR examination every year post-operatively in these patient groups.

Two studies compared transthoracic and transesophageal echocardiography (TTE, TEE) and CMR imaging techniques for post-operative control of patients. Cesare et al. (2000) used TEE and CMR in 29 patients with surgical repair of type A dissection to measure the diameter of the aortic root and of the distal anastomosis of the prosthesis, and periprosthetic thickness of the aortic wall. Concordance of the findings with both techniques compared to angiography as the reference was high (correlation coefficients of 0.93–0.84), and the inter-observer variability low. 3D-CE CMR was inferior to TEE in the assessment of periprosthetic wall thickness, but superior for the examination of the abdominal aorta and arterial side branches. The conclusion was that 3D-CE-CMR is a rapid and reliable technique in the postoperative evaluation of endoluminal alterations and side branches of the aorta with imaging results that are superior to transesophageal echocardiography. Dohmen et al. (2001) investigated 80 of 108 patients surviving type A dissection after surgical repair, and 62 of these patients had at least one of the four standard imaging procedures (all 62 with TTE, 53 with TEE, 51 with CT, 39 with CMR). The overall result was that CMR imaging and CT were superior to TEE in the evaluation of the aortic arch, whereas in the evaluation of flow profiles (including aortic insufficiency) and detection of residual re-entry sites TEE was superior to CMR and CT. With current high-resolution CMR techniques including CE-CMR and phase contrast mapping, it will be easy to obtain reliable functional data on aortic valve incompetence and flow within a residual false lumen and also to detect residual re-entry sites.

Bastounis et al. (1996) examined 104 patients with surgical prosthetic repair of abdominal aortic aneurysm, using color-coded Doppler and CMR imaging as well as CE-CT and digital subtraction angiography to detect the development of an aneurysm at the anastomosis site. Sensitivity was 100% for all four techniques, but specificity was 70% for Doppler, 60% for CE-CT, 85% for CE-CMR, and 100% for angiography. Combined Doppler echocardiography and CMR provided a 100% specific exclusion of an aneurysm at the anastomosis site. The conclusion was that regarding costs, safety, and availability of each imaging technique, color-coded Doppler is the method of choice for identifying aneurysms at the anastomosis site after surgical repair of an abdominal aortic aneurysm.

16.9 Myocardial Stem Cell Therapy

16.9.1 Animal Studies

CMR imaging is an emerging technique for controlling the fate of labelled stem cells and to assess their effect on the target organs. Several studies in experimental models have investigated the possibility for labelling and tracking stem cells in vitro and in vivo. Adler et al. (2009) proposed a CMR contrast-based on the paramagnetic agent gadolinium, to track the engraftment of embryonic stem cell-derived cardiovascular progenitor cells. Cardiovascular progenitor cells (ES-CPC) were labelled with GdFM-Cy3 by incubation, and a total of 50,000 GdFM-Cy3 labelled ES-CPCs or control ES-CPCs were injected into the myocardium of mice with and without myocardial infarction. In vitro studies demonstrated that GdFM-Cy3 was easily transfectable, non-toxic, stayed within cells after labelling, and could be visualized using CMR and fluorescence microscopy. In vivo studies confirmed the efficacy of the agent for the detection of cells transplanted into the hearts of mice after myocardial infarction. A correspondence between CMR and histology was observed. The conclusion of this study was that it is possible to identify and potentially track GdFM-Cy3 labelled ES-CPCs in mural infarct models via CMR. Wisenberg et al. (2009) established a model for in vivo tracking to monitor cell engraftment after autologous transplantation of bone marrow monocytes and stromal cells and measured concurrently infarct evolution and remodeling. In the study 22 dogs, 8 sham controls, 7 treated with autologous bone marrow monocytes, and 7 with stromal cells, were evaluated by both imaging of ^{111}Indium-tropolone labelled cells and late-gadolinium enhancement CMR for up to 12 wks after a 3 h coronary occlusion. Hearts were also examined using immunohistochemisty for capillary density and presence of PKH26 labelled cells. In vivo Indium imaging demonstrated an effective biological clearance half-life from the injection site of ~ 5 d, CMR demonstrated a pattern of progressive infarct shrinkage over 12 wks by 67–88 % of baseline values with monocytes producing a significant treatment effect. Relative infarct shrinkage was similar at 6 wks in all groups, when treatment effect became manifest. There was a trend towards an increase in capillary density with cell treatment. Foltz et al. (2006) correlated positive-contrast signal characteristics in the rabbit hind-limb with xenograft cell number of rat fibroblasts, bearing endocytosed 1 μm Bang's particles at different stages of Gd-DTPA administration, using 1 mm^2 in-plane resolution (2 min scans, 1.5 T). Linear regressions modelled satisfactorily the cell number dependencies of signal-to-noise (SNR) and area-of-enhancement ($r > 0.83$), over approximately a 50-fold fluctuation in cell number to a lowest detected limit of 25 k cells during Gd-DTPA administration. Gd-DTPA administration elevated the slopes of parameter regressions by four or more standard deviations. The conclusion of this paper was that linearities of parameter regression support continued evaluation of the feasibility of cell number quantification and cell fate characterisation in vivo by CE-CMR.

16.9.2 Human Studies

CMR imaging has also been used to assess changes in structure and function of the left ventricle following intracoronary administration of bone marrow stem cells. Meyer et al. (2006) reported that CMR performed 3.5 ± 1.5 d, 6 ± 1 mth and 18 ± 16 mths after PCI and intracoronary bone marrow cell transfer revealed an increase of global LV ejection fraction (LVEF) by 0.7 and 3.1 percentage points after 6 and 18 mths, respectively, compared to an increase of LVEF in the BMC transfer group by 6.7 and 5.9 percentage points (difference significant between the groups after 6 mths but not after 18 mths). The speed of LVEF recovery over the course of 18 mths was significantly higher in the BMC transfer group. In a second study of the same BOOST trial LVEF was again studied by CMR at 61 mths. LVEF decreased by 3.3 ± 9.5 % in the control group and by 2.5 ± 11.9 % in the BMC group ($p = 0.30$). Patients with infarct transmurality more than median appeared to benefit from BMC transfer throughout the 61 mths study period ($p = 0.040$). The conclusion was that a single intracoronary application of BMCs does not promote a sustained improvement of LVEF in patients with STEMI and with relatively preserved systolic function (Meyer 2009).

Dill et al. (2009) reported the results of serial CMR imaging for global LV-EF and end-diastolic (EDV) and end-systolic volumes (ESV) at baseline and after a follow-up of 12 mths in the REPAIR-AMI study. A total of 204 patients with STEMI and primary PCI were enrolled and randomly assigned to either BMC therapy or placebo after bone marrow aspiration. In the CMR substudy 54 patients completed serial CMR at baseline, 4 and 12 mths after enrolment (27 BMC, 27 placebo). At baseline there were no significant differences between the two groups with respect to LVEF, EDV and ESV. At 12 mths the treatment effect of BMC infusion on EF amounted to 2.8 absolute percentage points, the progression of EDV at 12 mths was less in the BMC group and unlike placebo, ESV did not increase. BMC administration was associated with a significantly improved EF, reduced EDV increase, and abrogation of ESV increase. Infarct size between the two groups was not assessed in this study.

In our own study on 42 patients with STEMI and acute PCI and reperfusion > 6 h after symptom onset the effect of bone marrow cell (BMC) therapy was assessed in a rigorous double-blind, randomized, placebo-controlled trial (Wöhrle

2010). The primary endpoint of LVEF and the secondary endpoint of changes in LVEDV index (EDVI) and ESV index (ESVI) and infarct size (IS) were quantitatively measured from serial CMR imaging. The baseline clinical and CMR parameters did not differ. Compared to baseline the difference in LVEF for the placebo group vs. BMC group was 1.7 ± 6.4% vs. – 0.9 ± 5.5% at 1 mth, 3.1 ± 6.0% vs. 1.9 ± 4.3% at 3 mths, and 5.7 ± 8.4% vs. 1.8 ± 5.3% at 6 mths (all not significant). No significant differences were found in the secondary endpoint, including IS and EDVI and ESVI. The conclusion was that using CMR imaging as the gold standard for reliable measurements of LV volumes and infarct size, no evidence of a positive effect of intracoronary BMC vs. placebo was observed.

16.10 Interventional and Surgical Treatment for Congenital Heart Disease

16.10.1 Tetralogy of Fallot (TOF)

CMR imaging has rarely been used for post-operative control in two main areas, the follow-up of patients with tetralogy of Fallot (TOF), and interventional treatment or surgical repair of aortic coarctation. Ho et al. (2007) used CMR imaging in 8 of 21 surgically corrected TOF patients with a mean age of 32.2 ± 12.4 yrs after a mean post-operative follow-up of 23.5 ± 12.1 yrs. These 8 patients showed dilated RVED volumes (RVEDVI 165.7 ± 34.8 ml/m^2), and a slightly reduced but preserved RV systolic function (EF 49.5 ± 5.7%). In the total cohort, 3 patients required pulmonary valve homograft replacement for severe pulmonary regurgitation, a common complication late in the course of surgically corrected TOF. Valsangiacomomo-Buechel et al. (2005) studied 20 of 28 patients with surgically corrected TOF and severe pulmonary regurgitation (PR) 5.6 ± 1.8 mths before and 5.9 ± 0.6 mth after pulmonary valve replacement (PVR) using CMR for assessing RV remodeling. Post-operative CMR demonstrated a significant reduction of RVEDVI from 189.8 ± 33.4 to 108.7 ± 25.8 ml/m^2 ($p < 0.001$), of RVESVI from 102.4 ± 27.3 to 58.2 ± 16.3 ml/m^2 ($p < 0.0001$), and of RV mass from 48.7 ± 12.3 to 35.8 ± 7.7 g/m^2 ($p < 0.0001$), whereas RV ejection fraction did not change significantly. It was concluded that prompt RV remodeling may be expected after performing PVR if RVEDV exceeds 159 ml/m^2, and early PVR prevents the detrimental complications of severe pulmonary regurgitation. Van Straten et al. (2004) reported similar results in 25 consecutive patients with surgically corrected TOF undergoing PVR, using CMR for assessing RV volumes and function before, at 7-mths, and at 19-mths follow-up. RVEDVI decreased from 166.9 ± 41.3 ml/m^2 before PVR to 113.5 ± 35.7 ml/m^2 ($p < 0.001$) at 7-mths and to 111.7 ± 41.1 ml/m^2 (n.s.) at 19-mths follow-up. RV ejection fraction corrected for pulmonary regurgitation (PR) improved from 25.0 ± 7.7% before surgery to 44.1 ± 11.9% ($p < 0.001$) at 7-mths and to 45.2 ± 11.1 (n.s.) at 19-mths follow-up. Of the 25 patients 11 had recurrent pulmonary regurgitation (PR) after PVR, while the other 14 did not. Improvement of RV ejection fraction was more marked in patients without PR. In a literature review of 19 studies on 1,070 patients Adamson et al. (2009) summarized that PVR after TOF repair has been shown to improve RV function and to offer symptomatic benefit, with reductions in RVEDV and RVESV and improvement in RV stroke volume in some retrospective reviews. Pulmonary valve replacement appears to result in improved clinical outcome and can be performed with low mortality.

16.10.2 Pulmonary Homograft Failure

Percutaneous pulmonary valve implantation (PPVI) has been recently introduced as a new treatment option for pulmonary homograft dysfunction in patients with congenital heart disease. Using CMR Romeih et al. (2009) found an early improvement of RV systolic function with a delayed improvement of diastolic RV function in 14 patients with PPVI. In a prospective study on 60 patients with homograft implantation (45 TOF, 15 with other congenital abnormalities) Nordmeyer et al. (2009a) described hemodynamic parameters of homograft failure at one year post-operative follow-up. A higher incidence of "eccentric" pulmonary forward flow pattern ($p < 0.001$), more acute "homograft distortion angle" ($p < 0.001$), larger relative "annular" size ($p < 0.01$), and a greater pre-homograft RVOT diameter ($p = 0.01$) with CMR was seen in patients with reduced homograft function. In a backward multivariate linear regression model "eccentric" pulmonary forward flow pattern and "homograft distortion angle" were independently associated with the degree of PR at 1 yr. It was concluded that these findings imply that mechanical factors may have an important impact on homograft performance.

16.10.3 Coarctation of the Aorta (CoA)

Plain balloon angioplasty or stenting is a valuable alternative to surgery (Figure 16-6) for treating patients with coarctation of the aorta (CoA). A recent report by Golden and Hellenbrand (2007) summarized the results of a multicenter (17 centers) registry on 588 stent placements, 580 of whom (98.6%) were successful; a total of 84 complications occurred in 69/588 (11.7%) cases, the most common being

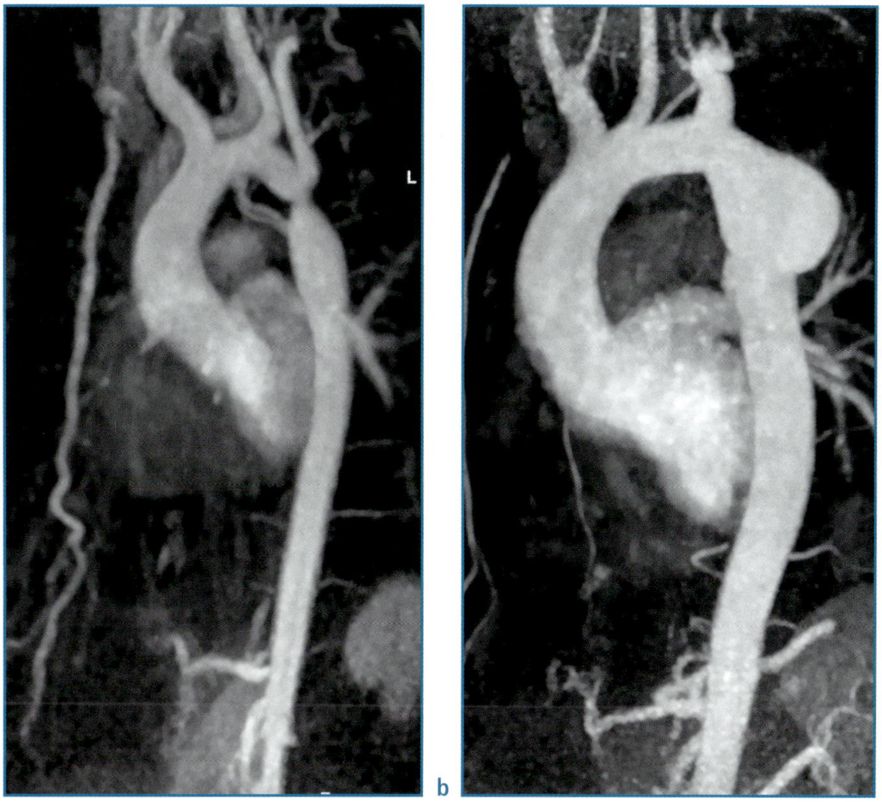

a b

Figure 16-6 Young patient with a significant coarctation of the aorta (a), and large aneurysm at the coarctation site 8 yrs after operative patch repair (b).

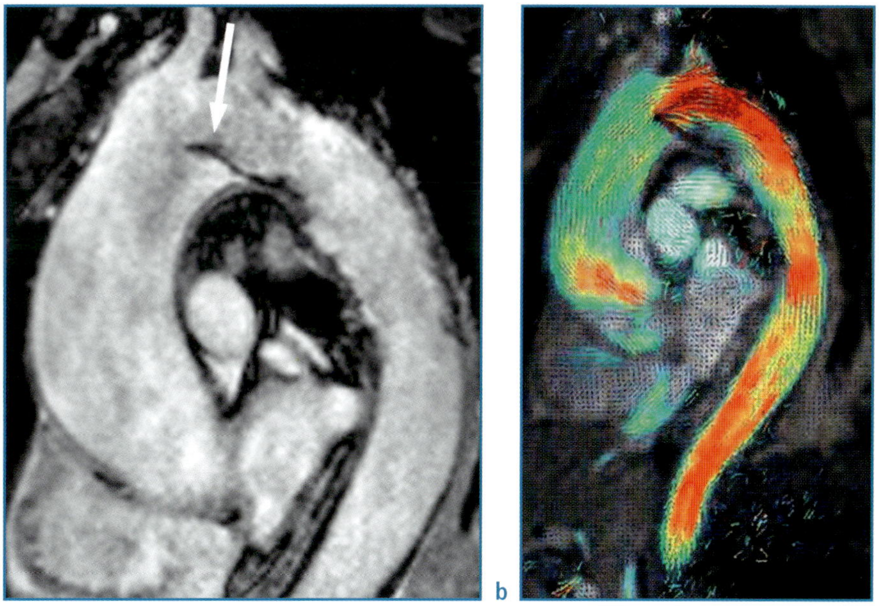

a b

Figure 16-7 Stentgraft in the aorta beginning at the arch between left carotid and subclavian artery for traumatic aortic rupture: Significant obstruction of the aortic lumen by the proximal inferior stent struts (arrow in (a)). Corresponding flow visualization in the aorta by a flow-sensitive 3D and 3-directional time-resolved GRE sequence with color-coded streamline and particle trace visualization at 3 T (b) showing disturbed laminar and high velocity flow at the obstruction site (high velocity stream lines: red approximately 4 m/s) continuing into the descending thoracic aorta (courtesy Prof. V. Rasche, Ulm).

femoral access vessel related (2.6%), aneurysm formation (2.2%), aortic dissection (1.5%), and cerebrovascular accident (1.0%). There were two procedure-related deaths (0.3%) recorded in the 16-yrs follow-up period, but the structural and functional results were not controlled by CMR imaging. There is one report on 19 consecutive patients with CoA, who were treated with balloon angioplasty, and where ultrasound or CMR was used for control. No patients had signs of aneurysm formation or deterioration of restenosis during follow-up of 20.2 ± 12.9 mths (Koerselman 2000).

A recent new application of CMR is comprehensive flow visualization in the aorta by a flow-sensitive 3D and 3-directional time-resolved GRE sequence with color-coded streamline and particle trace visualization at 3 T, which

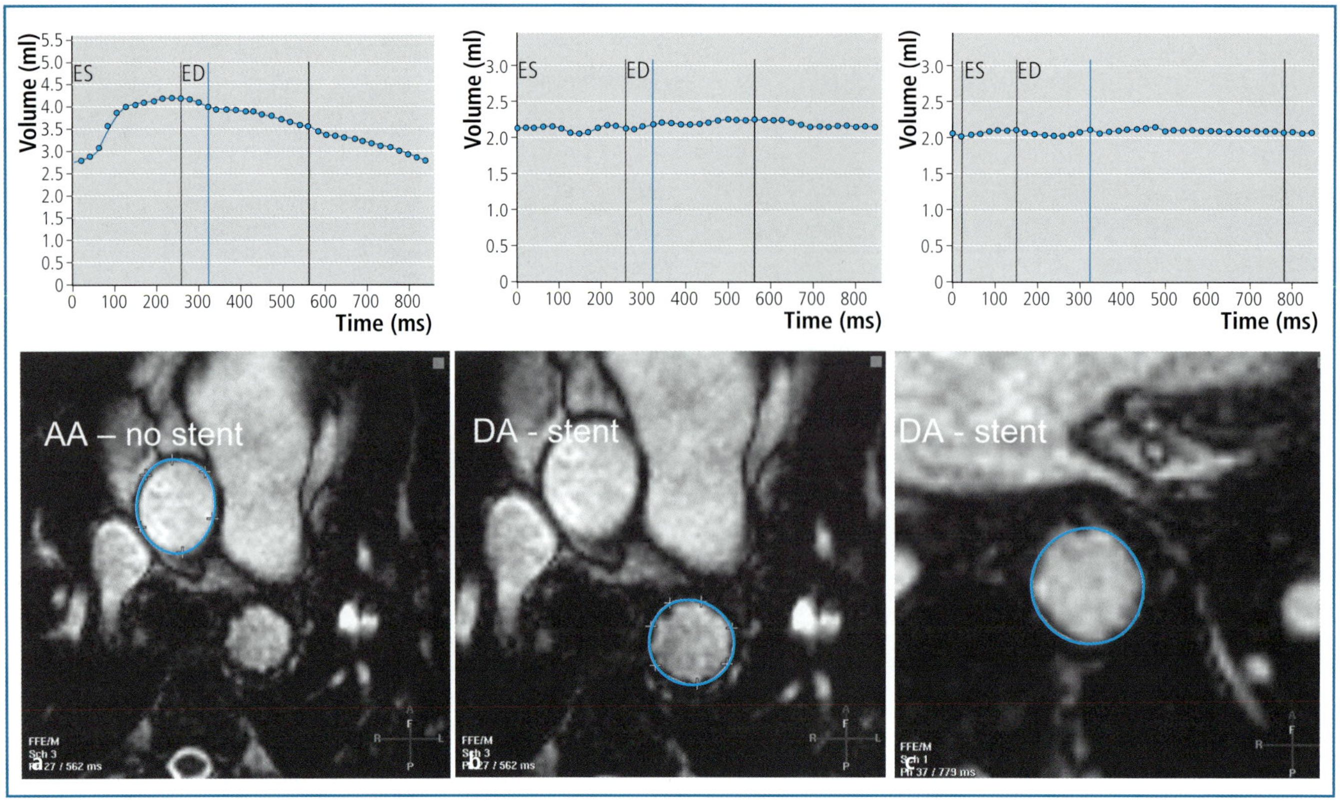

Figure 16-8 Analysis of regional aortic wall distensibility in the ascending aorta outside the stent (a), and at two different levels in the descending part within the stented aortic wall (b and c). Note virtually abolished distensibility (unchanged blood volume) within the stented areas compared with nearly normal distensibility (compliance) in the native aorta outside the stent. AA: ascending aorta; DA: descending aorta; ED: end-diastolic; ES: end-systolic (courtesy Prof. V. Rasche, Ulm).

provides regional physiological flow information and derived vessel parameters. This may be particularly interesting in patients with abnormal structures in the aorta and consecutive abnormal local flow characteristics, as shown by Frydrychowicz et al. (2008) for post-operative aneurysms in CoA, and by Rasche et al. (2009) in our institution for stenting of traumatic ruptures of the aortic arch, that in addition to abnormal regional flow (Figure 16-7) showed a blunted aortic distensibility at the edges of and within the stent-graft (Figure 16-8).

16.10.4 Summary and Conclusions

In conclusion, CMR imaging proves to be the imaging technique of choice for pre- and post-operative assessment of abnormal structure and function of the heart in congenital heart disease. In our institution CMR imaging is an indispensable part of the routine diagnostic work-up of patients with native as well as surgically palliated or corrected congenital heart disease.

16.11 Surgery for Adult Cardiovascular Disease

CMR imaging may be applied for post-interventional control of balloon angioplasty of stenosed pulmonary or mitral valves (Figure 16-9). However, CMR has more frequently been used for post-operative assessment of valve (Figure 16-10 and Figure 16-11) and aortic root replacement regarding complications or regression of left ventricular hypertrophy, as well as for LV aneurysmectomy and patch reconstruction of LV ventricular wall (Dor procedure). Fedriga et al. (1995) were able to detect 3 aneurysms of the ascending aorta, 3 dissections, and 3 false aneurysms in 10 patients (8 with aortic valve replacement = AVR), and found that CMR was superior to TEE and TTE in demonstrating these complications. Williams et al. (1999) found in a randomized study on 40 patients with implanted stentless vs. stented aortic bioprostheses an equal regression of LV muscle mass (LVMM) after 6 mths. After 36 mths reduction of LVMM was 38 % in the stentless vs. 20 % in the stented bioprosthesis group, indicating a better regression due to the larger implantation ring

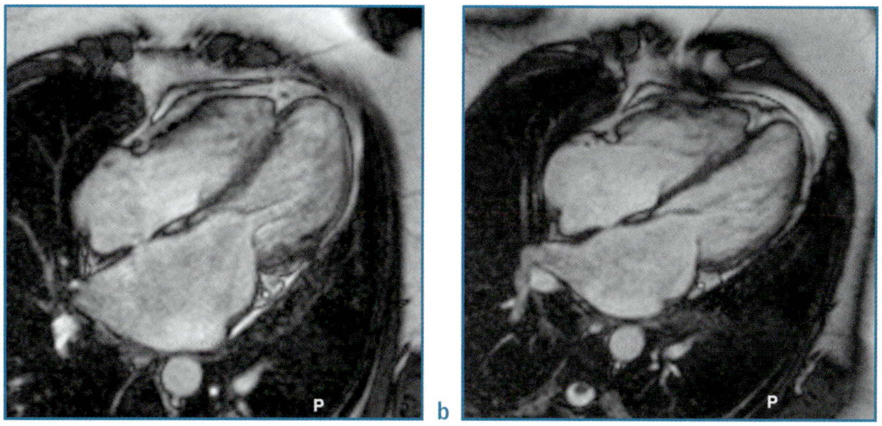

Figure 16-9 High-grade uncalcified mitral valve stenosis in a 4-ch view on cine-SSFP imaging at diastole before (a) and after balloon valvuloplasty (b). Significant improvement of degree of stenosis after interventional treatment (mitral valve area before 1.1 cm^2 and 2.9 cm^2 after balloon angioplasty).

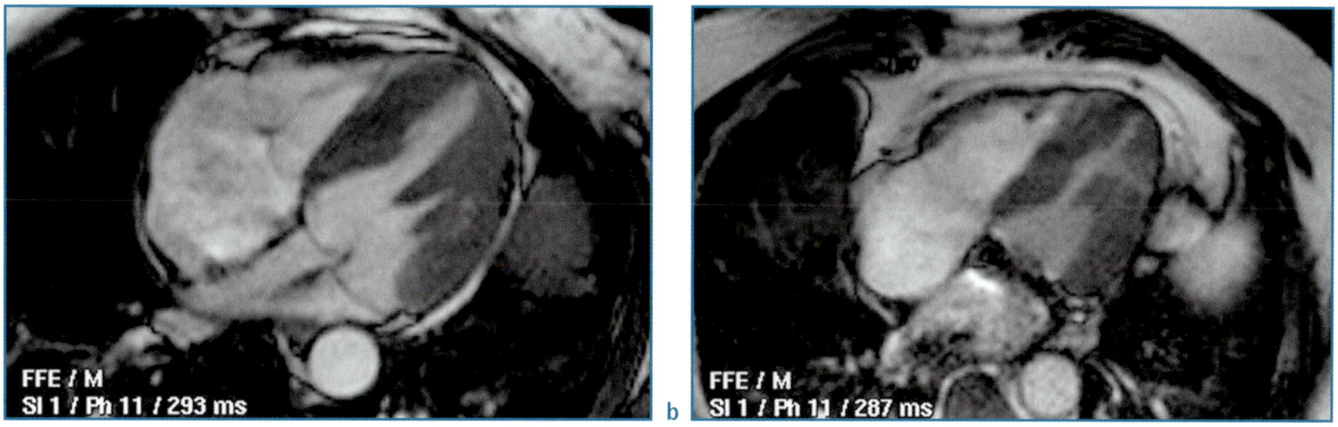

Figure 16-10 Cine-SSFP image in a 4-ch view at end-systole of a patient with a significant prolapse of the posterior mitral leaflet (flow void in (a)) before and after surgical repair of the mitral leaflet (b). Note the thickened mitral leaflets and mitral ring post-operatively; cine imaging revealed normal systolic and diastolic function of both mitral leaflets without significant residual mitral regurgitation (not shown here).

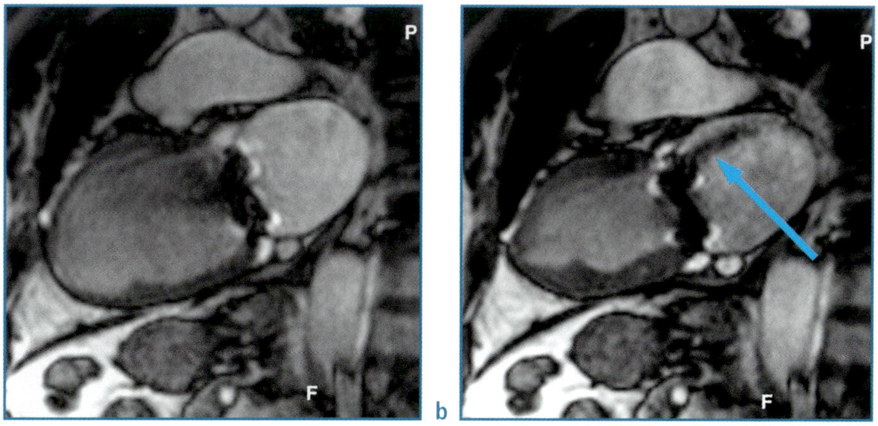

Figure 16-11 Cine-SSFP images in a 2-ch view in a patient with an implanted prosthetic valve in mitral position at end-diastole (a) and end-systole (b). In systole a significant regurgitant jet from the left ventricle to the left atrium is visible (arrow in (b)), indicating a significant paravalvular leakage. Note the enlarged left atrium and ventricle due to long-lasting mitral regurgitation of the patient.

of the stentless bioprostheses. Similar results were reported by Jasinski et al. (2004) in 16 patients randomly assigned to stentless and stented AVR. No segmental thickness reduction was observed in stented, but in stentless AVR early post-operative reduction of septal segments at the midventricular level was seen.

Schmid et al. (2002) reported on a rapid regression of LVMM in 42 consecutive patients with the Ross procedure for aortic stenosis, using CMR imaging. After 6 mths a significant reduction of LVMM near to normal values was observed. Carr-White et al. (1999) investigated RV volumes and function 6–35 mths after the Ross procedure (pulmonic

a b c d

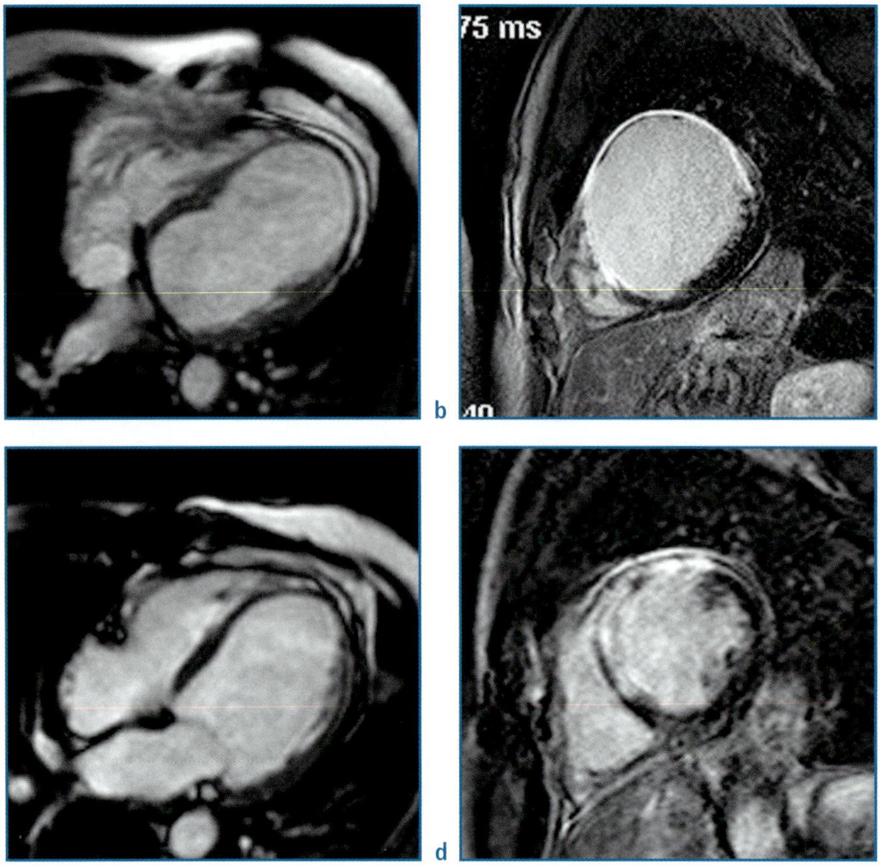

Figure 16-12 Surgical repair using the Dor procedure in a patient with a large left ventricular apical aneurysm following myocardial infarction with scarring and aneurysmic bulging of nearly the entire ventricular septum and apex of LV (short-axis view): Scar images in a 4-ch **(a)** and short-axis view **(b)** before **(top)** and after surgical repair **(bottom)**. Left ventricular remodeling **(c and d)** can be seen from the reduced left ventricular diameter and by the increase of left ventricular ejection fraction (from 16 % pre- to 36 % post-operatively) (courtesy Dr. J. Schwab, Nuremberg).

autocraft vs. aortic homograft), using CMR imaging. They found an increase in both end-systolic and end-diastolic RV volumes with an unchanged stroke volume indicating a similar slight impairment of RV longitudinal pump function. A recently introduced new technique is percutaneous pulmonary valve implantation (PPVI), that has been reported by Nordmeyer et al. (2009b) as an alternative treatment for right ventricle-pulmonary artery conduit failure. In 12 patients PPVI was successfully performed and RVOT gradient during catheterization and pulmonary regurgitant fraction on CMR fell after PPVI (gradient 34 ± 6 to 14 ± 3 mmHg, $p < 0.01$, regurgitant fraction 20 % ± 6 % to 2 % ± 1 %, $p < 0.05$). It was concluded that PPVI provides an effective transcatheter treatment strategy to prolong the life span of right ventricle-pulmonary artery conduits after the Ross procedure, reducing the reoperation burden on patients with aortic valve disease. Regarding the reliability of imaging procedures, Rajappan et al. (2003) demonstrated that CMR imaging was superior to M-mode echocardiography in assessing regression of LVMM after AVR in 39 patients with severe aortic stenosis. Changes in aortic distensibility after aortic root replacement have been studied by Melina et al. (2002). They found near-normal distensibility of the aortic wall in 15 patients (6 homografts, 9 xenografts) up to 1 yr after AVR, using CMR to assess percent change in aortic radius and pressure strain elastic modulus as indices of distensibility.

One large study by Dor et al. (2004) reported on the advantages of CMR imaging in assessing the effects of LV reconstruction with endoventricular circular patch plasty (EVCPP = Dor procedure) in patients with large LV aneurysms following acute myocardial infarction (example in Figure 16-12). Based on this center's 20 years of experience, the extreme value of CMR imaging was revealed for both pre-operative assessment of the abnormal morphology and function of the LV and post-operative control of the Dor procedure to non-invasively document the improvement of both LV structure and hemodynamics (EDDV, ESV, stroke volume, cardiac index). Therefore, CMR is the imaging technique of choice to reveal infarct size, localization of infarct scars, altered morphology of the ventricle, and to assess hemodynamic impairment after large myocardial infarctions. This is essential for optimal planning of a conservative or surgical strategy in these high risk patient populations.

16.12 Conclusions and Future Perspectives

Routine follow-up of interventionally and surgically treated patients includes clinical, electrocardiographic and echocardiographic techniques, sometimes cardiac catheterisation and coronary angiography, to control the success of an intervention and to diagnose early progression of disease. Based on recent reports CMR imaging should be chosen early in the routine evaluation of invasively treated patients, because it provides important informations on myocardial structure and function, the effect of revascularising techniques on myocardial perfusion, myocardial viability, and function or dysfunction of implanted devices can be assessed with high precision. Thus, with more widespread access to CMR this technique is the first-line non-invasive imaging modality for long-term follow-up of interventionally or surgically treated patients with a wide spectrum of cardiovascular diseases.

References

Adamson L, Vohra HA, Haw MP. Does pulmonary valve replacement post-repair of tetralogy of Fallot improve right ventricular function? Interact CardioVascular Thorac Surg 2009; 9: 520–7.

Adler ED, Bystrup A, Briley-Saebo KC et al. In vivo detection of embryonic stem-cell derived cardiovascular progenitor cells using Cy3-labeled gadofluorine M in murine myocardium. JACC Cardiovascular Imaging 2009; 2: 1114–22.

Anand I, McMurray J, Cohn JN et al. EARTH investigators. Long-term effects of darusentan on left-ventricular remodelling and clinical outcomes in the Endothelin A Receptor Antagonist Trial in heart Failure (EARTH): randomised, double-blind, placebo-controlled trial. Lancet 2004a; 364: 347–54.

Anand I, McMurray JJ, Whitmore J et al. Anemia and its relationship to clinical outcome in heart failure. Circulation 2004b; 110 (2): 149–54.

Attia C, Farhat F, Boussel L et al. Endovascular repair of lesions involving the descending thoracic aorta. Mid-term morphological changes. Interact Cardiovasc Thorac Surg 2008; 7: 595–9.

Bastounis E, Georgopoulos S, Maltezos C, Balas P. The validity of current vascular imaging methods in the evaluation of aortic anastomotic aneurysms developing after abdominal aortic aneurysm repair. Ann Vasc Surg 1996; 10: 537–45.

Bellenger NG, Rajappan K, Rahman SL et al. on behalf of the CHRISTMAS Study Steering Committee and Investigators. Effects of carvedilol on left ventricular remodelling in chronic stable heart failure: a cardiovascular magnetic resonance study. Heart 2004; 90 (7): 760–4.

Bello D, Shah DJ, Farah GM et al. Gadolinium cardiovascular magnetic resonance predicts reversible myocardial dysfunction and remodeling in patients with heart failure undergoing beta-blocker therapy. Circulation 2003; 108 (16): 1945–53.

Bernhardt P, Spiess J, Levenson B et al. Combined assessment of myocardial perfusion and late gadolinium enhancement in patients after percutaneous coronary intervention or bypass grafts. A multi-center study of an integrated cardiovascular magnetic resonance protocol. JACC Cardiovascular Imaging 2009; 2: 1292–300.

Bondarenko O, Beek AM, Nijveldt R et al. Functional outcome after revascularization in patients with chronic ischemic heart disease: a quantitative late gadolinium enhancement CMR study evaluating transmural scar extent, wall thickness and periprocedural necrosis. J Cardiovasc Magn Reson 2007; 9: 815–21.

Borgna-Pignatti C, Cappellini MD, De Stefano P et al. Cardiac morbidity and mortality in deferoxamine- or deferiprone-treated patients with thalassemia major. Blood 2006; 107: 3733–7.

Burgstahler C, Wöhrle J, Kochs M et al. Magnetic resonance imaging to assess changes in atrial and ventricular parameters after transcatheter closure of atrial septal defects. J Magn Reson Imag 2007; 25: 1136–40.

Carr-White GS, Kon M, Koh TW et al. Right ventricular function after pulmonary autograft replacement of the aortic valve. Circulation 1999; 100 (19 Suppl.): II36–41.

Cesare ED, Giordano AV, Cerone G et al. Comparative evaluation of TEE, conventional MRI and contrast-enhanced 3D breath-hold MRA in the post operative follow-up of dissecting aneurysms. Int J Card Imaging 2000; 16: 135–47.

Cheng ASH, Selvanayagam JB, Jerosch-Herold M et al. Percutaneous treatment of chronic total occlusions improves regional hyperemic myocardial blood flow and contractility. Insights from quantitative cardiovascular magnetic resonance imaging. J Am Coll Cardiol Inv 2008; 1: 44–53.

Dill T, Schächinger V, Rolf A et al. Intracoronary administration of bone marrow-derived progenitor cells improves left ventricular function in patients at risk for adverse remodeling after acute ST-segment elevation myocardial infarction: results of the Reinfusion of Enriched Progenitor cells And Infarct Remodeling in Acute Myocardial Infarction study (REPAIR-AMI) cardiac magnetic resonance imaging substudy. Am Heart J 2009; 157 (3): 541–7.

Dohmen G, Kuroczynski W, Dahm M et al. Value of echocardiography in patient follow-up after surgically corrected Type A aortic dissection. Thorac Cardiovasc Surg 2001; 49: 343–8.

Dong J, Dickfeld T, Dalal D et al. Initial experience in the use of integrated electro-anatomic mapping with three-dimensional MR/CT images to guide catheter ablation of atrial fibrillation. J Cardiovasc Electrophysiol 2006; 17: 459–66.

Dor V, Sabatier M, Montiglio F et al. Endovascular patch reconstruction of ischemic failing ventricle. A single center with 20 years experience. Advantages of magnetic resonance imaging assessment. Heart Failure Rev 2004; 9: 269–86.

Engellau L, Larsson EM, Albrechtsson U et al. Magnetic resonance imaging and MR angiography of endoluminally treated abdominal aortic aneurysms. Eur J Vasc Endovasc Surg 1998; 15: 212–9.

Fedriga E, Minorati D, Masini L et al. Magnetic resonance imaging in assessing the complications of cardiac surgery involving the ascending aorta. Radiol Med (Torino) 1995; 90: 238–43.

Foltz WD, Cunningham CH, Mutsaers AJ et al. Positive-contrast imaging in the rabbit hind-limb of transplanted cells bearing endocytosed superparamagnetic beads. J Cardiovasc Magn Reson 2006; 8 (6): 817–23.

Frydrychowicz A, Arnold R, Hirtler D et al. Multi-directional flow analysis by cardiovascular magnetic resonance in aneurysm development following repair of aortic coarctation. J Cardiovasc Magn Reson 2008; 10: 30.
Golden AB, Hellenbrand WE. Coarctation of the aorta: stenting in children and adults. Cath Cardiovasc Interv 2007; 69: 289–99.
Haulon S, Willoteaux S, Koussa M et al. Diagnosis and treatment of type II endoleak after stent placement for exclusion of an abdominal aortic aneurysm. Ann Vasc Surg 2001; 15: 148–54.
Ho KW, Tan RS, Wong KY et al. Late complications following tetralogy of Fallot repair: the need for long-term follow-up. Ann Acad Med Singapore 2007; 36: 947–53.
Jasinski MJ, Ulbrych P, Kolowca M et al. Early regional assessment of LV mass regression and function after stentless valve replacement: comparative randomized study. Heart Surg Forum 2004; 7: E 462–5.
Kahlert P, Eggebrecht H, Plicht B et al. Towards real-time cardiovascular magnetic resonance-guided transarterial aortic valve implantation: in vitro evaluation and modification of existing devices. J Cardiovasc Magn Reson 2010; 12: 58.
Klein C, Nagel E, Gebker R et al. Magnetic resonance adenosine perfusion imaging in patients after coronary artery bypass graft surgery. JACC Cardiovasc Imaging 2009; 2: 437–45.
Koerselman J, de Vries H, Jaarsma W et al. Balloon angioplasty of coarctation of the aorta: a safe alternative for surgery in adults: immediate and mid-term results. Cath Cardiovasc Interv 2000; 50: 28–33.
Kolandaivelu A, Lardo AC, Halperin HR. Cardiovascular magnetic resonance guided electrophysiology studies. J Cardiovasc Magn Reson 2009; 11 (1): 21.
Koos R, Altiok E, Mahnken AH et al. Evaluation of aortic root for definition of prosthesis size by magnetic resonance imaging and cardiac computed tomography: Implications for transcatheter aortic valve implantation. Int J Cardiol 2011; Feb 9 (Epub ahead of print).
Krittayaphong R, Laksanabunsong, Maneesai A et al. Comparison of cardiovascular magnetic resonance of late gadolinium enhancement and diastolic wall thickness to predict recovery of left ventricular function after coronary artery bypass surgery. J Cardiovasc Magn Reson 2008; 10: 41.
Lepore V, Lamm C, Bugge M, Larsson S. Magnetic resonance imaging in the follow-up of patients after aortic root reconstruction. Thorac Cardiovasc Surg 1996; 44: 188–92.
Lüscher TF, Ruschitzka F, Anand I et al. On behalf of the EARTH investigators. EARTH: Endothelin A Receptor Antagonist Trial in Heart Failure. Heart Drug 2001; 1: 294–8.
McGann CJ, Kholmovski EG, Oakes RS et al. New magnetic resonance imaging-based method for defining the extent of left atrial wall injury after ablation of atrial fibrillation. J Am Coll Cardiol 2008; 52: 1263–71.
Melina G, Rajappan K, Amrani M et al. Aortic distensibility after aortic root replacement assessed with cardiovascular magnetic resonance. J Heart Valve Dis 2002; 11: 67–74.
Meng J, Peters DC, Hsing JM et al. Late gadolinium enhancement of the esophagus is common on cardiac MR several months after pulmonary vein isolation: Preliminary observations. Pacing Clin Electrophysiol 2010; 33: 661–6.
Mesana TG, Caus T, Gaubert J et al. Late complications after prosthetic replacement of the ascending aorta: what did we learn from routine magnetic resonance imaging follow-up? Eur J Cardiothorac Surg 2000; 18: 313–20.
Meyer GP, Wollert KC, Lotz J et al. Intracoronary bone marrow cell transfer after myocardial infarction: 5-year follow-up from the randomized-controlled BOOST trial. Eur Heart J 2009; 30: 2978–84.
Meyer GP, Wollert KC, Lotz J et al. Intracoronary bone marrow cell transfer after myocardial infarction. Eighteen month's follow-up data from randomized, controlled BOOST (Bone marrow transfer to enhance ST-elevation infarct regeneration) trial. Circulation 2006; 113: 1287–94.
Modell B, Khan M, Darlison M et al. Improved survival of thalassemia major in the UK and relation to T2* cardiovascular magnetic resonance. J Cardiovasc Magn Reson 2008; 10: 42.
Moore NR, Parry AJ, Trottmann-Dickenson B et al. Fate of the native aorta after repair of acute type A dissection: a magnetic resonance imaging study. Heart 1996; 75: 62–6.
Mosquera VX, Herrera JM, Marini M et al. Mid-term results of thoracic endovascular repair in surgical high-risk patients. Interact Cardiovasc Thorac Surg 2009; 9: 61–5.
Nordmeyer J, Lurz P, Tsang VT et al. Effective transcatheter implantation after pulmonary homograft failure: a new perspective on the Ross operation. J Thorac Cardiovasc Surg 2009b; 138: 84–8.
Nordmeyer J, Tsang V, Gaudin R et al. Quantitative assessment of homograft function 1 year after insertion into pulmonary position: impact of in situ homograft geometry on valve competence. Eur Heart J 2009a; 30: 2147–54.
Nusser T, Höher M, Merkle N et al. Cardiac magnetic resonance imaging and transesophageal echocardiography in patients with transcatheter closure of patent foramen ovale. J Am Coll Cardiol 2006; 48: 322–9.
Oakes RS, Badger TJ, Kholmovski EG et al. Detection and quantification of left atrial structural remodeling with delayed-enhancement magnetic resonance imaging in patients with atrial fibrillation. Circulation 2009; 119: 1758–67.
Peters DC, Wylie JV, Hauser TH et al. Recurrence of atrial fibrillation correlates with the extent of post-procedural late gadolinium enhancement: a pilot study. JACC Cardiovasc Imaging 2009; 2 (3): 308–16.
Peters DC, Wylie JV, Hauser TH et al. Detection of pulmonary vein and left atrial scar after catheter ablation with three-dimensional navigator-gated delayed enhancement MR imaging: initial experience. Radiology 2007; 243: 690–5.
Piga A, Gaglioti C, Fogliacco E et al. Comparative effects of deferiprone and desferoxamine on survival and cardiac disease in patients with thalassemia major: a retrospective analysis. Haematologica 2003; 88: 489–96.
Prasad SK, Dargie HJ, Smith GC et al. Comparison of the dual receptor endothelin antagonist enrasentan with enalapril in asymptomatic left ventricular systolic dysfunction: a cardiovascular magnetic resonance study. Heart 2006; 92 (6): 798–803.
Rahimi K, Banning AP, Cheng AS et al. Prognostic value of coronary revascularisation-related myocardial injury: a cardiac magnetic resonance imaging study. Heart 2009; 95 (23): 1937–43.
Rajappan K, Bellenger NG, Melina G et al. Assessment of left ventricular mass regression after aortic valve replacement – cardiovascular magnetic resonance vs. M-mode echocardiography. Eur J CardioThorac Surg 2003; 24: 59–65.

Rasche V, Crelier G, Bornstedt A et al. Reconstruction of aortic flow pattern after thoracic stent graft implantation. In: Proceedings Annual Meeting ISMRM. Honolulu 2009; 3862.

Romeih S, Kroft LJ, Bokenkamp R et al. Delayed improvement of right ventricular diastolic function and regression of right ventricular mass after percutaneous pulmonary valve implantation in patients with congenital heart disease. Am Heart J 2009; 158: 40–6.

Schmid FX, Keyser A, Djavidani B et al. Left ventricular remodeling after pulmonary autograft aortic valve replacement: evaluation with color Doppler echocardiography and magnetic resonance imaging. Artif Organs 2002; 26: 444–8.

Schulz-Menger J, Strohm O, Waigand J et al. The value of magnetic resonance imaging of the left ventricular outflow tract in patients with hypertrophic obstructive cardiomyopathy after septal artery embolization. Circulation 2000; 101 (15): 1764–6.

Sherif MA, Abdel-Wahab M, Beurich HW et al. Hemodynamic evaluation of aortic regurgitation after transcatheter aortic valve implantation using cardiovascular magnetic resonance. EuroIntervention 2011; 7: 57–63.

Syed MA, Carlson K, Murphy M et al. Long-term safety of cardiac magnetic resonance imaging performed in the first few days after bare-metal stent implantation. J Magn Reson Imaging 2006; 24: 1056–61.

Taclas JE, Nezafat R, Wylie JV et al. Relationship between intended sites of RF ablation and post-procedural scar in AF patients, using late gadolinium enhancement cardiovascular magnetic resonance. Heart Rhythm 2009; 7: 489–96.

Tanner MA, Galanello R, Dessi C et al. Combined chelation therapy in thalassemia major for the treatment of severe myocardial siderosis with left ventricular dysfunction. J Cardiovasc Magn Reson 2008; 10 (1): 12.

Taylor AJ, Al-Saadi N, Abdel-Aty H et al. Elective percutaneous coronary intervention immediately impairs resting microvascular perfusion assessed by cardiac magnetic resonance imaging. Am Heart J 2006; 151: 891.e1–891.e7.

Telfer P, Coen PG, Christou S et al. Survival of medically treated thalassemia patients in Cyprus. Trends and risk factors over the period 1980–2004. Haematologica 2006; 91: 1187–92.

Teo KSL, Dundon BK, Molaee P et al. Percutaneous closure of atrial septal defects leads to normalisation of atrial and ventricular volumes. J Cardiovasc Magn Reson 2008; 10: 55.

Todd GJ, DeRose JJ, Martin EC. Complementary surgical/interventional techniques for nonresective management of "inoperable" aneurysms: a second look. Ann Vasc Surg 1998; 12 (3): 248–54.

Valeti US, Nishimura RA, Holmes DR et al. Comparison of surgical septal myectomy and alcohol septal ablation with cardiac magnetic resonance imaging in patients with hypertrophic obstructive cardiomyopathy. J Am Coll Cardiol 2007; 49 (3): 350–7.

Valsangiacomo-Buechel ER, Dave HH, Kellenberger CJ et al. Remodeling of the right ventricle after early pulmonary valve replacement in children with repaired tetralogy of Fallot: assessment by cardiovascular magnetic resonance. Eur Heart J 2005; 26: 2721–7.

Van der Laan MJ, Bartels LW, Viergever MA, Blankesteijn JD. Computed tomography vs. magnetic resonance imaging of endoleaks after EVAR. Eur J Vasc Endovasc Surg 2006; 32: 361–5.

Van Dockum WG, Beek AM, ten Cate FJ et al. Early onset and progression of left ventricular remodeling after alcohol septal ablation in hypertrophic obstructive cardiomyopathy. Circulation 2005; 111 (19): 2503–8.

Van Dockum WG, Knaapen P, Hofman MB et al. Impact of alcohol septal ablation on left anterior descending coronary artery blood flow in hypertrophic obstructive cardiomyopathy. Int J Cardiovasc Imaging 2009; 25 (5): 511–8.

Van Dockum WG, Kuijer JP, Götte MJ et al. Septal ablation in hypertrophic obstructive cardiomyopathy improves systolic myocardial function in the lateral (free) wall: a follow-up study using CMR tissue tagging and 3D strain analysis. Eur Heart J 2006; 27 (23): 2833–9.

Van Herwaarden JA, Muhs BE, Vincken KL et al. Aortic compliance following EVAR and the influence of different endografts: determination using dynamic MRA. J Endovasc Ther 2006; 13: 406–14.

Van Straaten A, Vliegen HW, Hazekamp MG et al. Right ventricular function after pulmonary valve replacement in patients with tetralogy of Fallot. Radiology 2004; 233: 824–9.

Williams RJ, Muir DE, Pathi V et al. Randomized controlled trial of stented and stentless aortic bioprostheses: hemodynamic performances at 3 years. Sem Thorac Cardiovasc Surg 1999; 11: 93–7.

Wisenberg G, Lekx K, Zabel P et al. Cell tracking and therapy evalution of bone marrow monocytes and stromal cells using SPECT and CMR in a canine model of myocardial infarction. J Cardiovasc Magn Reson 2009; 11: 11.

Wöhrle J, Merkle N, Mailänder V et al. Results of intracoronary stem cell therapy after acute myocardial infarction. Am J Cardiol 2010; 105: 804–12.

Wylie Jr. JV, Peters DC, Essebag V et al. Left atrial function and scar after catheter ablation of atrial fibrillation. Heart Rhythm 2008; 5 (5): 656–62.

17 Cardiac Tumors and Masses

Johannes Schwab and Vinzenz Hombach

17.1 Definition

Cardiac masses are characterized as any local tissue process that leads to a deformation of cardiac structures and occasionally to impairment of regional or global cardiac function. In addition, variants of normal cardiac structures are to be taken into account, which may be misinterpreted as a cardiac tumor.

17.2 Spectrum of Tumors

The spectrum of cardiac and extracardiac tumors comprises primary and secondary tumors, non-tumorous cardiac masses, and variants of normal cardiac structures. Primary tumors of the heart are rare across all groups with a prevalence of 0.001–0.03% in autopsy series, whereas secondary involvement of the heart through extracardiac tumors is 20–40 times more common. Despite rarity there are multiple histological types of primary cardiac tumors. When tumors primarily based in the pericardium such as mesotheliomas and teratomas are excluded, the overwhelming majority consists of mesenchymal tumors with a full spectrum of differentiation. About 75% of all primary cardiac tumors are benign, and include (in order of approximate decreasing occurrence) myxomas (around 50% of all benign tumors), rhabdomyomas, fibromas, papillary fibroelastomas, teratomas (these tumors can also demonstrate malignant features), hemangiomas, and lipomas. Very rare benign tumors include cystic tumor of the AV node (polycystic tumor), hamartoma (Purkinje tumor), plasma cell granuloma, neurilemmoma, gastrinoma, pheochromocytoma, and histicytoid tumors. Of the remaining 25% of cardiac tumors considered as malignant, the majority are sarcomas, followed by lymphomas.

17.3 Clinical Presentation

Clinical symptoms associated with most primary cardiac tumors are non-specific, and they often mimick far more commonly encountered disease entities. Many tumors present with mild and vague symptoms so that most routine work-ups will fail to identify the underlying process. This results in a delay in the disease diagnosis. Depending on the location, size, friability, mobility, and histologic type cardiac tumors can produce a variety of clinical findings, which can be divided into four general mechanistic categories: systemic manifestations, cardiac manifestations, embolic manifestations, and phenomena from metastatic disease.

Among the multitude of systemic phenomena patients may develop **constitutional symptoms** like fever, chills, malaise, fatigue, or weight loss, which may mimic those of several connective tissue diseases and vasculitis e.g. arthralgia, myalgia, muscle weakness, and Raynaud's phenomenon. Together with concomitant laboratory abnormalities like leuko- and thrombocytosis, anemia or thrombocytopenia and increased sedimentation rate, these phenomena are believed to result from secretory products released by the tumor and/or by necrotic parts of the tumor. Cardiac tumors can cause **systemic or pulmonary emboli** by parts of the tumor itself or thromboemboli released from or formed on the surface of the tumor. The propensity of a tumor to cause emboli depends largely on its localization (intramurally or intracavitary), and the type and friability of the intramural surface of the tumor. Primary tumors can embolize in any organ (coronary arteries, cerebral arteries, renal or periphereal arteries), resulting in ischemia, infarction, or delayed aneurysm formation. Sometimes emboli occur simultaneously in multiple organs or body sites. If embolectomy specimen is obtained, careful examination may reveal tumor emboli and confirm the clinical diagnosis of a central tumor within the cardio-circulatory system. Systemic emboli are typically caused by left-sided tumors, although right-sided tumors can also result in systemic emboli via a patent foramen ovale with concurrent right-to-left shunting.

Cardiac manifestations of primary tumors can result from direct mechanical interference with myocardial or valvular function, interruption of coronary blood flow, interference with the special conduction system (AV node, His bundle, bundle branches), or stimulation of pericardial fluid production. Partially or completely intramural tumors are typically asymptomatic, with mostly large intramural tumors located in or pressing on the major conduction pathways and potentially causing a variety of cardiac arrhythmias such as heart block, asystole or extrasystoles. Moreover, large intramural tumors may compress the cardiac cavities, obstruct the ventricular inflow or outflow tract, or contribute to mitral valve insufficiency. In contrast, tumors with a significant intracavitary component tend to cause more symptoms such as systemic emboli or hemodynamic problems. If tumors are mobile or pedunculated they can interfere with tricuspid or mitral valve opening and closure. Thus, left- or right-heart failure may occur in the case of hemodynamic compromise of tricuspid or mitral valve function, or outflow tract occlusion. Together with the aforementioned systemic or constitutional symptoms further investigations including imaging techniques should be initiated.

Metastatic disease may be the result of a primary malignant cardiac tumor with end-stage peripheral metastatic dissemination. Since most malignant cardiac tumors are detected in a late stage, metastatic disease may represent the initial clinical manifestation of a malignant cardiac tumor. There is a widespread spectrum of organ metastases, from cardiac angiosarcomas and rhabdomyosarcomas most commonly into the lung, brain and bone. However, metastases to the liver, lymph nodes, spleen, adrenal glands, and even the skin have been reported (for details see McManus 2012).

17.4 CMR Protocols

Using cine-SSFP sequences both morphology and function of the heart as well as possible hemodynamic compromise by a cardiac tumor can be assessed. If a pericardial tumor or mass is present, reduced or blunted regional myocardial contractility should be detected as a sign of infiltrative growth of the tumor into the pericardial sac. Some hints on the consistency of the tumor may be obtained from the relationship between signal intensities on T1- and T2-weighted imaging, as well as from susceptibility or chemical shift artifacts. Further informations on the fat content of the tumor/mass can be gained from fat suppression imaging. Black-blood sequences provide excellent information on anatomic and morphologic structures of the heart, valves, and pericardium. Contrast-enhanced imaging aims to assess blood perfusion of a given tumor, whereby contrast behaviour depends on perfusion and extent of the extracellular space. Most of the actual contrast media follow an extracellular distribution, and the contrast-enhanced signal intensity is mainly obtained from T1-weighted images. Perfusion of the tumor itself may be analyzed by first-pass perfusion studies using T1-weighted spoiled GRE sequences with a saturation-recovery prepulse. In order to increase tissue contrast and signal-to-noise ratio (SNR) an SSFP sequence with a saturation-recovery prepulse may be used. Using these sequences a time-signal intensity curve can be calculated, which may be qualitatively compared with first-pass perfusion of the myocardium, skeletal muscle, liver, or with the contrast passage through the LV cavum. Contrast enhancement may be imaged using T1-weighted spin echo sequences or inversion-recovery GRE sequences, as used for detection of myocardial scars following myocardial infarction. Tumor tissue with a large interstitial space, e.g. necrotic areas within the tumor, shows a strong enhancement (high signal intensity).

In general, the following **CMR imaging protocol** should be used:

- scout/survey with transversal planes covering the whole heart including the tumor/mass,
- cine-SSFP sequence, possibly combined with parallel imaging (SENSE) for assessing morphology and function,
- specially adapted sectional planes (two-perpendicular planes) through the tumor/mass using cine-SSFP sequences,
- T1-, T2- and PD-weighted black-blood sequences in the standard and tumor-adapted planes for anatomic and morphologic imaging, T2-images with and without fat suppression pulses,
- first-pass perfusion studies through the tumor/mass with concomitant assessment of perfusion through skeletal muscle or liver (appropriate FOV),
- contrast-enhanced imaging in the long- (2-ch, 4-ch) and short-axes, and through the tumor.

17.5 Differentiating Features

Certain CMR features allow differentiation between benign and malignant tumors or masses of the heart. These include location, size, border, calcification, and pericardial effusion. As a general rule, most cardiac tumors involving the right atrial wall are suspected to be malignant since the right atrial wall is an uncommon location for benign tumors. An exception to this rule is right atrial myxoma. Most benign tumors are small in comparison to malignant tumors, which are usually of considerable size and may sometimes fill an entire cardiac chamber. Some benign tumors particularly myxomas have a thin pedicle attaching their border to the myocardium, while malignant tumors are usually broad-based (O'Donnell 2009). The border of most benign tumors is smooth and well-defined without irregularities or infiltration, whereas malignant tumors tend to have more lobular, ill-defined borders and a tendency to invade the myocardium, pericardium, or the adjacent extracardiac structures (Araoz 1999, Siripornpitak 1997). Large foci of calcification are a characteristic feature of cardiac osteosarcoma, while some benign tumors such as myxomas or fibromas may contain small foci of calcification (Grebenc 2000). Pericardial effusion in the presence of cardiac tumor or mass makes it suspicious for malignancy (O'Donnell 2009). This has been confirmed by the study by Hoffmann et al. (2003), who suggested in 55 patients with cardiac masses that CMR characteristics were useful for distinguishing benign from malignant tumors (receiver-operator AUC was 0.90) based on tumor location, tissue characteristics, and presence of pericardial effusion.

Intracardiac thrombus is a common differential diagnosis for cardiac tumors. The detection of an intracardiac thrombus is essential for avoiding embolic events and to initiate anticoagulation. Echocardiography has limitations in detecting intracardiac thrombus due to a restricted imaging window, modest image reproducibility, and poor spatial and soft-tissue resolution, compared to CMR imaging (Gulati 2004). Contrast-enhanced CMR allows differentiation between thrombus and surrounding myocardium, because the thrombus is avascular and does not show contrast enhancement, unlike the vascularized myocardium (Barkhausen 2002). Only rarely do large chronic thrombi enhance peripherally and render differentiation from a malignant tumor very difficult. A further advantage of contrast-enhanced CMR is the detection of myocardial scars, which are an independent risk factor for intracardiac thrombus formation. Therefore, contrast-enhanced CMR appears to be very useful for thrombus detection.

17.6 Benign Cardiac Tumors

17.6.1 Myxoma

Prevalence

Myxomas account for 25–50 % of all primary cardiac tumors with an annual incidence of 0.5 per million population and most commonly present in adults 30–50 yrs of age, although they can occur from 1–83 yrs of age (McManus 2012). Of all cardiac myxomas, 65 % occur in women, and 4.5–10 % of cardiac myxomas are familial.

Pathology

Myxomas are benign tumors whose tumor cells most likely arise from multipotent mesenchymal cells that differentiate into several cell types like endothelial and fat cells. Hemorrhage, fibrosis, and calcification are frequently identified in the tumor, which is mostly sporadic in origin. The size of myxomas varies from 1–15 cm, with the most common locations being the left atrium (60–75 %), the right atrium (20–28 %), but rarely both atria or ventricles. If multiple tumors are present they may be part of Carney's triad syndrome (Muhm 1986). This autosomal dominant syndrome or complex consists of multiple cardiac or extracardiac myxomas, spotty skin pigmentation (e.g. blue nevi), endo-

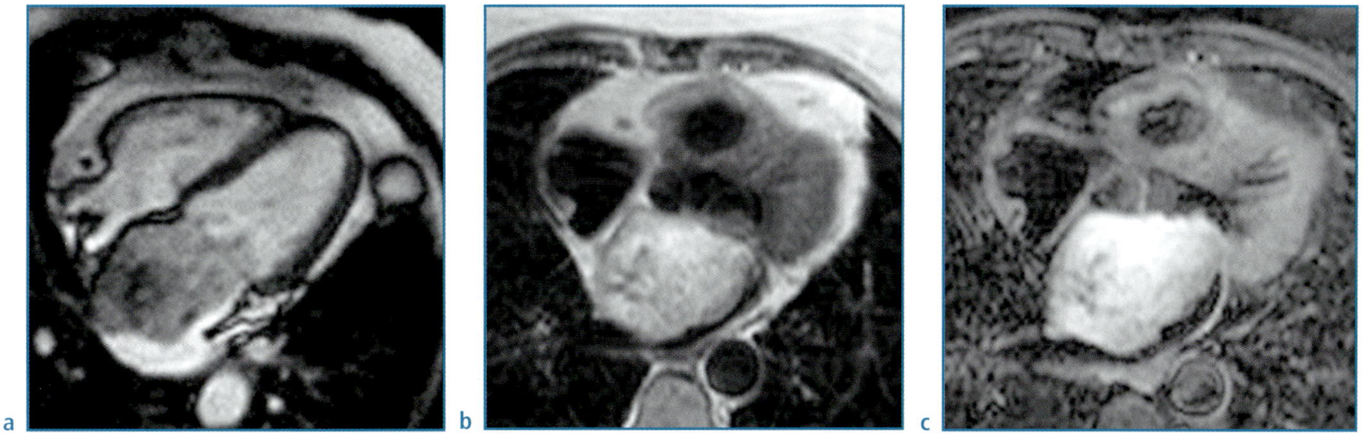

Figure 17-1 SSFP sequences: Large left atrial myxoma fixed at the interatrial septum with prolapse into the left ventricle on cine-SSFP imaging in a 4-ch view (a), T2-weighted black-blood imaging (b), and T2-weighted black-blood imaging with a fat suppression pulse (c) with heterogenous signal intensity of the myxoma. (b) and (c): short-axis views.

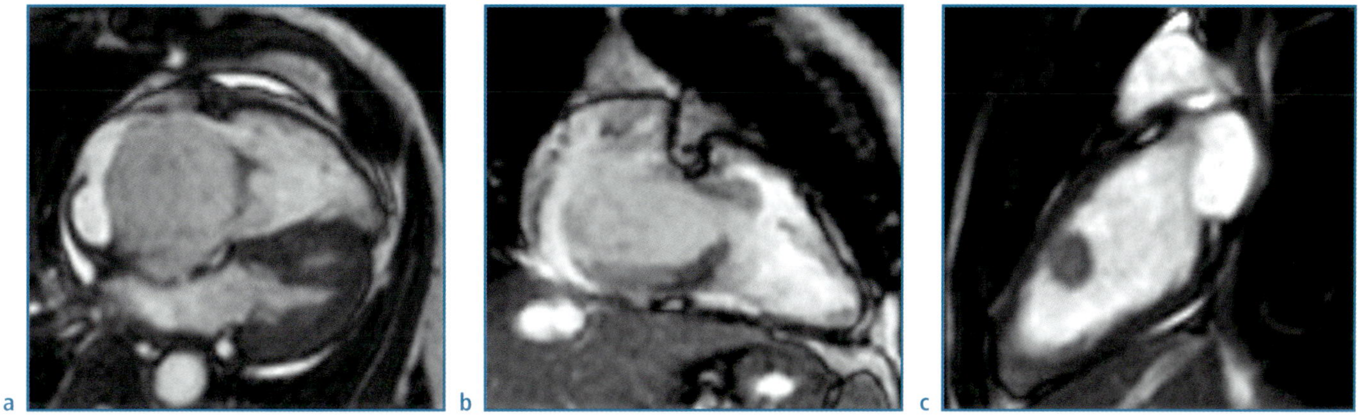

Figure 17-2 Large myxoma fixed at the right atrial site of the interatrial septum with prolapse into the right ventricle in a 4-ch (a) and 2-ch view (b). Atypical myxoma located at the anterior wall of the left ventricle in a 2-ch view (c).

crine hyperactivity, and other tumors such as testicular Sertoli cell tumor, psammomatous melanotic schwannoma, pituitary adenomas, and thyroid tumors (Wilkes 2006). Cardiac myxomas associated with Carney's syndrome show no age or gender predilection, can be single or multiple, can occur in any intracardiac location, and tend to recur with a rate of 20% after adequate surgical excision.

Clinical Presentation

Patients with symptomatic cardiac myxoma can have a variety of unspecific findings. The majority of patients will present with at least one of the typical triad of obstructive, embolic, or constitutional or systemic signs. Obstructive cardiac findings include dyspnea, dizziness, cough, pulmonary edema, and congestive heart failure as a result of mechanical obstruction of the mitral valve ring. Cardiac myxoma is the most common primary cardiac tumor to produce tumor emboli, which may occur in systemic and/or pulmonary circulation depending on its location and the patency of the foramen ovale. Constitutional and non-embolic findings secondary to cardiac myxoma include fever, fatigue, weight loss, arthralgia, myalgia, muscle weakness, and Raynaud's syndrome. Diagnosis is made by history (symptoms and signs), auscultation (eventually "tumor plop", pulmonary rales), ECG (left atrial enlargement, arrhythmias), and echocardiography (location, structure, and mobility of the tumor). For pre-operative assessment cardiac CT and most efficiently, CMR imaging should be used.

CMR Findings

Myxomas typically arise near the fossa ovalis of the interatrial septum, although some arise from free atrial walls and also, though rarely, from atrioventricular leaflets or ventricles (Figure 17-1 and Figure 17-2). Their contours are generally oval or round, sometimes lobulated with a smooth surface and narrow pedicle. On CMR images myxomas typically show a heterogenous appearance with intermediate signal intensity on T1-weighted and higher signal intensity on T2-weighted TSE sequences. If there are areas of subacute or chronic hemorrhage in the tumors, signal intensity may be high. To assess the mobility of the tumor and its attachment, cine-SSFP sequences should be used, particularly when a mobile left atrial myxoma protrudes into the mitral valve ring with subsequent obstruction. Due to their significant vascularization myxomas generally show moderate heterogenous enhancement after gadolinium injection.

Therapy

Treatment for symptomatic cardiac myxoma is prompt surgical resection of the tumor. Recurrence occurs in about 3% of cases, although the rate is higher with familial myxomas (between 3 mths and 14 yrs post-operatively).

17.6.2 Lipoma

Prevalence

The two most common fat-containing lesions in the heart are lipomatous interatrial septal hypertrophy (LHAS) and lipoma. Lipomas occur at any age with equal frequency in both sexes, but are observed most often in the middle and advanced ages. They constitute 8–12% of primary cardiac tumors.

Pathology

Lipomas are encapsulated and contain neoplastic mature fat cells with occasional fibrous connective tissue (fibrolipoma) and vacuolated brown fat (hibernoma-like). Areas of degeneration and radiographically apparent calcification may be present. Half of lipomas arise from the subendocardium and are relatively small, the other half are from either subepicardial (25%) or mid-myocardial layers (25%) (Grebenc 2000).

Clinical Presentation

Most cardiac lipomas are asymptomatic and typically present as incidental findings. But the tumor can produce a variety of symptoms depending on its location and size. Subendocardial lipomas with prominent intracavitary presence can interfere with mechanical function of the heart resulting in the clinical syndrome of heart failure. Subepicardial lipomas are usually asymptomatic, but large tumors may cause compression of the heart and produce pericardial effusion. Intramyocardial lipomas may interfere with the specialized conduction system in the heart and cause arrhythmias (e.g. AV block, supraventricular or ventricular extrasystoles). Diagnosis using conventional techniques (ECG, echocardiography) is difficult, even transesophageal echocardiography may detect location and size of the tumor, but may not be able to determine the tissue type because of the non-specific appearance of lipomas on ultrasound. Therefore, cardiac CT or preferentially CMR imaging should be used to clarify the diagnosis.

CMR Findings

Lipomas are preferentially located in the right atrium and the interatrial septum, with rare occurrence in the ventricles, and a size ranging from 1–8 cm in diameter. They usually have a homogenous signal on CMR images and have the same signal intensity as fat tissue, i.e. high signal intensity on T1- and lower signal intensity on T2-weighted TSE images. If cardiac lipoma is suspected a pre- and post-fat-saturated T1-weighted TSE sequence should be used, in which signal dropout is identified in the tumor in the fat-saturation sequence, confirming a fat-containing mass (Figure 17-3). Cine-CMR imaging using SSFP sequences should be used to localize the tumor, determine its size, and assess obstructive effects due to its size or location (e.g. on valves). Following gadolinium injection lipomas do not enhance (Kaplan and Rifkin 1989).

a
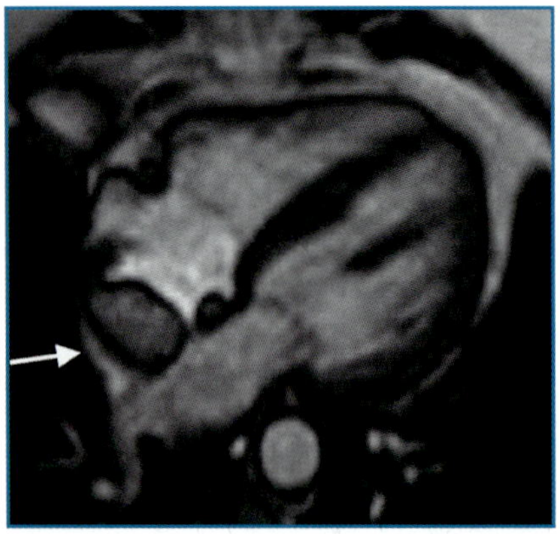
b
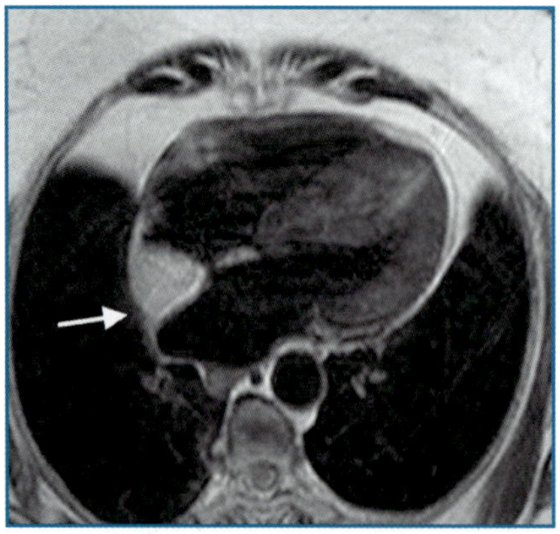
c
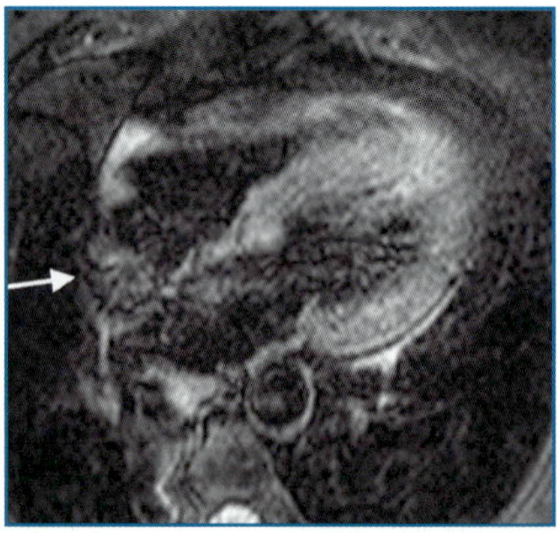

Figure 17-3 Right atrial lipoma (arrows) fixed at the roof and the interatrial septum in a 4-ch view with low signal intensity on SSFP (a), high signal intensity on black-blood (b), and signal void on fat suppression sequences (c).

Therapy

Symptomatic cardiac lipoma should be surgically resected, if location and size are appropriate for operation. The postoperative prognosis is excellent. CMR imaging may be the ideal technique to safely follow patients on conservative observation or after surgical treatment.

17.6.3 Papillary Fibroelastoma

Prevalence

This tumor is the third most common primary cardiac tumor with an incidence of up to 0.33% in autopsy series (2–33% of autoptic cases).

Pathology

Papillary fibroelastomas arise from endocardium with tumor sizes ranging from 2–70 mm with a mean diameter of about 10 mm. Macroscopically the tumor has been compared with the sea anemone because of its numerous and delicate papillary fronds. Papillary fibroelastoma is soft, white to tan (Grebenc 2000) and often friable with adherent thrombus, that is the likely source of embolic events. Histopathologically the tumor appears with narrow, elongated, avascular papillary fronds. Its surface is covered by a single layer of endothelial cells frequently presenting attached thrombi. The matrix of the papillary fronds consists of variable amounts of mucopolysaccharides, collagen, elastic fibers, and rare spindle cells resembling smooth muscle cells or fibroblasts.

Clinical Presentation

Most patients with papillary fibroelastoma are asymptomatic, but about half of the patients may present symptoms including angina, myocardial infarction, stroke, and dyspnea with cerebral emboli, and in rare instances subacute bacterial endocarditis. In contrast to cardiac myxoma, the embolic material from papillary fibroelastoma is considered to be fibrin or thrombus originating from the tumor surface. Fragments of the tumor itself have only rarely been found in the vessels involved. The incidence of embolic-type symptoms is about 6.6% within 1 yr follow-up (McManus 2012). Diagnosis may be made by history, symptoms, and transesophageal echocardiography, which may be sufficient in most cases. However, in unclear situations it is preferential to use CMR imaging to clarify the diagnosis.

CMR Findings

Papillary fibroelastomas are found in 80% of cases on aortic (37–45%) or mitral valves (15–25%), less commonly on the tricuspid (17%) or pulmonary valves (13%), or the left atrial or ventricular endocardium. On CMR images it typically appears as a small, round, homogenous mass, sometimes with a small pedicle that is usually attached to valvular structures (Figure 17-4). Cine-SSFP sequences may show a highly mobile, hypointensive mass with turbulent flow signal surrounding it. In T1-weighting signal intensity is intermediate and high in T2-weighted TSE images. Fat-saturation sequences differentiate papillary fibroelastoma from lipoma. The tumor does not show enhancement after injection of gadolinium, and in first-pass studies there is no perfusion. Both criteria may help to differentiate this benign tumor from a malignant tumor (Wintersprenger 2000).

Therapy

Treatment for papillary fibroelastoma is surgical excision with either reconstitution or, less commonly, replacement of the valve. Asymptomatic patients with small left-sided, nonmobile tumors should be cautiously observed, whereas patients with larger (≥ 1 cm) and/or mobile-type papillary fibroelastoma should be considered for excision. CMR

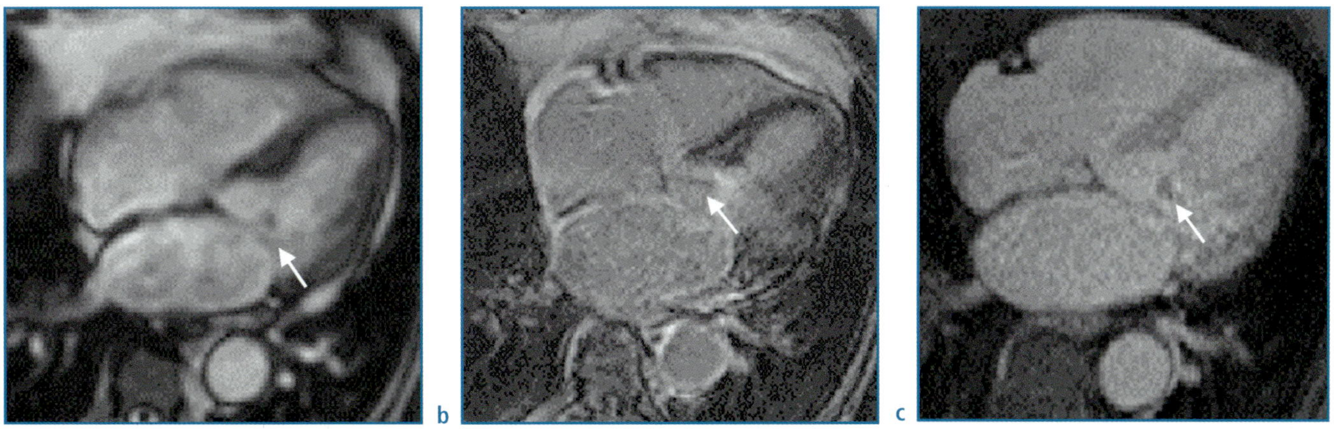

a b c

Figure 17-4 Left-sided papillary fibroelastoma (arrows) fixed at the anterior mitral leaflet imaged in a 4-ch view on a SSFP (a), T1-weighted (b), and gadolinium-enhanced sequence (c), depicted as a hypointense structure without contrast enhancement.

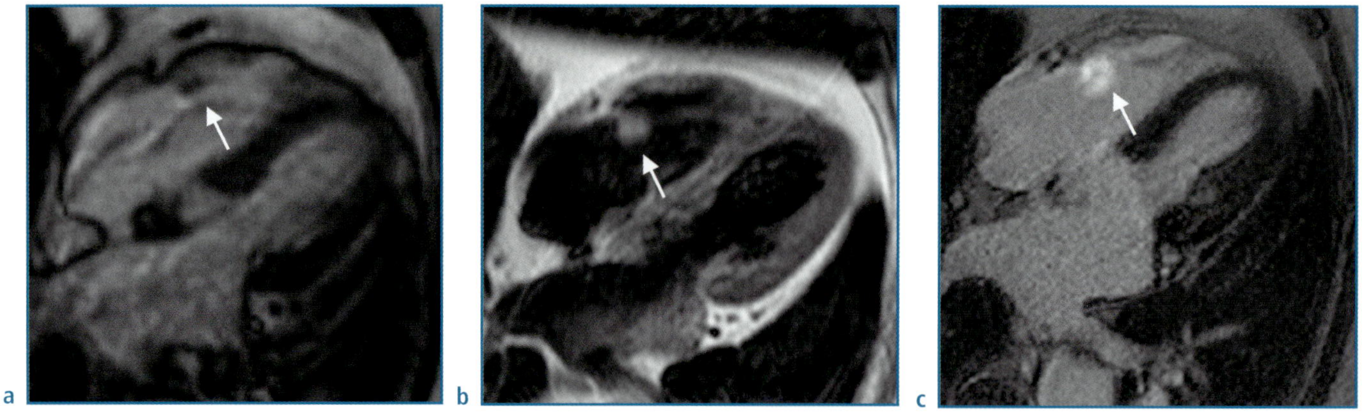

Figure 17-5 Fibroma (arrows) fixed at the lateral tricuspid leaflet in a 4-ch view on SSFP imaging (a), T2-weighted black-blood images (b), and a contrast-enhanced sequence (c), showing a low signal intensity in (a) and isointense signal in (b), but enhancement in the periphery with hypo-enhancement in the center of the tumor (c).

imaging may be the ideal technique to follow patients on conservative observation or after surgical treatment.

17.6.4 Fibroma

Prevalence

Cardiac fibromas are the second most common primary cardiac tumor in infants and children, about 90% of fibromas occur in children, although they may occur at any age up to 83 yrs. Some cases have been reported to be diagnosed prenatally by ultrasound (McManus 2012).

Pathology

Cardiac fibromas typically appear as solitary, rounded, intramural masses with a fibrous whorled cut surface. The tumor may be circumscribed or infiltrative with a pushing margin. The average size of the tumor is 5 cm, but lesions up to 10 cm have been reported. Histologically, cardiac fibromas show a proliferation of monomorphic fibroblasts with little or no cellular atypia. The degree of cellularity decreases with age, whereas the amount of collagen increases with age (Burke and Virmani 1996).

Clinical Presentation

Depending on size and location of the tumor patients may present with heart failure, chest pain, arrhythmias, syncope, and sudden cardiac arrest (the latter in 14% of patients, most commonly during childhood). Up to one third of patients may remain asymptomatic. In decreasing order symptoms are congestive heart failure in 21%, ventricular tachyarrhythmias in 13%, and atypical chest pain in 3.5% of cases (Parmley 1988). The ECG may reveal left or right ventricular hypertrophy, bundle branch block, AV block, and ventricular tachycardias. Using echocardiography cardiac fibroma appears as a solitary homogenous echogenic lesion. Diagnosis may be confirmed by cardiac CT or CMR imaging.

CMR Findings

The tumor typically appears as a solitary, well-defined mass in the myocardium, usually involving the interventricular septum or the left ventricular free wall, and often revealing central calcifications, which help to differentiate it from rhabdomyoma. CMR images of the tumor show characteristic inhomogenous or slightly hyperintensive signal intensities on T1-weighted and hypointensive signal on T2-weighted images in comparison to normal myocardium (Fujita 1994, O'Donnell 2009). Central calcifications may be represented by low signal areas in the tumor, which may be better imaged by cardiac CT. On gadolinium injection there is only slight or no enhancement compared to the surrounding normal myocardium due to the minimal vascular supply of cardiac fibromas. On T1-weighted images the tumor may show central hypointense areas with a well-demarcated isointense surrounding shell after gadolinium administration (Figure 17-5).

Therapy

In symptomatic patients complete surgical resection is recommended. Post-operative prognosis is generally good, although some surgical attempts in infants younger than 4 mths have resulted in death. Patients with very extensive tumors that are not entirely resectable can benefit from partial tumor excision. Cardiac fibromas remain stable in size for many years or may regress. CMR imaging may be the ideal technique to follow patients on conservative observation or after surgical treatment.

17.6.5 Rhabdomyoma

Prevalence

Cardiac rhabdomyoma is the most common primary tumor in infants and children, and about 80 % of tumors occur under 1 yr of age. Most tumors are diagnosed in neonates due to the routine use of prenatal ultrasound. Rare cases occur in adults, showing some phenotypic differences from the more-typically encountered fetal-type rhabdomyomas (McManus 2012).

Pathology

The tumor typically appears as a yellow-gray, firm, circumscribed lobulated mass with a size of 1–9 cm. Histologically the tumor is a well-demarcated lesion, composed of enlarged cells with clear cytoplasm and occasional "spider cells" (McManus 2012). Up to 50 % of cardiac rhabdomyomas are observed in combination with tuberous sclerosis (Bourneville-Pringle syndrome). This autosomal-dominant neurocutaneous dysplasia (phacomatosis) consists of glia proliferation, multiple calcified tumors of the brain ventricles, and multiple skin fibroadenomas (adenoma sebaceum, nevus Pringle). Clinical manifestations are epileptical seizures and oligophrenia.

Clinical Presentation

Type and severity of clinical symptoms depend on localisation and size of the tumor. Small intramural tumors often do not produce relevant symptoms, whereas larger intramural rhabdomyomas located within the interventricular septum may interfere with the specialized conduction system, resulting in complete AV block. Intramural rhabdomyomas may produce supraventricular or ventricular tachycardias, in some cases being the cause of sudden cardiac death. Intracavitary tumors may obstruct the ventricular cavum or the outflow tract with concomitant symptoms of heart failure.

CMR Findings

Cardiac rhabdomyomas are primarily (90 %) located in the ventricles with equal prevalence in the left and right ventricle. In 90 % of cases they are multiple, located intramurally and may be detected by CMR imaging given a minimal size of 1–2 mm (Rienmüller 1989). They mostly appear as solid and homogenous with low signal intensity on T1-weighted and slight hyperintensity on T2-weighted TSE images. They show typically minimal (Lundt 1989, Winkler and Higgins 1987) or no enhancement with gadolinium.

Therapy

Most cardiac rhabdomyomas show spontaneous regression before age 6. Therefore conservative clinical observation is mandatory in about 80 % of cases. In symptomatic patients with significant outflow tract obstructions, arrhythmias, or hypoxic spells, surgical excision with removal of the culprit portion of the tumor is sufficient. No recurrence has been reported for cardiac rhabdomyoma, and the prognosis is excellent. CMR imaging may be the ideal technique to follow patients on conservative observation or after surgical treatment.

17.6.6 Pheochromocytoma (Paraganglioma)

Prevalence

Cardiac pheochromocytomas (paragangliomas) are extremely rare neoplasms, the total prevalence is 0.07–0.3 % according to section statistics, and 2 of 1.0 million people according to epidemiologic data. Most lesions have been reported in adult patients with an age range of 18–85 yrs.

Pathology

Pheochromocytomas are primary benign tumors arising from neuroectodermal chromaffin cells primarily within the adrenal medulla and abdomen, but they may arise anywhere within the plexi of sympathetic adrenergic nerves. In the heart they are localized at the posterior left atrial wall, at the roof of the right atrium, at the interatrial septum, and along the coronary arteries, usually with a broad attachment to the corresponding walls of the heart. 80–90 % of all pheochromocytomas are located in the abdomen, and only 10–20 % are localized outside the adrenals. They are well-vascularized and their size may range between 3–8 cm. Histologically they are composed of nests of paraganglial cells surrounded by sustentacular cells.

Clinical Presentation

Patients may suffer from permanent or phasic secretion of catecholamines with consecutive symptoms like excessive sweating, headache, palpitations, tremulousness, chest pain, muscle weakness, and abdominal pain. Further signs are tachycardia, arterial hypertension, and weight loss. In some patients impaired left ventricular function may occur, possibly driven by left ventricular hypertrophy from associated hypertension, potential adverse effects of excess catecholamines on myocyte structure and contractility, and changes in coronary arteries including thickening of the media, potentially impairing blood flow to the myocardium. Diagnosis may be confirmed by demonstrating an increase in norepinephrine or epinephrine or its metabolites either in serum or blood. Quantitative 24 h urinary metanephrines are the most reliable screening procedures. Cardiac CT and CMR imaging are the preferred tools to detect cardiac pheochromocytoma and to confirm the diagnosis.

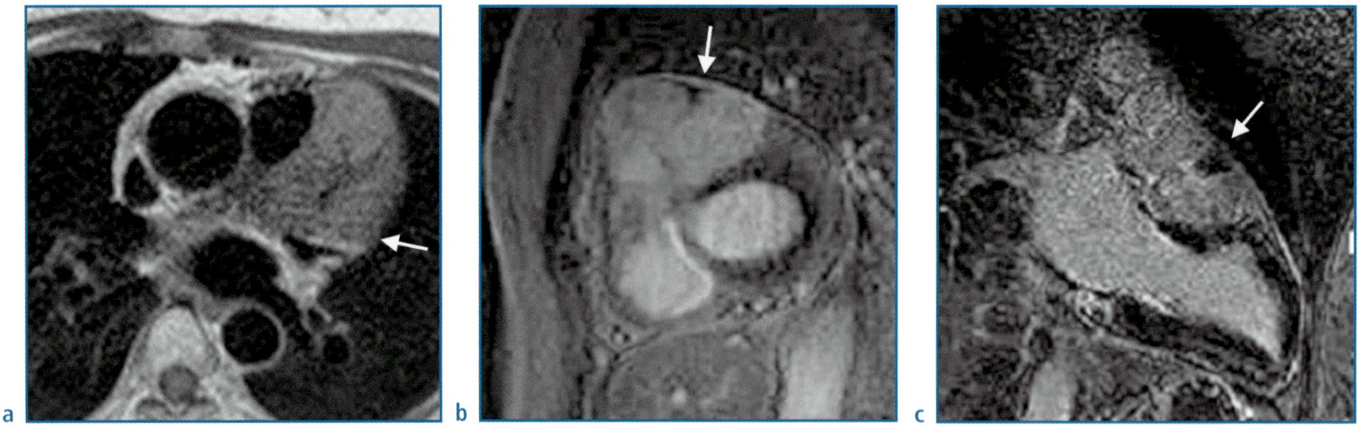

Figure 17-6 Pheochromocytoma (arrows) located within the sulcus interventricularis anterior in black-blood sequence and short-axis view (a), and with contrast enhancement after gadolinium injection in an axial (b) and 2-ch view (c).

CMR Findings

Using cine-SSFP sequences the size and intrapericardial location of the tumor(s) can be detected, appearing as single nodes or like a chord. Impaired left ventricular function can also be clearly assessed through cine-SSFP imaging, as can myocardial damage or scarring be detected by gadolinium studies. In T1-weighted TSE images the tumors are hypointensive, in T2-weighted images very hyperintensive. Following gadolinium injection the tumor(s) show strong, sometimes heterogenous hyperenhancement due to tumor necrosis (Figure 17-6).

Therapy

Definitive treatment of cardiac pheochromocytoma requires surgical resection of the lesion. It is usually successful and provides complete symptomatic relief. Because paragangliomas may be infiltrative, extensive resection of the atrial wall may be required for complete excision. CMR imaging may be the ideal technique to follow patients after surgical treatment.

17.6.7 Hemangioma

Prevalence

Primary benign vascular tumors of the heart are hemangioma, lymphangiomas, and hemangioendotheliomas. Lymphangiomas and hemangioendotheliomas are extremely rare tumors, whereas hemangioma is more common. It accounts for less than 2% of all cardiac neoplasms, but for 5–10% of primary benign cardiac tumors.

Pathology

Cardiac hemangiomas may originate from endocardium, epicardium, pericardium, or from ventricular myocardium including the interventricular septum. It may occur in any chamber, intracavitary, intramural, or as an epicardial/pericardial lesion with a size of 1–8 cm. Cardiac hemangiomas are classified into three subtypes: cavernous (composed of multiple thin-walled, dilated vessels), capillary (composed of smaller capillary-like vessels), and arteriovenous (composed of thick-walled dysplastic arteries, venous-like vessels, and capillaries). Intramural hemangiomas may be capillary, cavernous, or arteriovenous and may contain other tissue elements like fat or fibrous tissue. Endocardial hemangiomas are usually of capillary nature or mixed cavernous-capillary nature. They often present with a myxoid stroma and sparse inflammatory background (Grebenc 2000).

Clinical Presentation

Most affected patients are asymptomatic and the tumor is detected incidentally. Depending on the nature and location of the tumor, patients can present with chest pain, dyspnea on exertion, ventricular outflow tract obstruction, arrhythmias, right-sided heart failure, pericarditis and pericardial effusion, cerebral embolism, syncope, and sudden death. In some cases giant cardiac hemangiomas can results in Kasabach-Merrit syndrome characterized by multiple systemic and cardiac hemangiomas, recurrent consumptive thrombocytopenia, and coagulopathy (Brizard 1993).

CMR Findings

Intramural hemangiomas are often poorly circumscribed, spongy masses that appear hemorrhagic or congested. Endocardial-based hemangiomas are well-circumscribed, variably myxoid, soft masses (Grebenc 2000). CMR imaging shows that hemangiomas have an isointense or increased intensity on T1-weighted TSE images because of slow blood flow in the tumor. They are hyperintense on T2-weighted TSE images and show intense enhancement after injection of gadolinium contrast agents (Kemp 1996) due to the vascular nature of the tumor (Figure 17-7). Sometimes enhancement

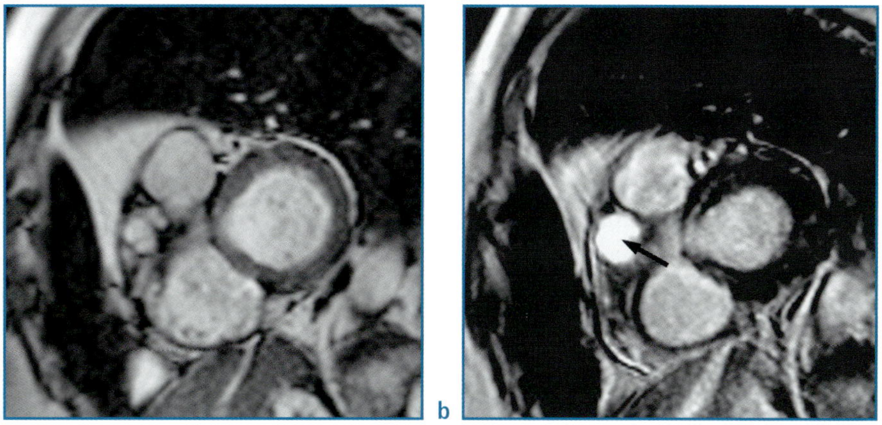

Figure 17-7 Intraepicardial hemangioma located within the corner of RVOT, aortic root and right atrium, with inhomogenous signal intensity on SSFP sequences (a) and bright enhancement after gadolinium injection on a T1-TFE-IR sequence (arrow) (b).

may be heterogenous because of calcifications or fibrous septa within the tumor (Seline 1990). A variant of hemangiomas, the cavernous hemangioma, does not show significant enhancement because of the very slow flow in the tumor.

Therapy

The tumor can be successfully excised, with surgical resection being the treatment of choice for symptomatic patients or in cases with uncertain diagnosis. The long-term outcome of patients with surgically treated symptomatic lesions is excellent (Brizard 1993). Sometimes spontaneous regression of the tumor may occur. Therefore faithful observation may be the treatment of choice, particularly in patients with large but asymptomatic hemangiomas, when surgical resection may be complex and potentially hazardous (Brizard 1993). CMR imaging may be the ideal technique to follow patients on conservative observation or after surgical treatment.

17.6.8 Teratoma

Prevalence

Pericardial teratoma is a rare, benign germ cell neoplasm that typically affects infants and children.

Pathology

Pericardial teratomas are usually right-sided masses, typically connected to one of the great vessels via a pedicle. Most cardiac teratomas are located within the pericardial sac and are rarely intramyocardial. The tumor contains derivatives of all three germ layers, with mature endodermal, mesodermal, and ectodermal elements; tissues discovered in pericardial teratomas include neuroglia, cartilage, skeletal muscle, liver, intestine, pancreas, and glandular tissue (Grebenc 2000).

Clinical Presentation

Patients present with respiratory distress, peripheral cyanosis, and heart failure secondary to pericardial compression or tamponade and compression of right-sided vascular structures such as the right atrium, superior vena cava, pulmonary artery, or aorta. Pericardial tamponade is a common cause of fetal death in affected patients.

CMR Findings

Like echocardiography, CMR imaging may show an intrapericardial heterogenous and complex multi-locular cystic mass. The mass is typically positioned at the right side of the heart, which may encase or compress the heart and the great vessels, frequently with associated pericardial effusion. Furthermore, CMR imaging will provide additional information on the relationship of the tumor to the great vessels, the normal myocardium, or other mediastinal structures. Signal intensity is heterogenous due to multiple tissue components of the tumor and foci of calcification.

Therapy

Patients with large intrapericardial teratomas usually require initial emergency and life-saving therapy with pericardiocentesis. In all cases urgent surgical resection is required because of the life-threatening nature of the lesion. Prognosis of surgically treated patients is generally good. CMR imaging may be the ideal technique to follow patients after surgical treatment.

17.7 Malignant Cardiac Tumors

About 25 % of all primary cardiac tumors are malignant and have already developed metastases in about 75 % of cases at the time of diagnosis. Preferred localisations of metastases are the lung, pleura, mediastinum, brain, bone, and the liver. About 95% of malignant tumors are different types of sarcomas; the remaining 5% are lymphomas or other rare malignant tumors. Of cardiac sarcomas the most common cell types are sarcoma (37% of cases), undifferentiated or unclassified sarcoma (24%), malignant fibrous histiocytoma (11–24%), leiomyosarcoma (8–9%), and osteosarcoma (3–9%). About 10% of surgically resected cardiac tumors are primary sarcomas (Grebenc 2000).

Typical features of malignant primary tumors of the heart are their manifestation in more than one cardiac chamber, extension into the pulmonary veins or arteries, broad attachment to the heart itself, necrosis in the lesion, extension beyond cardiac boundaries, and in many cases an hemorrhagic pericardial effusion with pericardial contrast enhancement. Another feature of a malignant cardiac tumor may be its intramural and intracavitary location.

17.7.1 Angiosarcoma

Prevalence

Primary cardiac angiosarcomas are the most common type of cardiac sarcoma in adults and account for 30–37% of all cases. Cardiac angiosarcomas typically occur in adults 30–50 yrs of age, but can occur between 2 and 80 yrs; a slight male predilection exists.

Pathology

Angiosarcomas are generally large, grossly hemorrhagic, multi-lobular, right atrial masses that spread along the epicardial surface, replace the right atrial wall, and may protrude into or fill the adjacent cardiac chambers (Grebenc 2000). Microscopically, angiosarcoma presents with irregular anastomosing vascular channels lined by atypical endothelial cells.

Clinical Presentation

The tumor may remain silent clinically for a long time. However, at initial presentation patients typically show advanced disease with 66–89% of patients demonstrating evidence of metastatic disease. Depending on localisation and size, intracavitary angiosarcomas induce in particular dyspnea, chest pain, arrhythmias, and evidence of congestive heart failure. Approximately 80–90% of cardiac angiosarcomas occur in the right atrium and involve the pericardium with consecutive symptoms from right-sided heart inflow obstructions or cardiac tamponade. Because of the general propensity of cardiac angiosarcoma to grow into the pericardium, pericardial effusion (most commonly hemorrhagic) and cardiac tamponade with dyspnea, tachycardia, hypotension etc. may be present. Less commonly, symptoms related to metastatic disease such as stroke-like neurologic symptoms due to cerebral metastases may occur. In about 25% of cases patients complain of precordial pain.

CMR Findings

CMR imaging typically demonstrates cardiac angiosarcomas as large, heterogenous, invasive right atrial masses. They are frequently associated with extensive pericardial involvement and hemorrhagic pericardial effusion. Signal intensity in these tumors is heterogenous because of their propensity for necrosis and hemorrhage. On T1-weighted TSE images angiosarcomas typically show low-signal intensity, whereas T2-weighted TSE images typically demonstrate increased signal intensity and central areas of hypointensity, consistent with necrosis and hemorrhage, as well as areas of moderate signal intensity in more peripheral regions (Best 2003). Because of their high vascularity angiosarcomas show a strong signal enhancement after i.v.-administration of gadolinium that is sometimes accompanied with linear signal enhancement along the vascular channels in the

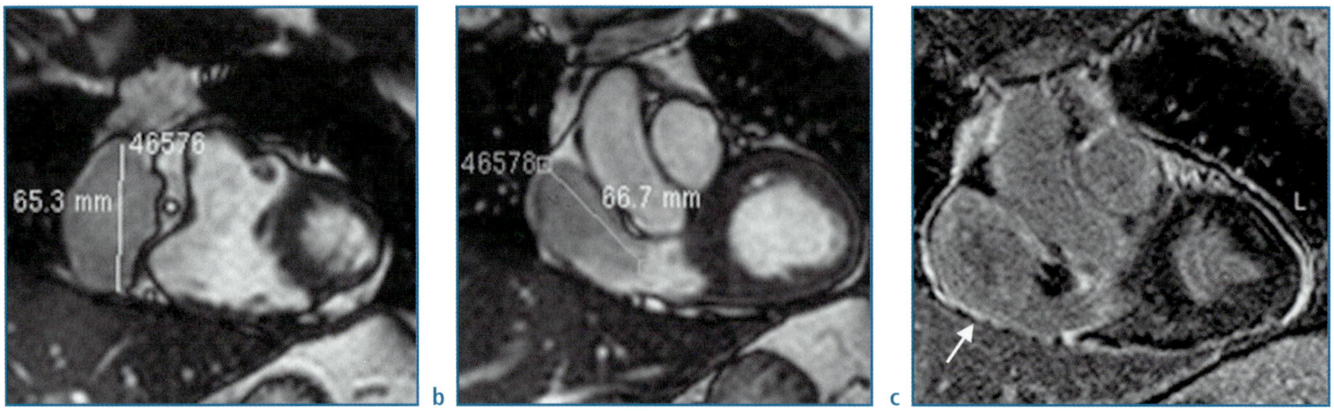

a b c

Figure 17-8 Short-axis views showing an angiosarcoma within the right atrium (diameter 6.6 cm) on a SSFP sequence **(a, b)**, and "sun-ray-phenomenon" after gadolinium injection on a T1-TFE-IR sequence (arrow) **(c)**.

tumor, known as the "sun ray phenomenon" (Yahata 1994) (Figure 17-8).

Therapy

Since primary cardiac sarcomas are highly aggressive lesions, they are uniformly fatal. However, aggressive surgery offers significant palliation of symptoms, caused by valvular and vascular obstruction, and improves survival. Complete tumor excision does not prevent local recurrence and metastatic disease, which occurs frequently and usually within one year. Heart transplantation has been performed in some cases but remains controversial in this setting. For patients with advanced disease, palliative treatment including the use of stents for SVC syndrome and for RVOT obstruction may help to improve the patient's short-term quality of life (McManus 2012). CMR imaging may be helpful to follow patients after surgical treatment and to detect early recurrence of the tumor with potential complications.

17.7.2 Rhabdomyosarcoma

Prevalence

Cardiac rhabadomyosarcoma is the most common primary sarcoma of the heart in children and the second most common malignant lesion in adults. Its manifestation is during second half of life, with a slight male predominance particularly in the pediatric population.

Pathology

These tumors are localized in any region of the myocardium with frequent infiltrative growth and/or protrusion into the cavities of the heart. Microscopically the tumor consists of primitive striated muscle fibers.

Clinical Presentation

Patients present with symptoms and findings of congestive heart failure, cardiac murmurs, arrhythmias, and constitutional symptoms with hypereosinophilia, hypertrophic osteoarthropathia, and polyarthritis. Intramural growth leads most commonly to arrhythmias, whereas intracavitary location with consecutive obstruction results in impairment of pump function, limitation of cardiac output on exercise, and pulmonary congestion (secondary pulmonary hypertension). Because rhabdomyosarcomas are aggressive neoplasms they have the tendency to produce local or distant metastases, most commonly to the lymph nodes and the lung.

CMR Findings

CMR imaging may present cardiac rhabdomyosarcomas as large, heterogenous, invasive intramural masses that eventually protrude into an atrial or ventricular cavity. On T1-weighted TSE images rhabdomyosarcomas show low-signal intensity, whereas T2-weighted TSE images demonstrate increased signal intensity. On gadolinium administration these lesions show a moderate to strong enhancement similar to normal ventricular myocardium.

Therapy

Because of its aggressive nature cardiac rhabdomysarcoma has a poor prognosis with patients surviving less than one year. The primary aim of treatment is complete surgical resection, but the highly infiltrative nature of the tumor often precludes such an attempt. The tumor also has a poor response to radiation and chemotherapy. CMR imaging may be helpful to follow patients after surgical treatment and to detect early recurrence of the tumor with potential complications. In selected cases heart transplantation may be considered if distant metastases are not detectable.

17.7.3 Leiomyosarcoma

Prevalence

Leiomyosarcoma represents about 8 % of cardiac sarcomas and affects patients during the fourth decade. The exact oncogenesis is unknown.

Pathology

This sarcoma is a malignant mesenchymal tumor that demonstrates smooth muscle differentiation. Approximately 70–80 % of leiomyosarcomas arise from the left atrium. They are sessile, lobulated, irregular masses, and multiple in 30 % of cases.

Clinical Presentation

Common clinical presentations include chest pain, dyspnea, atrial arrhythmias, pericardial effusion, and congestive heart failure.

CMR Findings

The tumor appears as an irregular lobulated mass most commonly attached to the posterior wall of the left atrium, with frequent invasion of the pulmonary veins. CMR images are non-specific with intermediate signal intensities of the tumor on T1-weighted and increased signal intensity on T2-weighted TSE images, and moderate gadolinium enhancement (Figure 17-9).

Therapy

The primary aim of treatment is complete surgical resection, but the infiltrative nature of this tumor often precludes such an attempt. The prognosis is generally poor with a high recurrence rate after surgical therapy. CMR imaging may be helpful to follow patients after surgical treatment and to

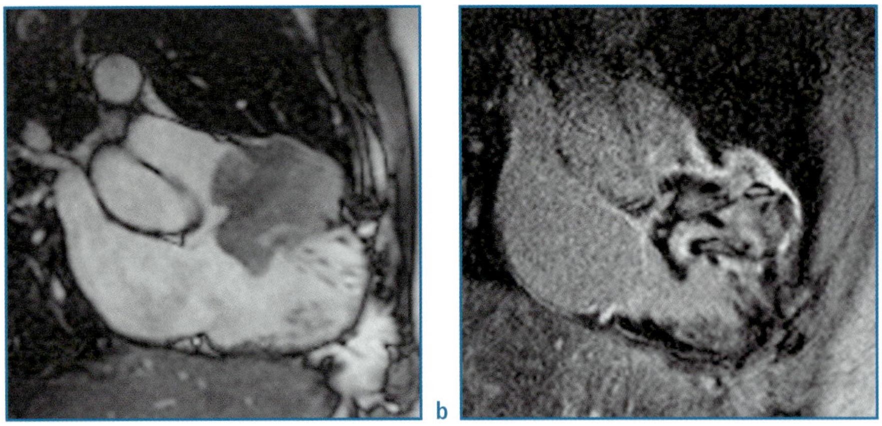

Figure 17-9 Recurrence of a surgically resected leiomyosarcoma within the right ventricle and RVOT (rv-long-axis view) with low signal intensity in a SSFP sequence (a), and irregular contrast enhancement after gadolinium injection (b).

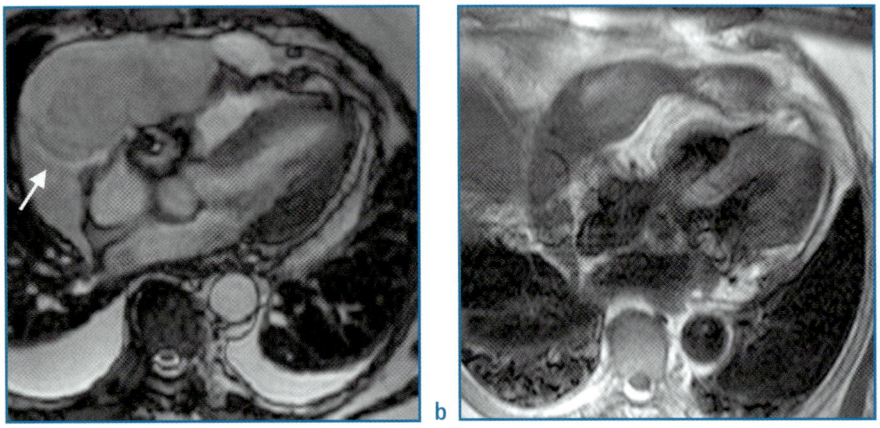

Figure 17-10 Large liposarcoma located on the entire wall of the right atrium in a 4-ch view on a SSFP (arrow) (a) and T1-weighted black-blood sequence (b) showing infiltrative growth of the tumor.

detect early recurrence of the tumor with potential complications (Figure 17-9).

17.7.4 Fibrosarcoma, Liposarcoma and Osteosarcoma

Prevalence

Fibrosarcoma represents about 5% of cardiac sarcomas, and liposarcoma is extremely rare, accounting for less than 1% of cardiac sarcomas. Cardiac osteosarcomas, however, make up about 3–9% of primary malignant cardiac tumors.

Pathology

These tumors arise from mesenchymal tissue. Like osteosarcoma and leiomyosarcoma, fibrosarcoma tends to occur in the left atrium, but may also be found in different cardiac chambers. Liposarcoma may occur in any cardiac chamber and may show pericardial and valve involvement (Figure 17-10). Primary liposarcomas are generally large with areas of necrosis and hemorrhage. Osteosarcoma commonly contains large foci of calcification, which are its most distinguishing imaging feature.

Clinical Presentation

Fibrosarcoma and osteosarcoma manifest mainly as congestive heart failure due to their preferred location in the left atrium. Liposarcoma may additionally cause valvular dysfunction.

CMR Findings

Fibrosarcomas demonstrate unspecific CMR findings with heterogenous signal intensity on T1-weighted TSE images without significant gadolinium enhancement. Liposarcomas appear as masses with heterogenous high signal intensity on T1-weighted TSE images and show mild gadolinium enhancement (Figure 17-11). Osteosarcoma shows a broad base of attachment and aggressive invasion of local vascular structures such as the pulmonary veins. In the central parts of the tumor, signal loss may be present due to foci of calcifications, which may be better imaged by cardiac CT.

Therapy

The primary aim of treatment is complete surgical resection, but the infiltrative nature of these tumors often precludes such an attempt. The prognosis of all tumors is

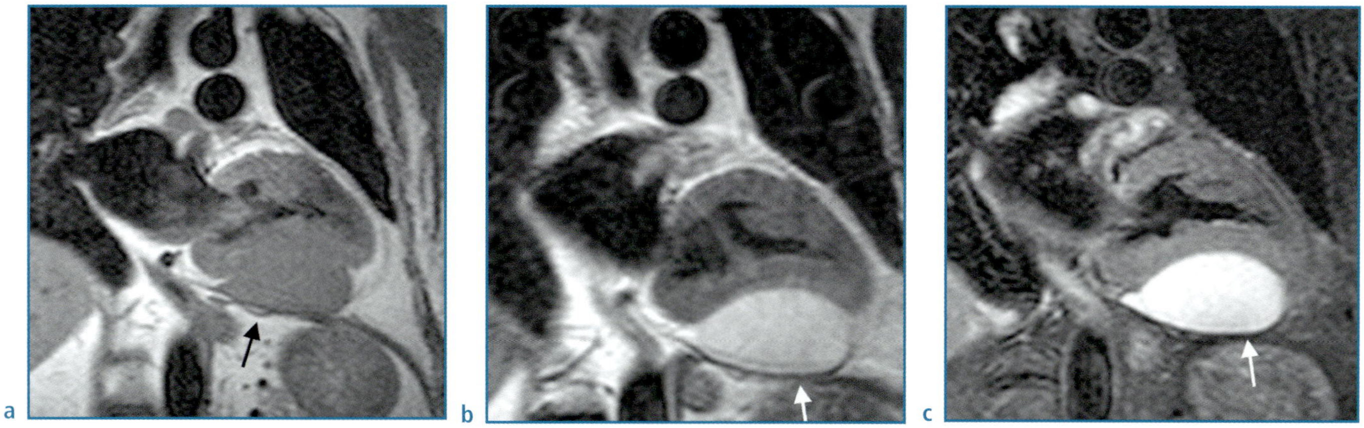

Figure 17-11 Liposarcoma at the inferior left ventricular wall infiltrating the diaphragm (arrows) in a 2-ch view with intermediate signal intensity on a T1-weighted black-blood sequence (a), and high signal intensity in a T2-weighted black-blood (b) and fat suppression sequence (c).

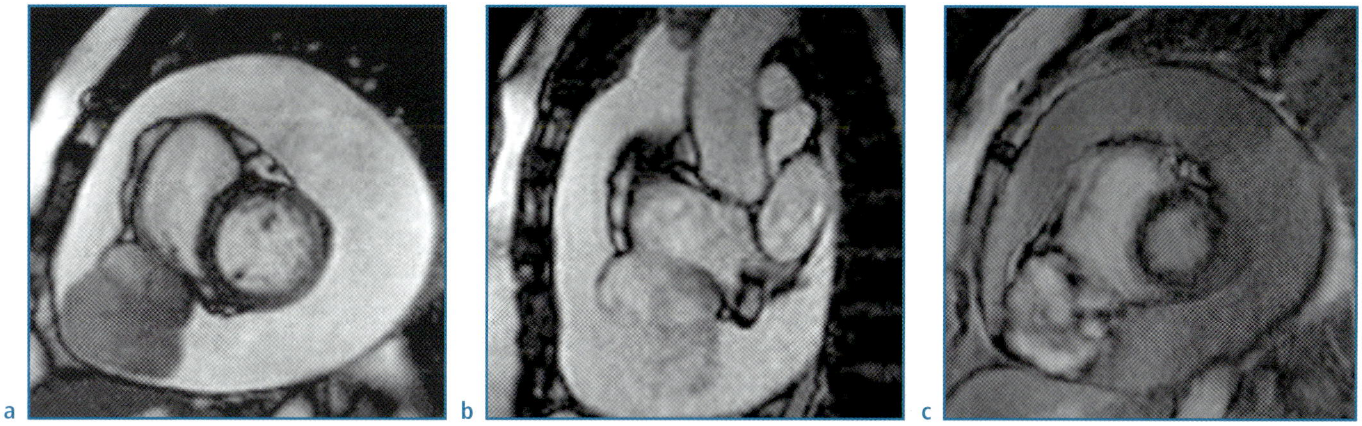

Figure 17-12 Fibromyxosarcoma on a SSFP sequence in a short-axis view (a) and a RVOT plane (b), and short-axis view on a T1-TFE inversion recovery sequence (c) shown as a heterogenous cardiac mass at the right ventricular diaphragmatic wall with a large pericardial effusion and heterogenous contrast enhancement.

generally poor with a high recurrence rate after surgical therapy. CMR imaging may be helpful to follow patients after surgical treatment and to detect early recurrence of the tumor with potential complications.

17.7.5 Malignant Fibrous Histiocytoma

Prevalence

Among the extremely rare avascular malignant tumors of the heart (undifferentiated sarcoma, myxosarcoma, synovial sarcoma) fibrous histiocytoma is the most common sarcoma.

Pathology

The tumor consists of a mix of malignant fibroblasts and histiocytes and sometimes myxoid areas. Its pathogenesis is unclear. Its preferred location is the left atrium with aggressive invasion into local thoracic vascular structures. The blood supply commonly arises from the coronary arteries.

Clinical Presentation

Depending on localization and size the tumor presents with unspecific chest pain, dyspnea, and signs of congestive heart failure.

CMR Findings

The location of the tumor is most commonly at the posterior wall of the left atrium, with an irregular tumor mass. In an advanced stage it infiltrates the atrial wall and the pericardium with subsequent hemorrhagic pericardial effusion. On T1-weighted images the tumor appears isointense, and shows a mild to moderate enhancement after administration of gadolinium (Figure 17-12).

Therapy

The primary aim of treatment is complete surgical resection, but the infiltrative nature of these tumors often pre-

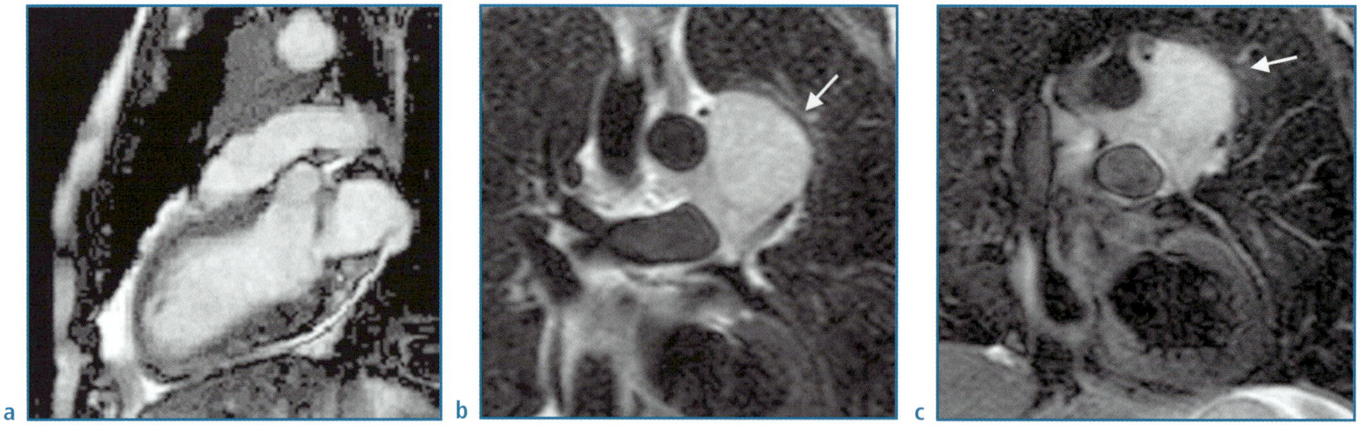

Figure 17-13 Malignant lymphoma (arrows) in a SSFP sequence in 2-ch (a) and a black-blood sequence without (b) and with fat suppression (c) in an axial view (b and c), characterized as a low signal intensity (a) and high signal intensity tumor (b and c) with infiltrative growth.

cludes such an attempt. The prognosis of all tumors is generally poor with a high recurrence rate after surgical therapy. CMR imaging may be helpful to follow patients after surgical treatment and to detect early recurrence of the tumor with potential complications.

17.7.6 Malignant Lymphoma

Prevalence

Although 16–28 % of patients with disseminated lymphoma have cardiac involvement, primary malignant lymphoma of the heart is extremely rare. It accounts for 1.3–2 % of primary cardiac tumors. The mean age at presentation is approximately 60 yrs (range 13–90 yrs) with a slight male predominance.

Pathology

Primary cardiac lymphomas are typically of the non-Hodgkin type and, by definition, involve only the heart or pericardium at the time of diagnosis with no evidence of extracardiac lymphoma. Cardiac lymphoma is an aggressive B-cell lymphoma, most commonly occurring in immunocompromised patients and particularly associated with AIDS. Cardiac lymphoma manifests with multiple, firm, white nodular masses with a fish-flesh, homogenous appearance, although foci of necrosis may occur (Grebenc 2000).

Clinical Presentation

Patients present with unresponsive, rapidly progressive heart failure (52 %), chest pain (17 %), constitutional symptoms (17 %), arrhythmias (12 %), superior vena cava syndrome, and cardiac tamponade (12 %). Most primary cardiac lymphomas are either diagnosed at autopsy, or are fatal soon after diagnosis (Grebenc 2000).

CMR Findings

The tumor usually arises from the right side of the heart, often from the right atrium, and is frequently accompanied by a large pericardial effusion. At presentation it is generally a large poorly marginated mass with variable morphology with either diffuse infiltration of the right atrium and/or ventricle or multiple nodules. The lesions are isointense to slightly hypointense relative to cardiac muscle on T1-weighted and isointense on proton density- and T2-weighted images. They further show heterogenous enhancement after administration of gadolinium (Figure 17-13).

Therapy

The prognosis of patients with primary cardiac lymphoma is very poor. Early diagnosis and treatment with chemotherapy may result in remission of the disease, palliation of pain, and longer survival. There is no evidence that surgery improves prognosis, although tumor debulking may be an effective palliative procedure (Nand 1991). Soon after initiation of chemotherapy patients may show a rapid deterioration due to tumor lysis with concomitant heart failure, arrhythmias, or even cardiac rupture. In some rare cases a complete remission of the disease has been observed following autologous stem cell transplantation (Porcar-Ramells 2002). CMR imaging may be extremely helpful to detect early life-threatening complications on chemotherapy, to follow patients after conservative treatment, and to detect early recurrence of the tumor with potential complications.

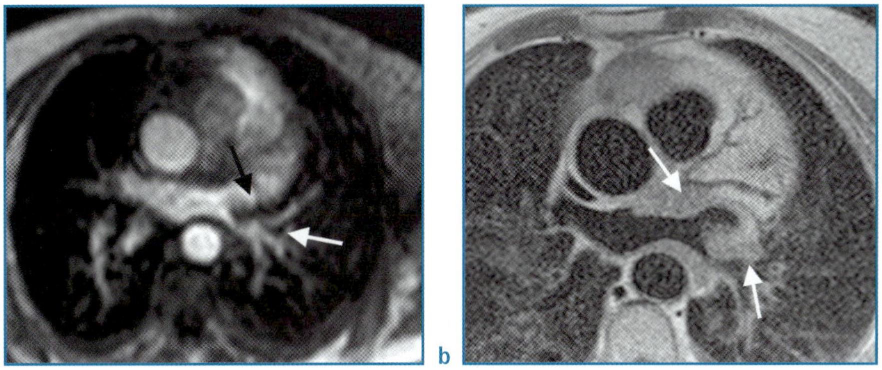

Figure 17-14 Metastasizing adenocarcinoma of the lung (bronchial carcinoma) in axial views on a SSFP (a) and T2-weighted black-blood sequence (b): The tumor is located around the left atrium with metastases (arrows) at the mouth of the left superior and inferior pulmonary veins.

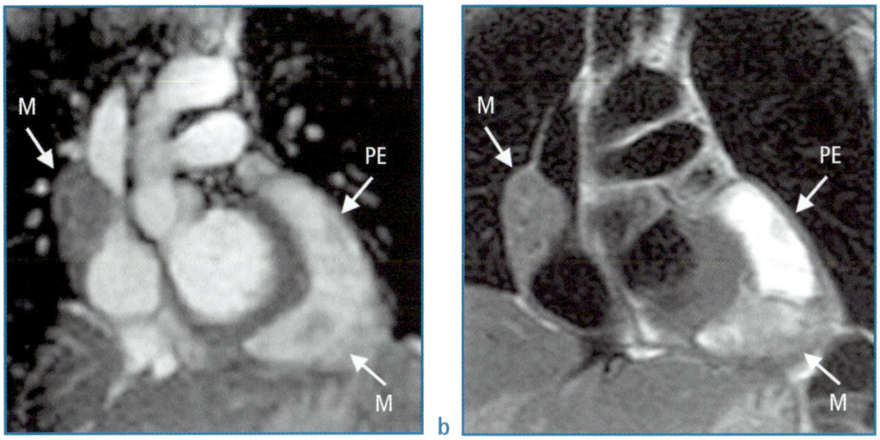

Figure 17-15 Metastasizing melanoma of the uvea in a coronal view using a SSFP (a) and proton density black-blood sequence (b) identified as a heterogenous mass (M) on top of the left ventricle and an isointense solid part in the superior caval vein (arrows, M), together with a pericardial effusion (PE).

17.8 Secondary Cardiac Tumors (Cardiac Metastasis)

Cardiac metastases are much more common than primary cardiac tumors (20–40 times). Their incidence on autopsy statistics is 1%, though metastases are rarely located solely in the heart. Also rarely does cardiac metastasis occur as the first clinical feature of malignancy, most patients with cardiac metastases are asymptomatic, and their diagnosis is generally made post-mortem. Cardiac metastasis may occur via one of the following four pathways: direct invasion (infiltration), transvenous extension, lymphatic extension, or hematogenous spread (Chiles 2001). The most common metastases to the heart and pericardium are from lung cancer (Figure 17-14) because of its proximity and the high prevalence of the tumor itself. The second most common metastasizing tumors are tumors of the breast, kidney, and esophagus, as well as lymphoma, leukemia, and melanoma (O'Donnell 2009).

Myocardial metastases are often associated with melanoma (50% of patients with disseminated melanoma show cardiac metastases post-mortem) (Figure 17-15) and with lymphoma and are suggestive of hematogenous spread. In patients with leukemia the heart is also frequently involved, leukemic infiltrations are localized between myocardial muscle cells and show massive deposits histologically. Renal cell carcinoma may spread via the inferior caval vein with tumor thrombus into the right atrium. Obliteration of a pulmonary vein may be suggestive of a bronchogenic carcinoma. Malignant pericardial effusion is the most common manifestation of metastasis, most likely through lymphatic spread or direct invasion from adjacent tissues such as lungs, lymph nodes, and breasts (O'Donnell 2009).

CMR imaging may be extremely helpful to demonstrate infiltration of the heart by an adjacent or peripheral tumor (Figure 17-16). The exact imaging of tumor invasion depth into the cardiac muscle or chamber is important for planning surgical resection. If the tumor has broken through the atrial or ventricular wall it is non-resectable in most cases. In addition, a pre-operative evaluation by coronary angiography is mandatory to demonstrate coronary arterial blood supply to the tumor. On CMR imaging most metastases show low signal intensity relative to cardiac muscle on T1-weighted and high-signal intensity on T2-weighted TSE images (Figure 17-17). Only melanoma appears bright on T1-weighted TSE images because of the paramagnetic effects of melanin. Almost all malignant metastatic lesions will show

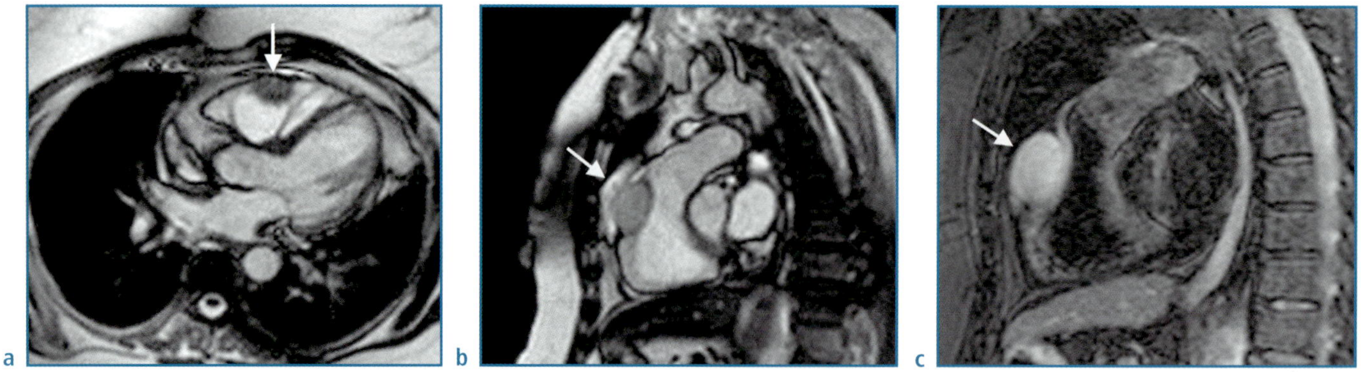

Figure 17-16 Metastasizing neuroendocrine carcinoma of the ileum using a SSFP sequence in a 5-ch (a) and RVOT plane view (b), as well as a black-blood sequence (c): The tumor appears as an isointense mass with impression of the free wall of the RVOT (arrows) in the SSFP sequence, and as a hyperintense mass in the black-blood sequence ((c), arrow).

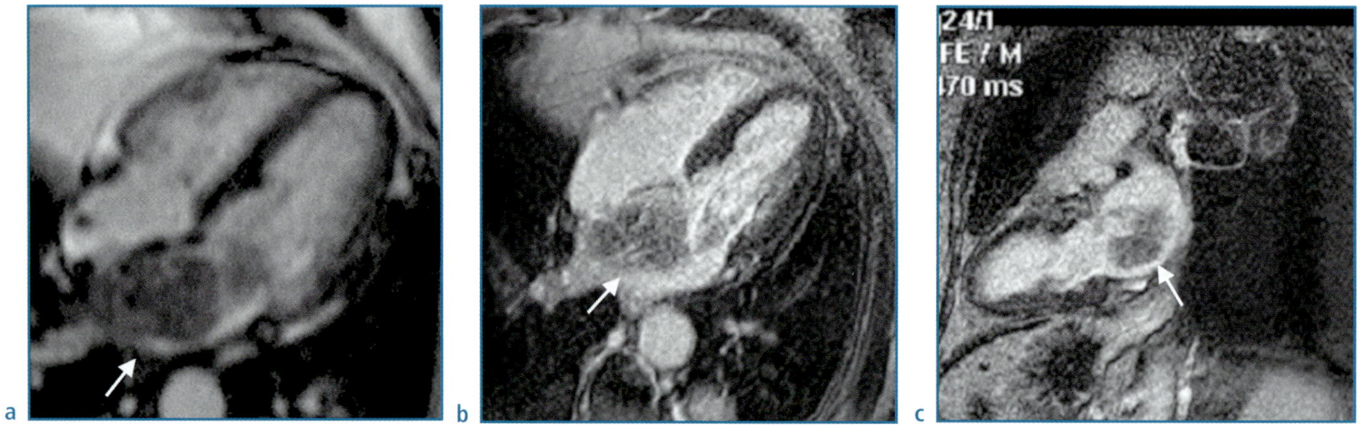

Figure 17-17 Metastasizing synovial carcinoma in a 4-ch view using a SSFP (a) and a black-blood sequence in a 4-ch (b) and 2-ch view (c): The tumor arises from the right upper pulmonary vein (a and b) and presents as a large rounded heterogenous mass within the left atrium (arrows).

modest to moderate enhancement after administration of gadolinium.

17.9 Non-Neoplastic Cardiac Masses

17.9.1 Intracardiac Thrombi

Etiology and Localization

Intracardiac thrombi are **the most common cardiac masses**; they occur in regions of slow flow and/or regional wall motion abnormalities:

- within the **left atrium** of patients with atrial fibrillation or mitral stenosis/incompetence and left atrial enlargement,
- within the **ventricles** (most commonly the left ventricle) in regions of hypo-akinesia (e.g. after myocardial infarction) or with generalized hypokinesia (e.g. dilated cardiomyopathy).

In the left atrium thrombi are attached to the lateral wall on a broad base as an immobile structure, or are located in the left atrial appendage (Figure 17-18a, b). Less commonly they may be mobile, or attached with a pedicle and may be mistaken as myxoma. Thrombi in the right atrium are most commonly found in patients with malignant hepatic or renal neoplasms or as a complication of SVC catheters (Figure 17-18c). Ventricular thrombi are immobile structures and have a broad-based attachment to the ventricular wall, most commonly they are located within the left ventricular apex or within a local aneurysm of the ventricular wall (Figure 17-19). The greatest clinical impact of intra-

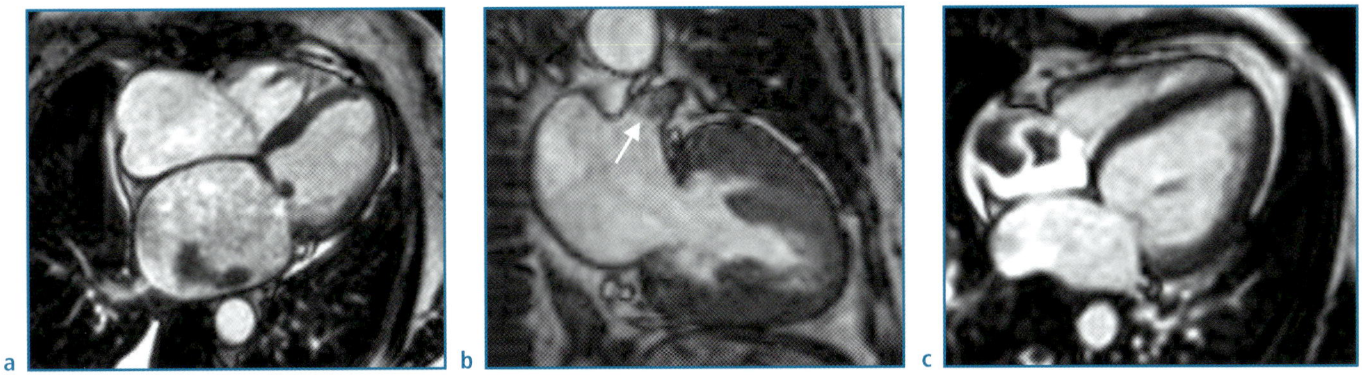

Figure 17-18 Thrombi in the enlarged left atrium (a) in a patient with high grade mitral stenosis, in the left atrial appendage ((b), arrow) in a patient with atrial fibrillation, and in the right atrium on the surface of a central venous catheter (c). The thrombi in (c) are partially fixed at the roof of the right atrium.

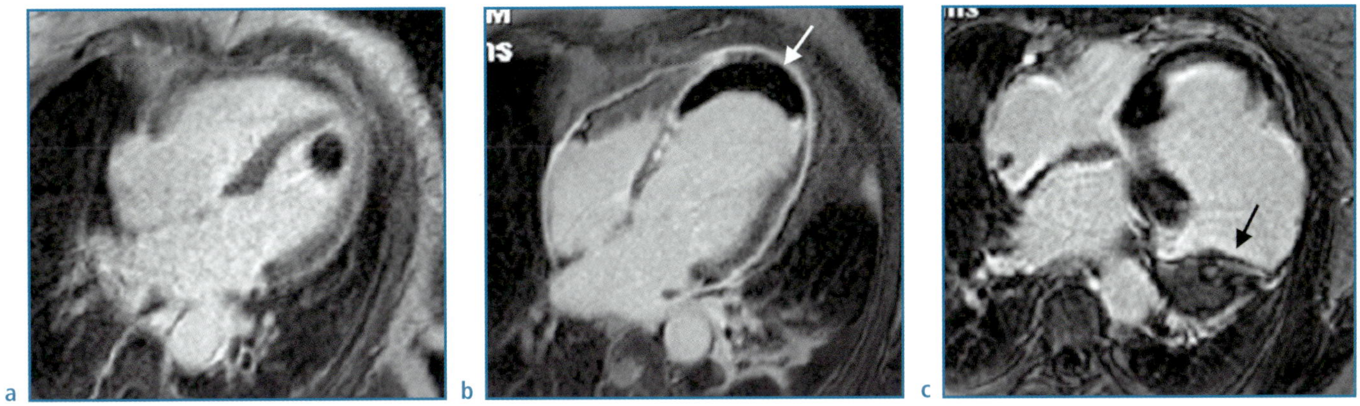

Figure 17-19 Left ventricular thrombi in 4-ch views using a T1-TFE-IR sequence after gadolinium injection: Small spherical thrombus in the left ventricular hypocinetic apex (a) following a small myocardial infarction. Broad-based large flat thrombus filling the whole left ventricular apex after an extensive acute anterior myocardial infarction ((b), arrow) with negative ventricular remodeling; and thrombus within a huge lateral ventricular post-infarction aneurysm ((c), arrow).

cardiac thrombi relates to systemic emboli into the cerebral, coronary, renal or lower leg arteries.

CMR Findings

CMR imaging is the most reliable imaging technique to diagnose intracardiac thrombi and to assess their location, size, and age. Fresh thrombi show a high signal intensity on T1- and T2-weighted TSE images, whereas chronic thrombi have low signal intensity on both T1- and T2-weighted images (due to the development of the paramagnetic substances methemoglobin and methemosiderin or superparamagnetic ferritin within the thrombus). Contrast-enhanced CMR allows differentiation between thrombus and surrounding myocardium (Figure 17-19), as the thrombus is avascular and does not show contrast enhancement, compared to the enhancing vascularized myocardium. Only rarely do large chronic thrombi enhance peripherally and make differentiation from a malignant tumor very difficult. On first-pass perfusion, thrombi do not enhance compared with the surrounding myocardium.

17.9.2 Cardiac Echinococcus Cysts

Etiology and Pathology

Echinococcus cyst involvement of the heart is very rare (0.5–2% of all clinical forms of this condition), but clinically significant. Echinoccosis is an infection in humans caused by the larval stage of the *Echinococcus granulosus* complex (dog form) or *Echinococcus multilocularis* (fox form). Echinococcus species have both intermediate and definite hosts, the definite hosts being canines that pass eggs in their feces. After ingestion of eggs, cysts develop in the intermediate hosts – sheep, cattle, humans, goats, horses – for the *Echinococcus granulosus* complex, and in mice and other rodents

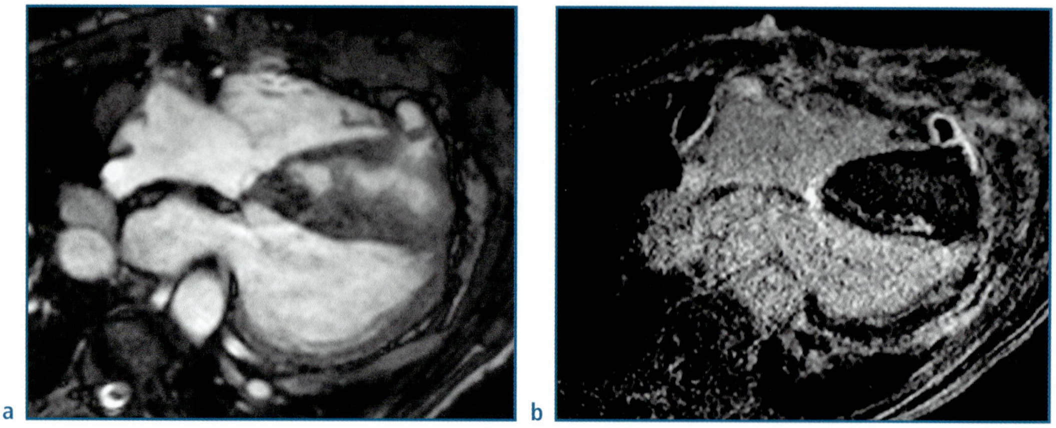

Figure 17-20 Large Echinococcus cyst in 4-ch views using an SSFP (a) and contrast-enhanced sequence (b): The heterogenous cystic mass appears with low signal intensity and daughter cysts within the interventricular septum (a) leading to a significant obstruction of the right ventricular cavum and outflow tract, and with enhancement of the boundary of the cyst to the normal septum with a small enhanced diverticulum within the right ventricular apex (b).

for the *Echinococcus multilocularis*. When a dog (*E. granulosus*) or fox (*E. multilocularis*) ingests infected meat containing cysts, the life cycle is completed.

Clinical Presentation

Patients with cardiac echinococcus are most commonly asymptomatic, sometimes they present with chest pain, arrhythmias, dyspnea on exertion (in case of large cysts with obstruction of cardiac chambers), and fatigue. In rare cases with pericardial involvement, pericardial tamponade may develop with severe dyspnea and heart failure. The diagnosis is confirmed by echocardiography, cardiac CT and particularly by CMR imaging. Treatment consists of chemotherapy (e.g. mebendazol), and/or surgical resection of large cysts obstructing the atrial or ventricular cavities or pericardial space with hemodynamic compromise. Recurrence rates may be high, and long-term prognosis is poor in most cases.

CMR Findings

CMR imaging may clearly detect location, size, and relationship of the cyst to the neighboring structures of the heart. One or several cysts may have different size, often being large with thick or thin wall and daughter cysts within the larger cysts. On T1-weighted TSE images signal intensity of the cysts is intermediate to low; in T2-weighted images signal intensity is high. After gadolinium injection the cysts may enhance (particularly their walls), which will facilitate their differentiation from the normal cardiac structures (Figure 17-20). CMR imaging is the ideal tool to follow patients with cardiac echinoccocus cysts regarding their growth, geometry, and hemodynamic compromise following medical or surgical treatment.

17.10 Normal Variants of the Heart

17.10.1 Lipomatous Hypertrophy of the Interatrial Septum (LHAS)

LHAS is pathogenetically a hypertrophy of pre-existing fat, but not a true neoplasm. It is often found in older and overweight patients and represents a fat accumulation within the interatrial septum in continuity with the epicardial fat. Since the fossa ovalis is spared from fat, LHAS often has a typical bilobed "dumbbell-shaped" or "camel-humped" appearance (Figure 17-21a). The lesion is rarely associated with symptoms, though sometimes atrial arrhythmias may be observed. On T1-weighted TSE images LHAS shows high signal intensity and lower signal intensity on T2-weighted images. Selective fat suppression techniques may be used (with signal drop out after fat saturation) to demonstrate the fatty nature and to differentiate LHAS from other non-lipomatous conditions.

17.10.2 Atrial Septal Aneurysm

This is defined as a diffuse or localized protrusion of the interatrial septum into the right or left atrium, or both, caused by bulging of the whole septum or the primary component of the septum through the fossa ovalis. It is an uncommon anomaly and may be associated with other congenital abnormalities (e.g. patent foramen ovale, atrial septal defects, or prolapse of the AV valves). Clinically systemic (sometimes paradoxic) pulmonary emboli may be observed, as well as atrial arrhythmias and palpitations. Diagnosis is usually made by echocardiography and CMR imaging (Figure 17-

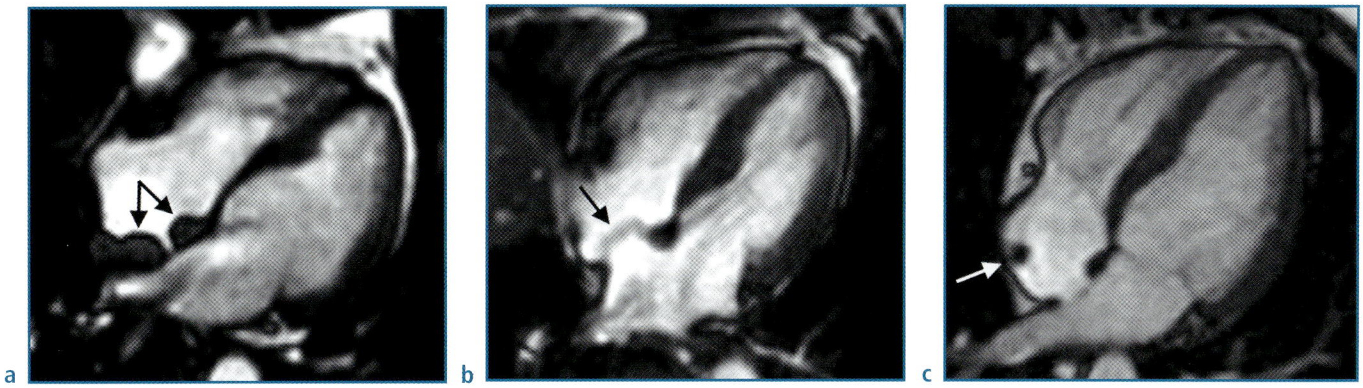

Figure 17-21 4-ch views with SSFP sequences: Lipomatous atrial septal hypertrophy with "camel-humped" appearance ((a), arrows), atrial septal aneurysm ((b), arrow), and prominent crista terminalis ((c), arrow).

21b). The latter technique is able to demonstrate the protrusion of the septum on cine-SSFP sequences together with slow-flow and signal-void within the aneurysm. Stagnant flow in SE-images may appear bright and may mimic a cardiac mass. The usual treatment for patients with systemic emboli is catheter-based implantation of an atrial septal occluder. CMR imaging is an ideal tool to follow patients after interventional treatment with an occluder.

17.10.3 Prominent Crista Terminalis

The crista terminalis courses as a fibromuscular band at the posterior wall of the right atrium between the entry of the SVC and IVC. On CMR imaging the crista terminalis, a particularly prominent crista, is routinely visible on black-blood and bright-blood MRI as a mural nodular or triangular structure adjacent to the lateral wall, which connects both caval veins (Figure 17-21c).

17.10.4 Chiari Network

The Chiari network is located in the right atrium and radiates from the crista terminalis to the IVC. Following regression of this structure single noduli may persist and may be visualized on standard CMR imaging and should not be mistaken as tumors.

17.11 Summary and Conclusions

CMR imaging has become a particularly valuable technique in the workup of suspected cardiac tumors. This is attributed to the optimal tumor characterization that may be achieved due to the different imaging sequences in combination with contrast enhancement studies, as well as to the unrestricted field of view and superior soft tissue characterization without ionizing radiation. The different imaging sequences follow a basis generic protocol; they allow optimum characterization of anatomy and tissue features of cardiac tumors and enable accurate assessment of their functional and hemodynamic impact (O'Donnel 2009). Therefore, CMR imaging should be routinely used early in the diagnostic process of suspected cardiac tumor, for follow-up of patients under treatment, and to detect early tumor recurrence.

References

Araoz PA, Eklund HE, Welch TJ et al. CT and MR imaging of primary cardiac malignancies. RadioGraphics 1999; 19: 1421–6.

Barkhausen J, Hunold P, Eggebrecht H et al. Detection and characterization of intracardiac thrombi on MR imaging. Am J Roentgenol 2002; 179: 1539–44.

Best AK, Dobson RL, Ahmad AR. Best cases from the AFIP: cardiac angiosarcoma. RadioGraphics 2003; 23: S141–S145.

Brizard C, Latremouille C, Jebara VA et al. Cardiac hemangiomas. Ann Thorac Surg 1993; 56: 390–6.

Burke A, Virmani R. Fascicle 16, 3rd series: Tumors of the heart and great vessels. In: Atlas of Tumor Pathology. Washington, DC: Armed Forces Institute of Pathology 1996.

Chiles C, Woodard PK, Gutierrez FR, Link KM. Metastatic involvement of the heart and pericardium: CT and MR imaging. RadioGraphics 2001; 21: 439–49.

Fujita N, Caputo GR, Higgins CB. Dignosis and characterization of intracardiac masses by magnetic resonance imaging. Am J Card Imaging 1994; 8: 69–76.

Grebenc ML, de Christenson MLR, Burke AP et al. Primary cardiac and pericardial neoplasms: radiologic-pathologic correlation. RadioGraphics 2000; 20: 1073–103.

Gulati G, Sharma S, Kothari SS et al. Comparison of echo and MRI in the imaging evaluation of intracardiac masses. Cardiovasc Intervent Radiol 2004; 27: 459–69.

Hoffmann U, Globits S, Schima W et al. Usefulness of magnetic resonance imaging of cardiac and paracardiac masses. Am J Cardiol 2003; 92: 890–5.
Kaplan KR, Rifkin MD. MR diagnosis of lipomatous infiltration of the interatrial septum. Am J Roentgenol 1989; 153: 495–500.
Kemp JL, Kessler RM, Raizada V et al. MR and CT appearance of cardiac hemangiomas. J Comput Assist Tomogr 1996; 20: 482–8.
Lund JT, Ehman RL, Julsrud PR et al. Cardiac masses. Assessment by MR. Am J Roentgenol 1989; 152: 469–75.
McManus B. Primary tumors of the heart. In: Bonow RO, Mann DL, Zipes DP, Libby P (eds.). Braunwald's Heart Disease. A Textbook of Cardiovascular Medicine. Elsevier Saunders 2012; 1638–50.
Muhm JR. General case of the day: Carney's triad. RadioGraphics 1986; 6: 914–6.
Nand S, Mullen GM, Lonchyna VA, Moncada R. Primary lymphoma of the heart. Prolonged survival with early systemic therapy in a patient. Cancer 1991; 68: 2289–92.
O'Donnell DH, Abbara S, Chaithiraphan V, Killeen RP et al. Cardiac tumors: optimal cardiac MR sequences and spectrum of imaging appearances. Am J Roentgenol 2009; 193: 377–87.
Parmley LF, Salley RK, Williams JP, Head GB. The clinical spectrum of cardiac fibroma with diagnosis and surgical considerations: non-invasive imaging enhances management. Ann Thorac Surg 1988; 45: 455–65.
Porcar-Ramells C, Clemente-Gonzalez C, Garcia-Pares D et al. Primary cardiac lymphoma: Cytological diagnosis and treatment with response to polychemotherapy and hematopoietic precursor autotransplant. An Med Interna 2002; 19: 305–9.
Rienmüller R, Lloret JL, Tiling R et al. MR imaging of pediatric cardiac tumors previously diagnosed by echocardiography. J Comput Assist Tomogr 1989; 13: 621–6.
Seline TH, Gross BH, Francis IR. CT and MR imaging of mediastinal hemangiomas. J Comput Assist Tomogr 1990; 14: 766–71.
Siripornpitak S, Higgins CB. MRI of primary malignant cardiovascular tumors. J Comput Assist Tomogr 1997; 21: 462–6.
Wilkes D, Charitakis K, Bassoon CT. Inherited disposition to cardiac myxoma development. Nat Rev Cancer 2006; 6: 157–65.
Winkler M, Higgins CB. Suspected intracardiac masses: evaluation with MR imaging. Radiology 1987; 165: 117–22.
Wintersprenger BJ, Becker CR, Gulbins H et al. Tumors of the cardiac valves: imaging findings in magnetic resonance imaging, electron beam computed tomography, and echocardiography. Eur Radiol 2000; 10: 443–8.
Yahata E, Endo T, Honma H et al. Sunray appearance of cardiac angiosarcoma with pericardial obliterations. Am Heart J 1994; 127: 468–71.

18 Pulmonary Circulation

Vinzenz Hombach

18.1 Physiology of Pulmonary Circulation

The lung has a double arterial blood supply from the pulmonary and bronchial arteries and a double venous drainage via the pulmonary and azygos veins. Blood from pulmonary arteries (PA) drains via the pulmonary veins (PV) into the left atrium (LA), while blood from the bronchial arteries drains via their capillary network and bronchial veins partly into the PV, but predominantly into systemic veins. This physiological right-to-left shunt amounts to 1% of cardiac output. The pulmonary circulation is characterized by high flow (transporting the entire right ventricular output), and by low pressure and low resistance. Its wide and thin-walled vessels reflect these hemodynamic features. Pulmonary perfusion is governed by reflex control, humoral mediator substances, and via the autonomic nervous system. **Hypoxia** is a powerful regional vasoconstrictor, and the hypoxic pulmonary vasoconstrictor response is an important adaptive mechanism in pulmonary physiology. Changes in the alveolar oxygenation affect the small pulmonary arteries and arterioles. A reduction in pulmonary artery blood volume occurs during hypoxia, with the small pulmonary arteries and arterioles being the main sites of vasoconstriction and increased resistance in the pulmonary circulation. **Adrenergic control** of pulmonary circulation is mainly governed by α-adrenergic receptors, though both α- and β-adrenergic receptors are expressed in the pulmonary vasculature. Excessive α_1-adrenergic receptor stimulation, e.g. by norepinephrine, appetite suppressants, or cocaine, produces smooth muscle cell contraction, proliferation, and growth. The α_1-adrenergic blocking agents, tolazoline and phentolamine, lower pulmonary vascular resistance in much that same way that β-adrenergic stimulation with isoproterenol does. However, β-adrenergic blockers do not have any effect on pulmonary vascular resistance. Acetylcholine is a potent relaxant of pulmonary arteries and arterioles, which transiently lowers pulmonary vascular resistance in patients with pulmonary arterial hypertension (i.e. with elevated vascular resistance). **Vascular mediators** such as prostaglandins, serotonin, and nitric oxide (by relaxation of resistance vessels), in addition to endothelin, thromboxane, and angiotensin II (by constriction of resistance vessels) are the most important regulators of pulmonary vascular resistance. Under normal conditions there is a balanced activity of these substances with an overall effect of low resistance and low pressure pulmonary flow (for further details see Rich 2012).

18.2 CMR Protocols

The aim of CMR imaging is to assess both morphology and function of the right ventricle (RV), the pulmonary arterial vessels, the pulmonary veins, the left ventricle including mitral valve function, flow in the great arteries, and to document damage or scarring in ventricular myocardium.

Therefore, the following **imaging protocol** should be used:

- scout/survey, with transversal planes covering the entire lung fields,
- cine-SSFP sequence with complete short- and long-axis planes, possibly combined with parallel imaging (SENSE) for assessing morphology and function (atria, ventricles, heart valves, regional and global systolic function, wall thickening, myocardial mass, intracardiac abnormal flow pattern),
- T1-, T2- and PD-weighted black-blood sequences in the standard planes for anatomic and morphologic imaging of cardiac structures (atrial and ventricular size, myocardium, great vessels, particularly the pulmonary artery and its branches),
- velocity-encoded cine-CMR (valvular dysfunction, intraventricular gradient, shunt calculation, diastolic function by transvalvular flow pattern),
- contrast-enhanced imaging in the long- (2-ch, 4-ch) and short-axes for LGE (myocardial damage, distribution pattern, extent, pericardial enhancement),
- contrast-enhanced T1w-GRE-angiography of the thoracic vessels, particularly of the right ventricle and the pulmonary arteries including their peripheral branches (exclusion of vessel pathology),
- optional: first-pass perfusion studies of the myocardium (to rule out significant CAD).

18.2.1 Right and Left Ventricular Volumes and Function

Assessment of right and left ventricular volumes and functional parameters provides basic information on cardiac involvement from lung disease. Right ventricular (RV) enlargement is one of the leading signs of hemodynamic overload. A reliable measurement of right ventricular volumes can only be obtained from a volumetric stack of short-axis slices. Common rotational models fail to represent the right ventricle adequately. Imaging should be performed in at least two perpendicular planes, especially for detecting and quantifying tricuspid regurgitation. Right ventricular muscular mass can be measured from short-axis slices, in addition to using volumetry of the outer and inner surfaces of ventricular myocardium. However, accuracy of volumetric assessment is lower than for the left ventricular myocardium because of the low wall thickness and occasional opposed-phase artifacts, with signal void at the border between myocardium and epicardial fat. Measurement of RV wall thickness can be achieved from basal short-axis slices at the inferior and anterior free wall of RV myocardium with clinically appropriate accuracy.

18.2.2 Velocity-Encoded Flow Mapping

To detect a left-to-right shunt as one possible cause of RV enlargement and myocardial hypertrophy, separate PC flow mapping should be performed in the pulmonary artery and the aorta. Volumetric assessment of shunts is less reliable due to tricuspid regurgitation present in most cases of RV overload. Generally, in the case of tricuspid regurgitation the gradient via the tricuspid valve can be measured using PC mapping of the backflow from the RV to the RA. This allows systolic pulmonary artery pressure to be calculated according to Bernoulli's formula. However, this approach may produce incorrect results due to the significant through-plane movement of the tricuspid valve, if an automatic slice tracking algorithm is not used. Interestingly, normal pulmonary intravascular blood volume may be quantified by VEC-PC flow analysis, as recently shown by Ugander et al. (2009) in 10 healthy volunteers. Blood flow in the pulmonary artery and pulmonary veins was quantified, and the difference in flow between both compartments was integrated to calculate the change in pulmonary blood volume throughout the cardiac cycle. The stroke volumes in the PA and the sum of PVs were 103 ± 6 ml and 95 ± 6 ml, respectively, pulmonary blood volume variation was 48 ± 5 ml, and expressed in percent of PA stroke volume 46 ± 3%. The maximum increase in pulmonary blood volume occurred 310 ± 12 ms after the R-wave of the ECG (32 ± 2% of the cardiac cycle). It was concluded that these findings have to be confirmed by larger studies to test the utility of pulmonary blood volume variation as a measure for identifying cardiac and pulmonary vascular disease.

18.2.3 Magnetic Resonance Angiography (MRA)

Using MRA significant morphological and functional information on the pulmonary artery and its peripheral branches including pulmonary veins can be obtained. Among the first groups, Paz et al. (1993) reported successful imaging of the pulmonary artery and its bifurcation using multi-planar spin echo sequences, with blood flow in the PA assessed by phase shift velocity mapping. Hatabu et al. (1996) used inversion recovery MRA (IR-MRA) with gadolinium to image the pulmonary artery and its peripheral subsegmental branches in 8 healthy volunteers. Pulmonary circulation time was 3.0–3.4 s, and a significant increase of signal intensity in the lung parenchyma from 4–7 s was seen. Goyen et al. (2001) reported imaging of the total pulmonary vascular tree within 4 s using dynamic acquisition of 3D data sets. In 3 healthy volunteers and 8 patients with dyspnea and known or suspected pulmonary arterial embolism, the whole pulmonary vascular tree was imaged down to the subsegment arteries. In 4 patients pulmonary emboli were detected in complete agreement with the standard technique of invasive pulmonary angiography.

The standard technique for imaging the whole pulmonary vascular compartments is **contrast-enhanced pulmonary angiography (CE-MRA)**. Because of the rapid pulmonary perfusion (transit) time, fast sequences with high temporal resolution up to a maximum of 4 s have to be used, if the arterial phase is to be documented without overlap by the venous phase. This can be achieved by fast gradient echo sequences (3D-technique, TR < 5 ms, TE < 2 ms) using surface multi-channel (5 channel) coils and parallel imaging (SENSE or SMASH, acceleration factor 2), i. e. ultrafast CE-MRA (spatial resolution: $1.2 \times 1.0 \times 1.6$ mm^3, acquisition/breath-hold period: 20–30 s). Using single sequences of less than 4 s, bolus tracking or bolus timing can be neglected if multiple dynamics are acquired. The plan scan of a 3D volume should include an AP infold correction and cover the entire lung fields. Predominant or exclusive **imaging of pulmonary veins** can be achieved by subtracting the pulmonary-arterial from the arteriovenous phase with the highest signal intensity (Schönberg 1998). In this study of 5 healthy controls, 8 patients with suspected pulmonary venous thrombosis, and 9 patients with tumor compression of pulmonary vessels, the large pulmonary veins including the segmental and subsegmental segments could be imaged without overlap of the pulmonary arteries. Thrombi were not detected in the pulmonary veins, but obstructions of pulmonary vessels by the malignant tumors were clearly depicted. Thus, ultrafast CE-MRA of the pulmonary arteries using subtraction techniques seems to be a valuable technique to accurately image pulmonary veins.

In principle, **five MRA techniques may be used for imaging pulmonary veins**:

- dynamic perfusion study with fractionated data acquisition of 3–5 data sets of 3.9 s (consecutive imaging of PA, PVs to LA and LV phase),
- single-bolus subtraction angiography: subtraction of the arterial phase from the peak image of the arteriovenous angiogram (= brightest vein signal) (3D-T1 w-TGE sequence, 8 successive 3D data sets of 2.9 s, coronal slab, spatial resolution $1.4 \times 1.9 \times 3.3$ mm^3),
- double-bolus correlation angiography: two contrast applications with low dose and high infusion rate (4 consecutive data sets of 6.28 s, 120 mm slab, spatial resolution $1.9 \times 1.4 \times 2.0$ mm^3, correlation analysis of two maximally anti-correlated pulmonary-arterial and -venous data sets resulting in a correlation angiogram of PAs and PVs),
- multi-fold acquisitions (= fractionated angiography): acquisition of several data sets within 15–20 s, interrupted by 5–10 s breathing,
- cine-phase contrast angiography or -mapping: quantification of PA or PV stenoses.

18.2.4 Technical Aspects

The survey/scout images may often detect central pulmonary artery abnormalities, masses, and possible abnormal pulmonary venous drainage. Using axial SSFP sequences (5–8 mm slice thickness, 1.5×1.5 mm^2 spatial resolution, one or several breath-holds) central parts of pulmonary arteries and veins can be quickly and accurately visualized. In addition to CE-MRA, continuous axial black-blood TSE-sequences, with a slice thickness of maximally 5 mm, are recommended for detecting intraluminal thrombi, dissections, or obstructing masses. These sequences provide a better vessel wall contrast, but slow-flow artifacts may occur in pulmonary vessels running parallel to the slice direction. Such artifacts may not be mistaken for intraluminal thrombi. To reach a safe diagnosis a second imaging plane has to always be acquired. When performing several breath-hold maneuvers a different end-expiratory level of the diaphragm including the thoracic organs has to be taken into account, which may result in overlapping or missed slices.

18.3 Pulmonary Arterial Hypertension (PAH)

Etiology and Pathophysiology

The prevalence of PAH is about 15 in 1.0 Mio population. *Idiopathic PAH* (IPAH) is more prevalent in women (female/male ratio 1.7 : 1) and was the most common type

Table 18-1 Revised WHO classification of pulmonary hypertension (PH).

1.	**Pulmonary arterial hypertension (PAH)**
1.1	Idiopathic PAH
1.2	Familial PAH
1.3	Associated with PAH (APAH):
1.3.1	Connective tissue disorder
1.3.2	Congenital systemic-to-pulmonary shunts
1.3.3	Portal hypertension
1.3.4	HIV infection
1.3.5	Drugs and toxins
1.3.6	Other (thyroid disorders, glycogen storage disease, Gaucher's disease, hereditary hemorrhagic teleangiectasia, hemoglobinopathies, chronic myeloproliferative disorders, splenectomy)
1.4	Associated with significant venous or capillary involvement:
1.4.1	Pulmonary veno-occlusive disease (PVOD)
1.4.2	Pulmonary capillary hemangiomatosis (PCH)
1.5	Persistent pulmonary hypertension of the newborn
2.	**Pulmonary hypertension with left heart disease**
2.1	Left-sided atrial or ventricular heart disease
2.2	Left-sided valvular heart disease
3.	**Pulmonary hypertension associated with lung diseases and/or hypoxemia**
3.1	Chronic obstructive pulmonary disease (COPD)
3.2	Interstitial lung disease
3.3	Sleep disordered breathing
3.4	Alveolar hypoventilation disorders
3.5	Chronic exposure to high altitude
3.6	Developmental abnormalities
4.	**Pulmonary hypertension due to chronic thrombotic and/or embolic disease (CTEPH)**
4.1	Thromboembolic obstruction of proximal pulmonary arteries
4.2	Thromboembolic obstruction of distal pulmonary arteries
4.3	Nonthrombotic pulmonary embolism (tumor, parasites, foreign material)
5.	**Miscellaneous**
sarcoidosis, histiocytosis X, lymphangiomatosis, compression of pulmonary vessels (adenopathy, tumor, fibrosing mediastinitis)	

in a French registry. *Familial PAH* (6–10% of patients with PAH) often results from a mutation in the bone morphogenetic protein receptor-2 (BMPR-2) and is inherited as an autosomal dominant disease with incomplete penetrance. PAH is also associated with connective tissue disorders (10% develop clinically apparent disease), congenital heart disease, drugs and toxins, HIV infection (incidence 0.5% of HIV infected individuals), portal hypertension (prevalence 2–6%), hemoglobinopathies (prevalence of 10% in sickle cell disease), and myeloproliferative disorders. Further forms of PAH are due to left heart disease, associated with lung disease, attributed to chronic thromboembolic disease, and miscellaneous etiologies (Table 18-1).

PAH is a syndrome resulting from restricted flow through the pulmonary arterial circulation, which leads to pathological increases in pulmonary vascular resistance (PVR) and ultimately to right heart failure. The predominant cause of increased PVR is loss of vascular lumen cross-section due to vascular remodeling produced by excessive cell proliferation and reduced rates of apoptosis. Excessive vasoconstriction plays a significant role in about 20% of patients. The PAH phenotype is characterized by endothelial dysfunction, a decreased ratio of apoptosis/proliferation in pulmonary artery smooth muscle cells, and a thickened disordered adventitia in which there is excessive activation of metalloproteinases (McLaughlin 2009). The RV and its function is a major determinant of functional capacity and prognosis in PAH. Over time RV hypertrophy and dilatation occur initiated by increased afterload (i.e. elevated PVR), and often followed by significant tricuspid regurgitation. The adequacy of RV's compensatory response with preservation of stroke volume is quite variable amongst individuals. It remains unclear why some right ventricles compensate while others decompensate, manifested by wall thinning and dilatation, and reduced RV ejection fraction (McLauglin 2009).

The **definition of pulmonary arterial hypertension** is based on hemodynamic criteria at resting conditions:

- **borderline PAH** = mean pulmonary artery pressure (PAP) of 21–25 mmHg,
- **manifest PAH** = mean PAP > 25 mmHg, pulmonary capillary wedge pressure < 15 mmHg and PVR > 3 Wood units.

Clinical Presentation

Patients present with dyspnea on effort and later on at rest, fatigue, exercise intolerance, chest pain, and in later stages with right heart failure including peripheral edema, and central and peripheral cyanosis. As cardiac output becomes fixed or eventually declines, patients may have episodes of syncope or near-syncope due to right heart failure. Physical examination reveals a large wave in jugular venous pulse, a low-volume carotid arterial pulse, a left parasternal RV heave, a systolic pulsation in the second left interspace by dilated, tense PA, an ejection click and systolic murmur in the same area, a closely split 2nd heart sound, and a 4th heart sound of RV origin. Further on signs of RV failure such as hepatomegaly, peripheral edema, and ascites may be present.

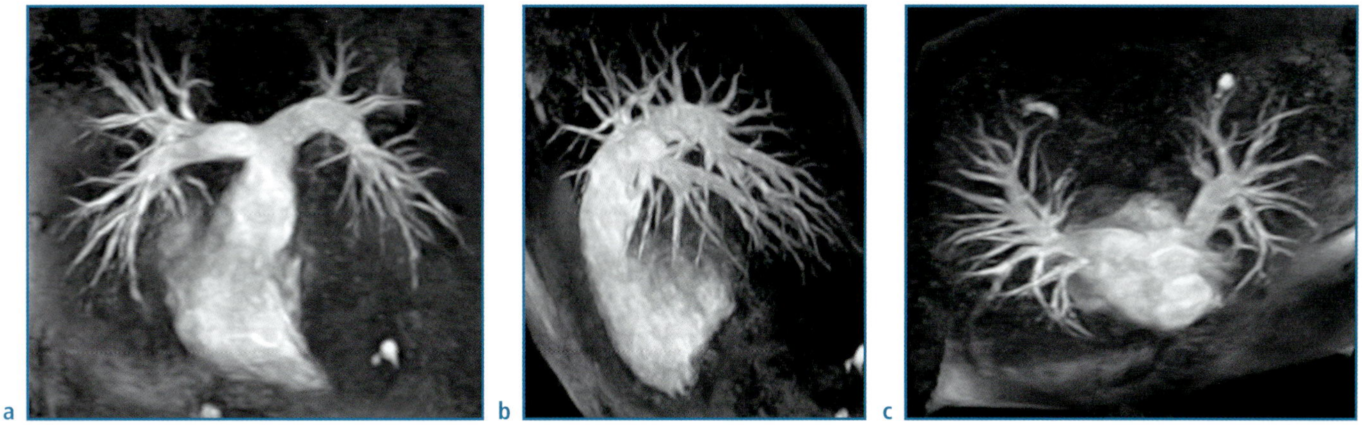

Figure 18-1 Contrast-enhanced magnetic resonance angiography (MRA) of the pulmonary arterial tree in a normal individual (one dynamic, flow-rate 4 ml/s) with MIP reconstruction in a coronal (a), sagittal (b), and transversal plane (c): Depiction of the right ventricle, both pulmonary arteries, and the entire subsegmental pulmonary arterial tree.

Diagnosis

Diagnosis is confirmed by chest X-ray (enlarged PA, marked tapering of peripheral arteries, encroachment of retrosternal air space), ECG (right axis deviation, RV hypertrophy, T-wave inversion), echocardiography (enlargement of RA and RV, normal or small LV dimensions, thickened interventricular septum), Doppler echocardiography (tricuspid regurgitation, estimation of systolic pulmonary pressure = relatively imprecise), lung scintigraphy (normal or diffuse patchy perfusion pattern), pulmonary angiography (central dilatation of PA, diffusely reduced peripheral vasculature), and cardiac catheterization (normal PCWP, increased mean PA pressure, normal or reduced cardiac output). Computed tomography is very helpful in diagnosing chronic thromboembolic PAH (visualization of peripheral thrombi, mosaic pattern of variable attenuation compatible with irregular pulmonary perfusion) or interstitial lung disease (high resolution CT scan) as a cause of PH. Most of these features can also be documented by CMR imaging (Figure 18-1, Figure 18-2, and Figure 18-3).

Therapy

Medical treatment includes digoxin, diuretics, anticoagulants, and vasodilator substances (calcium channel blockers, prostacyclins, endothelin receptor blockers, and phosphodiesterase type 5 inhibitors). In addition, treatment of the underlying disease (connective tissue diseases, congenital heart disease etc.) is crucial.

CMR Findings

Right Ventricle in PAH

RV end-diastolic (RVEDV) and end-systolic volumes (RVESV) are significantly increased in PH compared with controls, and RV ejection fraction, and cardiac output are significantly reduced (Hoeper 2001, Roeleveld 2004). Using CMR imaging LVEDV, LVESV, and LV peak filling rate (LVEDV per second) are significantly smaller in patients with PH compared to healthy controls (Hoeper 2001). The decreased LVEDV and LV stroke volume may be explained by the reduced RV stroke volume resulting from increased afterload with consecutive lower LV filling, and by interventricular septal bowing in systole and early diastole (i.e. right-to-left ventricular interaction and close relationship between LVEDV and stroke volume) (Gan 2006). Cine-CMR imaging may show that in the presence of increased RV systolic pressure the interventricular septum flattens and may bow towards the LV (Figure 18-2). Severe LV septal bowing has been considered to be associated with an unfavourable outcome. When expressing flattening of interventricular septum quantitatively as curvature, Roeleveld et al. (2005) found that a systolic PA pressure was proportional to septal curvature ($r = 0.77$, $p < 0.001$). Maximal distortion of the normal septal shape was found during the RV relaxation phase (leftward septum displacement due to pressure excess in the RV). Further a systolic PA pressure of > 67 mmHg may be expected if left ventricular septal bowing is seen. A further mechanism leading to LV volume reduction has been reported by Vonk-Noordegraaf et al. (2005), who using tagged MRI in patients with idiopathic PH could demonstrate a significant **interventricular asynchrony** caused by a longer RV systolic contraction time. This ventricular asynchrony decreased LV diastolic filling along with septal bowing and decreased RV function, resulting in a decreased LVEDV.

Exercise capacity of patients with PAH may also be correlated with RV function parameters. This was shown by Stevens et al. (2009) in 43 patients with PH, using a 6 min walk distance (6MWD) as a measure of functional class.

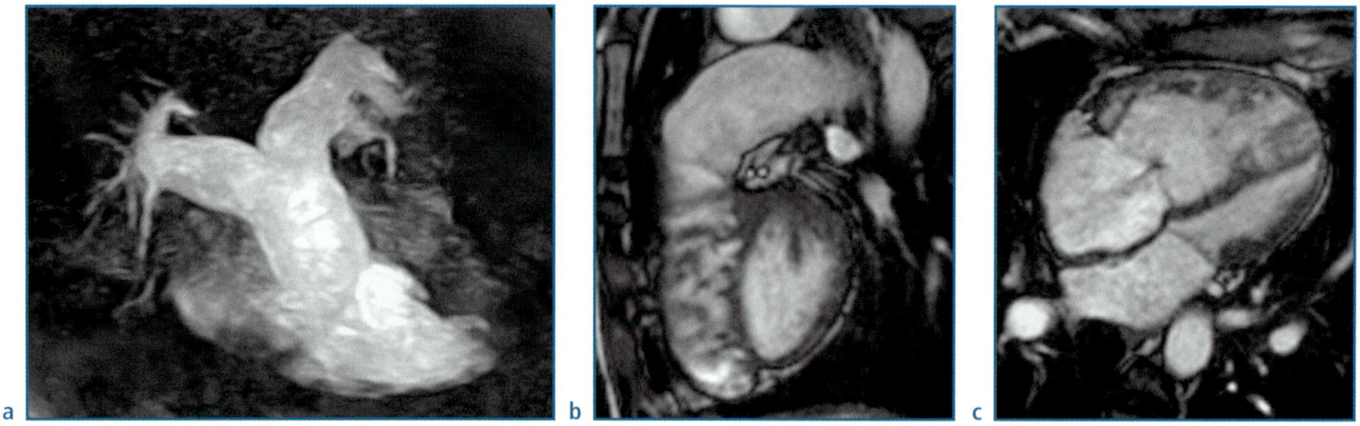

Figure 18-2 Contrast-enhanced MRA of the pulmonary arterial tree of a woman with idiopathic PAH in a coronal (a), sagittal (b), and 4-ch view (c). Note the dilated pulmonary trunk with a diameter of 38 mm (a and b), the dilated central pulmonary arteries with a diameter of 28 mm of the right and 30 mm of the left pulmonary artery (a), a considerable RV hypertrophy (b and c), and a flattened interventricular septum in systole (c) with a small tricuspid regurgitant jet due to chronic right ventricular pressure overload.

6MWD was correlated with PA eleasticity ($r = 0.41$, $p = 0.006$), PA average blood flow velocity ($r = 0.38$, $p = 0.014$), RV stroke volume index (RVSVI, $r = 0.41$, $p = 0.008$), LV stroke volume index (LVSVI, $r = 0.36$, $p = 0.080$), and RV stroke work index (RVSWI, $r = 0.37$, $p = 0.017$). It was concluded that stroke volume index, PA elasticity, and PA average blood flow velocity are novel CMR parameters associated with functional class in PAH. CMR can also be used to assess improvement in RV function in patients treated with vasodilators. Chin et al. (2008) demonstrated in 16 PAH patients that a 12 mths treatment with bosentan improved cardiac index, PVR, and 6MWD, together with a trend towards improvement in RV stroke volume. However no change in RV ejection fraction or RVEDV was seen. The conclusion is that CMR imaging may be valuable for determining response to therapy and prognosis in patients with PAH.

A more comprehensive evaluation of RV function in patients with PAH may be obtained by **RV pressure-volume curves.** This evaluation uses a combination of RV pressure measurements with MR compatible catheters and transducers and RV volume curves obtained instantaneously by cine-CMR (Kuehne 2004). In this study on 6 PAH patients (mean ± sd of PA pressure 57 ± 21 mmHg) and 6 controls, RV and LV stroke volumes and cardiac indices were significantly lower, despite higher RV ejection fraction and RV contractility. Using the same methodology of CMR-guided right-heart catheterization the same authors could show a reduction of PVR by nitric oxide inhalation (Kuehne 2005). The great advantage of this procedure is the reduction or elimination of X-ray radiation, added anatomic and functional information available with CMR, and the relative ease and accuracy of phase contrast magnetic resonance flow quantification. This may make the technique the method of choice for invasive measurement of PVR, though cost and availability of MR-compatible equipment may presently limit its use.

RV muscle mass (RVMM) was found to be significantly greater in patients with PAH compared to healthy volunteers as a consequence of increased pulmonary afterload (Figure 18-3), while the LVMM did not significantly differ (Katz 1993). Saba et al. (2002) used a **ventricular mass index** (VMI) > 0.6 (obtained by dividing RVMM by LVMM), with a sensitivity of 84% and specificity of 71%, for detecting PAH of various etiologies. However, Roeleveld et al. (2005) showed a much weaker correlation between VMI and mean PA pressure ($r = 0.56$). Still the VMI was found to be the best among five different CMR methods for estimating mean PA pressure.

RV diastolic dysfunction as an early sign of RV dysfunction is also present in patients with PAH and can be measured relatively easily by isovolumetric relaxation time (IVRT) (Gan 2007a). IVRT correlates positively with both RVMM and PVR, variables that are known to be of critical importance in the evaluation and prognosis of PAH. Moreover, IVRT improves in response to standard therapies known to decrease RV afterload, e.g. oral sildenafil (Michelakis 2002, Gan 2007a).

CMR contrast-enhanced imaging has revealed an interesting pattern of **RV hyperenhancement** (late gadolinium enhancement = LGE) in the study by Blyth et al. (2005) on 25 PAH patients. In 7 of 23 patients with LGE, hyperenhancement was limited to the RV insertion points but extended into the interventricular septum in the remaining 16 patients. In these 16 patients, septal LGE was associated with interventricular septum bowing. The extent of LGE correlated positively with RVEDV index, RVMM, mean PAP, and PVR and correlated inversely with RV ejection fraction. Similar results were reported by Junqueira et al. (2009), who found LGE in 13 of 20 PAH patients with RV dysfunction, hypertrophy and dilatation, 10 anterior and 12 inferior, all at the insertion points of the RV free wall into the interventricular septum. With the exception of disease duration, no significant correlations were found between LGE and RV ejection fraction or other hemodynamic variables. The true diagnostic and prognostic significance of LGE in patients with PAH and RV dysfunction has to be evaluated by larger prognostic studies.

Pulmonary Circulation

Velocity-encoded imaging of pulmonary arterial flow provides a description of changes or irregularities in the pulmonary blood flow in PAH patients. Kondo et al. (1992) reported highly inhomogenous velocity profiles, a large volume of retrograde flow, and decreased distensibility of the main PA. From the quantitative analysis of the profile of pulmonary blood flow non-invasive indices like acceleration time (time from onset of flow to the peak velocity) and acceleration volume have been derived to assess PVR. Peak blood flow velocity in the main PA was lower in patients with PAH and showed an inverse correlation with mean PA pressure and PVR (Mousseaux 1999). In another study by Bogren et al. (1989) distensibility of PA, measured as percent of maximal minus minimal cross-sectional area related to minimal area, was significantly lower in PAH patients compared to healthy individuals (8 vs. 23%). PA distensibility was also significantly greater during an acute vasodilator test with invasive hemodynamic evalution in responders (Jardim 2007). Proximal PA stiffness measured by CMR predicted mortality in patients with PH (Gan 2007b).

PA perfusion imaging using 3D dynamic CE-MRA is another valuable technique for assessing disease severity in patients with PAH. Ohno et al. (2007) reported significant differences in PA blood flow and mean transit time (MTT) between healthy and pulmonary hypertensive subjects, with good negative correlation between pulmonary blood flow and PVR and moderate correlation between MTT and PVR. For PAH patients in advanced stage, CE-MRA may show dilatation of pulmonary trunk as well as left and right PA, large proximal vessel calibre and diffuse, marked peripheral vessel tapering (Figure 18-2), with a delayed run-off of the contrast medium. In addition a dilated and hypertrophied RV with/without tricuspid regurgitation and reduced pump function can be demonstrated.

CMR Imaging for Control of Therapy

Although right heart catheterization remains the definitive assessment of PAH at present, the non-invasive evaluation of cardiac morphology and function and of pulmonary circulation is the promising new application of CMR imaging to monitor patient outcome under treatment. In a longitudinal CMR study van Wolferen et al. (2007) could show that RV dilatation, a decreased stroke volume, and LV diastolic volume were strong predictors of treatment failure and death at follow-up. Following lung transplantation changes in RV mass, function and pulmonary artery blood flow have been demonstrated by CMR imaging. In a small study Michelakis et al. (2003) demonstrated that, in 5 consecutive patients with Eisenmenger's syndrome, 50 mg sildenafil t.i.d. significantly reduced RV mass and increased RV stroke volume. In addition it lead to a reversal of pathological septal shift towards the LV. Roeleveld et al. (2004) reported in a prospective study on 11 PAH patients that prostacyclin significantly increased RV stroke volume as measured by PC flow mapping, which correlated well with WHO functional class and 6MWT. In a comparative study between bosentan and sildenafil, Wilkins et al. (2005) found that RV mass measured by CMR did not change 3 mths after bosentan treatment, whereas sildenafil reduced RV mass. It was also demonstrated by Van Wolferen et al. (2006), using CMR,

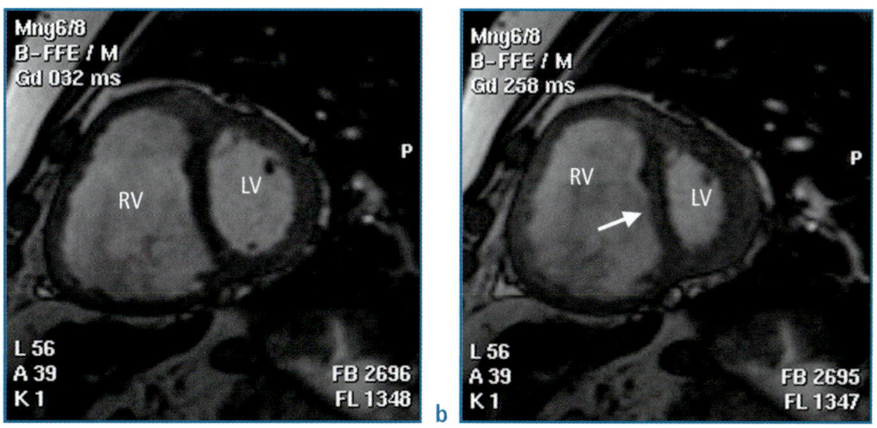

a b

Figure 18-3 Systolic bulging (arrow in (b)) of the interventricular septum in severe RV hypertrophy due to longstanding PAH; short-axis view in diastole (a) and systole (b). LV: left ventricle; RV: right ventricle.

that the addition of sildenafil reversed RV dilatation and hypertrophy in patients already receiving bosentan treatment. The results of the study by Chin et al. (2008) on 16 patients with PAH receiving bosentan treatment and showing improved CI, PVR and 6MWD, have already been discussed above.

In summary, CMR has emerged as the gold standard for detailed study of the RV and has become an established modality for the physiological assessment of PAH patients in cross-sectional studies, longitudinal follow-up studies and clinical trials of therapy (McLure and Peacock 2009).

18.4 Pulmonary Arterial Hypertension Associated with Significant Venous or Capillary Involvement

Etiology and Pathophysiology

Pulmonary veno-occlusive disease (PVOD) and pulmonary capillary hemangiomatosis (PCH) are two unusual and rare idiopathic disorders that manifest almost uniformly as PAH. The etiology of both diseases has not yet been identified. Since the earliest descriptions of PVOD and PCH there has been a debate as to whether these are two distinctive diseases or varied expressions of a single disorder (Frazier 2007). The estimated annual incidence of PVOD is 0.1–0.2 cases per million persons, and it affects patients in a wide age range, extending from 9 d to 60–70 yrs of age, with 30–50% of patients less than 20 yrs old. Furthermore, there is no sexual predilection (Frazier 2007). PCH is reported much less frequently, the range of affected individuals is also broad, from 2–71 yrs, with a mean age of 30 yrs.

Histopathologically PVOD is characterized by obstructive eccentric fibrous intimal pads in the pulmonary veins (PVs) and venules, and frequent arterialization of the PVs associated with alveolar capillary congestion. PCH is characterized by proliferation of capillary channels, predominantly within the alveolar walls, but also within the walls of bronchi and pulmonary vessels (Frazier 2007).

Clinical Presentation

The clinical manifestation of both PVOD and PCH are characterized by progressive dyspnea and fatigue, occasionally a progressive cough, chest pain, syncope, or digital clubbing. The presence of hemoptysis in 30% of PCH patients (absent in PVOD) and hemorrhagic pleural effusion in 25% of PCH patients (absent in PVOD), may help to differentiate both disorders.

Diagnosis

Diagnosis of associated PAH is made by clinical examination, chest X-ray, ECG, echocardiography, CMR, and right heart catheterization. The **gold standard** for assessing the diagnosis is a high resolution lung CT scan in order to detect an unsuspected capillary or post-capillary disorder that is otherwise obscured by impressive clinical features of PAH. The main CT features used to differentiate PVOD and PCH from mere PAH are presence of smooth septal lines, geographic or nodular ground-glass opacities, and pleural effusion. Except for assessing RV function, CMR imaging has no additional role in confirming the diagnosis of either PVOD or PCH.

Therapy

The only curative therapeutic option is lung or heart-lung transplantation. Pharmacological agents like diuretics, ACE-inhibitors, cardiac glycosides, or pulmonary vasodilators serve only as supportive care and as a bridge to transplantation.

18.5 Pulmonary Hypertension with Left Heart Disease

In the long-run all types of disorders of the left heart due to LV volume- or pressure overload or systolic or diastolic dysfunction may result in pulmonary hypertension (PH). Patients with PH and left heart disease may present with dyspnea on exercise, fatigue, and orthopnea or paroxysmal nocturnal dyspnea, and later on with symptoms of right heart failure. Diagnosis of primary left heart disease, as a cause of PH, is achieved by history, clinical examination, chest X-ray, ECG, and echocardiography including Doppler sonography, and if necessary by left- and right heart catheterization. CMR is a very valuable tool for assessing both type and hemodynamic consequences of left heart disease and the resulting consequences on RV function and pulmonary circulation. Therefore, in unclear situations CMR should be used to obtain valid results on diagnosis and disease severity, and provide valuable clues for selecting an effective medical or invasive treatment.

18.6 Pulmonary Arterial Hypertension Associated with Lung Disease and/or Hypoxemia

Diseases of the lung parenchyma such as chronic obstructive pulmonary disease (COPD), interstitial lung disease or adult cystic fibrosis are common causes of PAH. Most commonly, PAH in COPD patients has multiple causative factors, including pulmonary vasoconstriction caused by alveolar hypoxia, acedemia, hypercarbia, compression of pulmonary vessels by the high lung volume, loss of small vessels in the regions of emphysema and lung destruction, and increased cardiac output and blood viscosity from polycythemia secondary to hypoxia. The diagnosis of COPD should be considered in patients with chronic cough, sputum production, dyspnea, or history of exposure to disease risk factors. Cardiac involvement can be assessed by echocardiography and Doppler echocardiography, and by CMR imaging, which enables the assessment of both right and left heart function and pulmonary circulation. COPD and its severity are assessed by chest X-ray, lung function testing, and high resolution lung CT. It should be noted that there is a significant percentage of COPD patients with unrecognized left-sided chronic heart failure (CHF) (prevalence of up to 21 %), and of left ventricular dysfunction (prevalence of 10–46 %; Hawkins 2009). The value of CMR in identifying CHF in patients with COPD has been shown by Rutten et al. (2008). They used accurate and easily accessible morphologic and volume-based CMR-based measurements to identify previously unknown left-sided CHF in mild to moderate COPD patients (83 of 405 COPD patients = 20.5 %).

18.7 Pulmonary Arterial Hypertension due to Acute or Chronic Thrombotic and/or Embolic Disease

18.7.1 Acute Pulmonary Embolism (PE)

Etiology and Pathophysiology

Pulmonary embolism (PE) is part of a larger syndrome that includes the formation of thrombus and its distal consequences of embolization, arising from deep vein thrombosis (DVT) in the extremities and pelvic veins through acute pulmonary embolism (PE) or chronic thromboembolic disease (CTED), and leading in the final stages to CTEPH. DVT occurs for the first time in 100 per 100,000 persons each year (> 500 per 100,000 at ages of 80 yrs). High-risk categories of PE are individuals older than 75 yrs, with history of surgery plus morbid obesity, elective knee or hip replacement, factors like multiple traumas, stroke, hip-, pelvis- or femur fractures within the last 30 d, history of DVT/PE, family history of thrombosis, and additional risk factors such as CHF, MI, chronic lung diseases, or stroke history. PAH through acute PE develops via both mechanical obstruction and hypoxia-induced vasospasm.

Clinical Presentation

Depending on the extent and hemodynamic consequences of PE, patients present with acute dyspnea, chest pain, tachycardia, syncope, cardiopulmonary arrest, hemoptysis, and lower extremity edema as a sign of DVT.

Clinically, PE is divided into:
- massive (associated with shock and/or hypotension; systolic blood pressure < 90 mmHg),
- submassive (RV dysfunction identified by echocardiography), and
- small or non-massive (no systemic hypotension).

Diagnosis

Diagnosis is confirmed by:
- D-dimer assay, cardiac troponin,
- ECG (signs of acute RV pressure overload),
- vascular ultrasound (diagnosis of DVT and its sequelae),
- transthoracic echocardiography including Doppler techniques (RV enlargement and dysfunction, estimation of systolic pulmonary pressure by pressure gradient via the tricuspid valve),
- TEE (direct visualization of centrally located thrombi),
- nuclear ventilation/perfusion (V/Q) imaging (V/Q mismatch; high probability of PE with two or more large mismatched segmental defects), and
- computed tomography angiogram (CTA) that uses post-processing techniques like surface and volume 3D rendering of vessels, multi-planar reformatting, and MIP (CT positive for PE with completely or partially occluded vessel, mural defects at vessel wall, or central thrombus surrounded by contrast).

Pulmonary angiography remains the **gold standard** for diagnosis of PE, but because of its invasive nature it is less commonly used in clinical routine.

The **non-invasive gold standard** for assessing the diagnosis of PE is multi-detector CT (MDCT) with a sensitivity and specificity of 83 and 96 %, respectively. Sensitivity and specificity for performing a CT venogram with pulmo-

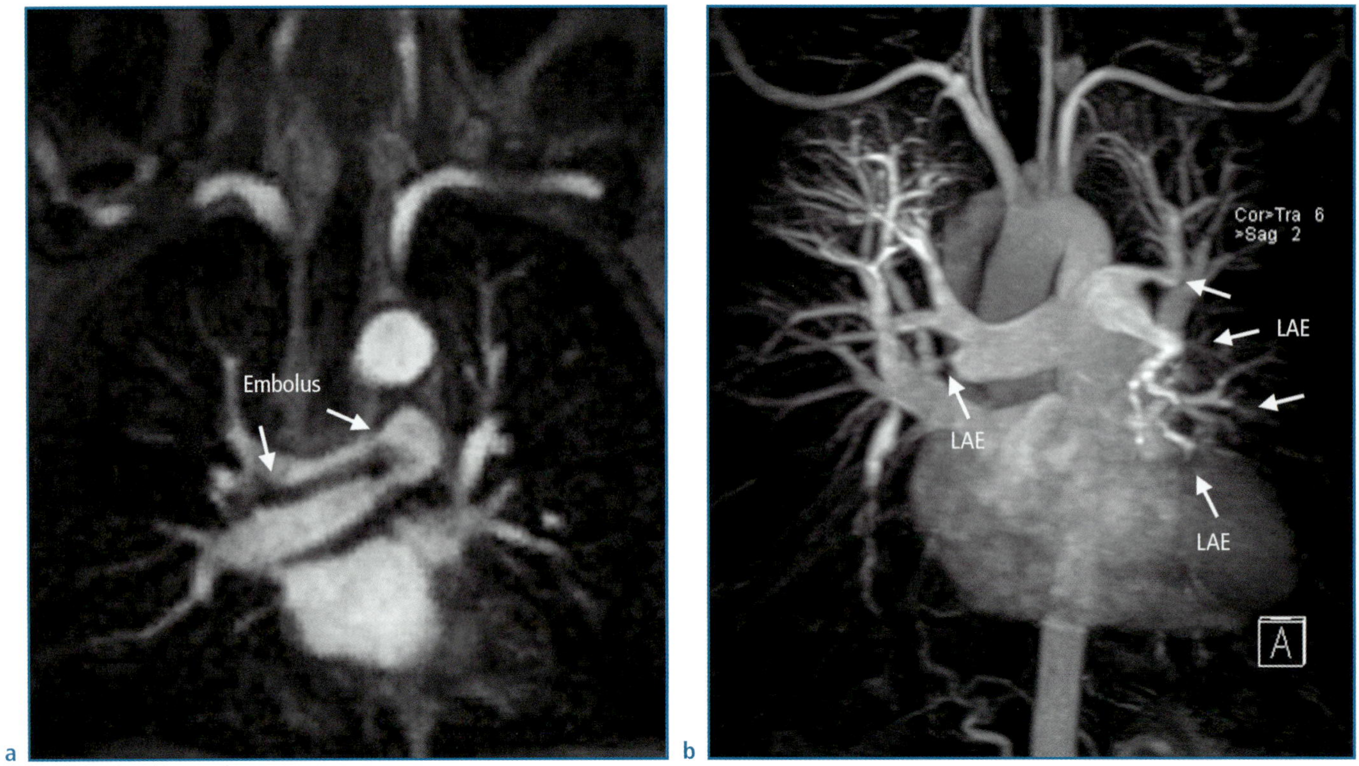

Figure 18-4 Large central pulmonary embolus in the main stem of the right pulmonary artery (a), and multiple small pulmonary emboli in segmental arteries on the right and particularly the left pulmonary arterial tree (arrows in (b)). LAE: pulmonary arterial embolus (Figure a by courtesy of Prof. J. Barkhausen, Lübeck; Figure b by courtesy of Prof. A. Buecker, Homburg/Saar).

nary CTA is 90 and 95 %, respectively. These are the findings reported from a large series of 824 patients studied by Stein et al. (2006). In contrast to MDCT, the clinical relevance of MRI for suspected PE is low at present because of its inferior spatial resolution, longer examination and breath-hold times, and reduced availability and experience of MR centers with PE imaging. However, there are potential advantages of MRI such as lower side effects from the MR-contrast media (nearly no renal and no thyroid side effects), no ionizing radiation (this may be relevant in certain patient groups such as young individuals and particularly for pregnant women etc.), recently achieved better spatial resolution, combination of angiography and perfusion, and availability of blood-pool contrast agents with the potential for alternative imaging modalities (navigator-gated MRI, time-resolved pulmonary MRA, high-resolution pulmonary MRA, whole-body MR venography).

There are two different approaches to pulmonary CE-MRA, either acquiring a 3D-volume data set of pulmonary vasculature (high, ideally isotropic spatial resolution, and parallel sub-millimeter imaging), or using time-resolved CE-MRA (less sensitive to incorrect bolus timing and motion artifacts, visualization of pulmonary perfusion). In a review paper Fink et al. (2007) reported that sensitivity and specificity of CE-MRA for detecting pulmonary embolism in 6 publications was 71–100 % and 92–100 %, respectively. The positive and negative predictive values were between 87–100 % and 57–100 %, respectively. When assessing pulmonary perfusion Ohno et al. (2004) compared the diagnostic accuracy of time-resolved CE-MRA with CTA and V/Q scans, and the sensitivity and specificity of the three modalities were 92 % vs. 83 % vs. 67 %, and 94 % vs. 94 % vs. 78 %, respectively, for the detection of PE. A combined protocol for pulmonary perfusion MR imaging and high-resolution CE-MRA provides a sensitivity and specificity of over 90 % and agrees closely with CTA (Kluge 2006). However, the PIOPED investigators (Stein 2010), who studied 371 individuals with suspected PE in 7 hospitals and their emergency services that employed pulmonary CE-MRA with or without venography, reported technically inadequate CE-MRA studies in 25 % of patients (range 11–52 %). This yielded a rate of 57 % for PE identification, while sensitivity and specificity of technically adequate MRA studies to diagnose PE was 78 and 99 %, respectively, and for adequate MRA and venography 92 and 96 %, respectively. The conclusion of this study was that pulmonary CE-MRA with/without MR venography to diagnose PE should only be used in experienced centers with a high performance rate and only in patients for whom standard tests are contraindicated. In most centers the actual policy is that MDCT is the first line diagnostic method for identifying PE, but centers experienced with CE-MRA (combined pulmonary vasculography and perfusion study) may use MRA as a valid alternative diagnostic method (example in Figure 18-4).

18.7.2 Chronic Thromboembolic Pulmonary Hypertension (CTEPH)

Etiology and Pathophysiology

PE either as a single episode or as a recurrent event is thought to be the initiating process of CTEPH, followed by progressive vascular remodeling. The thromboemboli fail to resolve adequately, undergo organization with incomplete recanalization, and are incorporated into the vascular wall in subsegmental, segmental or lobar vessels. The incidence of symptomatic CTEPH may be about 3 % within one and about 4 % at 2 yrs. An identifiable hypercoaculable status is found in only a minority of patients (lupus anticoagulant in 10–20 % of patients, inherited deficiencies of protein C or S, or antithrombin III in about 5 % of cases).

Clinical Presentation

Patients present with acrocyanosis, progressive dyspnea, pulmonary bruits (up to 10 %), signs of cor pulmonale, fatigue, and syncope or presyncope.

Diagnosis

Diagnosis is made by initial work-up (physical examination, pulmonary function testing, and chest radiography) to differentiate patients symptoms as cardiac, pulmonary, or pulmonary-vascular in origin, and thereafter by imaging techniques (echocardiography, ventilation-perfusion scanning, MDCT, and MRI). Echocardiography may reveal resting PAH from the Doppler velocity of tricuspid regurgitant jet, and examine overall cardiac anatomy for other causes (e.g. congenital heart disease). V/Q-scanning can reliably distinguish between large-vessel occlusive disease and small-vessel pulmonary vascular disease (a normal V/Q-scan virtually rules out CTEPH), but it has since been superseded by MDCT. CT angiography (CTA) shows luminal thrombi, organized mural thrombi, occlusions, and webs, as may be seen with conventional angiography. Moreover, high-resolution CT of the lungs shows a mosaic pattern that is virtually diagnostic for CTEPH. The only important mimic is air trapping seen in a variety of small-airway diseases. Bronchial artery dilatation, a well-recognized feature of CTEPH on conventional angiography, may also be detected by CTA. CE-MRA, as an established alternative to CTA, is ideally suited for examining young patients and those requiring serial assessment (e.g. for post-operative follow-up) to diagnose CTEPH. It shows the typical findings of intraluminal webs and bands, vessel cut-offs, and an organized central thrombus down to segmental levels. Pulmonary MRA has similar accuracy to V/Q scintigraphy in distinguishing between patients with CTEPH and idiopathic PAH. In addition, cine-MRI allows qualitative and quantitative assessment of ventricular function and exclusion of other causes for PAH. PC flow mapping can be used to measure flow in the aorta and right and left pulmonary artery, both before and after pulmonary thrombendarterectomy (PEA). In conclusion, pulmonary MRA has replaced conventional angiography as a surgical "road map" in patients with CTEPH considered for surgery. This method is ideally suited to monitor the success of PEA regarding vessel patency and recovery of RV function (D'Armini 2000, Kreithner 2004, Reesink 2007).

18.8 Diseases of the Pulmonary Vessels

18.8.1 Pulmonary Arterial Diseases

These include hypoplasia or atresia of pulmonary arteries, the pulmonary-arterial sling, the PA origin from the ductus arteriosus, and congenital arteriovenous fistulas (AVF). The former disorders are described elsewhere, here only AFV will be briefly discussed.

Arteriovenous Fistulas (AVF)

Congenital AVFs result in right-to-left shunt depending on their size and may lead to polyglobulia, cyanosis, finger clubbing, and in some cases to hemoptysis, paradoxical emboli, or brain abscess. Most patients present with Webler-Osler-Rendu syndrome (hereditary teleangiectasia), less frequently associated with further malformations of the bronchial tree, absent right lower lobe, or bronchiectasis. According to the number of supply or draining vessels, simple AVFs with one single artery and vein are differentiated from complex AVFs with several arteries and veins.

Diagnosis is made by chest X-ray (solitary or multiple pulsating rounded masses) and by pulmonary angiography including selective injections to document all fistulae for adequate planning of interventional (coiling) or surgical (resection) therapy. CMR imaging is also useful for detecting and assessing the size and location of AVFs (Figure 18-5), as well as to measure the amount of right-to-left shunting.

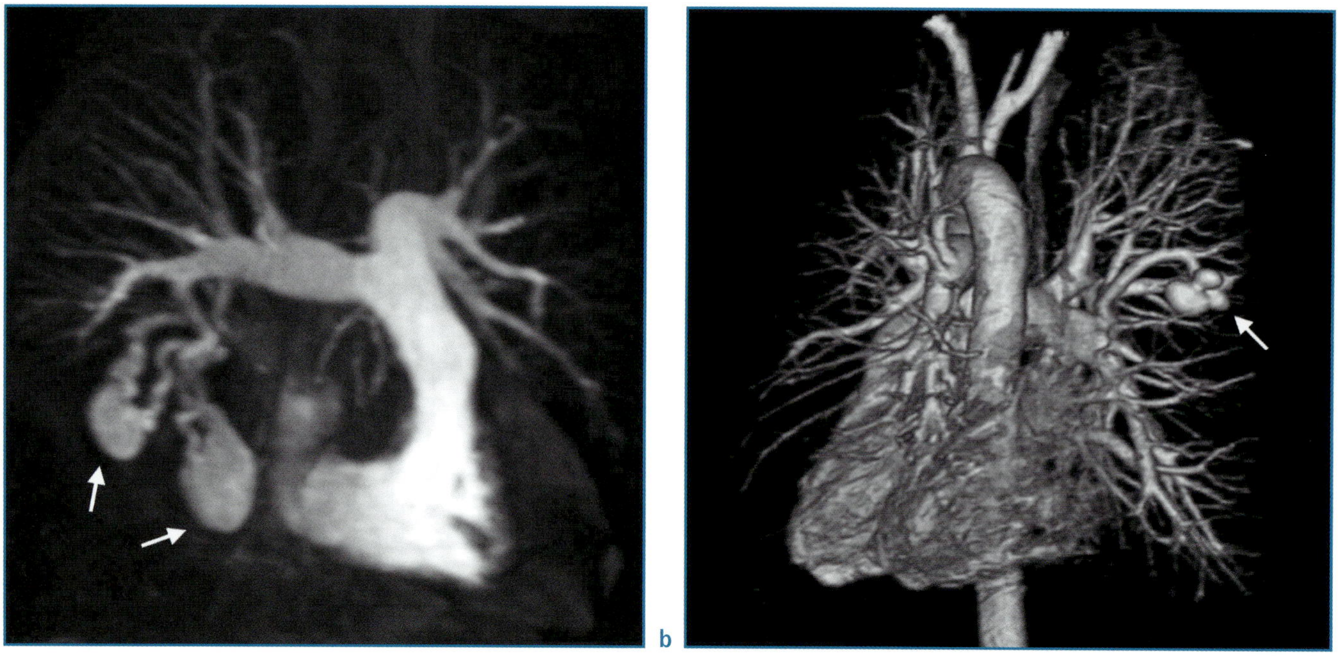

Figure 18-5 Two large arteriovenous fistulas (arrows) in the right lung in a contrast-enhanced MRA ((a), view from anterior) and in a volume-rendered angiogram ((b), view from posterior) (courtesy Prof. A. Buecker, Homburg/Saar).

Pulmonary Arterial Aneurysms

These disorders are rare and are observed most frequently in congenital heart disease (ASD, pulmonary stenosis), idiopathic with the very rare Hughes-Stovin syndrome (small or large aneurysms of the PAs and thrombi of the dural sinus and peripheral veins), and secondary with Morbus Behçet or Marfan's syndrome. Pseudoaneurysms may develop due to vessel wall lesions in the vicinity of a tuberculous caverna (Rasmussen pseudoaneurysm), through blunt or sharp thoracic trauma, by neoplasms, or as a complication of catheterizing the PAs. Diagnosis is made by conventional angiography, but both black-blood and particularly CE-MRA are able to assess the extent, localization, and relationship of the aneurysm to the surrounding tissue (Figure 18-6).

18.8.2 Pulmonary Venous Diseases

These include pulmonary venous varix nodes (dilated tubular confluens to the left atrium), congenital or acquired (iatrogenic) pulmonary vein (PV) stenoses, and the Scimitar syndrome. Acquired PV stenoses may be observed from tumor compression, or following PV ablation for atrial fibrillation (Figure 18-7). CMR imaging seems to be a useful

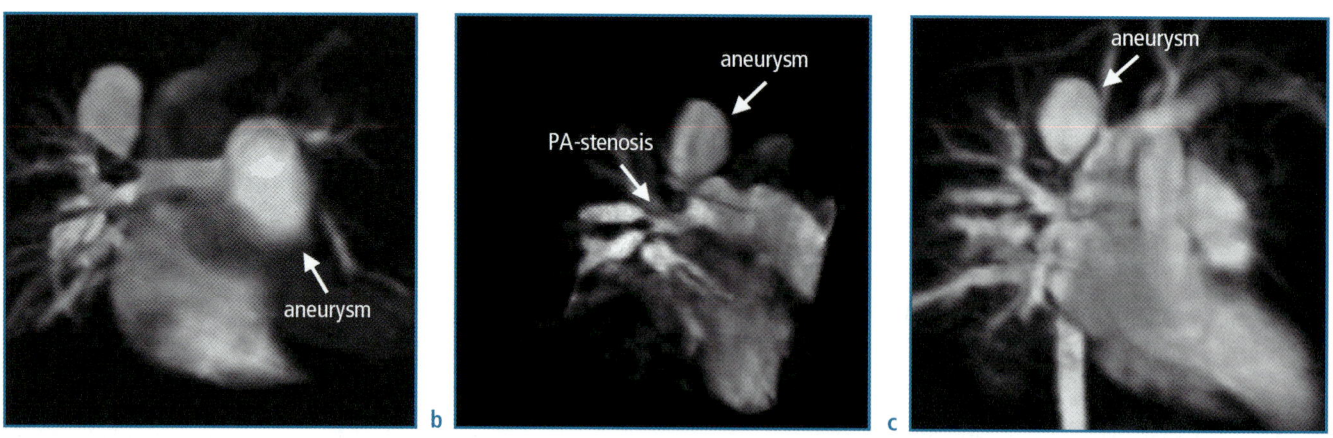

Figure 18-6 Aneurysm of the right pulmonary artery in a patient with Apitz-Beuren syndrome, coronal (a), sagittal (b), and oblique view (c) (courtesy Prof. J. Barkhausen, Lübeck).

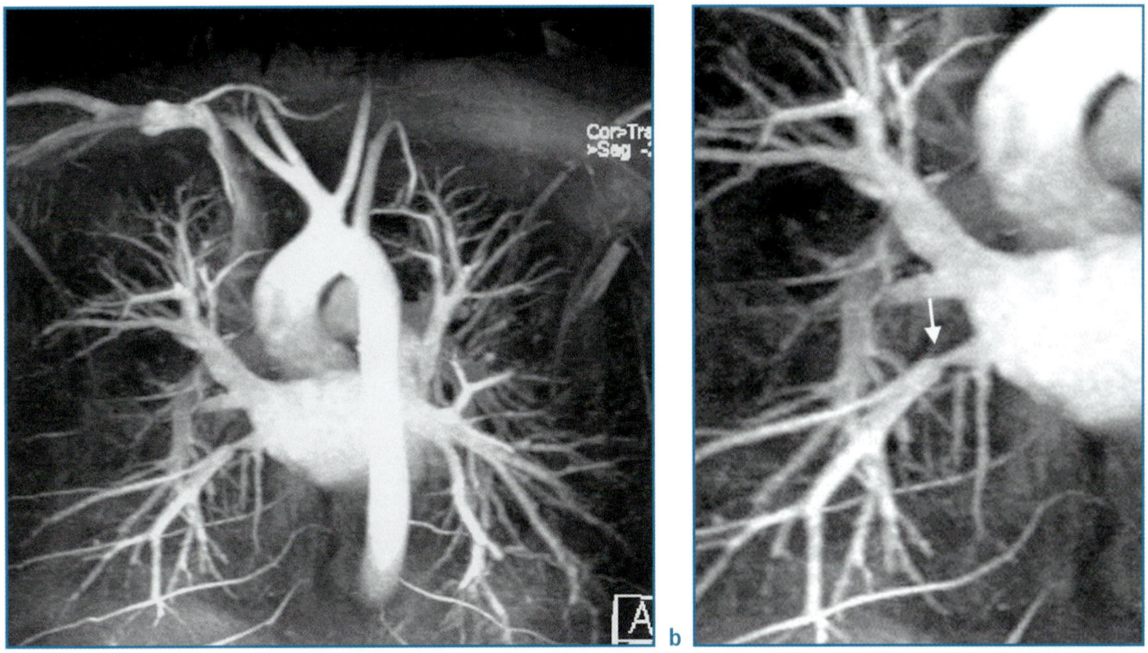

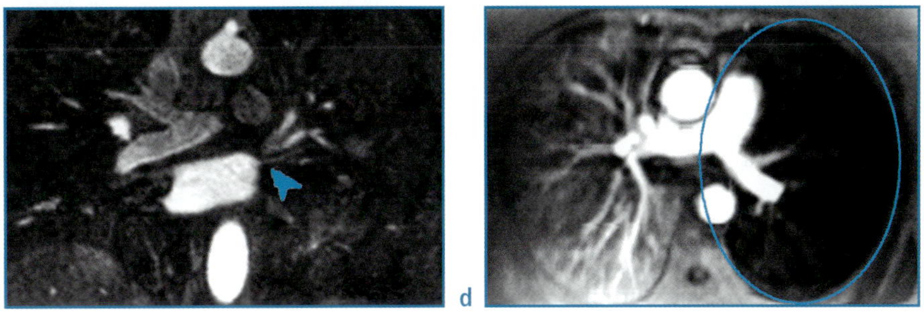

a b c d

Figure 18-7 Detection of a significant stenosis of the left inferior pulmonary vein (LLPV) in a contrast-enhanced MRA in a survey (a) and magnified dorsoventral view ((b), arrow) following radiofrequency ablation for atrial fibrillation. CE-MRA of the LLPV stenosis in an axial plane ((c), arrow), and severe perfusion defect on CE-MRA of the left lung ((d), circle) compared to the right lung (courtesy Prof. T. Dill, Bad-Nauheim).

technique for detecting significant PV stenoses following PV isolation. Dill et al. (2003) reported an incidence of relevant diameter reductions ≥ 25 % or stenosis of ≥ 50 % in 25 of 138 (18.1 %) treated veins 1 d and/or 3 mths after RF ablation. Arentz et al. (2005) observed 11 of 117 patients (9.4 %) with PV stenosis following RF ablation. None of these had PAH at rest, but 7 of these 11 patients developed PAH during exercise. Kluge et al. (2004) studied 51 of 110 patients after RF ablation (PV isolation or semicircular or focal ablation) with PV diameter reduction of ≥ 25 % or with clinical symptoms (i. e. dyspnea and cough), and found 20 of 21 perfusion defects using MR perfusion compared with SPECT perfusion as a reference. Perfusion decreased substantially in 21 of 25 areas (84 %) of PV stenoses ≤ 6 mm in diameter, compared to 2 of 180 areas (1.1 %) of PV stenoses > 6 mm in diameter. After PV balloon dilatation perfusion was restored partially after weeks, complete normalization was seen in 4 of 12 patients (33 %). Thus, CE-MRA and MR perfusion studies are valuable tools for long-term monitoring of patients after RF ablation for atrial fibrillation (Figure 18-7).

The **Scimitar syndrome** includes hypoplasia of the right lung, dextroposition of the heart, disorganized lung parenchyma, and abnormal vascularisation. The right lung is supplied in part by the right PA, in part by branches from the aorta, and an atypical pulmonary vein. All right-sided PVs drain into the inferior vena cava, or less frequently into a liver vein or the portal vein via a common confluens. Diagnosis is confirmed by chest X-ray (dextrocardia, volume reduction of the right lung, Scimitar-vessel production by the abnormal lower right PV or the common confluens vein), and most elegantly by CE-MRA (Figure 18-8).

18.9 Malformations of the Lung Parenchyma

18.9.1 Bronchopulmonary Sequestration

Etiology and Pathophysiology

A sequestration is generally defined as non-functioning lung tissue that is not in normal continuity with the tracheobronchial tree and derives its blood supply from systemic vessels. Bronchopulmonary sequestrations constitute approximately

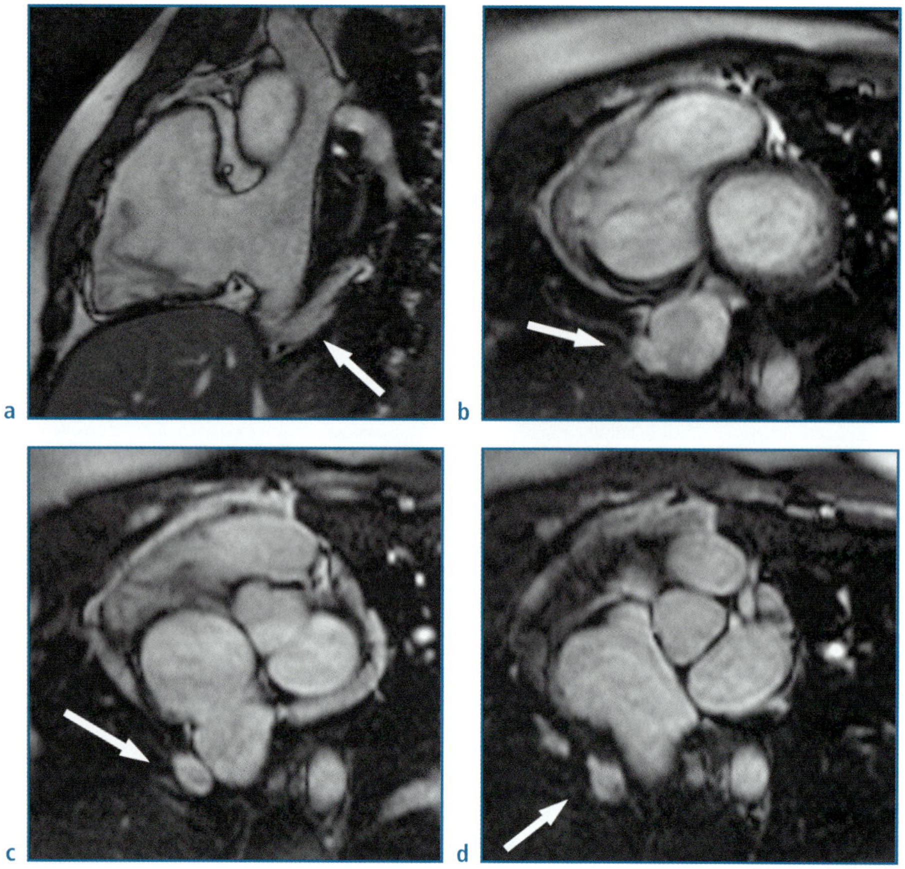

Figure 18-8 Scimitar syndrome in a contrast-enhanced MRA of the heart and pulmonary circulation in a 2-ch view (a), and three short-axis views beginning at the level of AV valves (b) to the atrial level (d). Note the abnormal Scimitar vein (arrows) draining into the inferior caval vein (a) and its course in the three axial planes (b–d). PC-flow mapping and volumetry resulted in a 20% left-to-right shunt.

0.15–6.4% of all congenital pulmonary malformations. Sequestrations may be either intralobar or extralobar. An **intralobar sequestration** shares the visceral pleural covering of an otherwise normal pulmonary lobe, with arterial supply from the aorta and venous draining via PVs. An **extralobar sequestration** is separated from normal lung by its own pleural covering, with arterial supply from the aorta and venous drainage via azygos or superior caval veins. Many variants of sequestration have been described and in many cases the distinction between intralobar and extralobar is unclear. The sequestration spectrum includes all anomalies in which there is abnormal connection between one or more of the four important components of lung tissue, i.e. tracheobronchial airway, lung parenchyma, arterial supply, and/or venous drainage.

Clinical Presentation

Intralobar sequestration accounts for about 75% of cases and almost always within the lower lobes (98% of cases). It is more common on the left and typically involves the posterobasal segment, with most lesions draining into the left atrium through the PVs. These lesions may remain asymptomatic for a long time and may manifest with recurrent cough and fever from infections. Minor hemoptysis is a common presenting complaint, usually in association with infection. **Extralobar sequestration** is commonly associated with other congenital malformations. In 63–77% of cases it occurs classically in the posterior costodiaphragmatic sulcus between the lower lobe and left hemidiaphragm, and less commonly, in the mediastinum or within or below the hemidiaphragm. It usually manifests in early infancy with respiratory distress and feeding difficulties, and is frequently detected when diagnosing associated congenital malformations.

Diagnosis

Diagnosis may be confirmed by:

- chest X-ray:
  - *intralobar*: intrapulmonary lesion involving the posterobasal segment of the left lower lobe, rarely the right lower lobe, homogenous opacity or patch of consolidation, sometimes areas of cavitation, cystic spaces with air fluid levels or completely air-filled, and a prominent vascular shadow seen as tubular or branching opacity,
  - *extralobar*: homogenous opacity in close relation to the posterior left hemidiaphragm, usually no cystic lesions, associated diaphragmatic hernia,

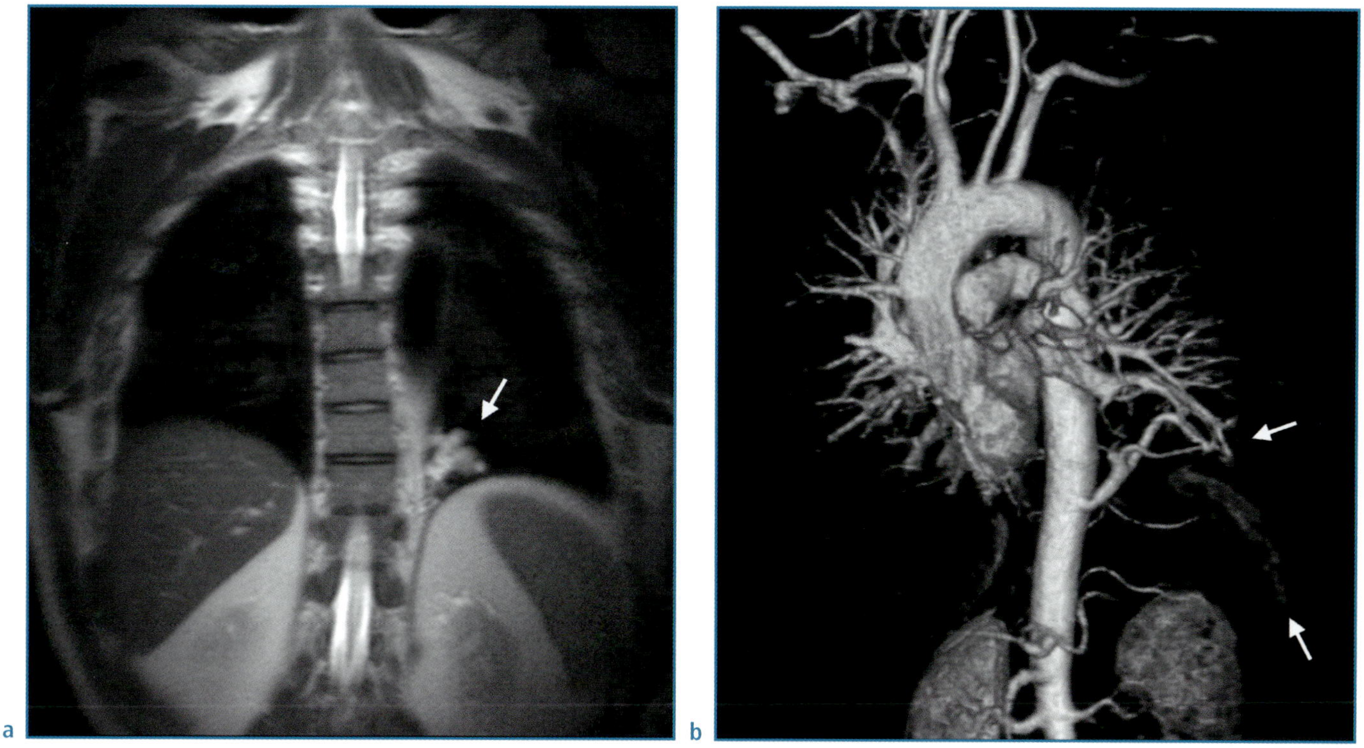

Figure 18-9 Detection of a lung sequester in a patient with recurrent bronchopulmonary infections, typically located in the posterior costo-diaphragmatic sulcus between the lower lobe and left hemidiaphragm (arrow in (a)). Volume rendering of the angiogram showed arterial supply of the sequester from the aorta with venous drainage via a pulmonary vein (intralobular sequestration, upper arrow in (b)) and a shadowy sequester (lower arrow in (b)) (courtesy Prof. A. Buecker, Homburg/Saar).

- angiography (depiction of arterial and venous anatomy),
- CT angiography (depiction of pulmonary parenchymal abnormality and of arterial and venous anatomy), and finally
- MRI (Abbey 2009).

The advantage of MRI over CT is its absence of radiation. Its multi-planar capability also provides an excellent visualization of the supplying systemic arterial anatomy as well as the pulmonary venous return and the relationship of the draining vein to the cardiac chambers (Figure 18-9). Moreover, MRI can show the cystic nature of many intralobar sequestrations and can depict hemorrhagic and solid components of the sequester (Abbey 2009).

18.9.2 Agenesia, Aplasia and Hypoplasia of Lung Parenchyma

Agenisia is defined as an absence of a complete lung with all associated structures (parenchyma, bronchi, and vessels), **aplasia** as absent lung parenchyma with rudimentary blind main bronchus, and **hypoplasia** as regularly developed main bronchus ending in a malformed cystic lobular lung parenchyma. Diagnosis is confirmed by chest X-ray and CT, MRI plays no diagnostic role.

References

Abbey P, Das CJ, Pangtey GS et al. Imaging in bronchopulmonary sequestration. J Med Imag Radiation Oncol 2009; 53: 22–31.

Arentz T, Weber R, Jander N et al. Pulmonary hemodynamics at rest and during exercise in patients with significant pulmonary vein stenosis after radiofrequency catheter ablation for drug resistant atrial fibrillation. Eur Heart J 2005; 26: 1410–4.

Blyth KG, Groenning BA, Martin TN et al. Contrast-enhanced cardiovascular magnetic resonance imaging in patients with pulmonary hypertension. Eur Heart J 2005; 26: 1993–9.

Bogren HG, Klipstein RH, Mohiaddin RH et al. Pulmonary artery distensibility and blood flow patterns: a magnetic resonance study of normal subjects and of patients with pulmonary arterial hypertension. Am Heart J 1989; 118 (5 Pt 1): 990–9.

Chin KM, Kingman M, de Lemos JA et al. Changes in right ventricular structure and function assessed using cardiac magnetic resonance imaging in bosentan-treated patients with pulmonary arterial hypertension. Am J Cardiol 2008; 101: 1669–72.

D'Armini AM, Cattadori B, Monterosso C et al. Pulmonary thrombendarterectomy in patients with chronic thromboembolic pulmonary hypertension: hemodynamic characteristics and changes. Eur J Card Thorac Surg 2000; 18: 696–702.

Dill T, Neumann T, Ekinci O et al. Pulmonary vein diameter reduction after radiofrequency catheter ablation for paroxysmal atrial fibrillation evaluated by contrast-enhanced three-dimensional magnetic resonance imaging. Circulation 2003; 107: 845–50.

Fink C, Ley S, Schoenberg SO et al. Magnetic resonance imaging of acute pulmonary embolism. Eur Radiol 2007; 17: 2546–53.

Frazier AA, Franks TJ, Mohammed TLH et al. Pulmonary veno-occlusive disease and pulmonary capillary hemangiomatosis. RadioGraphics 2007; 27: 867–82.

Gan CT, Holverda S, Marcus T et al. Right ventricular diastolic dysfunction and the acute effects of sildenafil in pulmonary hypertension patients. Chest 2007a; 132: 11–7.

Gan CT, Lankhaar JW, Marcus JT et al. Impaired left ventricular filling due to right-to-left ventricular interaction in patients with pulmonary arterial hypertension. Am J Physiol Heart Circ Physiol 2006; 290: H1528–H1533.

Gan CT, Lankhaar JW, Westerhof N et al. Non-invasively assessed pulmonary artery stiffness predicts mortality in pulmonary arterial hypertension. Chest 2007b; 132: 1906–12.

Goyen M, Laub G, Ladd ME et al. Dynamic 3DMR angiography of the pulmonary arteries in under four seconds. J Magn Reson Imaging 2001; 13: 372–7.

Hatabu H, Gaa J, Kim D et al. Pulmonary perfusion: qualitative assessment with dynamic contrast-enhanced MRI using ultra-short TE and inversion recovery turbo FLASH. Magn Reson Med 1996; 36: 503–8.

Hawkins NM, Petrie MC, Jhund PS et al. Heart failure and chronic obstructive pulmonary disease: diagnostic pitfalls and epidemiology. Eur J Heart Fail 2009; 11: 130–9.

Hoeper MM, Tongers J, Leppert A et al. Evaluation of right ventricular performance with a right ventricular ejection fraction thermodilution catheter and MRI in patients with pulmonary hypertension. Chest 2001; 120: 502–7.

Jardim C, Rochitte CE, Humbert M et al. Pulmonary artery distensibility in pulmonary arterial hypertension: a MRI pilot study. Eur Resp J 2007; 29: 476–81.

Junqueira FP, Macedo R, Coutinho Jr. AC et al. Myocardial delayed enhancement in patients with pulmonary hypertension and right ventricular failure: evaluation by cardiac MRI. Br J Radiol 2009; 82: 821–6.

Katz J, Whang J, Boxt LM et al. Estimation of right ventricular mass in normal subjects and in patients with primary pulmonary hypertension by nuclear magnetic resonance imaging. J Am Coll Cardiol 1993; 21: 1475–81.

Kluge A, Dill T, Ekinci O et al. Decreased pulmonary perfusion in pulmonary vein stenosis after radiofrequency ablation. Assessment with dynamic magnetic resonance perfusion imaging. Chest 2004; 126: 428–37.

Kluge A, Luboldt W, Bachmann G. Acute pulmonary embolism to the subsegmental level: diagnostic accuracy of three MRI techniques compared with 16-MDCT. Am J Roentgenol 2006; 187: W7–14.

Kondo C, Caputo GR, Masui T et al. Pulmonary hypertension: pulmonary flow quantification and flow profile analysis with velocity-encoded cine-MR imaging. Radiology 1992; 183: 751–8.

Kreitner KFJ, Ley S, Kauczor HU et al. Chronic thromboembolic pulmonary hypertension: pre- and post-operative assessment with breath-hold MR imaging techniques. Radiology 2004; 232: 535–43.

Kuehne T, Yilmaz S, Schulze-Neick I et al. Magnetic resonance imaging guided catheterisation for assessment of pulmonary vascular resistance: in vivo validation and clinical application in patients with pulmonary hypertension. Heart 2005; 91: 1064–9.

Kuehne T, Yilmaz S, Steendijk P et al. Magnetic resonance imaging analysis of right ventricular pressure-volume loops: in vivo validation and clinical application in patients with pulmonary hypertension. Circulation 2004; 110: 2010–6.

Magalang UJ, Richards K, McCarthy B et al. Continuous positive airway pressure therapy reduces right ventricular volume in patients with obstructive sleep apnea: a cardiovascular magnetic resonance study. J Clin Sleep Med 2009; 5 (2): 110–4.

Marcu CB, Beek AM, Van Rossum AC. Cardiovascular magnetic resonance imaging for the assessment of right heart involvement in cardiac and pulmonary disease. Heart Lung Circ 2006; 15 (6): 362–70.

Mauritz GJ, Marcus T, Boonstra A et al. Non-invasive stroke volume assessment in patients with pulmonary arterial hypertension: left-sided data mandatory. J Cardiovasc Magn Reson 2008; 10: 51.

McLaughlin VV, Archer SL, Badesch DB et al. ACC/AHA 2009 Expert Consensus Document on Pulmonary Hypertension. A Report of the American College of Cardiology Foundation Task Force on Expert Consensus Documents and the American Heart Association. Circulation 2009. doi: 10.1161/CIRCULATIONAHA.109.192230.

McLure LER, Peacock AJ. Cardiac magnetic resonance imaging for the assessment of the heart and pulmonary circulation in pulmonary hypertension. Eur Respir J 2009; 33: 1454–66.

Michelakis ED, Tymchak W, Lien D et al. Oral sildenafil is an effective and specific pulmonary vasodilator in patients with pulmonary arterial hypertension: comparison with inhaled nitric oxide. Circulation 2002; 105: 2398–403.

Michelakis ED, Tymchak W, Noga M et al. Long-term treatment with oral sildenafil is safe and improves functional capacity and hemodynamics in patients with pulmonary arterial hypertension. Circulation 2003; 108: 2066–9.

Mousseaux E, Tasu JP, Jolivet O et al. Pulmonary arterial resistance: non-invasive measurement with indexes of pulmonary flow estimated at velocity-encoded MR imaging – preliminary experience. Radiology 1999; 212: 896–902.

Ohno Y, Hatabu H, Murase K et al. Primary pulmonary hypertension: 3D dynamic perfusion MRI for quantitative analysis of regional pulmonary perfusion. Am J Roentgenol 2007; 188: 48–56.

Ohno Y, Higashino T, Takenaka D et al. MR angiography with sensitivity encoding (SENSE) for suspected pulmonary embolism: comparison with MDCT and ventilation-perfusion scintigraphy. Am J Roentgenol 2004; 183: 91–8.

Paz R, Mohiaddin RH, Longmore DB. Magnetic resonance assessment of the pulmonary arterial trunk anatomy, flow, pulsatility and distensibility. Eur Heart J 1993; 14: 1424–530.

Reesink HJ, Marcus T, Tulevski II et al. Reverse right ventricular remodeling after pulmonary endarterectomy in patients with chronic thromboembolic pulmonary hypertension: utility of magnetic resonance imaging to demonstrate restoration of the right ventricle. J Thorac Cardiovasc Surg 2007; 133: 58–64.

Rich S. Pulmonary hypertension. In: Bonow RO, Mann DL, Zipes DP, Libby P (eds.). Braunwald's Heart Disease. A Textbook of Cardiovascular Medicine. Elsevier Saunders 2012; 1696–718.

Roeleveld RJ, Marcus TJ, Boonstra A et al. A comparison of noninvasive MRI-based methods of estimating pulmonary artery pressure in pulmonary hypertension. J Magn Reson Imag 2005; 22: 67–72.

Roeleveld RJ, Vonk-Noordegraaf A, Marcus TJ et al. Effects of eprostenol on right ventricular hypertrophy and dilatation in pulmonary hypertension. Chest 2004; 125: 572–9.

Rutten FH, Vonken EJ, Cramer MJ et al. Cardiovascular magnetic resonance imaging to identify left-sided chronic heart failure in stable patients with chronic obstructive pulmonary disease. Am Heart J 2008; 156: 506–12.

Saba TS, Foster J, Cockburn M et al. Ventricular mass index using magnetic resonance imaging accurately estimates pulmonary artery pressure. Eur Resp J 2002; 20: 1519–24.

Schönberg SO, Knopp MV, Grau A et al. Ultrafast MRI phlebography of the lungs. Radiologe 1998; 38: 597–605.

Stein PD, Chenevert TL, Fowler SE et al. Gadolinium-enhanced magnetic resonance angiography for pulmonary embolism. A multi-center prospective study (PIOPED III). Ann Intern Med 2010; 152: 434–43.

Stein PD, Fowler SE, Goodman LR et al. Multi-detector computed tomography for acute pulmonary embolism. N Engl J Med 2006; 354: 2317–27.

Stevens GR, Lala A, Sanz X et al. Exercise performance in patients with pulmonary hypertension linked to cardiac magnetic resonance measures. J Heart Lung Transplant 2009; 28: 899–905.

Ugander M, Jense E, Arheden H. Pulmonary intravascular blood volume changes throughout the cardiac cycle in healthy volunteers studied by cardiovascular magnetic resonance measurements of arterial and venous flow. J Cardiovasc Magn Reson 2009; 11: 42.

Van Wolferen SA, Boonstra A, Marcus JT et al. Right ventricular reverse remodelling after sildenafil in pulmonary arterial hypertension. Heart 2006; 92 (12): 1860–1.

Van Wolferen SA, Marcus JT, Boonstra A et al. Prognostic value of right ventricular mass, volume, and function in idiopathic pulmonary arterial hypertension. Eur Heart J 2007; 28: 1250–7.

Vonk-Noordegraaf A, Marcus TJ, Gan CT et al. Interventricular mechanical asynchrony due to right ventricular pressure overload in pulmonary hypertension plays an important role in impaired left ventricular filling. Chest 2005; 128 (Suppl.): 628S–630S.

Wilkins MR, Paul GA, Strange JW et al. Sildenafil vs. endothelin receptor antagonist for pulmonary hypertension (SERAPH) study. Am J Respir Crit Care Med 2005; 171: 1292–7.

19 Diseases of the Thoracic and Abdominal Aorta

Christina Heilmaier, Florian Vogt and Jörg Barkhausen

19.1 Introduction

The spectrum of diseases affecting the thoracic and abdominal aorta is broad, reaching from congenital anomalies such as coarctation of the aorta or double aortic arch, to disorders of connective-tissue metabolism such as Marfan's syndrome, inflammatory infiltration of the vessel wall to atherosclerotic diseases. These disorders may result in thickening of the aortic wall, aortic dilatation or dissection, sometimes taking a fulminating course requiring rapid and reliable diagnostic evaluation.

19.2 MRI Techniques

MR imaging (MRI) and MR angiography (MRA) techniques have been firmly established as robust clinical diagnostic modalities for the evaluation of all relevant diseases of the thoracic and abdominal vasculature. Contrast-enhanced 3D MR angiography nowadays is one of the standard practice tools with ever-increasing flexibility for luminography of the thoracic and abdominal aorta and its major branches. Continuing improvements in hardware and software had a significant impact on image quality and acquisition time, overcoming former barriers such as motion and the time required for high quality diagnostic studies.

New ultra-fast gradient systems and parallel imaging techniques allow acquisition time reduction while maintaining or improving spatial resolution. Furthermore, the introduction of strategies for enlarging the effective MRI image area, like multi-station and continuously moving table techniques, have pushed high-spatial resolution MRA from a limited to a rather unlimited field of view (FOV) imaging modality. In addition to improving the reliability for acquiring high-spatial resolution arterial-phase images within a large FOV, high frame rate examinations are able to depict filling patterns in cases of dissections, endoleaks and other complex contrast dynamics in 3D.

Cine-MR imaging can be performed to evaluate blood flow through structures, e. g. real-time assessment of intimal flap movement in aortic dissection, delineating the relationship to branch vessels and possible occlusion of these during systolic or diastolic phase (Figure 19-1). In addition, differentiation between true and false lumen or possible thrombus and slow-flowing blood can be easily achieved. Cine-MR imaging can also be used specifically to assess valvular and cardiac function. Cine phase contrast imaging on the other hand, helps to determine flow velocity and direction. Dark blood and post-contrast T1-weighted sequences have shown to be very supportive in diagnosis of intramural hematoma and inflammatory disease of the aorta.

19.2.1 MR Angiography (MRA)

High-spatial resolution contrast-enhanced MRA is an established non-invasive imaging technique for assessing aortic aneurysm, aortic dissection, intramural hematomas, pene-

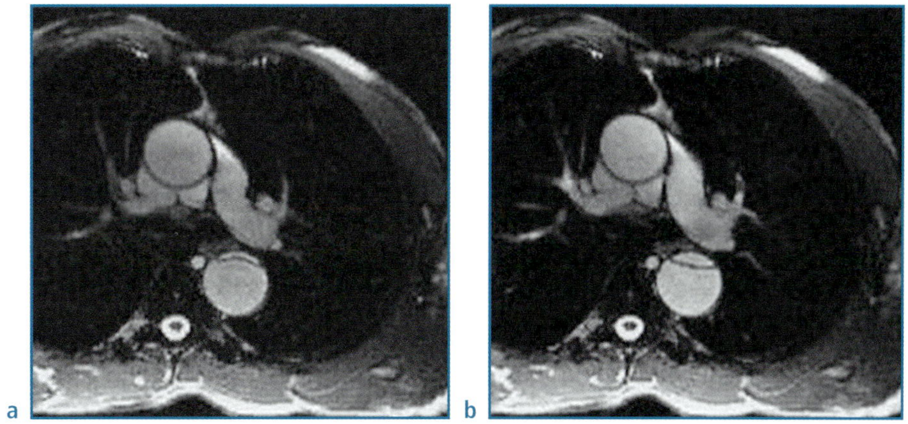

Figure 19-1 Cine-SSFP sequence in a patient with acute aortic dissection. Images acquired at systole (a) and diastole (b) demonstrate movement of the dissection membrane during cardiac cycle.

trating ulcerative plaques or vasculitis. Although many institutions utilize CTA as the primary imaging tool in an acute clinical setting, contrast-enhanced 3D MRA is increasingly favored in the more stable patient and follow-up assessment of these pathologies. The technique is based on a 3D Fourier transform gradient recalled (GRE) sequence using rapid radiofrequency pulsing. Optimization of MRA is related to rapid data collection to overcome respiratory and cardiac motion artifacts, especially in the thoracic region. Thus, the fastest available sequences with minimal repetition and echo times should be chosen. The partition dimensions (i. e. partition thickness, matrix size and FOV) should be chosen to achieve the smallest possible voxel size to allow for sufficient spatial coverage of the target vessel within a single breath-hold. Section thickness should be adjusted to be between 0.5 and 2 mm to ensure full coverage of the vascular system under consideration and still permit multi-planar reformations. Imaging time can be further decreased using partial Fourier imaging, decreased phase-encoding steps, and a rectangular FOV. Widening bandwidth and the implementation of newer parallel imaging techniques also enable faster scanning, although this causes a reduction in SNR. The use of multi-array surface coils and the introduction of 3 T systems have advanced the performance of magnetic resonance and counteracted the problem of reduced SNR.

It is well-recognized that, to ensure high image quality in 3D MRA, the contrast must be near or at the peak concentration in the vasculature of interest when acquiring the central phase-encoding views of the MRA. To facilitate the timing of the contrast bolus different contrast agent injection strategies have been developed, including test bolus, fluoroscopic or automatic triggering. However, exact timing of contrast application remains most crucial and inadequate timing may affect image quality in different ways: venous overlap, ringing artifacts, or insufficient signal within the vessels of interest.

The use of non-enhanced MRA strategies in the depiction of vasculature structures may be an alternative non-invasive approach to assess or screen for aortic disease, e. g. in patients with end-stage renal disease who are at high risk for developing gadolinium-based contrast material-related complications (i. e. nephrogenic systemic fibrosis), difficult venous access or during pregnancy.

Free-breathing cardiac and respiratory gated non-enhanced 3D steady-state free precession (SSFP) MRA using non-selective radiofrequency excitation has been shown to be a promising novel technique in the non-contrast assessment of major vessels. The sequence is characterized by balanced gradients in all three directions, ensuring maximum recovery of the transverse magnetization. The image contrast with SSFP is determined by favourable T2*/T1 properties that are nearly independent from blood flow. The main advantage of this sequence is related to its high signal of fluids. This results in high contrast delineating vessels seen as bright structures, while at the same time outlining all other morphology. The short time of repetition and echo time reduce susceptibility artifacts and lead to extremely short data acquisition times.

19.2.2 Time-Resolved MRA

Even if technically perfect, standard high-spatial resolution MRA techniques only provide static morphologic information and hold the risk of incorrect bolus timing resulting in a suboptimal arterial contrast or venous overlay. To overcome these limitations time-resolved contrast-enhanced 3D MRA techniques have been introduced and received considerable attention recently owing to their ability for providing a dynamic complement for a variety of clinical indications (Figure 19-2). These techniques incorporate various advantages compared to conventional static MRA techniques – incorrect bolus timing is almost impossible resulting in an improved arterialvenous discrimination with reduced a 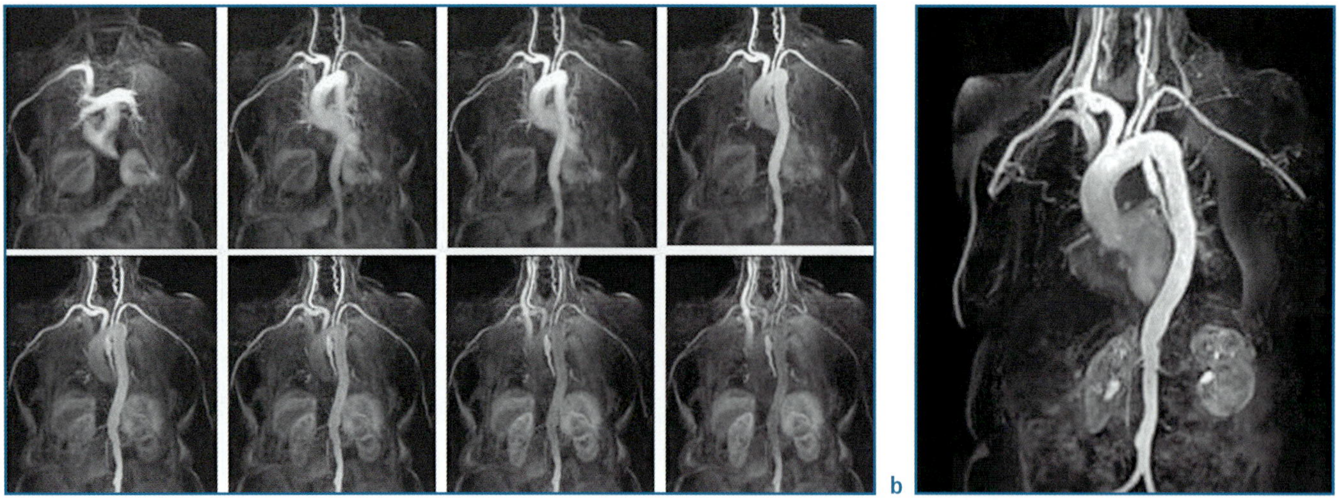 b

Figure 19-2 Combined high-temporal resolution magnetic resonance angiography (MRA) (a) followed by high-spatial resolution MRA (b) in a patient with acute aortic dissection. High-temporal resolution MRAs show slow filling of the false lumen with delayed and prolonged enhancement compared to the true lumen.

venous overlay, minimized sensitivity to motion artifacts, and additional diagnostic information from the dynamic assessment of contrast-enhancement and tissue perfusion.

A number of various k-space sampling techniques have been described to accelerate acquisition of 3D MRA images. These techniques, although differing in their image reconstruction routines, have in common that some parts of the k-space are updated more often than others, leading to an effective shortening of the acquisition time of each 3D data set. With the introduction of parallel acquisition techniques, acquisition time per 3D data set was also noticeably reduced. Complementary improvements in gradient hardware, pulse sequences, or computational power further reduced scan and reconstruction times to seconds or less for a series of undersampled 3D data sets. In clinical practice this acceleration allows rapid sequential acquisitions within a single breath hold and leads to an improvement of spatial and/or temporal resolution of MRA. Studies can be performed with an administration of a small amount of gadolinium-based contrast agent within the range of only 3–5 ml. Therefore, if necessary, the dynamic MRA can easily be combined with a standard high-resolution MRA.

Especially in the event of aortic dissection, time-resolved MRA can correctly characterize true and false lumen as well as the origin of the branch vessels. The temporal resolution of the MRA allows rapid visualization of the contrast agent bolus transit within the true and the false lumen and provides additional information compared to the static MRA. These finding can have impact on therapy planning such as for example endovascular stent-graft repair.

Furthermore, time-resolved MRA has been shown to have potential in assessing functional abnormalities in patients with congenital heart disease with respect to define intra- or extra-cardiac shunts or post-surgical leaks. Time-resolved MRA is not only able to evaluate functional abnormalities of the arterial system; it may also be useful for depicting central venous abnormalities.

19.2.3 Whole-Body MRA

In most patients the thoracic and abdominal aorta can be assessed in one examination using a large FOV and dedicated surface coils providing high spatial resolution. Thus, all pathologies of the aorta can be depicted accurately without the necessity of dividing the examination into several discrete partial examinations by moving the patient table together with the table relative to the imaging volume. However, it is well-known that the prevalence of peripheral arterial occlusive disease is elevated in many patients with thoracic and abdominal aortic abnormalities as e.g. aneurysms or dissection. Additionally, aortic diseases may affect the supra-aortic arteries.

Different treatment options are available for aortic diseases, ranging from conservative pharmacological treatment and catheter-based interventions up to surgical methods with remodeling of the vessels or bypass surgery. For treatment planning, all listed procedures have in common that they rely on initial diagnostic imaging to assess the degree and extent of additional arterial disease. In this respect there is widespread agreement that imaging of the arterial system with depiction of the entire course of the aorta and its branches is desirable. In the light of this problem the potential of whole-body MRA seems to be reasonable.

Recent developments in MR hardware and software, such as dedicated whole-body MR systems with specially

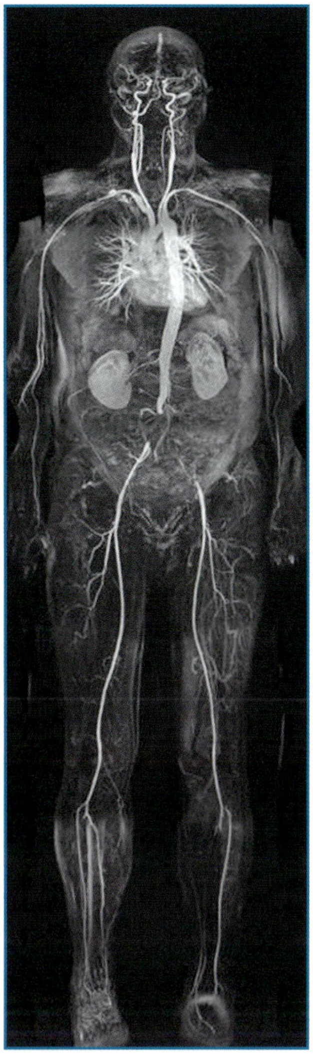

Figure 19-3 Whole-body magnetic resonance angiography in a patient suffering from Leriche syndrome. Images were acquired using continuous moving table technique providing one seamless field of view.

designed surface coils, the movement to higher field strength and the implementation of parallel acquisition techniques (PAT), have helped to overcome the restriction to body parts and only one FOV with a maximum of 50 cm.

The whole-body MRA (Figure 19-3) concept is today based on two strategies: the acquisition of 4–5 slightly overlapping 3D sets in immediate succession using an automatic moving table technique in between or the data acquisition during continuous table movement in a manner more comparable to computed tomography angiography (CTA), creating a seamless FOV. The new technique with continuous table movement promises to be a technique easily applicable for imaging without the need for planning different steps and FOV positioning, thereby reducing examination time considerably. Both whole-body MRA approaches have also shown to be a reliable single-dose MRA technique in combination with a high-spatial and high-temporal resolution MRA providing good image quality. Despite the use of single-dose contrast agent, large field of view coverage and dynamic images can be acquired.

19.3 Diseases of the Thoracic Aorta

Originating from the left ventricular outflow tract the aorta runs distally to the aortic bifurcation, where it splits into the right and left common iliac (sciatic) artery. With regard to its course, it is subdivided in four sections: the ascending aorta, the aortic arch, the descending thoracic aorta as well as the descending abdominal aorta.

The aortic root, which represents the initial portion of the ascending aorta, contains the aortic bulb that bears the three cusps of the aortic valve and tapers at the sinotubular junction to become a part of the ascending aorta. The coronary arteries arise directly distal of the aortic valve and originate at the left and right coronary sinuses (of Valsalva), which are accompanied by a third, non-coronary sinus.

On its way through the thorax the aorta has an initial upward and backward course, before it runs to the left to continue its way down parallel to the vertebral spine to the aortic hiatus in the diaphragm to proceed distally as the abdominal aorta. While the supra-aortic vessels, which are often point of anatomic variants, branch from the aortic arch, the bronchial arteries, spinal arteries, and smaller arterial branches arise from the descending thoracic aorta.

19.3.1 Aortic Aneurysm (Aneurysma Verum)

In healthy subjects the thickness of the aortic wall measures less than 4 mm. The vessel diameter, however, depends on various factors such as the site of measurement, the age and sex of the patient as well as on the individual's physical activity. For example, normal values for females are usually approximately 10 % lower than for men, and subjects with a high level of physical labour have larger aortic diameters than individuals with predominantly sedentary activities. Normal diameter values are 2.3–3 cm for the aortic annulus, 3–3.7 cm for the sinus of Valsalva, and 2.5–3.5 cm for the proximal ascending aorta. More precisely, the aortic diameters should be given in relation to the body surface area with a normal range of values of 1.4–2.1 cm/m^2 for the ascending aorta and 1.0–1.6 cm/m^2 for the descending aorta.

Etiology and Pathogenesis

The aortic diameter usually grows 1–2 mm over a 10-yrs period as part of a physiologic process that comes along with ageing. In addition, aortic enlargement may occur due to congenital diseases (e.g. Marfan's syndrome, Ehlers-Danlos syndrome, bicuspid aortic valve) or be due to an acquired disease, with classic atherosclerotic risk factors such as arterial hypertension representing the major predisposing factor.

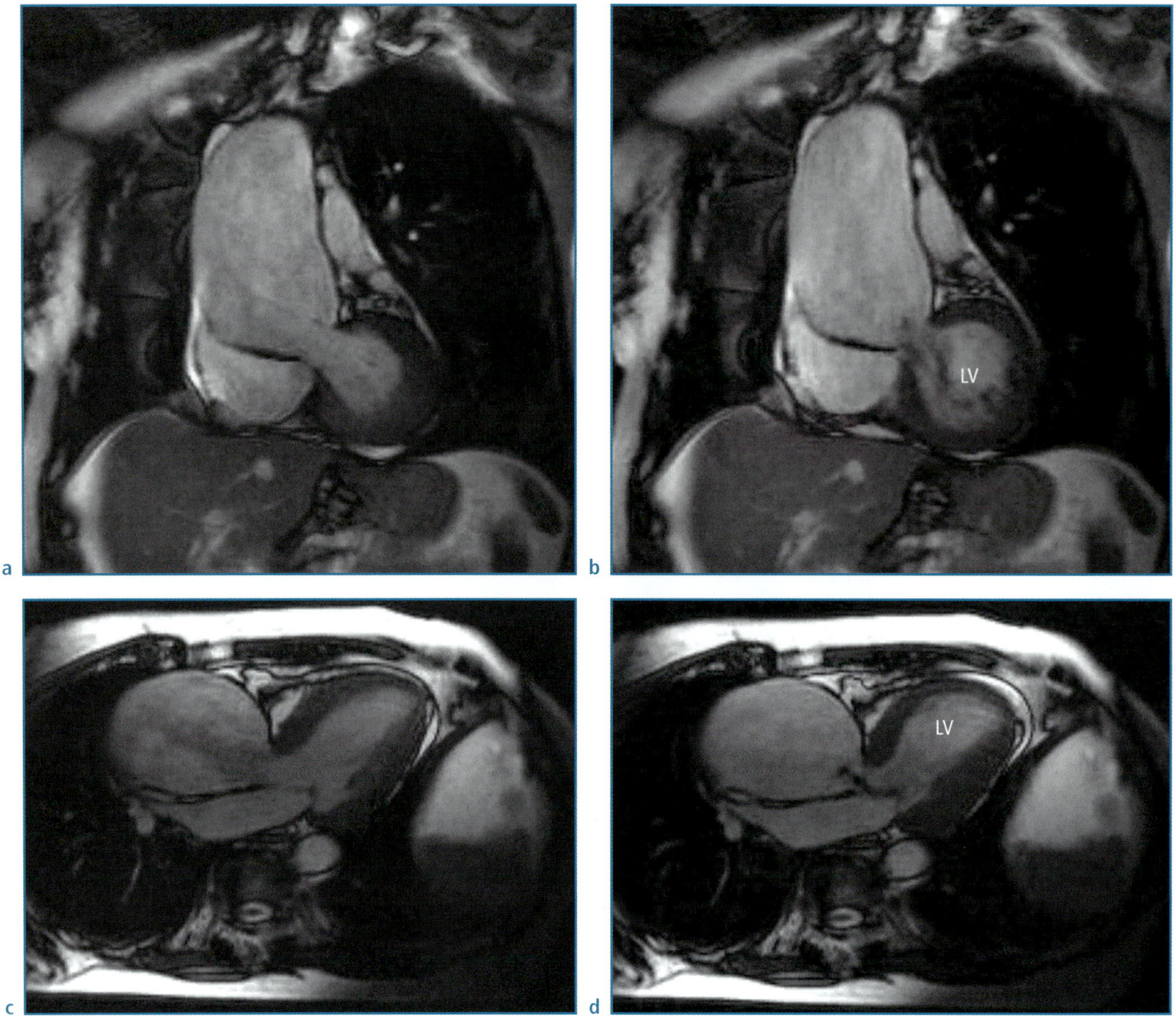

Figure 19-4 Large aneurysm of the ascending aorta with accompanying aortic regurgitation in a 62-yrs-old patient. Cine-SSFP sequence in the coronal plane (a, b) and in the 3-ch view (c, d). Diastolic jet through the aortic valve in the coronal plane (b) and 3-ch view (d). LV: left ventricle.

If the diameter exceeds normal values (> 3.5 cm for the ascending aorta, > 3 cm for the descending aorta), it is initially called aortic ectasia. When the diameter is larger than 4 cm it is described as an aortic aneurysm (Figure 19-4 and Figure 19-5). Around one-third of the aortic aneurysms occur in the thoracic aorta with the remaining two-thirds developing in the abdominal part of the descending aorta.

A true aneurysm involves all wall layers and is distinguished on the basis of the dilatation shape as fusiform (spindle-shaped) and saccular (pouch-shaped). Contrary to that a pseudoaneurysm does not affect all wall layers but has at least partially penetrated the vessel wall, often only kept together by a fibrous capsule. A pseudoaneurysm might be of traumatic, infectious, or iatrogenic etiology or can emerge as a complication of a penetrating aortic ulcer.

Clinical Presentation

Typically aortic aneurysms do not cause any symptoms and are detected incidentally, e.g. in context of diagnostic procedures related to other diseases. If not yet discovered, aneurysms may first become apparent in case of aneurysm dissection, which usually causes unbearable pain and displays a medical emergency.

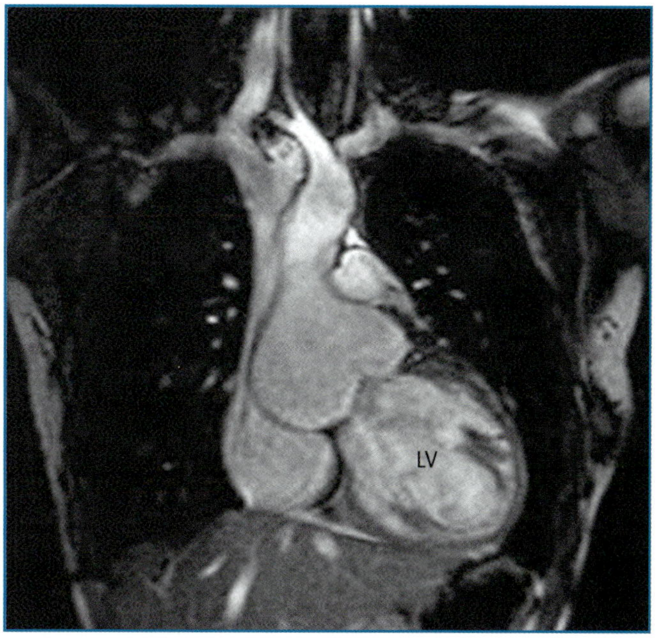

Figure 19-5 12-yrs-old patient suffering from Marfan's syndrome with large aneurysm of the aortic bulb. LV: left ventricle.

Therapy

To avoid rupture or dissection, surgical treatment should be considered if the maximum diameter of the ascending aortic aneurysm exceeds 5 cm or if it grows by more than 1 cm per year. However, associated changes such as a severe aortic regurgitation with dilatation of the left ventricle may warrant an earlier surgical intervention.

Compared to the ascending aorta surgical therapy of aneurysms within the aortic arch and the descending aorta is usually more elaborate; therefore, indication for operative treatment is usually withheld until the diameter of the aneurysm measures more than 6.5 cm or until the aneurysm grows by more than 1 cm per year. Surgical options encompass either open surgery or endovascular aortic stent grafting with the latter recently having established itself as a significantly less invasive alternative to the open surgery.

Aneurysms, which do not yet need treatment, should be monitored on a regular basis with the diameter of the aneurysms defining the follow-up intervals. For example, aneurysms exceeding 5 cm, in which surgical intervention is so far not indicated, should be initially rechecked frequently, such as every 3 mths. After a sequence of follow-ups with no change in the maximum diameter of the aneurysm the intervals may increase. To guarantee comparability of the results, great care should be taken to measure the maximum diameter of the aneurysm at the same site as in previous follow-ups. Therefore, the maximum diameter of the aorta should be measured perpendicular to the main direction of blood flow making use of the centerline method, which might be hampered in the case of aortic elongation and kinking.

Imaging Results

The **examination protocol** includes several MR imaging techniques aiming at different diagnostic informations:

- 3D-CE-MRA: assessment of the extent and diameter of the aortic aneurysm by imaging of ascending aorta, aortic arch, and descending aorta to the bifurcation,
- cine-SSFP sequences: assessment of a concomitant aortic valve insufficiency,
- PC-mapping: quantification of a concomitant aortic valve insufficiency,
- dark blood turbo spin echo sequences: assessment and quantification of aortic wall thickness, checking for presence of intraluminal thrombi and intramural/periaortal hematoma,
- T1-weighted turbo spin echo- or gradient echo sequences after contrast media application: assessment of contrast uptake of the aortic wall, especially in cases of inflammatory aortic disease.

19.3.2 Dissecting Aneurysm

Nowadays a dissection of the aorta is subsumed with other acute diseases of the aorta as "acute aortic syndrome". This syndrome is characterized by acute chest pain and is the most frequent acutely life-threatening condition after acute myocardial ischemia.

According to the **Svensson classification**:

- a classic aortic dissection with formation of a true and false lumen (*class 1 dissection*),
- an intramural hematoma (*class 2 dissection*),
- a circumscribed dissection (*class 3 dissection*),
- a penetrating aortic ulcer (*class 4 dissection*), as well as
- a traumatic/iatrogenic dissection (*class 5 dissection*)

can be distinguished and constitute subcategories of an acute aortic syndrome.

A class 1 dissection is characterized by a longitudinal separation of the aortic wall layers leading to blood flow within the vessel wall and to the consequent creation of a false lumen between the intima and adventitia. The tear is frequently (approximately 65 % of cases) localized directly distal of the aortic valve or in close proximity to the origin of the left subclavian artery, at the level of the aortic isthmus, with the dissection being circumscribed, or extending to the aortic bifurcation or to the iliac arteries, often involving aortic branches. The incidence is estimated to be 5–15 per 100,000 populations per year with the peak age between 50 and 70 yrs, if the dissection is not caused by Marfan's syndrome. Males are 3 times more often affected than females.

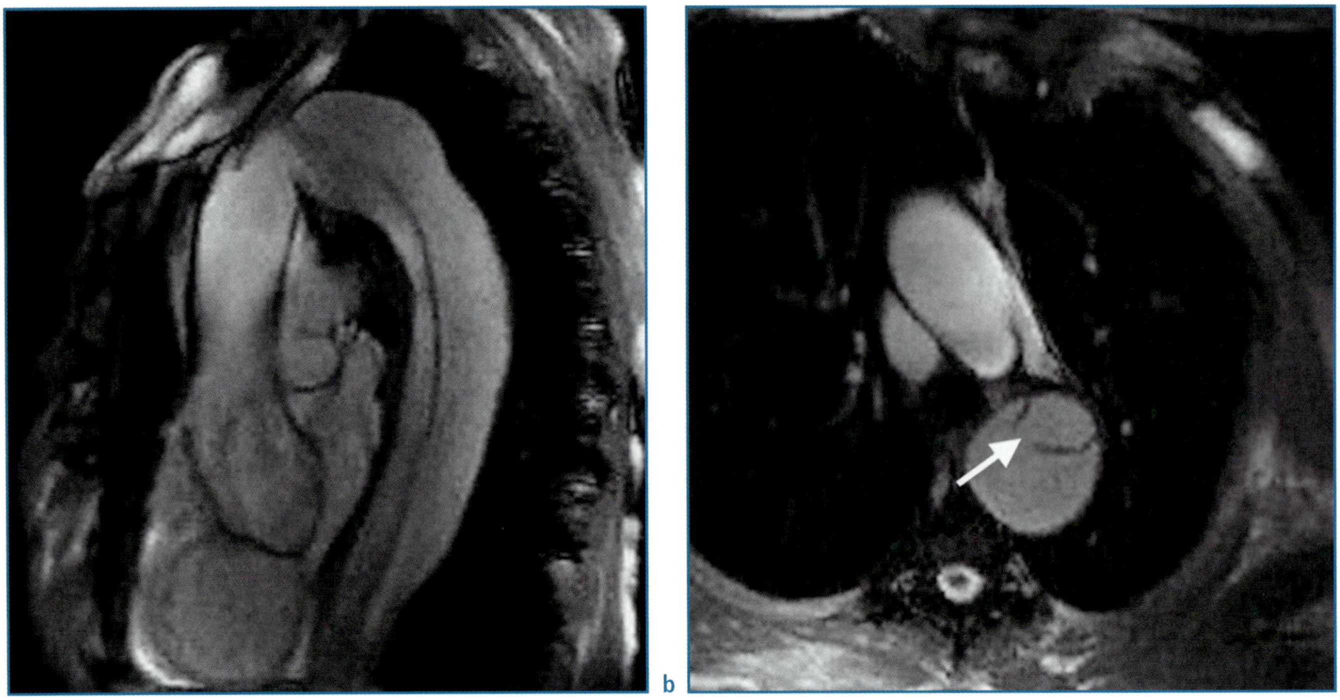

Figure 19-6 Dissection of the descending aorta with high-grade compression of the true lumen caused by the false lumen in a 67-yrs-old patient. Parasagittal cine-SSFP sequence (a), axial cine-SSFP sequence (b) at the level of the entry (white arrow).

Etiology and Pathogenesis

In most cases an aortic dissection is caused by aortic sclerosis with arterial hypertension being the prime risk factor. However, it can also be due to cystic media-necrosis in patients suffering from Marfan's or Ehlers-Danlos syndrome or be due to a direct trauma.

Aortic dissections can be distinguished according to the **Stanford classification** taking into account the involvement of the ascending aorta, while the location of the tear can be neglected:

- **Type A**: a dissection involving the ascending aorta, which may be circumscribed or expansive,
- **Type B**: a dissection confined to the descending aorta (Figure 19-6 and Figure 19-7).

This distinction is of great clinical importance as involvement of the aorta ascendens (type A-dissection) requires immediate surgical intervention because of its high mortality rate. Contrary to that type B-dissections are often not an emergency and allow for a conservative or interventional treatment.

Clinical Presentation

In up to 15% of the patients the aortic dissection is painless. However, the most common symptom reported is a sudden, unbearable pain located between the scapulae that does not subside spontaneously or after application of nitroglycerin. Due to its severity the pain almost always induces strong vasovagal reactions such as vomiting or sweating. In case of a type A-dissection an incomplete coaptation of the aortic valve cusps may be the result of a disruption of the aortic bulb geometry, ultimately leading to an aortic regurgitation. This is present in up to 70% of the patients with type A-dissection. As a consequence of the regurgitation an acute left heart failure accompanied by pulmonary edema might occur. Rarely do other symptoms such as a cerebrovascular accident, neuropathy or paraplegia caused by ischemia, or sudden cardiac death emerge due to an acute aortic dissection. Another, possible life-threatening complication of a type A-dissection is a pericardial tamponade, requiring rapid intervention by means of pericardiocentesis and insertion of drainage.

Therapy

As mentioned before, an acute type A-dissection is accompanied with high lethality and requires immediate surgical intervention with insertion of a prosthesis and replacement of the aortic valve in case of a concomitant aortic valve insufficiency. The utmost urgency of an operation is stressed by high mortality rates, in the event of conservative treatment, with about 25% in the first 24 h, about 75% in the first 4 wks, and exceeding 90% in the first year after the type A-dissection. Contrary to that, conservative therapy is warranted after initial stabilization of patients suffering from an acute type B-dissection. Due to the development of

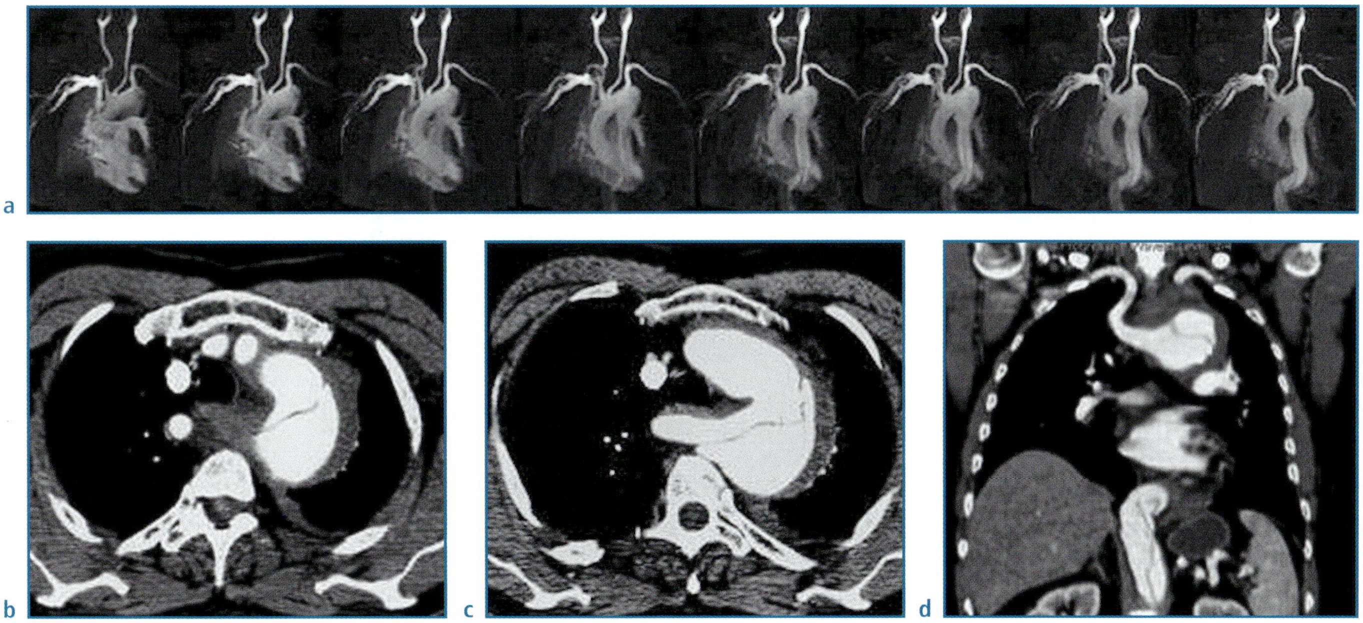

Figure 19-7 78-yrs-old patient with dissection of the descending thoracic aorta and aberrant right subclavian artery originating from the false lumen. Coronal MIPs of subsequent time frames showing delayed contrast filling **(a)** of right subclavian artery, corresponding axial CT images **(b, c)** and coronal MPR **(d)** confirms aberrant right subclavian artery.

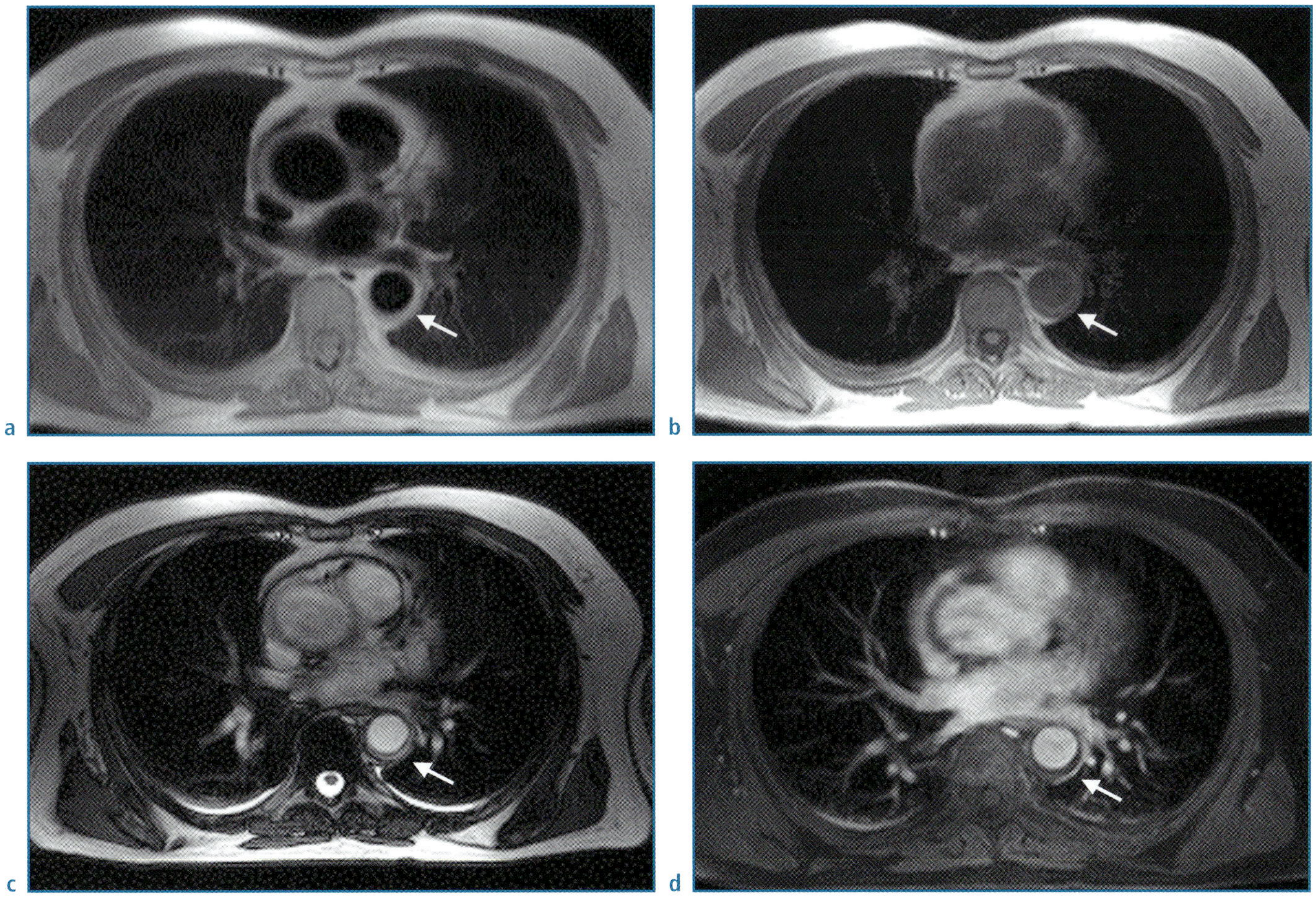

Figure 19-8 Intramural hematoma (arrow) in a 57-yrs-old patient. All sequences show a thickening of the vessel wall. The hyperintensity of the aortic wall as seen in the unenhanced T1w and SSFP sequences is due to hemorrhage within the wall. Single-shot TSE **(a)**, T1w-TSE **(b)**, SSFP **(c)** and T1w sequence **(d)** after gadolinium administration.

percutaneous stent grafts open surgery in case of a type B-dissection is hardly necessary nowadays, allowing for a gentle treatment of the dissection.

Imaging Results

The **CMR imaging protocol** aims at different diagnostic informations:

- 3D-CE-MRA: depiction of the type of dissection as well as involvement of aortic branches; here, special attention should be paid to the expansion of the dissection membrane into the supra-aortal branches; additionally, imaging of the true and false lumen, as well as of the entry and re-entry, if applicable; determination of the supply of the branch arteries by the true or false lumen,
- cine-SSFP sequences: assessment of a concomitant aortic regurgitation and of left ventricular function; imaging and evaluation of the fluctuation of the dissection membrane: an intimal flap might lead to static occlusion at the origin of a visceral artery, thereby causing a malperfusion syndrome,
- follow-up: both patients with a type A- and B-dissection should be rechecked on a regular basis.

19.3.3 Intramural Hematoma and Penetrating Ulcer

A classic dissection can be the result of several preceding diseases such as an intramural hematoma (IMH, Svensson class 2-dissection) (Figure 19-8) or a penetrating aortic ulcer (PAU, Svensson class 4-dissection) (Figure 19-9 and Figure 19-10), which might be present long before the dissection evolves. It is estimated that between 16 and 36% of all IMH progress to a classic dissection.

Etiology and Pathogenesis

An IMH is usually caused by the same predisposing factors as for the dissection itself, with arterial hypertension being the major risk factor. In most cases the IMH occurs due to an acute bleeding from ruptured vasa vasorum in the aortic media, leading to blood accumulation within the aortic wall. Contrary to a classic dissection the blood is confined to the aortic wall and does not communicate with the true aortic lumen. The IMH may be either localized or may involve the aorta in its full length. An intramural hematoma of the ascending aorta may extend to the pulmonary artery.

A PAU is typically the outcome of massive aortic sclerosis, which leads to the formation of atherosclerotic plaques that progressively erode the aortic wall. These erosions can spread to the media and adventitia after having penetrated the internal elastic membrane, and may result in a classic dissection, in a pseudoaneurysm, or in a (confined) aortic rupture. If erosions affect the vasa vasorum, an intramural

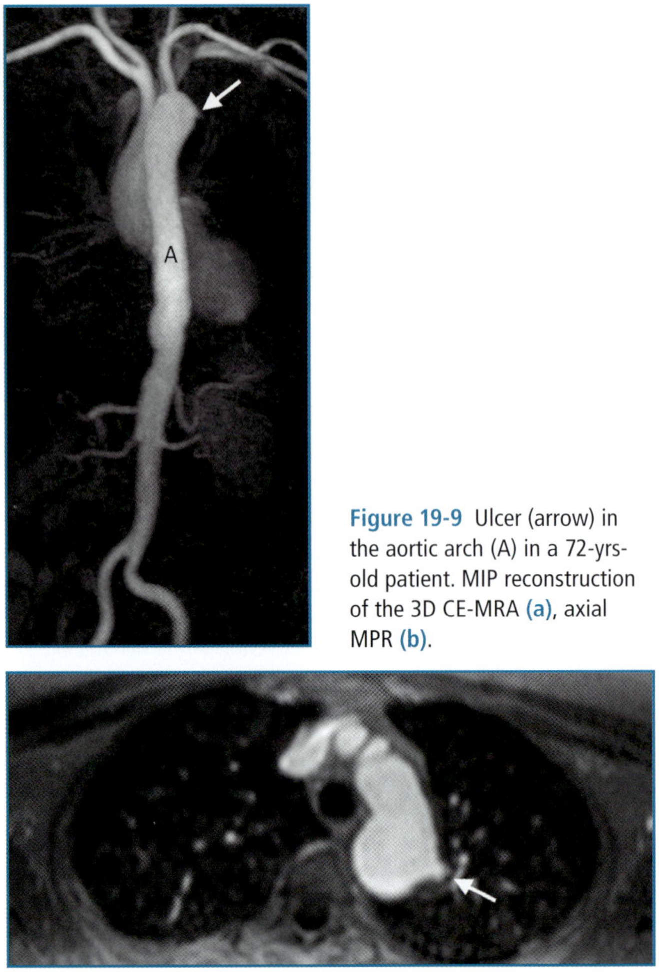

a

b

Figure 19-9 Ulcer (arrow) in the aortic arch (A) in a 72-yrs-old patient. MIP reconstruction of the 3D CE-MRA (a), axial MPR (b).

hemorrhage may occur. It is usually localized and represents an unfavourable prognostic sign. The main risk factors for progression include ectasia of the aorta as well as involvement of the ascending aorta that comes along with a poor prognosis.

Clinical Presentation

Similar to patients diagnosed with an acute aortic dissection, some patients with IMH or PAU may be completely without any discomfort, while others report on unbearable pain or other symptoms similar to those from a dissection. Thus, it is sometimes not possible to distinguish between either of the diseases on the basis of their clinical presentation.

Therapy

As a consequence of the worse prognosis that accompanies conservative treatment and in analogy to type A-dissection, IMH involving the ascending aorta should undergo surgical replacement. An affection of the descending aorta, however, allows for less invasive therapy by means of insertion of a stent graft.

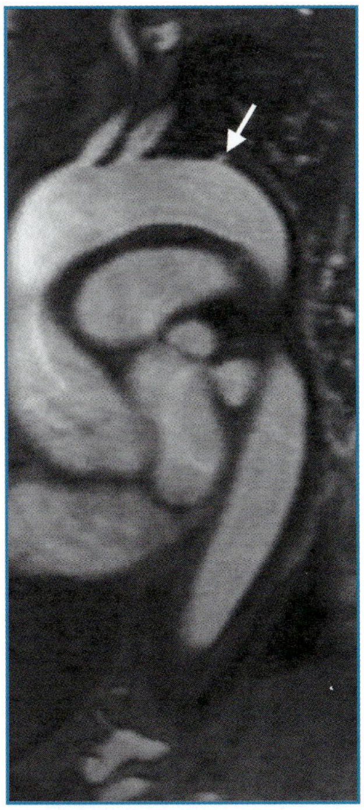

a

Figure 19-10 66-yrs-old patient. The parasagittal MPR **(a, b)** of the 3D CE-MRA shows a small ulcer (arrow) in the aortic arch **(a)** without signs of a dissection at the level of the left atrium in the axial MPR **(b)**.

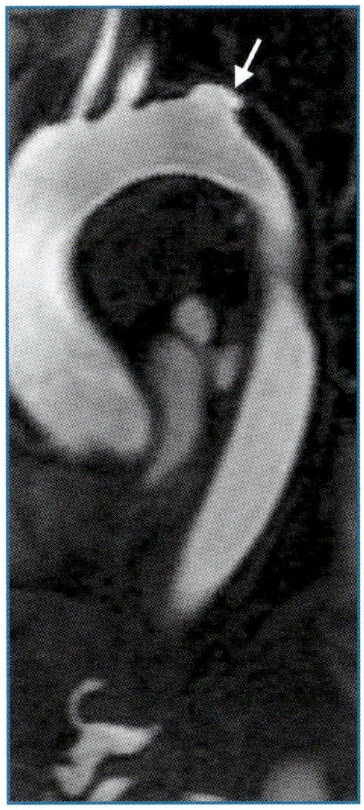

c

The same patient at a control examination 3 wks later **(c, d)** with significant progression of the ulcer in the aortic arch **(c)** actually showing aortic dissection and a false lumen (arrow) at the level of the left atrium **(d)**.

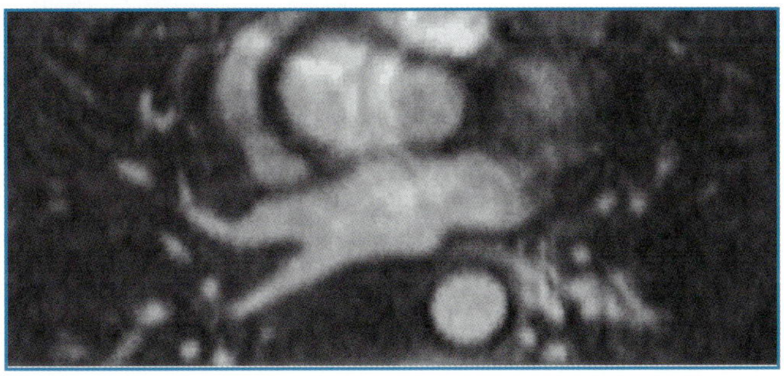

b

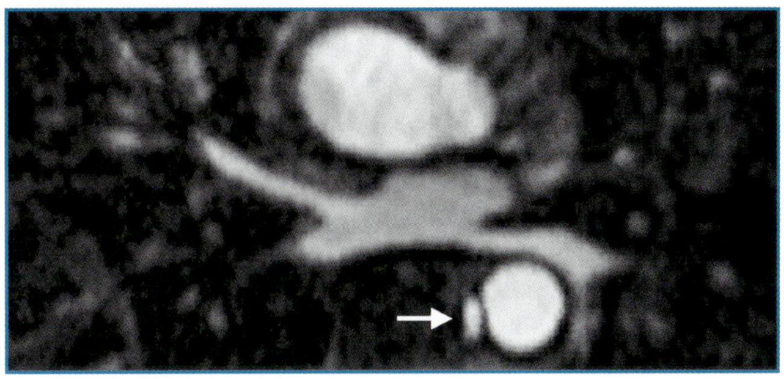

d

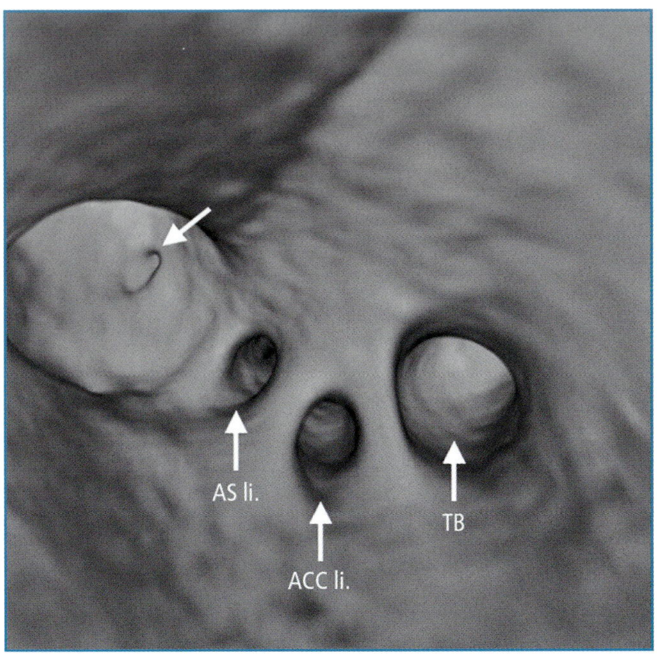

e

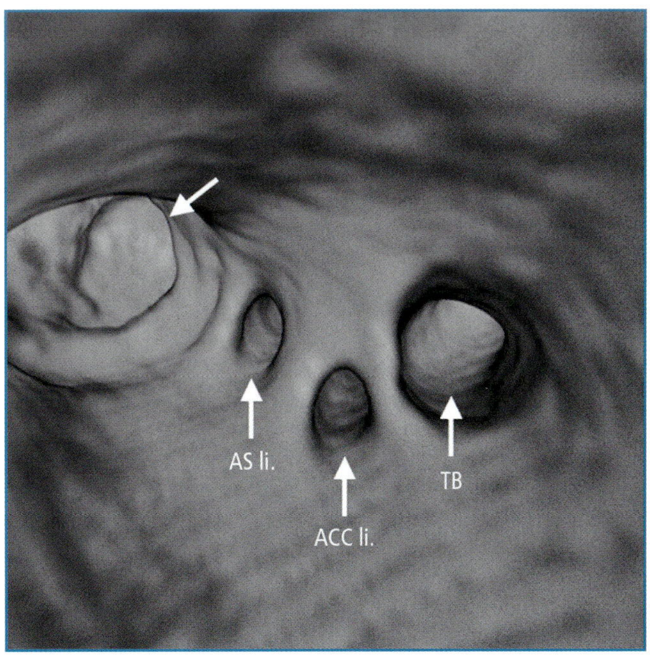

f

"Fly-through" imaging **(e, f)** of the aortic ulcer at the initial examination (diagonal arrow in **(e)**) and in the course of the disease **(f)**. ACC li.: left common carotid artery; AS li.: left subclavian artery; TB: brachiocephalic trunk.

Imaging Results

The **examination protocol** includes several MR imaging techniques aiming at different diagnostic informations:

- 3D-CE-MRA: if clinical information does not suggest the presence of an IMH, it can be easily missed in the MRA; this is due to the fact that the circular or semicircular swelling of the aortic wall may be difficult to delineate (especially in the arterial phase) as the aortic wall and the surrounding tissue are usually hypointense, while only the lumen displays a strong signal; in contrast, a PAU can be easily detected in the MRA because it typically presents as a contrast-filled crater of variable size that is located outside the boundaries of the aortic lumen and that is accompanied by significant atherosclerosis; especially in case of a PAU, the entire aorta should be scanned because PAU often involves multiple aortic segments,
- dark blood turbo spin echo (TSE) sequences: ECG-gated dark blood TSE-sequences should always be acquired if there are clinical hints suggesting the presence of an IMH; they not only enable imaging of the wall swelling but allow for detection of blood within the central part of the aortic wall; in addition to that these sequences are useful for estimating the age of intramural blood (*fresh hemorrhage*: high signal intensity in T2-weighted sequences; *subacute hemorrhage*: high signal intensity both on T1- and T2-weighted images due to the formation of methemoglobin),
- cine-SSFP sequences: especially if the existence of an IMH is suspected, cine-SSFP sequences should be included in the analysis because they are well-suited for demonstrating the degree of aortic wall thickening.

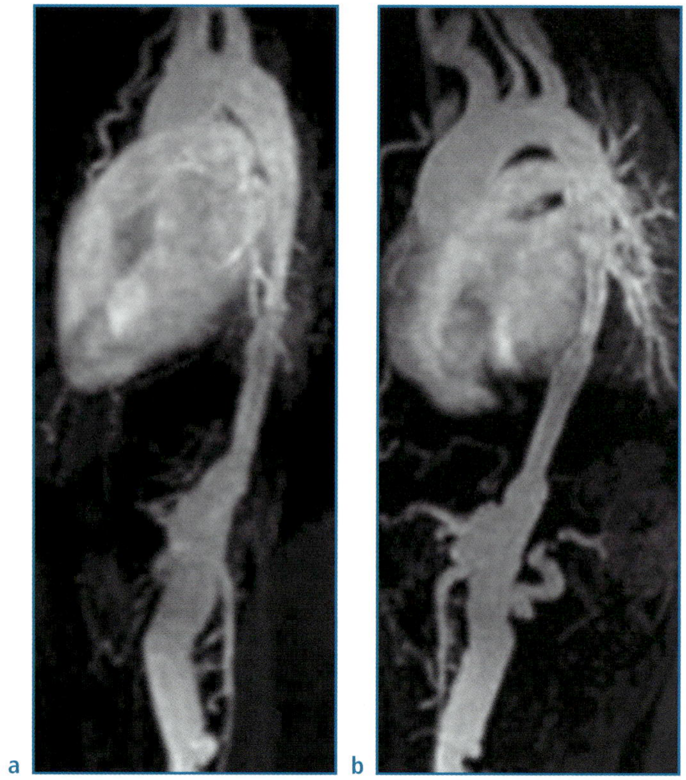

Figure 19-11 59-yrs-old patient with Takayasu arteritis and distinct irregularities of the outline and caliber of the abdominal aorta. Lateral projection of the magnetic resonance angiogram (MRA) (a), latero-anterior projection of the MRA (b).

19.4 Aortitis

Aortitis is the generic term for diseases accompanying an inflammatory infiltration of the aortic wall.

Etiology and Pathogenesis

In consideration of its etiology **three main forms** can be differentiated:

- the infectious syphilitic aortitis,
- the infectious non-syphilitic aortitis, as well as
- the non-infectious aortitis.

Nowadays, infectious syphilitic aortitis is mainly found in immune-compromised patients (e.g. HIV), while infectious non-syphilitic aortitis is predominantly detected in patients with a pre-existing aneurysm with staphylococcus aureus or gram-negative bacteria, such as salmonella or proteus species, being the causative agents. The non-infectious aortitis usually occurs in the context of autoimmune or rheumatologic disorders (e.g. systemic lupus erythematosus, Behçet disease) or is accompanied by a giant-cell arteritis or Takayasu arteritis (Figure 19-11). Regardless of the underlying cause "mycotic" aneurysms may develop due to the inflammatory infiltration of the aortic wall with consequent weakening of the wall structure. These "mycotic" aneurysms characteristically have an atypical configuration and show rapid growth.

Clinical Presentation

Most patients do not report on any symptoms directly attributed to the aortitis but mention discomfort caused by their underlying illness.

Therapy

In the event of aneurysm formation, as a consequence of the aortitis, prosthetic replacement of the aorta may be necessary. Otherwise emphasis lies on the treatment of the underlying disease.

Imaging Results

The **CMR imaging protocol** aims at different diagnostic informations:

- 3D-CE-MRA: imaging of the affected aortic segment and its branches,
- dark blood turbo spin echo sequences: assessment of the aortic wall and evaluation of its thickness,
- dark blood turbo spin echo sequences or gradient echo sequences after application of contrast media: assessment of contrast uptake of the thickened aortic wall,
- follow-up: all patients should be followed-up by MRI, regardless if they are treated conservatively (anti-inflammatory or anti-bacterial therapy) or surgically; in both cases the MRI provides important information on the effectiveness of the chosen therapy.

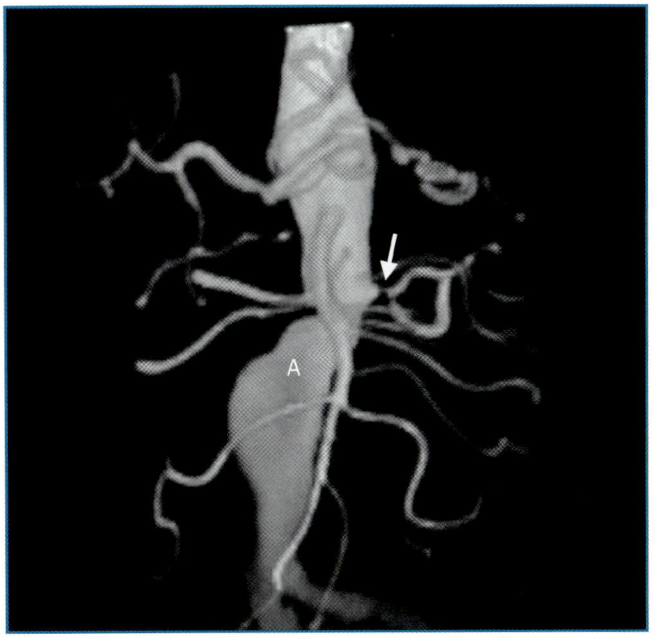

Figure 19-12 Infrarenal aneurysm of the abdominal aorta in a 59-yrs-old patient. Incidental finding of three renal arteries on both sides with stenosis of the early-branching main renal artery on the left side (arrow). A: aneurysm.

19.5 Diseases of the Abdominal Aorta

The abdominal aorta originates directly distal of the aortic hiatus located in the diaphragm and runs distally to the aortic bifurcation, where it divides into the left and right common iliac (sciatic) artery. On its way down it emits important branches including the celiac trunk, the superior and inferior mesenteric artery, as well as the renal arteries.

19.5.1 Aneurysm

An aneurysm of the abdominal aorta is a common disease and can be found in 5–7% of patients older than 65 yrs. In most cases it is fusiform-shaped and begins just below the origin of the renal arteries. It often ends proximal of the aortic bifurcation but may also involve the bifurcation and/or the renal arteries.

Etiology and Pathogenesis

The development of an aneurysm of the abdominal aorta (Figure 19-12) can be due to several reasons, although in most cases it is induced by atherosclerosis and/or arterial hypertension. In addition to that genetic, environmental, hemodynamic or immunological causes play a major role in the formation of an aneurysm.

Clinical Presentation

Most aneurysms of the abdominal aorta are detected incidentally and are asymptomatic. However, especially in younger patients the aneurysm can cause pain located in the hypogastrium or in the groin. Complications may arise if the aneurysm is partially filled with a thrombus, which may lead to embolic disease of the legs. Similar to the thoracic aorta, the appearance of new, unbearable pain may be a first hint of a rupture of the aneurysm, requiring immediate diagnosis and therapeutic intervention.

Therapy

If of small size (< 5 cm) an observant proceeding is eligible as no significant difference can be detected between conservative therapy and an early surgical intervention. Consequently, most asymptomatic aneurysms do not undergo operative procedures until they have exceeded 5 cm or have grown by more than 0.5–1 cm per year. The percutaneous insertion of a stent graft is only possible if an adequate aortic segment distal of the renal arteries is available. The segment must not be affected by the aneurysm and offer enough space for anchoring of the graft.

Imaging Results

The **CMR imaging protocol** aims at different diagnostic informations:

- 3D-CE-MRA: imaging of the abdominal aorta and its branches as well as of the iliac and femoral arteries in order to assess the extent of the aneurysm; special attention should be paid not only to the distance of the aneurysm to the renal arteries but also to concomitant vessel stenoses,
- T1-weighted turbo spin echo- or gradient echo sequences with fat saturation after application of contrast media:

measurement of the maximum diameter of the aneurysm, which might be difficult in the MRA as here only the lumen supplied with blood, not the thrombosed lumen, can be easily delineated; assessment of inflammatory changes in the surrounding tissue as an indicator of an inflammatory aneurysm of the abdominal aorta; imaging of a paraaortal leak, if applicable,

- follow-up: MRI is well-suited for the follow-up of patients who underwent conservative, interventional or surgical treatment and enables the determination of the exact diameter of the aneurysm and assessment of the function of the stent graft and prosthesis, respectively.

19.5.2 Inflammatory Aneurysm

An inflammatory aneurysm (Figure 19-13) is a special form of an aneurysm of the abdominal aorta and comprises up to 15% of the patients, who undergo surgical treatment for abdominal aneurysm. It is mainly located in the infrarenal segment of the aorta with only 8% lying proximal of the renal arteries. The inflammatory aneurysm may involve aortic branches as well, illustrated by the fact that the renal arteries are affected in almost 40% of cases.

Etiology and Pathogenesis

The exact etiology of inflammatory aneurysms is not cleared yet. The pathophysiological process comprises fibrosis of the periaortal tissue with lymphocytic and plasmacellular infiltration of the adventitia as well as callosity of the aortic wall, which communicates with the dorsal parts of the peritoneum.

Clinical Presentation and Therapy

Most patients do not report any symptoms caused by the inflammatory aneurysm itself, but notice discomfort due to the underlying disease. If diagnosis of an inflammatory aneurysm is established the affected segment should be excised and be replaced by a prosthesis.

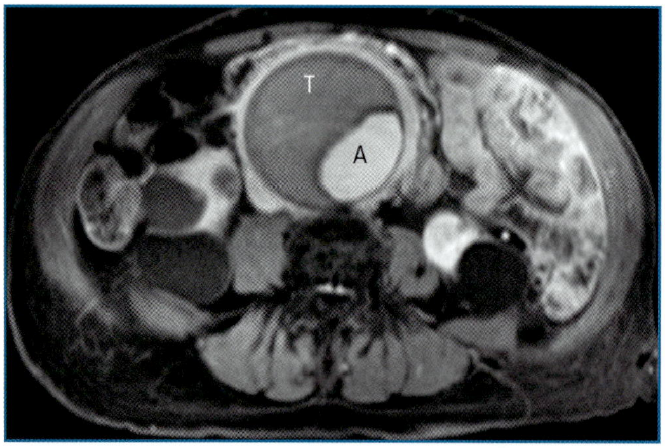

Figure 19-13 Axial plane of a 3D gradient echo sequence in a 78-yrs-old patient with inflammatory aneurysm of the abdominal aorta and extensive contrast enhancement of the aortic wall and surrounding tissue. A: perfused lumen; T: thrombus-filled lumen.

Imaging Results

The **CMR imaging protocol** aims at different diagnostic informations:

- 3D-CE-MRA: as in case of a classic abdominal aneurysm the aim of the MRA is to image the abdominal aorta with its branches as well as the iliac and femoral vessels; it should not only help to determine the extent of the aneurysm and its distance to the renal arteries but should also give information on concomitant vessel stenoses,
- T1-weighted turbo spin echo- or gradient echo sequences with fat saturation after application of contrast media: imaging of the surrounding tissue with regard to inflammatory changes; measurement of the maximum diameter of the aneurysm, which may be difficult in the MRA, in which the thrombosed lumen of the aorta is not displayed,
- follow-up: again both, in patients undergoing conservative or surgical therapy, regular follow-ups are necessary, which can be done by duplex sonography and/or MRI.

19.5.3 Leriche Syndrome

A Leriche syndrome is a special form of an atheromatous aortoiliac disease and means a complete occlusion of the infrarenal aorta with or without involvement of the iliac arteries (Figure 19-14).

Etiology and Pathogenesis

In general, an acute occlusion of the infrarenal aorta can be differentiated from a chronic disease. While an acute occlusion may be caused by trauma, thromboembolic disease, thrombosis of an aneurysm, or a pre-existing ulcerating plaque, the chronic form is usually caused by atherosclerotic lesions. Rarely, does a chronic occlusion occur in the context of a Takayasu arteritis or as a consequence of a congenital hypo- or dysplastic disease.

An acute occlusion may lead to a life-threatening situation with ischemia of both legs as no collateral vessels are present. The ischemic syndrome comes along with unbearable pain, pallor, paresthesias, as well as paralysis, requiring immediate (surgical) treatment.

Clinical Presentation

The side and degree of symptoms depends on the existence and location of collateral vessels. In some cases this collateral system is very well-developed, preventing the appearance of symptoms despite extensive vessel occlusion.

Nevertheless up to 90% of the patients suffer from a bilateral claudicatio of the calf or of the pelvic girdle and

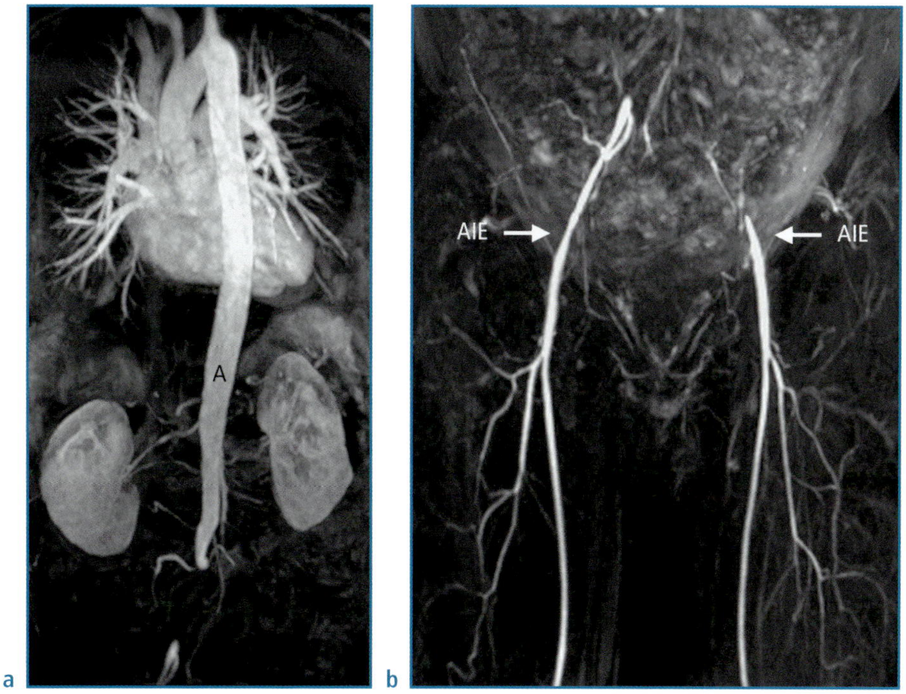

Figure 19-14 High-resolution magnetic resonance angiography in a 59-yrs-old patient suffering from Leriche syndrome. Abdomino-pelvic level (a), femoral level (b). A: aorta; AIE: external iliac (sciatic) artery.

thighs. An erectile dysfunction can be found in 20% of the affected men; other symptoms such as abdominal pain during walking are rare.

Therapy

In addition to an acute occlusion, a surgical treatment is warranted in case of chronic disease with severe clinical symptoms and/or if one or both renal arteries are involved. In these patients reconstruction of the aorta and iliac (sciatic) arteries is necessary, which might include the insertion of a bypass. Patients with a well-developed collateral system and who do not sustain a significant impairment of their quality of life can be treated observantly.

Imaging Results

The **CMR imaging protocol aims at two goals**:

- 3D-CE-MRA: imaging of the aortic occlusion and assessment of the collateral system:
  - subclavian artery → internal thoracic artery → superior epigastric artery → inferior epigastric artery → external iliac (sciatic) artery ("Winslow pathway"),
  - abdominal aorta → lumbar artery → iliolumbal artery → internal iliac (sciatic) artery → external iliac (sciatic) artery,
  - abdominal aorta → posterior intercostal artery → lumbar artery → circumflex iliac artery → external iliac (sciatic) artery,
  - abdominal aorta → superior mesenteric artery → Riolan's anastomosis → inferior mesenteric artery → superior and inferior rectal artery → inferior pudendal artery → internal iliac (sciatic) artery → external iliac (sciatic) artery,
  - abdominal aorta → testicular (ovarian) artery → anterior scrotal artery → external iliac (sciatic) artery,
  - median sacral artery → lateral sacral artery → internal iliac (sciatic) artery → external iliac (sciatic) artery,
- follow-up: regardless if treated conservatively, interventionally (PTA or stent) or surgically, all patients require regular follow-ups that can be performed using MRI.

19.6 Conclusions and Future Perspectives

MR imaging and MR angiography allow for non-invasive assessment of all vascular territories. However, in an acute setting with clinically unstable patients, e.g. aortic dissection, computed tomography (CT) is the method of first choice, due to availability, short examinations times, and excellent patient access during the examination. On the other hand MR imaging provides morphologic and functional information without any radiation. Therefore, cardiovascular MR imaging must be considered the best diagnostic test in stable patients and for follow-up examinations.

Magnetic resonance imaging has improved significantly within the last decade, and this process is not yet over. High-field MRI combined with accelerated CMR using zonal, parallel and prior knowledge driven imaging methods, will further improve spatial and temporal resolution without increasing scan time. Time-resolved 3D contrast-enhanced MRA provides additional dynamic information and avoids any timing issues and venous overlay. Therefore, this technique will definitively replace standard MRA in the near future.

20 Diseases of the Cerebral and Peripheral Arteries

Mathias Goyen and Christoph U. Herborn

20.1 Cerebral Arteries

20.1.1 Extracranial MRA

Digital subtraction angiography (DSA) has been the gold standard for diagnosis of carotid disease for many years and has also been used for treatment decisions in the NASCET and ESC trials. The risks associated with DSA regarding ischemic attacks, stroke, the inherent invasiveness as well as the limitations due to projection variation and interobserver variability have motivated the development of less invasive cross-sectional imaging modalities. Magnetic resonance angiography (MRA) offers both two-dimensional (2D) and three-dimensional (3D) techniques that can either be used with or without paramagnetic contrast material for an accurate assessment of carotid artery disease (Leclerc 1998, Remonda 1998, Wintersperger 2000, Serfaty 2000, Barbier 2001). Injection of an intravenous contrast bolus of gadolinium shortens the T1 of the blood. Further, larger flip angles can be used to generate a stronger signal with improved background suppression and less signal saturation. Contrast-enhanced (CE)-MRA provides morphological information over a substantial length of the neck arteries beginning at the origin and extending up to the circle of Willis. For CE-MRA fast scan times and adequate timing, based on a test bolus, are required to avoid venous overprojection of the jugular veins. Currently available CE-MRA methods acquire a high-contrast arterial signal in the first 10 s, falling within the time window of arterial enhancement. Acquisition is continued, however, to increase the resolution of the depicted arteries. The high spatial resolution obtained allows excellent visualization of near-occlusions of the brain-feeding arteries. Flow-related artifacts are also strongly diminished.

Non-contrast-enhanced MRA techniques include time-of-flight (TOF) and phase contrast (PC) methods. While the former can be used for the precise display of the carotid arteries, the latter is mainly used for hemodynamic information, e.g. flow velocity. Both techniques rely on their inherent flow sensitivity and are thus not only time-consuming but also prone to pitfalls associated with slow flow, turbulence, and motion of the patient during data acquisition. Considering these potential drawbacks, contrast-enhanced (CE) 3D MRA is an ideal candidate for a proper, time-effective assessment of carotid artery morphology. The high vascular signal due to T1-shortening of the blood pool caused by paramagnetic contrast agents and the insensitivity to flow artifacts are significant advantages of 3D CE-MRA, which can be acquired in virtually any plane in order to optimally display stenotic disease of the extracranial carotid artery (Phan 2001, Huston 2001, Catalano 2001, Randoux 2001, Remonda 2002, Townsend 2003, Parmar 2005, Yang 2005, Frydrycowitz 2006). Using the latest invents of MRI, such as higher field strength and parallel acquisition, submillimeter spatial resolution can be attained in all three dimensions. As a result, even subtle changes of the carotid artery wall including eccentric stenosis can be detected and accurately assessed.

Technique

As a consequence of the relatively short arterial venous recirculation time in the supra-aortal vasculature, and venous contamination of the jugular veins that could obscure the carotid bulb, 3D CE-MRA of the carotids is very demanding. Therefore, precise timing of the contrast bolus is mandatory and also the key element for data acquisition. In order to prevent venous overlay, the passage of the contrast bolus is monitored with a fast 2D fluoroscopic sequence of the aortic arch. When the bolus arrives in the aortic arch the patient is immediately instructed to take a deep breath and hold it during acquisition of the 3D data set. With a range of 15 s and reasonable spatial resolution, it covers the great vessels from the aortic arch to the Circle of Willis. The 3D MRA can be acquired in the coronal or sagittal plane, with preference given to acquisition in the coronal plane due to the concomitant display of both carotid arteries. In case of known disease to a single side, a sagittal acquisition may be used instead for optimal in-plane spatial resolution.

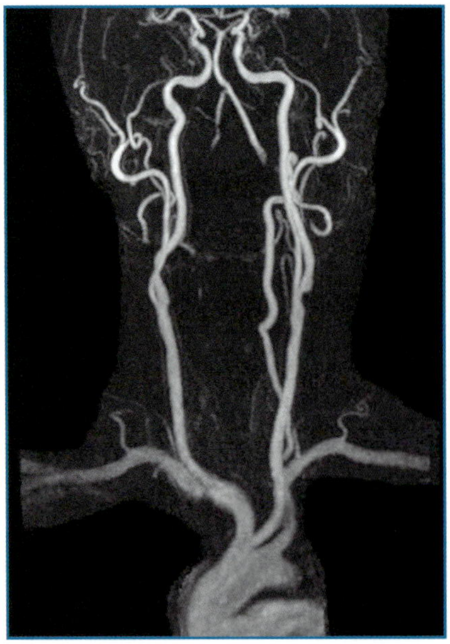

Figure 20-1 Maximum intensity projection (MIP) of a 3D contrast-enhanced magnetic resonance angiography study of the carotid arteries showing a high-grade stenosis (> 70 %) of the left internal carotid artery.

Typical technical parameters of the 3D CE-MRA sequence for optimal spatial resolution 512 or higher include:

- TR < 5 ms,
- TE < 2 ms,
- flip angle = 30–45°,
- matrix > 256.

The protocol should always include a native mask sequence for later image subtraction. With new k-space filling techniques, such as TRICKS or TREAT, time-resolved 3D CE-MRA permits a distinct differentiation between arterial and venous filling using contrast material. Post-processing techniques for a 3D CE-MRA data set includes image subtraction, multi-planar reformatting, maximum intensity projection, and volume rendering, just to mention a few techniques. All of these methods provide a thorough and diligent evaluation of carotid artery disease. However, 3D CE-MRA is a mere display of the vessel lumen. In order to fully exploit the possibilities of MRI with regard to the vessel wall, it might be of interest to add 2D spin echo sequences to the protocol in order to analyze the composition of plaque or the relation between intima-media thickness.

After image acquisition, maximum intensity projections can be reconstructed. The maximum intensity projection images can be projected in any plane to provide multiple views of the vascular anatomy. With the large "reach" of CE-MRA even the origin of the common carotid arteries can be visualized. Furthermore, 3D-TOF, 3D-PC and CE-MRA can be used to demonstrate anatomical variation in the internal carotid arteries (ICAs) and vertebral arteries (VBAs) such as vascular elongation, or kinking and coiling. For ICA stenosis measurements, a series of studies comparing the diagnostic performance of MRA techniques relative to the gold standard, intraarterial digital subtraction angiography, were carried out. Most recent studies showed high sensitivities and specificities especially for CE-MRA in the detection of a stenosis of > 70 % according to the North American Symptomatic Carotid Surgery Trial criteria (Figure 20-1). The high resolution of CE-MRA allows extracranial sources of collateral circulation to be visualized, such as the arterial connections between the branches of the external carotid artery and the intracranial vasculature. With respect to the VBA the variable origin of these arteries can be demonstrated, as well as the dominance of a single vertebral artery, hypoplasia of a vertebral artery or the presence of a subclavian steal syndrome (Clevert 2006, Fenchel 2006, Nael 2006a, Nael 2006b, Hahnel 2006, Sumi 2007, Layton 2007, Lell 2007).

Indications

Carotid Bifurcation Disease

Carotid bulb disease is the leading cause of ischemic attacks to the brain and stroke the major cause of considerable morbidity and mortality in the developed world. The results of the NASCET and ESCT have clearly shown that symptomatic patients suffering from stenotic disease compromising more than 70% of the vessel lumen significantly benefit from carotid endarterectomy. Hence, accurate measurements of stenosis severity are very important in determining the need for therapy in these patients (Figure 20-2). The aforementioned advantages of 3D CE-MRA, such as high signal from the vascular bed, reduced sensitivity to artifacts, large anatomical coverage, and time-effectiveness, make this technique an ideal method for an exact display of stenotic changes of the carotid arteries.

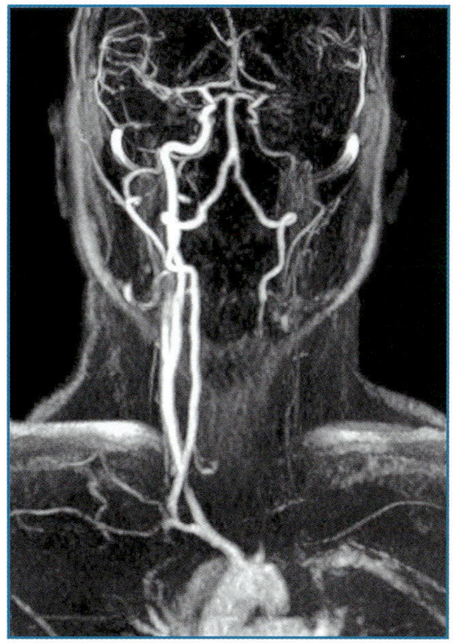

Figure 20-2 Total occlusion of both the left internal carotid artery and the ipsilateral vertebral artery can be recognized on this MIP of a contrast-enhanced magnetic resonance angiography study of the supra-aortal arteries.

Arch Vessel Disease

Atherosclerotic disease of the arch vessels is rare, but it may be an important cause of cerebrovascular pathology. The left subclavian artery is more frequently involved than the right, and stenotic disease tends to include the origins of the vertebral arteries. In the case of hypoperfusion to the arm due to high-grade stenosis of the proximal subclavian artery, retrograde flow in the ipsilateral vertebral artery, especially during exercise, causes subclavian steal syndrome. While 3D CE-MRA nicely demonstrates the localization and degree of stenotic disease affecting the subclavian artery, additional phase contrast velocity measurements or time-resolved 3D CE-MRA can display and quantify retrograde flow in the vertebral artery (Figure 20-3).

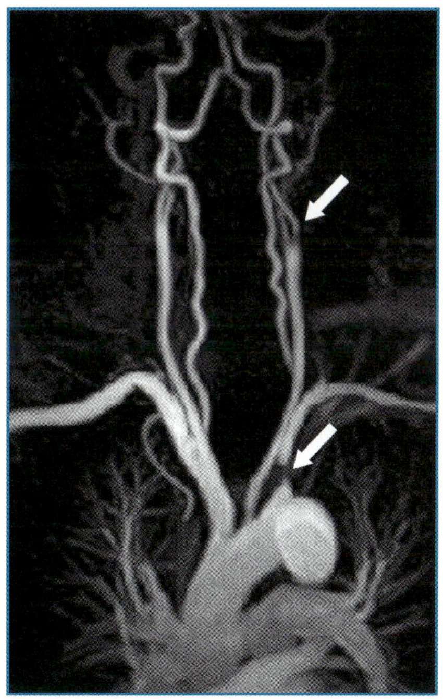

Figure 20-3 This study displays two high-grade stenoses of the left carotid bifurcation and left subclavian artery, respectively (arrows).

Vertebral Artery Disease

The tortuous anatomy of the vertebral arteries, which leads to in-plane saturation of spins has always hampered the quality of non-contrast MRA images. These difficulties have been eliminated with the introduction of 3D CE-MRA. This technique permits an accurate display of the entire course of the vertebral arteries. However, even with 3D CE-MRA, respiratory motion at the thoracic inlet level can reduce image quality of the vertebral artery origins.

20.1.2 Intracranial MRA

Prior to the advent of non-invasive vascular imaging techniques, DSA played a major role in the diagnosis of intracranial vasculature diseases. Today, MRA has become the standard in the diagnosis of most cerebral vascular pathologies, but certain intrinsic technical limitations still restrict its application to the diagnosis of arterial and venous vessel stenosis and cerebral aneurysms. For the pre-interventional evaluation of intracranial vascular malformations, DSA still remains the reference technique. Evaluation of the normal arterial and venous circulation is typically achieved using different methodological approaches. In large part, this is due to the overall complexity of the intracranial vascular system and to the rapid (5–6 s) circulation time.

For morphological evaluation of the intracranial arteries and veins **three MRA methods** are currently available:
- time-of-flight (TOF)-MRA,
- phase contrast (PC)-MRA, and
- contrast-enhanced (CE)-MRA.

Time-of-Flight (TOF)-MRA

Currently, the arterial circulation is most often studied using TOF-MRA. This non-invasive technique allows the visualization of the major intracranial arteries and peripheral branches in a relatively short time (3–5 min). It also generally does not require the use of contrast agent. The TOF method achieves visualization of the arterial lumen by measuring the inflow of fresh (unsaturated) blood through an image section with pre-saturated static tissue. Either two-dimensional (2D) or three-dimensional (3D) TOF-MRA techniques can be performed. In 2D TOF-MRA thin slices are acquired one after another, reducing the saturation effects of the MR pulses on the blood and increasing the sensitivity for arterial inflow. Consequently, 2D TOF-MRA is suited to visualize slow flow, relative to 3D TOF in which a larger imaging volume is acquired simultaneously. In general, with 3D TOF-MRA a larger trajectory of arteries is visualized with a high spatial resolution and a high signal-to-noise ratio (SNR). A drawback of TOF-MRA-based techniques is the potential occurrence of flow void artifacts, due to turbulence of the blood flow, that arise distal to a severe arterial stenosis (Figure 20-4a, b).

Nevertheless, its major limitation is that the distal arterial branches are often not optimally displayed on maximum intensity projection (MIP) reconstructions due to the progressive saturation of these vessels during image acquisition. The result is an overall reduction of diagnostic confidence, which could partly be overcome by the introduction of magnets operating at 3.0 T field strength.

Phase Contrast (PC)-MRA

While TOF-MRA depends on the refreshment of inflowing blood into a slice, PC-MRA employs the phase shift in the signal that is induced by the flowing blood. This phase shift is proportional to the velocity and a direct correlation with signal intensity is present. Therefore, small vessels can be clearly visualized with PC-MRA, even with slow flowing blood. PC-MRA is applicable for both 2D and 3D acquisition. 2D PC-MRA is especially valuable as a survey scan, and phase velocity maps can be constructed for quantitative measurements of blood volume (ml/min) flowing through a vessel. A disadvantage of 3D PC-MRA is the relatively long acquisition time and the presence of venous overprojection.

Contrast-Enhanced (CE)-MRA

One of the first attempts to increase the quality of MRA images of the intracranial circulation was to combine the 3D TOF-MRA technique with the intravenous infusion of gadolinium contrast agent. While this technique improved visualization of the more distal portions of the intracranial arterial circulation, the relatively long acquisition times (between 8 and 10 min/volume acquisition) and the rapid distribution of contrast agent resulted in the concomitant display of cerebral arteries and veins. Additionally, the presence of contrast agent in the capillary-venous compartment was shown to lead to increased signal intensity of the surrounding brain. Recently, the introduction of stronger gradients and the development of ultrafast sequences (acqui-

a 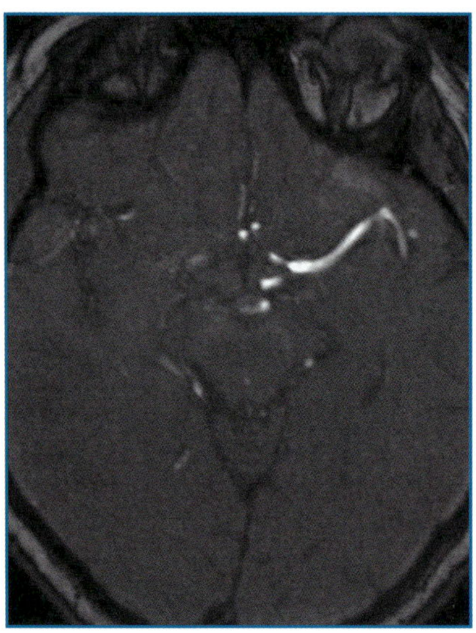 b 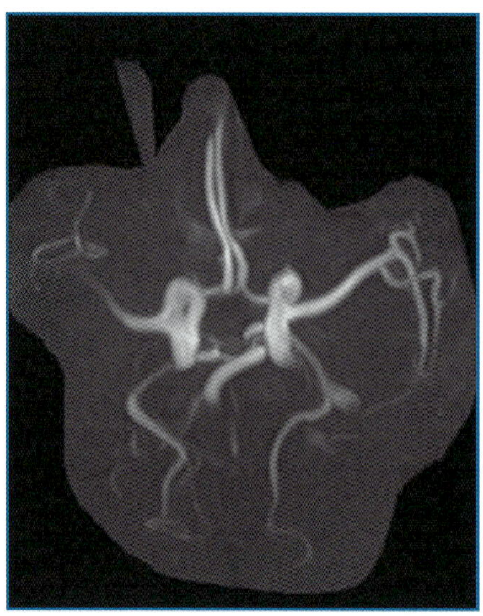

Figure 20-4 Source image **(a)** of the 3D TOF-MRA of the intracranial arteries showing a subtotal occlusion of the right medial cerebral artery (MCA), which can also be appreciated on the MIP of the same data set **(b)**.

sition times of 20–50 s as opposed to 8–10 min), has enabled 3D CE-MRA to be applied for the diagnosis of intracranial vascular pathologies. The technique, which requires a rapid intravenous injection of gadolinium contrast agent, has been shown to be more sensitive and more selective than previous techniques. These results have been realized partly through recent developments in k-space sampling, in which the central portion of the k-space is the first to be acquired. Elliptically centric encoded acquisitions must be timed precisely to the arrival of contrast agent in the circle of Willis in order to minimize enhancement of the venous vasculature, which might obscure arterial pathology. Although the overall scan time ranges from 20–50 s, with elliptical centric phase ordering the center of the k-space is filled very efficiently during the initial seconds of the scan. This permits a more selective visualization of major intracranial arteries without major venous overlay.

Time-Resolved MRA

More recently other "time-resolved" 3D CE-MRA techniques have been proposed which permit a high temporal resolution of approximately 1 s, while still maintaining adequate spatial resolution. Among these new techniques are those referred to as TRICKS and CENTRA. As an alternative to 3D CE-MRA a 2D thick-slice MR-DSA (2D MR-DSA) approach can be employed. This method combines a series of 2D CE thick slices, each frame lasting 1–2 s, with subtraction of precontrast images from subsequent contrast-enhanced images. These techniques are currently utilized for the study of cerebral aneurysms and for the assessment of cerebrovascular occlusive diseases.

MRA of Intracranial Aneurysms

Although 2D MR-DSA is available these days, 3D TOF-MRA is currently a widely employed technique for the detection of intracranial aneurysms (Wikstrom 2008, Hnatiuk 2008). However, 3D TOF-MRA is prone to underestimating the size of aneurysms due to spin saturation effects. For this reason 3D CE-MRA is increasingly being considered as the technique of choice for the study of large and giant aneurysms. Moreover, it has the inherent advantage over other techniques in facilitating depiction of the aneurysm from numerous projections following MIP reconstruction. A widely accepted application of MRA is in the follow-up of coiled aneurysms. Several studies have been performed that have demonstrated the feasibility and sensitivity of 3D TOF-MRA in the detection of aneurysm recanalization. Recently, the use of techniques with very short TR and TE have permitted marked reductions of artifacts. Moreover, the use of 3D CE-MRA with elliptic centric acquisition seems to have greater sensitivity compared to 3D TOF-MRA in demonstrating aneurysm patency.

MR Imaging of Intracranial Venous Circulation

Basic MRI combined with MRA has shown a very high sensitivity for the detection of cerebral venous thrombosis, as applied towards the investigation of intracranial venous circulation. For accurate confirmation of the presence and extent of a venous thrombosis, 3D PC-MRA techniques are generally preferred to TOF-MRA sequences, which may be disturbed by artifactual metahemoglobin from a subacute thrombus. The use of 3D fast GE T1-weighted CE-MRA has recently been proposed as a more sensitive technique for the evaluation of dural sinuses, particularly in those regions (transverse sinuses, posterior part of superior sagittal sinus, transverse-sigmoid junction) where TOF-MRA techniques, and to a lesser extent PC-MRA techniques, are troublesome due to saturation or complex flow. Although this technique appears promising, there is currently little information available concerning its application in pathological series when compared to unenhanced MRA techniques. Whereas unenhanced MRA acquisitions can differentiate between occlusion and focal stenosis of large sinuses, it may be difficult to rule out stenosis in cases of normal variants or sinus hypoplasia. In these cases diagnosis may be improved with the use of 3D CE-MRA.

Indications

In summary, using the different MRA techniques the following **intracranial pathologies** can be investigated:

- anatomic variants of the carotid arteries and the arteries of the circle of Willis,
- cerebral arteriovenous malformations,
- stenoses or occlusions of the intracerebral arteries (cerebrovascular occlusive disease) including concomitant collateral circulation,
- intracranial aneurysms (most frequently at the base of the brain),
- cerebral venous thrombosis (particularly in the posterior part of the superior sagittal sinus, the transverse sinuses, or the transverse-sigmoid junction).

Summary and Conclusions

Contrast-enhanced MR angiography is presently an established technique for visualization of the carotid arteries and other vessels of the supra-aortic vasculature. Although challenging because of the rapid arterialvenous circulation time, its advantages including the development of ultrafast imaging sequences, the possibility of acquiring large imaging volumes from the carotid bifurcation to the intracranial territory, and the absence of the various drawbacks associated with unenhanced MRA techniques, have resulted in the routine use of CE-MRA in daily clinical practice. Although CE-MRA of the intracranial vasculature has yet to be routinely accepted, its use is becoming more widespread. In particular, the development of stronger gradients and the development of elliptically centric encoded sequences have proven beneficial for the evaluation of aneurysm patency and cerebral arteriovenous malformations on CE-MRA. The advantage of ultrafast intracranial CE-MRA is the feasibility of attaining selective visualization of major intracranial arteries without significant venous contamination.

20.1.3 Perfusion

Techniques

Cerebral perfusion provides the basis for the delivery of oxygen and nutrients the brain needs to maintain function. Various MR techniques allow the anatomy and hemodynamics of brain tissue perfusion to be investigated. In addition to depicting the anatomy of the circle of Willis, the currently available TOF- and CE-MRA methods can demonstrate the branching vessels of the circle of Willis and detect steno-occlusive lesions in the proximal parts of the anterior cerebral artery (ACA), medial cerebral artery (MCA), and posterior cerebral artery (PCA) (Figure 20-5). Recently, MR flow territory imaging methods have been introduced which allow for the extension of the distal branches of the ACA, MCA and PCA to be visualized. These methods are different implementations of arterial spin labeling (ASL). In ASL-MRI the protons of the arterial water in the feeding vasculature of the brain are magnetically labeled and used as an endogenous tracer. A labeling delay allows the labeled arterial water protons to flow through the arterial vascular tree and exchange with the unlabeled brain tissue water. The subsequent change in tissue magnetization is restricted to the flow territory of the labeled artery. The first selective ASL methods were based on the use of a local surface coil, with selective labeling of a single ICA achieved through the low penetration depth of this surface coil. Another selective ASL approach is based on angulation of a labeling slab to reach selectivity for a single ICA. Planning of these labeling slabs is based on anatomical MRA scans of the brain vasculature. In patients with cerebrovascular disease, selective ASL can demonstrate a decreased flow territory with the presence of steno-occlusive disease as well as an increased flow territory with the presence of compensatory collateral flow. In addition to flow territory measurements, the regional cerebral blood flow (CBF) contribution of each individual artery can be obtained.

Measurement of Regional Cerebral Blood Flow (CBF)

For measurements of the regional CBF (ml/min/100 g tissue), a method with injection of gadolinium, dynamic susceptibility contrast MRI, or an ASL-MRI approach as described above can be used. Dynamic susceptibility contrast MRI monitors the first passage of a bolus of intravenously injected contrast agent through the brain tissue. The presence of contrast agent results in a decay of the signal in a T2*-weighted image. This allows for the time evolution of the contrast agent concentration to be monitored through dynamic image acquisition of the brain. Quantification of the perfusion parameters requires measurements of the characteristics of the injected bolus. This is called arterial input function (AIF) determination and is defined as the evolution in time of the contrast agent in the brain-feeding arteries. After correction of the passage through the brain tissue for the AIF, the response function is obtained. This response

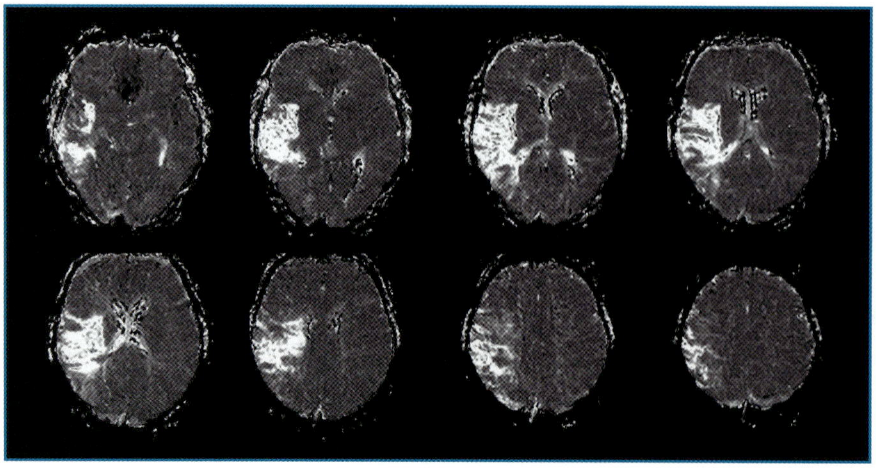

Figure 20-5 Perfusion examination of the same patient as in Figure 20-4 accurately shows the infarct area in the region of the right medial cerebral artery (MCA).

function reflects the hemodynamic properties of the microvasculature. From this response function both the CBF and several timing parameters for the contrast passage as well as blood volume can be calculated. Even with the acquisition of the AIF, further dispersion of the contrast bolus will occur from the arteries in the neck towards the microvasculature. This dispersion will result in uncertainties with respect to CBF quantification, especially in patients with steno-occlusive disease and delayed collateral flow.

20.2 Peripheral Arteries

20.2.1 General Aspects

Peripheral vascular occlusive disease (PVOD) is caused by the generalized systemic process of atherosclerosis, and is often associated with additional manifestations in other arteries throughout the body. Atherosclerotic lesions, such as stenosis or aneurysms, frequently arise at sites of complex flow (e.g. branching points) and sites of mechanical stress on the vessel (e.g. adductor canal). Non-contrast-enhanced techniques, especially time-of-flight MRA, have been shown to be particularly helpful in displaying infrapopliteal arteries, but these methods are limited by their inherently long acquisition time and sensitivity to artifacts. The advent of 3D CE-MRA allows for a fast, comprehensive and reliable display of the peripheral arterial system in case of suspected PVOD (Hany 1997, Rofsky 2007a, Rofsky 2007b, Vosshenrich 1997, Boos 1998, Reimer 1998, Shetty 1998, Winterer 1999, Westenberg 1999, Visser 2000, Goyen 2000, Lenhart 2000, Koelemay 2001, Ruehm 2001).

20.2.2 Contrast-Enhanced MRA

3D CE-MRA of the peripheral vasculature can be performed at a single station of a dedicated region (Figure 20-6) or at several concomitant and slightly overlapping stations in order to cover a larger anatomic field (Figure 20-7). Such multi-station approaches are carried out by giving a single injection of contrast material and following with a series of 3D data acquisitions, which chase the bolus down to the legs (bolus chase technique). Usually up to three overlapping stations are acquired with this method. Each station is examined as fast as possible with reasonable spatial resolution in order to avoid venous overlap in the more peripheral territory. The patient is placed supine in the scanner and the legs are positioned horizontally in order to minimize the anteroposterior volume of the data set, which in turn reduces acquisition time. Dedicated peripheral phased-array lower extremity coils guarantee optimal signal quality. After

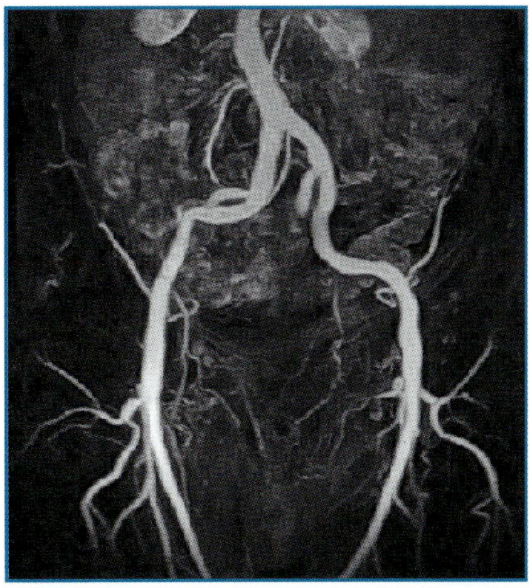

Figure 20-6 Atherosclerotic remodeling of the iliac arteries demonstrated by the MIP of this 3D contrast-enhanced magnetic resonance angiography of the pelvic arterial vasculature.

acquisition of 2D scout images, the course and localization of the arteries under investigation can be determined for the 3D CE-MRA examination. Plain mask images can be used for subtraction after contrast enhancement, which leads to vastly reduced background signal and improved conspicuity especially of smaller vessels. The three stations comprise the lower abdominal aorta, the iliac arteries and the upper and lower leg arteries in a single examination. While spatial resolution is lower for the upper two stations, the most distal station mandates highest spatial resolution as the diameter of the run-off arteries is rather small.

Typical technical parameters of peripheral 3D CE-MRA include:

- TR < 7 ms,
- TE < 3 ms,
- flip angle = 30–40°,
- field of view: 40–50 cm,
- matrix 512.

The data set is collected in the coronal plane. In order to improve the quality of the most distal station with regard to avoidance of venous contamination and increased signal from the arterial bed, two modifications of the method have recently been introduced. The first is bilateral venous compression with subsystolic pressures at the level of the upper thigh reduces arteriovenous recirculation time and thereby prolongs the acquisition window for the lower leg arteries. The pressure (usually between 40–60 mmHg) is kept constant throughout the examination and is fairly well-tolerated. Another elusive option to avoid venous overlay is to start with one third of the contrast bolus for a single station 3D CE-MRA of the lower legs, providing optimal display of the

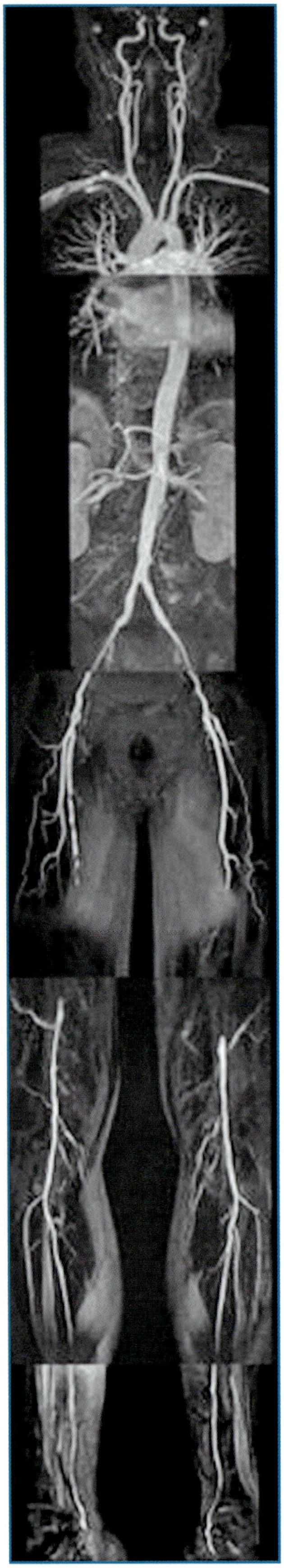

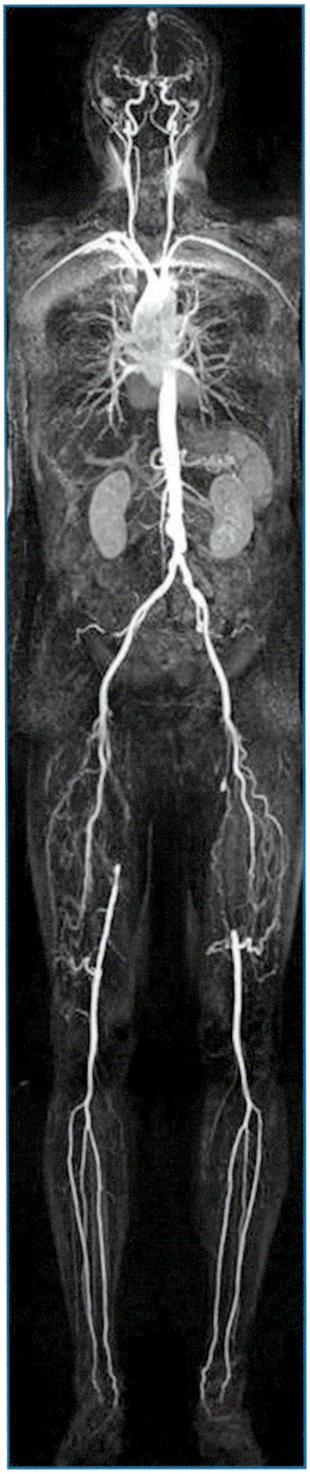

arteries. After a short break the aortoiliac and upper leg arteries are examined using a two-station protocol with the remaining contrast material. This technique is called hybrid-MRA.

20.2.3 Whole-Body 3D Contrast-Enhanced MRA

As atherosclerosis affects virtually the entire arterial tree, the advent of whole-body 3D CE-MRA has opened the door for a systemic imaging technique for a systemic disease: Chasing the contrast bolus with 4–5 contiguous fields of view from head to toe leads to total coverage of the entire arterial tree, with exception of the coronary arteries, in just over 1 min acquisition time. Such an approach permits a most comprehensive evaluation of the extent of atherosclerosis not only in patients suffering from claudication but also in asymptomatic subjects in a supposedly healthy screening population. However, whole-body 3D CE-MRA is still restricted to few MR systems and its clinical value is currently under clinical investigation (Carroll 2001, Foo 2001, Schoenberg 2001, Maki 2002, Goyen 2002).

20.2.4 Indications for CE-MRA in Peripheral Arterial Diseases

Peripheral Vascular Occlusive Disease (PVOD)

The manifestation and extent of peripheral vascular occlusive disease (PVOD) can accurately be assessed with 3D CE-MRA in a very reasonable examination time. In comparison to DSA, 3D CE-MRA reaches sensitivities and specificities between 92 and 100 %, respectively. In patients with aortoiliac disease, 3D CE-MRA can accurately determine the length of a stenotic or occluded segment and thereby help to identify patients for angioplasty or vascular surgery. Proper assessment of lower leg disease remains more complicated due to substantial variations in contrast travel time in patients with occlusive disease (Figure 20-8). Time-resolved 3D CE-MRA might be an option in these cases (Wang 2002, Hood 2002,

Figure 20-7, left Whole-body 3D magnetic resonance angiography (MRA) study demonstrating bilateral occlusions of the superficial femoral artery; whole-body MRA images can be acquired in slightly more than 1 min.

Figure 20-8, right Collateral flow due to occlusion of the superficial femoral artery in both legs is properly displayed on the 3D contrast-enhanced whole-body magnetic resonance angiogram.

Goyen 2002, Herborn 2003, Hentsch 2003, Meaney 2003, Loewe 2003, Leiner 2003, Steffens 2003, Winterer 2003, Herborn 2004a, Herborn 2004b, Herborn 2004c, Quick 2004, Ho 2004, Bilecen 2004, Leiner 2004, de Vries 2005, Krause 2005, Meissner 2005, Pereles 2005, Zenge 2006, Kressler 2006, Ersoy 2006, Tongdee 2006, Goyen 2006, Li 2006, Dellegrottaglie 2007, Kramer 2007, Brauck 2007, Vogt 2007, Nael 2007a, Nael 2007b, Ruhl 2008, Vahl 2008, Berg 2009).

Bypass Grafts

Since non-contrast-enhanced MRA techniques are more prone to artifacts associated with metal clips that can mimic stenotic lesions in patients with bypass grafts, these techniques have been fully replaced by 3D CE-MRA. The latter has proven in many studies to be a reliable diagnostic tool for assessing bypass graft patency.

Arteriovenous Malformations (AVM)

Arteriovenous malformations are benign neoplasms in the soft tissue that can cause complications due to spontaneous hemorrhage or local extension. 3D CE-MRA can detect AVMs or fistulas of the extremities and might help in distinguishing feeding and draining vessels by demonstrating early filling during a multiphase examination. Thereby fast flow AVMs might be separated from hemangiomas or capillary malformations with slow flow. Additional sequences, in particular short tau inversion recovery (STIR), in various planes help to fully analyze the extent of the lesion and potential involvement with surrounding structures (e.g. muscle or bone).

References

Cerebral Arteries

Barbier C, Lefevre F, Bui P et al. Contrast-enhanced MRA of the carotid arteries using 0.5 T: comparison with selective digital angiography. J Radiol 2001; 82: 245–9.

Catalano C, Laghi A, Pediconi F et al. Magnetic resonance angiography with contrast media in the study of carotid arteries. Radiol Med (Torino) 2001; 101: 54–9.

Clevert DA, Johnson T, Michaely H et al. High-grade stenoses of the internal carotid artery: comparison of high-resolution contrast-enhanced 3D MRA, duplex sonography and power Doppler imaging. Eur J Radiol 2006; 60: 379–86.

Fenchel M, Nael K, Ruehm S et al. Isotropic high spatial resolution magnetic resonance angiography of the supra-aortic arteries using two-dimensional parallel imaging (iPAT2) at 3 T: a feasibility study. Invest Radiol 2006; 41: 545–52.

Frydrychowicz A, Bley TA, Winterer JT et al. Accelerated time-resolved 3D contrast-enhanced MR angiography at 3 T: clinical experience in 31 patients. Magma 2006; 19: 187–95.

Hahnel S, Nguyen-Trong TH, Rohde S et al. 3.0 T contrast-enhanced MR angiography of carotid artery stents: in vitro measurements as compared with 1.5 T. J Neuroradiol 2006; 33: 75–80.

Hnatiuk B, Emery DJ, Wilman AH. Effects of doubling and tripling the spatial resolution in standard 3D contrast-enhanced magnetic resonance angiography of carotid artery disease. J Magn Reson Imaging 2008; 27: 71–7.

Huston 3rd J, Fain SB, Wald JT et al. Carotid artery: elliptic centric contrast-enhanced MR angiography compared with conventional angiography. Radiology 2001; 218: 138–43.

Layton KF, Huston 3rd J, Cloft HJ et al. Specificity of MR angiography as a confirmatory test for carotid artery stenosis: is it valid? Am J Roentgenol 2007; 188: 1114–6.

Leclerc X, Martinat P, Godefroy O et al. Contrast-enhanced three-dimensional fast imaging with steady-state precession (FISP) MR angiography of supraaortic vessels: preliminary results. Am J Neuroradiol 1998; 19: 1405–13.

Lell M, Fellner C, Baum U et al. Evaluation of carotid artery stenosis with multi-section CT and MR imaging: influence of imaging modality and post-processing. Am J Neuroradiol 2007; 28: 104–10.

Nael K, Michaely HJ, Villablanca P et al. Time-resolved contrast-enhanced magnetic resonance angiography of the head and neck at 3.0 T: initial results. Invest Radiol 2006a; 41: 116–24.

Nael K, Ruehm SG, Michaely HJ et al. High spatial-resolution CE-MRA of the carotid circulation with parallel imaging: comparison of image quality between 2 different acceleration factors at 3.0 T. Invest Radiol 2006b; 41: 391–9.

Parmar H, Sitoh YY, Hui F. Normal variants of the intracranial circulation demonstrated by MR angiography at 3 T. Eur J Radiol 2005; 56: 220–8.

Phan T, Huston 3rd J, Bernstein MA et al. Contrast-enhanced magnetic resonance angiography of the cervical vessels: experience with 422 patients. Stroke 2001; 32: 2282–6.

Randoux B, Marro B, Koskas F et al. Carotid artery stenosis: prospective comparison of CT, three-dimensional gadolinium-enhanced MR, and conventional angiography. Radiology 2001; 220: 179–85.

Remonda L, Heid O, Schroth G. Carotid artery stenosis, occlusion, and pseudo-occlusion: first-pass, gadolinium-enhanced, three-dimensional MR angiography – preliminary study. Radiology 1998; 209: 95–102.

Remonda L, Senn P, Barth A et al. Contrast-enhanced 3D MR angiography of the carotid artery: comparison with conventional digital subtraction angiography. Am J Neuroradiol 2002; 23: 213–9.

Serfaty JM, Chirossel P, Chevallier JM et al. Accuracy of three-dimensional gadolinium-enhanced MR angiography in the assessment of extracranial carotid artery disease. Am J Roentgenol 2000; 175: 455–63.

Sumi T, Sumi M, Van Cauteren M et al. Parallel imaging technique for the external carotid artery and its branches: comparison of balanced turbo field echo, phase contrast, and time-of-flight sequences. J Magn Reson Imaging 2007; 25: 1028–34.

Townsend TC, Saloner D, Pan XM, Rapp JH. Contrast material-enhanced MRA overestimates severity of carotid stenosis, compared with 3D time-of-flight MRA. J Vasc Surg 2003; 38: 36–40.

Wikstrom J, Ronne-Engstrom E, Gal G et al. Three-dimensional time-of-flight (3D TOF) magnetic resonance angiography (MRA) and contrast-enhanced MRA of intracranial aneurysms treated with platinum coils. Acta Radiol 2008; 49: 190–6.

Wintersperger BJ, Huber A, Preissler G et al. MR angiography of the supraaortic vessels. Radiologe 2000; 40: 785–91.

Yang CW, Carr JC, Futterer SF et al. Contrast-enhanced MR angiography of the carotid and vertebrobasilar circulations. Am J Neuroradiol 2005; 26: 2095–101.

Peripheral Arteries

Berg F, Bangard C, Bovenschulte H et al. Hybrid contrast-enhanced MR angiography of pelvic and lower extremity vasculature at 3.0 T: Initial experience. Eur J Radiol 2009; 70: 170–6.

Bilecen D, Jager KA, Aschwanden M et al. Cuff-compression of the proximal calf to reduce venous contamination in contrast-enhanced stepping-table magnetic resonance angiography. Acta Radiol 2004; 45: 510–5.

Boos M, Lentschig M, Scheffler K et al. Contrast-enhanced magnetic resonance angiography of peripheral vessels. Different contrast agent applications and sequence strategies: a review. Invest Radiol 1998; 33: 538–46.

Brauck K, Maderwald S, Vogt FM et al. Time-resolved contrast-enhanced magnetic resonance angiography of the hand with parallel imaging and view sharing: initial experience. Eur Radiol 2007; 17: 183–92.

Carroll TJ, Korosec FR, Swan JS et al. The effect of injection rate on time-resolved contrast-enhanced peripheral MRA. J Magn Reson Imaging 2001; 14: 401–10.

Dellegrottaglie S, Sanz J, Macaluso F et al. Technology insight: magnetic resonance angiography for the evaluation of patients with peripheral artery disease. Nat Clin Pract Cardiovasc Med 2007; 4: 677–87.

de Vries M, Nijenhuis RJ, Hoogeveen RM et al. Contrast-enhanced peripheral MR angiography using SENSE in multiple stations: feasibility study. J Magn Reson Imaging 2005; 21: 37–45.

Ersoy H, Zhang H, Prince MR. Peripheral MR angiography. J Cardiovasc Magn Reson 2006; 8: 517–28.

Foo TK, Ho VB, Hood MN et al. Preferential arterial imaging using gated thick-slice gadolinium-enhanced phase contrast acquisition in peripheral MRA. J Magn Reson Imaging 2001; 13: 714–21.

Goyen M, Herborn CU, Kroger K et al. Total-body 3D magnetic resonance angiography influences the management of patients with peripheral arterial occlusive disease. Eur Radiol 2006; 16: 685–91.

Goyen M, Heuser LJ. Improved peripheral MRA using multi-velocity-encoding phase contrast-enhanced MRA techniques. Acta Radiol 2000; 41: 139–41.

Goyen M, Quick HH, Debatin JF et al. Whole-body three-dimensional MR angiography with a rolling table platform: initial clinical experience. Radiology 2002; 224: 270–7.

Goyen M, Ruehm SG, Debatin JF. MR angiography for assessment of peripheral vascular disease. Radiol Clin North Am 2002; 40: 835–46.

Goyen M, Ruehm SG, Debatin JF. MR-angiography: the role of contrast agents. Eur J Radiol 2000; 34: 247–56.

Hany TF, Debatin JF, Leung DA, Pfammatter T. Evaluation of the aortoiliac and renal arteries: comparison of breath-hold, contrast-enhanced, three-dimensional MR angiography with conventional catheter angiography. Radiology 1997; 204: 357–62.

Hentsch A, Aschauer MA, Balzer JO et al. Gadobutrol-enhanced moving-table magnetic resonance angiography in patients with peripheral vascular disease: a prospective, multi-centre blinded comparison with digital subtraction angiography. Eur Radiol 2003; 13: 2103–14.

Herborn CU. Peripheral contrast-enhanced 3D MRA with 1.0 M gadobutrol. Eur Radiol 2004a; (14 Suppl. 5): M23–25.

Herborn CU, Goyen M, Quick HH et al. Whole-body 3D MR angiography of patients with peripheral arterial occlusive disease. Am J Roentgenol 2004b; 182: 1427–34.

Herborn CU, Lauenstein TC, Ruehm SG et al. Intraindividual comparison of gadopentetate dimeglumine, gadobenate dimeglumine, and gadobutrol for pelvic 3D magnetic resonance angiography. Invest Radiol 2003; 38: 27–33.

Herborn CU, Vogt FM, Waltering KU et al. Optimization of contrast-enhanced peripheral MR angiography with mid-femoral venous compression (VENCO). Rofo 2004c; 176: 157–62.

Ho CF, Wu MH, Wu HM et al. Comparison of auto-moving table contrast-enhanced 3-D MRA and iodinated contrast-enhanced DSA for evaluating the lower-extremity arteries. J Chin Med Assoc 2004; 67: 511–20.

Hood MN, Ho VB, Foo TK et al. High-resolution gadolinium-enhanced 3D MRA of the infrapopliteal arteries. Lessons for improving bolus-chase peripheral MRA. Magn Reson Imaging 2002; 20: 543–9.

Koelemay MJ, Lijmer JG, Stoker J et al. Magnetic resonance angiography for the evaluation of lower extremity arterial disease: a meta-analysis. Jama 2001; 285: 1338–45.

Kramer H, Michaely HJ, Matschl V et al. High-resolution magnetic resonance angiography of the lower extremities with a dedicated 36-element matrix coil at 3 T. Invest Radiol 2007; 42: 477–83.

Krause U, Kroencke T, Spielhaupter E et al. Contrast-enhanced magnetic resonance angiography of the lower extremities: standard-dose vs. high-dose gadodiamide injection. J Magn Reson Imaging 2005; 21: 449–54.

Kressler B, Spincemaille P, Prince MR, Wang Y. Reduction of reconstruction time for time-resolved spiral 3D contrast-enhanced magnetic resonance angiography using parallel computing. Magn Reson Med 2006; 56: 704–8.

Leiner T, de Vries M, Hoogeveen R et al. Contrast-enhanced peripheral MR angiography at 3.0 T: initial experience with a whole-body scanner in healthy volunteers. J Magn Reson Imaging 2003; 17: 609–14.

Leiner T, Nijenhuis RJ, Maki JH et al. Use of a three-station phased array coil to improve peripheral contrast-enhanced magnetic resonance angiography. J Magn Reson Imaging 2004; 20: 417–25.

Lenhart M, Herold T, Volk M et al. Contrast media-enhanced MR angiography of the lower extremity arteries using a dedicated peripheral vascular coil system. First clinical results. Rofo 2000; 172: 992–9.

Li W, Vu AT, Tutton S et al. Scoutless stepping-table peripheral contrast-enhanced MR angiography. J Magn Reson Imaging 2006; 23: 235–41.

Loewe C, Cejna M, Schoder M et al. Contrast material-enhanced, moving-table MR angiography vs. digital subtraction angiography for surveillance of peripheral arterial bypass grafts. J Vasc Interv Radiol 2003; 14: 1129–37.

Maki JH, Wilson GJ, Eubank WB, Hoogeveen RM. Utilizing SENSE to achieve lower station sub-millimeter isotropic resolution and minimal venous enhancement in peripheral MR angiography. J Magn Reson Imaging 2002; 15: 484–91.

Meaney JF. Magnetic resonance angiography of the peripheral arteries: current status. Eur Radiol 2003; 13: 836–52.

Meissner OA, Rieger J, Weber C et al. Critical limb ischemia: hybrid MR angiography compared with DSA. Radiology 2005; 235: 308–18.

Nael K, Fenchel MC, Kramer U et al. Whole-body contrast-enhanced magnetic resonance angiography: new advances at 3.0 T. Top Magn Reson Imaging 2007a; 18: 127–34.

Nael K, Ruehm SG, Michaely HJ et al. Multi-station whole-body high-spatial-resolution MR angiography using a 32-channel MR system. Am J Roentgenol 2007a; 188: 529–39.

Pereles FS, Collins JD, Carr JC et al. Accuracy of stepping-table lower extremity MR angiography with dual-level bolus timing and separate calf acquisition: hybrid peripheral MR angiography. Radiology 2006; 240: 283–90.

Quick HH, Vogt FM, Maderwald S et al. High spatial resolution whole-body MR angiography featuring parallel imaging: initial experience. Rofo 2004; 176: 163–9.

Reimer P, Landwehr P. Non-invasive vascular imaging of peripheral vessels. Eur Radiol 1998; 8: 858–72.

Rofsky NM, Johnson G, Adelman MA et al. Peripheral vascular disease evaluated with reduced-dose gadolinium-enhanced MR angiography. Radiology 1997a; 205: 163–9.

Rofsky NM, Purdy DE, Johnson G et al. Suppression of venous signal in time-of-flight MR angiography of the lower extremities after administration of gadopentetate dimeglumine. Radiology 1997b; 202: 177–82.

Ruehm SG, Goyen M, Barkhausen J et al. Rapid magnetic resonance angiography for detection of atherosclerosis. Lancet 2001; 357: 1086–91.

Ruhl KM, Katoh M, Langer S et al. Time-resolved 3D MR angiography of the foot at 3 T in patients with peripheral arterial disease. Am J Roentgenol 2008; 190: 360–4.

Schoenberg SO, Londy FJ, Licato P et al. Multi-phase multi-step gadolinium-enhanced MR angiography of the abdominal aorta and run-off vessels. Invest Radiol 2001; 36: 283–91.

Shetty AN, Bis KG, Vrachliotis TG et al. Contrast-enhanced 3D MRA with centric ordering in k-space: a preliminary clinical experience in imaging the abdominal aorta and renal and peripheral arterial vasculature. J Magn Reson Imaging 1998; 8: 603–15.

Steffens JC, Schafer FK, Oberscheid B et al. Bolus-chasing contrast-enhanced 3D MRA of the lower extremity. Comparison with intraarterial DSA. Acta Radiol 2003; 44: 185–92.

Tongdee R, Narra VR, McNeal G et al. Hybrid peripheral 3D contrast-enhanced MR angiography of calf and foot vasculature. Am J Roentgenol 2006; 186: 1746–53.

Vahl AC, Geselschap J, Montauban van Swijndregt AD et al. Contrast-enhanced magnetic resonance angiography vs. intra-arterial digital subtraction angiography for treatment planning in patients with peripheral arterial disease: a randomised controlled diagnostic trial. Eur J Vasc Endovasc Surg 2008; 35: 514–21.

Visser K, Hunink MG. Peripheral arterial disease: gadolinium-enhanced MR angiography vs. color-guided duplex US – a meta-analysis. Radiology 2000; 216: 67–77.

Vogt FM, Herborn CU, Parsons EC et al. Diagnostic performance of contrast-enhanced MR angiography of the aortoiliac arteries with the blood pool agent Vasovist: initial results in comparison to intra-arterial DSA. Rofo 2007; 179: 412–20.

Vosshenrich R, Fischer U, Kopka L, Grabbe E. MR angiography of the pelvic-leg blood vessels: current status and perspectives. Aktuelle Radiol 1997; 7: 14–8.

Wang Y, Chen CZ, Chabra SG et al. Bolus arterial-venous transit in the lower extremity and venous contamination in bolus chase three-dimensional magnetic resonance angiography. Invest Radiol 2002; 37: 458–63.

Westenberg JJ, Wasser MN, van der Geest RJ et al. Scan optimization of gadolinium contrast-enhanced three-dimensional MRA of peripheral arteries with multiple bolus injections and in vitro validation of stenosis quantification. Magn Reson Imaging 1999; 17: 47–57.

Winterer JT, Laubenberger J, Scheffler K et al. Contrast-enhanced subtraction MR angiography in occlusive disease of the pelvic and lower limb arteries: results of a prospective intraindividual comparative study with digital subtraction angiography in 76 patients. J Comput Assist Tomogr 1999; 23: 583–9.

Winterer JT, Strecker R, Lohrmann C et al. Background suppression using magnetization preparation for contrast-enhanced 3D MR angiography of the pelvic and lower leg arteries. Rofo 2003; 175: 28–31.

Zenge MO, Vogt FM, Brauck K et al. High-resolution continuously acquired peripheral MR angiography featuring partial parallel imaging GRAPPA. Magn Reson Med 2006; 56: 859–65.

21 Incidental Findings at Cardiac Magnetic Resonance Imaging

Sandra Pauls and Christian Schumann

21.1 Prevalence

When evaluating the heart and great vessels by CMR, the cardiac magnetic resonance imaging field of view includes the thorax and upper abdomen. Therefore, CMR scans can detect findings that are incidental to the initial indication for which an examination was requested. The prevalence of non-cardiac pathology in clinical CMR has not been well-described, and the prevalence varies in a wide range depending on the age of the patient cohort studied.

McKenna et al. (2008) investigated 132 voluntary participants with a mean age of 74.2 yrs (range, 61–89 yrs; 127 males and 5 females) using CMR with 7 sequences. All images were retrospectively reviewed by a radiologist, specifically assessing for non-cardiac findings. Visualised abnormalities were noted and categorized according to clinically significant findings, intermediate significant findings, and clinically insignificant findings. Clinically significant findings were defined as those requiring further clinical or radiological work-up, moderately significant findings as those that may affect patient care depending on medical history of symptoms, and clinically insignificant were the remaining findings. In 107 of 132 participants (81 %) extracardiac findings were detected, with 63 (78 %) having multiple findings. 17 % of these incidental findings were potentially clinically significant, necessitating further work-up. Among different slice orientation and MR imaging sequences the SSFP coronal localizer, the SSFP axial localizer, and short-access SSFP cine oblique sequences were more sensitive in detecting incidental findings ($p = 0.013$ vs. four other sequences). It was concluded that this high percentage of incidental findings may be related to the patient age in the cohort examined. In conclusion, it was suggested to look beyond the heart when reviewing cardiac MRI studies and to carefully assess the entire field of view for abnormalities.

Chan et al. (2009) reported significantly lower rates of incidental findings in the 1,534 patients (62 % male, age 50 ± 15 yrs) in clinical CMR studies performed between 2002 and 2006. All studies had been interpreted by both a staff cardiologist (level III trained in CMR) and a board-certified radiologist (with fellowship training in CMR). A total of 116 (7.6 %) studies had at least one non-cardiac finding. These findings included 55 major findings, e. g. lymphadenopathy, lung abnormalities, mediastinal masses, in 48 distinct reports (prevalence of 3.1 %), and 74 minor findings, e. g. small pleural effusions, liver cysts, renal cysts, in 70 distinct reports (prevalence of 4.6 %). The majority (62 %) of major findings, ultimately deemed to be new and clinically important/significant, were previously only known in 8 findings in 6 of 1,534 reports (0.4 %). The age of those with non-cardiac pathology was greater (54 ± 16 yrs vs. 49 ± 16 yrs, $p < 0.001$). It was concluded that in this large series of consecutive clinical CMR studies interpreted by both staff cardiologists and radiologists, non-cardiac pathology was uncommonly reported, and new major findings were detected in < 0.5 % of reports.

Several studies have investigated this issue regarding other cardiac imaging modalities. Horton et al. (2002) looked at 1 326 screening electron-beam computer tomography studies and found that 7.8 % had significant extra-cardiac pathology. In a similar trial of 1,812 EBCT exams, Hunold et al. (2001) found that 53 % of the patients had visible non-coronary pathology, including cardiac abnormalities. However 67 % of these abnormalities were extra-cardiac in origin. 9.3 % of the 2,055 total extra-coronary findings required further diagnostic testing. In conclusion, the prevalence of clinically significant incidental findings varies between 3.1 and 17.4 % in regular CMR studies.

21.2 Significance of CMR versus Multi-Detector CT Imaging

Compared with MRI, multi-detector-row CT is the imaging technique of choice for diagnosing diseases of the thorax, because it has greater spatial resolution and captures the entire chest. CMR sequences are also not optimized for non-cardiac pathology. In addition, CT imaging is much faster than CMR and is generally more available than CMR. The advantage of MR imaging is its higher soft tissue contrast that is better in detecting infiltrations and involvement of neighbouring structures, and its biologically inert imaging modality. Multi-detector-row CT and PET-CT are the imaging techniques of choice for staging of lung cancer. MRI is only indicated for demonstrating infiltration of the mediastinum, thoracic wall, or diaphragm by a given tumor. A special indication for MRI is to assess the topographic relationship of a pancoast tumor to the spinal canal or to the brachial plexus. Multi-detector-row CT is also the imaging technique of choice for staging of malignant lymphoma and detecting metastases of the lungs. Therefore, the primary clinical significance of CMR imaging is to carefully look at processes outside the heart to detect incidental non-cardiac pathology requiring further diagnostic work-up. Therefore the entire field of view should be routinely and carefully assessed for non-cardiac abnormalities.

21.3 Topographic Distribution

Non-cardiac abnormalities should be localized and classified according to their **topographic appearance** into:

- masses and tumours in the mediastinum,
- diffuse diseases of the mediastinum,
- diseases of the lung,
- diseases of the tracheobronchial tree,
- diseases of the pleura,
- diseases of the thoracic wall.

21.4 Anterior Mediastinal Masses

Among the **masses of the anterior mediastinum** are the **4 Ts**:

- retrosternal goiter (**th**yreoidea),
- thymus hyperplasia/tumors (**th**ymus),
- teratoma (**te**ratoma), and
- **te**rrible lymphoma (malignant non-Hodkin lymphoma), as well as abdominal Morgagni's hernia.

Retrosternal **struma** (goiter) commonly shows a continuous connection with the normal thyroid gland, and has the same signal intensity (SI) as the thyroid itself. SI of the struma is isointense to skeletal muscle in T1-weighted (T1w)-images, and has a high SI in T2-weighted (T2w)-images. After gadolinium administration it shows a strong enhancement. In addition, focal lesions (adenoma) or regressive changes (cysts, calcifications) are frequently encountered. In struma nodosa, SI of parenchyma and adenomas is reduced in T1w- and increased in T2w-images.

The thymus is usually large in infants and reaches the lateral contours of the mediastinum on both sides; it regresses by the age of 30. Following severe stress, e.g. burning, polytrauma, large surgical procedures, or diseases like hyperthyreosis or Morbus Addison the thymus may again proliferate (rebound phenomenon). In myasthenia gravis **thymus hyperplasia** is present in about 65 % of cases; however, in only 25 % is it large enough to be detected by magnetic resonance imaging (MRI). The SI of normal thymus tissue is slightly higher than skeletal muscle in T1w-, and higher than fat or muscle in T2w-images. Benign or malignant **thymomas** are rare, showing up as a rounded mass with a smooth surface and frequent calcifications, but rarely with cystic alterations. The SI is low in T1w sequences and high but inhomogenous in T2w sequences. **Thymus carcinoma** shows similar SI and reveals frequent invasive growth and remote metastases.

Germ cell tumors are encountered in the second to fourth decade, with more than 90 % located in the anterior mediastinum and constituting about 10–15 % of all tumors in this region. **Teratoma** is the most common benign tumor (80 %), while the remaining 20 % of malignant tumors include **seminoma** (30–40 %), **embryonic carcinoma** (10 %), **malignant teratoma** (10 %), and **chorion carcinoma** (5 %). Teratoma contains all three germ layers with fat, cysts, soft tissue, and calcifications. The SI is low or intermediate in

T1w- and intermediate to high in T2w-images. Benign teratomas are smooth with sharp boundaries and contain fat and calcifications, while malignant tumors show infiltration into the neighboring structures. **Seminoma** has a homogenous inner structure without fat, cysts or calcifications; SI is low in T1w- and intermediate to high in T2w-images.

Hodgkin lymphoma may occur in the anterior mediastinum. The tumors are rounded and homogenous; SI is low in T1w- and intermediate to high in T2w-sequences with little enhancement on gadolinium administration.

Adenoma of the **parathyroid gland** is rare and is the most frequent cause of primary hyperparathyroidism (85%) compared to 10% with diffuse hyperplasia, 5% with multiple adenomas, and 1% with carcinoma. The adenomas are small with only a few millimeters in diameter. Their SI is low in T1w- and high in T2w-images and shows a strong enhancement after gadolinium injection. Thus, MRI is the diagnostic method of choice to detect and localize parathyroid adenomas.

21.5 Middle Mediastinal Masses

Masses within the middle mediastinum include:

- lymph node diseases:
  - malignant non-Hodkin lymphoma,
  - lymph node metastases,
  - Castleman lymphoma,
  - sarcoidosis, and
  - inflammatory lymphadenopathies like tuberculosis, and by bacteria, fungi, or viruses,
- centrally located lung cancer,
- aortic aneurysms, and
- cysts (bronchogenic, pericardial).

The most frequent masses in the middle mediastinum are processes originating from lymph nodes, including primary malignant lymphomas, lymph node metastases, or inflammatory lymph node processes. **Malignant non-Hodkin lymphomas** are the most common malignant lymphomas in this region and are characterized by discontinuous dissemination, involvement in unusual lymph node tracts (mammaria interna, cardiophrenic etc.) and the posterior mediastinum, and extranodal manifestations. These masses are most commonly homogenous without cysts, bleeding, or calcifications. SI in T1w-images is low and iso- to hyperintense in T2w-sequences, with lymphomas showing a strong enhancement after gadolinium injection. **Sarcoidosis** involves lymph nodes in a bilateral symmetric pattern together with a significant bi-hilar lymphadenopathy, and in later stages infiltration of the lung parenchyma (Figure 21-1 and Figure 21-2). SI is low in T1w- and intermediate to hyperintense in T2w-images, but MRI does not aid in differentiating between the many types of lymphomas. **Inflammatory lymphadenopathies** (tuberculosis, histiocytosis, coccidiomycosis, bacterial, viral) are also most commonly located in the middle mediastinum, but do not show specific MRI characteristics.

Aortic aneurysm presents with typical dilatation of the aorta with or without dissection or aortic regurgitation. Aortic aneurysms are well-visualized by bright-blood and black-blood sequences, and CE-MRA is the method of choice to confirm the diagnosis. **Cysts** in the middle mediastinum include bronchogenic or pericardial cysts. They are all benign and usually asymptomatic. SI of cysts is low in T1w- and high in T2w-images, and there is no enhancement following gadolinium injection. Only inflammatory cysts may show an enhancement within the wall of the cyst.

a
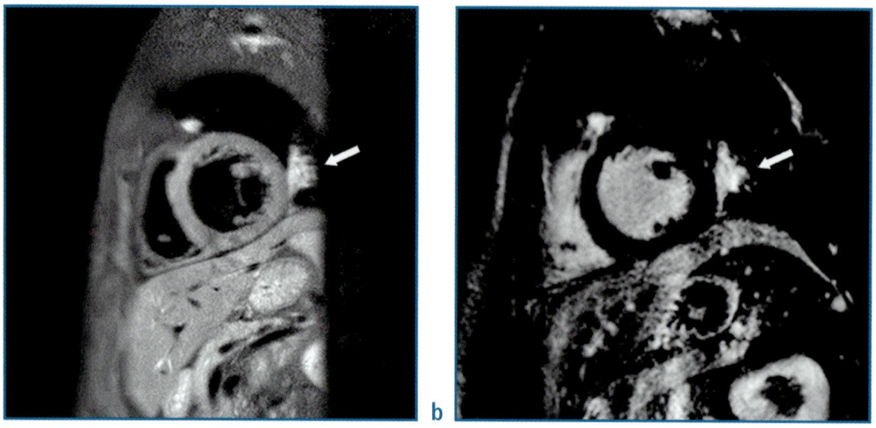
b

Figure 21-1 28-yrs-old male patient with known sarcoidosis. T2-TSE (a) and IR-TFE images (b) show paracardial sarcoid pulmonary infiltration (arrows).

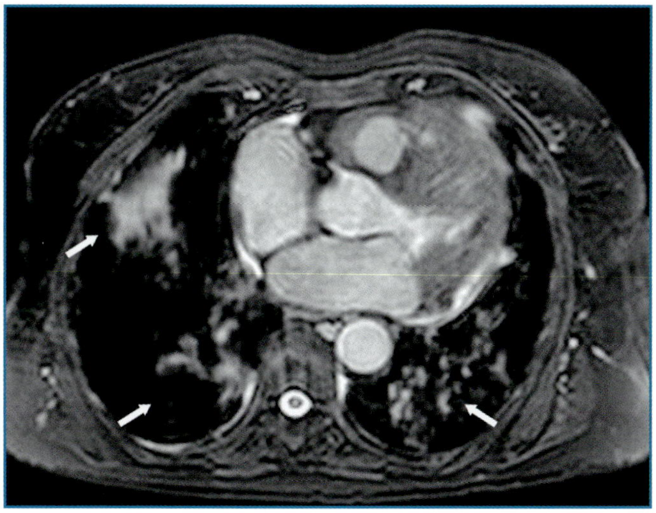

Figure 21-2 56-yrs-old female patient with known sarcoidosis: Diffuse infiltration of the peripheral lung fields (arrows).

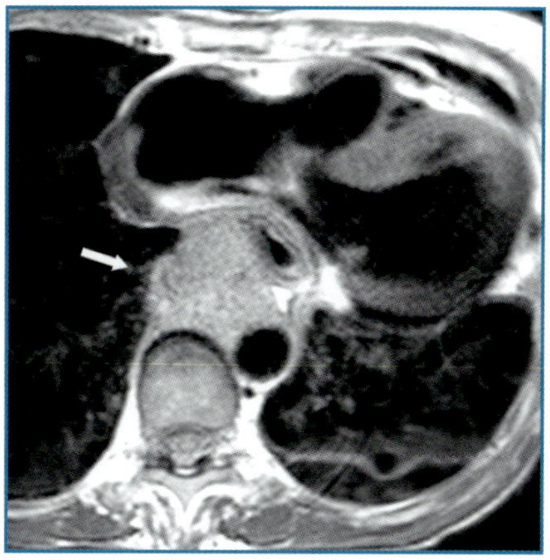

Figure 21-3 67-yrs-old female patient with an incidental finding: Solid mass of the dorsal mediastinum (arrow). Histology revealed a carcinoma of the distal esophagus.

21.6 Posterior Mediastinal Masses

Masses within the posterior mediastinum include:

- esophageal diseases:
  - carcinoma,
  - leiomyoma,
  - varices,
  - duplicated esophagus,
- neurogenic tumors:
  - neurofibroma,
  - schwannoma,
  - neuroblastoma,
  - ganglioneuroma,
  - ganglioblastoma,
- extramedullary hematopoiesis (e.g. in sickle cell anemia, spherocytosis or thalassemia),
- cysts (neuroenteric, meningocele, pseudocysts of the pancreas), and
- hernia (Bochdalek hernia, hiatal hernia).

Carcinoma of the esophagus shows an early tumor expansion into the mediastinum, lymph nodes, and distal metastases (Figure 21-3). MRI typically reveals a diffuse thickening of the esophageal wall in the tumor region with infiltration into the surrounding tissue, and a pre-stenotic dilatation of the esophagus proximally to the tumor. SI is low in T1w- and iso- to hyperintense in T2w-sequences, with a moderate enhancement after gadolinium injection. **Neurogenic tumors** are typically located in the posterior mediastinum; SI is slightly hyperintense in T1w- and high in T2w-images. A strong enhancement after gadolinium injection is seen. **Extramedullary hematopoiesis** is located in the liver, spleen, and in lymph nodes; in the mediastinum paravertebral lobulated soft-tissue-like masses may be detected on both sides of the spinal cord below the level of the 6th vertebral body. SI is low in T1w- and high in T2w-images. **Cysts** include duplication of the esophagus (connection with the esophagus), neurenteric cysts (connection with esophagus and the meninges), meningoceles (associated with a defect of the vertebral body), and pseudocysts of the pancreas (following pancreatitis). Cysts typically show low SI in T1w- and high SI in T2w-images.

21.7 Diffuse Mediastinal Diseases

Diffuse diseases of the mediastinum include:

- mediastinal lipomatosis (idiopathic, obesity, Cushing's disease),
- diffuse acute mediastinitis (perforation of the esophagus, centrally located lung cancer, trauma), and
- fibrosing mediastinitis (idiopathic likewise Ormond's disease, post-infections from tuberculosis, lues, or histoplasmosis, and following treatments such as radiation or methysergide medication).

Mediastinal lipomatosis is commonly seen in general obesity (50% of cases), with long-lasting Cushing's disease, or on maintained corticoid treatment. SI is typically high in both T1w- and T2w-images, and signal loss occurs on fat suppression sequences. **Diffuse mediastinitis** is commonly seen with perforation of the esophagus (heavy vomiting, perforation of an esophageal tumor, following endoscopy), and MRI shows an edema and inflammatory infiltration of mediastinal fatty tissue (Figure 21-4), sometimes with a

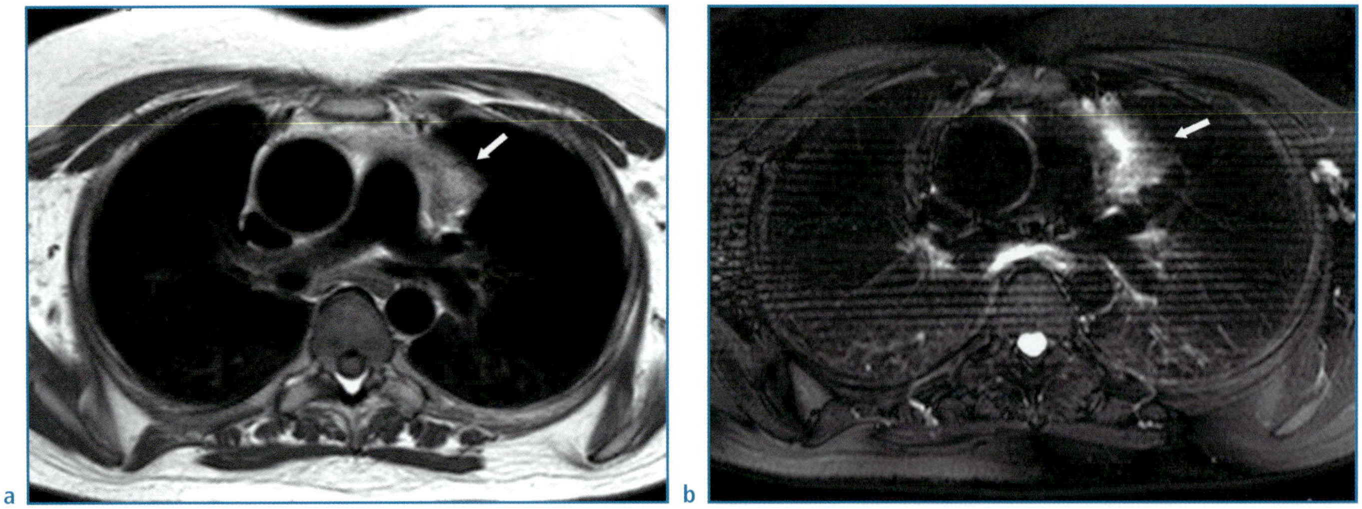

Figure 21-4 32-yrs-old female patient with mediastinitis: Masses are located antevertebrally and next to the pulmonary trunk (arrow, (a)). The inversion-recovery image on the right side shows diffuse contrast enhancement of the mass (arrow, (b)).

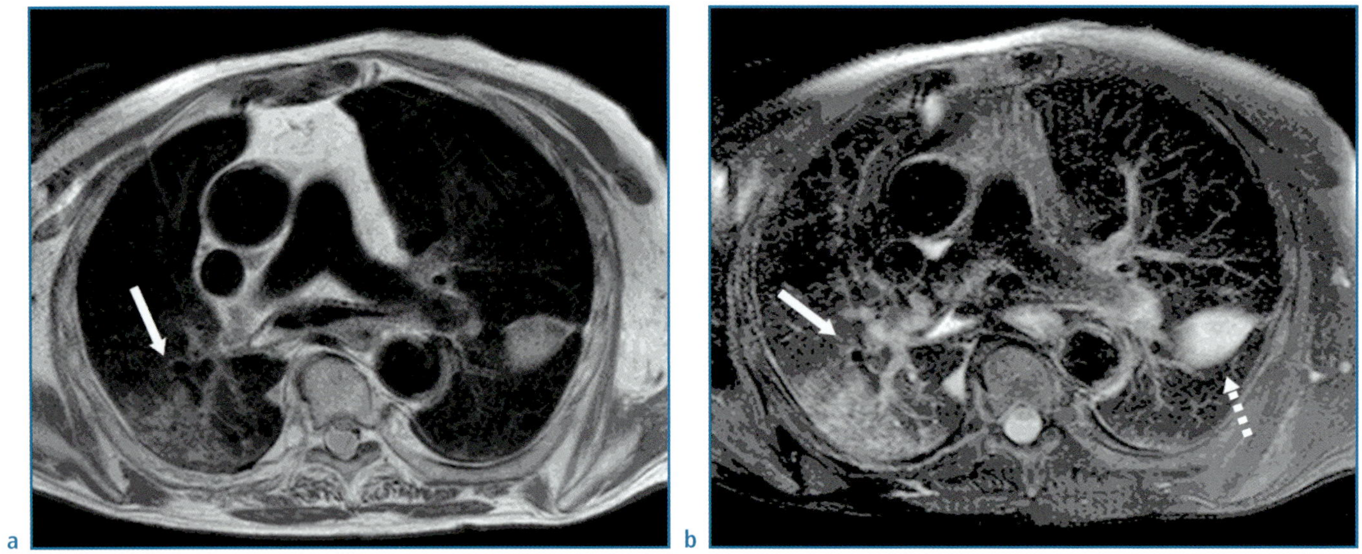

Figure 21-5 46-yrs-old male patient with right sided pneumonia (arrows): On the left side encapsulated pleural effusion (dashed arrow). T2-TSE without (a) and with fat saturation (b).

necrotic core and strong enhancement in the border zone. Most commonly secondary phenomena such as pleural effusion, atelectasis of the adjacent lung parenchyma, and diaphragmatic elevation are present. **Fibrosing mediastinitis** may be idiopathic or be caused by infection (tuberculosis, lues, histoplasmosis, fungi), or after treatment (radiation, mythysergide medication). SI is heterogenous in T1w- and unusually low in T2w-images.

21.8 Diseases of the Lung Parenchyma

Diseases of the lung parenchyma include:

- incidental pneumonia (Figure 21-5),
- pulmonary sequestration (extralobular, intralobular),
- bronchogenic cysts,
- arteriovenous fistulas,
- congenital cystic adenomatoid malformations (CAM), and
- metastases from breast cancer, lung cancer, thyroid carcinoma, malignant melanoma, or sarcoma.

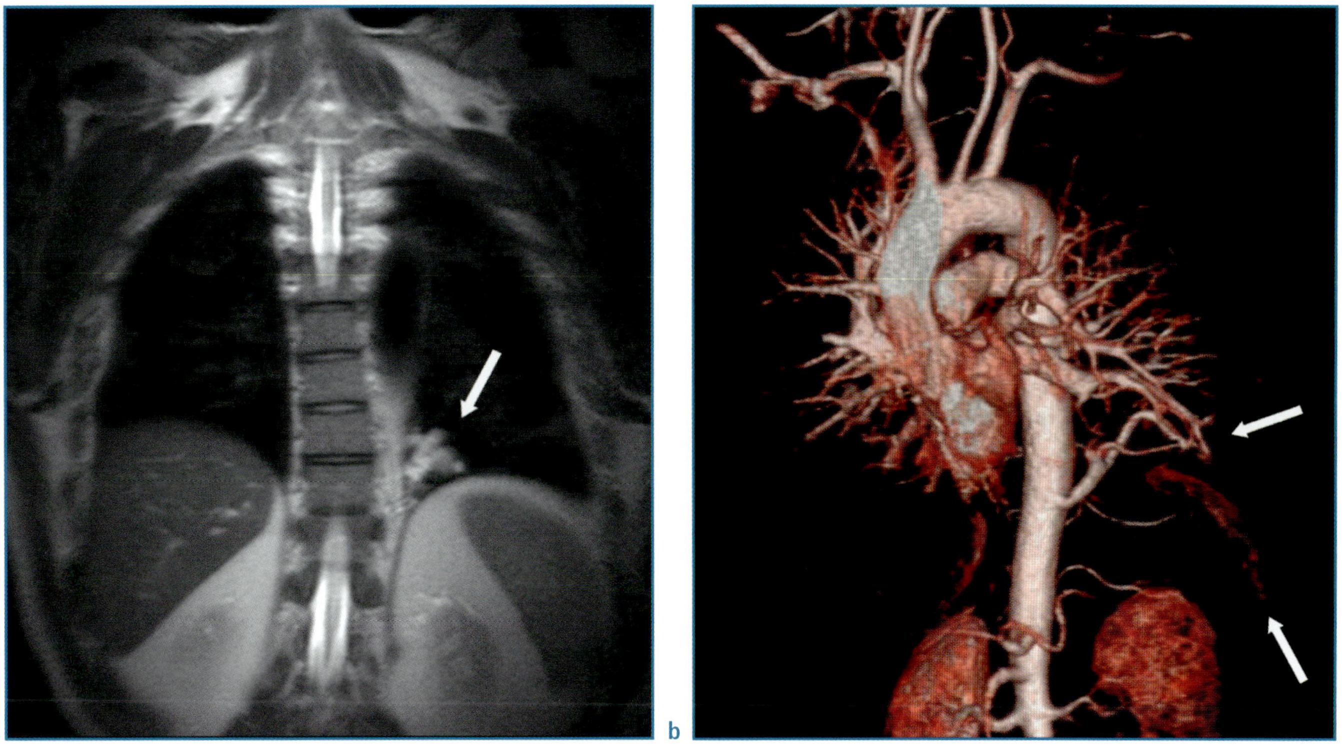

a b

Figure 21-6 56-yrs-old male patient with recurrent bronchopulmonary infections, showing pulmonary sequestrum at the typical posterobasal location on the left side (arrow, (a)). The volume-rendered reconstruction nicely shows arterial supply from the aorta and venous outflow via a pulmonary vein (= intralobar sequestration) (arrow, (b)) (courtesy Prof. A. Buecker, Homburg/Saar).

In **pulmonary sequestration** lung tissue is dissected from the tracheobronchial system, with the sequestrum most commonly localized in the left posterobasal lower lobe (65% of cases) (Figure 21-6), or the right lower lobe (35% of cases). In the rarer extralobar sequestration, tissue is surrounded by its own visceral pleura, and is frequently associated with other congenital cardiovascular or gastrointestinal malformations. Its aberrant arterial supply originates from the aorta, and venous outflow is provided via the inferior vena cava or azygos veins. The more common intralobar sequestration, as an isolated malformation, lacks its own pleura, the arterial inflow originates from the aorta, but the venous outflow is provided via pulmonary veins. MRI is able to detect the aberrant artery originating from the aorta or the aortic branches. The SI is high in both T1w- (impaction by mucus) and T2w-images, and these lesions show enhancement after gadolinium injection at the same time as in the aorta.

Bronchogenic cysts are smooth, rounded or oval fluid containing lesions that show low to moderate SI in T1w-images (depending on the composition of the fluid), high SI in T2w-sequences and no contrast enhancement. **Arteriovenous fistulas** appear as rounded unifocal or multi-focal lesions with isointense SI in T1w- and hyperintense SI in T2w-images. **Congenital cystic adenomatoid malformation** (CAM) is a malformation of lung parenchyma consisting of immature bronchoid and adenomatoid structures, most commonly localized in the lower lobes of the lung.

CAM presents as:

- **type 1** with one or more large cysts,
- **type 2** with several smaller cysts, and
- **type 3** with multiple microscopic cysts.

Its SI is low in T1w-sequences, and diagnosis is confirmed by CT imaging.

Metastases of the lung parenchyma from breast cancer, lung cancer, renal cell carcinoma, thyroid carcinoma, or sarcoma appear as single or multiple rounded lesions with sharp demarcations. Central liquefactions in metastases are rare (only in squamous cell carcinoma or sarcoma), but are more frequent after cytostatic therapy. SI is low in T1w- and iso- to hyperintense in T2w-images and do not show significant contrast enhancement (Figure 21-7). Only in the presence of hemorrhagic lesions (chorion carcinoma), fat (liposarcoma), or melanin (malignant melanoma) is SI high in T1w-images.

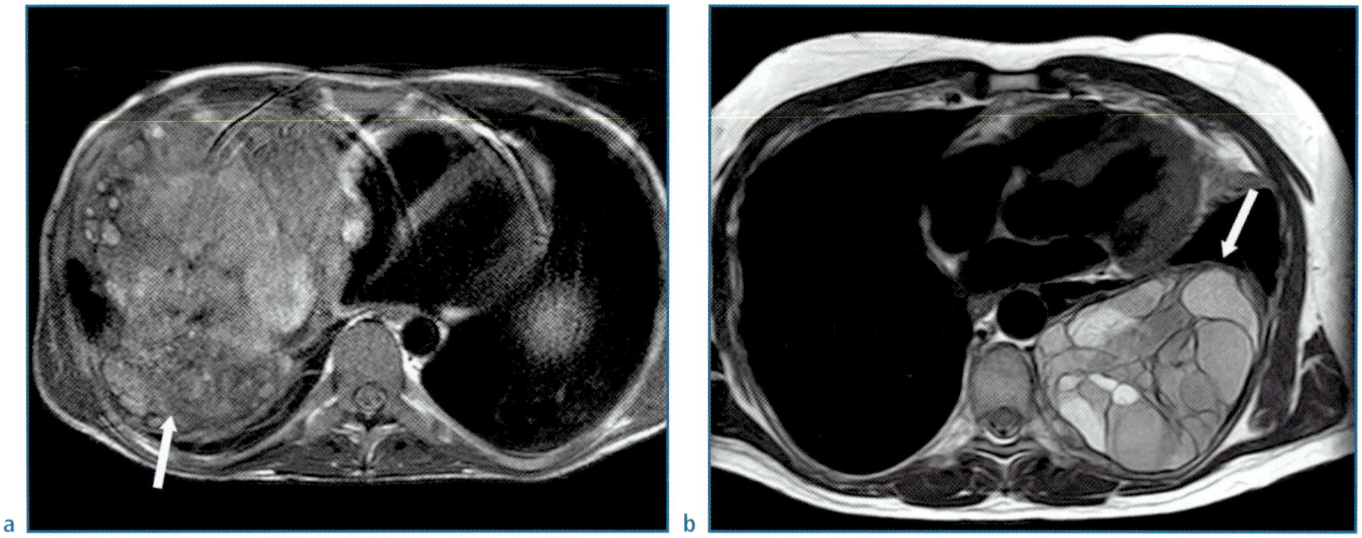

Figure 21-7 T2-weighted images of two different patients with teratocarcinoma of the testis: Images show extensive metastasis of the lung (arrows, (a and b)).

21.9 Tracheobronchial Diseases

Tracheobronchial diseases include:

- circumscribed processes of the trachea like strictures or tumors:
  - papillomas,
  - papillomatosis,
  - carcinoma,
  - infiltrative tumors from bronchi, esophagus, thyroid, and
  - malignant lymphoma,
- diffuse processes such as:
  - diffuse dilatation (bronchomegaly), or
  - diffuse stenoses (from amyloidosis, Wegener's granulomatosis, sarcoidosis, colitis ulcerosa, polychondritis), and
- diseases of the bronchi (bronchial cysts, bronchiectasis, bronchial carcinoma).

Morbus Wegener with tracheobronchial manifestation, may induce a concentric or eccentric thickening of the tracheal wall extending several centimeters, most commonly beginning at the subglottic level. **Amyloidosis** manifests not only with diffuse involvement of the lung parenchyma, but also with a diffuse or localized deposition in the wall of the central airways with secondary obstructions of trachea and bronchi. Similar diffuse thickening of the tracheobronchial walls may be induced by recurrent polychondritis, tracheobronchopathia osteochondroplastica, colitis ulcerosa, and sarcoidosis. MRI cannot differentiate between these various lesions.

Primary **tumors of the trachea** are rare, the most common benign tumors are papillomas, either isolated or presenting as papillomatosis. The most common primary malignant tumors of the trachea are squamous carcinoma or adenocystic carcinoma (in 95% of cases). Tumors of the trachea show a low SI in T1w-images, and iso- to hyperintense SI in T2w-sequences, and a variable degree of contrast enhancement. A differentiation of these tumors cannot be made by MRI despite the fact that the extent and infiltrative nature of the lesions can be reliably assessed. **Lung cancer** (LC) is the most frequent malignant tumor with the highest mortality in western countries. LC may present with different types including non-small cell carcinoma (squamous cell carcinoma, adenocarcinoma, large cell carcinoma in about 80% of cases), and small cell carcinoma (about 20% of cases). LC may present as a single nodule (Figure 21-8) or

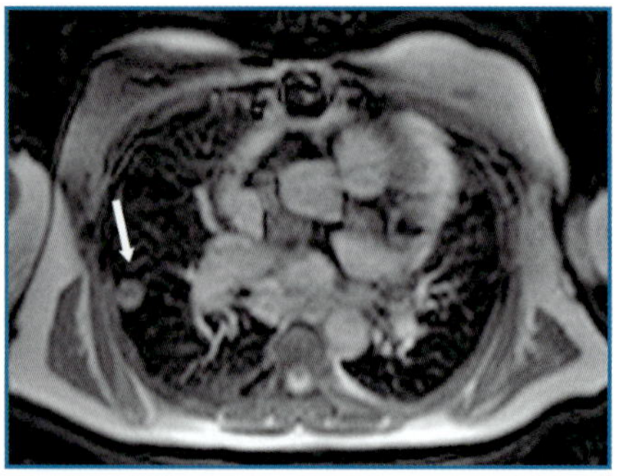

Figure 21-8 70-yrs-old female patient referred for adenosine stress perfusion. Additional finding of a solitary pulmonary nodule of the right middle lobe (arrow); histology after resection of the tumor revealed a non-small cell lung cancer (NSCLC).

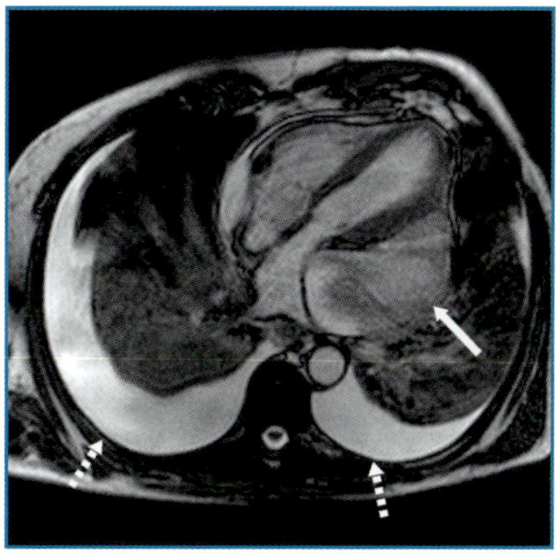

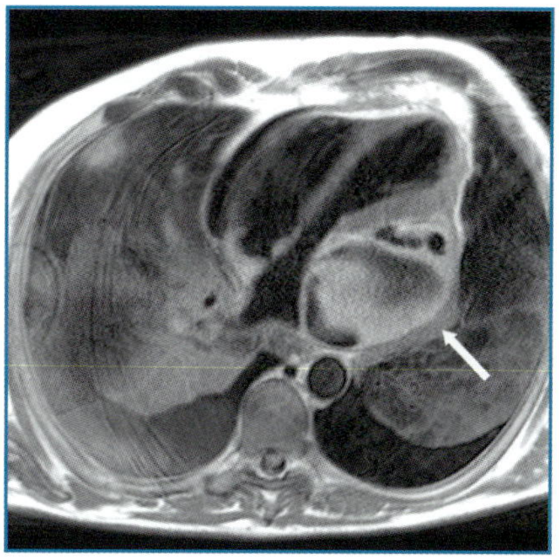

Figure 21-9 53-yrs-old patient with lung cancer and functional mitral stenosis due to infiltration of the pericardium by the tumor (arrows, (a and b)). This resulted in a smaller pericardial and extensive pleural effusion (dashed arrows in (a)).

a mass of different size and irregular border. Located in the center or periphery of the thorax (Figure 21-9), it causes local infiltration including regional ipsilateral and/or contralateral lymph node metastases, and atelectasis. SI of the tumor is low in T1w- and high in T2w-images with variable significant contrast enhancement. Central necrosis occurs most frequently in squamous cell carcinoma. Hilar or mediastinal lymph node metastases present with MRI signal intensities similar to LC.

Carcinoid is a typical tumor of the gastrointestinal tract (90 % of cases). Among the bronchopulmonary tumors carcinoid is rare (about 1–4 % of all tumors). Pulmonary carcinoid originates endobronchially in the central bronchial tree (80–90 % of cases), preferentially at bronchial branching, and causing bronchial obstruction with atelectasis or regional post-stenotic pneumonia. In MRI the tumor appears as an endobronchial lesion with a smooth surface and distal obstruction of the bronchus. The tumor may contain calcifications with susceptibility artifacts in the MRI, central liquefactions, however, are rare. SI of the tumor is typically low in T1w- and high in T2w-images, with strong enhancement after gadolinium injection.

Adenocystic carcinoma is a rare tumor, most frequently evolving from the tracheobronchial tree, and showing a growth tendency slower than that of lung cancer. It cannot be differentiated from lung cancer by MRI because of similar shape and signal behaviour. **Sarcoma** of the trachea presents in different histologic types (leiomyosarcoma, fibrosarcoma, chondrosarcoma, liposarcoma, malignant fibrous histiocytoma) and is also very rare. At the time of tumor detection they may be as large as 10 cm in diameter. **Leiomyosarcoma** may be differentiated in MRI by its polypoid shape, unilateral location, and contrast enhancement.

21.10 Diseases of the Pleura

Diseases of the pleura include:
- incidental pneumothorax (Figure 21-10),
- tumors:
  - benign (benign fibrous tumor, lipoma, fibroma, asbestos-induced round atelectasis),
  - malignant (pleural mesothelioma, carcinosis of the pleura, infiltration by non-Hodgkin lymphoma),
- effusion (exudate, transudate, hemorrhagic effusion, chylothorax),
- fibrosis (endstage of several pleural diseases), and
- asbestos-induced plaques.

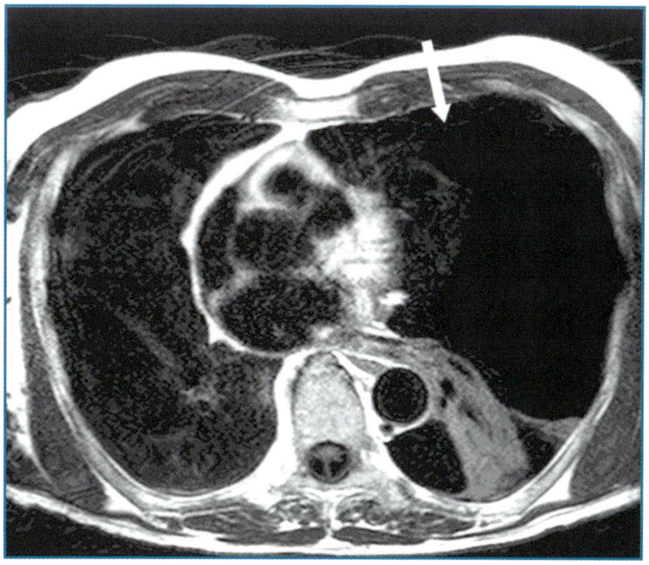

Figure 21-10 46-yrs-old patient with pneumothorax and complete collapse of the left lung (arrow) with concomitant shift of the heart to the right. This symptomatic patient was referred for adenosine stress perfusion because of chest pain (angina pectoris).

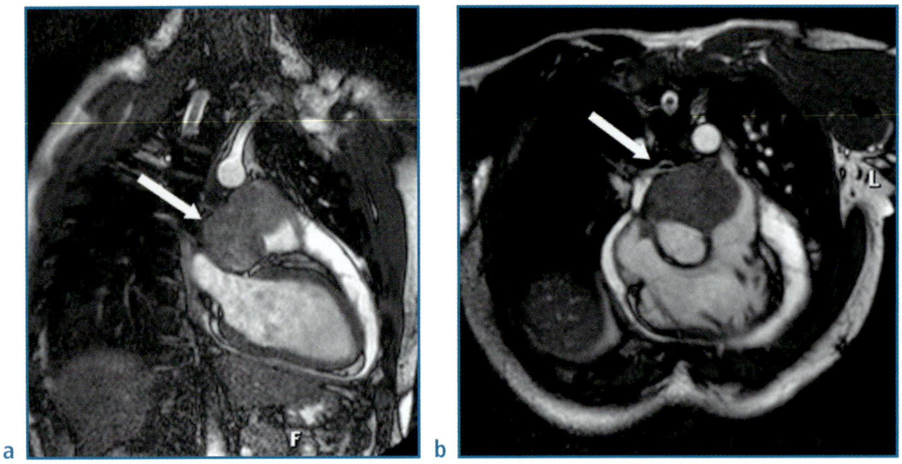

Figure 21-11 31-yrs-old male patient with a primitive neuroectodermal tumor (PNET) located in the mediastinum (arrows). This mass presents homogenously in SSFP sequences, signal intensity is comparable to that of myocardium, 2-ch view (a), axial view (b).

Benign fibrous tumor of the pleura is rare (10% of all pleural neoplasms) and not associated with exposure to asbestos. Occasionally, patients present with extrapulmonary symptoms like osteoarthropathy, finger clubbing, watch-glass nails, or hypoglycemia. SI is low in T1w- and higher in T2w-images, with strong enhancement after gadolinium injection. **Lipoma** and **fibroma** are rare and only occasionally detected. **Round atelectasis** may occur with exposure to asbestos, but also with other fibrosing diseases of the pleura by folding of lung parenchyma. Its diameter is typically 2–7 cm, showing a sharp border and usually localized at the posterior aspect of both lower lobes of the lung. Bronchi and vessels extending into the lesion show a curvilinear course (comet-like structure), that is well-visualized by spin echo sequences together with a strong enhancement of the infolded lung after gadolinium injection.

Pleural mesothelioma is most commonly caused by exposure to asbestos. The tumor shows a nodular or diffuse thickening or mass within the pleural space and the mediastinum, extending into the interlobar cleft. In progressive stages infiltration of the mediastinum, pericardium, ribs, and lymph nodes is present together with remote metastases in the adrenals, kidneys, or the lung. On MRI an extended pleural effusion is present, and parietal nodular lesions show low SI in T1w- and high SI in T2w-images together with an inhomogenous enhancement after gadolinium injection. Sometimes the whole lung is engrafted by the tumor without deviation of the mediastinum to the contralateral site even despite a large pleural effusion resulting from hemithorax fettering.

Pleural metastases or **carcinosis** from an extrapleural malignant tumor (lung cancer, breast cancer, and malignant lymphoma) are more commonly detected than pleural mesothelioma. In 10% of cases the primary tumor cannot be identified for the pleural metastasis/carcinosis. The metastatic masses present with irregular, nodular thickening of the pleura with low SI in T1w- and high SI in T2w-images, along with strong enhancement after gadolinium injection. These lesions cannot be differentiated from mesothelioma. **Lymphoma** involvement of the pleura is more frequently observed in non-Hodgkin than in Hodgkin lymphoma. In most cases circumscriptive, rarely diffuse, solid lesions are frequently found associated with thoracic or pulmonic lymph nodes. SI in MRI is similar to that described for lymphomas of the mediastinum.

Pleural effusion may be differentiated into transudates and exudates, and both are associated with different diseases (*transudate* due to heart failure, liver cirrhosis, nephrotic syndrome, atelectasis; *exudate* by infection or malignant diseases [Figure 21-9 and Figure 21-11]; *empyema* due to bacteria within a parapneumonic exudate). Accumulation of lymph fluid is called chylothorax (due to obstructed lymph vessels or malignant lymphoma), while blood accumulation is called hematothorax (due to trauma or malignant disease). SI is low in T1w- and high in T2w-images without enhancement after gadolinium administration (exept with empyema). MRI cannot differentiate between the different types of pleural effusion.

Diffuse **pleural thickening** is caused by diffuse fibrosis and represents the endstage of different pleural lesions (pleuritis, pleural empyema, hematothorax, and asbestos-associated pleuritis). **Pleural plaques** are the most common manifestation of asbestos-associated pleural lesions in about 20–60% of exposed individuals with a latency of 15–20 yrs. SI in pleural fibrosis or plaques is low in T1w- and iso- to hyperintense in T2w-images with no enhancement after gadolinium injection.

21.11 Diseases of the Thoracic Wall

Diseases of the thoracic wall include:

- primary tumors:
  - benign (chondroma, fibrous dysplasia, Morbus Paget, atheroma, lipoma, fibroma, hemangioma, lymphangioma, neurinoma, neurofibroma),
  - malignant (primitive neuroectodermal tumor [PNET], plasmocytoma, fibrosarcoma, malignant fibrous histiocytoma, rhabdomyosarcoma, and desmoid tumor),
- secondary tumors from infiltration (lung cancer, breast cancer, malignant lymphoma), and
- metastases (lung cancer, breast cancer, renal cell carcinoma, thyroid carcinoma).

Primary tumors of the thoracic wall are rare and include benign and malignant tumors. The malignant **PNET** occurs primarily in infants and adolescents. SI is low in T1w- and iso- to hyperintense in T2w-images; malignant tumors often show infiltrative growth into the neighboring structures (Figure 21-11). **Secondary tumors** infiltrating the thoracic wall include lung cancer, breast cancer, malignant lymphoma, and metastases. MRI is able to reliably detect whether the tumor is confined to the surface of the lung or is infiltrating the thoracic wall. This is particularly important for tumors located in the apex of the lung (**"pancoast tumor"**), near the diaphragm, or the spinal canal. Infiltration of the thoracic wall by **breast cancer** is similarly detectable by MRI, as is infiltration by a malignant lymphoma. **Metastases** (Figure 21-12) of the thoracic wall most often originate from lung cancer, breast cancer, renal cell carcinoma, thyroid carcinoma, or plasmocytoma. SI is low in T1w- and iso- to hyperintense in T2w-images. Tumors containing fat (lipoma, liposarcoma) can be differentiated by fat suppression sequences, and vascularized tumors (hemangioma) may be diagnosed by strong enhancement after gadolinium injection.

21.12 Diseases of the Upper Abdomen

Diseases of the upper abdomen include:

- diseases of the liver (cysts, tumors like hemangioma, focal nodular hyperplasia, adenoma, hepatocellular carcinoma, cholangiocarcinoma, and inflammatory processes like abscesses),
- lesions of the spleen (cysts, tumors like lymphoma, angiosarcoma, fibrosarcoma, leiomyosarcoma, malignant teratoma, and metastases),
- pancreatic diseases (cysts, cystic adenoma or carcinoma, adenocarcinoma, lymphoma),
- diseases of the stomach (hiatal hernia, carcinoma), and
- diseases of the kidneys (cysts, renal cell carcinoma).

Since most of these lesions are only visualized on the scout images for CMR (Figure 21-13) without detailed imaging protocols using the whole spectrum of sequences and weighting (T1w, T2w, PDw), a further detailed diagnostic differentiation has to be performed in a second step using other imaging modalities.

21.13 Summary and Conclusions

Due to the large field of view, at least in initial scout images, CMR can detect findings that are incidental to the initial indication for which an examination was requested. The prevalence of non-cardiac pathology in clinical CMR varies

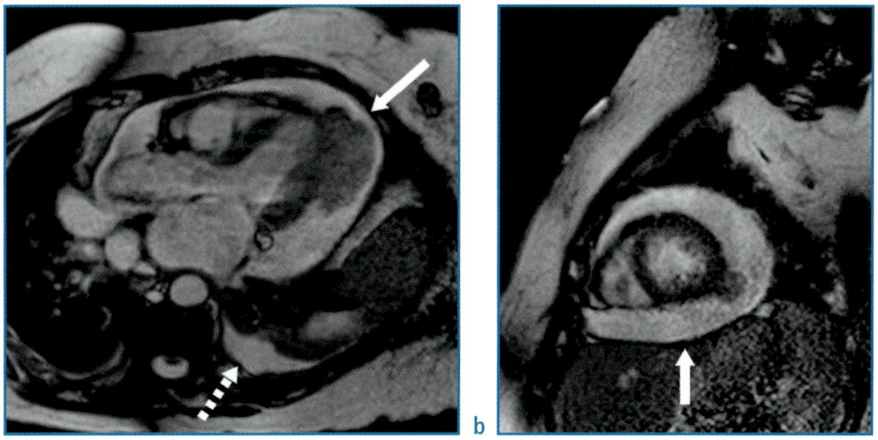

a b

Figure 21-12 76-yrs-old female patient with a known melanoma of the right leg: CMR was performed as a control for a newly diagnosed pericardial effusion and showed an epicardial metastasis (arrow, (a)) with large malignant pericardial effusion (arrow, (b)), and small pleural effusion (dashed arrow, (a)).

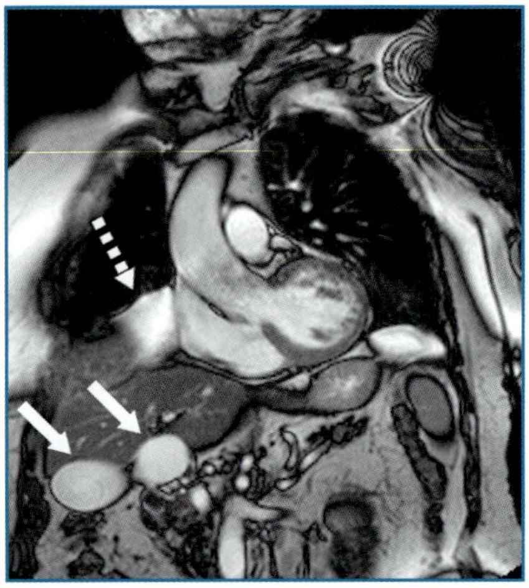

Figure 21-13 65-yrs-old female patient with an incidental finding of multiple liver cysts (white arrows) and a pericardial cyst (dashed arrow).

in a wide range depending on the age of the patient cohort studied. Several papers have reported a prevalence of clinically significant incidental findings between 3.1 % and 17.4 % in regular CMR studies. As a consequence, further diagnostic steps have to be undertaken to clarify the real nature of such an incidental finding. Compared with MRI multi-detector-row CT is the imaging technique of choice for further diagnosing diseases of the thorax. This is due to its greater spatial resolution and ability to capture the entire chest. CMR sequences are also not optimized for non-cardiac pathology. In addition, CT imaging is much faster than CMR, and is generally more available than CMR. But nevertheless, it remains mandatory that the entire field of view should be routinely and carefully screened in CMR images for non-cardiac abnormalities so as not to miss clinically relevant extracardiac diseases that may be harmful in the further course of the individual patient.

References

Chan PG, Smith MP, Hauser TH et al. Noncardiac pathology on clinical magnetic resonance imaging. J Am Coll Cardiol Imag 2009; 2: 980–6.

Horton KM, Post WS, Blumenthal RS, Fishman EK. Prevalence of significant noncardiac findings on electron-beam computed tomography coronary artery calcium screening examinations. Circulation 2002; 106: 532–4.

Hunold R, Schmermund A, Seibel RM et al. Prevalence and clinical significance of accidental findings in electron-beam tomographic scans for coronary artery calcifications. Eur Heart J 2001; 22: 1748–58.

McKenna DA, Laxpati M, Colletti PM. The prevalence of incidental findings at cardiac MRI. Open Cardiovasc Med J 2008; 2: 20–5.

Part III

Innovative and Experimental Imaging Techniques

22 High-Field Cardiac Magnetic Resonance

Matthias Stuber and Peter R. Luijten

22.1 Basic Principles – Why Higher Fields?

Signal-to-noise (SNR) is theoretically proportional to the field strength of the static magnetic field B_0 in magnetic resonance spectroscopy (MRS) and imaging (MRI). Therefore, high-field systems, of which both 3 T and more recently 7 T systems have been approved by the FDA for human use, may be exploited to enhance SNR for many cardiovascular applications. An enhanced SNR leads to improved detail visibility, will support the acquisition of higher spatial and temporal resolution images and abbreviated scanning times may be among the benefits. Concomitant with this SNR benefit, an increased spectral resolution will be advantageous for both MRS and MRI as well as the potential generation of contrast using susceptibility effects. However, there are not only advantages but also challenges associated with higher field strength. Increased susceptibility at tissue borders, shortened T2*, enhanced B_1 inhomogeneity, an increase of the specific absorption rate (SAR) that is not linear but quadratic with the magnetic field strength, B_0 homogeneity compromised by tissue interfaces and amplified artifactual signals overlaid to the ECG are among the technical challenges that remain to be addressed. Especially at 7 T, a major focus is currently on the development of new hardware components and related MR methods since these are neither fully established and developed nor are they commercially available. Therefore, a direct translation of established cardiovascular protocols from lower to higher field strengths is not straightforward and careful adaptations of the hardware, scanning protocols and MR methods is a mandatory first step.

22.2 Challenges for Imaging at High Fields

22.2.1 Specific Absorption Rate (SAR)

The electric component of the RF excitation field will induce currents in conductive tissue, which result in heat when dissipated in the body. This energy deposition and its concomitant heat generation is an important safety aspect of high-field imaging. As heat generation scales with the electrical field squared, power deposition prescribes substantial constraints in pulse sequence design at higher magnetic field strengths. The energy deposition, expressed as the specific absorption rate (SAR), represents the average energy dissipated in the body per unit time and mass. Current guidelines will restrict the maximum SAR to 4 and 3 W/kg averaged over the body and head, respectively, while local maxima in SAR (averaged over 10 g of tissue) have to be within the 10 W/kg for head and trunk and 20 W/kg for the extremities (International Commission on NON-Ionizing Radiation

Protection 2004). For many relatively low flip angle gradient echo sequences this restriction will hardly limit the potential applications at high-field strength. However, for more RF demanding sequences with large flip angles (steady state free precession applications and black-blood fast spin echo sequences) alternative sequences will have to be designed to overcome the SAR limitations particularly at 7 T. The first feasibility studies using a single element radiofrequency transmit coil by van Elderen et al. (2009) resulted in the first human coronary images at 7 T within the prescribed SAR limits. However, before the full potential of ultra high-field strengths can be exploited, in depth research of optimized pulse sequences will be required.

22.2.2 B_1 Inhomogeneities

One of the most challenging aspects of whole-body applications at ultra field strengths is to overcome the inhomogeneous nature of the RF excitation field over the field of view. At higher frequencies, the penetration depth of the B_1^+ field decreases requiring more RF power which may result in inacceptable high SAR levels. A second effect that occurs at higher field strengths is directly related to the reduction in wavelength in going from 1.5 and 3.0 T to 7 T. Interference effects will cause non-uniformity in signal intensity or may even result in total signal annihilation in some regions due to complete destructive interference of the B_1^+ field when using RF-waves at 7 T that may reach a wavelength of approximately 11 cm for the proton resonance frequency (Schick 2005). Using single excitation coils some of the B_1^+ inhomogeneity may be alleviated by using adiabatic pulses for excitation and refocusing. However, these pulses introduce even more SAR restrictions and the applied B_1^+ fields may be insufficient to create pulses with sufficient adiabatic behavior to overcome the unwanted inhomogeneities.

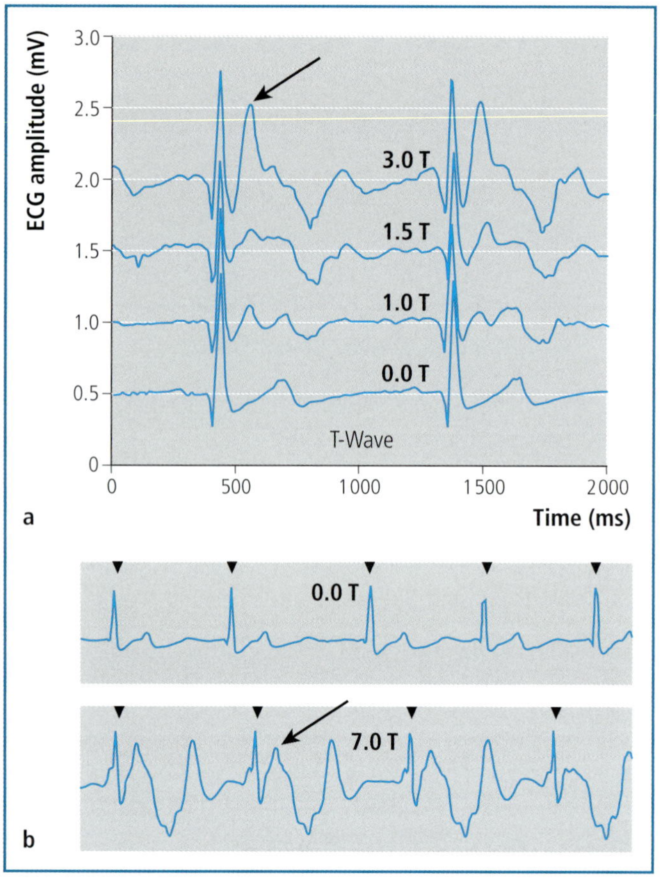

Figure 22-1 The magnetohydrodynamic effect increases as a function of the magnetic field strength and artifactually augments the T-wave of the ECG (arrows). This may adversely affect R-wave triggering/gating and therefore image quality at higher magnetic field strength. ECG traces recorded at 0.0, 1.0, 1.5 and 3 T are shown in **(a)**, while those obtained at 0.0 and 7 T are shown in **(b)**. The use of sophisticated ECG hard and software is mandatory at high-field strength and acoustic methods have been established as a potential alternative to circumvent that problem (from Fischer et al. Magn Reson Med 1999; 42 (2): 361–70 and Snyder et al. Magn Reson Med 2009; 61 (3): 517–24; with permission of John Wiley and Sons, New York, USA).

22.2.3 Magnetohydrodynamic Effect

The relative signal insensitivity of MR on the one hand and the rapid motion of the heart on the other hand make real-time volumetric data acquisition with sufficient temporal and spatial resolution impractical. While this paradigm will have to be revisited at higher field strength as new software and hardware is being developed, sufficient spatial and temporal resolution as well as volumetric coverage is currently obtained using k-space segmentation. However, this critically depends on the assumption that the geometry of the heart is absolutely identical for the acquisition of each k-space segment. For these reasons, sophisticated motion suppression strategies that suppress intrinsic and extrinsic cardiac motion are required. To suppress intrinsic motion of the heart, ECG gating or triggering has been shown to be very effective. However, at higher magnetic field strength, the magnetohydrodynamic effect is amplified and leads to an artifactual voltage that is added to the ECG signal (Figure 22-1). Since this effect depends on the blood-flow velocity in the great vessels, these artifacts are typically most pronounced during ventricular systole and an artifactual augmentation of the T-wave is the result (Figure 22-1, arrows). Therefore, the distinction between R-wave and T-wave of the ECG is particularly challenging and consistent triggering to the R-wave in consecutive cardiac cycles may no longer be guaranteed. While sophisticated vector ECG approaches have been developed to address this problem at 1.5 T and 3 T (Fischer 1999), they may no longer suffice at 7 T (Snyder 2009). Therefore, creative solutions such as the "MRI stethoscope" have been proposed (Frauenrath 2009). This presents a promising alternative to currently available techniques for cardiac gating of (ultra)high-field MRI. Its intrinsic insensitivity to interference from electromagnetic fields renders it suitable for clinical imaging because of its excellent trigger reliability, even at 7.0 T. However, its performance in patients with valvular insufficiency for example remains to be defined.

22.3 Dedicated Developments

22.3.1 Multi-Transmit Options and B_1 Shimming

As described above, the creation of RF-waves that will generate homogenous body images at magnetic fields of 3 T and more specifically 7 T (or even higher) is far from trivial. Even for an organ as small as a prostate a uniform excitation over the region of interest cannot be performed using a single (body) birdcage excitation coil. Figure 22-2 shows the B_1^+ distribution using a single quadrature body coil at 7 T. New coil and excitation concepts have recently been introduced that utilize multiple (independent) amplifiers and antennae at the same time (Vaughan 2009). These new approaches provide numerous additional degrees of freedom (phase, amplitude, pulse shapes) that can be manipulated to not only create a more homogeneous B_1^+ field, but also to reduce SAR at the same time. At 3.0 T this technology ("B_1 shimming") already has been introduced to improve image quality on clinical platforms using a dual transmit configuration, whereas at 7.0 T these approaches have become an absolute requirement for obtaining diagnostically acceptable images in the human body (van den Bergen 2007). Multi-transmit applications for cardiac imaging are still in its infancy. However, to fully leverage increased signal and contrast to noise at higher field strengths, these parallel excitation schemes will become a pre-requisite and a challenging research area for years to come. Local SAR reduction, a more homogeneous excitation field and local excitation will be among the techniques that will benefit cardiovascular applications.

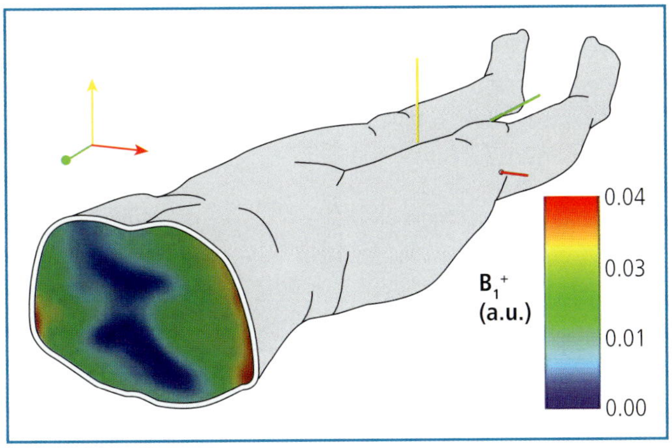

Figure 22-2 A simulation of the B_1^+ distribution in arbitrary units in the torso using a quadrature body coil at 7 T. The simulation clearly shows severe destructive interference and lack of RF penetration towards the center of the body (courtesy C. A. T. van den Berg and A. Andreychenko, University of Utrecht).

22.4 Clinical Benefit

22.4.1 Global Function

Steady-state with free precession (SSFP) techniques (Oppelt 1986) have rapidly been adopted by clinical and research MR centers for functional cardiac imaging. Hereby, local contractility of the myocardium, ventricular volume and mass are measures that are qualitatively and quantitatively assessed (Salton 2002). Using SSFP techniques at 1.5 T, a major advantage in SNR and contrast-to-noise ratio (CNR) is obtained and the resulting improved endocardial border definition facilitates automated or semiautomated contouring. However, short TR is mandatory to minimize flow artifacts, banding artifacts and signal voids due to local field inhomogeneities. While these challenges have successfully been addressed at 1.5 T, an increase in both B_0 and B_1 inhomogeneity as well as SAR constraints are among the major impediments for functional SSFP cardiac imaging at higher field strength. However, careful adaptation of the RF excitation angles, higher order shimming and modifications of the imaging protocol to the changed physical boundary conditions have already successfully been implemented (Schär 2004) at 3 T as displayed in Figure 22-3. In Figure 22-3, SENSE-abbreviated long-axis (Figure 22-3a), 4-chamber (Figure 22-3b) and short-axis functional images acquired at different anatomical levels (Figure 22-3c, d, e) using an SSFP sequence are shown. A high visual contrast between the ventricular blood-pool and the signal-attenuated myocardium is obtained. To minimize adverse effects of B_0 inhomogeneity, localized higher-order shimming was utilized (Schär 2004). In accord with these findings, recent volunteer studies demonstrated that imaging at 3 T using 2D cine-SSFP provides substantially higher SNR and CNR compared with imaging at 1.5 T, offering overall good image quality (Gutberlet 2005, 2006). Michaely et al. (2006) also reported a similar SNR gain for functional cardiac cine image at 3 T. In this study, spoiled gradient echo (GRE) sequences seemed to benefit more from the higher field strength, being less

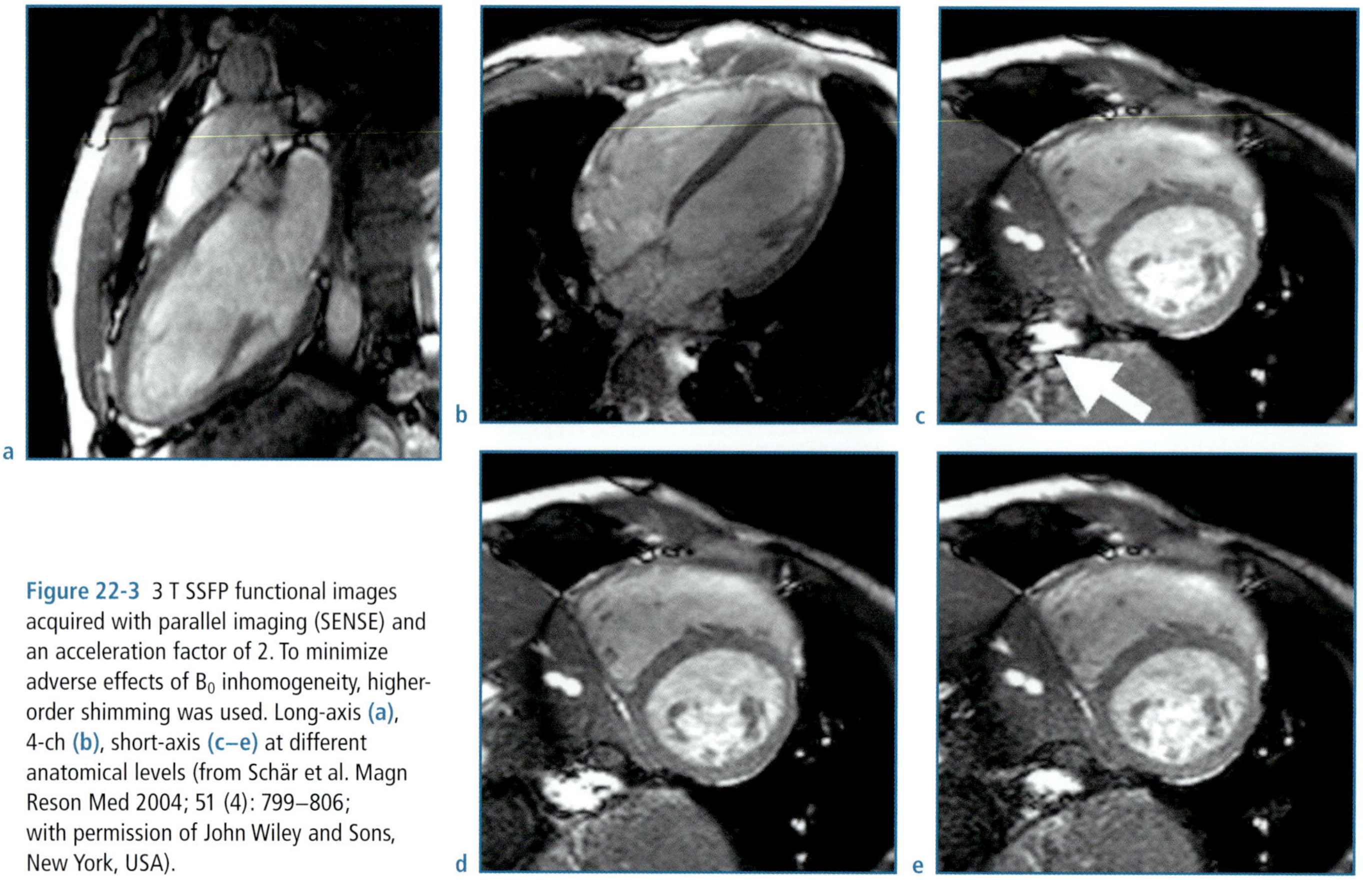

Figure 22-3 3 T SSFP functional images acquired with parallel imaging (SENSE) and an acceleration factor of 2. To minimize adverse effects of B_0 inhomogeneity, higher-order shimming was used. Long-axis **(a)**, 4-ch **(b)**, short-axis **(c–e)** at different anatomical levels (from Schär et al. Magn Reson Med 2004; 51 (4): 799–806; with permission of John Wiley and Sons, New York, USA).

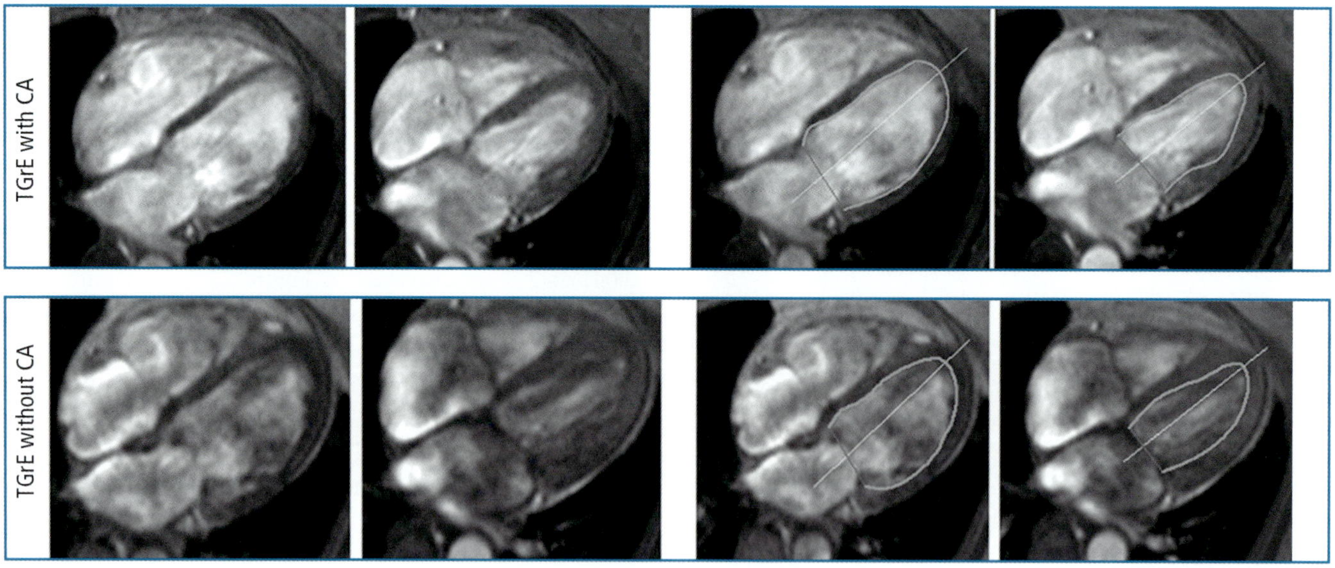

Figure 22-4 Identical 4-ch view acquired with post-contrast **(upper row)** and pre-contrast **(bottom row)** segmented k-space gradient echo cine imaging in the same patient at 3 T. LV endocardial contours were traced manually at end-diastole **(left)** and end-systole **(right)** to calculate LV volumes and LV ejection fraction according to area-length method. The image quality and endocardial contour delineation clearly suffers from saturation effects before contrast agent administration (from Hamdan et al. J Cardiovasc Magn Reson 2007; 9 (6): 845–53; with permission of Taylor and Francis, London, U.K.).

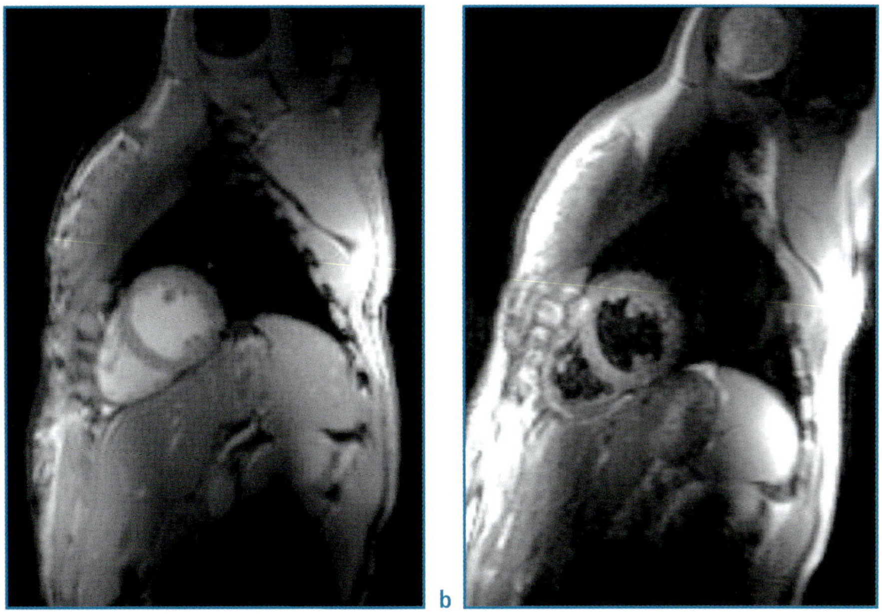

Figure 22-5 Segmented k-space gradient echo cine (a) and fast spin echo (b) images in a short-axis orientation obtained from the same healthy adult subject at 7 T. As expected, gradient echo imaging leads to a bright-blood contrast while fast spin echo imaging results in a dark blood contrast (from Snyder et al. Magn Reson Med 2009; 61 (3): 517–24; with permission of John Wiley and Sons, New York, USA). a b

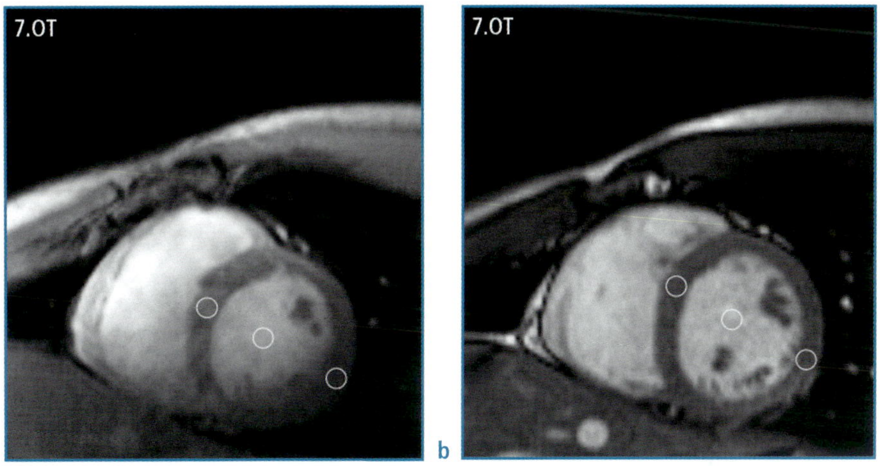

Figure 22-6 Example of a mid-ventricular end-diastolic short-axis image of the same healthy adult subject at 7 T using an RF-spoiled gradient echo sequence (a) and at 1.5 T using a balanced steady-state gradient echo sequence (b). Region of interests (ROIs) indicate the locations for signal analysis for this particular study. Due to the use of a local surface transmit/receive coil at 7 T, both signal and contrast drop with the distance from the coil (from Brandts et al. Magn Reson Med 2010; 64 (5): 1471–7; with permission of John Wiley and Sons, New York, USA). a b

affected by artifacts when compared to SSFP pulse sequences. Maroules et al. (2008) also found that SENSE imaging at 3 T is a reproducible technique for assessing RV and LV structure and function. Detection of inducible wall motion abnormalities by dobutamine MRI confers a significantly increased risk of cardiac events and has substantial incremental value over clinical risk factors and the detection of resting wall motion abnormalities (Jahnke 2007). In studies where improvement in regional contractility after revascularisation served as the gold standard, dobutamine MRI at 1.5 T had a sensitivity of 94% and specificity of 90% for detecting hibernating myocardium (Camici 2008). Kelle et al. (2008) recently demonstrated that dobutamine stress CMR at 3 T is similarly accurate for depiction of significant coronary disease.

In general and at higher magnetic field strength, conventional segmented k-space gradient echo cine sequences are quite robust and provide an excellent fall-back with or without extracellular contrast agents while the use of extracellular contrast agents improves the image quality for the assessment of LV volumes mainly in the long-axis orientation (Hamdan 2007) (Figure 22-4).

The early feasibility of human cardiac MRI at 7 T was demonstrated by Snyder and colleagues (2009). High-resolution cine segmented k-space gradient echo (Figure 22-5a) and fast spin echo images (Figure 22-5b) have been acquired with an eight-channel local transceiver array in conjunction with a dedicated local B_1 shimming technique.

In a very recent study also conducted at 7 T, Brandts et al. (2010) determined the ability of 7 T cardiac MRI to quantitatively assess left ventricular volumes, mass, and function from cine short-axis series and left ventricular diastolic filling from velocity-encoded MRI in 10 healthy subjects in comparison to 1.5 T (Figure 22-6). In this early study they found that imaging at 7 T MRI was successful in 80 % of the examinations. Assessment of left ventricular volumes, function, and mass at 7 T showed good agreement with 1.5 T (no significant differences between variables describing volumes, function, and mass with intraclass correlation coefficients ranging from 0.77–0.96). Transmitral stroke volume and the ratio between early and atrial peak filling rate showed strong agreement at both field strengths (no significant differences between stroke volumes and filling ratios with intraclass correlation coefficients 0.92 for stroke volumes and 0.77 for peak filling ratios). It was concluded that the assessment of left ventricular volumes, function, and flow was feasible at 7 T and that standardized MRI protocols provide similar quantitative results when compared with 1.5 T.

22.4.2 Regional Function

MR myocardial tagging has shown to be a useful tool for the assessment of local myocardial motion in healthy and diseased states (McVeigh 1996). While fading of the tags limits access to diastolic myocardial motion for most of the contemporary tagging sequences, this fading of the tags is T1 dependent. However, at higher field strength, T1 of myocardium is increased which results in a reduced fading of the tags throughout the cardiac cycle. Together with the expected increase in SNR secondary to the higher field strength, this attenuated fading may result in a higher temporal resolution and a more accurate identification of the tags, which will facilitate access to subtle changes in myocardial motion throughout the cardiac cycle. A recent study in healthy adult subjects has confirmed the increase of CNR at 3 T for myocardial tagging techniques (Gutberlet 2006). Together with the increase in SNR, this has been attributed to a prolonged T1 of the myocardium at 3 T.

In contrast to conventional tagging, strain encoded MR imaging (SENC) uses tag surfaces that are not orthogonal, but rather parallel to the image plane (Osman 2001). Implementation of SENC on higher fielded systems may increase the spatial and temporal resolution of this technique (Hamdan 2009) (Figure 22-7), thereby enhancing its sensitivity to detect systolic and diastolic dysfunction in patients with heart failure (Korosoglou 2008), and ischemic disorders in patients with coronary artery disease (Ibrahim 2008). In addition, such stimulated echo-based techniques suffer from an intrinsic SNR loss of 50 % or more. However, at higher magnetic field strength, this relative loss can be compensated while the prolonged T1 affords an additional SNR benefit (Hamdan 2009).

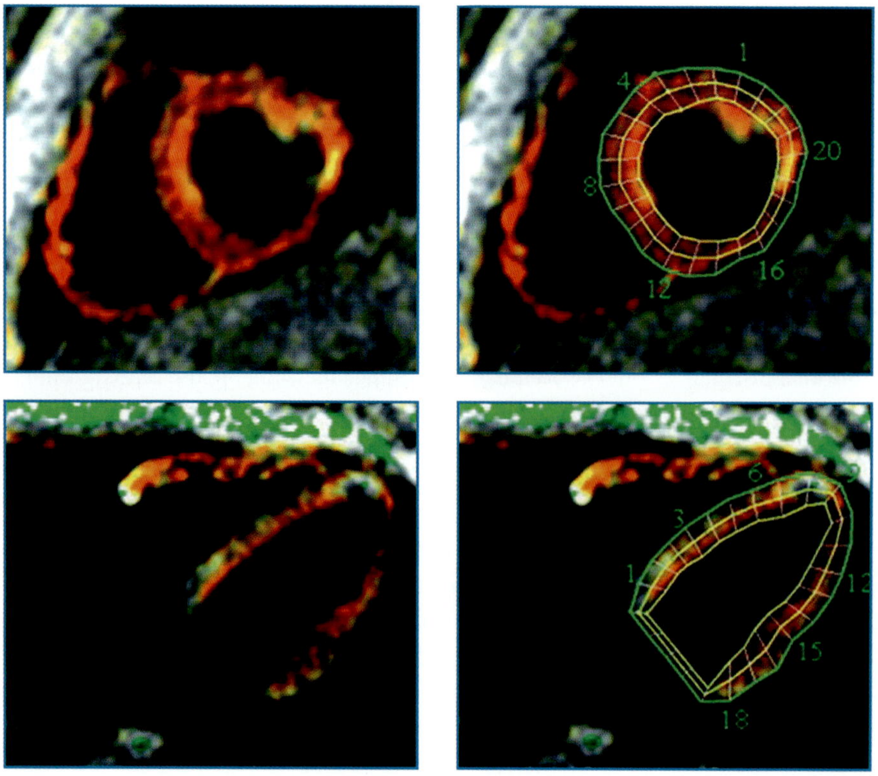

a

b

Figure 22-7 End-systolic strain images in a short-axis **(a)** and a 4-ch view **(b)** obtained with the stimulated echo-based SENC imaging sequence at 3 T. The magnitude of tissue contraction is color-coded and goes from white (chest wall, liver: no contraction) to yellow and red indicative of contraction in the heart (from Hamdan et al. J Magn Reson Imaging 2009; 29 (4): 799–808; with permission of John Wiley and Sons, New York, USA).

22.4.3 Coronary Angiography

The first international multicenter trial on coronary MRA suggests that non-endogenous contrast-enhanced navigator gated and corrected free-breathing coronary MRA becomes a valuable tool for the non-invasive assessment of significant proximal coronary artery disease (Kim 2001). However, reading of distal segments and branching vessels was not included in this study and the overall specificity and detail visibility of the method remains to be improved. Therefore, a higher spatial resolution approaching that of multi-slice computed tomography (ca. 500 μm) may be required. It is expected that the higher SNR secondary to a higher field strength would allow for a further improved spatial resolution, which will support isotropic resolution and access to more distal or branching vessels. However, not only advantages but also potential challenges have to be considered at higher field strength as already mentioned. Therefore a first study investigating the feasibility of in vivo human coronary MRA at higher field strength was performed (Stuber 2002). Hereby, the 1.5 T technique used in the multicenter trial (Kim 2001) was adopted and adaptations were made to account for the changed physical boundary conditions at 3 T. Vector ECG (VECG) technology was used (Fischer 1999), and a body transmit coil together with a prototype 6-element cardiac phased-array surface receive coil was employed. Imaging was performed using a 3D segmented k-space gradient echo imaging sequence using a T2-prep and a spectrally selective fat saturation for endogenous contrast enhancement (Botnar 1999), and a 2D selective real-time navigator for respiratory motion suppression during free breathing (McConnell 1997). To minimize the sensitivity of the navigator 2D selective RF pulse to ΔB_0 and T2* effects, the number of revolutions in excitation k-space was reduced (from n = 12 at 1.5 T) to n = 8 so as to shorten the excitation duration. To suppress contamination of the navigator with spurious signal originating from higher order components (aliasing) concentric with the central 2D selective excitation, a local receive coil positioned over the sternum was selectively employed for navigator signal reception. Segmented k-space gradient echo imaging with 10 RF excitations (TR = 8.2 ms; TE = 2.4 ms) per RR interval (acquisition window = 82 ms) was performed. The RF excitation angles were constant (25°) and adapted to account for the prolonged blood-T1 at 3.0 T (~ 1,600 ms) (Noeske 2000). In-plane resolution was 0.6–0.7 × 0.6–1.0 mm² and the slice thickness was 3 mm. The average scan duration for each free-breathing 3D acquisition was ~ 7 min with an average navigator efficiency of 55%. In all cases, no major susceptibility artifacts were seen in the vicinity of the left or the right proximal to mid coronary arterial segments. In selected healthy adult subjects (Ustun 2007), high spatial resolution images with a voxel size of 0.3 × 0.3 × 1.5 mm could be obtained at 3 T (Figure 22-8).

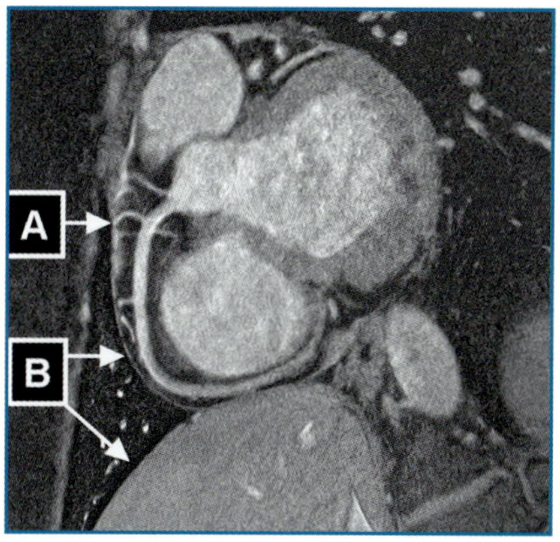

Figure 22-8 3 T image of a right coronary artery with a small voxel size of 0.3 × 0.3 × 1.5 mm. Scanning time was about 10 min during free breathing. Note the visibility of the small-diameter branching vessels (A) and the excellent border definition of the pericardium and the lung liver interface (B) indicative of the quality of the motion suppression that can be obtained (from Ustun et al. Am J Roentgenol 2007; 188 (3): W283–90; with permission of the American Roentgen Ray Society, Leesburg, USA).

In a subsequent patient study comparing 1.5 T and 3 T coronary MRA for the identification of significant luminal coronary artery disease with X-ray coronary angiography as the gold standard, the gain in SNR and CNR at 3 T vs. 1.5 T did not translate into improved accuracy for the detection of coronary lesions (Sommer 2005). This has been attributed in part to the presence of intrinsic and extrinsic motion artifacts, to susceptibility-related local magnetic field variations, and to off-resonance effects, which adversely affect T2-preparation among other things. In response, an adiabatic version of the T2-preparation has been developed mainly to suppress artifacts originating from B_1 inhomogeneity and off-resonance. This technique provides a significantly improved definition of the coronary arteries at 3 T (Nezafat 2006) (Figure 22-9). Using this methodology, it has been shown that anomalies and variants of the coronary arteries can successfully be evaluated at 3 T (Gharib 2008).

Further volunteer studies demonstrated the feasibility of a radial sampling technique to acquire 3D coronary artery images at 3 T within a single breath hold. The combination of a radial k-space acquisition, parallel imaging and interleaved sliding window reconstruction provided good SNR and high coronary vessel sharpness (Bi 2005). In a head-to-head comparisons of coronary MRA at 3 T vs. 1.5 T in healthy subjects, SNR, CNR and vessel sharpness were reported to be substantially higher at 3 T (Nayak 2004, Bi and Li 2005). Furthermore, recent studies convincingly demonstrated that coronary MRA at 3 T in conjunction with slow infusion of gadolinium contrast agents and seg-

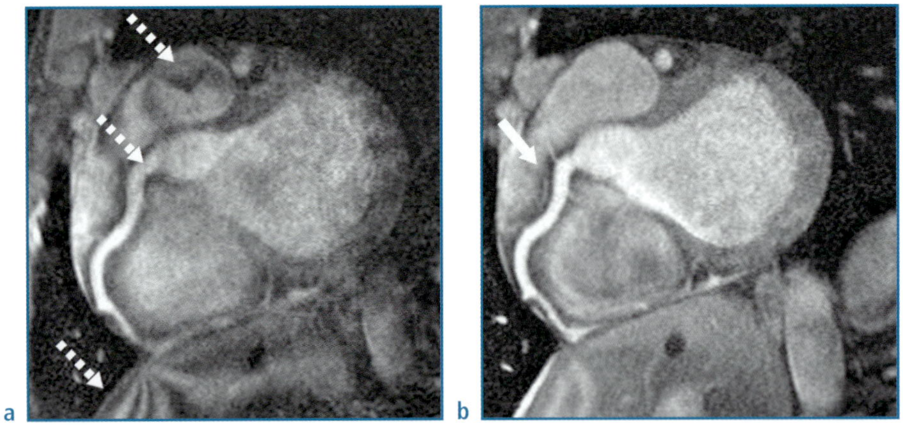

Figure 22-9 3 T image of the right coronary artery obtained in a healthy adult subject with a conventional (a) and an adiabatic (b) T2-prep for endogenous contrast enhancement. Signal uniformity in the regions of the dashed arrows is significantly improved with the adiabatic variant of the T2-prep (b) (from Nezafat et al. Magn Reson Med 2006; 55 (4): 858–64; with permission of John Wiley and Sons, New York, USA).

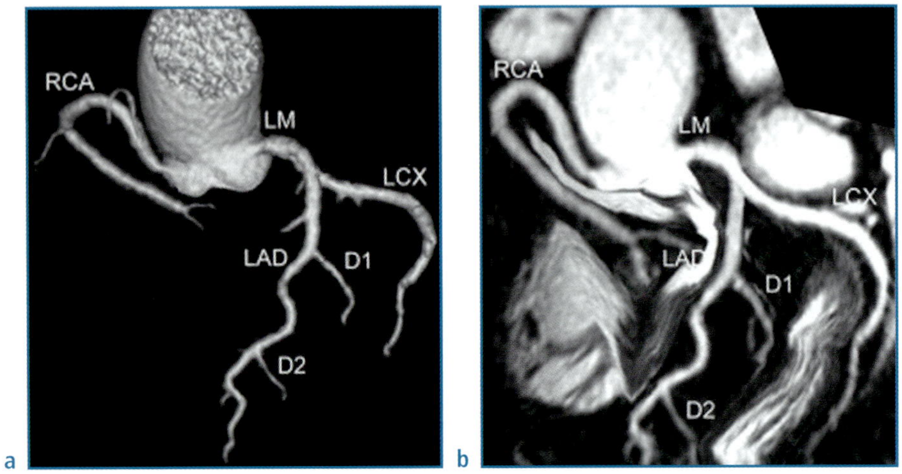

Figure 22-10 3 T contrast-enhanced whole-heart CMRA images of a 71-yrs-old woman with normal coronary arteries. Volume-rendered image (a) provides an overview of coronary anatomy and clearly depicts the right coronary artery (RCA), left anterior descending artery (LAD), and diagonal branches (D1, D2). Curved multi-planar reformation image (b) shows the left main artery (LM), LAD, left circumflex artery (LCX), and RCA (from Yang et al. J Am Coll Cardiol 2009; 54 (1): 69–76; with permission of Elsevier Inc., Amsterdam, The Netherlands).

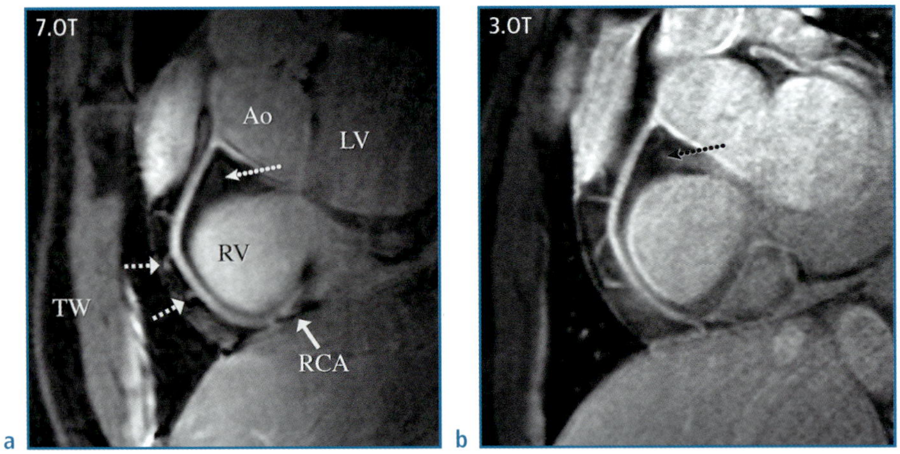

Figure 22-11 7 T (a) vs. 3 T (b) coronary MRA obtained with identical scanning times in the same healthy adult subject. A signal drop more distant from the anterior transmit/receive coil is evident on the 7 T image. Small branching vessels can be seen on the 7 T image in the region of the dashed arrows. Ao: ascending aorta; LV: left ventricle; RCA: right coronary artery; RV: right ventricle (from van Elderen et al. Radiology 2010; 257 (1): 254–9; with permission of the Radiological Society of North America, Oak Brook, USA).

mented k-space gradient echo signal readout can significantly improve the depiction of major coronary arteries with high SNR in healthy volunteers (Bi 2007). This 3 T technique was subsequently translated into the patient setting where it was used to prospectively evaluate the diagnostic performance of 3.0 T contrast-enhanced (0.2 mmol/kg gadobenate dimeglumine) whole-heart coronary magnetic resonance angiography in 69 patients with suspected coronary artery disease (Yang 2009) (Figure 22-10). In this study, coronary MRA acquisition time was 9 ± 2 min. The technique correctly identified significant CAD in 32 patients and correctly ruled out CAD in 23 patients. The sensitivity, specificity, and accuracy for detecting significant stenoses were 91.6, 83.1, and 84.1 %, respectively, on a per-segment basis. It was concluded that contrast-enhanced 3 T whole-heart coronary MRA allows for the accurate detection of coronary artery stenosis with high sensitivity and moderate specificity.

At 7 T, first human coronary MRA in vivo data were reported by van Elderen and colleagues (2009). In this study, the feasibility to obtain free-breathing navigator gated and corrected fat suppressed segmented k-space gradient echo images of the right coronary artery was demonstrated using a single transmit-receive coil element with the 2D selective navigator localized at the base of the left ventricle. While the right coronary artery could clearly be visualized in several subjects, the left coronary system cannot be adequately visualized and T2-preparation with an adiabatic T2-prep is currently not possible due to SAR constraints. However, and with a more advanced transmit-receive coil design (van Elderen 2009), the same authors directly compared 3 T and 7 T right coronary MRA in the healthy adult subjects and demonstrated that at 7 T, the right coronary artery is visualized with better-defined vessel borders and higher SNR when compared to 3 T acquisitions with identical acquisition duration (Figure 22-11). However, limited depth penetration of the coil and inability to generate blood-myocardium contrast secondary to SAR constraints are still limiting factors and currently preclude the visualization of the left coronary system.

22.4.4 Coronary Vessel Wall Imaging and Plaque Visualization

Several studies at 1.5 T have already demonstrated the ability to visualize the coronary vessel wall in both healthy and diseased states (Fayad 2000). Later positive arterial remodeling of the coronary artery vessel wall was documented in patients with established but non-significant coronary artery disease at 1.5 T (Kim 2002). In patients with type 1 diabetes, the same author also demonstrated that the quantitative coronary vessel wall thickness is significantly increased in patients with nephropathy (Kim 2007). However, the ultimate goal would not only be the coronary vessel wall thickness measurement but also the differentiation between plaque components and consequently the identification of vulnerable plaque (Fayad 2000). Still, this may necessitate a significantly improved spatial resolution. At higher field strength, a further step in this direction is expected. Due to the relatively small size of the coronary vessel wall (~ 1 mm), the central location within the thorax, and constant movement due to intrinsic and extrinsic myocardial motion, coronary vessel wall imaging is among the technically most challenging topics in cardiovascular MR to the present date.

At 3 T, navigator-gated and real-time motion corrected cross-sectional views of the RCA were obtained in 6 healthy adults by Botnar and colleagues (2003). The MR pulse sequence consisted of a dual-inversion black-blood prepulse with the inversion delay (TI) (Fleckenstein 1991) adapted for the prolonged T1 of blood (TI ~ 700 ms at 60 bpm, dual-inversion and data collection every other heartbeat) at 3 T. The 2D segmented k-space gradient echo imaging sequence was immediately preceded by the 2D selective navigator pulse, a frequency selective fat suppression prepulse, and a NAV-restore prepulse (Stuber 2001) for optimization of navigator performance in the presence of a nonselective inversion of the magnetization. Other imaging parameters included TE = 2.3 ms, TR = 8 ms, RF excitation angle = 30°, 10 RF excitations per RR interval, NSA = 2, FOV = 360 mm, image matrix = 512 × 512 resulting in an in-plane resolution of 0.7 × 0.7 mm and a slice thickness of 5 mm. Although a relatively SNR inefficient black-blood segmented k-space gradient echo imaging sequence was used, these data demonstrated feasibility of 3 T coronary MR vessel wall imaging.

Recently, the potential of black-blood turbospin echo sequences for the visualization of the coronary artery wall at 3 T has been demonstrated in volunteer studies (Koktzoglou 2005, Priest 2005). In these studies, the higher SNR at 3 T supported a clear visualization of the coronary vessel wall both during a single breath-hold (Koktzoglou 2005) and using navigator gating (Koktzoglou 2005, Priest 2005). Particularly the use of adiabatic pulses for both inversion and re-inversion (Priest 2005) has been reported to be robust to off-resonance and RF inhomogeneity (Figure 22-12). However, substantial improvements in resolution and image quality are still required in order to evaluate the composition of coronary atherosclerotic plaques, and the spatial resolution of MRI even at higher magnetic field strength may never be sufficient for the visualization of the fibrous cap. However, with targeted contrast agents that highlight specific plaque components, this may not be mandatory.

22.4.5 Perfusion and Late Enhancement

Both perfusion and late enhancement imaging require administration of extracellular contrast agents. Given the fact that gradient echo techniques with short echo times were applied successfully for both modalities at 1.5 T, no major impediments are expected from a sequence standpoint at 3 T. Previous in vitro studies demonstrated a higher contrast enhancement by gadolinium contrast agents at higher field strengths (Rinck and Muller 1999). First volunteer studies recently confirmed these findings. In a study involving 12 healthy subjects, the assessment of myocardial perfusion and viability at 3 T substantially increased SNR,

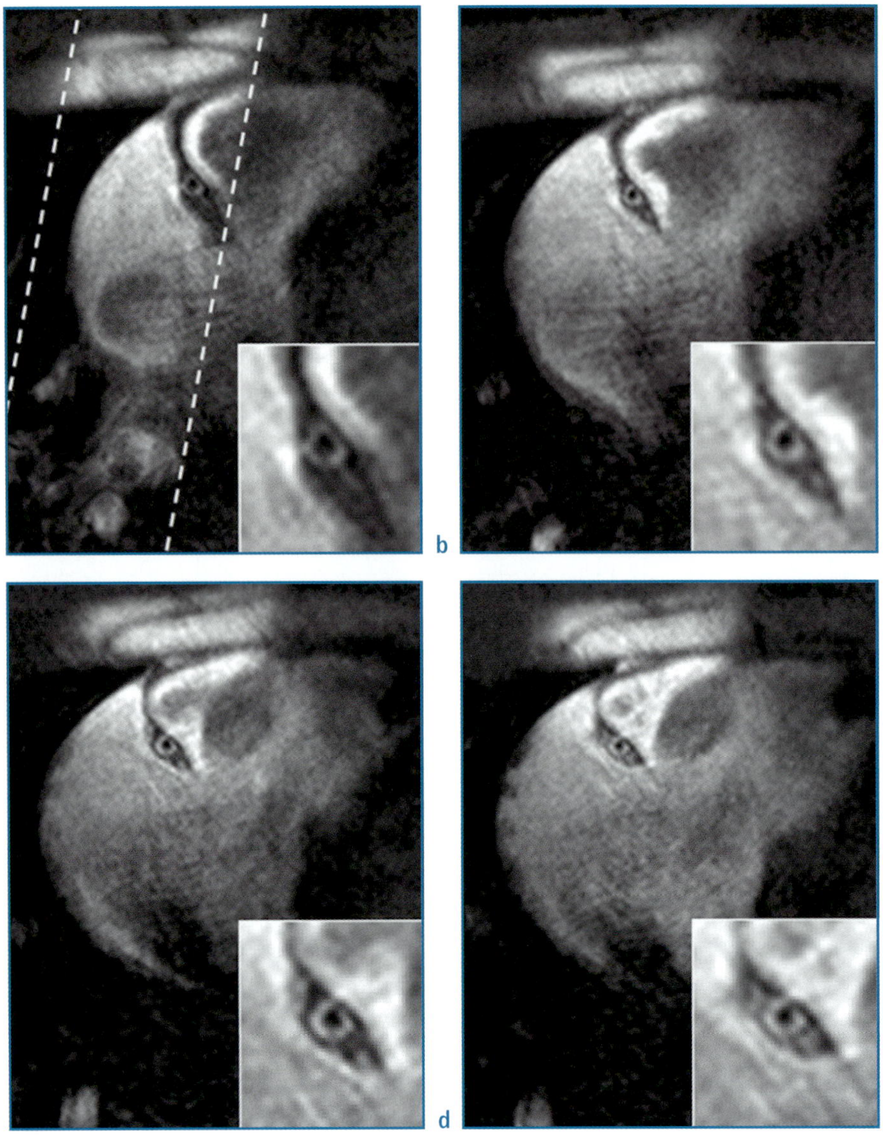

a b c d

Figure 22-12 3 T coronary vessel wall imaging. Cross-sectional images from different positions along the RCA (a–d) of a healthy volunteer. The coronary vessel wall is shown enlarged in the inserts. The dashed lines in slice (a) indicate the boundaries of the re-inversion slab (from Priest et al. Magn Reson Med 2005; 54 (5): 1115–22; with permission of John Wiley and Sons, New York, USA).

CNR and overall image quality compared with imaging at 1.5 T (Gutberlet 2006). Consistent with these findings, the use of 3 T MR imaging was reported to significantly increase contrast and image quality in first-pass myocardial perfusion imaging for different gadolinium doses (Araoz 2005) and to reduce subendocardial dark rim artifacts (Strach 2007) when compared with perfusion imaging at 1.5 T. This suggests that lower doses of contrast may be used at 3 T. Similarly, Cheng et al. (2007a) recently demonstrated that perfusion CMR at 3 T has superior diagnostic performance for identifying both single- and multi-vessel coronary artery disease, when compared with 1.5 T. Visual assessment of perfusion CMR at 3 T had high sensitivity (98%) and negative predictive value (94%) for significant coronary disease, indicating the potential of the technique as a screening tool. More recent studies have confirmed the excellent diagnostic performance of perfusion CMR for detecting significant coronary disease at 3 T (Gebker 2008, Meyer 2008). Delayed hyperenhancement MRI may benefit from the higher field strength because of multiple reasons. First, an improved SNR and CNR will improve delineation of the infarct borders. Second, the prolonged T1 of the myocardium helps to increase the difference in signal between normal and hyperenhanced myocardium. Nevertheless, the increased B_1 inhomogeneity at higher field strength may lead to non-uniform signal nulling. However, the use of adiabatic RF pulses may provide a relatively simple solution (Gutberlet 2006). Similar to lower field strengths, the phase-sensitive inversion-recovery sequence (Kellman 2002) is a powerful technique that has already been successfully applied at 3 T (Huber 2006, Cochet 2007).

Using the conventional two-dimensional segmented k-space inversion-recovery gradient echo pulse sequence, Cheng et al. (2007b) found excellent agreement in measurements of mass and transmural extent of hyperenhanced myocardium between 1.5 and 3 T. However, due to the prolonged T1 of the myocardium, image acquisition at 3 T should be triggered to every other cardiac cycle to allow for adequate relaxation of the magnetization between successive inversion pulses. This study also demonstrated, that the optimal inversion delay time to null the signal of normal myocardium needs to be longer at 3 T for the same dose of contrast agent, due to the increased T1 relaxation time associated with the higher field strength. Multiple studies have found that using this pulse sequence at 3 T provided improved image quality, SNR and CNR, compared with 1.5 T (Gutberlet 2006, Klumpp 2006).

22.4.6 Spectroscopy

Increase in both signal-to-noise and chemical shift dispersion are the main drivers for increasing the magnetic fields strength for spectroscopy applications. For proton (^{1}H) and fluorine (^{19}F) spectroscopy, the same impediments at high-field strengths in terms of B_1^+ inhomogeneity and SAR constraints will apply as described for proton imaging at these field strengths. For most other nuclei that may be of interest in biomedical research such as phosphorus (^{31}P), carbon (^{13}C), oxygen (^{17}O) and sodium (^{23}Na) the resonance frequencies are substantially lower, which alleviates the B_1^+ homogeneity and SAR constraints to some extent. However, several challenges remain. The more restricted bandwidth at higher frequencies related to the available RF power may be insufficient to cover the increased chemical shift dispersion of the different metabolites. This also restricts the use of slice selection for spatial localization as the chemical shift artifact may result in large spatial shifts for different chemical compounds. Many of the RF sequences in spectroscopy use adiabiatic excitation and refocusing, which introduce substantial SAR limitations. Quantitative cardiac ^{31}P-spectroscopy at 3 T using adiabatic pulses (Figure 22-13) has been shown to promise better quantification at 3 T from improved signal-to-noise ratios and spectral resolution compared with 1.5 T (El-Sharkawy 2009). Saturation effects as well as T2-decay effects due to the use of small-angle adiabatic pulses to compensate for inhomogeneous B_1 surface coil excitation have been taken into account. T1 values at 3.0 T have been reported as well: 6.8 and 5.4 s for PCr and ATP in calf muscle respectively and 5.8 and 3.1 s in myocardium.

^{31}P-spectrosopy at 3 T has been used to study the in vivo cardiac energetics in normal myocardium and hypertrophic cardiomyopathy (Shivu 2010). Reduced PCr/ATP levels in the myocardium are reported for patients suffering from dilated cardiomyopathy. Recently, a saturation transfer method was introduced to quantify creatine kinase forward rate constants at 3 T (Schär 2010).

An important confounding factor in comparing SNR's between 1.5 T, 3.0 T and higher field strengths in ^{31}P- and ^{13}C-spectroscopy is the use of proton decoupling. Proton decoupling at high-field is extremely SAR sensitive and may not be feasible for broadband applications. Additionally, in the case of proton decoupling of ^{31}P in vivo spectroscopy, SNR may benefit substantially from nuclear overhauser enhancement magnetization transfer from water protons to the ^{31}P-resonances at lower field strengths. At higher field strengths, where relaxation may be less dominated by di-

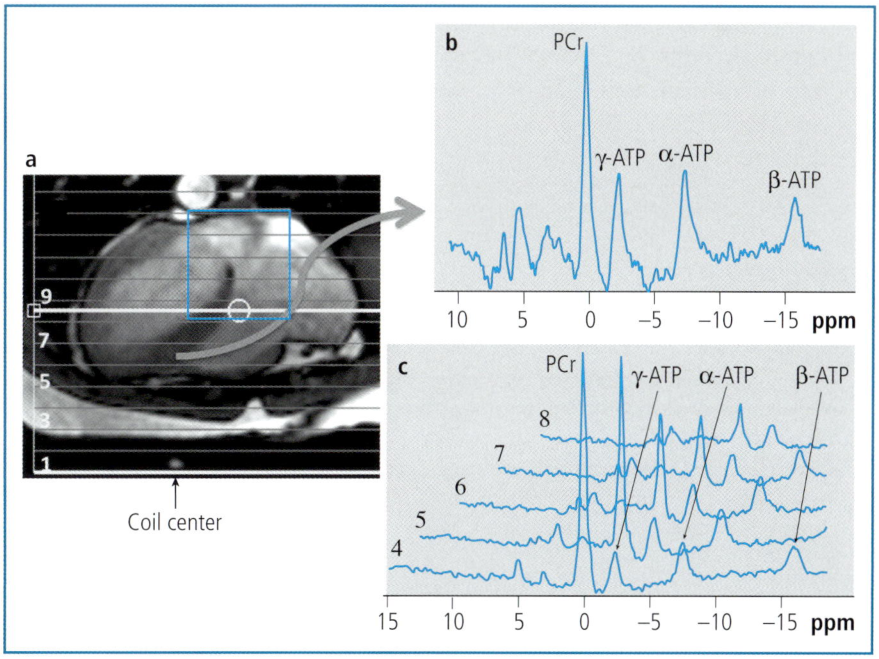

Figure 22-13 Axial image of the heart (a) of a healthy volunteer annotated to show the locations of cardiac-gated ^{31}P-spectra (b, c) obtained from one-dimensional chemical shift imaging (1D CSI; 1 cm resolution) at 3 T. The spectra are used for metabolite quantification and are acquired almost fully-relaxed (TR = 12 s) in about 5 min with adiabatic half-passage excitation (adapted from El-Sharkawy et al. 2009; courtesy P. A. Bottomley, Baltimore, USA). ATP: adenosine triphosphate; PCr: phosphocreatine.

polar coupling and other mechanism may become more prominent (e.g. chemical shift anisotropy contributions that scale with B_0^2), decoupling may become less efficient on top of the increased power requirements. More research is warranted to reveal the clinical potential of this technology, e.g. by introducing parallel acquisition scheme's for these applications as earlier introduced for high resolution proton imaging.

22.5 Conclusions and Future Perspectives

With state-of-the-art 3 T hardware, software, and methodology, high-quality images can be acquired in all the major areas of contemporary cardiovascular MRI.

The benefits associated with the higher field-strength have already been documented for many applications and areas, where 3 T already outperforms 1.5 T in terms of image quality, have clearly been identified in direct quantitative comparisons. However, the outcome of patient studies together with new scientific findings will ultimately define the added value of 3 T when compared to 1.5 T.

In contrast, cardiovascular MR at 7 T is clearly in its infancy and its use is currently mainly limited to academic research centers only. Transmit/receive coils still have to be custom built, B_0 and B_1 inhomogeneity are amplified and SAR limitations are a major constraint that put an emphasis on the development of new and innovative sequences and cardiac specific methodology. For these reasons, the short-term focus at 7 T will clearly be on technical developments before new cardiovascular scientific findings can be obtained and before strengths and weaknesses of 7 T cardiovascular MR will be defined more clearly in volunteer and patient studies.

References

Araoz PA, Glockner JF, McGee KP et al. 3 T MR imaging provides improved contrast in first-pass myocardial perfusion imaging over a range of gadolinium doses. J Cardiovasc Magn Reson 2005; 7 (3): 559–64.

Bi X, Carr JC, Li D. Whole-heart coronary magnetic resonance angiography at 3 T in 5 min with slow infusion of Gd-BOPTA, a high-relaxivity clinical contrast agent. Magn Reson Med 2007; 58 (1): 1–7.

Bi X, Li D. Coronary arteries at 3.0 T: Contrast-enhanced magnetization-prepared three-dimensional breathhold MR angiography. J Magn Reson Imaging 2005; 21 (2): 133–9.

Bi X, Park J, Larson AC et al. Contrast-enhanced 4D radial coronary artery imaging at 3.0 T within a single breath-hold. Magn Reson Med 2005; 54 (2): 470–5.

Botnar RM, Stuber M, Danias PG et al. Improved coronary artery definition with T2-weighted free-breathing 3D-coronary MRA. Circulation 1999; 99 (24): 3139–48.

Botnar RM, Stuber M, Lamerichs R et al. Initial experiences with in vivo right coronary artery human MR vessel wall imaging at 3 T. J Cardiovasc Magn Reson 2003; 5 (4): 589–94.

Brandts A, Westenberg JJ, Versluis MJ et al. Quantitative assessment of left ventricular function in humans at 7 T. Magn Reson Med 2010; 64: 1471–7.

Camici PG, Prasad SK, Rimoldi OE. Stunning, hibernation, and assessment of myocardial viability. Circulation 2008; 117 (1): 103–14.

Cheng AS, Pegg TJ, Karamitsos TD et al. Cardiovascular magnetic resonance perfusion imaging at 3 T for the detection of coronary artery disease: a comparison with 1.5 T. J Am Coll Cardiol 2007a; 49 (25): 2440–9.

Cheng AS, Robson MD, Neubauer S, Selvanayagam JB. Irreversible myocardial injury: assessment with cardiovascular delayed-enhancement MR imaging and comparison of 1.5 and 3.0 T – initial experience. Radiology 2007b; 242 (3): 735–42.

Cochet A, Lalande A, Walker PM et al. Comparison of the extent of delayed-enhancement cardiac magnetic resonance imaging with and without phase-sensitive reconstruction at 3.0 T. Invest Radiol 2007; 42 (6): 372–6.

El-Ibrahim SH, Weiss RG, Stuber M et al. Stimulated-echo acquisition mode (STEAM) MRI for black-blood delayed hyper-enhanced myocardial imaging. J Magn Reson Imaging 2008; 27 (1): 229–38.

El-Sharkawy A, Schär M, Ouwerkerk R et al. Quantitative Cardiac ^{31}P-spectroscopy at 3 T using adiabatic pulses. Magn Reson Med 2009; 61: 785–95.

Fayad ZA, Fuster V, Fallon JT et al. Non-invasive in vivo human coronary artery lumen and wall imaging using black-blood magnetic resonance imaging. Circulation 2000; 102 (5): 506–10.

Fischer SE, Wickline SA, Lorenz CH. Novel real-time R-wave detection algorithm based on the vectorcardiogram for accurate gated magnetic resonance acquisitions. Magn Reson Med 1999; 42 (2): 361–70.

Fleckenstein JL, Archer BT, Barker BA et al. Fast short-tau inversion-recovery MR imaging. Radiology 1991; 179 (2): 499–504.

Frauenrath T, Hezel F, Heinrichs U. Feasibility of cardiac gating free of interference with electro-magnetic fields at 1.5 T, 3.0 T and 7.0 T using an MR-stethoscope. Invest Radiol 2009; 44 (9): 539–47.

Gebker R, Jahnke C, Paetsch I et al. Diagnostic performance of myocardial perfusion MR at 3 T in patients with coronary artery disease. Radiology 2008; 247 (1): 57–63.

Gharib AM, Ho VB, Rosing DR et al. Coronary artery anomalies and variants: technical feasibility of assessment with coronary MR angiography at 3 T. Radiology 2008; 247 (1): 220–7.

Gutberlet M, Noeske R, Schwinge K et al. Comprehensive cardiac magnetic resonance imaging at 3.0 T: feasibility and implications for clinical applications. Invest Radiol 2006; 41 (2): 154–67.

Gutberlet M, Schwinge K, Freyhardt P et al. Influence of high magnetic field strengths and parallel acquisition strategies on image quality in cardiac 2D CINE magnetic resonance imaging: comparison of 1.5 T vs. 3.0 T. Eur Radiol 2005; 15 (8): 1586–97.

Hamdan A, Kelle S, Schnackenburg B, Fleck E, Nagel E. Improved quantitative assessment of left ventricular volumes using TGrE approach after application of extracellular contrast agent at 3 T. J Cardiovasc Magn Reson 2007; 9 (6): 845–53.

Hamdan A, Thouet T, Kelle S et al. Strain-encoded MRI to evaluate normal left ventricular function and timing of contraction at 3.0 T. J Magn Reson Imaging 2009; 29 (4): 799–808.

Huber A, Bauner K, Wintersperger BJ et al. Phase-sensitive inversion recovery (PSIR) single-shot TrueFISP for assessment of myocardial infarction at 3 T. Invest Radiol 2006; 41 (2): 148–53.

Ibrahim el-SH, Weiss RG, Stuber M et al. Identification of different heart tissues from MRI C-SENC images using an unsupervised multi-stage fuzzy clustering technique. J Magn Reson Imaging 2008; 28 (2): 519–26.

International Commission on NON-Ionizing Radiation Protection. Medical magnetic resonance (MR) procedures: protection of patients. Health Physics 2004; 87: 197–216.

Jahnke C, Nagel E, Gebker R et al. Prognostic value of cardiac magnetic resonance stress tests: adenosine stress perfusion and dobutamine stress wall motion imaging. Circulation 2007; 115 (13): 1769–76.

Kelle S, Hamdan A, Schnackenburg B et al. Dobutamine stress cardiovascular magnetic resonance at 3 T. J Cardiovasc Magn Reson 2008; 10: 44.

Kellman P, Arai AE, McVeigh ER, Aletras AH. Phase-sensitive inversion recovery for detecting myocardial infarction using gadolinium-delayed hyperenhancement. Magn Reson Med 2002; 47 (2): 372–83.

Kim WY, Astrup AS, Stuber M et al. Subclinical coronary and aortic atherosclerosis detected by magnetic resonance imaging in type 1 diabetes with and without diabetic nephropathy. Circulation 2007; 115 (2): 228–35.

Kim WY, Danias PG, Stuber M et al. Coronary magnetic resonance angiography for the detection of coronary stenoses. N Engl J Med 2001; 345 (26): 1863–9.

Kim WY, Stuber M, Börnert P. Three-dimensional black-blood cardiac magnetic resonance coronary vessel wall imaging detects positive arterial remodeling in patients with nonsignificant coronary artery disease. Circulation 2002; 106 (3): 296–9.

Klumpp B, Fenchel M, Hoevelborn T et al. Assessment of myocardial viability using delayed enhancement magnetic resonance imaging at 3.0 T. Invest Radiol 2006; 41 (9): 661–7.

Koktzoglou I, Simonetti O, Li D. Coronary artery wall imaging: initial experience at 3 T. J Magn Reson Imaging 2005; 21 (2): 128–32.

Korosoglou G, Youssef AA, Bilchick KC et al. Real-time fast strain-encoded magnetic resonance imaging to evaluate regional myocardial function at 3.0 T: Comparison to conventional tagging. J Magn Reson Imaging 2008; 27 (5): 1012–8.

Maroules CD, McColl R, Khera A, Peshock RM. Interstudy reproducibility of SSFP cine magnetic resonance: impact of magnetic field strength and parallel imaging. J Magn Reson Imaging 2008; 27 (5): 1139–45.

McConnell MV, Khasgiwala VC, Savord BJ et al. Comparison of respiratory suppression methods and navigator locations for MR coronary angiography. Am J Roentgenol 1997; 168 (5): 1369–75.

McVeigh ER. MRI of myocardial function: motion tracking techniques. Magn Reson Imaging 1996; 14 (2): 137–50.

Meyer C, Strach K, Thomas D et al. High-resolution myocardial stress perfusion at 3 T in patients with suspected coronary artery disease. Eur Radiol 2008; 18 (2): 226–33.

Michaely HJ, Nael K, Schoenberg SO et al. Analysis of cardiac function – comparison between 1.5 T and 3.0 T cardiac cine magnetic resonance imaging: preliminary experience. Invest Radiol 2006; 41 (2): 133–40.

Nayak KS, Cunningham CH, Santos JM, Pauly JM. Real-time cardiac MRI at 3 T. Magn Reson Med 2004; 51 (4): 655–60.

Nezafat R, Stuber M, Ouwerkerk R et al. $B_{(1)}$-insensitive $T(2)$-preparation for improved coronary magnetic resonance angiography at 3 T. Magn Reson Med 2006; 55 (4): 858–64.

Noeske R, Seifert F, Rhein KH, Rinneberg H. Human cardiac imaging at 3 T using phased array coils. Magn Reson Med 2000; 44 (6): 978–82.

Oppelt A et al. FISP – a new fast MRI sequence. Electromedica 1986; 54: 15–8.

Osman NF, Sampath S, Atalar E, Prince JL. Imaging longitudinal cardiac strain on short-axis images using strain-encoded MRI. Magn Reson Med 2001; 46 (2): 324–34.

Priest AN, Bansmann PM, Kaul MG et al. Magnetic resonance imaging of the coronary vessel wall at 3 T using an obliquely oriented re-inversion slab with adiabatic pulses. Magn Reson Med 2005; 54 (5): 1115–22.

Rinck PA, Muller RN. Field strength and dose dependence of contrast enhancement by gadolinium-based MR contrast agents. Eur Radiol 1999; 9 (5): 998–1004.

Salton CJ, Chuang ML, O'Donnell CJ et al. Gender differences and normal left ventricular anatomy in an adult population free of hypertension. A cardiovascular magnetic resonance study of the Framingham Heart Study Offspring cohort. J Am Coll Cardiol 2002; 39 (6): 1055–60.

Schär M, El-Sharkawy A, Weiss RG, Bottomley PA. Triple repetition time saturation transfer (TRiST) ^{31}P-spectroscopy for measuring human creatine kinase reaction kinetics. Magn Reson Med 2010; 63: 1493–501.

Schär M, Kozerke S, Fischer SE, Boesiger P. Cardiac SSFP imaging at 3 T. Magn Reson Med 2004; 51 (4): 799–806.

Schick F. Whole-body MRI at high-field: technical limits and clinical potential. Eur Radiol 2005; 15 (5): 946–59.

Shivu GN, Abozguia K, Phan TT et al. ^{31}P magnetic resonance spectroscopy to measure in vivo cardiac energetic in normal myocardium and hypertrophic cardiomyopathy: Experiences at 3 T. Eur J Radiol 2010; 73: 255–9.

Snyder CJ, DelaBarre L, Metzger GJ et al. Initial results of cardiac imaging at 7 T. Magn Reson Med 2009; 61 (3): 517–24.

Sommer T, Hackenbroch M, Hofer U et al. Coronary MR angiography at 3.0 T versus that at 1.5 T: initial results in patients suspected of having coronary artery disease. Radiology 2005; 234 (3): 718–25.

Strach K, Meyer C, Thomas D et al. High-resolution myocardial perfusion imaging at 3 T: comparison to 1.5 T in healthy volunteers. Eur Radiol 2007; 17 (7): 1829–35.

Stuber M, Botnar RM, Fischer SE et al. Preliminary report on in vivo coronary MRA at 3 T in humans. Magn Reson Med 2002; 48 (3): 425–9.

Stuber M, Botnar RM, Spuentrup E et al. Three-dimensional high-resolution fast spin echo coronary magnetic resonance angiography. Magn Reson Med 2001; 45 (2): 206–11.

Ustun A, Desai M, Abd-Elmoniem KZ et al. Automated identification of minimal myocardial motion for improved image quality on MR angiography at 3 T. Am J Roentgenol 2007; 188 (3): W283–90.

Van den Bergen B, van den Berg CAT, Bartels LW, Lagendijk JJW. 7-T body MRI: B_1 shimming with simultaneous SAR reduction. Phys Med Biol 2007; 52: 5429–41.

Van Elderen SGC, Versluis MJ, Webb AG et al. Initial results on in vivo human coronary magnetic resonance angiography at 7 T. Magn Reson Med 2009; 62: 1379–84.

Vaughan TT, Snyder CJ, DelaBarre LJ et al. Whole-body imaging at 7 T: preliminary results. Magn Reson Med 2009; 61: 244–8.

Yang Q, Li K, Liu X et al. Contrast-enhanced whole-heart coronary magnetic resonance angiography at 3.0 T: a comparative study with X-ray angiography in a single center. J Am Coll Cardiol 2009; 54 (1): 69–76.

23 Cardiac Magnetic Resonance Imaging in Small Animal Models

Volker Herold, Karl-Heinz Hiller and Peter M. Jakob[1]

23.1 Introduction

Over the past decade, transgenic and knockout rodent models, in particular mouse models, have played a major role in cardiac research, since they have significantly advanced our understanding of individual genes and the basic mechanism involved in heart disease. It was the understanding of the mammalian genome, which allowed for the increased generation of animal models for complex human cardiac diseases, which now are ready to use for studying cardiovascular development, changes, and function. Since disease models play an important role of transgenic modeling of the murine heart, it is now of paramount importance to analyze these phenotypes in vivo by collecting anatomical, functional and metabolic information simultaneously over time with non-invasive imaging modalities. Therefore, there is clearly a great demand in cardiac research for imaging modalities that can provide this information in vivo in a longitudinal and three-dimensional fashion without limitations by depth resolution.

Among the different non-invasive imaging techniques available, cardiac magnetic resonance imaging (CMRI) is currently one of the modalities of choice (Hoit 2001), since MRI has a **number of characteristics** that makes it an ideal candidate for a broad range of imaging tasks:

- extraordinary three-dimensional capabilities,
- superb contrast abilities and spatial resolution combined with a high temporal resolution, and
- a high safety profile since no harmful ionizing radiation is applied.

This allows for repeated experiments in the same animal, and thus CMRI offers for the repetitive characterization of animal models at different time points. This is important, since interindividual variances are avoided and thus less animals are required to fulfill statistical significance. Another advantage is the non-invasive nature of MRI in monitoring the progression of a chronic disease and regression during therapy.

Cardiac MRI has evolved as a powerful diagnostic tool in humans over the past 20 years. Most of the MRI techniques originally developed for cardiac imaging in humans have been adapted and optimized for rodent imaging in a "1 : 1-fashion". In fact, the development of feasible methods for CMRI in small animals was always lacking behind the

1 Acknowledgment: The authors would like to thank the Deutsche Forschungsgemeinschaft (SFB 688) and the Bundesministerium für Bildung und Forschung (Projekt 01EZ0816) for financial support.

achievements made in cardiac MRI of humans, since tremendous efforts had to be spent to extend the possibilities of MRI for small animal cardiac investigations encountering much smaller pixel sizes. MRI at this more microscopic level (also called MR microscopy [MRM]) is based on the same physical principles as its clinical counterpart MRI : MR microscopy, which can loosely be defined as MRI in the spatial resolution regime beyond 100 μm, is now increasingly exploited to provide anatomical and functional information in (transgenic) animal models, with the focus of revealing anatomical and physiological changes during disease progression or in response to potential therapeutic treatment. Depending on the technique used, slice-based as well as true 3D image sets can be obtained, with resolution of 100 μm in all dimensions in living animals and 10 μm isotropic in fixed specimens, with the possibility to view images of whole animals or organs in arbitrary planes. This extension of MRI to MR microscopy, however, required a significant increase in spatial resolution in all three dimensions accompanied by a severe signal reduction. Overcoming this deficit required the development of technology specific to MRM – strong magnets, dedicated receiver coils and chains, strong gradient sets, image acquisition sequences, and finally biological support for small animals in high magnetic fields. In addition, a whole arsenal of CMRI and MR spectroscopy methods known from human applications had to be adopted and further developed for in vivo cardiac studies in rodents.

These techniques include:

- cine-CMR for assessment of LV size, shape, global LV function and wall thickening,
- techniques for quantifying regional wall motion,
- techniques for assessing myocardial microcirculation,
- ^{1}H- and ^{31}P-MR spectroscopy for metabolism, and
- (targeted) contrast-enhanced techniques for detecting myocardial infarction and molecular imaging applications.

In the following sections, these methods are described and their application to rodent studies in normal physiology and in pathophysiology are reviewed.

23.2 MR-Hardware and Animal Preparation for CMRI in Small Animals

As one scales proton MR imaging from the human dimension down to the microscopic dimension of a rodent several challenges and limitations with respect to signal-to-noise ratio (SNR), spatial resolution and scan time emerge. A simple comparison of the typical heart weight of mice (~ 300 mg) and of humans (~ 300 g) demonstrates that in order to resolve the same relative anatomical details, the rodent image must be acquired with a voxel volume approximately 1,000-times smaller than that of a human, delivering a factor 1,000 reduced MR-signal strength. In order to combat the reduced MR-signal strength met in rodent imaging, most research groups are using horizontal or vertical high-field magnet systems with a small-bore specifically designed for small animal applications. The driving force for using high-fields strengths between 4.7 T and 17.6 T stems from the primary advantage that the SNR increases (approximately linearly) with the field strength, which allows higher spatial resolution to be achieved. In addition, even so no single field strength is widely assumed optimal for MRI of the rodent heart, higher field strength provide increased spectral resolution, however, at the prize of increased susceptibility artifacts.

For completeness, it should be mentioned, that CMRI in rodents can also be implemented using pre-existing clinical whole-body MRI systems with 1.5–3.0 T (Brockmann 2007), which offers an interesting alternative to dedicated small animal systems, since they provide sufficient image quality in applications which do not require extremely high temporal or spatial resolution. In many applications small animal imaging protocols on clinical MR scanners can be realized in scan times comparable to those used for human examinations using optimized RF coils that improve the signal reception and dedicated pulse sequences.

Various optimized radiofrequency (RF) coils, being the key-players in the SNR game, with high filling factors and sensitivities are required in small animal CMRI (Haase 2000) such as surface coils, volume coils (e.g. birdcage coils) and more recently phased array coils (Gareis 2007). In particular, the concept of phased array coils has become increasingly important, since it allows to distribute the high SNR performance of their small component surface coils over a larger area covered by the entire array, with no increase in imaging time. Thus, this phased arrays can be used to boost image quality within the same acquisition time or are the "coils-of-choice" whenever parallel imaging capabilities are of importance (see Chapter 1). Today, phased array coils for mice and rats with 4–16 coil elements are commercially available for pure animal and clinical MR systems.

Finally, dedicated small animal MRI systems are equipped with high performance gradients which are typically 10–50 times stronger than those of a clinical system (200–1,000 mT/m), which allow to achieve the same "anatomical resolution" in rodents compared to humans. In addition, they enable the use of fast imaging sequences, which make it possible to image rapidly time-resolved physiological and pharmacological events. In this context, it should be mentioned that various MR pulse sequences can be used for CMRI. However, the "working-horses" on high-field systems are currently T1-weighted gradient echo methods, which easily can be adapted for dynamic imaging delivering 2D-cine movies with an inplane resolution of 200 μm in less than 1 min.

The determination of normal and abnormal cardiovascular function in murine animal models is not only challenging because of the reduced cardiac size but also due to rather short cardiac cycles. In small animals, typical heart rates are between 300–400 beats/min in rats and 500–600 beats/min in mice. Thus the typical length of the cardiac mouse cycle is only one tenth of that of a human. To minimize motion related artifacts, reliable ECG and respiratory gating or navigation is mandatory to obtain high-quality time-resolved cardiac images. Different gating strategies have been reported using direct or indirect detection methods. Direct detection methods sense heart and respiratory motion using, for example, the ECG signal (Rommel 2000) as double trigger unit with optimized gating strategies (Cassidy 2004), or pneumatic (Minard 1998), fiberoptic (Brau 2002), piezoelectric (McKibben and Reo 1992), infrared (Lemieux and Glover 1996) or inductive sensors (Fishbein 2001). Indirect detection methods exploit additional navigator MR signals as a measure for data acceptance (Wang 1996). The detection of a clear and precise ECG signal without disturbances from RF- or gradient-switching pulses is an important prerequisite for almost any small animal cardiac application, including cine-CMR, quantification of MR relaxation times, perfusion via spin labeling or pulse wave velocities. All these applications require the exact timing of the image data acquisition. In general, CMRI requires the rodents to be immobilized and thus anesthesized. To avoid negative chronotropic and inotropic effects, inhalative anesthetics such as isoflurane or i.v. anesthetics such as propofol are commonly used and given via nose cone or tail vein catheter and allow for short induction and recovery times (Kober 2005, Ruff 1998a). While under anesthesia, the temperature of the animals must be kept constant at 37 °C using either warm airflow, and circulating water or electrical heating pads, since the temperature inside the magnet core is only in the 15–20 °C range. In general, the vital functions of the animals during anesthesia have to be carefully controlled.

23.3 Structural and Functional Analysis in Small Animals

23.3.1 Cine-CMR – Myocardial Volumes, Function and Mass

Cine-CMR techniques, first established in humans, have also become the working horse for almost every small animal cardiac study, since it is an information-rich tool to quantify cardiac morphology and function (Franco 1998, Manning 1990, Rudin 1991, Ruff 1998, Slawson 1998, Wiesmann 2000). In cine-CMR techniques the imaging process is synchronized with the cardiac cycle and thus can be extended over many cardiac cycles by employing ECG-gating or navigator gating, see previous section. Gated, single-phase spin echo and multi-phase gradient echo techniques allow for the accurate determination of important cardiac parameters in rodents. The list of cardiac parameters, which can be extracted from the complete coverage of the heart using bright blood cine images comprises left ventricle (LV) mass, wall thickness and wall thickening, LV volume for each cardiac phase, and in addition end-diastolic volume (EDV), end-systolic volume (ESV), stroke volume, cardiac output, and ejection fraction (EF). Typically, these short-axis cine-CMRs in rodents are performed on high-field magnets (> 4.7 T) using ECG/respiratory triggered segmented gradient echo sequences. The maximal acquisition window per frame should be in the range of 6–8 ms, in order to allow for 12–16 image frames being acquired to cover the whole cycle. Spatial in plane resolution for volumetry should be in the range of 100–150 μm for mice, which have a wall thickness of approximately 1 mm, and not more than 250 μm for rats, which have a wall thickness of up to 2 mm. The slice thickness is typically around 1 mm for mice and 1–2 mm for rats. In order to cover the entire LV from the base to the apex by contiguous short-axis slices, the acquisition of 10–20 slices is necessary.

Other **typical imaging parameters** are as follows:
- flip angle 30–40°,
- echo time 1–3 ms,
- repetition time 5–8 ms,
- field of view: 30 mm^2,
- image matrix 128–256 × 128–256.

For RF excitation and MR-signal reception a rodent-size adapted and homogeneous volume coil (e.g. a birdcage coil) is used.

For data processing, the size of the myocardial and ventricular compartments can be determined by semiautomated segmentation in the short-axis slice images covering the entire heart. Therefore, for all slices, endocardial borders

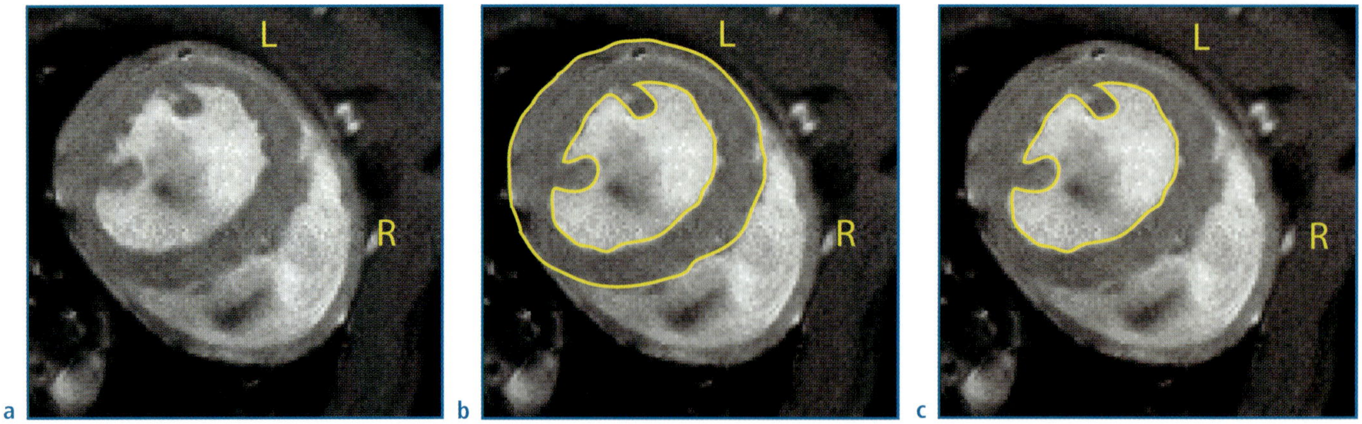

Figure 23-1 End-diastolic frame (short-axis view) of a mouse heart (a). Segmentation of the left ventricular myocardium (b) and LV volume (c). L: left ventricle; R: right ventricle.

in both end-diastolic and end-systolic frames have to be delineated. These borders can be clearly distinguished by exploiting the high contrast between the flowing ventricular blood and the myocardial tissue. The derived compartment areas are multiplied with the slice thickness to determine the myocardial and ventricular slice volumes.

Ventricular volumes are calculated as follows:

- stroke volume (SV) = end-diastolic volume (EDV) – end-systolic volume (ESV),
- ejection fraction (EF) = SV / EDV and
- cardiac output (CO) = SV multiplied by heart rate.

Myocardial masses can be calculated from the multiplication of the total volumes with the specific density of the myocardium (1.05 g/cm^3) (considering the myocardial tissue density to be constant).

Volumes and masses are calculated with similar reproducibility and accuracy as known from human MR studies. Compared to autopsy data, MRI determined cardiac masses and volumes were in excellent agreement. Applying this technique (Figure 23-1), LV morphology and function can be accurately assessed (Franco 1998, Nahrendorf 2003a, Ruff 1998b) and hypertrophic changes can be quantified (Siri 1997, Slawson 1998).

Cine-CMR also allows in a parallel fashion to the LV the quantification of right ventricular (RV) volumes and function (Wiesmann 2002). This is important because gene-targeted mouse models of cardiomyopathy may also develop remodeling of the right heart. The assessment of RV function is more difficult than it is for the LV, due to the complex geometry. Consistent with human physiology, Wiesmann et al. showed higher RV end-diastolic and end-systolic volumes compared to LV volumes in wild type mice (Wiesmann 2002). In mice with LV heart failure due to myocardial infarction, significant structural and functional changes of the RV could be demonstrated. These mice developed a RV dysfunction caused by ligation of the left anterior descendent coronary artery.

Using the cine-CMR technique, serial assessment of LV cardiac structure and function was reliable and accurate also in neonatal, juvenile, and adult growth stages (Wiesmann 2000). Considering the fact that transgenic mice may develop an early phenotype or even may die within the first days of life, cine-CMR may give new insights into the underlying pathophysiology in these models and also allow to follow-up changes during growth by serial measurements in the same animal. Cine-CMR also allows accurate and reproducible serial measurements of cardiac output and stroke volume when compared to thermodilution derived data (Franco 1999). Nahrendorf et al. (2003a, 2003b) also demonstrated the feasibility of the in vivo determination of myocardial infarct size. In this study, myocardial infarct size was calculated for each slice by dividing the sum of the endocardial and epicardial circumferences occupied by the infarct with significant thinning and akinesia or dyskinesia during systole by the sum of the total epicardial and endocardial circumferences of the LV.

23.3.2 Regional Wall Motion Analysis

Imaging methods for the visualization and quantitative assessment of the intramyocardial wall motion, such as myocardial tagging or motion-encoded phase contrast imaging, were originally developed for humans and are now also available for rodent applications. By directly visualizing non-invasively myocardial motion patterns and regional functional parameters such as myocardial strain, a detailed evaluation of the pathophysiological state of the heart of small animals has become possible.

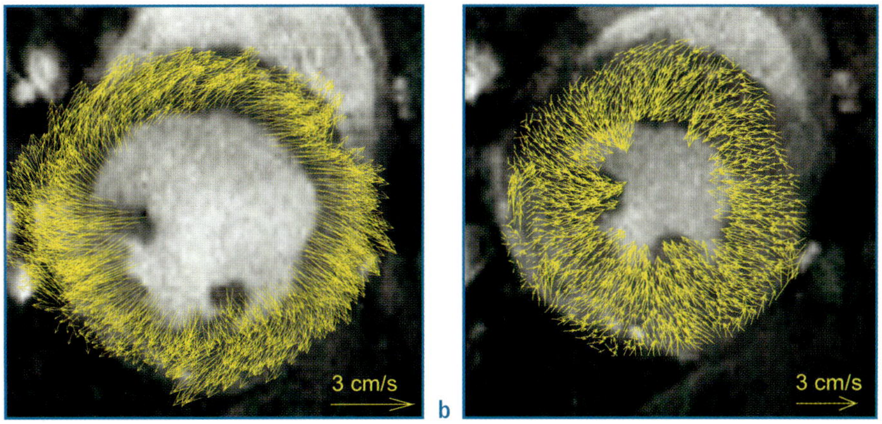

Figure 23-2 Representative cine images of the mouse heart with overlaid vector maps obtained by an ECG triggered PC-cine method. Diastolic time frame (a), systolic time frame (b).

The basic principle behind myocardial tagging and variations there of (see also Chapter 1), is to place a "tag"-mark of saturated spins on the myocardium via spatially selective RF-saturation pulses and to track the displacement of these "tag"-marks over time via cine-CMR. Spatial modulation of magnetization (SPAMM) "tagging" provided the first non-invasive approach to investigate myocardial motion patterns (Axel and Dougherty 1989, Epstein 2002, Zhou 2003). Post-processing the deformation pattern of the imprinted tagging grid at different cardiac cycles enables to estimate myocardial wall motion and determining strain values. However early tagging methods were limited by low tagging resolution allowing for less than three taglines covering the myocardial wall (when imaging the murine heart for instance). The limited resolution of the motion information thus hampers the calculation of myocardial wall strain. To improve the tag resolution, different tagged images can be generated with a spatial shifted tagging grid (Stuber 1999). The combination of two tagged images with shifted tagging grids thus can double the resolution of motion information.

To obtain motion information beyond the resolution of an imprinted tagging grid the combination of SPAMM with an additional unencoding gradient module called displacement encoding with stimulated echoes (DENSE) was proposed (Aletras 1999, Gilson 2004, Gilson 2005). This method delivers accurate pixelwise displacement information of the murine myocardium at different phases of the heart cycle. Tagging methods as well as the DENSE sequences make use of a dedicated preparation module which translates displacement information into a deformation of the tagging grid or representative phase values (DENSE), respectively.

To directly encode motion information on a pixelwise resolution phase contrast (PC) imaging allows the assessment of velocity values for each moving voxel (Streif 2003). Velocity encoding is achieved by using short bipolar gradient pulses leading to a phase accumulation proportional to the velocity of the moving isochromats. Modulus images are not affected by motion encoding gradients. To clear the phase values carrying the velocity information from phase distortions caused by additional effects such as B_0 field inhomogeneities and RF penetration effects usually two datasets with different motion encoding gradients have to be acquired. Velocity values for each voxel can then be extracted by subtracting the according pair of phase data. Due to the short velocity encoding module (bipolar gradient) and due to the intrinsic high resolution of the velocity maps tissue motion can be visualized at very high temporal and spatial resolutions (Figure 23-2). This wall motion imaging technique was initially investigated in mice using a 2D approach at 7 T (Streif 2003) and more recently using a 3D approach at 17.6 T (Herold 2006). These studies demonstrated pixel-wise measurements of LV myocardial velocities, which provide higher spatial resolution of functional parameters than tagging. These studies also characterized normal wall velocities in mice and demonstrated the ability to detect reduced wall velocities in mice after myocardial infarction (MI).

23.3.3 Myocardial Perfusion and Blood Volume

The quantification of myocardial microcirculatory parameters such as perfusion (P) or regional blood volume (RBV) is crucial for the evaluation of different forms of heart disease, since impairments in microcirculation affect cardiac function.

Cardiac perfusion, a parameter quantifying myocardial blood supply, is defined as the amount of blood, which flows per unit time within the cardiac tissue normalized to the mass or volume of this tissue. The current clinical approach for MR cardiac perfusion imaging is contrast-enhanced first-pass perfusion MRI, where a bolus of an MR contrast agent is applied intravenously, and the kinetics of the signal enhancement in the myocardial tissue and the blood of the

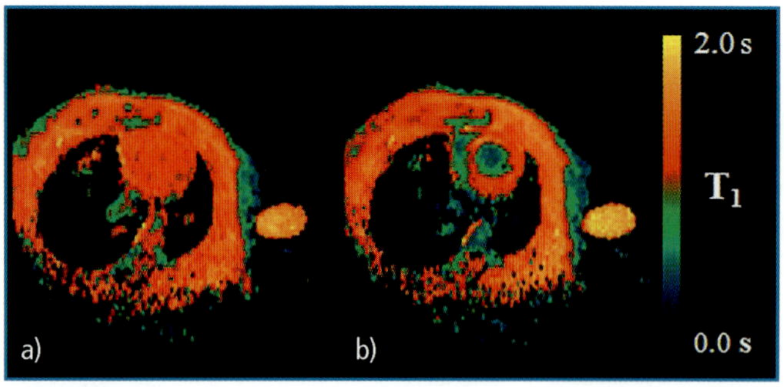

Figure 23-3 T1 maps of a rat $T1_{nsel}$ (a), $T1_{sel}$ (b). Images are acquired in a short-axis view.

LV is measured dynamically. The analysis of the first-pass of the contrast agent through the myocardium via tracer-kinetic modeling provides all the required information about perfusion and regional blood volume in the heart. The translation of this bolus-tracking method to small animals, however, is hampered by the rapid heart rate and small size of the mammal heart. In small rodents, cardiac cycles are in the order of 100–200 ms only, which precludes successful image acquisition with sufficient spatial resolution and SNR within one heart beat. For this and other reasons, MRI bolus tracking methods are rather uncommon in small animal cardiac perfusion imaging.

As a versatile alternative, arterial spin labeling (ASL) techniques for quantifying myocardial perfusion have been established for small animal studies, which do not require an exogenous contrast agent (Detre 1992). Instead, this method exploits the water signal of flowing blood as an endogenous tracer via magnetic labeling. In this technique, also called spin labeling, the effect of perfusion is detected by measuring its effect on the observed myocardial tissue T1 relaxation time.

In detail, two series of images are acquired at various delay times after either a *non-selective* (global, $_{nsel}$) or *slice-selective* ($_{sel}$) spin inversion pulse (= spin labeling pulses), so that the T1 relaxation of the magnetization can be tracked in the detection slice of interest. These two sets of images can then be used to estimate the myocardial tissue T1 relaxation times, $T1_{nsel}$ and $T1_{sel}$ (Figure 23-3). With the global inversion pulse, the magnetization of water spins perfusing the slice is inverted, similar to the magnetization of the tissue in the slice. Thus the inflowing spins have no effect on the T1 relaxation time of the slice being imaged and the global inversion measurement gives the intrinsic T1 relaxation of the tissue $T1_{nsel}$.

In contrast, for the slice selective inversion experiment, only the tissue spins within the detection slice are effected by the inversion pulse, whereas the blood water spins outside the detection slice are not inverted and thus in thermal equilibrium. Once these spins enter the detection slice due to perfusion, the mixing of non-inverted flowing and inverted spins in the detection slice modifies the apparent relaxation time $T1_{sel}$ and thus creates flow-related contrast. In fact, non-inverted flowing spins cause an apparent and measurable acceleration of the relaxation, thus that $T1_{sel} < T1_{nsel}$, and reflect information about the perfusion in this area. Myocardial perfusion P in ml/g/min can be calculated by the following equation first described by Detre et al. (1992):

$P/\lambda = 1 / T1_{sel} - 1 / T1_{nsel}$, where λ is the blood/tissue partition coefficient.

The major difficulty of the spin labeling approach is related to the small differences between the T1 values of the global and the slice selective measurements (in the order of 3–5 %). Therefore each relaxation time measurements needs to be perfectly synchronized with the heart cycle using an efficient ECG trigger unit, since the perfusion calculation requires the exact knowledge of the timing of each image with respect to the inversion pulse. In addition, a high magnetic field strength is favorable for spin labeling imaging. High-field strengths not only push the intrinsic SNR, but supplementary provide also longer inflow observation times, since T1 increases with the field strength. Dedicated transmit-receive coil setups are also required. In particular, to assure global spin inversion within the whole mouse, a size-adapted homogeneous RF transmit coil has to be provided (Streif 2005). The ASL technique has been successfully validated against microspheres in rat myocardium (Waller 2000) and was used to quantify perfusion in the non-infarcted myocardium of a MI mouse model (Streif 2005). In this study a significantly decreased perfusion 4 wks after MI was found. Reduced myocardial blood flow was detected as a significant marker for development of systolic dysfunction in hypertrophied hearts (Maestri 2003, Waller 2008). Also the effect of different types of anesthesia on myocardial blood flow in mice was studied (Kober 2005) and a strong response of blood flow to higher isoflurane concentrations was observed. Myocardial perfusion imaging was also used for phenotypic characterization of transgenic mice. In a creatine kinase double knockout $CK^{-/-}$ mice, the deletion of the creatine kinase enzyme system leads to left ventricular hypertrophy and dilatation of the left ventricle. Nahrendorf et al. (2006) found a significantly reduced myocardial perfusion in these mice, which was inversely correlated to left ventricular mass and might be caused by reduced capillary density (Nahrendorf 2006).

Another useful parameter quantifying blood supply in the myocardium is regional blood volume (RBV), which is defined as the volume of blood inside a unit volume or mass of myocardial tissue, and mainly reflects the volume of myocardial capillaries. However, RBV in rodents cannot be determined by first-pass techniques, for all the imaging con-

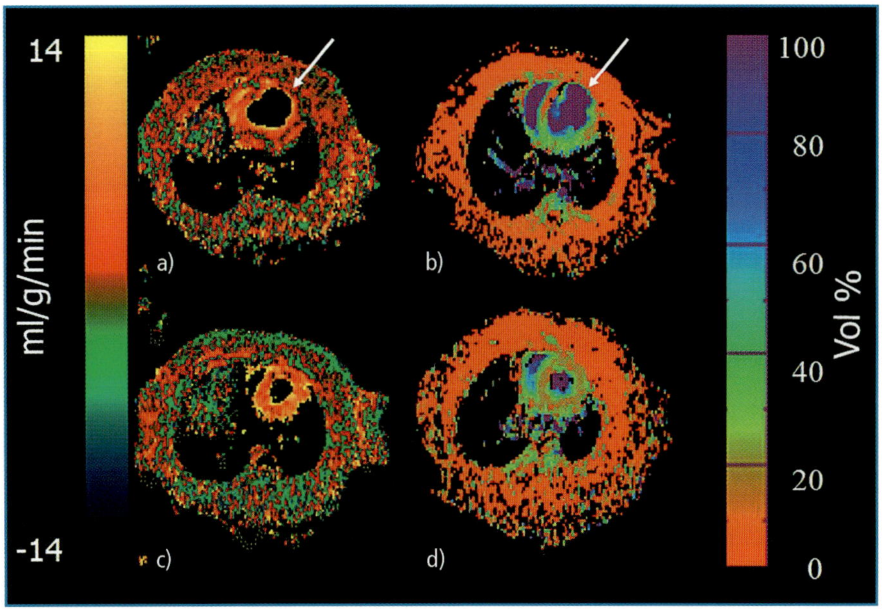

Figure 23-4 Perfusion (expressed in ml/g/min) (a, c) and RBV maps (expressed in %) (b, d) of an animal 8 wks after myocardial infarction (a, b) and a control animal (c, d). Images are acquired in a short-axis view. In the infarcted rat heart, the scar (arrow) and left ventricular dilatation are clearly visible.

straints mentioned above. As a versatile alternative, techniques exploiting the T1-enhancement effect of intravascular MR contrast agents in combination with T1-mapping procedure can be employed. The underlying concept is that an intravascular contrast agent, even when confined to the intracapillary space, spreads its enhancement effect on T1 relaxation to the extravascular space due to transcapillary spin exchange. Thus, only a small volume fraction of intracapillary blood filled with contrast agent is sufficient to significantly accelerate the T1 in the myocardium as a characteristic function of RBV. RBV may be determined from slice selective T1 experiments by measurement of $1/T1_{sel}$ before and after application of the intravascular contrast agent (CA), which can be described as follows:
$RBV / \lambda\ (1 / T1_{CA\ sel} - 1 / T1_{sel}) / (1 / T1_{CA\ blood} - 1 / T1_{blood})$, where λ is the blood/tissue partition coefficient, CA = contrast agent.

Values for $T1_{blood}$ were obtained from the left ventricular heart chamber of $T1_{nsel}$ maps (Waller 2000).

The T1 of changes in blood and myocardial tissue before and after the injection of the intravascular contrast media can be measured via the T1 mapping procedure described above.

Waller et al. (2001) used this method to quantify regional blood volume by application of Gd-DTPA-albumin as an intravascular contrast agent. In a serial rat heart study the basal regional blood volume at rest increased significantly after 8 wks after myocardial infarction (MI) and remained elevated after 16 wks compared with sham-operated rats, while myocardial blood flow was reduced. The results indicate that significant microvascular changes occur during cardiac remodeling (Figure 23-4). But, looking at the maximum RBV under stress conditions, induced by application of adenosine, the RBV_{max} appears to be independent from the degree of hypertrophy (Waller 2008).

23.3.4 Measurement of Blood Flow in Aorta and Coronary Arteries

Blood flow measurements in the great vessels such as the aorta or the pulmonary artery are mainly based on phase contrast imaging methods. By using a PC-cine method (see Chapter 1), time resolved 1D and 2D velocity maps can be generated. 2D-in-plane encoding strategies with flow encoding gradient along the read- and phase-encoding direction are applied to visualize the velocity distribution along a certain section of the vessel. This allows for the detection of the peak velocity for example when examining a stenotic jet. However for small vessels partial volume effects are likely to occur due to large voxel sizes compared to the vessel wall diameter. Using a 1D-through-plane encoding strategy (Feintuch 2007) allows to determine more accurately the cross-sectional flow profile (Figure 23-5). By integrating the volume flow for all time frames during the cardiac cycle, total blood volume ejected during a single heartbeat can be calculated. This method is commonly used for the calculation of right ventricular (RV) and left ventricular (LV) outputs. By determining the regurgitant fraction of flow across the aortic or pulmonary valve this method also allows to evaluate the degree of valvular insufficiency.

Due to the reduced vessel diameter in small animal studies partial volume effects also potentially impair the accuracy of volumetric flow calculation. However high-field MR microscopic imaging with strong gradient fields allows

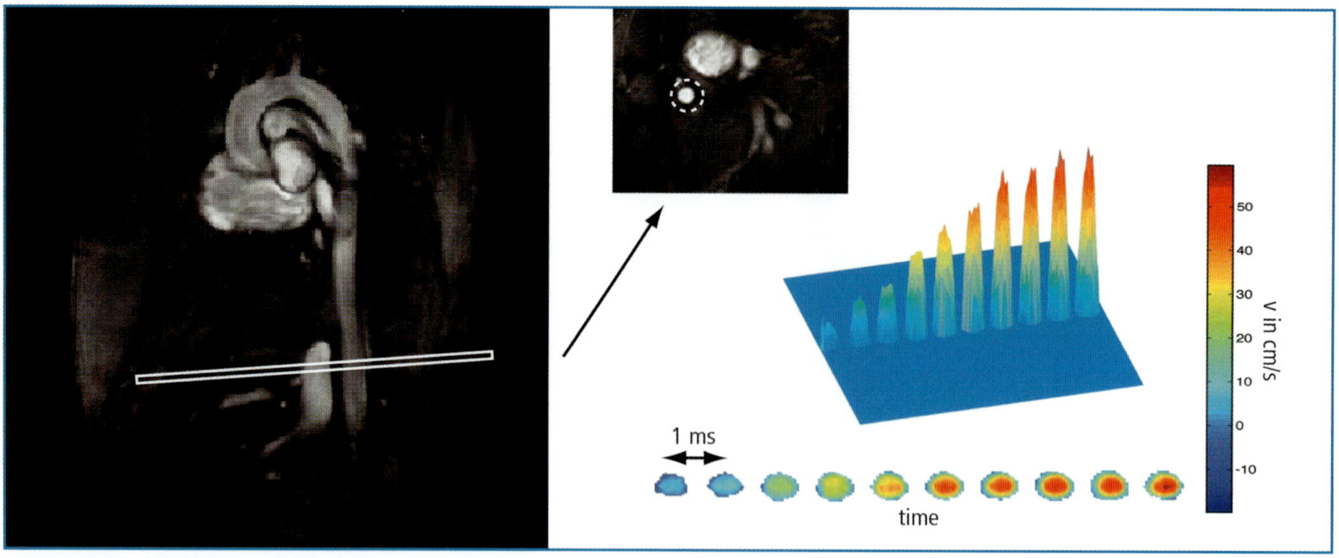

Figure 23-5 Through-plane flow measurement in the abdominal murine aorta of the early systolic flow-pulse with PC-cine imaging and an interleaved acquisition to improve the temporal resolution.

for volumetric flow quantification in the murine aorta with a relative error less than 3%. In addition misalignment between the direction of flow and the flow encoding direction of less than 15% causes errors for the flux calculation of less than 5% (Herold 2009).

Due to the cyclic nature of phase values only a certain velocity window leading to phase accumulations in the limit of $\pm\,\pi$ can be measured without ambiguity. Thus upper limits of the expected blood flow velocities should be known prior to the MR measurement to ensure an optimized exploitation of the provided phase range.

When studying the blood flow in the coronary system in small animals sequences with a very high spatiotemporal resolution are necessary. Phase contrast methods using motion-encoding gradients are hardly suitable to realize sufficient short echo times with high spatial encoding gradients. Moreover, 2D or 3D PC-cine acquisition requires the acquisition of several motion encoded and ECG triggered data sets which leads to long measurement times (several averages are necessary to achieve sufficiently high SNR at a high spatial resolution). Long measurement times however often lead to temporal shifts of the trigger pulse due to variations of the heart cycle and thus affect the accuracy of the velocity calculations.

In this context time-of-flight acquisition schemes based on gradient echo sequences with very short echo times have proven to be more suitable to estimate blood flow velocity even in the coronary arteries of mice (Cochet 2010, Parzy 2009).

23.3.5 Vessel Wall and Atherosclerosis Imaging

Morphological Imaging

MR sequences based on a spin echo design have emerged to become the gold standard when investigating the morphology of the vessel wall in small animals. Since high-field MR systems are widely used in small animal imaging, gradient echo designs have increasingly to deal with susceptibility artifacts, which can be avoided when using spin echo methods. Moreover the short cardiac cycles of small animals enable to implement an intrinsic black-blood contrast with cardiac triggered spin echo sequences. Therefore data acquisition has to be gated to occur during systole (i.e. when blood flow velocity is at its maximum) such that excited, fast flowing blood is not refocused during acquisition and thereby generating images with black-blood contrast (Figure 23-6). Using further a multi-slice acquisition scheme allows to cover an entire section of the vessel with various image slices without increasing the total measurement time to generate a 3D visualization of the morphological structure. During each cardiac cycle typically one k-space line for one slice of the 3D slice package is acquired (Herold 2009). The repetition time can then be calculated by the formula (when omitting respiratory gating): TR = number of slices × RR (duration of one cardiac cycle). The balance between TR and TE is crucial for the image contrast behavior and can be used to identify different plaque compartments. The Table 23-1 gives some guidelines how to emphasize the MR signal of different plaque regions with multi-contrast imaging (Itsko-

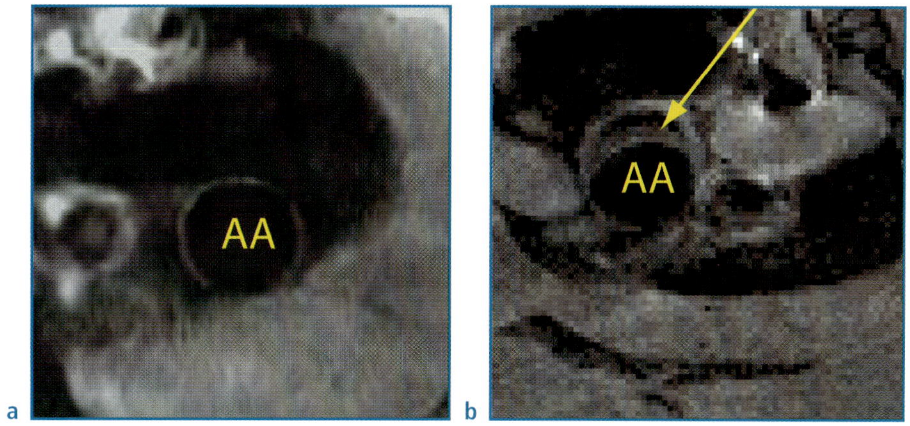

Figure 23-6 Black-blood contrast spin echo image of the murine ascending aorta (AA). Visualization of the healthy vessel wall (a), atherosclerotic plaque (arrow) (b).

Table 23-1 Contrast behavior of different atherosclerotic plaque regions.

	T1-Weighting	PD-Weighting	T2-Weighting
thrombus	+ ⟷ +/–	– ⟷ +/–	– ⟷ +/–
lipid core	+	+	–
fibrous tissue	+/–	+	+/– ⟷ +
calcium	–	–	–
TE/TR*	10 ms/500 ms	10 ms/2,000 ms	30 ms/2,000 ms

+: hyperintense; –: hypointense; * B_0 field: 9.4 T.

vich 2004). TR can be customized by adjusting the slice number of the multi-slice data set.

Functional Imaging

Arterial stiffening caused by the accumulation of fibrous plaque is assumed to be an indicator of response to therapies aimed at modification of endothelial function. The pulse-wave velocity (PWV) has proven to be an independent predictor of cardiovascular risk in certain cases of cardiovascular diseases, as it is known to increase with increasing arterial stiffness.

In recent years MRI has shown the ability to estimate functional parameters such as the PWV in small animal models in particular in mice (Herold 2009, Zhao 2009). Basic motion sensitive sequences such as PC-cine methods are applied to temporally determine the systolic upstroke of the flow pulse at high temporal resolution.

Most commonly this method is applied at two locations along the flow path. By dividing the distance between the two locations along the flow path by the difference of the pulse wave arrival times at the same locations, the PWV can be estimated. This approach is known as the transit-time (TT) method and gives an estimate for the *averaged PWV* along the propagation pathway (Mohiaddin 1993). A further approach uses 1D in-plane-flow encoding to determine the systolic upstroke at multiple regions of interest (ROIs) along the blood vessel. Therefore the imaging slice has to be oriented so that the flow propagation path of the vessel coincides with the flow encoding direction. By plotting the distance of each ROI against the pulse wave arrival times, the PWV can be estimated as the slope of this plot (Figure 23-7).

In mice the systolic upstroke of the flow pulse generally lasts less than 10–15 ms. Thus a high temporal resolution at 1 ms is crucial to accurately determine the starting time of each flow pulse. Using an interleaved acquisition scheme as described by Herold et al. (2009) allows to measure the flow pulse at a sufficiently high sampling rate to estimate the PWV.

A third approach allows to estimate the PWV *at a defined position*. This method makes use of the assumption that the early systolic pulse wave can be regarded as reflectionless. Then the *local PWV* can be estimated by measuring the blood volume flow Q(t) and the cross-sectional area A(t). Using the expression for the characteristic impedance and the wave equation for inviscid flow, the PWV can then be described as (Vulliémoz et al. 2002):

$$PWV = \frac{dQ}{dA}.$$

Thus, to calculate the local PWV the early systolic flow pulse has to be sampled at a high temporal and spatial resolution. PC-cine sequences applied in high-field imaging with through-plane flow encoding have shown to deliver sufficiently high accuracy in spatial and temporal resolution to allow the local PWV estimation in small animals such as mice (Herold 2009).

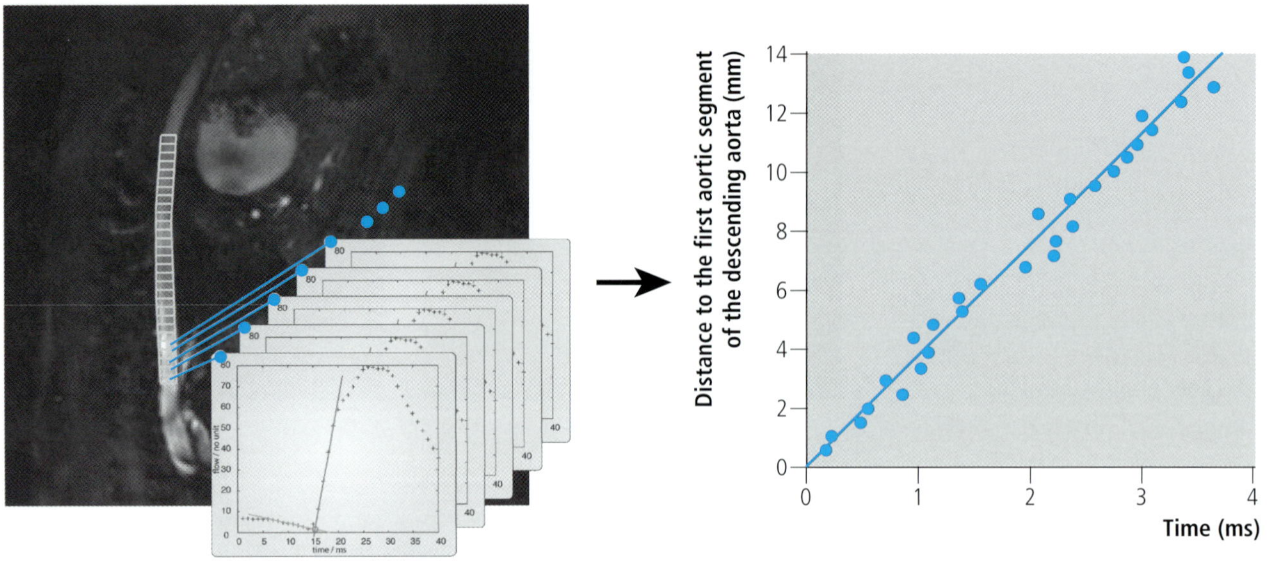

Figure 23-7 Schematic overview of the multi-site transit time method to estimate the mean pulse wave velocity (PWV) along the murine aorta. Plotting the time arrival times of the beginning systolic flow pulse over the distance to the first ROI allows the calculation of the PWV.

23.4 Contrast-Enhanced and Molecular MRI

Despite MRIs various endogenous sources of contrast and corresponding diagnostic options, there is still an urgent need for additional exogenous contrast materials, which artificially emphasize contrast. The driving force behind the use of additional contrast agents in cardiac research is, to enhance the contrast between normal and pathological cardiac tissue. Contrast agents commonly used in MRI (see also Chapter 3) are chemical structures rich in unpaired electrons, i. e. be paramagnetic. These paramagnetic centers provide an additional pathway for relaxation by altering (in general: shortening!) the relaxation times of protons that come in close proximity to the contrast agent. The most important candidates for transmitting this paramagnetic effect are e. g. molecular oxygen, ions and complexes of transition metals (Fe^{2+}, Fe^{3+}, Mn^{2+}, Mn^{3+}) or of lanthanides (Gd^{3+}, Ho^{3+}). For instance, *paramagnetic* gadolinium (Gd) complexes such as Gd (Gd-DTPA) reduce primarily T1-values of the tissues by penetrating the extracellular space, whereas *superparamagnetic* iron oxides, which have 2–3 orders of magnitude higher susceptibility over conventional paramagnetic ions, reduce primarily T2-values of the tissues and can be detected at significantly lower concentrations.

23.4.1 Late Enhancement

One important milestone in the area of contrast-enhanced cardiac MRI was laid by the so-called "delayed contrast-enhanced MRI or late enhancement MRI" of the heart, which allows for improved myocardial infarction (MI) detection and MI size estimation. This technique has meanwhile become the **clinical gold standard** for human applications and was adapted and validated successfully for studying infarction development and LV remodeling in animal models. In this approach, first 0.1–0.6 mmol/kg Gd-DTPA are injected intravenously as a T1-shortening contrast agent and in a second step, 10–20 min after injection, highly T1-weighted short-axis gradient echo images are acquired. With this setup, meaningful images can be obtained, where contrast-enhanced regions of the myocardium highlight the non-viable infarct zones. This enhancement represents the accumulation of gadolinium in the extracellular space, due to the loss of membrane integrity in the infarcted tissue. Since this technique allows for assessing accurately infarct size, extent, and borders, it can be used in a longitudinal fashion to study post-infarct remodeling processes during days/weeks after experimental MI (Simonetti 2001).

Manganese (Mn^{2+})-enhanced MRI (MEMRI) based on the T1-shortening effect of Mn^{2+} is another interesting alternative for myocardial infarction imaging, exploiting the fact that Mn^{2+} as a Ca^{2+}-antagonist is actively pumped into viable myocytes through voltage-gated Ca^{2+} channels. It has been shown in a post-infarct mouse model, that several minutes after injection of $MnCl_2$ infarcted and noninfarcted myocardial tissue showed a distinct signal enhancement, which allows for infarct volume determination (Hu 2004).

23.4.2 Molecular MRI

Another research area, where (targeted) exogenous contrast agents are of paramount importance, arises in the fast growing field of molecular imaging. In general, molecular imaging can be defined as the "in vivo characterization and measurement of biological processes at the cellular and molecular level" and aims to image molecular abnormalities associated with diseases. MRI appears very attractive for molecular imaging, since current MRI protocols already provide anatomic, functional and biochemical information in excellent image quality.

Molecular MRI, which can be principally performed by using (actively or passively) targeted exogenous MRI-contrast agents, has the major potential to detect target structures beyond the resolution limit of current MRI techniques. In the following some exemplary small animal applications of molecular MRI in the field of cardiovascular imaging will be presented.

Imaging of Atherosclerosis

Typical targets for molecular imaging of atherosclerosis are e.g. macrophages, fibrin, glycoprotein receptors, VCAM1, ICAM and MMPs. Usually in addition to the target structure an antibody or peptide is linked with nanoparticles, which are significantly para/superparamagnetic or will be loaded with paramagnetic or superparamagnetic materials.

Detection of Thrombosis

Thrombosis is a pathological marker of many kinds of cardiovascular diseases, like myocardial infarction, stroke or pulmonary embolism. Specific molecular MRI bears the potential to be a method for early diagnostics. One method is visualization of the coagulation factor XIII activity, which reflects the status of acute thrombosis. Therefore a coated iron oxide particle (CLIO) is bound to a factor XIII specific peptid. This contrast agent binds itself to factor XIII in the thrombus, which now becomes visible by MRI (Jaffer 2002).

USPIO-Labeling of Macrophages

The use of ultrasmall supraparamagnetic iron oxide particles (USPIO) allows the detection of regions with high macrophage activity elsewhere in the organism. The imaging contrast results from the iron induced magnetic field inhomogeneities. Thus, cellular labeling of macrophages by intravenous injection of USPIO results in darkening (signal void) of the target tissue on the MR images. The USPIO uptake is depending on particle size (Pratten and Lloyd 1986). These contrast agents are taken up by incorporation (phagocytosis) into the macrophages of the immune system and can be visualized in atherosclerotic plaques (Dardzinski 2001, Ruehm 2001). Recently new MRI methods were developed to image magnetically labeled cells with positive contrast using dedicated pulse sequences (Cunningham 2005). Advantages of this positive contrast methods are the minor dependence on partial volume effects and spatial resolution.

Imaging of Angiogenesis

Angiogenesis plays an important role in detection and therapy of cardiovascular and oncologic diseases. To visualize angiogenesis of tumours, for example, $\alpha_v\beta_3$-integrin antibodys are used, because $\alpha_v\beta_3$-integrin is highly expressed in activated neovascular cells and is absent in quiescent cells. The $\alpha_v\beta_3$-integrin antibodys were linked to either Gd-DTPA-based complexes (Anderson 2000, Winter 2003), liposomes or nanoparticles to localize the angiogenic endothelium. Angiogenesis is also associated with atherosclerosis and could be localized by use of $\alpha_v\beta_3$-integrin nanoparticles in hyperlipidemic New Zealand White rabbits (Winter 2003).

Imaging of Apoptosis

One area, where mouse models are used for testing novel targeted myocardial contrast agents, is imaging of apoptosis or programmed cell death. One of the earliest events in apoptosis is the redistribution of phosphatidylserine (PS) from the inner to the outer leaflet of the cell membrane, which makes PS an attractive and specific target for molecular imaging. Certain proteins (e.g. annexin-V), which bind tightly and with high specificity to PS, can be used to monitor cardiac apoptosis.

In one recent study, annexin-V labeled cross-linked iron oxide nanoparticles injected 20 min after coronary occlusion were used for imaging apoptosis in the reperfused infarcted beating mouse heart in vivo (Sosnovik 2005). Cardiac images obtained after injection of the targeted contrast agent showed a clear signal loss in the coronary territory associated with the ligated artery. This effect was proven to due to the presence of the targeted contrast agent, since iron oxide nanoparticles are very effective in decreasing signal intensity in T2/T2*-weighted MR images.

In another study, annexin-V was linked to Gd-DTPA coated liposomes with a diameter of 40 nm as a "positive" T1 relaxation marker. MRI experiments in the isolated rat heart revealed that after acute myocardial infarction followed by reperfusion, this contrast agent allows for the specific detec-

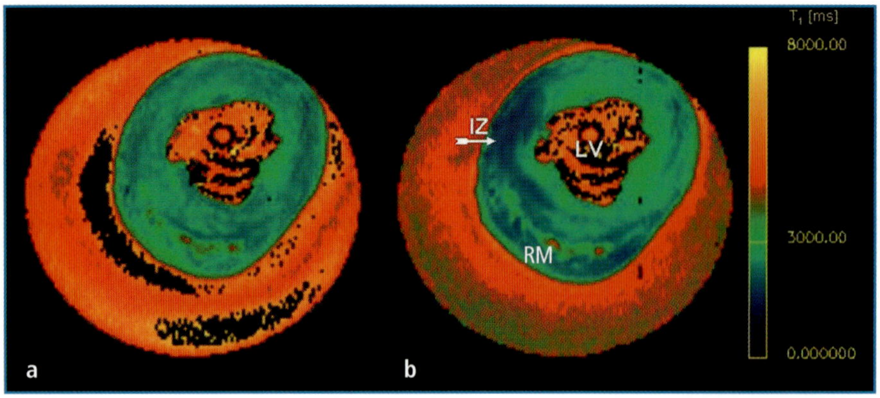

Figure 23-8 T1 maps representing an isolated rat heart (short-axis view) after left coronary occlusion followed by reperfusion before **(a)** and post **(b)** Gd-annexin V infusion. IZ: ischemic zone; LV: left ventricle; RM: remote myocardium (control area).

tion of apoptosis (Figure 23-8). In contrast to the remote myocardium the T1 time was shortened by this targeted contrast agent in the ischemic region (Hiller 2006).

23.5 Conclusions and Future Perspectives

An impressive arsenal of cardiac MRI and MRS at field strengths of 1.5 T up to 17.6 T have been adopted from human protocols and successfully applied for applications in rodents including the estimation of LV size and wall thickness, global and regional LV function, perfusion, and late enhancement infarction imaging. The non-invasive and quantitative nature of MRI makes it an ideal tool for phenotyping transgenic mice models, which is so far only hampered by its relatively high costs, complexity and limited availability.

Wishes for the future include:

- realtime CMRI in rodents,
- high throughput screening and cardiac phenotyping of large quantities of living transgenic mice, and
- finally more effcient targeted contrast agents with much higher relaxivity for molecular MRI.

References

Aletras AH, Ding S, Balaban RS, Wen H. DENSE: displacement encoding with stimulated echoes in cardiac functional MRI. J Magn Reson 1999; 137 (1): 247–52.

Anderson SA, Rader RK, Westlin WF et al. Magnetic resonance contrast enhancement of neovasculature with alpha(v)beta(3)-targeted nanoparticles. Magn Reson Med 2000; 44 (3): 433–9.

Axel L, Dougherty L. Heart wall motion: improved method of spatial modulation of magnetization for MR imaging. Radiology 1989; 172 (2): 349–50.

Brau ACS, Wheeler CT, Hedlund LW, Johnson GA. Fiber-optic stethoscope: a cardiac monitoring and gating system for magnetic resonance microscopy. Magn Reson Med 2002; 47 (2): 314–21.

Brockmann MA, Kemmling A, Groden C. Current issues and perspectives in small rodent magnetic resonance imaging using clinical MRI scanners. Methods 2007; 43 (1): 79–87.

Cassidy PJ, Schneider JE, Grieve SM et al. Assessment of motion gating strategies for mouse magnetic resonance at high magnetic fields. J Magn Reson Imaging 2004; 19 (2): 229–37.

Cochet H, Montaudon M, Laurent F et al. In vivo MR angiography and velocity measurement in mice coronary arteries at 9.4 T: assessment of coronary flow velocity reserve. Radiology 2010; 254 (2): 441–8.

Cunningham CH, Arai T, Yang PC et al. Positive contrast magnetic resonance imaging of cells labeled with magnetic nanoparticles. Magn Reson Med 2005; 53 (5): 999–1005.

Dardzinski BJ, Schmithorst VJ, Holland SK et al. MR imaging of murine arthritis using ultrasmall superparamagnetic iron oxide particles. Magn Reson Imaging 2001; 19 (9): 1209–16.

Detre JA, Leigh JS, Williams DS, Koretsky AP. Perfusion imaging. Magn Reson Med 1992; 23 (1): 37–45.

Epstein FH, Yang Z, Gilson WD et al. MR tagging early after myocardial infarction in mice demonstrates contractile dysfunction in adjacent and remote regions. Magn Reson Med 2002; 48 (2): 399–403.

Feintuch A, Ruengsakulrach P, Lin A et al. Hemodynamics in the mouse aortic arch as assessed by MRI, ultrasound, and numerical modeling. Am J Physiol Heart Circ Physiol 2007; 292 (2): H884–H92.

Fishbein KW, McConville P, Spencer RG. The lever-coil: a simple, inexpensive sensor for respiratory and cardiac motion in MRI experiments. Magn Reson Imaging 2001; 19 (6): 881–9.

Franco F, Dubois SK, Peshock RM, Shohet RV. Magnetic resonance imaging accurately estimates LV mass in a transgenic mouse model of cardiac hypertrophy. Am J Physiol 1998; 274 (2 Pt 2): H679–H83.

Franco F, Thomas GD, Giroir B et al. Magnetic resonance imaging and invasive evaluation of development of heart failure in transgenic mice with myocardial expression of tumor necrosis factor-alpha. Circulation 1999; 99 (3): 448–54.

Gareis D, Wichmann T, Lanz T et al. Mouse MRI using phased-array coils. NMR Biomed 2007; 20 (3): 326–34.

Gilson WD, Yang Z, French BA, Epstein FH. Measurement of myocardial mechanics in mice before and after infarction using multislice displacement-encoded MRI with 3D motion encoding. Am J Physiol Heart Circ Physiol 2005; 288 (3): H1491–H7.

Gilson WD, Yang Z, French BA, Epstein FH. Complementary displacement-encoded MRI for contrast-enhanced infarct detection and quantification of myocardial function in mice. Magn Reson Med 2004; 51 (4): 744–52.

Haase A, Odoj F, von Kienlin M et al. NMR probeheads for in vivo applications. Concepts Magn Res 2000; 12: 361–88.

Herold V, Mörchel P, Faber C et al. In vivo quantitative three-dimensional motion mapping of the murine myocardium with PC-MRI at 17.6 T. Magn Reson Med 2006; 55 (5): 1058–64.

Herold V, Parczyk M, Mörchel P et al. In vivo measurement of local aortic pulse-wave velocity in mice with MR microscopy at 17.6 T. Magn Reson Med 2009; 61 (6): 1293–9.

Herold V, Wellen J, Ziener CH et al. In vivo comparison of atherosclerotic plaque progression with vessel wall strain and blood flow velocity in apoE$^{(-/-)}$ mice with MR microscopy at 17.6 T. MAGMA 2009; 22 (3): 159–66.

Hiller K-H, Waller C, Nahrendorf M et al. Assessment of cardiovascular apoptosis in the isolated rat heart by magnetic resonance molecular imaging. Mol Imaging 2006; 5 (2): 115–21.

Hoit BD. New approaches to phenotypic analysis in adult mice. J Mol Cell Cardiol 2001; 33 (1): 27–35.

Hu TC-C, Bao W, Lenhard SC et al. Simultaneous assessment of left-ventricular infarction size, function and tissue viability in a murine model of myocardial infarction by cardiac manganese-enhanced magnetic resonance imaging (MEMRI). NMR Biomed 2004; 17 (8): 620–6.

Itskovich VV, Samber DD, Mani V et al. Quantification of human atherosclerotic plaques using spatially enhanced cluster analysis of multi-contrast-weighted magnetic resonance images. Magn Reson Med 2004; 52 (3): 515–23.

Jaffer FA, Tung CH, Houng AK et al. MRI of blood coagulation factor XIII activity using a novel derivatized caged iron oxide nanoparticle (F13-CLIO). Mol Imaging 2002; 1: 217–8.

Kober F, Iltis I, Cozzone PJ, Bernard M. Myocardial blood flow mapping in mice using high-resolution spin labeling magnetic resonance imaging: influence of ketamine/xylazine and isoflurane anesthesia. Magn Reson Med 2005; 53 (3): 601–6.

Lemieux SK, Glover GH. An infrared device for monitoring the respiration of small rodents during magnetic resonance imaging. J Magn Reson Imaging 1996; 6 (3): 561–4.

Maestri R, Milia AF, Salis MB et al. Cardiac hypertrophy and microvascular deficit in kinin B2 receptor knockout mice. Hypertension 2003; 41 (5): 1151–5.

Manning WJ, Wei JY, Fossel ET, Burstein D. Measurement of left ventricular mass in rats using electrocardiogram-gated magnetic resonance imaging. Am J Physiol 1990; 258 (4 Pt 2): H1181–H6.

McKibben CK, Reo NV. A piezoelectric respiratory monitor for in vivo NMR. Magn Reson Med 1992; 27 (2): 338–42.

Minard KR, Wind RA, Phelps RL. A compact respiratory-triggering device for routine microimaging of laboratory mice. J Magn Reson Imaging 1998; 8 (6): 1343–8.

Mohiaddin RH, Firmin DN, Longmore DB. Age-related changes of human aortic flow wave velocity measured non-invasively by magnetic resonance imaging. J Appl Physiol 1993; 74 (1): 492–7.

Nahrendorf M, Hiller K-H, Hu K et al. Cardiac magnetic resonance imaging in small animal models of human heart failure. Med Image Anal 2003a; 7 (3): 369–75.

Nahrendorf M, Hu K, Fraccarollo D et al. Time course of right ventricular remodeling in rats with experimental myocardial infarction. Am J Physiol Heart Circ Physiol 2003b; 284 (1): H241–H8.

Nahrendorf M, Streif JU, Hiller KH et al. Multi-modal functional cardiac MRI in creatine kinase-deficient mice reveals subtle abnormalities in myocardial perfusion and mechanics. Am J Physiol Heart Circ Physiol 2006; 290 (6): H2516–H21.

Parzy E, Miraux S, Franconi J-M, Thiaudière E. In vivo quantification of blood velocity in mouse carotid and pulmonary arteries by ECG-triggered 3D time-resolved magnetic resonance angiography. NMR Biomed 2009; 22 (5): 532–7.

Pratten MK, Lloyd JB. Pinocytosis and phagocytosis: the effect of size of a particulate substrate on its mode of capture by rat peritoneal macrophages cultured in vitro. Biochim Biophys Acta 1986; 881 (3): 307–13.

Rommel E, Kuhstrebe J, Wiesmann F et al. A double trigger unit for ECG and breath triggered mouse heart imaging. MAGMA 2000; 11: 250–5.

Rudin M, Pedersen B, Umemura K, Zierhut W. Determination of rat heart morphology and function in vivo in two models of cardiac hypertrophy by means of magnetic resonance imaging. Basic Res Cardiol 1991; 86 (2): 165–74.

Ruehm SG, Corot C, Vogt P et al. Magnetic resonance imaging of atherosclerotic plaque with ultrasmall superparamagnetic particles of iron oxide in hyperlipidemic rabbits. Circulation 2001; 103 (3): 415–22.

Ruff J, Wiesmann F, Hiller KH et al. Influence of isoflurane anesthesia on contractility of mouse heart in vivo. MAGMA 1998a; 6: 169–75.

Ruff J, Wiesmann F, Hiller KH et al. Magnetic resonance microimaging for non-invasive quantification of myocardial function and mass in the mouse. Magn Reson Med 1998b; 40 (1): 43–8.

Simonetti OP, Kim RJ, Fieno DS et al. An improved MR imaging technique for the visualization of myocardial infarction. Radiology 2001; 218 (1): 215–23.

Siri FM, Jelicks LA, Leinwand LA, Gardin JM. Gated magnetic resonance imaging of normal and hypertrophied murine hearts. Am J Physiol 1997; 272 (5 Pt 2): H2394–H402.

Slawson SE, Roman BB, Williams DS, Koretsky AP. Cardiac MRI of the normal and hypertrophied mouse heart. Magn Reson Med 1998; 39 (6): 980–7.

Sosnovik DE, Schellenberger EA, Nahrendorf M et al. Magnetic resonance imaging of cardiomyocyte apoptosis with a novel magneto-optical nanoparticle. Magn Reson Med 2005; 54 (3): 718–24.

Streif JUG, Herold V, Szimtenings M et al. In vivo time-resolved quantitative motion mapping of the murine myocardium with phase contrast MRI. Magn Reson Med 2003; 49 (2): 315–21.

Streif JUG, Nahrendorf M, Hiller K-H et al. In vivo assessment of absolute perfusion and intracapillary blood volume in the murine myocardium by spin labeling magnetic resonance imaging. Magn Reson Med 2005; 53 (3): 584–92.

Stuber M, Fischer SE, Scheidegger MB, Boesiger P. Toward high-resolution myocardial tagging. Magn Reson Med 1999; 41 (3): 639–43.

Vulliémoz S, Stergiopoulos N, Meuli R. Estimation of local aortic elastic properties with MRI. Magn Reson Med 2002; 47 (4): 649–54.

Waller C, Hiller K-H, Kahler E et al. Serial magnetic resonance imaging of microvascular remodeling in the infarcted rat heart. Circulation 2001; 103 (11): 1564–9.

Waller C, Hiller K-H, Pfaff D et al. Functional mechanisms of myocardial microcirculation in left ventricular hypertrophy: a hypothetical model of capillary remodeling post-myocardial infarction. Microvasc Res 2008; 75 (1): 104–11.

Waller C, Kahler E, Hiller K-H et al. Myocardial perfusion and intracapillary blood volume in rats at rest and with coronary dilatation: MR imaging in vivo with use of a spin-labeling technique. Radiology 2000; 215 (1): 189–97.

Wang Y, Rossman PJ, Grimm RC et al. Navigator-echo-based real-time respiratory gating and triggering for reduction of respiration effects in three-dimensional coronary MR angiography. Radiology 1996; 198 (1): 55–60.

Wiesmann F, Frydrychowicz A, Rautenberg J et al. Analysis of right ventricular function in healthy mice and a murine model of heart failure by in vivo MRI. Am J Physiol Heart Circ Physiol 2002; 283 (3): H1065–H71.

Wiesmann F, Ruff J, Engelhardt S et al. Dobutamine-stress magnetic resonance microimaging in mice: acute changes of cardiac geometry and function in normal and failing murine hearts. Circ Res 2001; 88 (6): 563–9.

Wiesmann F, Ruff J, Hiller K-H et al. Developmental changes of cardiac function and mass assessed with MRI in neonatal, juvenile, and adult mice. Am J Physiol Heart Circ Physiol 2000; 278 (2): H652–H7.

Winter PM, Caruthers SD, Kassner A et al. Molecular imaging of angiogenesis in nascent Vx-2 rabbit tumors using a novel alpha(nu)beta3-targeted nanoparticle and 1.5 T magnetic resonance imaging. Cancer Res 2003; 63 (18): 5838–43.

Winter PM, Morawski AM, Caruthers SD et al. Molecular imaging of angiogenesis in early-stage atherosclerosis with alpha(v) beta3-integrin-targeted nanoparticles. Circulation 2003; 108 (18): 2270–4.

Zhao X, Pratt R, Wansapura J. Quantification of aortic compliance in mice using radial phase contrast MRI. J Magn Reson Imaging 2009; 30 (2): 286–91.

Zhou R, Pickup S, Glickson JD et al. Assessment of global and regional myocardial function in the mouse using cine and tagged MRI. Magn Reson Med 2003; 49 (4): 760–4.

24 Cardiac Magnetic Resonance Spectroscopy

Cameron Holloway, Kieran Clarke and Stefan Neubauer[1]

24.1 Introduction

Significant advances in cardiac magnetic resonance imaging (MRI) over the last decade have allowed this technique to become established and routinely used in clinical cardiology and research. The signal obtained in MRI comes from a single nucleus, ^{1}H, contained in both water (H_2O) and fat (-CH_2 and -CH_3). In contrast, cardiac magnetic resonance spectroscopy (MRS) is a multi-nuclear technique, where signals can be obtained from a variety of other biologically interesting nuclei that have the property of nuclear spin, i.e. they have an odd number of protons, neutrons, or both. MRS is the only known method that allows the non-invasive study of myocardial metabolism without the external administration of radioactive tracer molecules (as in positron emission tomography). Table 24-1 shows an overview of the atomic nuclei that can be detected using MRS. Those of particular importance in metabolic imaging include: ^{1}H, ^{13}C, ^{23}Na and ^{31}P. Although ^{31}P has been most extensively used, ^{1}H- and novel ^{13}C-hyperpolarisation techniques are rapidly expanding areas in MRS.

A technique to non-invasively assess cardiac metabolism would provide a powerful tool in clinical cardiac imaging, however MRS has not yet fulfilled this role. The two fundamental limitations that have prevented widespread clinical applications are the relatively low concentrations of metabolites, which are many orders of magnitude lower than the ^{1}H-nuclei of water and fat molecules (Table 24-1) and the low sensitivity of the nuclei compared to the signal from ^{1}H obtained in MRI. Overcoming these physical limitations is necessary before MRS can become a clinically useful tool. The direct consequence is that, while in principle, MR spectroscopy of the human heart can be performed, the spatial and temporal resolution of MRS is many times lower than that of MRI. Whilst cardiac MRS can provide multinuclear metabolic assessment, high resolution imaging is not currently possible and therefore has not become established in clinical cardiology. Future advances (see below) may eventually allow this to be achieved.

Since the first recorded ^{31}P-MR spectrum from an isolated perfused heart by the Radda's group in 1977, MRS has become a well-established method in experimental cardiology and numerous studies have reported various aspects of myocardial metabolism with this method. An introduction to the experimental applications of MRS is important for a clinical textbook, as it can be used to explain basic principles

1 Acknowledgment: The thanks of the authors go to a variety of colleagues of the last 10 years: Meinrad Beer, Andrew Blamire, Lowri Cochlin, Jennifer Crilley, Sairia Dass, Yaso Emmanuel, Jane Francis, Lucy Hudsmith, Andy Johnson, Saul Myerson, Matthew Robson, George Radda, Chris Rodgers, Juergen Schneider, Michaela Schuermann-Freestone, Joseph Suttie, Peter Styles, Damian Tyler, Matthias Spindler, Hugh Watkins, Frank Wiesmann.

Table 24-1 Nuclei of interest for MRS examination of the myocardium.

Nucleus	Natural abundance	Relative MR sensitivity	Myocardial tissue concentrations	Relative signal intensity compared to H_2O
^{1}H	99.98 %	1	H_2O: 110 M, up to ~ 90 mM	1:1,200
^{31}P	100 %	0.066	PCr: up to ~ 20 mM	1:80,000
^{13}C	1.1 %	0.016	^{13}C-labeled compounds: several mM	1:100,000,000
^{23}Na	100 %	0.093	intracellular: ~ 11 mM extracellular: 140 mM	1:100,000

used to define experimental research findings. Additionally, it illustrates the considerable potential of the method for future clinical applications, should the technical limitations of MRS be overcome.

24.2 Physics of MR Spectroscopy

The nucleus that has been most commonly examined in MR spectroscopy is ^{31}P, with a considerable amount of work performed on animal models, specifically using isolated buffer-perfused rat heart. The basic principles of MRS (the physical principles are described in much greater detail, for example, by Gadian 1995) can be explained using ^{31}P-MRS of the isolated heart model as an example. However, the same fundamental principles also apply to other nuclei. In MRS experiments, an MR spectrometer is required, which consists of a high-field superconducting magnet in a vertical or horizontal position, with a bore diameter of between 5 cm and 1 m. The magnet strength is currently up to 7 T in a clinical setting and 18 T for pre-clinical studies. The bore of the magnet contains a nucleus-specific probe, or radiofrequency (RF) coil, which allows a RF pulse to excite the nuclear spins, and receives MRS signals. The experiment is controlled by a central computer, which also controls the gradients of the magnet, the radiofrequency transmitters and receivers. In an MRS experiment, the magnetic field is first homogenised with the help of so-called shim gradients ("shimming"). Shimming is particularly important in MRS, compared with conventional MR imaging, because MRS places higher demands on field homogeneity than MRI. To excite the nuclei under examination, a signal (RF pulse) with a specific radiofrequency (dependent on the field strength) is transmitted to the heart through the RF coil. The resulting MR signal, the free induction decay (FID), is then digitally stored. The FID describes the relationship between time and signal intensity, and typically shows an exponential signal decay over time. Following the acquisition of the FID, signal is converted using a mathematical manipulation, the "Fourier transformation", into an MR spectrum. This spectrum describes the relationship between resonance frequency and signal intensity, allowing quantification of metabolites. One of the major limitations of MRS is its low sensitivity, and therefore a large number of FIDs must be recorded to obtain an MR spectrum with a sufficient signal-to-noise ratio (SNR).

The **number of acquisitions required** (signal averaging) for sufficient signal depends on several factors, including:

- the concentration of the metabolite in the organ being studied,
- the "filling factor" (calculated as the mass of the investigated object size relative to the coil),
- the natural occurrence of the investigated isotope,
- the relative MR sensitivity of the metabolite (Table 24-1),
- the flip angle and
- the pulse repetition time (TR).

For an experiment on perfused rat hearts, at 7–12 T, typically 104–200 FIDs are recorded to obtain sufficient signal. In MRS, when selecting pulse angles and repetition times, the effects of partial saturation of different spin populations (resonances) have to be considered: a full (unsaturated) MR signal of a particular nucleus is only available if the nucleus is excited from a fully relaxed state, that is, if time of at least 5 × T1 has passed since the last signal excitation (for example, the T1 of phosphocreatine at 7 T is about 3 s so a TR of at least 15 is needed and the T1 of phosphocreatine at 1.5 T approximately 4.4 s so a TR of 22 is required). Fully relaxed spectra can therefore only be obtained for long TR times, resulting in impractically long acquisition times. However, the FID is an exponential signal intensity drop, so most information can be acquired at the beginning of the FID. Shorter TR can produce spectra with higher SNR's for a given acquisition time, however, part of the signal is lost in these spectra by saturation effects (partially saturated spectra). Because the T1 times of ^{31}P-metabolites, such as phosphocreatine and ATP, are significantly different (the T1 of phosphocreatine is about 2–3 times longer than the T1 of

ATP), the degree of partial saturation of different ^{31}P-resonances also varies. Therefore, a correction factor must be applied for the partially saturated spectra. These factors are determined individually for each metabolite by comparing fully relaxed and partially saturated spectra. In practice, TR times and flip angles are chosen to achieve acceptable measurement times at 20–50 % saturation of the phosphocreatine resonance.

Figure 24-1 shows a typical ^{31}P-spectrum of an isolated beating rat heart, recorded in 5 min at 7 T, with a TR of 1.93 s and a flip angle of 45°. The ^{31}P-spectrum shows resonances corresponding to the three ^{31}P-nuclei of ATP (γ, α and β), phosphocreatine (PCr), inorganic phosphate (Pi) and monophosphate esters (MPE). Although the heart muscle contains significantly more ^{31}P-metabolites, further ^{31}P-resonances are not visible, because ^{31}P-nuclei concentrations must be above a certain threshold (about 0.6 mM) and be free in solution to be measurable. In contrast, immobile ^{31}P-metabolites, for example the phosphates bound to the cell membrane, do not have a measurable MR signal due to their very short T2 times, such metabolites contribute only to the broad "baseline hump" of ^{31}P-spectra. In MR spectroscopy the term "chemical shift" describes the phenomenon whereby different metabolites resonate at different frequencies and so can be distinguished from each other. The "chemical shift" is quantified in parts per million (ppm) and displayed on the x-axis of a spectrum (as in Figure 24-1). The physical explanation for this chemical shift phenomenon, which leads to spreading of the resonance frequencies, is that different nuclei within a molecule (e.g. γ-, α- and β-ATP) behave differently depending on the interaction with their surrounding chemical environment, which slightly alters the local magnetic field strength. Metabolites in a ^{31}P-spectrum are seen over a range of about 30 ppm.

In animal ^{31}P-MRS experiments quantification of intracellular pH is possible using the chemical shift between the position of inorganic phosphate, which is pH sensitive, relative to phosphocreatine. After saturation correction, experimental quantification of ^{31}P-spectra is performed by determining the area under each resonance, which is directly proportional to the amount of each ^{31}P-nucleus in the body, and therefore individual resonances are quantified by the integration of their area. This is typically achieved with the help of "Lorentzian line fit" algorithms. Relative metabolite concentrations can be calculated directly via these algorithms (the ratio of phosphocreatine/ATP). Determination of absolute concentrations of phosphorus metabolites is possible *in vivo* only by comparison of the resonances with those of an external ^{31}P-concentration standard. The most commonly used standard for this purpose is phenylphosphonate, which produces an additional resonance in the ^{31}P-spectrum. Given the challenges with measuring absolute metabolite concentrations in humans, relative levels are more often assessed in practice.

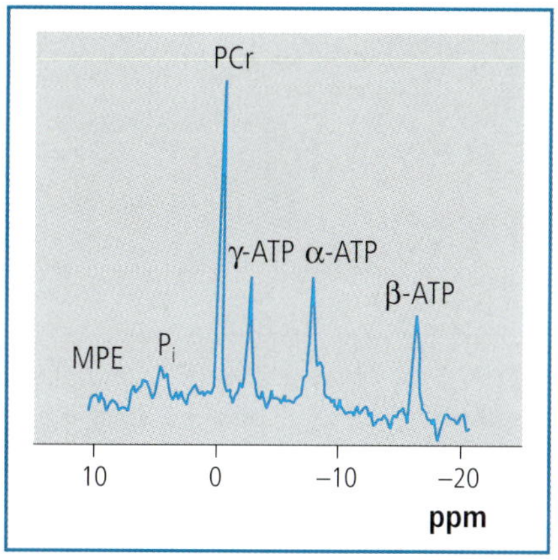

Figure 24-1 ^{31}P-MR spectrum of an isolated buffer-perfused rat heart, recorded in 5 min at 7 T. ATP: adenosine triphosphate; MPE: monophosphate esters; PCr: phosphocreatine; P_i: inorganic phosphate.

A key advantage of MRS is the non-invasive nature of the method. This is in contrast to destructive methods used to obtain the same data, as occurs in traditional biochemical assays in which the tissues must be extracted and frozen. Given MRS is non-destructive, serial spectral acquisitions are possible, allowing for sequential determination of myocardial energy metabolism in experimental and clinical settings. This becomes important when determining the effect of substrate supply to the heart or to monitor the effect of hypoxia or inotropic stimulation during an experiment. In contrast to wet chemical analysis, each heart can be used as its own control and therefore the number of experiments required for a protocol is drastically reduced.

Most clinical MRS studies have been carried out at a field strength of 1.5 T, although recent studies have included work at 3 T, with a 2-fold better SNR for spectra at the higher field strength, bringing clinical applications closer to reality. Overall, there is promise of better sensitivity with the emergence of even higher field strength magnets, such as 7 T.

24.3 Experimental Studies

24.3.1 ^{31}P-MRS Studies

^{31}P-MRS allows the continuous study of myocardial energy metabolism during an experiment (see above regarding the metabolites seen in a ^{31}P-spectrum). ATP is the fuel for all energy consuming reactions in the cell, whereas phosphocreatine (PCr), the other major energy-rich phosphate compound, serves as a reservoir of energy.

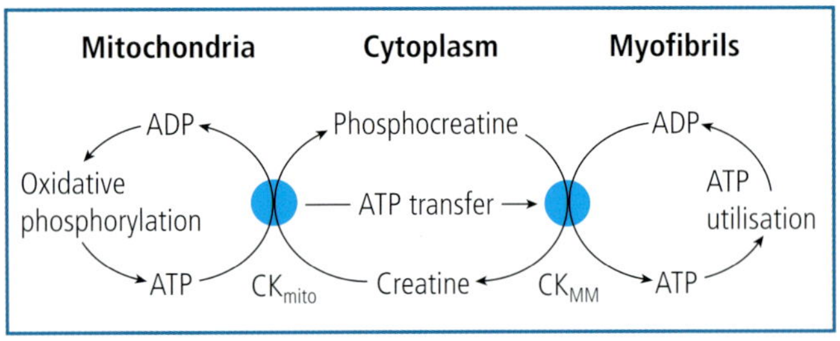

Figure 24-2 Creatine kinase – phosphocreatine energy transport mechanism ("energy shuttle"). Details are described in the text. ADP: adenosine diphosphate; ATP: adenosine triphosphate.

PCr has at least **two additional functions**:

- Phosphocreatine serves as an energy transport molecule in the creatine kinase/phosphocreatine "energy shuttle" (Neubauer 2007; Figure 24-2). A high-energy phosphate bond is transferred to ADP to form ATP within the mitochondria. This high energy phosphate bond can then be transferred from ATP to creatine, where phosphocreatine and ADP are formed. This reaction is catalyzed by the mitochondrial isoenzyme of creatine kinase. Phosphocreatine, a much smaller molecule than ATP, then diffuses through the cytosol to the sites of ATP utilization, especially the myofibrils, where the reverse reaction occurs and ATP is consumed for contraction. This reaction is catalyzed by the myofibril-bound MM-creatine kinase isoenzyme. The free creatine then diffuses back to the mitochondria. This "energy shuttle" is essential for cells with high energy consumption, because the low concentration of free cytosolic ADP (40–80 μM) is insufficient to provide adequate diffusion capacity back to mitochondria, whereas free creatine concentrations are at least two orders of magnitude higher than free ADP.
- The second crucial cellular function of phosphocreatine and creatine kinase is to keep the free cytosolic ADP concentration low. The concentration of free ADP cannot be determined directly, but can be calculated using the creatine kinase equilibrium equation:

  $$\text{ADP} = \frac{([\text{ATP}] \times [\text{creatine}])}{([\text{phosphocreatine}] \times [\text{H}^+]\ \text{Keq})}$$

  ADP concentrations are therefore also related to the intracellular hydrogen ion concentrations and the equilibrium constant, Keq, of the creatine kinase reaction.

A low free cytosolic ADP concentration is essential for the maintenance of normal contractile function, since ADP directly determines the free energy of ATP hydrolysis (ΔG, kJ/mol), which is a measure of the energy that is released on ATP hydrolysis:

$$\Delta G_{ATP} = \Delta G_0 + RT \ln (\text{ADP} \times \text{inorganic phosphate}) / \text{ATP}.$$

ΔG_0 is the standard free energy at 37 °C and $[Mg^{2+}]$ of 1 mM. R is the universal gas constant and T is the temperature [K]. Normally ΔG is in the order of −58 kJ/mol. Various intracellular enzymes, such as the SR-Ca^{2+}-ATPase stop functioning if the ΔG is below a certain threshold of about −52 kJ/mol.

Inorganic phosphate is formed in the hydrolysis of ATP: ATP ⟷ ADP + Pi. Inorganic phosphate accumulation occurs when ATP hydrolysis exceeds ATP utilization, which happens, for example, during ischemia.

^{31}P-MRS has found widespread applications in investigations of myocardial energy metabolism under different pathophysiological conditions. In the isolated perfused heart, the effects of perfusion with various metabolic substrates can be investigated. For example, phosphocreatine concentrations are higher when hearts are perfused with pyruvate and/or free fatty acids as substrates, or with blood (PCr/ATP ratio ~ 1.5–2.0), than for perfusion with glucose as the sole substrate (PCr/ATP ratio ~ 1.3; Ingwall 1982). ATP remains stable over a wide range of cardiac loads, as the equilibrium constant of the creatine kinase reaction favours ATP synthesis over phosphocreatine synthesis by a factor of approximately 100. This is why in all forms of myocardial stress, including ischemia, ATP remains constant initially, but phosphocreatine decreases. Therefore, the PCr/ATP ratio is a sensitive indicator of the energy state of the myocardium. The PCr/ATP ratio has been used in numerous ^{31}P-MRS studies to examine changes in myocardial energy metabolism during ischemia and reperfusion (e.g. Clarke 1987). In addition to studies on ischemic heart, hypoxia/reperfusion studies can be carried out on isolated perfused heart. These complement studies of ischemia, as only the oxygen supply is interrupted, while maintaining perfusion and substrate supply. Figure 24-3 shows an example of changes in cardiac energy metabolism during a control phase, hypoxia and reoxygenation: after 30 min of hypoxia, the ATP resonance is at ~ 50 % of the starting value and phosphocreatine is reduced to ~ 80 %, with accumulation of inorganic phosphate. During reoxygenation there is complete recovery of inorganic phosphate, partial restoration of phosphocreatine content, while ATP does not recover. We have shown (Neubauer 1989) that, when hearts are pre-treated with a calcium antagonist, attenuation of these changes in energy metabolism occurs: verapamil protects the heart against the effects of the hypoxic insult. An important experimental study by Clarke et al. (1987) showed that changes in energy metabolism occurred very fast after the onset of ischemia. The decrease in phosphocreatine and the increase of inorganic phosphate were among the earliest metabolic changes during myocardial ischemia, which occurred even seconds after the start of ischemia, while the changes of ATP and intracellular pH were observed later, within minutes. This study described summation of individual spectra, where a temporal resolution of 12 s was achieved, demonstrating that

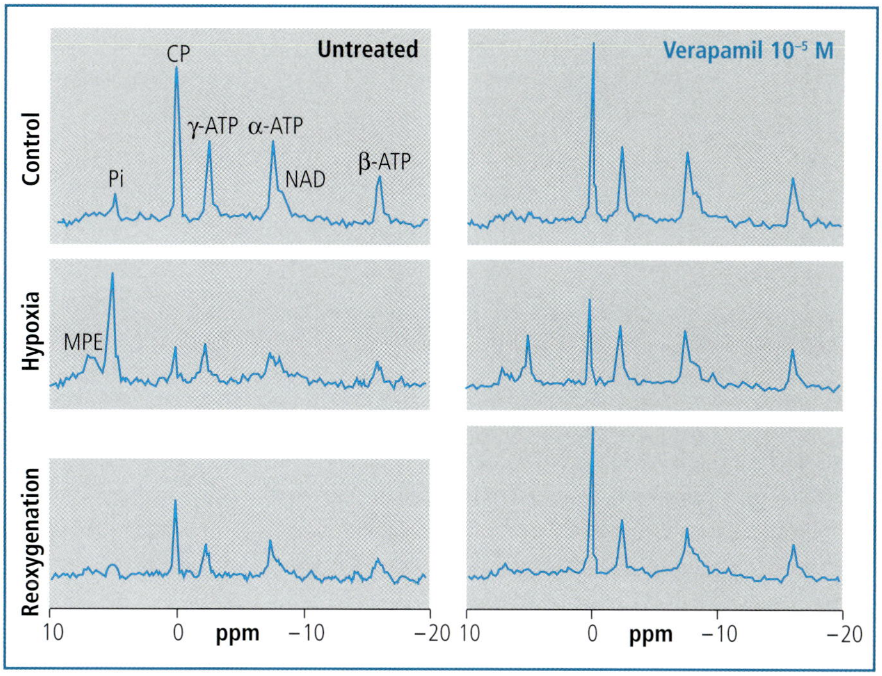

Figure 24-3 ^{31}P-MR spectra of an untreated perfused rat heart and a heart that has been pre-treated with verapamil (control phase, after 30 min hypoxia and after 30 min reoxygenation). Further details in the text. ATP: adenosine triphosphate; CP: creatine phosphate, synonymous with phosphocreatine; MPE: monophosphate ester; NAD: nicotine adenine dinucleotide; Pi: inorganic phosphate (modified from Neubauer and Ingwall 1989).

if it were possible to detect changes in energy metabolism in the human heart with high temporal and spatial resolution, we would be able to detect myocardial ischemia using metabolic imaging within seconds after its inception. Currently this is not possible using any diagnostic method.

^{31}P-MRS technology has the ability to directly determine the rate and speed of chemical reactions *in vivo*, for which the saturation transfer (or magnetization transfer) method is used (e.g. Neubauer 1995). This method is suitable to use on the heart, to quantify the creatine kinase and ATP synthesis reactions. Bittl et al. (1985) showed that the velocity of the creatine kinase reaction, a parameter for the extent of the ATP transfer from the mitochondria to the myofibrils, correlated closely with cardiac work. During reperfusion after ischemia, we showed (Neubauer 1988) the creatine kinase reaction rate correlated closely with the recovery of mechanical function. This could have important applications in human heart, especially in heart disease (see below).

Experimental ^{31}P-MRS studies have contributed significantly to the understanding of the role of energy metabolism in heart failure. Various experimental models of heart failure have been studied, including the hypertensive rat, the Syrian cardiomyopathic hamster, furazolidone-induced cardiomyopathy and, as the clinically most relevant model, chronic coronary artery ligation in the rat and the pig heart. The myocardium in heart failure is chronically energy deficient, regardless of the etiology, and this manifests as a characteristic phenotype: reduced phosphocreatine concentrations and unchanged or slightly reduced (up to 30% less) ATP levels. Additionally inorganic phosphate remains unchanged or slightly increased, and significantly impaired creatine kinase kinetics is observed. Furthermore, the total creatine content is reduced (in order to maintain the ΔG_{ATP}, as is the mitochondrial creatine kinase activity), while fetal BB-and MB-creatine kinase isoenzymes increase. These changes may contribute to the reduction of contractile reserve in heart failure, presumably by the inability of the failing heart to maintain high ΔG_{ATP} values during inotropic stimulation. Horn and colleagues (2001) clearly demonstrated a causal role of energy metabolism in the chronically failing rat heart. They found that after treating rats with a creatine analogue (β-guanidinopropionate) for 2 mths, phosphocreatine was depleted by 85%, as measured by ^{31}P-MRS. Under these conditions, rats with chronically impaired energy metabolism were not capable of maintaining normal ATP levels, which was not the case for infarcted control hearts not treated with β-guanidinopropionate. Interestingly, pre-treatment with β-guanidinopropionate (pre-depletion of phosphocreatine levels before coronary ligation) led to 100% 24h mortality after myocardial infarction, in comparison with standard 40% mortality in this model. These results show that failing hearts with massively depleted phosphocreatine levels cannot maintain normal ATP metabolism and that high levels of phosphocreatine are needed to survive the stress of acute myocardial infarction. This demonstrates the important role of the creatine kinase/phosphocreatine systems for acute and chronic myocardial stress. Results of such experimental ^{31}P-MRS investigations led directly to clinical ^{31}P-MRS studies on human heart failure (see below).

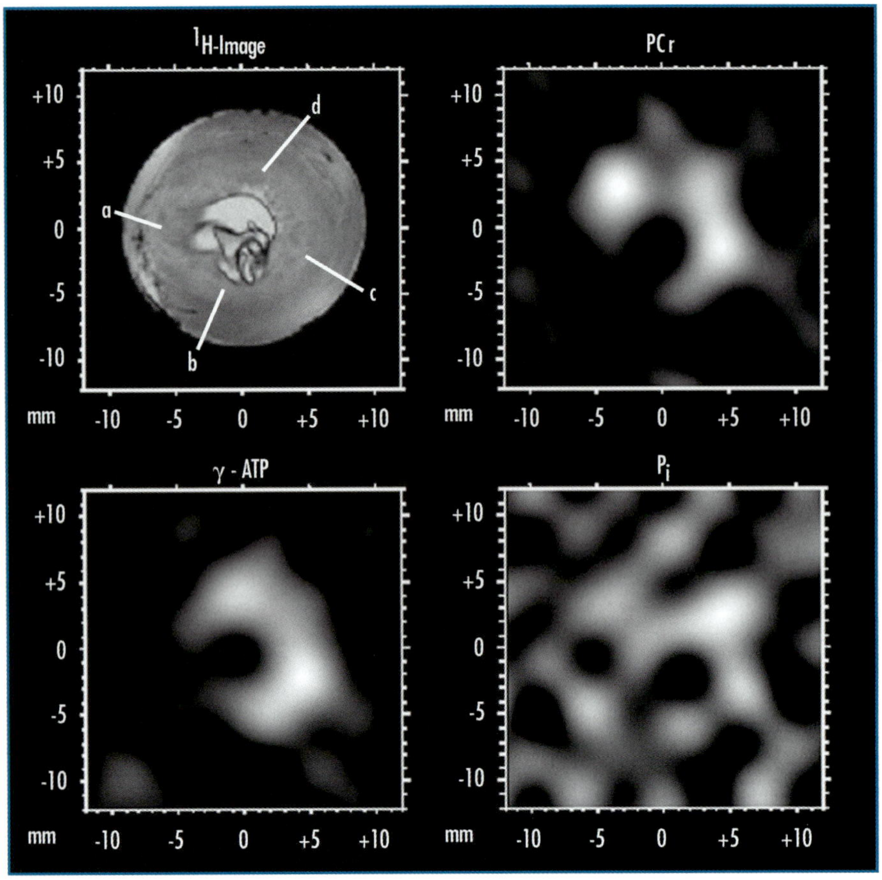

Figure 24-4 Midequatorial layer of a 3D ^{31}P-chemical shift imaging experiment on the isolated, chronically infarcted rat heart (12 T, nominal voxel size 54 μl). The ^{1}H-image above **(top left)** shows little contrast for the infarcted area in the anterior wall (a), compared to normal myocardium (b–d). The ^{31}P-metabolite images show, however, the infarcted area as an area of complete signal loss phosphocreatine (PCr) **(top right)** and γ-ATP **(bottom left)**. Inorganic phosphate (Pi) cannot be depicted with sufficient resolution due to its low concentration **(bottom right)** (from Kienlin et al. Magn Reson Med 1998; 39: 731–41; with permission of John Wiley and Sons, New York).

Most of the early experimental ^{31}P-MRS studies in animals did not use additional localization techniques, with surface coils providing only rough localization of the area of interest. However 2D and 3D localized spectroscopic imaging techniques now allow a non-invasive measurement of regional heterogeneity of myocardial energy metabolism (Figure 24-4). For example, on large animals (dogs and pigs) Zhang et al. (1995) showed that with ^{31}P-MRS it is possible to obtain different spectra within layers of the myocardial wall, from endocardium to epicardium, allowing assessment of the transmural heterogeneity of energy metabolism. These studies indicated that during myocardial stress, energetic changes are more pronounced in the subendocardium compared with the epicardium.

24.3.2 Other MRS-Detectable Nuclei (^{1}H, ^{13}C, ^{23}Na)

The **^{1}H-MR nucleus** shows the highest sensitivity of all MR detectable nuclei, as well as having a high natural abundance in the body (Table 24-1). In principle, many metabolites can be detected by ^{1}H-MRS, as this nucleus is present in an enormous number of metabolites. The most relevant ^{1}H containing metabolites that can be detected include creatine, lactate, carnitine, taurine and the -CH_3 and -CH_2 resonances in lipids. ^{1}H-MRS has proved to be a robust non-invasive method to detect total creatine content and, when measured in the conjunction with high energy phosphates assessed by ^{31}P-MRS, it provides a more complete assessment of cardiac metabolism, including calculation of free ADP (Bottomley 2001). Furthermore, ^{1}H-MRS can be used to non-invasively measure oxymyoglobin and deoxymyoglobin resonances (tissue oxygen levels). A major consideration when performing ^{1}H-MRS is the use of pulse sequences to suppress the hugely dominant signal from water molecules. Furthermore, the complex ^{1}H-spectrum shows many overlapping resonances, many of which remain to be defined. In addition to determination of creatine levels in the human heart, myocardial lipid levels can be detected, which may be of interest in obesity, diabetes and during dietary intervention studies. The high sensitivity of ^{1}H-MRS means it has substantial potential for clinical applications.

The **^{13}C-nucleus** has a low natural abundance (~ 1%). Therefore, cardiac ^{13}C-MRS experiments must use ^{13}C-labeled substances, such as 1-^{13}C-glucose. These labelled compounds are typically added to the perfusate or directly infused into a coronary artery. Such experiments allow determination of substrate utilisation and enable determination of key enzyme activities or flow through metabolic pathways. For example, the rate of the citric acid cycle, pyruvate dehydrogenase, or the β-oxidation of fatty acids can be determined using ^{13}C-MRS. ^{13}C-studies have investigated intermediary metabolism in animal models of myocardial ischemia and heart failure.

Clinical applications in heart have not yet been reported, owing to **fundamental methodological limitations**, including:

- the sensitivity of ^{13}C-MR nucleus is too small for a practical spatial resolution at a realistic measurement time,
- high concentrations of exogenous ^{13}C-labelled substrates are required, and
- *in vivo* studies require ^{13}C-labeled substances to be directly infused into a coronary artery.

Hyperpolarised ^{13}C-MRS (see below) may offer a solution to these problems.

^{23}Na-MRS is the only non-invasive method to allow the assessment of changes in the intra- and extracellular sodium content during myocardial injury (Kohler 1991). Maintenance of the sarcolemmal Na^+ concentration gradient (~ 140 mM extracellular, compared with ~ 10 mM intracellular) is a fundamental requirement for normal cardiac function. During membrane depolarisation Na^+ enters cardiomyocytes via the fast Na^+ channels and is removed by the sarcolemmal Na^+/K^+-ATPase. The ^{23}Na-spectrum of the heart shows a single resonance, which represents the entire Na^+ signal. A distinction between intra- and extracellular Na^+ pools can be made using "shift reagents", such as (DyTTHA) 3 or (TmDOTP) 5, added to the perfusate. These chelate complexes of high molecular weight distribute in the extracellular space, but cannot cross the cell membrane. Sodium in the immediate vicinity of such shift reagents undergoes a chemical shift of its resonance frequency ("down field"; Figure 24-5). This method has been used experimentally to determine the mechanism of intracellular Na^+ accumulation during ischemia reperfusion and the mechanisms of ventricular fibrillation, which follows an increase in intracellular Na^+ concentrations (Clarke 1998). Although potentially interesting for use in human heart, no studies have reported use of ^{23}Na-MR shift reagents for clinical studies and no such agents are licenced. Experimental MR imaging of the total ^{23}Na-content (not using shift reagents) was first reported by DeLayre et al. (1981). During acute ischemia, an increase in total myocardial ^{23}Na-MRI signal was observed (see above) and there was formation of intra- and extracellular edema. Furthermore, we showed (Horn 2001) that the total Na^+ signal during chronic scar formation after myocardial infarction in the rat model remains elevated, as there is an expansion of the extracellular space within the scar (Figure 24-5), and the area of increased ^{23}Na-signal

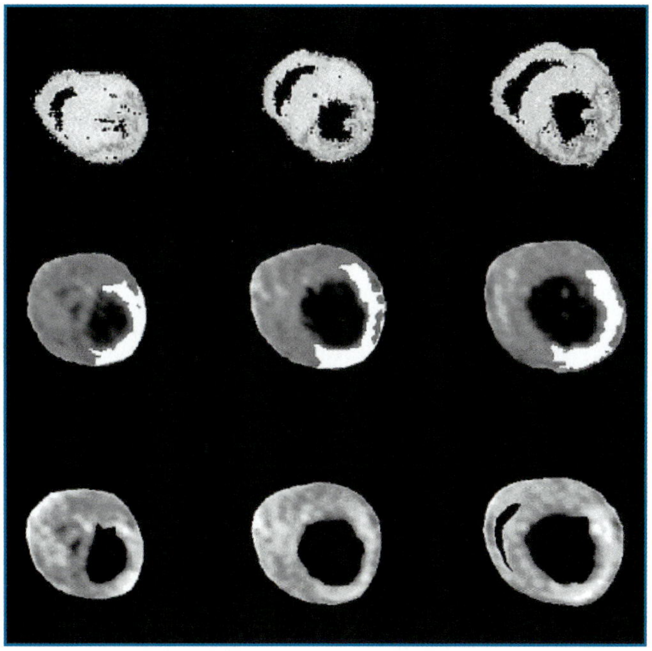

Figure 24-5 Three adjacent layers of 3D ^{23}Na-MRI experiments on isolated rat hearts 4 wks after myocardial infarction **(bottom row)**. Shown is the segmented image. Regions showing a signal of more than two standard deviations above the mean ^{23}Na-signal are shown in white, these are used for infarct size determination **(middle row)**. Corresponding histological sections with infarct staining **(top row)**. The size of the area with increased ^{23}Na-signal intensity correlated closely with histological scar size ($r = 0.91$, $p < 0.0001$) (from Horn et al. Magn Reson Med 2001; 45: 756–64; with permission of John Wiley & Sons, New York).

correlated closely with the infarct size on histology. In contrast, the ^{23}Na-content in hibernating or stunned myocardium is not increased. Therefore, ^{23}Na-MR provides a non-invasive assessment of myocardial viability without the need for external contrast agents, such as gadolinium used to determine patterns of late enhancement. Due to the relatively high sensitivity of the ^{23}Na-nucleus, and its short T1 time, ^{23}Na-MR imaging of the human myocardium is possible (see below). We also reported (Weidensteiner 2002) imaging of intracellular Na^+ using ^{23}Na-MR chemical shift imaging in perfused heart, where acute coronary occlusion led to a regional 60–110% increase in Na^+ signal within the ischemic region.

24.3.3 Hyperpolarised ^{13}C-Studies

Innovative hyperpolarisation techniques are perhaps the most promising development in MRS in the last decade, allowing massive increases (5 orders of magnitude) in spectroscopic signal to detect molecules with low abundance. Even in the strongest magnets, there is relatively low nuclear spin under usual conditions, underlying the low sensitivity of MR. Ways of increasing the polarization of nuclear spins includes increasing the magnetic field strength, decreasing the temperature or specific hyperpolarization techniques, for example dynamic nuclear polarization (DNP). In DNP, radicals are frozen with a ^{13}C-containing substance and irradiated close to the electron resonance frequency in a high magnetic field, improving the sensitivity of ^{13}C-MR spectroscopy many orders of magnitude. The resultant "hyperpolarized" solution has an enhanced ^{13}C-MR signal that can be used for determination of metabolites and enzyme kinetics in fundamental metabolic pathways of substrate metabolism. To date, this technique has been limited to research applications. Asssessment of pyruvate and its metabolites, including lactate, alanine and bicarbonate, have been possible in *in vivo* animal hearts. Merritt et al. (2008) used isolated rat hearts and investigated changes in both ^{31}P-MRS and hyperpolarized ^{13}C-pyruvate and -alanine. Using a multinuclear approach this study demonstrated that after 10 min of global ischemia, there was inhibition of carbohydrate oxidation during the first minute of reperfusion and during reperfusion pyruvate dehydrogenase flux was essentially zero, but recovered within 20 min in reversibly-injured myocardium. We can speculate that if this technique were suitable for use in humans, it would have the potential to provide real-time metabolic assessment in heart failure patients and to monitor response to therapies. An enormous amount of information can be gained from these techniques and rapid developments in hyperpolarisation methods will occur in the coming years.

24.3.4 Experimental Studies in Genetically Altered Mice

In recent years, there has been increased interest in experimental MRS, mainly due to the development and testing of genetically engineered mice. Transgenic technology has allowed generation of new mouse strains, in which key metabolic regulators are either eliminated (knockout) or are overexpressed. These new models may provide greater understanding of cardiac metabolic regulatory mechanisms in the intact and chronically failing heart. MRS is an ideal technique for studying the metabolic consequences of genetic alterations in the perfused heart. *In vivo* methods for MR spectroscopy in mice are currently being developed by a number of groups.

The combined assessment of cardiac metabolism and myocardial function with MRI and MRS in the anesthetized mouse *in vivo* has been performed with near physiological heart rates of ~ 600/min. These studies, by Chacko et al. (2000), were carried out with a 1D-CSI localization method at 4.7 T. For the adult mouse a phosphocreatine/ATP ratio was reported at 2.0 ± 0.2, which is in agreement with results for human myocardium. Left ventricular ejection fraction determined by MRI was 65 ± 7%. This combined method has the potential to investigate cardiac function and metabolism in new genetically engineered mouse models. The finding of comparable phosphocreatine/ATP ratios for the hearts of humans and mice suggests that the mouse represents a clinically relevant model for studies of myocardial energy metabolism.

Weiss et al. (2002) demonstrated that mice with transgenic overexpression of the creatine transporter had increased levels of creatine and phosphocreatine, but the heart cannot keep the augmented creatine pool adequately phosphorylated, so that free ADP levels rose and thus, pure metabolic intervention led to heart failure.

The GLUT4 protein is a sarcolemmal insulin-sensitive glucose transporter, which is responsible for a substantial proportion of glucose uptake in the heart. Mice with a "knockout" of GLUT4 developed severe left ventricular hypertrophy and a 30% decrease in systolic function. ^{31}P-MRS studies of these mice *in vivo* surprisingly showed unchanged ATP, with a ~ 60% increase in phosphocreatine and total creatine. The molecular mechanisms that might explain this unusual finding of increased phosphocreatine and creatine concentrations after GLUT4 overexpression remain to be clarified by further studies.

^{1}H-MRS can also be used for phenotype characterization, helping our understanding of the metabolic consequences of genetic manipulation. The myoglobin-knockout mouse (Merx 2001), for example, shows a complete lack of myoglobin signal using ^{1}H-MRS. It is foreseeable that, in the coming years, the number of research centers using a combination of MR imaging and MR spectroscopy for noninvasive phenotype characterization in genetically engineered mice will significantly increase.

24.4 Clinical Studies

24.4.1 Methods for Clinical Cardiac Spectroscopy

Cardiac MR spectroscopy in humans has been limited almost exclusively to the study of the ^{31}P-nucleus. Significant technical challenges remain before cardiac spectroscopy can be adopted as a clinical method. To be clinically feasible, the total time for both MR imaging and spectroscopy should be less than 1 h. This constraint limits the time for signal acquisition in spectroscopy. The difficulties in overcoming respiratory and cardiac motion in spectral acquisition have been partially addressed by navigator sequences (which track diaphragm motion), and by ECG-triggering, respectively. However, these techniques increase the scanning time required. The field strength of clinical MR systems is considerably less than that used in animal work. Given that the signal from MRS is directly proportional to the strength of the magnet, 1.5 and 3 T scanners, which are currently used for human MRS, have considerable limitations compared with the field strength used for pre-clinical work (up to 18 T). The heart lies anatomically behind a layer of chest wall muscle, which creates a strong ^{31}P-signal that must be suppressed when examining myocardium with MRS. This makes the use of localization methods necessary. Typical localization techniques for spectroscopy in humans include cardiac DRESS (depth-resolved surface coil in vivo spectroscopy), rotating frame, 1D-CSI (chemical shift imaging), ISIS (image-selected in vivo spectroscopy) and 3D-CSI. MRS studies are usually performed in the prone position, with the heart positioned over the surface coil, which theoretically improves the heart-to-coil distance and increases the sensitivity. However, this position can be uncomfortable and may increase motion artifacts. Phased array coils are now being used by some groups to improve signal sensitivity. For most spectroscopic localization methods, first a series of ^{1}H-scout images is acquired, which then allows positioning of the spectroscopic volumes, or voxels. Due to the low sensitivity of ^{31}P-MRS voxel sizes are typically in the order of 30 ml.

A typical ^{31}P-MR spectrum of a healthy volunteer is shown in Figure 24-6.

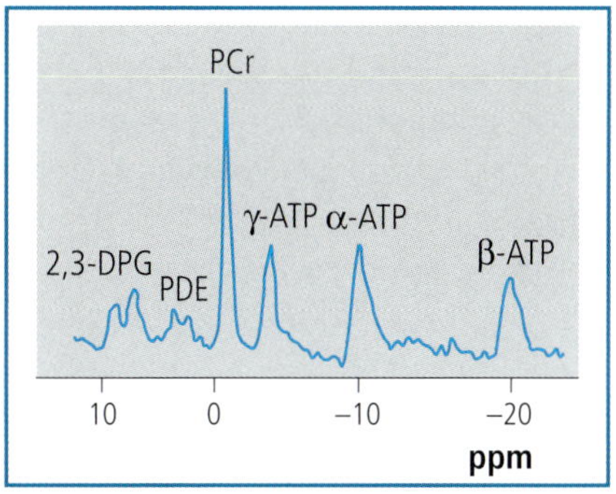

Figure 24-6 An example of a cardiac ^{31}P-MR spectrum in a healthy subject. ATP: adenosine triphosphate; DPG: diphosphoglycerate; PCr: phosphocreatine; PDE: phosphodiesters.

> Compared with the rat heart, the SNR is lower, and there are **two additional resonances** identified:
> - 2,3-diphosphoglycerate (2,3-DPG), which is attributed to blood contamination, and
> - phosphodiesters (PDE), signal from cell membrane and serum phospholipids.

The 2,3-diphosphoglycerate resonance overlaps with the signal from inorganic phosphate and for this reason pH in human ^{31}P-MR spectra are impossible to measure with current MRS applications.

Although absolute quantification of PCr and ATP is possible in human ^{31}P-spectra, the relative proportions of phosphocreatine/ATP and phosphodiester/ATP ratios (i.e. calculated as the ratios of resonance areas) are more often reported. The phosphocreatine/ATP ratio provides an index of the energetic status of the myocardium (see Chapter 24.3.1). The importance of the phosphodiester/ATP ratio is unclear, and is unaltered in myocardial diseases. ^{31}P-spectra from humans must be corrected for the effects of partial saturation, according to the principles described for experimental heart MRS. At 1.5 T, the T1 of phosphocreatine is ~ 4.4 ± 0.5 s and the T1 of ATP is ~ 2.4 ± 0.4 s. Experimental studies have shown that ^{31}P-T1s may not change in myocardial disease. ^{31}P-spectra also require a correction factor for the blood contamination. Blood contributes signal to the ATP, 2,3-diphosphoglycerate and phosphodiester resonances in the human heart. Since human blood spectra have an ATP/2,3-diphosphoglycerate area ratio of ~ 0.11 and a phosphodiester/2,3-diphosphoglycerate ratio of ~ 0.19, a correction factor can be applied to cardiac ^{31}P-MRS to correct for the blood contamination (Neubauer 1992). ^{31}P-metabolite ratios in the blood can change with disease state, a fact that should be considered when correcting for blood contamination. It is hoped that blood correction of heart spectra will become unnecessary if voxel sizes can be sufficiently reduced to achieve voxels largely uncontaminated by blood. For the measurement of resonance areas in human heart spectra, Lorentzian line fit algorithms are applied in the time or frequency domain.

Absolute quantification of phosphocreatine and ATP is technically complicated, but can add significantly to the evaluation by ^{31}P-MRS, especially when a simultaneous decrease in phosphocreatine and ATP occurs, for example, in non-viable myocardium. In principle, total ^{31}P-metabolite concentrations can be determined from a ^{31}P-standard signal, and measurement of myocardial mass. An alternative method uses the simultaneous recording of a ^{1}H-spectrum, which is used to calibrate the ^{31}P-signal against the total tissue water concentration. Meininger et al. (1999) introduced an advanced localization technique, known as spectral localization with optimum point spread function (SLOOP). This technique allowed the acquisition of a volume of arbitrary shape, which allowed the voxel of interest to be shaped to the myocardium, reducing contamination from adjacent tissue. This method provides absolute quantification of high energy phosphates with high accuracy, however it is technically challenging to implement.

In the long run, the combination of ^{31}P- and ^{1}H-MRS applications for cardiac spectroscopy to measure energy metabolism will be crucial to allow additional parameters, including free ADP and ΔG of ATP hydrolysis, to be measured, as recently described for studies in dogs. Another highly relevant area of energy metabolism in human myocardium, which has enormous potential, is the ability to measure the extent of the ATP transfer from ATP production sites, the mitochondria, to the site of ATP utilization, the myofibrils. As described above, this can be measured in the isolated perfused heart using the saturation transfer method. The same methods have not been possible in human myocardium, as such a measurement would take several hours. However, Bottomley et al. (2002) introduced the "four-angle saturation transfer" (FAST) method, which allowed measurement of CK flux in human heart in about 30 min. The calculated creatine kinase rate constant for the healthy human myocardium measured with this method was 0.29 ± 0.06 s. The method has now found initial applications in clinical studies (Weiss 2001).

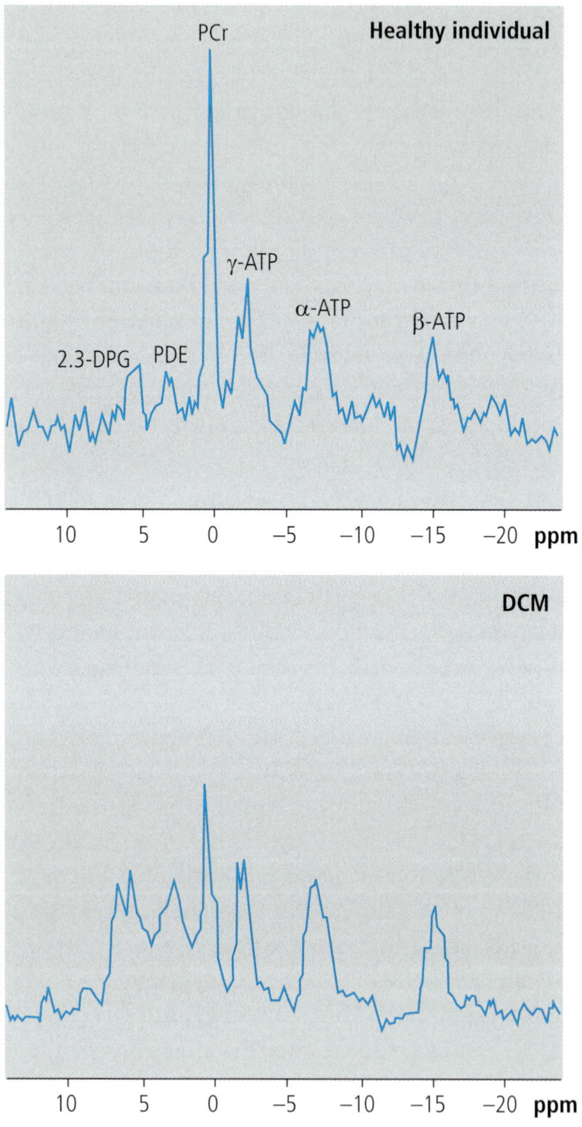

Figure 24-7 An example of a ^{31}P-MR cardiac spectrum from a patient with heart failure **(bottom)**, with reduced PCr/ATP ratio compared with a normal ^{31}P-MR spectrum **(top)**. Both spectra are from the interventricular septum in a mid-ventricular slice. ATP: adenosine triphosphate; DPG: diphosphoglycerate; PCr: phosphocreatine; PDE: phosphodiesters (modified from Neubauer et al. 1995).

Spectral signal falls dramatically with increasing distances from the ^{31}P-surface surface coils, which has meant that it was previously impossible to determine cardiac metabolism in the posterior wall of the human myocardium. Pohmann et al. (2001) reported a novel acquisition technique, using ^{31}P-chemical shift imaging, in healthy subjects at 2 T. Acquisition weighting significantly reduced signal contamination between adjacent voxels and allowed the measurement of ATP and phosphocreatine in the human heart with a spatial resolution of 16 ml and an acquisition time of 30 min, and the posterior wall could be imaged for the first time.

With increased magnet strength, acquisition time can be reduced. We demonstrated at 3 T that acquisition of ^{31}P-MRS is possible within 8 min (Hudsmith 2009), which makes acquisition of resting, exercise and recovery spectra possible within the same examination. Despite these technical advances in MRS acquisition, substantial technical developments are still required for MRS to become a practical and clinically relevant method in cardiology practice. Progress in coil design, sequence development and the implementation of MRS at higher field strength will determine whether MRS fulfils the promise of clinical relevance. Significant effort is also required to develop a generally accepted technical standard that can be used in different centers, enabling comparison of MRS results between sites.

24.4.2 Normal Values for ^{31}P-Spectroscopy

In the healthy human heart, the phosphocreatine/ATP ratio is approximately 1.8, but numerous different methods used to acquire the spectra data likely account for the large differences in "normal" reported values, which have varied from 1.1–2.4. This again highlights the need to develop generally accepted methodological standards. With the SLOOP method for measuring absolute concentrations, we have reported (Neubauer 1989) normal values for phosphocreatine concentrations (9.0 ± 1.2) and ATP concentrations (5.3 ± 1.2 mmol/kg) wet weight. These measurements agree with data obtained in animal studies. Köstler et al. (2006) were the first to demonstrate a relationship with cardiac energetics and age, where in 30 healthy volunteers decreased PCr and ATP were demonstrated in older healthy volunteers, but the differences in metabolic concentrations between sexes were not significant. See Figure 24-7 for a normal ^{31}P-MRS spectrum, compared to a patient with reduced PCr/ATP.

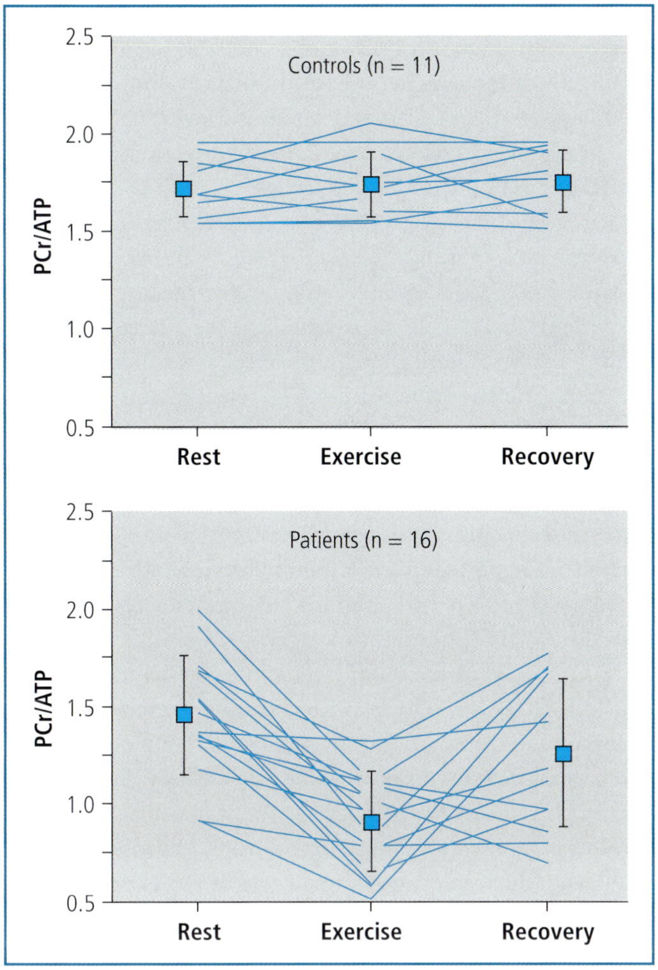

Figure 24-8 PCr/ATP ratios at rest, during exercise (handgrip) and recovery for healthy subjects (controls) **(top)** and patients with LAD stenosis **(bottom)**. The PCr/ATP ratio under stress decreases in patients, but not in healthy subjects (modified from Weiss et al. 1990).

24.4.3 Coronary Heart Disease

Coronary heart disease may potentially see the greatest benefit from MRS in detecting metabolic derangement in ischemic myocardium and for measuring myocardial viability.

Biochemical Ergometry

A decrease in phosphocreatine and an increase in inorganic phosphate are amongst the earliest metabolic changes that occur during myocardial ischemia. In fact, these alterations occur within a few seconds after the ischemic insult. Thus, the ability to measure these metabolites in human myocardium with high temporal and spatial resolution would create an ideal test, with a high sensitivity for detecting stress-induced myocardial ischemia, without contrast or radiation. Such a biochemical stress test would allow demonstration of the biochemical consequences of regional myocardial ischemia at rest, during exercise and recovery. Whilst high resolution metabolic imaging for MRS is not yet technically feasible, the principle of the method has been demonstrated in selected patients with large anterior wall ischemic areas: Weiss et al. (1990) and Buchthal et al. (2000) (Figure 24-8 and Figure 24-9) showed that in patients with severe LAD stenosis, the phosphocreatine/ATP ratio was normal at rest, but during exercise (with a 30–35 % increase in myocardial workload) the PCr/ATP ratio decreased (from 1.5 ± 0.3 to 0.9 ± 0.2), and returned to normal values during recovery. After revascularization (angioplasty or bypass surgery) phosphocreatine/ATP ratios did not alter during exercise. These results were confirmed by Yabe et al. (1994), and this group also showed that a decrease in the phosphocreatine/ATP ratios only occurred in patients with reversible defects on thallium scans, presumably indicating viable myocardium, but did not change in patients with fixed thallium defects, presumably indicating necrotic myocardium. In the latter case, the phosphocreatine/ATP ratios were already reduced at rest. If a method with high temporal and spatial resolution were to become feasible, it would become an attractive tool for the clinical diagnosis of cardiac ischemia. Such a technique could also be used to document the effectiveness of revascularization and to determine the efficacy of anti-anginal drug therapy.

Another important clinical application of ^{31}P-MRS exercise testing was reported by Buchthal et al. (2000): the pathophysiological mechanism of exercise-induced angina in women with normal coronary arteries has been a contentious topic, and microvascular dysfunction with associated tissue ischemia is a likely cause. In the study by Buchthal, such subjects showed a 29 ± 5 % decrease in the phosphocreatine/ATP ratio under increased workload, despite having normal coronary arteries. This study provides direct evidence for stress-induced myocardial ischemia in a subset of women with angina pectoris and normal coronary arteries.

Myocardial Viability

The second potential clinical application of ^{31}P-MRS in patients with coronary heart disease is the assessment of myocardial viability. Akinetic, non-contractile myocardium, which is supplied by a stenosed coronary artery, can be nonviable, where revascularization, via angioplasty or bypass, does not lead to an improvement of function. Alternatively, akinetic myocardium can be viable (morphologically and biochemically hibernating or stunned). Hibernating myocardium reduces its contractility to minimize energy consumption, to balance the discrepancy between oxygen supply and demand. Stunned myocardium shows a transient dysfunction, despite reperfusion after a reversible ischemic event. Both biochemical and ^{31}P-MRS studies in animal

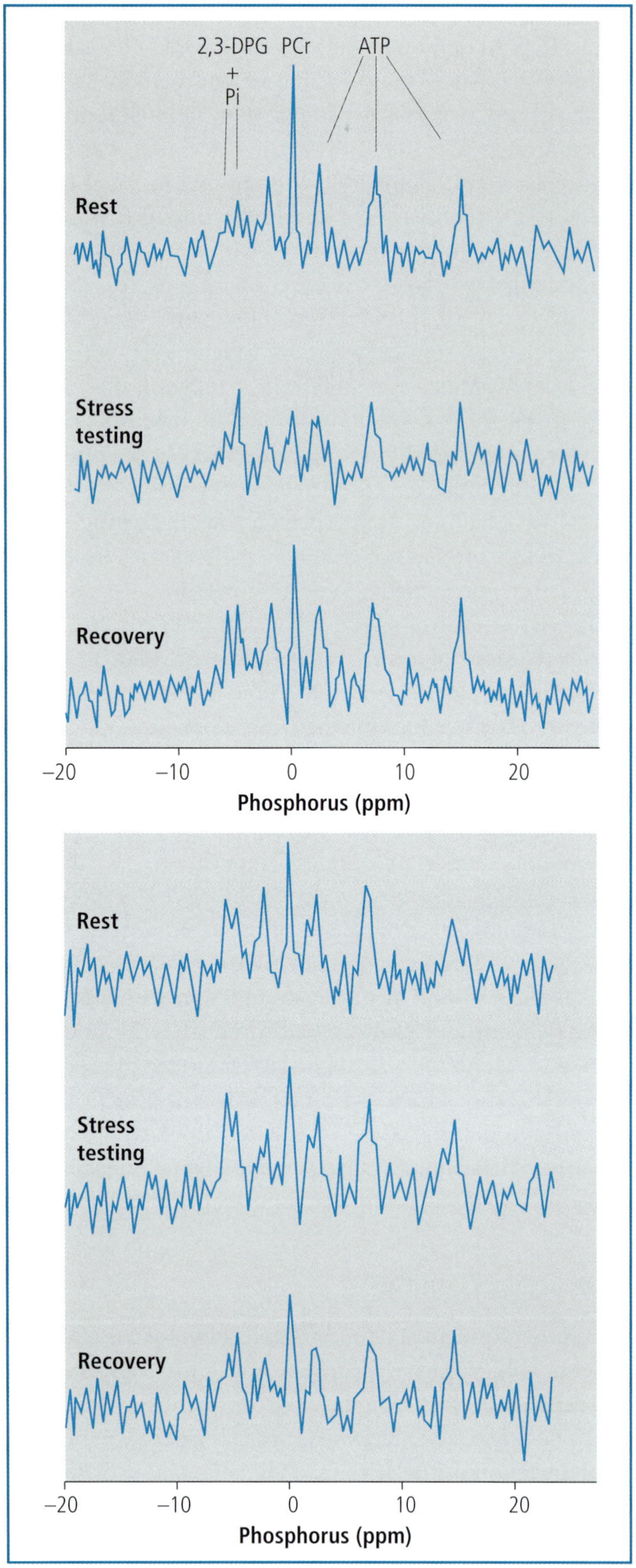

Figure 24-9 Results of ^{31}P-MR spectroscopy for two women with angina pectoris and coronary stenosis of less than 20 % luminal narrowing. Example **(top)** shows a significant decrease in the PCr/ATP ratio by 27 % during exercise. Example **(bottom)** shows no change. 2,3-DPG: 2,3-diphosphoglycerate; PCr: phosphocreatine; Pi: inorganic phosphate (modified from Buchthal et al. 2000).

models have clearly shown that myocardial scar tissue contains minimal concentrations of ATP (< 1 %), whilst stunned and hibernating myocardium show almost normal ATP levels. A non-invasive method for measuring the absolute concentrations of ATP with high temporal and spatial resolution should therefore be an ideal technique for assessing myocardial viability. Few clinical studies have published on this topic so far: Kalil-Filho et al. (1997) studied 29 patients, 4 and 39 d after anterior myocardial infarction. All patients initially showed akinesia of the anterior myocardium, however, later on a complete recovery of myocardial function. The phosphocreatine/ATP ratios remained normal in stunned myocardium (1.51 ± 0.17 vs. 1.61 ± 0.18 in volunteers), before and after the recovery of mechanical function (1.51 ± 0.17 compared with 1.53 ± 0.17). These results were confirmed by Beer et al. (2000), although this group also studied patients with non-viable infarction, which showed no recovery after 6 mths, and the ^{31}P-spectra showed a complete loss of phosphocreatine signal in the infarcted myocardium. These initial studies illustrate the principle of the method. However, significant technical advances would be necessary to achieve a clinically reliable method to determine myocardial viability in individuals. In addition to ^{31}P-MRS, localised ^{1}H-MRS has applications in assessing myocardial viability, via the determination of total creatine content. Scar tissue shows almost complete loss of total creatine. Due to the higher sensitivity of ^{1}H-MR and the higher concentration of hydrogen nuclei in creatine, which is ~ 30 times higher than ^{31}P-concentration of ATP, the resolution of the ^{1}H-MRS is significantly better than ^{31}P-MRS, currently ~ 1 ml. As with ^{31}P-MR, significant methodological complexities exist for ^{1}H-MRS, which must be overcome before this method can become clinically applicable.

As described above, ^{23}Na-MR imaging allows the assessment of myocardial viability without the application of external intravenous contrast, with increased myocardial ^{23}Na-signal in both acute myocardial necrosis and in chronic infarct scar. The ^{23}Na-nucleus has the second highest resolution of all MR detectable nuclei for imaging. This is due to the high natural abundance, the relatively high MR sensitivity (9.3 % of the ^{1}H-nucleus), the high tissue concentration (~ 140 mmol extracellular, intracellular ~ 10 mmol) and the short T1 (~ 30 ms at 1.5 T), which allows short TR times. ^{23}Na-MRI has allowed measurement of total sodium content in human myocardium with a resolution of 392 µl using an ECG-triggered 3D gradient echo sequence (FLASH), with an acquisition time of ~ 1 h (Figure 24-10). We were able to apply this method to patients with subacute (8 d) and chronic (over 6 mths) myocardial infarction (Sanstede 2001), and reported on the first ^{23}Na-MR images of the infarcted human heart. All patients after subacute infarction, and 12/15 patients with chronic infarction, showed areas of

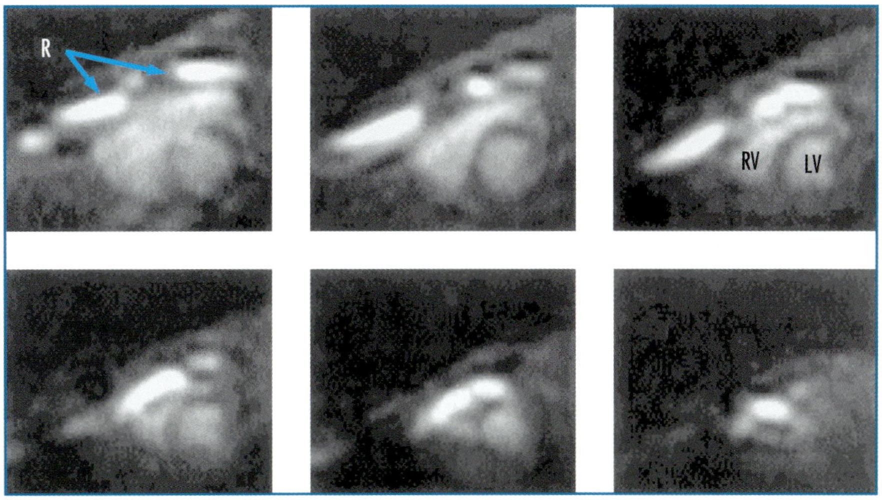

Figure 24-10 ^{23}Na-MRI of the human heart. Six consecutive short-axis slice, ECG-gated FLASH images, heart-healthy volunteer. Layer resolution 3.5 × 7 mm, acquisition time 49 min. LV: left ventricle; R: rib; RV: right ventricle (from Pabst et al. Magn Reson Med 2001; 45: 164–6; with permission of John Wiley & Sons, New York).

increased sodium signal, which correlated significantly with regional wall motion abnormalities. Further improvements of the spatial resolution of ^{23}Na-MRI using stronger gradients, improved MR coils and higher field strengths, as well as the generation of sodium concentration maps are important prerequisites for a clinically practical implementation of ^{23}Na-MRI to assess myocardial viability.

Therefore, in principle ^{31}P-MRS, ^{1}H-MRS and ^{23}Na-MRI provides a range of diagnostic approaches, which could play an important role in the assessment of myocardial viability.

Unlike current diagnostic methods for assessment of viability, including dobutamine-stress echocardiography, thallium scanning, and positron emission tomography, MRS methodology has **fundamental advantages**:

- it is radiation free,
- requires no intravenous substances, no physical or pharmacological stress and
- it uses intrinsic contrast to distinguish between viable and non-viable myocardium.

Furthermore, the mechanisms of image contrast in MRS are fully understood, whereas this is not the case for other MRI techniques, for example Gd-DTPA late enhancement. Despite these advantages, a significant improvement in the temporal and spatial resolution of the techniques is required (see above) before widespread clinical application becomes feasible.

24.4.4 Valvular Heart Disease

Animal studies have demonstrated impairment of myocardial energy metabolism in advanced left ventricular hypertrophy. Accordingly, clinical studies on patients with left ventricular hypertrophy due to aortic stenosis or incompetence (Conway 1991) have shown reduced phosphocreatine/ATP ratios (1.10 ± 0.32, compared with 1.50 ± 0.20 in normal volunteers), but only if these patients had clinical signs of heart failure. For asymptomatic patients with valve disease, the phosphocreatine/ATP ratios were unchanged. In patients with aortic valve disease, we (Neubauer 1997) demonstrated a reduction of phosphocreatine/ATP ratio only for NYHA classes III and IV, but not for NYHA classes I and II. For a similar degree of heart failure, the derangement of energy metabolism in aortic stenosis (pressure overload) was more pronounced than for aortic incompetence (volume overload). Decreased PCr/ATP ratios also correlated with left ventricular end-diastolic pressure and with end-diastolic wall stress (Neubauer 1997). Using SLOOP for absolute quantification, patients with aortic stenosis had unchanged absolute ATP levels and phosphocreatine concentrations reduced 28 %. ^{31}P-MRS can also be used to study the time course of recovery of myocardial energy metabolism after the regression of hypertrophy following heart valve replacement: patients with aortic stenosis were studied using MRS before and 40 wks after valve replacement (Beyerbacht 2001). During that time, the PCr/ATP ratios increased from 1.28 ± 0.17 to 1.44 ± 0.14 (compared with healthy subject ratios of 1.43 ± 0.14). Therefore, normalisation of myocardial energy metabolism occurred 9 mths after valve replacement surgery. It is conceivable that ^{31}P-MRS may in the future provide clinically relevant information on the optimal timing for valve replacement. However, a long-term prospective clinical study is required to clarify this.

24.4.5 Hypertension and Athletes

Only three MRS studies have been reported in patients with left ventricular hypertrophy due to chronic hypertension. Lamb et al. (1999) showed that the PCr/ATP ratios in patients with hypertension, both at rest and during dobutamine-stress, are reduced. Furthermore, the PCr/ATP correlated inversely with indices of diastolic function, including the E deceleration. In contrast, two other studies (Okada 1998, Beer 2002) showed no significant changes in myocardial energy metabolism in hypertension. This discrepancy is probably due to differences in patient populations, such as the severity and duration of hypertension, because animal data have clearly shown that myocardial energy metabolism is impaired by prolonged hypertension. In patients with advanced hypertensive heart disease, ^{31}P-MRS may be suitable to follow the regression of hypertrophy and associated improvements in energy metabolism during treatment with different antihypertensive drugs.

Interestingly, there are differences between "physiological" ("athlete's heart") and "pathological" forms of hypertrophy, with the former having a normal myocardial PCr/ATP both at rest and during exercise (Pluim 1998). This is consistent with experimental studies in rats that were exercised regularly and showed no difference in the cardiac PCr/ATP ratio after training (Spencer 1997). The molecular mechanisms for these energetic differences are not well understood, so is an important area for future studies.

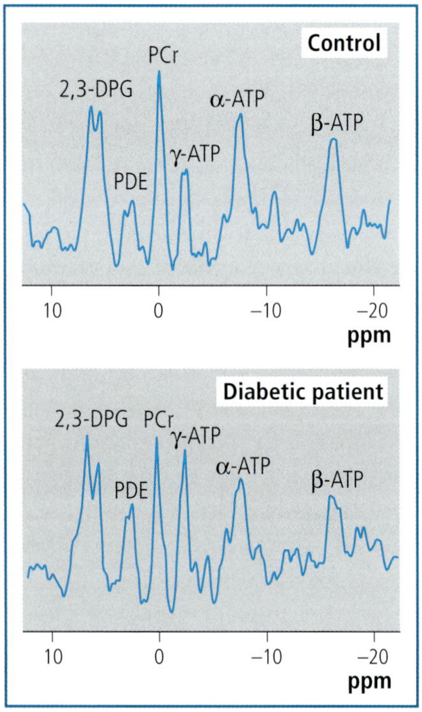

Figure 24-11 Typical cardiac ^{31}P-MR spectra from a normal control **(top)** and a patient with type 2 diabetes **(bottom)**, showing lower PCr/ATP ratio in the patient. ATP: adenosine triphosphate; DPG: diphosphoglycerate; PCr: phosphocreatine; PDE: phosphodiesters (modified from Scheuermann-Freestone et al. 2003).

24.4.6 Diabetes, Obesity and Diets

Patients with diabetes have impaired cardiac function and low cardiac PCr/ATP ratios, which is unrelated to the duration of diabetes and independent of microvascular dysfunction, suggesting a metabolic etiology (Figure 24-11). Scheuermann-Freestone (2003), Shivu (2010b) and others have found that patients with diabetes and normal systolic function, PCr/ATP was reduced. The Lamb and Szczepaniak groups (Reingold 2005, van der Meer 2007), amongst others, have pioneered much of the ^{1}H-MRS work measuring cardiac lipid concentrations and have demonstrated elevated levels in patients with diabetes with reduced myocardial triglycerides after a low calorie diet. Similar studies in heart failure patients are awaited. These studies demonstrate that ^{1}H- and ^{31}P-MRS can be used to determine the metabolic relationships in heart diseases and also show the potential of this technique to help determine the influence of substrate modulation, via diet and drugs, on the heart.

24.4.7 Heart Failure

Animal studies consistently show reduced phosphocreatine and total creatine levels and a significant reduction of the creatine kinase reaction velocity in heart failure due to chronic coronary ligation. Initial clinical studies using ^{31}P-MRS, where patients were not stratified for the severity of heart failure, did not find a significant reduction of myocardial PCr/ATP ratios. Hardy et al. (1991) were first to demonstrate a significant decrease in myocardial PCr/ATP ratios in patients with symptomatic heart failure, from both ischemic and non-ischemic etiologies. In patients with dilated cardiomyopathy, we showed that the decrease in the PCr/ATP ratio correlated closely with the clinical severity of heart failure according to the NYHA class and with left ventricular ejection fraction (Neubauer 1992). Importantly, we showed that decreases of PCr/ATP only occur for the higher grades and symptomatic stages of heart failure.

In heart failure, there is a reduction in phosphocreatine, with ATP levels also falling in more advanced disease. This means that PCr/ATP levels will be reduced in heart failure patients, but may be underestimating the true changes in high energy phosphate levels in advanced heart failure. By using the SLOOP technique, which allows absolute quantification of metabolites, we investigated patients with heart failure due to dilated cardiomyopathy (with an average ejection fraction of 18% [Beer 2002]). Absolute phosphocreatine concentrations were reduced by 51%, with ATP concentrations reduced by 35%, and an overall 25% reduction in PCr/ATP. Thus, non-invasive ^{31}P-MRS detected decreased ATP levels in heart failure and that the true extent of the change of energy metabolism is underestimated by phosphocreatine/ATP ratios. This demonstrates the importance of absolute quantification for determining the energetic status in heart failure.

ATP turnover rates may be the most sensitive indicators of abnormal cardiac ^{31}P-energetics in heart failure. Accordingly, using image-guided 4-angle saturation transfer (FAST) ^{31}P-MRS quantification of CK flux, Bottomley et al. (2002) directly measured ATP flux via the creatine kinase (CK) reaction in normal and failing human hearts. They found an 18 % reduction in cardiac PCr concentration in heart failure patients compared with healthy controls, with no reduction in ATP levels. However, in contrast, ATP turnover rates via CK were substantially reduced by 50 %, compared with those in healthy controls. Additionally, this group has also shown in hypertrophied hearts with maintained left ventricular function 30 % reduced CK flux. Thus, these results show that measures of ATP turnover rates are the most sensitive indicators of energetic abnormalities in the heart.

Multiple studies have demonstrated the key pathophysiological role of impaired energy metabolism in heart failure. An analysis of clinical heart failure studies over the past 20 years has clearly shown that medical treatments which increase energy cost of myocardial contraction, such as positive inotropes that stimulate β-adrenoreceptors or phosphodiesterase inhibitors, increase mortality, despite short-term improvement of cardiac output. On the other hand, any form of energetically favourable treatment of chronic heart failure, such as β-blockers, ACE-inhibitors or angiotensin II receptor blockers, results in improved prognosis. For this reason, it would be highly attractive to study the early myocardial energetic response of the failing heart to new forms of drug therapy. It is conceivable that the phosphocreatine/ATP ratio, or absolute concentrations of phosphocreatine and ATP, show meaningful surrogate parameters of mortality. This hypothesis needs to be systematically examined. Our initial observation (Neubauer 1992) was that six patients with dilated cardiomyopathy under standard drug therapy (ACE-inhibitors, digitalis, diuretics, 4/6 β-blockers) showed an increase in the phosphocreatine/ATP ratio from 1.51 ± 0.32 to 2.15 ± 0.27 in parallel with clinical recompensation. However, the first reported treatment study using ^{31}P-MRS was in patients with Friedreich's ataxia. Friedreich's ataxia is a primarily neurological disorder that often leads to the development of cardiomyopathy due to a defect in the mitochondrial protein frataxin, which has insufficient mitochrondrial respiratory activity and increased toxicity from free radicals. Lodi et al. (2001) reported that patients with Friedreich's ataxia, who were on a cocktail of antioxidants (coenzyme Q and vitamin E) treated over 6 mths had an increase in myocardial phosphocreatine/ATP ratio from 1.34 ± 0.59 to 2.02 ± 0.43, which shows that myocardial

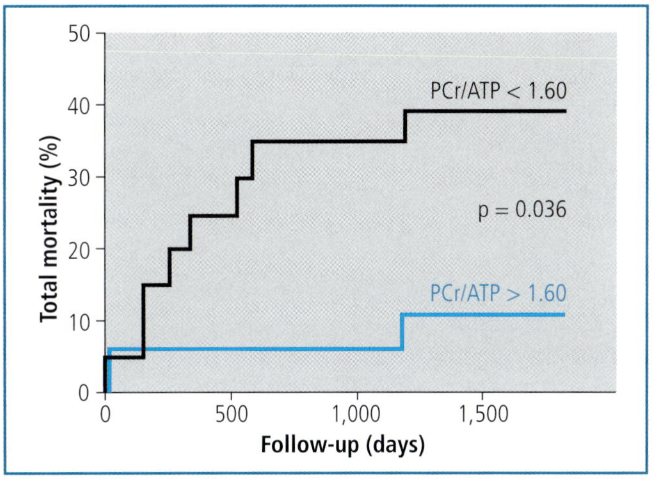

Figure 24-12 Kaplan-Meier life table analysis for total mortality in dilated cardiomyopathy. Classification of patients into two groups, divided according to the myocardial PCr/ATP ratio (< 1.6 vs. > 1.6). Patients with an initial low PCr/ATP showed an increased overall mortality over the study period of 2.5 yrs (modified from Neubauer et al. 1997).

energy metabolism was significantly improved by chronic antioxidant treatment. Heart failure patients with ischemic and non-ischemic cardiomyopathies, treated with a substrate modulator, trimetazidine, which switches energy metabolism from fatty acid to glucose oxidation, had a 33 % improvement in PCr/ATP from 1.35 ± 0.33 to 1.80 ± 0.50 (Fragasso 2006). This randomised, double-blind, cross-over study in twelve heart failure patients, already on standard heart failure therapy, suggests promising results for this drug and other potential therapies that may modulate myocardial substrate metabolism.

In addition to therapeutics, a recent study (Beer 2008) investigating the effects of exercise training on myocardial function and energetics in dilated cardiomyopathy found improvement in left ventricular end-systolic volume and ejection fraction, however no change in cardiac PCr/ATP levels. The authors concluded that the absence of deterioration in myocardial energetics suggested that the exercise training was not energy-costly to the myocardium, supporting exercise therapy in dilated cardiomyopathy.

In line with the concept that energetically favourable forms of medical therapy improve long-term prognosis of heart failure, we reported that phosphocreatine/ATP ratios could provide prognostic information on the life expectancy of patients with heart failure, which goes beyond the information on clinical and hemodynamic parameters. In patients with dilated cardiomyopathy, we demonstrated that the myocardial phosphocreatine/ATP ratios predict the long-term life expectancy more accurately than left ventricular ejection fraction or NYHA class (Neubauer 1997; Figure 24-12).

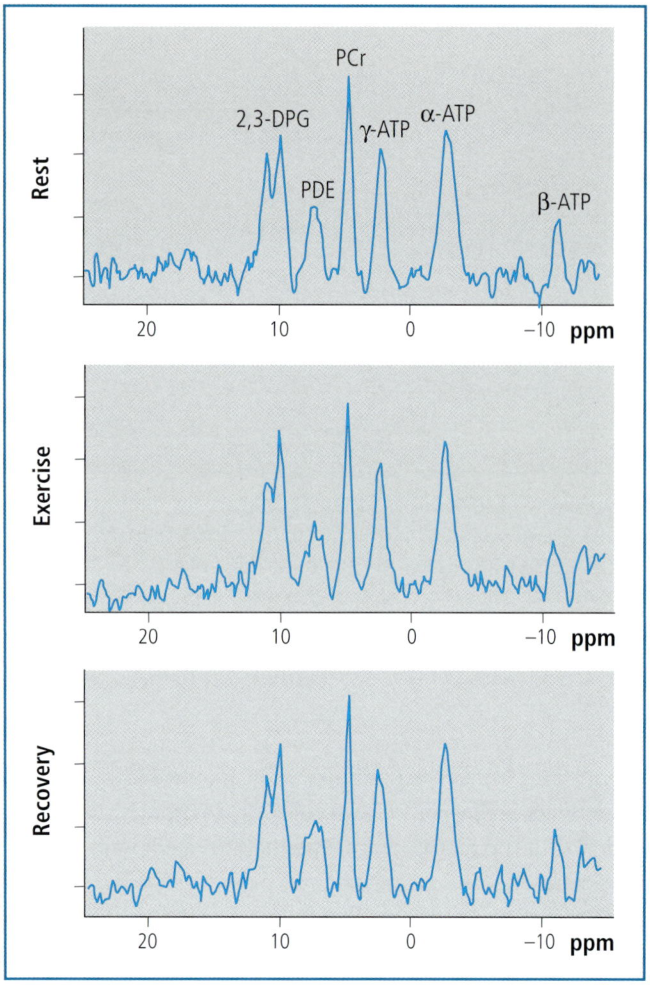

Figure 24-13 Typical cardiac ^{31}P-spectra from a male healthy volunteer at rest, during exercise and on recovery. ATP: adenosine triphosphate; DPG: diphosphoglycerate; PCr: phosphocreatine; PDE: phosphodiesters (modified from Hudsmith et al. 2009).

Therefore, ^{31}P-MRS might in future be used to assess the prognosis of patients with heart failure. However, determination of the creatine kinase reaction velocity in heart failure may be an even more relevant parameter. We have shown (Neubauer 1988) using the magnetization (saturation) transfer method, the rate and velocity of the creatine kinase reaction, a measure of ATP transfer from mitochondria to myofibrils, can be measured *in vivo*. Additionally, Bittl et al. (1987) demonstrated that creatine kinase reaction velocity correlated with cardiac workload. We have shown that the creatine kinase reaction also correlates with the recovery of mechanical function after ischemia.

Moreover, recently Phan et al. (2009) showed that patients with heart failure and normal systolic function have abnormalities in cardiac energy metabolism, suggesting an energetic basis for diastolic heart failure. In this study cardiac PCr/ATP was reduced in 37 patients with heart failure and preserved systolic function, vs. control subjects (1.57 ± 0.52 vs. 2.14 ± 0.63), indicating reduced energy reserves. We have recently shown (Hudsmith 2009) that PCr/ATP is not reduced during exercise in normal subjects (Figure 24-13). Studies are required to determine whether further reductions in PCr/ATP occur during exercise in patients with heart failure.

24.4.8 Heart Transplantation

Animal studies by Fraser et al. (1990) suggested that ^{31}P-MRS may be suitable for the detection of organ rejection after heart transplantation. Therefore, it was hoped that MRS could provide a non-invasive measure of the extent of graft rejection, and thus eliminate the need for repetitive endomyocardial biopsies. Clinical studies could not confirm this (Bottomley 1991). Although the phosphocreatine/ATP ratios were reduced in transplanted hearts with histological signs of rejection, there were no correlations with the histological severity of rejection. In the first weeks after transplantation, ^{31}P-MRS showed a transient decrease in the phosphocreatine/ATP ratios as an inevitable result of peri-operative myocardial ischemia (van Doddenburgh 1999). Measurement of resting phosphocreatine/ATP ratios therefore cannot be used for the diagnosis of transplant rejection. However, it is conceivable that the measurement of absolute concentrations of ATP and phosphocreatine would be more powerful. Cardiomyocyte mass will be reduced as part of rejection, and this could lead to a reduction of the absolute concentrations of phosphocreatine and ATP despite unchanged metabolite ratios. The transplanted heart typically develops transplant vasculopathy, and Evanochko et al. (2002) speculated that a biochemical stress test with ^{31}P-MRS could be a sensitive indicator of rejection. With the help of ^{31}P-MRS at rest and during exercise, 25 patients were examined after heart transplantation. During stress there was a $26 \pm 4\%$ decrease of the phosphocreatine/ATP ratio. A reliable non-invasive diagnostic test for the accurate prediction of rejection would be clinically relevant.

24.4.9 Genetic Heart Muscle Disease

Potentially one of the most promising clinical applications of cardiac spectroscopy is the non-invasive phenotype characterisation of cardiomyopathies caused by specific gene defects. While this field of work is in its infancy, in principle it is conceivable that certain genetic defects can be identified using a specific metabolic profile, which is non-invasively detectable using MRS. The few published studies on this have focused on hypertrophic cardiomyopathy (HCM). HCM in most, if not all cases, is due to well-characterized genetic mutations, which typically lead to a significant increase in left ventricular wall thickness and a structural disarray of the myofibrils. Experimental studies using transgenic mouse models of HCM have shown an impairment of myocardial energy metabolism (Spindler 1998). In line with these findings, studies in patients with HCM have consistently demonstrated reduced phosphocreatine/ATP ratios in hypertrophied myocardium. The largest clinical group of patients with HCM has been investigated by Jung et al. (1998), who reported significantly reduced phosphocreatine/ATP ratios in young, asymptomatic patients, which indicates a degree of deterioration of energy metabolism during the early stages of the disease process. In a subsequent study (Jung 2000) these authors reported that HCM patients with a clear family history (with an inherited genetic defect) showed a more pronounced reduction of the phosphocreatine/ATP (1.81 ± 0.28) than patients with no family history (2.10 ± 0.39). The majority of this work has been at 1.5 T, although studies at high-field strength are emerging. In a recent study by Shivu et al. (2010a) at 3 T, 37 healthy controls and 26 patients with HCM had significantly reduced PCr/ATP compared with controls (1.42 ± 0.51 and 2.11 ± 0.57). In the future, larger patient populations with HCM will need to be identified, and genetic defects investigated, in order to systematically evaluate the hypothesis of metabolic phenotype characterization using ^{31}P-MRS. Such studies should also include the measurement of the regional absolute concentrations of ATP and phosphocreatine, because a regional loss of cardiomyocytes in HCM would be undetectable in measuring metabolite ratios. Combined ^{1}H- and ^{31}P-MRS investigations should allow clarification of whether a reduced phosphocreatine in HCM is due to relative myocardial ischemia (if there is normal total creatine content) or due to a loss of total creatine, the latter phenomenon is typical of other forms of hypertrophy.

An interesting study has been performed in muscular dystrophy (Becker's disease), an X-linked inherited disease associated with loss or altered expression of dystrophin in cardiac and skeletal muscle, which can lead to the development of muscular dystrophy, cardiomyopathy and heart failure (Crilley 2000). Both patients (phosphocreatine/ATP ratio of 1.55 ± 0.33) as well as apparently healthy female carriers (1.37 ± 0.25) showed significantly decreased phosphocreatine/ATP ratios (healthy subjects 2.44 ± 0.33) although all the carriers and most of the patients showed normal left ventricular function (Crilley 2000). This suggests that a disorder of energy metabolism may causally contribute to the development of contractile dysfunction.

24.5 Conclusions and Future Perspectives

MR spectroscopy is a technique different from any other non-invasive method, which has allowed the study of many aspects of metabolism in healthy and diseased hearts. As described in this chapter, the methodology provides varied information that could theoretically be of high clinical relevance in cardiology. This raises the question of why cardiac spectroscopy has not yet been established in clinical cardiology practice and also whether this will ever be the case in the future, or whether the method will remain a research tool for specialized academic centers. The main obstacles to the implementation of cardiac MRS in routine cardiology practise has been, and remains, that it is a tool of significant technical complexity with limited signal and resolution. Major technical advances are needed to improve the spatial resolution of ^{31}P-examinations from the current ~ 25 ml to ~ 1 ml voxel sizes. At the same time, the temporal resolution must improve from 20–30 min acquisition time, to more acceptable acquisition times, such as 3–5 min. Equally important is to record MR spectra with high SNR's, minimal variability (< 5%) and with high reproducibility. Finally, a standardization of acquisition, signal processing and quantification of spectra is essential, and appropriate protocols should be developed in coming years. Should it be possible to meet all these conditions, then clinical cardiologists could be given a powerful and non-invasive measurement tool that would be applicable to many clinical problems, resulting in entirely new clinical algorithms for the benefit of patients.

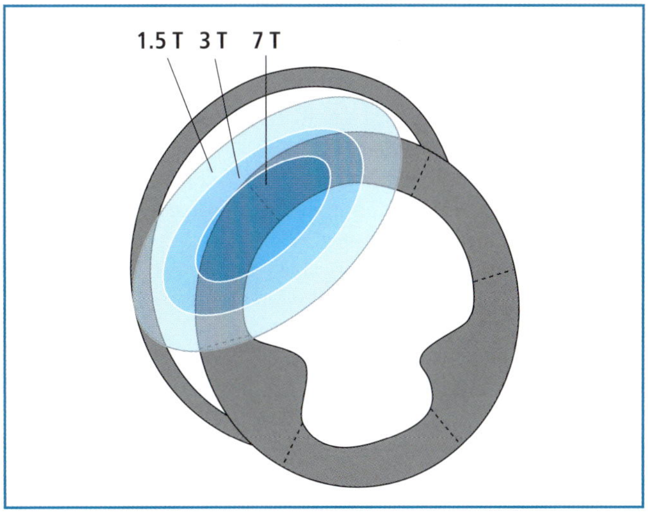

Figure 24-14 Improved resolution of MRS voxel sizes with increasing field strength: 1.5 T, 3 T, and 7 T. A schematic short-axis view of the left ventricle with voxel position and sizes at 1.5, 3, and 7 T is shown (modified from Hudsmith et al. 2009).

The authors believe that with a large-scale development effort in coming years, which focuses on coil design, sequence design and high-field magnets (Figure 24-14), these aims might be achievable, so that high-resolution metabolic imaging can form part of the routine diagnostic approach to patients with ischemic heart disease, heart failure, valvular disease and genetic cardiomyopathies.

References

Beer M, Sandstede J, Landschutz W et al. Altered energy metabolism after myocardial infarction assessed by ^{31}P-MR spectroscopy in humans. Eur Radiol 2000; 10 (8): 1323–8.

Beer M, Seyfarth T, Sandstede J et al. Absolute concentrations of high-energy phosphate metabolites in normal, hypertrophied, and failing human myocardium measured non-invasively with $^{(31)}$P-SLOOP magnetic resonance spectroscopy. J Am Coll Cardiol 2002; 40 (7): 1267–74.

Beer M, Wagner D, Myers J et al. Effects of exercise training on myocardial energy metabolism and ventricular function assessed by quantitative ^{31}phosphorus magnetic resonance spectroscopy and magnetic resonance imaging in dilated cardiomyopathy. J Am Coll Cardiol 2008; 51 (19): 1883–91.

Beyerbacht HP, Lamb HJ, van Der Laarse A et al. Aortic valve replacement in patients with aortic valve stenosis improves myocardial metabolism and diastolic function. Radiology 2001; 219 (3): 637–43.

Bittl JA, Ingwall JS. Reaction rates of creatine kinase and ATP synthesis in the isolated rat heart. A ^{31}P-NMR magnetization transfer study. J Biol Chem 1985; 260 (6): 3512–7.

Bottomley PA, Ouwerkerk R, Lee RF, Weiss RG. Four-angle saturation transfer (FAST) method for measuring creatine kinase reaction rates in vivo. Magn Reson Med 2002; 47 (5): 850–63.

Bottomley PA, Weiss RG. Non-invasive localized MR quantification of creatine kinase metabolites in normal and infarcted canine myocardium. Radiology 2001; 219 (2): 411–8.

Bottomley PA, Weiss RG, Hardy CJ, Baumgartner WA. Myocardial high-energy phosphate metabolism and allograft rejection in patients with heart transplants. Radiology 1991; 181 (1): 67–75.

Buchthal SD, den Hollander JA, Merz CN et al. Abnormal myocardial ^{31}phosphorus nuclear magnetic resonance spectroscopy in women with chest pain but normal coronary angiograms. N Engl J Med 2000; 342 (12): 829–35.

Chacko VP, Aresta F, Chacko SM, Weiss RG. MRI/MRS assessment of in vivo murine cardiac metabolism, morphology, and function at physiological heart rates. Am J Physiol Heart Circ Physiol 2000; 279 (5): H2218–H24.

Clarke K, Cross HR, Keon CA et al. Cation MR spectroscopy (^{7}Li, ^{23}Na, ^{39}K and ^{87}Rb). MAGMA 1998; 6 (2–3): 105–6.

Clarke K, O'Connor AJ, Willis RJ. Temporal relation between energy metabolism and myocardial function during ischemia and reperfusion. Am J Physiol 1987; 253 (2 Pt 2): H412–H21.

Conway MA, Allis J, Ouwerkerk R et al. Detection of low phosphocreatine to ATP ratio in failing hypertrophied human myocardium by ^{31}P-magnetic resonance spectroscopy. Lancet 1991; 338 (8773): 973–6.

Crilley JG, Boehm EA, Rajagopalan B et al. Magnetic resonance spectroscopy evidence of abnormal cardiac energetics in Xp21 muscular dystrophy. J Am Coll Cardiol 2000; 36 (6): 1953–8.

DeLayre JL, Ingwall JS, Malloy C, Fossel ET. Gated ^{23}sodium nuclear magnetic resonance images of an isolated perfused working rat heart. Science 1981; 212 (4497): 935–6.

Evanochko WT, Buchthal SD, den Hollander JA et al. Cardiac transplant patients response to the $^{(31)}$P-MRS stress test. J Heart Lung Transplant 2002; 21 (5): 522–9.

Fragasso G, Perseghin G, De Cobelli F et al. Effects of metabolic modulation by trimetazidine on left ventricular function and phosphocreatine/adenosine triphosphate ratio in patients with heart failure. Eur Heart J 2006; 27 (8): 942–8.

Fraser Jr. CD, Chacko VP, Jacobus WE et al. Early ^{31}phosphorus nuclear magnetic resonance bioenergetic changes potentially predict rejection in heterotopic cardiac allografts. J Heart Transplant 1990; 9 (3 Pt 1): 197–204.

Gadian DG. NMR and its applications to living systems. 2. ed. New York: Oxford University Press 1995.

Hardy CJ, Weiss RG, Bottomley PA, Gerstenblith G. Altered myocardial high-energy phosphate metabolites in patients with dilated cardiomyopathy. Am Heart J 1991; 122 (3 Pt 1): 795–801.

Horn M, Weidensteiner C, Scheffer H et al. Detection of myocardial viability based on measurement of sodium content: A $^{(23)}$Na-NMR study. Magn Reson Med 2001; 45 (5): 756–64.

Hudsmith LE, Tyler DJ, Emmanuel Y et al. $^{(31)}$P cardiac magnetic resonance spectroscopy during leg exercise at 3 T. Int J Cardiovasc Imaging 2009; 25 (8): 819–26.

Ingwall JS. Phosphorus nuclear magnetic resonance spectroscopy of cardiac and skeletal muscles. Am J Physiol 1982; 242 (5): H729–H44.

Jung WI, Hoess T, Bunse M et al. Differences in cardiac energetics between patients with familial and nonfamilial hypertrophic cardiomyopathy. Circulation 2000; 101 (12): E121.

Jung WI, Sieverding L, Breuer J et al. ^{31}P-NMR spectroscopy detects metabolic abnormalities in asymptomatic patients with hypertrophic cardiomyopathy. Circulation 1998; 97 (25): 2536–42.

Kalil-Filho R, de Albuquerque CP, Weiss RG et al. Normal high energy phosphate ratios in "stunned" human myocardium. J Am Coll Cardiol 1997; 30 (5): 1228–32.

Kohler SJ, Perry SB, Stewart LC et al. Analysis of ^{23}Na-NMR spectra from isolated perfused hearts. Magn Reson Med 1991; 18 (1): 15–27.

Kostler H, Landschutz W, Koeppe S et al. Age and gender dependence of human cardiac phosphorus metabolites determined by SLOOP ^{31}P-MR spectroscopy. Magn Reson Med 2006; 56 (4): 907–11.

Lamb HJ, Beyerbacht HP, van der Laarse A et al. Diastolic dysfunction in hypertensive heart disease is associated with altered myocardial metabolism. Circulation 1999; 99 (17): 2261–7.

Lodi R, Hart PE, Rajagopalan B et al. Antioxidant treatment improves in vivo cardiac and skeletal muscle bioenergetics in patients with Friedreich's ataxia. Ann Neurol 2001; 49 (5): 590–6.

Meininger M, Landschutz W, Beer M et al. Concentrations of human cardiac phosphorus metabolites determined by SLOOP ^{31}P-NMR spectroscopy. Magn Reson Med 1999; 41 (4): 657–63.

Merritt ME, Harrison C, Storey C et al. Inhibition of carbohydrate oxidation during the first minute of reperfusion after brief ischemia: NMR detection of hyperpolarized $^{13}CO_2$ and $H^{13}CO_3$. Magn Reson Med 2008; 60 (5): 1029–36.

Merx MW, Flogel U, Stumpe T et al. Myoglobin facilitates oxygen diffusion. FASEB J 2001; 15 (6): 1077–9.
Neubauer S. The failing heart – an engine out of fuel. N Engl J Med 2007; 356 (11): 1140–51.
Neubauer S, Hamman BL, Perry SB et al. Velocity of the creatine kinase reaction decreases in post-ischemic myocardium: a ^{31}P-NMR magnetization transfer study of the isolated ferret heart. Circ Res 1988; 63 (1): 1–15.
Neubauer S, Horn M, Naumann A et al. Impairment of energy metabolism in intact residual myocardium of rat hearts with chronic myocardial infarction. J Clin Invest 1995; 95 (3): 1092–100.
Neubauer S, Horn M, Pabst T et al. Cardiac high-energy phosphate metabolism in patients with aortic valve disease assessed by ^{31}P-magnetic resonance spectroscopy. J Investig Med 1997; 45 (8): 453–62.
Neubauer S, Ingwall JS. Verapamil attenuates ATP depletion during hypoxia: ^{31}P-NMR studies of the isolated rat heart. J Mol Cell Cardiol 1989; 21 (11): 1163–78.
Neubauer S, Krahe T, Schindler R et al. ^{31}P-magnetic resonance spectroscopy in dilated cardiomyopathy and coronary artery disease. Altered cardiac high-energy phosphate metabolism in heart failure. Circulation 1992; 86 (6): 1810–8.
Okada M, Mitsunami K, Inubushi T, Kinoshita M. Influence of aging or left ventricular hypertrophy on the human heart: contents of phosphorus metabolites measured by ^{31}P-MRS. Magn Reson Med 1998; 39 (5): 772–82.
Phan TT, Abozguia K, Nallur Shivu G et al. Heart failure with preserved ejection fraction is characterized by dynamic impairment of active relaxation and contraction of the left ventricle on exercise and associated with myocardial energy deficiency. J Am Coll Cardiol 2009; 54 (5): 402–9.
Pluim BM, Lamb HJ, Kayser HW et al. Functional and metabolic evaluation of the athlete's heart by magnetic resonance imaging and dobutamine stress magnetic resonance spectroscopy. Circulation 1998; 97 (7): 666–72.
Pohmann R, von Kienlin M. Accurate phosphorus metabolite images of the human heart by 3D acquisition-weighted CSI. Magn Reson Med 2001; 45 (5): 817–26.
Reingold JS, McGavock JM, Kaka S et al. Determination of triglyceride in the human myocardium by magnetic resonance spectroscopy: reproducibility and sensitivity of the method. Am J Physiol Endocrinol Metab 2005; 289 (5): E935–E9.
Sandstede JJ, Pabst T, Beer M et al. Assessment of myocardial infarction in humans with $^{(23)}$Na-MR imaging: comparison with cine MR imaging and delayed contrast enhancement. Radiology 2001; 221 (1): 222–8.
Scheuermann-Freestone M, Madsen PL, Manners D et al. Abnormal cardiac and skeletal muscle energy metabolism in patients with type 2 diabetes. Circulation 2003; 107 (24): 3040–6.
Shivu GN, Abozguia K, Phan TT et al. $^{(31)}$P magnetic resonance spectroscopy to measure in vivo cardiac energetics in normal myocardium and hypertrophic cardiomyopathy: Experiences at 3 T. Eur J Radiol 2010a; 73 (2): 255–9.
Shivu GN, Phan TT, Abozguia K et al. Relationship between coronary microvascular dysfunction and cardiac energetics impairment in type 1 diabetes mellitus. Circulation 2010b; 121 (10): 1209–15.
Spencer RG, Buttrick PM, Ingwall JS. Function and bioenergetics in isolated perfused trained rat hearts. Am J Physiol 1997; 272 (1 Pt 2): H409–H17.
Spindler M, Saupe KW, Christe ME et al. Diastolic dysfunction and altered energetics in the alphaMHC403/$^{+}$ mouse model of familial hypertrophic cardiomyopathy. J Clin Invest 1998; 101 (8): 1775–83.
van der Meer RW, Diamant M, Westenberg JJ et al. Magnetic resonance assessment of aortic pulse wave velocity, aortic distensibility, and cardiac function in uncomplicated type 2 diabetes mellitus. J Cardiovasc Magn Reson 2007; 9 (4): 645–51.
Van Dobbenburgh JO, De Groot MC, De Jonge N et al. Myocardial high-energy phosphate metabolism in heart transplant patients is temporarily altered irrespective of rejection. NMR Biomed 1999; 12 (8): 515–24.
von Kienlin M, Rosch C, Le Fur Y et al. Three-dimensional ^{31}P-magnetic resonance spectroscopic imaging of regional high-energy phosphate metabolism in injured rat heart. Magn Reson Med 1998; 39 (5): 731–41.
Weidensteiner C, Horn M, Fekete E et al. Imaging of intracellular sodium with shift reagent aided $^{(23)}$Na-CSI in isolated rat hearts. Magn Reson Med 2002; 48 (1): 89–96.
Weiss RG, Bottomley PA. Clinical cardiac magnetic resonance spectroscopy. 1. ed. Philadelphia: Churchill Livingstone 2001.
Weiss RG, Bottomley PA, Hardy CJ, Gerstenblith G. Regional myocardial metabolism of high-energy phosphates during isometric exercise in patients with coronary artery disease. N Engl J Med 1990; 323 (23): 1593–600.
Weiss RG, Chatham JC, Georgakopolous D et al. An increase in the myocardial PCr/ATP ratio in GLUT4 null mice. FASEB J 2002; 16 (6): 613–5.
Yabe T, Mitsunami K, Okada M et al. Detection of myocardial ischemia by ^{31}P-magnetic resonance spectroscopy during handgrip exercise. Circulation 1994; 89 (4): 1709–16.
Zhang J, Duncker DJ, Xu Y et al. Transmural bioenergetic responses of normal myocardium to high workstates. Am J Physiol 1995; 268 (5 Pt 2): H1891–H905.

25 Interventional Cardiovascular Magnetic Resonance Imaging

Maythem Saeed and Mark W. Wilson

25.1 Introduction

Over the past decade, interventional cardiovascular magnetic resonance (ICMR) imaging has emerged as a new technology representing the next major advancement in diagnostic and therapeutic intervention imaging. The rapid evolution of minimally invasive cardiovascular interventions is shaping the demand for high temporal and spatial resolution imaging that offers safety, accuracy, flexibility and functionality. ICMR imaging refers to the rapid acquisition, reconstruction, and display of images. It also describes the ultimate requirements for monitoring therapeutic interventions. ICMR imaging can form the basis of minimally invasive surgeries and image-guided interventions that offer improved patient management and cost effectiveness.

X-ray fluoroscopy has been routinely used to guide cardiovascular interventions because it provides high spatial and temporal resolution, however, patients with ischemic or congenital heart disease require repeated exposures to ionizing radiation and iodinated contrast agents. In general, the accumulative radiation exposure to patients presents a significant risk such as development of solid tumors and infertility, which limits its use in long or repeated interventional procedures (Lindholt 2003, Kuon 2008, Frush 2003, McFadden 2002, Bacher 2005, Brenner 2001). More specifically, cardiovascular structure, function, perfusion and viability cannot be inferred under X-ray fluoroscopy. The lack of contrast between viable and non-viable myocardium limits the usefulness of X-ray fluoroscopy for delineating peri-infarction zone, measuring infarct size or determining the distance between the endovascular catheter and the target on 2D images (Peters 2006), which leads to blind delivery of local therapies to the regions of interest (infarct and border zone) (Saeed 2006b, Saeed 2008a). Therefore, another minimally invasive imaging technique without the above limitation is needed to perform interventional cardiovascular procedures. The recently developed ICMR imaging techniques allow frame rates comparable to those achieved with X-ray fluoroscopy. Soft tissue visualization, multiple contrast mechanisms and 3D tomographic imaging were quickly recognized as valuable features of MR imaging that could provide essential information on cardiovascular structure, function, perfusion and viability to the interventionist during the procedure (Axel 1997, Osman 1999, Jaquier 2007). To ease and enhance the transition from interventional X-ray fluoroscopy to ICMR imaging, two aspects of the technology need to be developed: namely customized interventional MR scanners with a larger diameter bore and shorter in length than standard scanners and MR friendly instruments.

25.2 Basic Principles

The physics of MR imaging dictate that optimal image quality is achieved when the magnet, gradients, and RF coils can closely surround the patients, which may be difficult or uncomfortable for both the interventionist and the patient. Available ICMR imaging systems are characterized by the compromise between patient access, speed of data acquisition and display and image qualities (Shellock 2002).

> ICMR imaging is now possible because of **major advancements** in a variety of fields:
> - data acquisition,
> - data transfer,
> - image reconstruction and
> - interactive control and display.

Advances also include highly uniform magnetic fields, rapidly changeable magnetic field gradients, multi-channel receivers and advanced computing systems.

The speed of a given MR imaging technique is determined by how quickly this spatial encoding may be performed and how fast the corresponding image (k-space) data can be acquired. Actively shielded, strong, fast-switching gradients and fast electronics have allowed the intervals for data acquisition and the intervals between data acquisition periods to be significantly reduced. Most of real-time sequences achieve their high speeds by maximizing the switching rates of gradients and RF pulses. Real-time MR images may be obtained orders of magnitude faster than with conventional sequences.

New MR scanners provide real-time steady-state free precession (SSFP), true fast imaging with steady-state precession (trueFISP), balanced fast field echo (bFFE), or fast imaging employing steady-state acquisition (FIESTA) capability with interactive graphic slice prescription during continuous scanning (Busse 2001). Different vendors will have similar imaging sequences. SSFP imaging yields high signal-to-noise ratio (SNR), fast image acquisition, high spatial resolution and high contrast between tissue and blood due to T2/T1-weighting (Duerk 1998). SSFP acquisitions have been performed using traditional rectilinear, radial (Peters 2003), and spiral (Spielman 1995) k-space trajectories. Keyhole imaging and view-sharing have also been used to enhance temporal resolution during real-time imaging (Shankaranarayanan 2001). While parallel imaging techniques (Pruessmann 1999) offer other means to increase temporal resolution, the reduction in SNR may impart too severe a penalty for many interventional procedures. Real-time images are typically acquired without cardiac or respiratory gating to obtain the highest possible frame rate.

For serial characterization of the efficacy of local therapies, a variety of conventional MR imaging sequences have been used. Cine-MR imaging has been used for the measurements of global function, while tagged or DENSE and velocity-encoded MR imaging are used for the determination of regional 3D strain (Axel 1997, Osman 1999, Hundley 1999, Aletras 1999). Furthermore, previously acquired delayed contrast-enhanced MR imaging for infarct localization can also be used to target local injections to regions surrounding the infarction (Saeed 2005, Saeed 2007, Saeed 2008a, Saeed 2008b).

25.3 Hardware and Software

Different MR scanner designs are available for interventional procedures, namely open scanner, short-bore scanner and hybrid systems (Hushek 2008). The open MR scanners use weak magnetic fields and low gradient strength; therefore, they offer low image quality and slow switching speeds. Wacker et al. (2005) observed that a 1.0 T closed-bore scanner halved the procedure time during stent deployment compared to a 0.2 T open-bore scanner.

Current interventional scanners partially fulfill the requirements of therapeutic procedures that require more advanced functionality, including real-time multi-slice acquisition and 3D display of the endovascular catheter and surrounding tissues.

> MR venders introduced **two distinct XMR systems**:
> - X-ray source and MR scanner with patient transport between the two systems on a sliding table, and
> - an X-ray modality implanted between two halves of MR scanner (double doughnut), without the need for patient transport.

> The **advantages of XMR systems** are:
> - patients must not undergo two separate scans and movement between them which may cause problems with soft tissue registration,
> - unlike X-ray fluoroscopy system, the combined system permits evaluation of the impact of interventional procedures using MR monitoring,
> - it permits rapid deployment of catheters, and efficient execution of the desired interventions without the obligation of using MR friendly catheters and equipment, and
> - it reduces radiation exposure (Muthurangu 2004).

A protocol has been developed that fuses the images from X-ray and MR imaging to determine source location from one modality and soft-tissue boundaries (Saikus 2009).

In 2001 the first XMR system with a fully functional catheterization laboratory was installed at the University of California, San Francisco. This short-bore MR scanner (1.57 m, 1.5 T, Intera I/T; Philips Medical Systems, Best, The Netherlands) is equipped with full cardiovascular features and located in a room adjacent to the catheterization lab, equipped with an X-ray C-arm with an acquisition rate of 30 frames/s (Integris V5000), in-room displays and sliding tabletop for patient movement between the two scanners. Monitoring and patient support equipment, such as blood pressure systems, ECG monitor, infusion pumps, and contrast injectors are MR-compatible and can be placed inside the 5-Gauss line within the scanner room, while non-MR-compatible equipment, such as ventilator, anesthesia machine and hemodynamic monitoring systems as well as interventional ferromagnetic catheters and devices must be placed outside the scanner room.

25.4 Catheter Tracking and Interventional Devices

In contrast to ultrasound, X-ray fluoroscopy and computed tomography visualization of interventional catheters and devices has been difficult on MR imaging. Therefore, ICMR imaging requires customized catheters, guide-wires and devices with adequate reference markers to visualize and locate the devices. At the present time, there are three approaches, namely passive, active and magnetically steerable, for tracking and navigating endovascular catheters.

It should be noted that most commercially available endovascular guide-wires, endovascular catheters and devices are MR incompatible (ferromagnetic) and cause image distortion. The factors that affect the magnitude of distortion are the magnetic field strength, the materials and design of the devices, and spatial orientation of the device relative to the magnetic field geometry (Klemm 2000, Kuehne 2003). Studies showed that stents containing non-ferromagnetic materials cause less image distortion than ferromagnetic stents (Kuehne 2002, Kuehne 2003, Buecker 2004). While commercially available nitinol devices are desirable because they are visible on MR images and are non-ferromagnetic, there remains the potential problem of radiofrequency heating in surrounding tissue (Konings 2000, Nitz 2001). Furthermore, ferromagnetic materials create large susceptibility artifact, making them useless for MR-guided procedures, while nickel-titanium alloys (nitinol, amplatzer septal occluder), platinum (coils and stents), gold, copper, nonbraided catheters and plastic have less susceptibility artifact (Kuehne 2003). As an alternative, a fiberglass-based guidewire with a tip impregnated with dysprosium oxide rings has been proposed (Bakker 1998). Later, Mekle et al. (2006, 2009) introduced a new synthetic MR friendly polymer-based guidewire for peripheral vascular interventions. Investigators demonstrated the dilatation of an artificial stenosis in phantoms and in the carotid artery, aorta, and iliac arteries of swine using polymer-based guidewire (Mekle 2009).

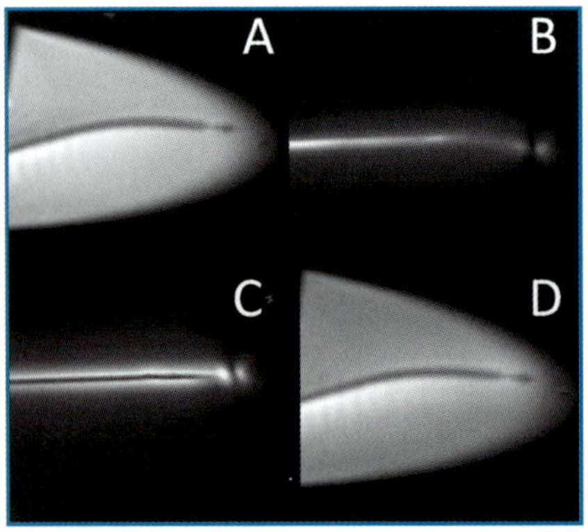

Figure 25-1 MR images of an active catheter with multiple coils placed in water bath. Only the external surface coil elements were active (A), only the catheter coil was active (B), only the catheter tip microcoil was active (C). Both surface coil elements and active catheter coil are contributing to the image (D). This active catheter was used later for transendocardial delivery of angiogenic agents (from Saeed M, Martin AJ, Lee RJ et al. MR guidance of targeted injections into border and core of scarred myocardium in pigs. Radiology 2006; 240 (2): 419–26; with permission of Radiological Society of North America, Inc.).

25.4.1 Passive Catheter Tracking

Passive catheter tracking relies on magnetic susceptibility artifacts. These artifacts are related to displacement of fluids (water protons by the catheter) and differing magnetic susceptibility. Catheter or background blood signals can be altered using MR contrast media. MR contrast media plays an important role in cases of passive catheter tracking and defining the target. The T1-shortening caused by the circulating blood-pool agent is known to prevent flow artifacts because the steady-state is reached earlier thus improving the catheter for faster tracking (Maes 2005, Martin 2003).

Bakker et al. (1997) were the first to use the passive tracking approach for steering in human basilica veins of healthy volunteers. They used dysprosium markers mounted on 3F non-braided catheters for endovascular tracking and were able to reliably visualize these catheters. Later, this passive approach was adapted by Manke et al. (2000) and Razavi et al. (2003) in patients.

25.4.2 Active Catheter Tracking

This approach relies on specially designed microcoils, current running through wire loops and self-resonant radiofrequency circuits (Flask 2001) (Figure 25-1). The use of microcoils provides robust tracking of the catheter shaft and tip that allows for tracking and targeting of the region of interest (Saeed 2006, Bock 2004). The coils pick up signal during slice excitation and generate frequency-encoded recall echos.

These echoes can be detected in 3D at a spatial resolution of approximately 1 mm. Active tracking has great potential because it allows the catheter shaft or guidewire to be visualized and the imaging plane to be automatically adapted to the moving catheter.

Quick et al. (2002) used antennas for active catheter tracking and imaging of the abdominal aorta, superior mesenteric artery, renal arteries, hepatic artery and celiac trunk. They were able to simultaneously visualize the vascular tree, catheter shaft and tip during imaging. Hillenbrand et al. (2006) made an active catheter using copper wire mounted on conventional 5F catheters for characterizing aortic and iliac arterial walls. The drawback of this technique is that both the catheter and the background anatomy can not be simultaneously visualized (Figure 25-2). Moreover, the safety issue of these devices is still a major concern. The long, conductive nature of the metallic braid creates a safety hazard in the MR environment, as the braided shaft can interact with incident RF energy and the electric field transmitted from the RF coil (Konings 2000, Nitz 2001, Park 2007). The methods for mitigating the potential for heating include using unbraided catheters, insulating the conductive structure, limiting the RF power to which it is exposed, and altering its interaction with the RF energy source (Kocaturk 2009).

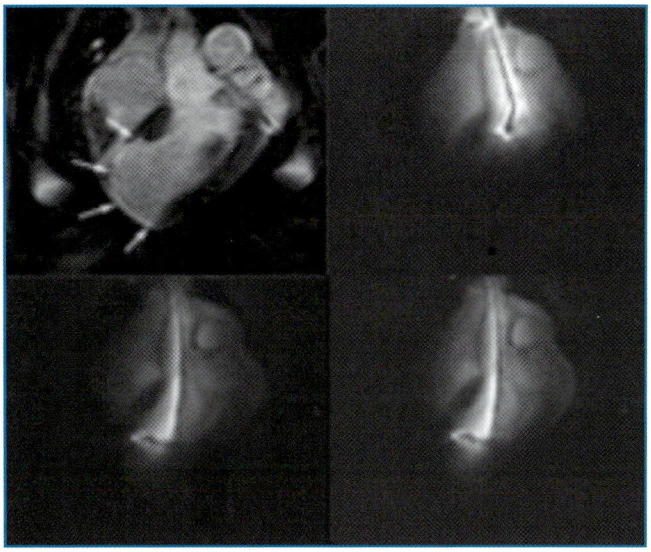

Figure 25-2 Selected delayed contrast-enhanced MR **(top, left)** and MR fluoroscopic images show heart with the infarction and the navigation of the active endovascular catheter in the ascending aorta **(top, right)** and LV chamber **(bottom)**, respectively. Note that the background anatomy can not be simultaneously visualized on MR fluoroscopy using only the active catheter.

25.4.3 Magnetic Catheter Steering

In addition to the imaging advantages of MR imaging, the strong homogeneous magnetic (B_0) field inside the MR imaging scanner provides a unique opportunity for catheter tip steering by remote control (Demas 2007). A small magnetic moment created by application of electrical current to copper coils on the catheter tip result in alignment with the direction of the B_0 field. If three such coils are placed on the catheter tip, then remote controlled deflection can be achieved in 3D. Low levels of current supplied to the catheter coils also permits active visualization of the catheter tip, which otherwise can be difficult to see in the MR environment. In addition to improved catheterization at low power levels, this technology also permits deposition of thermal energy for ablation of tissues at higher power levels.

Roberts et al. (2002) developed a laser lathe lithography technique to synthesize catheters tipped with copper coils in up to three orthogonal axes. Real-time MR imaging has been used to visualize the tip of a magnetic catheter in phantoms and in situ using a clinical MR scanner (Roberts 2002, Settecase 2007) (Figure 25-3). This technology allows for more efficient navigation of small, tortuous blood vessels, which are currently difficult to catheterize due to build-up of friction at the many vascular bends between the femoral access site and target blood vessels.

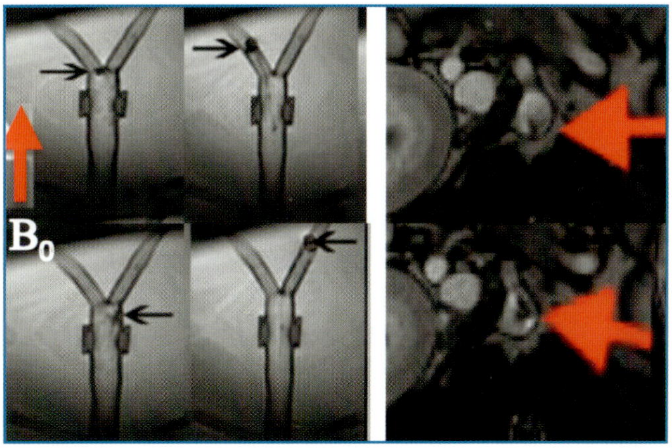

Figure 25-3 Dynamic coronal MR images of a 2.5 F two-axis (saddle and helical) coil-tipped catheter deflected and advanced up the left **(top, left block)** and right **(bottom, left block)** of a phantom (B_0-bore of magnet). Right block shows the catheter in the superior mesenteric artery (large arrows).

25.5 Endovascular Interventions

Clear distinction between blood, vascular wall and surrounding soft tissue are major features of MR imaging. ICMR imaging adds other important features such as catheter visualization and movement as well as a 3D display or visualization of the regions of interest (Saeed 2006a). MR-guided endovascular catheters have been used in preclinical and clinical studies for dilatation of the aorta, pulmonary, coronary, renal, iliac and femoral arteries (Saeed 2006b, Kuehne 2003, Paetzel 2004, Paetzel 2005, Omary 2000, Manke 2001) and for delivering genes in the vascular wall (Yang 2006).

MR-guided endovascular intervention has been used for angioplasty. In 1997 the first human study showed excellent visualization of an endovascular catheter labeled with five dysprosium ring markers (Bakker 1997). In this study, investigators did not use guide wires during the movement of the catheter in the cephalic vein of healthy volunteers. Later, MR-guided percutaneous transluminal angioplasty was successfully used in 13 patients with iliac stenosis (Manke 2001) and in 15 patients with femoral and popliteal artery stenosis (Paetzel 2005). Both the guidewire and balloon were visible on real-time MR imaging, and the balloon was placed correctly to cover the entire stenosis. Balloon dilatation was used to reduce the degree of stenosis and there was no complication. MR-guided endovascular intervention has been used for delivery of stents in large and small blood vessels of experimental animals (Saeed 2006b, Wacker 2005, Kuehne 2003, Raval 2005, Spuentrup 2002, Buecker 2000, Dion 2000). A few investigators performed vascular stenting in patients under MR guidance (Paetzel 2005, Manke 2001). Post-interventional MR imaging showed the localization and function of the stents.

MR-guided endovascular intervention has been used for vascular valve placement. This technology may also play an important role in the replacement of insufficient aortic or pulmonic valves (Kuehne 2001, Kuehne 2002, Kuehne 2003). MR imaging offers quantitative assessment of the regurgitate fraction before and after valve stent placement. Pulmonary artery stents have been accurately implanted across the pulmonary valve (Kuehne 2001, Kuehne 2002, Kuehne 2003). Kuehne et al. (2004a) have demonstrated successful implantation of a self-expanding stent valve in the aorta via percutaneous access under MR-guidance. Visualization of both coronary ostia during stent implantation allowed optimal positioning and flow assessment. A different MR approach has been recently described to guide the placement of a prosthetic aortic valve in the beating heart via direct apical access (McVeigh 2006).

25.6 CMR-Guided Catheterization and Interventions in Congenital Heart Disease

Interventions in children and adults with congenital heart disease are more complex and challenging than in patients with acquired heart disease, thus require special attention due to anatomical variability. The interventions are currently performed under X-ray guidance and transesophageal echocardiography. A variety of MR-guided interventions have been successfully used in congenital heart diseases including placing transjugular, intrahepatic portosystemic stents, radiofrequency ablation, aortic coarctation, ASD and cardiac catheterization. Other indications for diagnostic cardiac catheterization in pediatric cardiology are abnormalities of the pulmonary arteries and the aortic arch. Both abnormalities can be repaired and assessed on MR imaging and angiography, respectively (Kong 2002, Holmqvist 2001, Godart 2002, Ohno 2002).

Investigators were successful in placing transjugular intrahepatic portosystemic stents (Kee 1999) and using radiofrequency ablation under MR-guidance (Lardo 2000). As with other interventional procedures, accurate localization of the catheter tip in relation to surrounding soft tissue structures is critical for ablation of arrhythmias. Furthermore, knowledge of RF lesion size and location relative to existing abnormal tissue or additional lesions improve success rate in complex patients. More recent developments include the design of a two-wire electrophysiology catheter that simultaneously records intracardiac ECG and receives an MR signal for active catheter tracking. Lardo et al. (2000) demonstrated in a pre-clinical study that a non-magnetic RF ablation catheter can be navigated under MR guidance to the atrial free wall and right ventricular apex.

Several clinical studies (Peters 2007, Reddy 2008, McGann 2008) showed the capability of direct visualization of **atrial scar tissue** on contrast-enhanced MR imaging that results from RF ablation. This finding allows further insight into the mechanism of this procedure, and a direct comparison of the electrophysiologic results with the anatomical data. Yokokawa et al. found that contrast-enhanced and T2-weighted MR imaging can demonstrate the evolution of edema and infarct after RF ablation of the cavotricuspid isthmus (Yokokawa 2011).

Coarctation of the aorta is the most common congenital vascular disease. It is characterized by a stenosis and maldevelopment with hyperplasia of the descending aortic arch. One of the more attractive potential uses for MR-guidance is stent repair of coarctation. In a preclinical study, an aortic stent was delivered under MR-guidance and demonstrated the significant increase in aortic flow and the decrease in collateral flow after coarctation repair, using velocity-encoded cine-MR imaging (Saeed 2006b) (Figure 25-4). In 2006, Krueger et al. performed the first MR-guided study using balloon angioplasty for treating aortic coarctation lesions, in 5 patients. This was an important first clinical step toward completely MR-guided treatment of this congenital lesion.

Atrial septal defect (ASD) is another congenital defect common in children, leading to heart failure and pulmonary

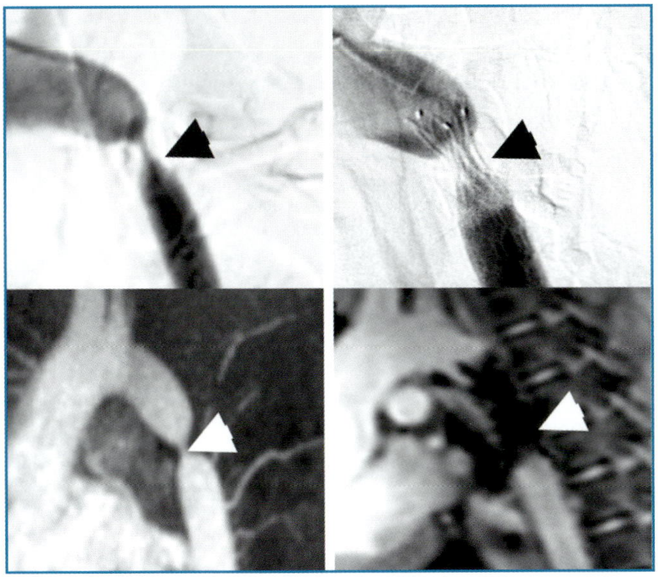

Figure 25-4 Contrast-enhanced X-ray fluoroscopy scans **(top)** and CE-MRA **(bottom)** showing the aortic coarctation in dogs before **(left)** and after **(right)** the deployment of the nitinol stents (arrow heads). Note that the lumen of the stent is visible on X-ray fluoroscopy, but not on MR imaging. The stents restored the flow (measured by VENC-MR imaging) and phasic blood pressure (measured by a pressure transducer) in the aorta (from Saeed M, Henk CB, Weber O et al. Delivery and assessment of endovascular stents to repair aortic coarctation using MR and X-ray imaging. J Magn Reson Imaging 2006; 24 (2): 371–8; this material is reproduced with permission of John Wiley & Sons, Inc.).

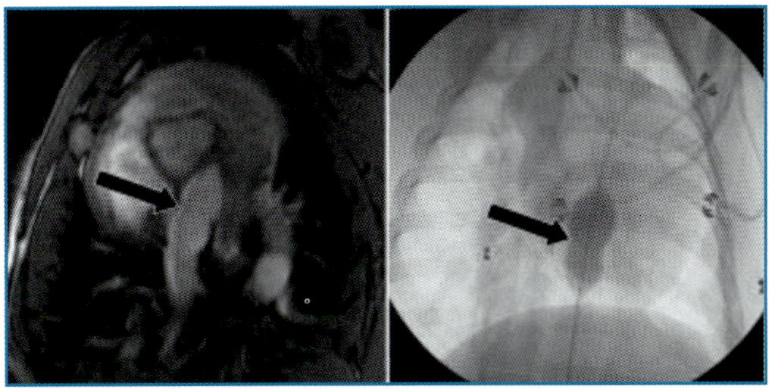

Figure 25-5 Balloon sizing of ASD on a MR image **(left)**, inflated with MR contrast medium, and a X-ray image **(right)**, inflated with CT contrast medium. Note the close estimate of the waist diameter (arrows), representing the stretched ASD diameter (from Schalla S, Saeed M, Higgins CB et al. Balloon sizing and transcatheter closure of acute atrial septal defects guided by magnetic resonance fluoroscopy: assessment and validation in a large animal model. J Magn Reson Imaging 2005; 21 (3): 204–11; with permission of John Wiley & Sons, Inc.).

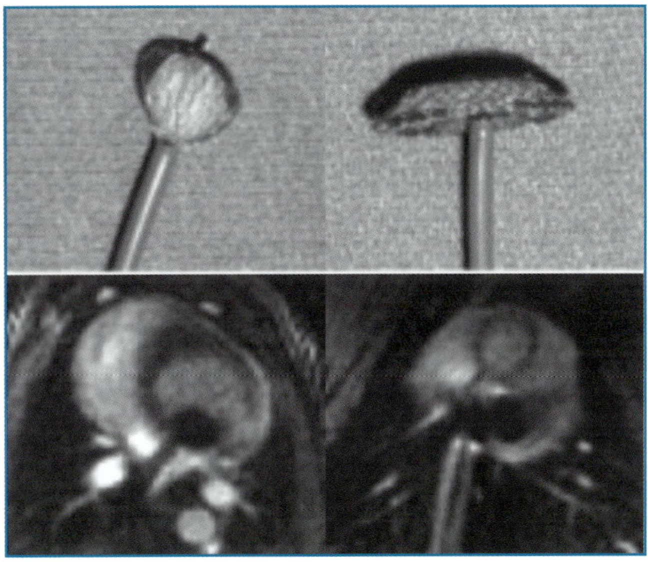

Figure 25-6 Simulation of deployment of the septal occluder device in vitro **(top)**, and corresponding selected real-time MR images in vivo **(bottom)**. The device was easily detected as a signal void on real-time MR images. The closure device was advanced inside the delivery sheath until the folded first disk appeared **(left)** followed by the release of the second disk in the right atrium **(right)** (from Schalla S, Saeed M, Higgins CB et al. Balloon sizing and transcatheter closure of acute atrial septal defects guided by magnetic resonance fluoroscopy: assessment and validation in a large animal model. J Magn Reson Imaging 2005; 21 (3): 204–11; with permission of John Wiley & Sons, Inc.).

hypertension. MR imaging has the capability to provide reliable diagnosis of ASD with extremely high sensitivity (Kersting-Sommerhoff 1990). Percutaneous transcatheter delivery of ASD occluder has been successfully performed under X-ray guidance (Omeish 2001). For ICMR imaging, ASD occluders are made of a nitinol mesh (Schalla 2003), but these devices still produce some artifacts that extend beyond the device dimensions and make assessment of chamber volumes problematic. Substantial experience has been obtained in animal models where real-time MR imaging was used for delivery of ASD closure (Buecker 2002a, Buecker 2002b) and sizing of the ASD (Schalla 2005) (Figure 25-5).

Buecker et al. (2002b) successfully implanted a prototype nitinol double-disk septal occluder in the atrial septum. Repositioning was required due to initial malposition and limited septal visualization. Later a commercial nitinol snare coaxial catheter system was used for delivery of AGA septal occluders (Schalla 2005). Advancement of the delivery system through the IVC to the right atrium and through the septum into the left atrium was monitored using real-time MR imaging (Figure 25-6).

Schalla et al. (2003) simulated clinical-grade pediatric diagnostic catheterization in an animal model with an atrial septal defect and combined the invasive pressure and oxygen measurements with a velocity-encoded MR sequence. In this study both right and left heart catheterization was performed using an active tracking catheter with a hockey stick shape and single tip receiver coil. All chambers and vessels

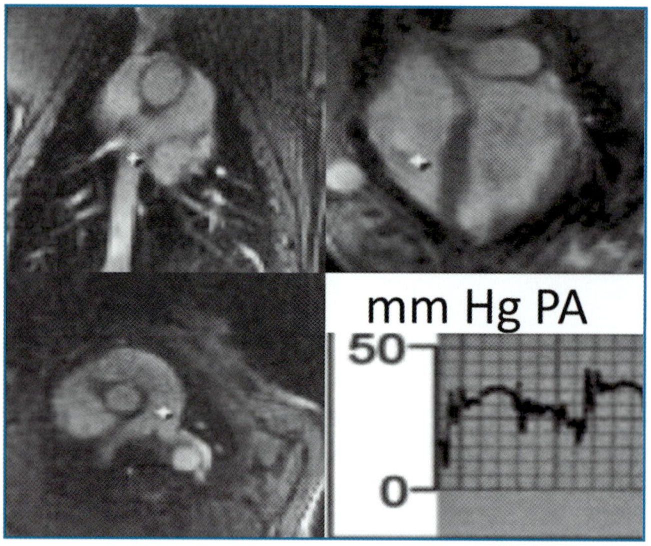

Figure 25-7 Selected real-time MR images show different planes for right atrium and ventricle cardiac catheterization. The images show the plane used for catheter steering to IVC-RA **(top, left)**. The image plane was then switched to a cardiac 4-ch (long-axis) view **(top, right)** to steer the catheter across tricuspid valve into RV. To advance catheter into PA, PA plane **(bottom, left)** was acquired for positioning of catheter into main PA. A PA pressure curve in mmHg is shown **(bottom, right)** (from Schalla S, Saeed M, Higgins CB et al. Magnetic resonance-guided cardiac catheterization in a swine model of atrial septal defect. Circulation 2003; 108 (15): 1865–70; with permission of Lippincott, Williams & Wilkins, Inc.).

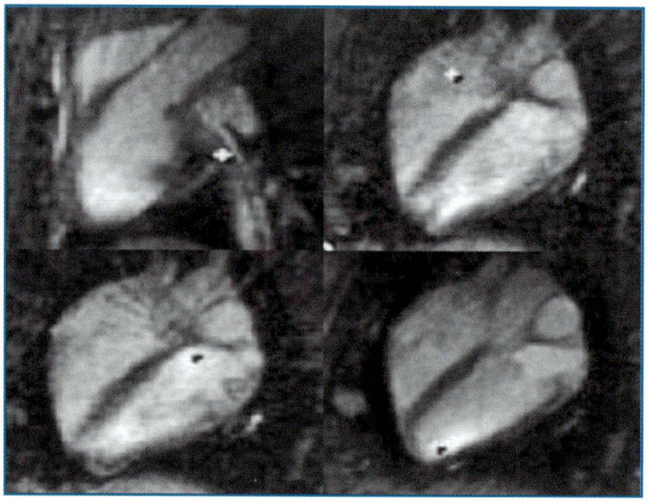

Figure 25-8 Selected real-time MR images show antegrade catheterization of LV (femoral venous/transseptal access). The images show advancement of tracking catheter from IVC **(top, left)** into RA **(top, right)**, transseptally into LA **(bottom, left)**, and LV **(bottom, right)**. Catheter tip is detected as a cross (from Schalla S, Saeed M, Higgins CB et al. Magnetic resonance-guided cardiac catheterization in a swine model of atrial septal defect. Circulation 2003; 108 (15): 1865–70; with permission of Lippincott, Williams & Wilkins, Inc.).

of interest were easily entered using both antegrade and retrograde approaches. The catheter tip and background anatomy were imaged using real time imaging (Figure 25-7 and Figure 25-8). The proposed technique can be used for measurements of blood pressure, oxygen saturation, and flow to define the severity of valvular or vascular stenosis and to characterize ventricular diastolic and systolic function and pulmonary vascular resistance.

Measurements of flow from velocity-encoded MR imaging and blood pressure from the catheter were used to calculate pulmonary resistance. The flow and resistance data obtained from Fick and MR cardiac catheterization methods were in excellent agreement (Razavi 2003, Schalla 2003), suggesting accurate physiologic data can be obtained on MR imaging.

A recent study in 10 patients and 5 volunteers showed that ICMR imaging is suited to guide flow directed catheters for measurement of invasive pulmonary artery pressures (Kuehne 2005). Pulmonary vascular flow volumes were measured with the velocity-encoded cine-MR imaging. Pulmonary pressure was measured through flow directed catheters guided into the pulmonary artery under MR-guidance. The results indicate that MR imaging is a promising tool for measurement of pulmonary vascular resistance in patients with different degrees and forms of pulmonary hypertension (Kuehne 2005). MR-guided cardiac catheterization has also been performed in humans using passive tracking of CO_2-filled balloon catheters (Razavi 2003, Kuehne 2004b).

The ICMR imaging has also been used in connecting cardiac chambers and blood vessels. In a swine study, Arepally et al. (2006) connected right and left atrium by puncturing the interatrial septum using an active Brockenbrough-style needle. Similar approaches could be applied in the future to more challenging geometry and more elaborate procedures. In a preliminary clinical study in seven patients, Dick et al. (2005) conducted trans-septal puncture and balloon septostomy using the MR-guided approach.

25.7 ICMR-Guided Gene and Stem Cell Delivery

Current treatments for myocardial ischemia due to coronary stenosis include pharmacologic drugs and revascularization using percutaneous transluminal coronary angioplasty, stenting or bypass grafting. However, there are an increasing number of patients who have persistent chronic angina, despite having multiple previous coronary revascularization procedures. These patients are not candidates for further

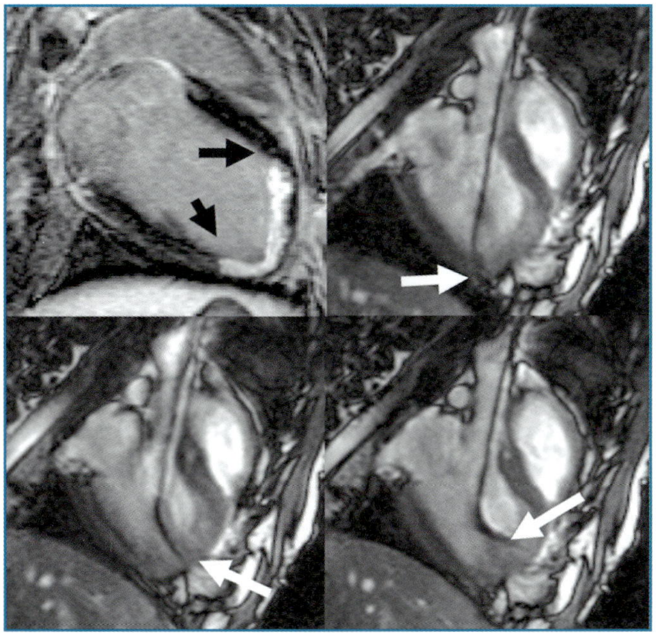

Figure 25-9 Selected delayed contrast-enhanced MR image (top, left) shows the target (infarct and border zone, black arrows). Other real-time MR images show the navigation of the endovascular catheter (arrows) in the LV chamber and the sites of injections of hepatocyte growth factor gene (VM202) in the target. Both surface coil elements and passive catheter are contributing to the images (from Saeed M, Martin A, Jacquier A et al. Permanent coronary artery occlusion: cardiovascular MR imaging is platform for percutaneous transendocardial delivery and assessment of gene therapy in canine model. Radiology 2008; 249 (2): 560–71; with permission of Radiological Society of North America, Inc.).

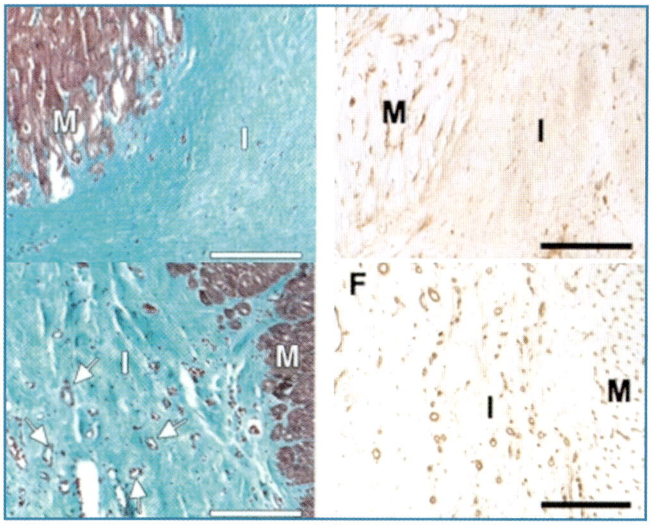

Figure 25-10 Micrographs of infarctions received transendocardially under MR-guidance either plasmid-LacZ (control, top) or plasmid-VEGF (therapy, bottom). Masson trichrome (left) and isolectin B4 (right) stained infarct scar and vascular endothelial cells blue and brown, respectively. Note the new vascularization in plasmid-VEGF animal at 7 wks (arrows), suggesting success of delivery and effectiveness of the gene in revascularizing ischemically injured myocardium. F: fibrosis; I: infarct scar; M: normal myocardium (from Saeed M, Martin A, Jacquier A et al. Permanent coronary artery occlusion: cardiovascular MR imaging is platform for percutaneous transendocardial delivery and assessment of gene therapy in canine model. Radiology 2008; 249 (2): 560–71; with permission of Radiological Society of North America, Inc.).

such revascularization procedures because of diffuse distal vessel disease with poor angiographic run-off, lack of available conduits or unacceptably high peri-operative risk. Furthermore, surgical strategies are impractical in end-stage patients because these strategies increase morbidity and limit the feasibility of repeat administrations (Klein 2007).

The **advantages of local delivery of angiogenic genes and cell therapies** are:

- targeting only the diseased region,
- delivering high local dose,
- eliminating a high systemic dose and side effects, and
- reducing the chance of angiogenesis or arteriogenesis in hidden tumor sites especially in elderly patients.

In early clinical studies local intramyocardial delivery of angiogenic growth factors or genes was used in combination with coronary artery bypass grafting (Allen 1999, Laham 1999, Simon 2000, Simonetti 2002, Ruel 2002, Kleinman 2003, Stamm 2007). Furthermore, MR imaging offers unique and accurate data on cardiac structure, function, and perfusion at both the gross and cellular levels. MR contrast media empowered MR imaging by delineating the target (infarct) and defining the sites of injected materials.

Gene therapy is an exciting area of modern medicine and may be a more straightforward approach to angiogenesis and myogenesis than stem cells considering the environmental and procedural limitations. Therapeutic genes can be delivered to cells in vivo by means of viral or nonviral vectors. Recent MR-guided studies (Saeed 2008a, Saeed 2011) demonstrated the success of catheter-based transendocardial injection of vascular endothelial growth factor gene and hepatocyte growth factor gene (Figure 25-9). In these studies, cine, tagged, velocity-encoded, perfusion and delayed contrast enhancement MR sequences documented the beneficial effects of vascular endothelial growth factor gene and hepatocyte growth factor gene on LV architecture, function, perfusion and viability. Histopathology showed angiogenesis in dogs treated with plasmid-VEGF gene, confirming the success of MR-guided transendocardial delivery (Figure 25-10). Another MR study (Pearlman 2000) showed the increased collateral blood flow in infarcted myocardium after injecting vascular endothelial growth factor. Thus, non-invasive evaluation of physiologic parameters is sensitive for detecting the potential benefits of locally delivered angiogenic genes. Clinical trials, however, have shown that adenoviruses carry a risk of evoking the immune response and this risk must be overcome before MR-guided therapy delivery is clinically applicable (Raper 2003).

Stem cells are a potential candidate for treatment of ischemic heart disease. Recently, investigators used MR-guided procedure to deliver labeled stem cells to infarcted myocardium (Budde 2009, Kraitchman 2003). Most laboratories used iron-oxide MR contrast media that enable the visualization of the cells as dark spots on MR images as a consequence of the largely dominant T2* effects induced by the presence of the magnetic particles (Budde 2009, Kraitchman 2003, Arbab 2005). Follow-up imaging several weeks later showed hypoenhanced artifact indicative of migration of stem cells with in the infarction. MR imaging was used to evaluate changes in LV remodeling following the delivery of cellular therapy (Amado 2005, Arai 2006, Moelker 2006, Grauss 2008, Hashemi 2008, Ziebart 2008). Amado et al. (2006) have been able to identify a time-dependent recovery of local contractility associated with the appearance of new tissue resulting from transplantation of allogeneic stem cells in a pig model of myocardial infarct.

Recent randomized clinical trials demonstrated the safety of bone marrow mononuclear treatment after intracoronary injection using MR imaging (Bartunek 2005, Janssens 2006). Promising clinical results from intracoronary delivery of autologous bone marrow derived stem cells and progenitor cells showed improved myocardial function (Wollert 2004, Bartunek 2005, Schächinger 2006a, Schächinger 2006b, Dill 2009). Schächinger et al. (2006a) studied the efficacy of bone marrow derived progenitor cells using intracoronary route in patients with acute myocardial infarct and in patients at risk for adverse remodeling after acute ST segment elevation myocardial infarct and found sustained improvement in LV ejection fraction (Schächinger 2006a, Dill 2009). The proposed mechanisms of protection by stem cells include angiogenesis via the release of angiogenic factors, myogenesis, cytoprotection via the release of paracrine factors, recruitment of stem cells and suppression of inflammation (Dimmeler 2009).

25.8 Summary

X-ray fluoroscopy has been routinely used to guide endovascular and cardiac catheterization, but it has several limitations that make it suboptimal. Currently, MR vendors are investing in designs tailored toward cardiovascular interventional systems, which can be continuously upgraded. Technological advances have allowed MR imaging to provide 3D images, excellent soft-tissue contrast, multi-planar views, and dynamic imaging in a single imaging session and to guide interventional cardiovascular procedures. Balloon inflation, stent placement, valvar replacement, atrial septal defect closure, radiofrequency ablation and local gene and cell delivery have been shown to be feasible in pre-clinical studies. Translation of cardiac catheterization under MR-guidance to the clinical setting has been slow due to limited availability of MR-friendly catheters, wires, and devices worldwide. MR-guidance of gene or stem cell therapy represents a new discipline whose systematic development will foster minimally invasive interventional procedures and will hasten the identification and deployment of effective new therapies for revascularization. Interventional cardiovascular MR imaging enables a substantially reduced level of invasiveness compared with open-chest surgery, potentially resulting in treatment on an outpatient basis, rapid patient recovery, and cost savings to the health care system.

References

Aletras AH, Ding S, Balaban RS, Wen H. DENSE: displacement encoding with stimulated echoes in cardiac functional MRI. J Magn Reson 1999; 137: 247–52.

Allen KB, Dowling RD, Fudge TL et al. Comparison of transmyocardial revascularization with medical therapy in patients with refractory angina. N Engl J Med 1999; 341: 1029–36.

Amado LC, Saliaris AP, Schuleri KH et al. Cardiac repair with intramyocardial injection of allogeneic mesenchymal stem cells after myocardial infarction. Proc Natl Acad Sci USA 2005; 102: 11474–9.

Amado LC, Schuleri KH, Saliaris AP et al. Multi-modality non-invasive imaging demonstrates in vivo cardiac regeneration after mesenchymal stem cell therapy. J Am Coll Cardiol 2006; 48: 2116–24.

Arai T, Kofidis T, Bulte JW et al. Dual in vivo magnetic resonance evaluation of magnetically labeled mouse embryonic stem cells and cardiac function at 1.5 T. Magn Reson Med 2006; 55: 203–9.

Arbab AS, Yocum GT, Rad AM et al. Labeling of cells with ferumoxides-protamine sulfate complexes does not inhibit function or differentiation capacity of hematopoietic or mesenchymal stem cells. NMR Biomed 2005; 18: 553–9.

Arepally A, Karmarkar PV, Weiss C, Atalar E. Percutaneous MR imaging-guided transvascular access of mesenteric venous system: study in swine model. Radiology 2006; 238: 113–8.

Axel L. Non-invasive measurement of cardiac strain with MRI. Adv Exp Med Biol 1997; 430: 249–56.

Bacher K, Bogaert E, Lapere R et al. Patient-specific dose and radiation risk estimation in pediatric cardiac catheterization. Circulation 2005; 111: 83–9.

Bakker CJ, Hoogeveen RM, Hurtak WF et al. MR-guided endovascular interventions: susceptibility-based catheter and near-real-time imaging technique. Radiology 1997; 202: 273–6.

Bakker CJ, Smits HF, Bos C et al. MR-guided balloon angioplasty: in vitro demonstration of the potential of MRI for guiding, monitoring, and evaluating endovascular interventions. J Magn Reson Imaging 1998; 8: 245–50.

Bartunek J, Vanderheyden M, Vandekerckhove B et al. Intracoronary injection of CD133-positive enriched bone marrow progenitor cells promotes cardiac recovery after recent myocardial infarction: feasibility and safety. Circulation 2005; 112: 178–83.

Bock M, Volz S, Zuhlsdorff S et al. MR-guided intravascular procedures: real-time parameter control and automated slice positioning with active tracking coils. J Magn Reson Imaging 2004; 19: 580–9.

Brenner D, Elliston C, Hall E, Berdon W. Estimated risks of radiation-induced fatal cancer from pediatric CT. Am J Roentgenol 2001; 176: 289–96.

Budde MD, Frank JA. Magnetic tagging of therapeutic cells for MRI. J Nucl Med 2009; 50: 171–4.

Buecker A, Adam GB, Neuerburg JM et al. Simultaneous real-time visualization of the catheter tip and vascular anatomy for MR-guided PTA of iliac arteries in an animal model. J Magn Reson Imaging 2002a; 16: 201–8.

Buecker A, Neuerburg JM, Adam GB et al. Real-time MR fluoroscopy for MR-guided iliac artery stent placement. J Magn Reson Imaging 2000; 12: 616–22.

Buecker A, Spuentrup E, Grabitz R et al. Magnetic resonance-guided placement of atrial septal closure device in animal model of patent foramen ovale. Circulation 2002b; 106: 511–5.

Buecker A, Spuentrup E, Ruebben A et al. New metallic MR stents for artifact-free coronary MR angiography: feasibility study in a swine model. Invest Radiol 2004; 39: 250–3.

Busse RF, Riederer SJ. Steady-state preparation for spoiled gradient echo imaging. Magn Reson Med 2001; 45: 653–61.

Demas V, Herberg JL, Malba V et al. Portable, low-cost NMR with laser-lathe lithography produced microcoils. J Magn Reson 2007; 189: 121–9.

Dick AJ, Raman VK, Raval AN et al. Invasive human magnetic resonance imaging: feasibility during revascularization in a combined XMR suite. Catheter Cardiovasc Interv 2005; 64: 265–74.

Dill T, Schachinger V, Rolf A et al. Intracoronary administration of bone marrow-derived progenitor cells improves left ventricular function in patients at risk for adverse remodeling after acute ST-segment elevation myocardial infarction: results of the Reinfusion of Enriched Progenitor cells And Infarct Remodeling in Acute Myocardial Infarction study (REPAIR-AMI) cardiac magnetic resonance imaging substudy. Am Heart J 2009; 157: 541–7.

Dimmeler S, Zeiher AM. Cell therapy of acute myocardial infarction: open questions. Cardiology 2009; 113: 155–60.

Dion YM, Ben El-Kadi H, Boudoux C et al. Endovascular procedures under near-real-time magnetic resonance imaging guidance: an experimental feasibility study. J Vasc Surg 2000; 32: 1006–14.

Duerk JL, Lewin JS, Wendt M, Petersilge C. Remember true FISP? A high SNR, near 1 s imaging method for T2-like contrast in interventional MRI at 2 T. J Magn Reson Imaging 1998; 8: 203–8.

Flask C, Elgort D, Wong E et al. A method for fast 3D tracking using tuned fiducial markers and a limited projection reconstruction FISP (LPR-FISP) sequence. J Magn Reson Imaging 2001; 14: 617–27.

Frush DP, Donnelly LF, Rosen NS. Computed tomography and radiation risks: what pediatric health care providers should know. Pediatrics 2003; 112: 951–7.

Godart F, Labrot G, Devos P et al. Coarctation of the aorta: comparison of aortic dimensions between conventional MR imaging, 3D MR angiography, and conventional angiography. Eur Radiol 2002; 12: 2034–9.

Grauss RW, van Tuyn J, Steendijk P et al. Forced myocardin expression enhances the therapeutic effect of human mesenchymal stem cells after transplantation in ischemic mouse hearts. Stem Cells 2008; 26: 1083–93.

Hashemi SM, Ghods S, Kolodgie FD et al. A placebo controlled, dose-ranging, safety study of allogenic mesenchymal stem cells injected by endomyocardial delivery after an acute myocardial infarction. Eur Heart J 2008; 29: 251–9.

Hillenbrand CM, Jesberger JA, Wong EY et al. Toward rapid high resolution in vivo intravascular MRI: evaluation of vessel wall conspicuity in a porcine model using multiple imaging protocols. J Magn Reson Imaging 2006; 23: 135–44.

Holmqvist C, Hochbergs P, Bjorkhem G et al. Pre-operative evaluation with MR in tetralogy of fallot and pulmonary atresia with ventricular septal defect. Acta Radiol 2001; 42: 63–9.

Hundley WG, Hamilton CA, Thomas MS et al. Utility of fast cine magnetic resonance imaging and display for the detection of myocardial ischemia in patients not well suited for second harmonic stress echocardiography. Circulation 1999; 100: 1697–702.

Hushek SG, Martin AJ, Steckner M et al. MR systems for MRI-guided interventions. J Magn Reson Imaging 2008; 27: 253–66.

Jacquier A, Higgins CB, Martin AJ et al. Injection of adeno-associated viral vector encoding vascular endothelial growth factor gene in infarcted swine myocardium: MR measurements of left ventricular function and strain. Radiology 2007; 245: 196–205.

Janssens S, Dubois C, Bogaert J et al. Autologous bone marrow-derived stem-cell transfer in patients with ST-segment elevation myocardial infarction: double-blind, randomised controlled trial. Lancet 2006; 367: 113–21.

Kee ST, Rhee JS, Butts K et al. MR-guided transjugular portosystemic shunt placement in a swine model. J Vasc Interv Radiol 1999; 10: 529–35.

Kersting-Sommerhoff BA, Diethelm L, Stanger P et al. Evaluation of complex congenital ventricular anomalies with magnetic resonance imaging. Am Heart J 1990; 120: 133–42.

Klein HM, Ghodsizad A, Marktanner R et al. Intramyocardial implantation of $CD133^+$ stem cells improved cardiac function without bypass surgery. Heart Surg Forum 2007; 10: E66–E9.

Kleinman NS, Patel NC, Allen KB et al. Evolving revascularization approaches for myocardial ischemia. Am J Cardiol 2003; 92: 9N–17N.

Klemm T, Duda S, Machann J et al. MR imaging in the presence of vascular stents: A systematic assessment of artifacts for various stent orientations, sequence types, and field strengths. J Magn Reson Imaging 2000; 12: 606–15.

Kocaturk O, Saikus CE, Guttman MA et al. Whole shaft visibility and mechanical performance for active MR catheters using copper-nitinol braided polymer tubes. J Cardiovasc Magn Reson 2009; 11: 29.

Kong H, Gu X, Titus JL et al. Creation of an intra-atrial communication with a new amplatzer shunt prosthesis: preliminary results in a swine model. Catheter Cardiovasc Interv 2002; 56: 267–71.

Konings MK, Bartels LW, Smits HF, Bakker CJ. Heating around intravascular guidewires by resonating RF waves. J Magn Reson Imaging 2000; 12: 79–85.

Kraitchman DL, Heldman AW, Atalar E et al. In vivo magnetic resonance imaging of mesenchymal stem cells in myocardial infarction. Circulation 2003; 107: 2290–3.

Krueger JJ, Ewert P, Yilmaz S et al. Magnetic resonance imaging-guided balloon angioplasty of coarctation of the aorta: a pilot study. Circulation 2006; 113: 1093–100.

Kuehne T, Saeed M, Higgins CB et al. Endovascular stents in pulmonary valve and artery in swine: feasibility study of MR imaging-guided deployment and post-interventional assessment. Radiology 2003; 226: 475–81.

Kuehne T, Saeed M, Moore P et al. Influence of blood-pool contrast media on MR imaging and flow measurements in the presence of pulmonary arterial stents in swine. Radiology 2002; 223: 439–45.

Kuehne T, Saeed M, Reddy G et al. Sequential magnetic resonance monitoring of pulmonary flow with endovascular stents placed across the pulmonary valve in growing swine. Circulation 2001; 104: 2363–8.

Kuehne T, Yilmaz S, Meinus C et al. Magnetic resonance imaging-guided transcatheter implantation of a prosthetic valve in aortic valve position: Feasibility study in swine. J Am Coll Cardiol 2004a; 44: 2247–9.

Kuehne T, Yilmaz S, Schulze-Neick I et al. Magnetic resonance imaging guided catheterisation for assessment of pulmonary vascular resistance: in vivo validation and clinical application in patients with pulmonary hypertension. Heart 2005; 91: 1064–9.

Kuehne T, Yilmaz S, Steendijk P et al. Magnetic resonance imaging analysis of right ventricular pressure-volume loops: in vivo validation and clinical application in patients with pulmonary hypertension. Circulation 2004b; 110: 2010–6.

Kuon E. Radiation exposure in invasive cardiology. Heart 2008; 94: 667–74.

Laham RJ, Sellke FW, Edelman ER et al. Local perivascular delivery of basic fibroblast growth factor in patients undergoing coronary bypass surgery: results of a phase I randomized, double-blind, placebo-controlled trial. Circulation 1999; 100: 1865–71.

Lardo AC, McVeigh ER, Jumrussirikul P et al. Visualization and temporal/spatial characterization of cardiac radiofrequency ablation lesions using magnetic resonance imaging. Circulation 2000; 102: 698–705.

Lindholt JS. Radiocontrast induced nephropathy. Eur J Vasc Endovasc Surg 2003; 25: 296–304.

Maes RM, Lewin JS, Duerk JL, Wacker FK. Combined use of the intravascular blood-pool agent, gadomer, and carbon dioxide: a novel type of double-contrast magnetic resonance angiography (MRA). J Magn Reson Imaging 2005; 21: 645–9.

Manke C, Nitz WR, Djavidani B et al. MR imaging-guided stent placement in iliac arterial stenoses: a feasibility study. Radiology 2001; 219: 527–34.

Manke C, Nitz WR, Lenhart M et al. Stent angioplasty of pelvic artery stenosis with MRI control: initial clinical results. Rofo 2000; 172: 92–7.

Martin AJ, Weber OM, Saeed M, Roberts TP. Steady-state imaging for visualization of endovascular interventions. Magn Reson Med 2003; 50: 434–8.

McFadden SL, Mooney RB, Shepherd PH. X-ray dose and associated risks from radiofrequency catheter ablation procedures. Br J Radiol 2002; 75: 253–65.

McGann CJ, Kholmovski EG, Oakes RS et al. New magnetic resonance imaging-based method for defining the extent of left atrial wall injury after the ablation of atrial fibrillation. J Am Coll Cardiol 2008; 52: 1263–71.

McVeigh ER, Guttman MA, Lederman RJ et al. Real-time interactive MRI-guided cardiac surgery: aortic valve replacement using a direct apical approach. Magn Reson Med 2006; 56: 958–64.

Mekle R, Hofmann E, Scheffler K, Bilecen D. A polymer-based MR-compatible guidewire: a study to explore new prospects for interventional peripheral magnetic resonance angiography (ipMRA). J Magn Reson Imaging 2006; 23: 145–55.

Mekle R, Zenge MO, Ladd ME et al. Initial in vivo studies with a polymer-based MR-compatible guide wire. J Vasc Interv Radiol 2009; 20: 1384–9.

Moelker AD, Baks T, van den Bos EJ et al. Reduction in infarct size, but no functional improvement after bone marrow cell administration in a porcine model of reperfused myocardial infarction. Eur Heart J 2006; 27: 3057–64.

Muthurangu V, Taylor A, Andriantsimiavona R et al. Novel method of quantifying pulmonary vascular resistance by use of simultaneous invasive pressure monitoring and phase contrast magnetic resonance flow. Circulation 2004; 110: 826–34.

Nitz WR, Oppelt A, Renz W et al. On the heating of linear conductive structures as guide wires and catheters in interventional MRI. J Magn Reson Imaging 2001; 13: 105–14.

Ohno Y, Hatabu H, Takenaka D et al. Contrast-enhanced MR perfusion imaging and MR angiography: utility for management of pulmonary arterio-venous malformations for embolotherapy. Eur J Radiol 2002; 41: 136–46.

Omary RA, Frayne R, Unal O et al. MR-guided angioplasty of renal artery stenosis in a pig model: a feasibility study. J Vasc Interv Radiol 2000; 11: 373–81.

Omeish A, Hijazi ZM. Transcatheter closure of atrial septal defects in children and adults using the Amplatzer Septal Occluder. J Interv Cardiol 2001; 14: 37–44.

Osman NF, Kerwin WS, McVeigh ER, Prince JL. Cardiac motion tracking using CINE harmonic phase (HARP) magnetic resonance imaging. Magn Reson Med 1999; 42: 1048–60.

Paetzel C, Zorger N, Bachthaler M et al. Magnetic resonance-guided percutaneous angioplasty of femoral and popliteal artery stenoses using real-time imaging and intra-arterial contrast-enhanced magnetic resonance angiography. Invest Radiol 2005; 40: 257–62.

Paetzel C, Zorger N, Bachthaler M et al. Feasibility of MR-guided angioplasty of femoral artery stenoses using real-time imaging and intraarterial contrast-enhanced MR angiography. Rofo 2004; 176: 1232–6.

Park SM, Kamondetdacha R, Nyenhuis JA. Calculation of MRI-induced heating of an implanted medical lead wire with an electric field transfer function. J Magn Reson Imaging 2007; 26: 1278–85.

Pearlman JD, Laham RJ, Simons M. Coronary angiogenesis: detection in vivo with MR imaging sensitive to collateral neocirculation – preliminary study in pigs. Radiology 2000; 214: 801–7.

Peters DC, Lederman RJ, Dick AJ et al. Undersampled projection reconstruction for active catheter imaging with adaptable temporal resolution and catheter-only views. Magn Reson Med 2003; 49: 216–22.

Peters DC, Wylie JV, Hauser TH et al. Detection of pulmonary vein and left atrial scar after catheter ablation with three-dimensional navigator-gated delayed enhancement MR imaging: initial experience. Radiology 2007; 243: 690–5.

Peters TM. Image-guidance for surgical procedures. Phys Med Biol 2006; 51: R505–R40.

Pruessmann KP, Weiger M, Scheidegger MB, Boesiger P. SENSE: sensitivity encoding for fast MRI. Magn Reson Med 1999; 42: 952–62.

Quick HH, Kuehl H, Kaiser G et al. Inductively coupled stent antennas in MRI. Magn Reson Med 2002; 48: 781–90.

Raper SE, Chirmule N, Lee FS et al. Fatal systemic inflammatory response syndrome in a ornithine transcarbamylase deficient patient following adenoviral gene transfer. Mol Genet Metab 2003; 80: 148–58.

Raval AN, Telep JD, Guttman MA et al. Real-time magnetic resonance imaging-guided stenting of aortic coarctation with commercially available catheter devices in swine. Circulation 2005; 112: 699–706.

Razavi R, Hill DL, Keevil SF et al. Cardiac catheterisation guided by MRI in children and adults with congenital heart disease. Lancet 2003; 362: 1877–82.

Reddy VY, Schmidt EJ, Holmvang G, Fung M. Arrhythmia recurrence after atrial fibrillation ablation: can magnetic resonance imaging identify gaps in atrial ablation lines? J Cardiovasc Electrophysiol 2008; 19: 434–37.

Roberts TP, Hassenzahl WV, Hetts SW, Arenson RL. Remote control of catheter tip deflection: an opportunity for interventional MRI. Magn Reson Med 2002; 48: 1091–5.

Ruel M, Laham RJ, Parker JA et al. Long-term effects of surgical angiogenic therapy with fibroblast growth factor 2 protein. J Thorac Cardiovasc Surg 2002; 124: 28–34.

Saeed M, Henk CB, Weber O et al. Delivery and assessment of endovascular stents to repair aortic coarctation using MR and X-ray imaging. J Magn Reson Imaging 2006a; 24: 371–8.

Saeed M, Martin A, Jacquier A et al. Permanent coronary artery occlusion: cardiovascular MR imaging is platform for percutaneous transendocardial delivery and assessment of gene therapy in canine model. Radiology 2008a; 249: 560–71.

Saeed M, Martin A, Ursell P et al. MR assessment of myocardial perfusion, viability, and function after intramyocardial transfer of VM202, a new plasmid human hepatocyte growth factor in ischemic swine myocardium. Radiology 2008b; 249: 107–18.

Saeed M, Martin AJ, Lee RJ et al. MR guidance of targeted injections into border and core of scarred myocardium in pigs. Radiology 2006b; 240: 419–26.

Saeed M, Saloner D, Do L et al. Cardiovascular magnetic resonance imaging in delivering and evaluating the efficacy of hepatocyte growth factor gene in chronic infarct scar. Cardiovasc Revasc Med 2011; 12 (2): 111–22.

Saeed M, Saloner D, Martin A et al. Adeno-associated viral vector-encoding vascular endothelial growth factor gene: effect on cardiovascular MR perfusion and infarct resorption measurements in swine. Radiology 2007; 243: 451–60.

Saeed M, Saloner D, Weber O et al. MRI in guiding and assessing intramyocardial therapy. Eur Radiol 2005; 15: 851–63.

Saikus CE, Lederman RJ. Interventional cardiovascular magnetic resonance imaging: a new opportunity for image-guided interventions. JACC Cardiovasc Imaging 2009; 2: 1321–31.

Schächinger V, Erbs S, Elsasser A et al. Intracoronary bone marrow-derived progenitor cells in acute myocardial infarction. N Engl J Med 2006a; 355: 1210–21.

Schächinger V, Erbs S, Elsasser A et al. Improved clinical outcome after intracoronary administration of bone-marrow-derived progenitor cells in acute myocardial infarction: final 1-year results of the REPAIR-AMI trial. Eur Heart J 2006b; 27: 2775–83.

Schalla S, Saeed M, Higgins CB et al. Magnetic resonance-guided cardiac catheterization in a swine model of atrial septal defect. Circulation 2003; 108: 1865–70.

Schalla S, Saeed M, Higgins CB et al. Balloon sizing and transcatheter closure of acute atrial septal defects guided by magnetic resonance fluoroscopy: assessment and validation in a large animal model. J Magn Reson Imaging 2005; 21: 204–11.

Settecase F, Sussman MS, Wilson MW et al. Magnetically-assisted remote control (MARC) steering of endovascular catheters for interventional MRI: a model for deflection and design implications. Med Phys 2007; 34: 3135–42.

Shankaranarayanan A, Wendt M, Aschoff AJ et al. Radial keyhole sequences for low field projection reconstruction interventional MRI. J Magn Reson Imaging 2001; 13: 142–51.

Shellock FG, Crues 3rd. JV. MR Safety and the American College of Radiology. White Paper. Am J Roentgenol 2002; 178: 1349–52.

Simon M, Bonow RO, Chronos NA et al. Clinical trials in coronary angiogenesis: issues, problems, consensus: An expert panel summary. Circulation 2000; 102: E73–E86.

Simonetti O, Lucarini G, Brancorsini D et al. Immunohistochemical expression of vascular endothelial growth factor, matrix metalloproteinase 2, and matrix metalloproteinase 9 in cutaneous melanocytic lesions. Cancer 2002; 95: 1963–70.

Spielman DM, Pauly JM, Meyer CH. Magnetic resonance fluoroscopy using spirals with variable sampling densities. Magn Reson Med 1995; 34: 388–94.

Spuentrup E, Ruebben A, Schaeffter T et al. Magnetic resonance-guided coronary artery stent placement in a swine model. Circulation 2002; 105: 874–9.

Stamm C, Kleine HD, Choi YH et al. Intramyocardial delivery of $CD133^+$ bone marrow cells and coronary artery bypass grafting for chronic ischemic heart disease: safety and efficacy studies. J Thorac Cardiovasc Surg 2007; 133: 717–25.

Wacker FK, Hillenbrand C, Elgort DR et al. MR imaging-guided percutaneous angioplasty and stent placement in a swine model comparison of open- and closed-bore scanners. Acad Radiol 2005; 12: 1085–8.

Wollert KC, Meyer GP, Lotz J et al. Intracoronary autologous bone-marrow cell transfer after myocardial infarction: the BOOST randomised controlled clinical trial. Lancet 2004; 364: 141–8.

Yang X, Atalar E. MRI-guided gene therapy. FEBS Lett 2006; 580: 2958–61.

Yokokawa M, Tada H, Koyama K et al. The change in the tissue characterization detected by magnetic resonance imaging after radiofrequency ablation of isthmus-dependent atrial flutter. Int J Cardiol 2011; 148: 30–5.

Ziebart T, Yoon CH, Trepels T et al. Sustained persistence of transplanted proangiogenic cells contributes to neovascularization and cardiac function after ischemia. Circ Res 2008; 103: 1327–34.

26 Cardiovascular Computed Tomography

Martin Hoffmann, Sabine Wuchenauer, Horst Brunner and Oliver Klass

26.1 Introduction

Cardiovascular computed tomography (CT) is the accepted standard of reference for non-invasive aortic and pulmonary angiography imaging, it has replaced invasive methods for the detection of pulmonary embolism and aortic dissection. During the last decade we have seen another non-invasive angiographic application to be proposed for CT. The rapid rise of coronary CT angiography from a research application to a robust, widely embraced clinical tool has few parallels in modern medicine. We currently observe a multitude of indicators that CT angiography has the potential to become a pivotal cornerstone in cardiovascular disease management. It therefore deserves the highest level of attention, which has culminated in a dedicated CT chapter of this primarily MR oriented textbook. The chapter is written to emphasize aspects of cardiovascular CT imaging with supplemental and competitive potential for MR imaging of the heart.

26.2 Basic Principles and Technology

In order to provide a suitable tool for non-invasive coronary imaging sub-millimeter spatial resolution has to be coupled with sufficient temporal resolution for artifact free images. The first generation of CT scanners to achieve this was based on electron-beam deflection to sweep stationary tungsten target rings to produce X-rays (Lipton 1984). The fastest version of this type of EBT scanner the "e-Speed" was optimized for a temporal resolution of 33 ms per cross-sectional image (Budoff 2003). But the complicated and expensive technology provides only limited tube power. Larger cone angles of homogenous X-rays cannot be produced to illuminate a large area detector behind a patient. This is the reason why excellent temporal resolution of EBT cannot be coupled with sufficient spatial resolution nor with short breath-hold durations for the completion of image acquisition.

The cost efficient technology that initiated the rapid development of cardiac CT is based on multi-detector technology (Bastarrika 2009). The original "Hounsfield" CT scanner consisted of a single detector row mounted on one side of the patient with an X-ray tube on the opposite side of the patient (Hounsfield 1973, Hounsfield 1976). The set-up was rotated around the patient to reconstruct cross-sectional images. In the late 90ies a second detector row was added to this setup to simultaneously acquire cross-sectional images at different longitudinal planes along the body (Kramer 1998). In 1998 another set of detector rows was added to arrive at a 4 detector row array (Ohnesorge 2000). This initiated an exponential growth of detector rows arriving at up to 320 simultaneous detector rows with a 16 cm long detector array at present (Dewey 2009). Such a large detector allows to cover the cardiac volume within a single rotation. Very efficient acquisitions from a single cardiac cycle can be obtained. The only disadvantage of this setup is the limited temporal resolution due to a limited tube power to illuminate the large cone angle. The rotation time of the 16 cm detector setup is currently limited to 350 ms. Half a rotation is necessary for a complete reconstruction of the dataset. In other words the temporal resolution of the 16 cm detector system is only 175 ms. Other vendors have therefore constructed CT gantry setups which compromise on detector size and temporal resolution. An 8 cm detector setup with a high power tube allows rotational times of up to 270 ms, the fastest value achieved in current systems (Klass 2010). The rotation time of the gantry can be easily increased, provided that sufficient peak tube power will be available in the upcoming years. The system is no longer mounted on conventional ball bearings to rotate the heavy gantry but sits on air bearing cushions. This allows to rotate the 1–2 ton heavy gantry at very high speeds. The typical temporal resolution at helical scan modes of this set-up is 67–135 ms utilizing so-called multi-cycle retrospective gating modes. Multiple successive heart beats are combined for temporal resolution values beyond half a gantry rotation. This does very effectively reduce the temporal window length for reconstruction down to less than 67 ms. But multi-cycle reconstructions succeed to improve temporal resolution at certain heart rate ranges only (Hoffmann 2005a). The multi-cycle reconstruction does not work satisfactorily with a single tube and detector setup due to two cyclic processes (gantry rotation and cardiac cyclic motion) interfering with one another. Dual source gantry setups with two tubes and detectors mounted in 90° phase shift on the gantry ring have been created in order to obviate this deficiency (Flohr 2006). The fastest currently available machine rotates at gantry speeds of 280 ms and reduces the temporal resolution window to a length of 70 ms irrespective of heart rate (Lell 2009).

The typical scan mode for almost all CT scan acquisitions since the early 90ies is helical or spiral. That means the patient is propagated through the gantry on a sliding table at various speeds. For cardiac scanning an ECG signal is recorded in relation to the scan propagation. The table speed is reduced (low pitch settings) in order to acquire a complete cardiac cycle at any given longitudinal z-axis position (Hoffmann 2005a). Retrospective gating without any "dose saving" measures is not ideally suited for cardiac imaging. This is simply due to the fact that cardiac imaging requires phase or cardiac cycle correlation. If phase correlation is coupled with another cyclic process like the rotation of the scanner gantry, one cyclic process has to wait for the other. In other words, helical CT imaging with ECG registration has to guarantee that the rotating CT gantry will capture at least one complete cardiac cycle at any given z-axis position. This results in a tremendous reduction of the acquisition speed with a very slow table feed. Without any tube current modulation or other measures to reduce the dose exposure this would result in a huge amount of redundant tissue exposure. Only a fraction of this dataset (centered on the phase of interest) is subsequently used for image reconstruction. But tube current modulations have proven not very effective in dose reduction and amount to 50% savings at best (Hoffmann 2005a). Since the advent of non-invasive coronary angiography utilizing CT the clinical value of the modality has almost never been questioned. Criticism has concentrated on the very high dose exposure of CT imaging per se (Brenner and Hall 2007) and cardiac CT imaging especially (Einstein 2007). The dose exposure for retrospective helical gating is in the range of 10–18 mSv (Hausleiter 2009, Klass 2010). This compares very unfavorably to catheter angiography reported with dose exposures in the range of 5–8 mSv (Dewey 2009).

The very high dose exposure associated with helical cardiac CT has stimulated a quest for a more effective solution. For the large area detectors with a detector width of > 4 cm the standard acquisition mode of helical propagation is no longer used as the routine protocol for cardiac acquisitions. It has been replaced by much more dose efficient prospectively gated acquisition modes (Bastarrika 2009). For a detector size of 16 cm the scanner rotates at the level of the heart and a single X-ray exposure shoot is placed at the presumably most quiescent phase of the cardiac cycle (mid-diastolic or diastasis for heart rates < 65 bpm, and end-systolic for higher heart rates). For smaller detectors a so-called step and shoot mode is applied, e.g. for an 8 cm detector a total of 3 heart beats is needed (Klass 2010). The scanner acquires the upper part of the cardiac volume in heart beat one, than travels to the lower part of the cardiac volume in heart beat two and completes the acquisition in heart beat three. This scan mode is much more dose efficient compared to retrospective techniques, most of the coronary angiography scans can be completed at a cumulative dose exposure of 1–4 mSv today. One disadvantage of axial acquisition techniques is that a functional cine sequence cannot be reconstructed. This may preclude the functional evaluation of non-coronary cardiac structures. The helical scan will therefore remain first choice for valvular or ventricular functional CT imaging provided that contraindications for MR exist and MR imaging should be considered as the mainstay modality for such purposes.

26.2.1 Heart Rate Reduction and Vasodilatation

Even with the latest generation of CT scanners (64-slice, 256-slice and 320-slice MDCT) it is recommended to slow the heart rate by the administration of β-blockers or ion-channel blockers such as ivabradine. Some of the most recent scanner generations equipped with rapid rotational gantries or dual-source technology are able to render diagnostic image quality at higher (i. e. > 75–80 bpm) heart rates (Lell 2009). But both image quality and efficiency of dose saving protocols is always compromised without the use of heart rate reduction. Heart rate reduction can be efficiently achieved by oral administration of medication 1–2 h prior to the examination, i.v. injection on the CT table or a combination of both. Heart rate reduction not only reduces the amount of motion artifacts in the acquisition window but also allows to efficiently lower radiation dose exposure. Both high-pitch helical scanning with dual source scanners and prospective axial gating techniques with single source large area detectors require low heart rates (< 65 bpm) to provide good image quality at maximum dose savings. For a full chest coverage with the intention of triple-rule-out scanning the dose exposure can be as high as 20 mSv with standard helical scanning at higher heart rates. With the use of efficient dose reduction techniques that require heart rates of less than 65 bpm the effective dose can be efficiently reduced to 4 mSv, equivalent to non-gated scan acquisition (Sommer 2010). The application of sublingual nitroglycerine immediately before scanning results in increased diameters of the coronary arteries and substantially improves evaluability (Klass 2009).

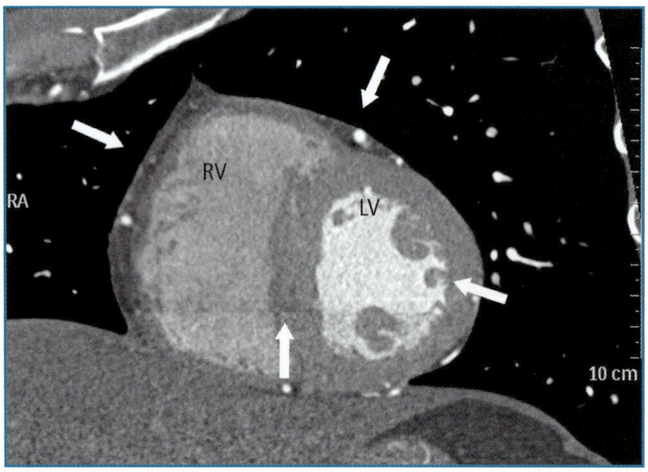

Figure 26-1 Multi-planar reformation in short-axis orientation. The high density contrast bolus injection has arrived in the coronary artery circulation (bright white round spots on the epicardial surface represent cross-sectional cuts of the coronary arteries, arrows). The tail of the bolus is located in the left ventricle with a high attenuation in the cavum. Filling defects are induced by papillary muscles and myocardial trabecularization. The right ventricle is contrasted against surrounding septal and free wall myocardium due to the addition of 10–20 % contrast agent to the saline flush. LV: left ventricle; RV: right ventricle.

26.2.2 Breath Holding and Positioning

It is important to practice **inspiratory breath holding** with the patient on the CT table before scanning.

> This has a number of **important beneficial effects**:
> - patients familiarize with the breath holding instruction and duration,
> - the physician or technologist can ensure that patients perform adequately with no residual motion during the short acquisition time, and
> - the heart rate varies between rest and breath holding, allowing to adjust the β-blocker dosage.

26.2.3 Contrast Injection

There are various injection protocols that can be applied to coronary CTA. Some parameters are even vendor specific. It is beyond the scope of this book chapter to offer details. However, there are a number of common principles that are important to review. The intravenous line is ideally of large bore and should be placed in the right antecubital fossa. The right side is preferred for a shorter distance to the heart and avoids the passage of dense contrast past the ostium of the left internal mammary artery (LIMA) and the great vessels via the left innominate vein. This avoids streak artifacts to interfer with diagnostic image quality. High flow rates typically in the range of 5–7 ml/s are needed. Larger patients generally require faster flow rates (and larger overall volumes) to achieve the same opacification as in smaller patients. Dual-head injection pumps are standard for cardiac CT. This allows to follow the initial phase of contrast injection with a saline chaser flush. Contrast is washed out of the veins and the right atrium and ventricle. This avoids artifacts and enhances the contrast in the descending right coronary artery. Some investigators supplement the saline flush with 10–20% of contrast agent in order to achieve low contrast opacification of the right side of the heart (Klass 2009). This allows the evaluation of right ventricular function and morphology (Figure 26-1).

26.2.4 Best Phase Selection

The initial reconstruction of images for coronary CTA datasets is usually performed in mid- to late-diastole (so-called diastasis) in which the heart is most quiescent. Late-diastole is usually less appropriate due to atrial contraction generating coronary tree motion. This holds true especially for the AV groove sections of the RCA and the LCX. One exception to this rule is atrial fibrillation with absent atrial contraction, for these an end-diastolic phase selection renders best image quality. The field of view of the axial source stack is limited to the cardiac structures in order to maximize in plane spatial resolution. Slice thickness is 0.6–1 mm in the majority of cases. Most centers and vendors recommend to reconstruct axial images with an overlap in longitudinal z-axis direction. The first step of image analysis is devoted to the detection of coronary motion artifacts. If motion blurring is found additional phase reconstructions are necessary. Late-systolic reconstructions may be helpful at higher heart rates (typically > 70 bpm) if coronary artery motion cannot be otherwise eliminated for various diastolic reconstructions (Hoffmann 2005a). During the image analysis the interpreter may need to jump back and forth between different phases because residual segmental motion may vary for the different coronary territories. In the presence of high density objects (such as stents or calcium) interpretation of the adjacent lumen may be difficult. This problem can be somewhat alleviated with the use of sharper high-contrast filters.

26.3 Coronary Artery Calcifications and Plaque Imaging

26.3.1 Calcium Scoring

Cardiac risk assessment is either based on traditional risk factors (diabetes, smoking etc.) or on biomarkers (e.g. hs-CRP) that should add up to an accurate prediction of foreseeable cardiovascular events in an asymptomatic patient. The shortcomings of this approach are all to often highlighted by major cardiac events occurring in presumably low-risk candidates. The estimated number of 785,000 previously asymptomatic Americans to have an acute coronary event as the initial manifestation of coronary artery disease in 2010 is a testimony of the failure of conventional risk assessment models (Lloyd-Jones 2010). Consequently, there has been a focus on markers of subclinical atherosclerosis that may be utilized for risk assessment of individuals, rather than extrapolating from risk factors that reflect trends in large groups of patients in epidemiologic studies. The most powerful of these subclinical markers is coronary artery calcium (CAC).

Most coronary events occur in the territory of coronary arteries that do not demonstrate prior high-grade stenosis. Although atherosclerotic plaque is invariably present as a substrate for an acute coronary event, significant stenosis is not necessary (Libby 2005). However, complications of atherosclerotic plaque such as rupture or erosion with subsequent thrombus formation are important events leading to acute coronary syndrome. Many different factors including plaque composition, hemodynamics, endothelial function, and blood thrombogenicity may influence which plaque induces a hemodynamically significant event. Nonetheless, there is a strong relation between the extent of coronary plaque burden and the risk of a coronary event. Since atherosclerosis is the only disease process associated with calcification of the coronary arteries, the degree of coronary calcification as demonstrated by CT is predictive of the overall burden of atherosclerotic plaque (Greenland 2004). This prediction will only be outperformed by the detection of both calcified and non-calcified components of the plaque load on the coronary territory of an individual patient. The detection of calcium in the coronary territory is possible without the use of contrast in a low dose CT scan while the detection and separation of calcified and non-calcified plaque territories is only possible on contrast-enhanced CT coronary angiography scans.

Calcium scoring is based on the identification of high-density material within the coronary circulation on a non-contrast CT scan. Both EBT and MDCT have been used for evaluation of coronary calcium. The largest databases are available for EBT. However, a strong linear association is present between calcium scoring as provided by EBT and MDCT (r value 0.96–0.99) (Stanford 2004). The current literature therefore suggests that MDCT is comparable to EBT for coronary calcium screening (Becker 2001). The effective radiation dose from a calcium scoring examination is in the range of 1.0–1.8 mSv (Hunold 2003). This compares favorably to the expected dose of helical MDCT cardiac angiography and nuclear stress tests (both in the range of 10–18 mSv).

Calcium scoring is a simple test that should take no more than 5 min. Electrocardiogram (ECG) leads are placed on the patient. A CT scout image is obtained to determine the location of the heart. A prospective ECG-gated scan with 3 mm slice thickness is then obtained from the level of the carina through the bottom of the heart. To obtain an accu-

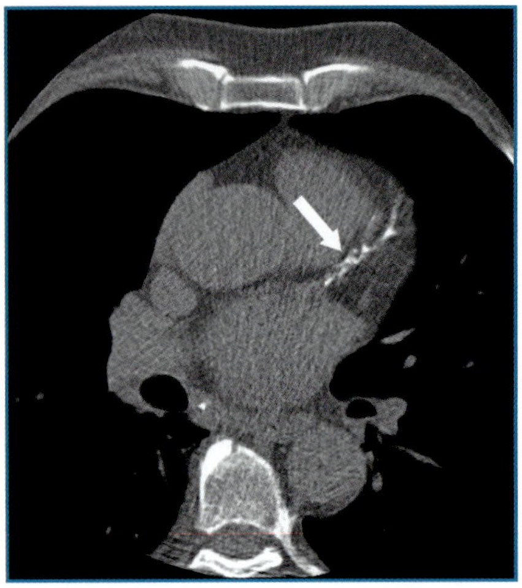

a

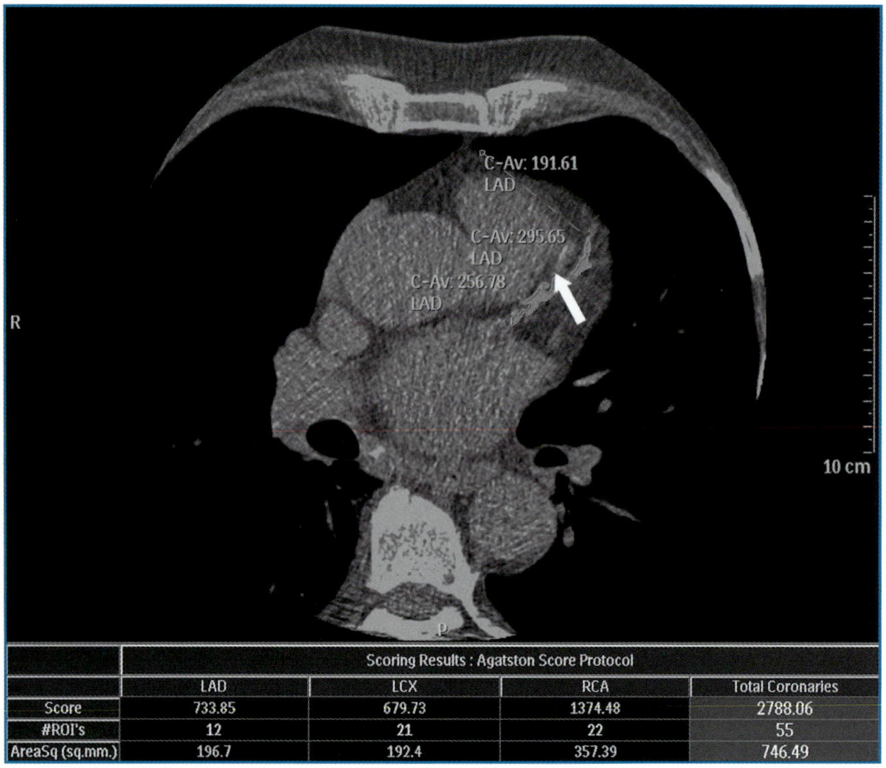

	LAD	LCX	RCA	Total Coronaries
Score	733.85	679.73	1374.48	2788.06
#ROI's	12	21	22	55
AreaSq (sq.mm.)	196.7	192.4	357.39	746.49

b

Figure 26-2 Non-contrasted axial or transverse slice at the level of the left anterior descending artery (a) shows bright spots representing coronary artery wall calcifications (arrow). The calcifications (arrow) are automatically processed according to the Agaston method with total calcium score (b).

rate calcium score, calcification of the coronary artery wall must be distinguished from calcifications involving other parts of the heart, especially the annulus of the aortic and the mitral valve.

Once the location of coronary calcium is identified on a CT examination, an automated program is used to compute a calcium score (Figure 26-2). The Agatston method has been tradionally utilized to score the amount of coronary calcium with CT (Agatston 1990). For each focus of calcified coronary plaque, plaque area and maximum attenuation are measured on each CT slice. An attenuation cofactor is assigned to each plaque based on CT attenuation measured in Hounsfield units (HU). The cofactor is assigned as 1 for 131–200 HU, 2 for 201–300 HU, 3 for 301–400 HU and 4 for greater than 400 HU. The area of each plaque is multiplied by the appropriate attenuation cofactor to achieve a calcium score. The scores of all the individual plaques in all vessels are summed to obtain a single total Agatston calcium score for risk analysis.

The Agatston method does have its shortcomings: Modern CT units are capable of sub-millimeter resolution, but the attenuation cofactors are determined at 3 mm slice thickness. This renders susceptibility for partial volume averaging due to adjacent high density structures. Both volumetric and mass scores have been proposed to overcome this deficiency, but with the large amount of data published based on the Agatston method most clinicians continue to use it.

Coronary calcium scores are generally divided into:

- normal (no calcium),
- mildly elevated (1–100),
- moderately elevated (101–400), or
- severely elevated (> 400).

As the level of coronary calcium increases, the risk of significant stenosis is higher, but there is not a one-to-one correlation. Calcium scoring is most useful as a risk assessment tool for adults who are at intermediate risk of coronary disease based on a Framingham risk score that demonstrates a 10–20 % risk of coronary events in the next 10 yrs (Hecht 2006). Patients with a low Framingham risk score combined with other well-established risk factors, such as an elevated C-reactive protein, metabolic syndrome, obesity, or a family history of premature coronary disease, may also benefit from calcium scoring. In these patients, calcium scoring may elevate patients into a higher risk category and demonstrate a need for aggressive medical therapy. Furthermore, knowledge of the calcium score may increase patient compliance.

26.3.2 Non-Calcified Plaque Imaging

One of the unique abilities of contrast attenuated CT coronary angiography is that it allows for non-invasive visualization of nonstenotic, noncalcified coronary plaque. For quite a while it was considered possible with conventional CT technology to separate the lipid-rich and fibrous components of a plaque lesion. But both partial volume averaging due to insufficient spatial resolution and contrast uptake of the non-calcified plaque components were found to induce an amount of variability to impede this ambition (Cademartiri 2005, Halliburton 2006). Nevertheless, a comparison to intravascular ultrasound (the standard of reference for the detection and quantification of coronary plaque lesions) has shown promising results to detect non-calcified and calcified plaque components on CT coronary angiography imaging. The feasibility of the method for therapy monitoring with the surrogate markers of plaque progression or regression has been positively tested (Lehman 2009). Quantification strategies based upon current CT technology rely on the volumetric assessment of calcified and non-calcified plaque components.

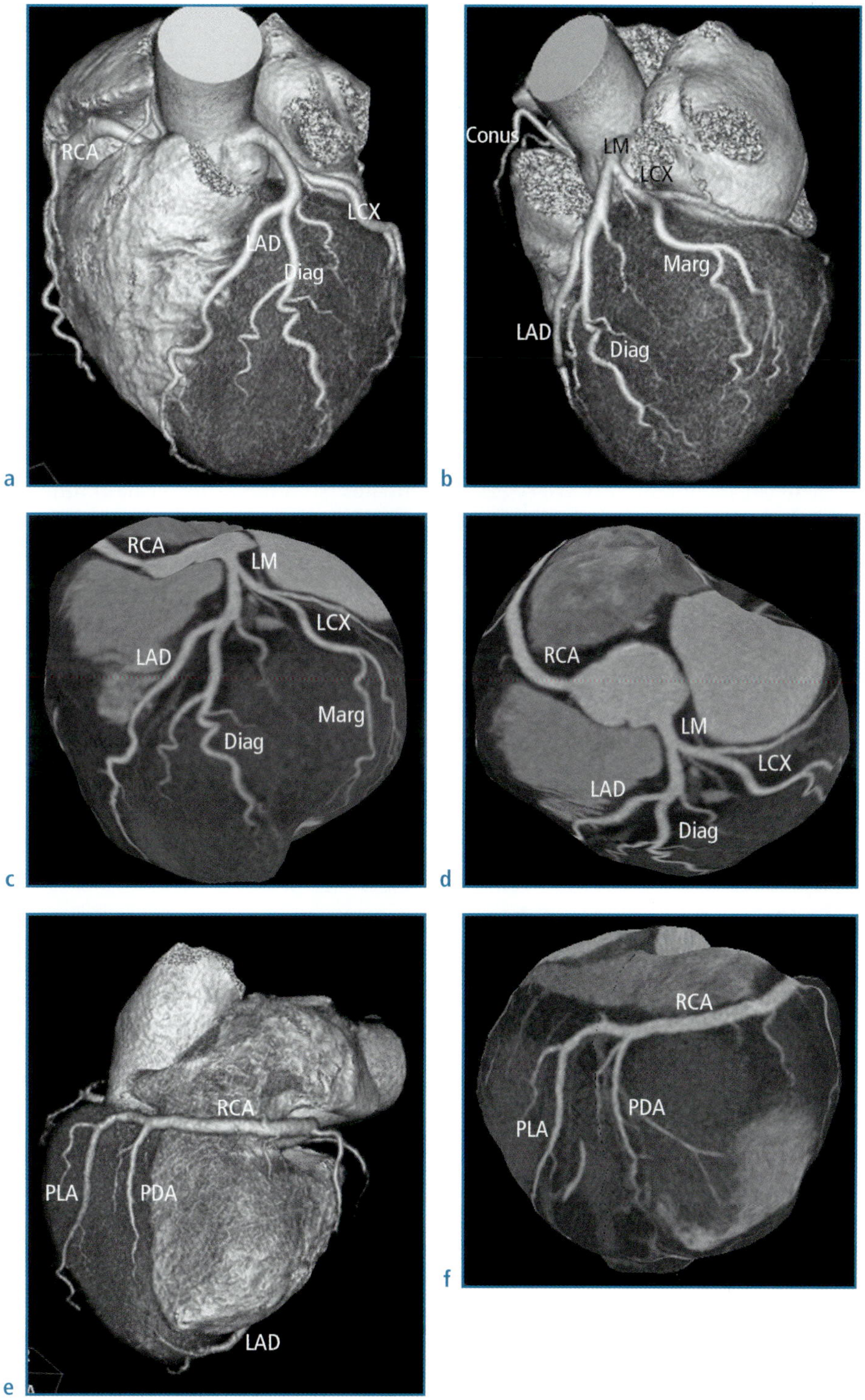

Figure 26-3 Volume rendering of the heart in anteroposterior orientation (a) with a cranial tilt. The left main (LM) and left anterior descending (LAD) coronary artery are displayed with all branches (Diag: diagonal branches). The proximal part of the left circumflex (LCX) and right coronary artery (RCA) are also projected. The volume rendering of Figure a is tilted in left anterior oblique (LAO) direction (b). This projection shows marginal branches (Marg) of the left circumflex artery. The conus branch (Conus), a small proximal side branch of the RCA is also seen. Maximum intensity projection (MIP) (c) with a thickness of 3 mm is projected along the epicardial surface of the heart (so-called "globe view"). This allows to visualize the epicardial vessels in their true anatomical orientation. The globe view is rotated in LAO and cranial tilt orientation. All major branches of the left coronary artery are projected. Globe view (d) with a reverse spider view resemblance. The left main and proximal branches are seen along with the main stem of the RCA. Volume rendering projecting the inferior surface of the heart (e) with the peripheral branches of the RCA. The posterior descending artery (PDA) and posterolateral (PLA) branches are seen along with the peripheral part of the LAD curving around the apex of the heart. Globe view (f) with same projection as in Figure e.

26.4 CT Coronary Angiography

26.4.1 Coronary Anatomy

The RCA originates from the right sinus of Valsalva (Figure 26-3d). The first RCA branch is the conus branch, which supplies the myocardium of the right ventricular outflow tract (RVOT). Occasionally the conus branch may have a separate ostium. The RCA supplies the anterior free wall of the right ventricle with side branches and gives rise to the acute marginal branches that run along the angle of the anterior and inferior RV free wall. The RCA is dominant in the majority of cases (~ 80 %). Dominance is determined by the branch that supplies the inferior and part of the posterolateral myocardium of the left ventricle. Two branches originate from the crux cordis (the point of the inferior cardiac surface where the ventricles and the atria meet in a cross like configuration). The posterior descending artery (PDA) runs along the inferior interventricular groove and the posterior left ventricular (PLV) branch supplies the inferior and part of the posterolateral myocardium (Figure 26-3e, f). In cases of left dominance the RCA does not reach the crux and both PLV and PDA are supplied by the left circumflex artery (LCX). The AV nodal branch usually originates from the crux region.

The left main coronary artery (LM) originates from the left sinus of Valsalva (Figure 26-3a, d) in a more cranial position compared to the RCA ostium. A bifurcation within 2 cm of its origin gives rise to the left anterior descending (LAD) and the LCX branch. Sometimes three separate branches with the intermediate artery originating between the LAD and the LCX can be discerned.

The LAD runs in the anterior interventricular groove and supplies the septum with perforators branching in perpendicular fashion. Diagonal branches supply the anterior LV wall (Figure 26-3a, b, c). The distal LAD commonly wraps around the apex, where it may form collaterals to the PDA.

The LCX runs in the left (or posterior) atrioventricular groove and gives rise to obtuse marginal branches and posterolateral branches (Figure 26-3b, c). If the PDA and PLV arise from the LCX, the system is considered left dominant. Co-dominance is present if both the RCA and the LCX provide branches to the PDA territory.

26.4.2 Clinical Role of CT Coronary Angiography

The most important role for cardiac CT is to detect stenoses in the coronary arteries that likely will be hemodynamically significant and therefore will be the cause of the patient's symptoms (Figure 26-4 and Figure 26-5). The standard of reference against which CT has been extensively tested is conventional catheter-based coronary angiography (Hoffmann 2005b).

Computed tomography angiography is an excellent tool for visualization of both calcified and noncalcified plaque, and subsequently for the assessment of coronary stenosis induced by negative remodeling plaque lesions encroaching upon the lumen size. Because CTA obtains a volumetric data set, vessels may be visualized in any desired orientation. Each coronary segment may be rotated into multiple orientations to visualize the vessel lumen and plaque. Although

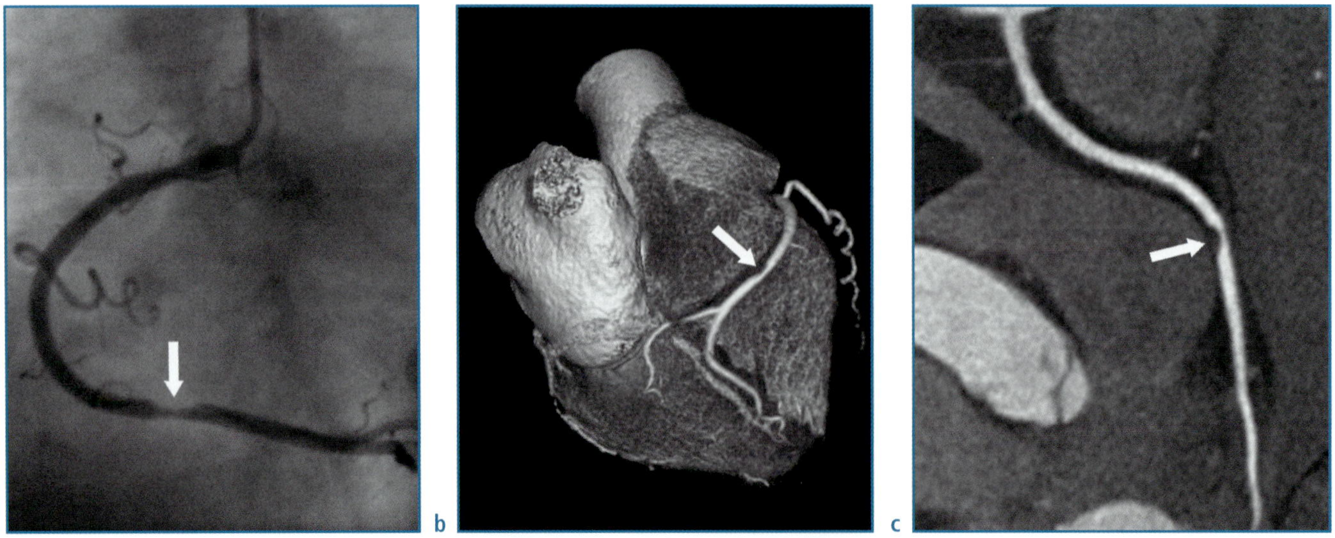

a b c

Figure 26-4 Left anterior oblique projection of the RCA (a) shows high grade stenosis (arrow) in segment 3. The volume rendered CT image (b) shows the stenosis (arrow) in good correlation to the invasive angiogram. The curved multi-planar reformat (c) demonstrated a large non-calcified plaque to induce the lumen narrowing (arrow).

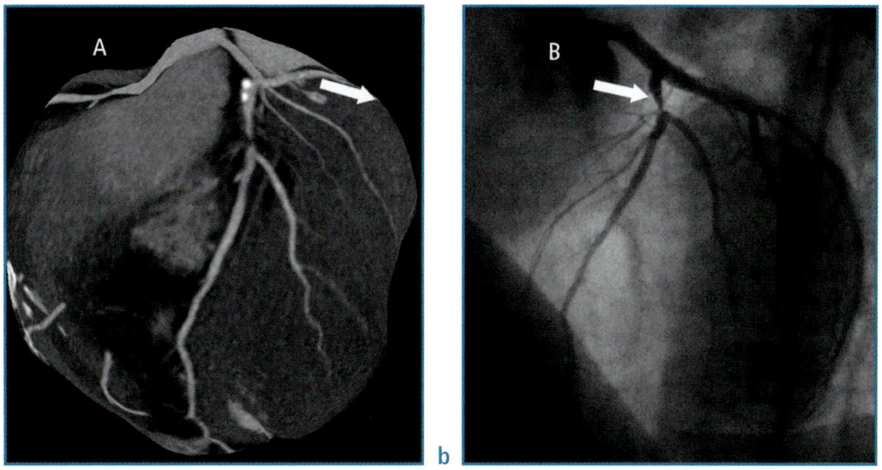

Figure 26-5 CT globe view (a) demonstrating a high grade stenosis (arrow) of the LAD. This correlates well with the invasive angiogram (b) (arrow). The two calcifications (bright spots in (a) do not induce a relevant lumen narrowing.

a b

selective catheter angiography is the accepted standard of reference for coronary lumen assessment it only provides a finite set of 2D projections. The so-called foreshortening effect that may induce incomplete segmental coverage on two-dimensional catheter angiography is not apparent on three-dimensional CT angiography data sets. But CT compared to catheter angiography falls behind for both spatial and temporal resolution.

CT coronary angiography outperforms MR-based techniques in terms of robustness and spatial resolution (Schuijf 2006). The typical image acquisition time for current generation CT scanners is from one single cardiac cycle to a total of three cardiac cycles. This speed cannot be achieved with any other currently available non-invasive technology.

From a clinical standpoint the most valuable CT image for the individual patient is that of normal coronaries. If CT clearly shows the absence of coronary artery stenoses, any further testing is not necessary. This statement is based on a multitude of single and multi-center studies comparing the accuracy of CT coronary angiography with invasive catheter angiography (Budoff 2008, Garcia 2006, Meijboom 2008, Miller 2008). It has been consistently shown that CT has a high sensitivity and consequently high negative predictive value to rule out coronary artery stenosis. The discriminative power of CT coronary angiography is dependent on the pre-test likelihood of disease in an individual patient. The method performs best in symptomatic patients with an intermediate pre-test likelihood of CAD (Meijboom 2007). The pre-test likelihood is assessed based upon gender, age and clinical presentation according to the standards published in 1979 (Diamond and Forrester 1979). For patients with a high likelihood CT performance is compromised by false positive findings mainly due to calcium plaque oversizing or blooming artifacts. It has therefore been proposed to rely on ischemia testing or catheter angiography for patients with a high likelihood and apply CT testing for the intermediate group only.

Acute Chest Pain

Cardiac and gated chest CT imaging offer the possibility to rule out coronary artery disease, acute aortic dissection and pulmonary embolism on a single contrast-enhanced chest CT scan. This application is based on the so-called triple-rule-out protocol (White and Kuo 2007). Both thoracic aortic and coronary angiography rely on the same contrast material timing. It is therefore easy to combine both applications in a single scan by simply extending the scan range to cover both the aortic and coronary territory. Contrast administration has to be modified for the additional pulmonary arterial assessment. This is either achieved with a substantially longer contrast agent injection or a second phase added to the initial rapid injection of contrast for systemic arterial enhancement. The second phase, the so-called long contrast bolus tail for pulmonary opacification is injected at lower rates than the first phase and may be composed of saline and contrast agent fractions from a dual head injector. With this protocol patients with acute chest pain and clinical uncertainty of its origin may be evaluated to rule out the big three life threatening entities.

Many million patients are evaluated each year for acute chest pain in the emergency department. Despite standardized protocols and high vigilance, between 2 and 6% of patients are erroneously discharged with missed myocardial infarction (Chinnaiyan 2009). CT coronary angiography with its high negative predictive value should be well-suited in this subset of patients to rule out obstructive coronary artery disease and thereby safely discharge them with a favorable prognosis. This hypothesis has been verified by first clinical trial results showing superior performance of a

CT-based approach to patients with a low to intermediate risk for an acute coronary syndrome. CT coronary angiography was superior in comparison to the standard of care based upon either serial biomarkers or myocardial perfusion testing. High risk patients with either ST elevation myocardial infarction or non-ST elevation myocardial infarction are perceived as contraindications for CT coronary imaging and should undergo invasive coronary angiography directly. In association with an application for acute chest pain triage CT coronary angiography has undergone some initial cost effectiveness testing. First results indicate that CT imaging is superior to nuclear stress testing in the management of suspected CAD patients with a low to intermediate risk profile (Khare 2008).

Stents

Evaluation of coronary artery stents with CT coronary angiography remains challenging. The visualization of the in-stent lumen suffers from the same high-density artifacts as the exact lumen delineation adjacent to high density calcified plaques. In addition to that beam hardening with streak artifacts may occur in the vicinity of thick stent struts composed of certain metal alloys. Various so-called catalogue papers have been published testing the suitability of stent materials for CT imaging (Maintz 2009). It was found that thin strut bare metal stents composed of cobalt-chromium alloys are more suitable than drug-eluting stents mounted mostly on high density stainless steel backbones.

In addition to the stent material the most important determinator of stent lumen visibility is the size of the in-stent lumen. Proximal stents with a lumen size of 3 mm or greater are interpretable, if the achieved image quality is of good to excellent quality (i. e. low noise level, absent motion or respiratory artifacts). The reported accuracy to detect in-stent stenosis for segments deemed to be evaluable ranges from 75–95 %. Because these numbers are not great and given the fact that many stents are not evaluable at all, in-stent lumen imaging with CT should be discouraged for clinical decision making with currently available CT technology.

Bypass Grafts

Imaging of patients with bypass grafts by CT angiography has been possible since the early days of both electron beam and multi-detector CT. The relative large diameter and little motion of saphenous vein grafts results in reliably good image quality, compared to the native coronary arteries. Imaging of arterial grafts and especially mammary pedicle grafts is much more demanding due to the comparably smaller size and metal artifacts induced by the clipping of side branches during the harvesting process.

Recent studies have shown that graft occlusion and stenoses can be detected with high diagnostic accuracy close to 100 % (Weustink 2009). However, complete assessment of patients after aortocoronary bypass grafting should include both bypass grafts and native coronary arteries. The diagnostic accuracy in the distal run-off region, though small in diameter, and in the distal anastomosis region is still acceptable (Figure 26-6), but both native coronary arteries proximal to the bypass anastomosis and non-grafted vessel branches are not sufficiently well-covered. The much lower accuracy in these vessel territories is well-explained by a very high likelihood of calcified plaques and stents to be present. In summary, whereas CT coronary angiography may compete with invasive angiography for the grafts and distal run-off segments, invasive angiography is still needed to confirm or refute CT findings for the proximal segments

a b
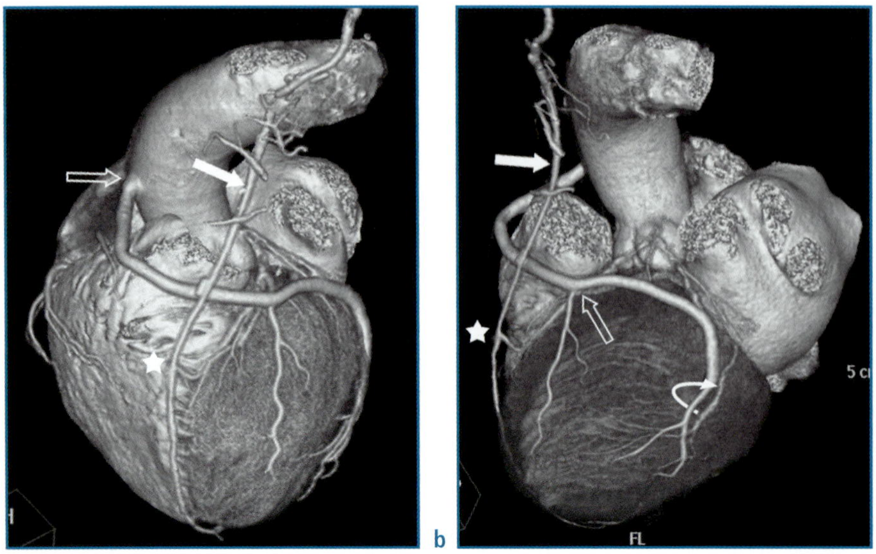

Figure 26-6 Follow-up scan after coronary artery bypass grafting (CABG). The left mammary pedicle was distally anastomosed to the LAD and is patent (large arrow in (a) and (b)). The pedicle is too short and induces traction on the coronary artery with a triangular configuration of the LAD at the distal anastomotic site (asterisk in (a) and (b)). A venous graft was proximally inserted into the ascending aortic root (open arrow in (a)). The graft was anastomosed in side-to-side fashion to the diagonal branch (open arrow in (b)) and in end-to-side fashion to the large marginal branch of the LCX (curved arrow in (b)). All segments of this bypass graft are patent with non-obstructed proximal and distal anastomosis sites.

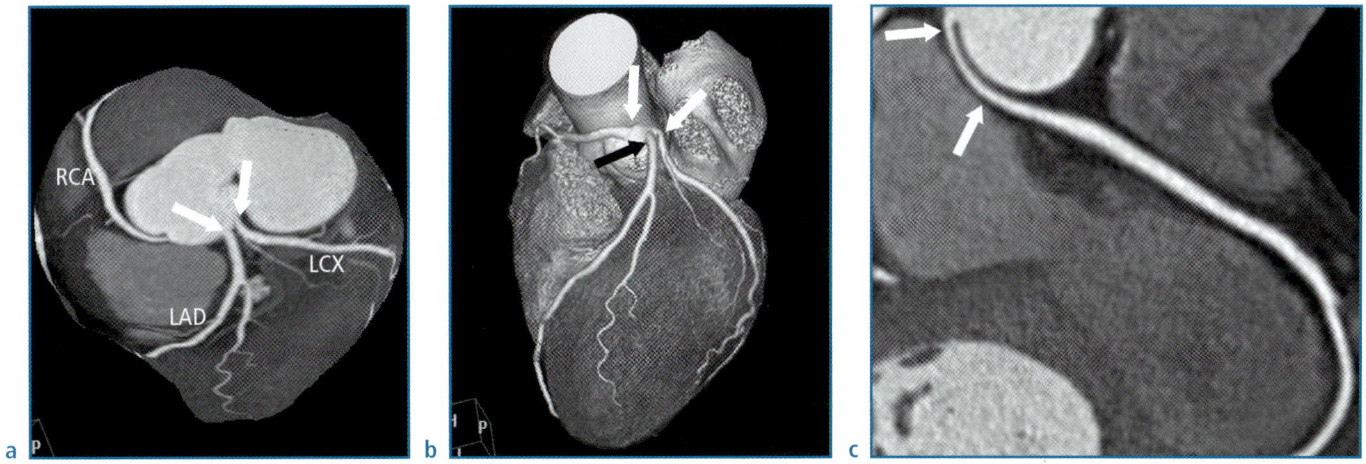

Figure 26-7 Patient with absent left main coronary artery and malignant anomaly of the right coronary artery. The globe view (a) shows separate ostia for the LAD and LCX (arrows). The RCA originates from the left coronary sinus but the ostium is not displayed without overlay in this rendering. The volume rendering (b) demonstrates nicely the anatomical relation of three separate ostia in the wall of the left sinus of Valsalva (arrows). A curved multi-planar reformat (c) along the RCA shows the lumen narrowing of the main stem and proximal segment. This view also highlights the section of the RCA impinged between the pulmonary trunk and the aortic root (arrows). LAD: left anterior descending artery; LCX: left circumflex artery; RCA: right coronary artery.

and non-grafted segments of coronary vessels after bypass grafting. Invasive catheter angiography will therefore not be replaced by CT angiography at the current level of technology.

On the other hand, CT is very valuable for the planning of reoperation and may show pathology not readily apparent on invasive angiograms, it should therefore be perceived as supplemental rather than competitive to catheterization angiography. Occluded grafts may be completely invisible on CT angiograms with the exception of an out-pouching of the proximal aortic anastomosis site. It is therefore important to correlate the graft number and location from the original cardiac surgical report (OR) with the findings on post-CABG CT angiograms. A mismatch usually indicates a graft occlusion. This especially applies to sequential grafts with more than one distal anastomosis. Such grafts may have one proximal anastomosis to the aorta and one or multiple side-to-side anastomoses to various coronary vessels with one end-to-side anastomosis as the final distal insertion. Without OR report correlation an occlusion of the distal segment of such grafts may be easily missed.

Another potential complication post-CABG surgery is the formation of aneurysms. Unlike invasive angiography, CT has the advantage to delineate the graft lumen and potentially present mural thrombus. CT is also superior to invasive angiograms for the planning of reoperations. It allows to visualize both aortic root calcifications and retrosternal space width and content. Bypass grafts running next to the sternal wire loops or the retrosternal surface are at great risk to be severed during the re-dissection for repeat surgical access. Occasionally the space between the right ventricular wall and the sternum may be extremely tight, which increases the risk of RV rupture during the opening of the chest. The morphologic information of gated chest CT has proven to be very valuable for re-do cardiac surgery (Kamdar 2008, Khan and Yonan 2009). It significantly reduces the risk of re-operative complications.

Coronary Anomalies and Fistula

Congenital anomalies of the coronary arteries are found in approximately 1–2% of the general population. A number of imaging modalities are suitable to detect and classify coronary anomalies, including MRI, CT and invasive angiography. Today, cardiac CT is considered the standard of reference for this application. The main reason for this is that CT can readily depict the proximal coronary arteries in a three-dimensional dataset with high isovolumetric spatial resolution and high contrast, and at the same time shows the surrounding structures (Shi 2004). Although magnetic resonance is promising, it is less robust and technically more challenging.

CT has proven in multiple studies to show the origin of abnormal vessels and its course (Figure 26-7 and Figure 26-8). When determining the benign vs. malignant character of a coronary anomaly, it is important to determine whether the abnormal coronary artery passes between the pulmonary trunk and the ascending aorta (Figure 26-7c). Those anomalies with segments passing between the two great vessels are usually considered to be at risk of compression and sudden cardiac death. There is consensus that passage of the left main with right sided origin between the aorta

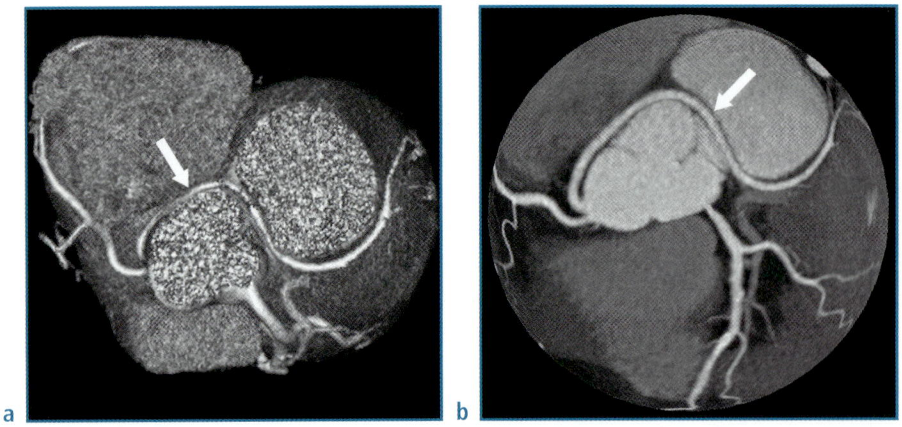

Figure 26-8 Typical benign coronary anomaly with the left circumflex artery branching of the right coronary sinus and passing with it's main stem in the back of the aorta (arrows on volume rendering (a) and globe view (b)) – no impingement between the left atrial roof and the aorta.

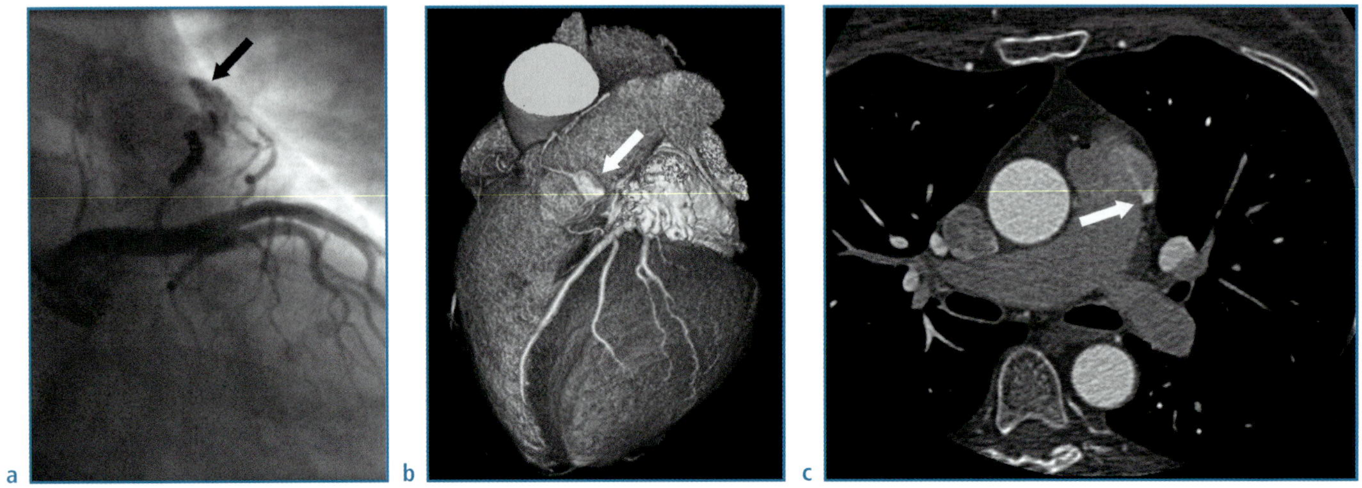

Figure 26-9 Coronary angiography with contrast injection into the left coronary artery (a) accurately demonstrates the side branches of the LM and LAD supplying a fistula network but fails to show the drainage site (arrow). The volume rendering of the cardiac CT scan (b) shows the drainage site with an out-pouching (arrow) of the pulmonary artery trunk on top of the fistula drainage ostium. The cross-sectional transverse slice at the drainage site level (c) shows a bright contrast jet directed in retrograde fashion onto the pulmonary valve. The fistula was occluded with coil-packing of the pulmonary artery out-pouching introduced via the pulmonary artery (not shown).

and the pulmonary artery constitutes a malignant coronary anomaly.

Based on the data from the Cleveland Clinic study benign coronary anomalies are more prevalent than malignant coronary anomalies (Yamanaka and Hobbs 1990). The most common variant is an absent left main with separate ostia for the LAD and the LCX from the left sinus of Valsalva (Figure 26-7a, b). The second most common variant is an anomalous LCX with origin from the right sinus or the RCA main stem (Figure 26-8a, b). This variant usually courses in the back of the aorta. The most common malignant variant are left sided origin of the RCA and right sided origin of the left coronary artery or the LAD.

Variations of coronary anomalies very frequently visualized by CT are coronary fistula formations (Figure 26-9). They become clinically apparent with symptoms mimicking CAD with excertional angina, and are most often identified with coronary steal syndromes on invasive angiograms. The types most often found are fistulas to the pulmonary main stem with feeders from the right conus branch, the left coronary artery and mediastinal branches of the aorta. The most extreme form of a coronary artery fistula is the partial Bland-White Garland syndrome with part of the coronary tree arising from the pulmonary arterial circulation. In this situation retrograde flow in the anomalous coronary artery will ensue with syncope or angina resulting from antegrade flow at higher pulmonary pressure.

26.5 CT of Cardiac Structure and Function

CT imaging has a relatively high spatial resolution, and a high contrast between the blood pool and other tissues can be achieved after the injection of an iodinated contrast agent. CT has the ability to provide high-resolution morphologic imaging of the heart and adjacent thoracic vessels (Figure 26-10). With a contrast administration regimen including a dense bolus for the left cardiac structures followed by a saline flush supplemented with a low fraction of contrast agent, both the left and right sided cardiac cavities can be well discerned against the myocardium and the epicardial fat pad (Figure 26-1). Clinically, however, CT imaging does not play a very prominent role for this indication. Both echocardiography and magnetic resonance imaging (MRI) can provide all relevant information in most clinical situations.

Quantitative analysis of cardiac chamber geometry and ventricular function is an essential part of a complete cardiac evaluation. MRI is currently considered the standard of reference for ventricular global and regional function analysis. As part of a retrospectively gated cardiac imaging study CT can provide an anatomically precise evaluation of chamber morphology and function, along with a detailed assessment of coronary and valvular anatomy. Global LV functional parameters calculated from CT datasets acquired utilizing > 64 detector technology correlate well with MRI in daily clinical practice (van der Vleuten 2009). They may be considered interchangeable. However, MRI datasets are acquired without any ionizing radiation dose and no need to administer contrast agents. Functional CT data are only available utilizing high dose retrospective helical ECG-gating or continuous acquisition of a full cardiac cycle utilizing a 16 cm detector. Modern dose saving technology allows morphologic coronary and cardiac imaging at a dose exposure of 1–4 mSv. Both high-pitch helical scanning and prospectively gated coronary CT angiography restrict dose exposure to one quiescent cardiac phase without acquisition of the full cardiac cycle in order to achieve substantial dose reductions. Functional cardiac analysis is not permitted by these technologies. In other words, CT functional data require a dose exposure in the range of 10–20 mSv almost 10 times the dose we acquire from natural sources during a full year. Such a high dose exposure is not warranted for the purpose of functional and morphologic cardiac analysis, which can be achieved with other modalities at the same level of accuracy. But contraindications for MRI preclude imaging in patients with the majority of pacemakers, intracardiac defibrillators (ICD) or cardiac resynchronization systems (CRT). MDCT derived functional analysis constitutes a viable alternative for this subset of patients. One restriction though applies for CT functional imaging, the flow sensitivity that is clinically very useful for both echocardiography and MRI cannot be achieved with CT imaging.

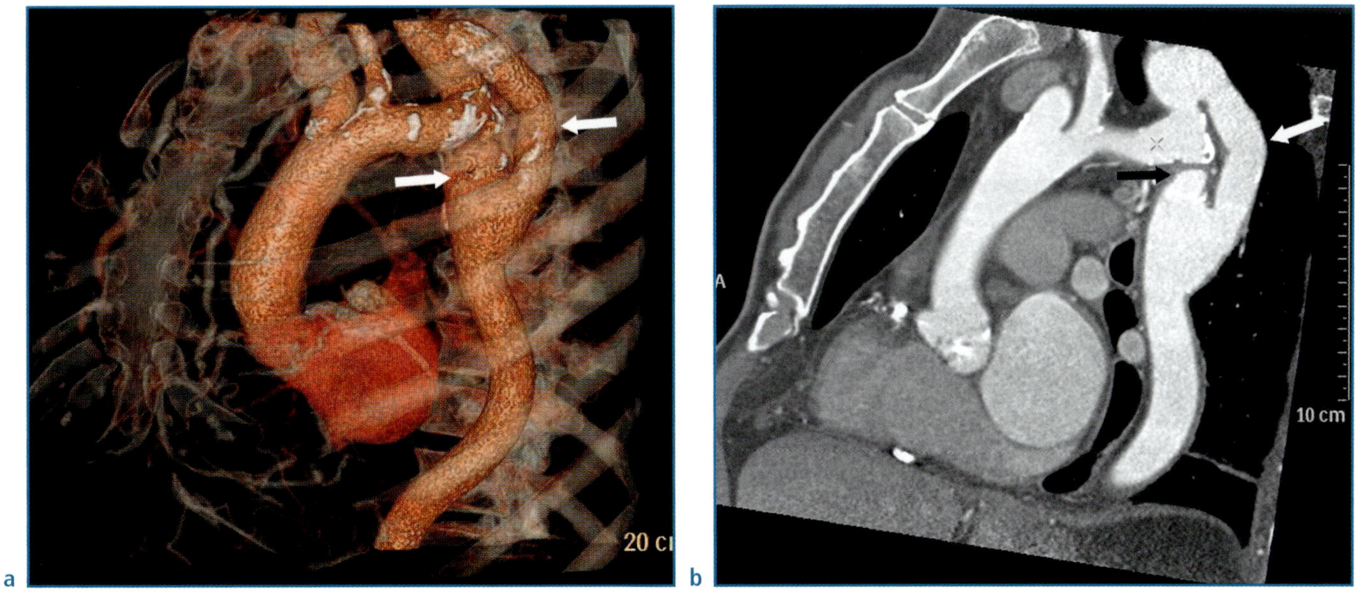

Figure 26-10 Thoracic morphology scans show congenital coarctation with a complete occlusion of the native aorta (small arrows in (a), (b)). The coarctation was surgically treated with an extra-anatomical bypass (large arrows in (a), (b)).

26.6 Myocardial Perfusion and Viability

Myocardial perfusion is one of the most important prognostic indicators for patient outcome in the management of CAD. The comprehensive assessment of myocardial perfusion and morphologic coronary artery evaluation has been shown to provide incremental diagnostic value over either technique alone (van Werkhoven 2009). So far image fusion of two modalities (e.g. nuclear perfusion testing and coronary CT angiography) was necessary to provide the comprehensive morphology and function assessment. CT, though, has the potential to achieve the coveted goal of a stand-alone modality providing both morphology and function of a stenotic lesion. At the time of this writing no vigorous clinical trials testing the diagnostic accuracy of CT-based perfusion scanning have been completed, but first feasibility trials indicate the potential of both snapshot CT perfusion (Figure 26-11) and first-pass imaging with rapid successive frame acquisition (George 2009). Initial dose exposure calculations for the additional CT perfusion scanning render values in the range of 5–10 mSv, which compares very favorably to nuclear stress testing but very unfavorably to the 0 mSv of MRI perfusion imaging. Clinical trials are ongoing to establish the best perfusion imaging modality to be combined with CT coronary angiography.

The determination of myocardial viability is playing an increasing role in predicting the success of revascularization therapy. Delayed contrast-enhanced imaging with MR detects accumulation of gadolinium-based chelates in areas of myocardial necrosis after infarction. The same principles may apply to cardiac CT, since iodine-based intravenous contrast material has similar kinetics as gadolinium chelates. Low kilovoltage (e.g. 80 kVp) protocols have been shown to result in better iodine contrast differentiation and the additional radiation dose exposure for performing viability imaging with CT was quantified at 3.8 mSv in females and 2.8 mSv in males. But the contrast sensitivity of MRI easily outperforms CT imaging for the purpose of viability testing, this was validated in trials showing a systematic underestimation of the true infarct size by CT compared with MRI (Nieman 2008). MR imaging with superior gadolinium contrast sensitivity is therefore considered the standard of reference for this application.

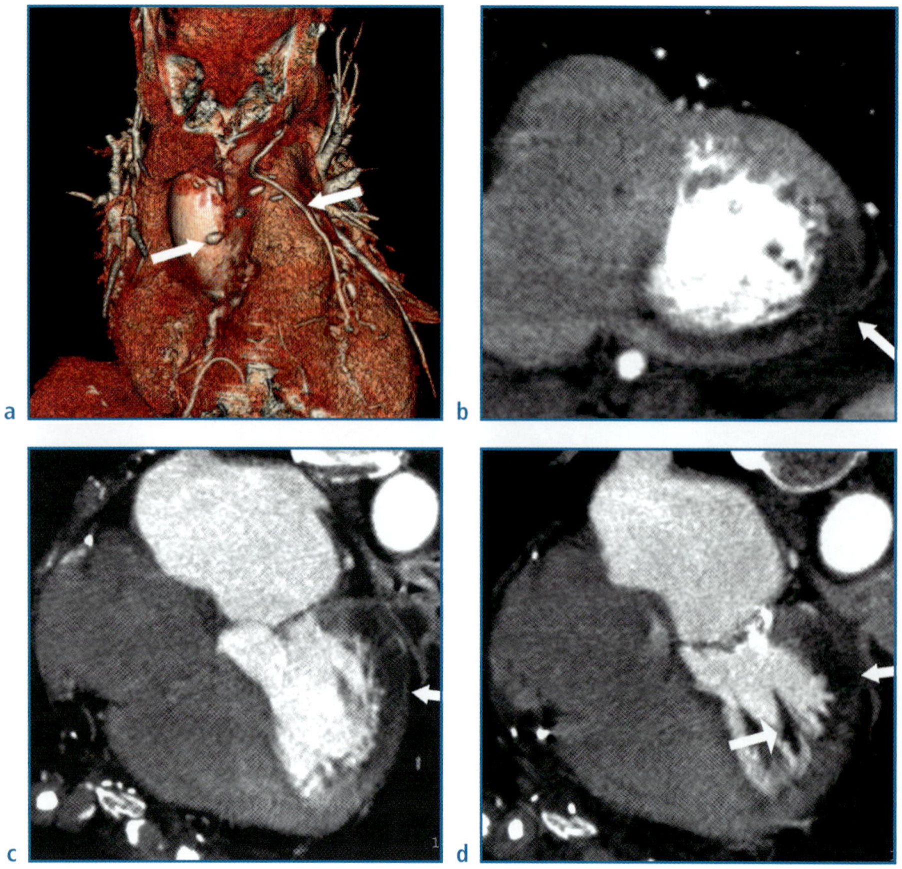

Figure 26-11 Patients presents 6 d post-surgery with suspected graft occlusion. A high-grade left main stenosis with acute lumen occlusion initiated the aortocoronary bypass grafting. The mammary pedicle (thick arrow) to the LAD is patent, but the venous graft to the LCX (thin arrow in (a)) is occluded. This induced acute ischemia in the LCX territory as apparent on the early enhancing snapshot images oriented along short-axis planes (b) and long-axis planes in mid-ventricular position (c) and papillary muscle coverage (d). The large hypodense perfusion defect in the lateral wall (arrows in (b–d)) also affects the papillary muscular structures (thin arrow in (d)).

26.7 Pericardial Disease

The pericardium is usually embedded in epi- and pericardial fat that separates the pericardial layers from the myocardium. CT imaging shows a very low density or attenuation of fat (0 to ~ 100 HU) which is easily contrasted against both myocardium and pericardium (both ~ 50 HU). This allows to discern a thin line of normal thickness pericardium (range between 1–2 mm) against the myocardium if the epicardial fat layer is this enough. It usually appears as a thin line and is best delineated on the anterior surface of the heart (Breen 2001).

Visualization of the pericardium is relevant for various congenital and acquired conditions. Congenital absence of the pericardium can be complete or partial. The condition is infrequent, and patients are usually asymptomatic. A CT scan can be helpful in establishing the absence or presence of a segment of pericardium, but lack of visualization of the pericardium, especially on the posterior surface, is not a sufficient criterion for making the diagnosis.

The normal pericardial thickness is 1–2 mm on high resolution CT scans, pericardial thickening of more than 4–6 mm, even if only localized can be helpful in suspected constriction. Thickened pericardium can be found in many situations, including the early post-operative period, uremia, rheumatic heart disease, and sarcoidosis or as a consequence of radiation therapy. It does not constitute proof of constriction per se. Constrictive pericarditis is associated with calcifications in the late to chronic course of the disease, CT imaging is very well-suited to delineate the calcified pericardium even without contrast administration (Figure 26-12).

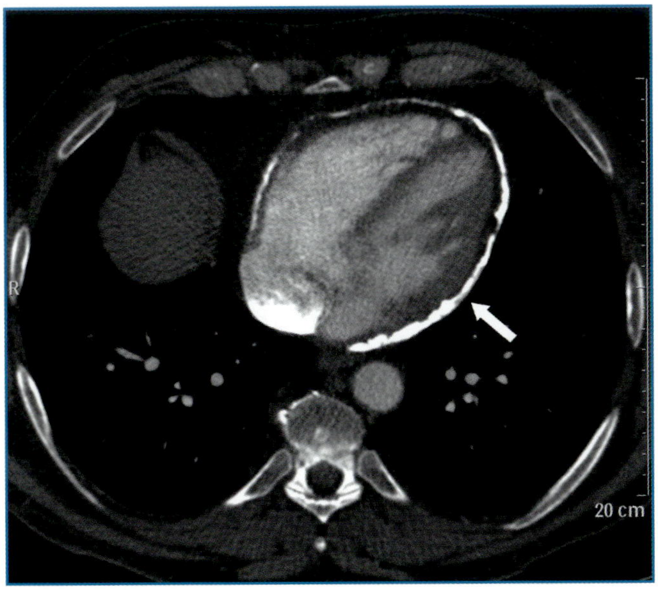

Figure 26-12 Constrictive pericarditis: A non-gated thoraco-abdominal CT acquired for non-cardiac purposes shows the calcified pericardium (arrow) surrounding the ventricles and part of the atria.

Pericardial fluid can be reliably detected on CT images. Though echocardiography is the first line modality for this purpose, CT imaging may be supplemental in cases of limited acoustic windows. Other findings easily discerned on high resolution CT images are pericardial, bronchogenic cysts or teratomas. Primary neoplasms of the pericardium are infrequent but can be the reason for thickened pericardium on CT scans. The density of a pericardial effusion can be indicative of its origin, a serous fluid effusion would be close to the density of water (0–20 HU) while a bloody pericardial effusion would be measured around 50 HU.

26.8 Diagnosis of Cardiac Masses

Echocardiography is the first line modality for the detection of cardiac masses. But both MRI and CT may supplement the echo findings with additional information because of their ability to visualize cardiac morphology without the restriction of acoustic windows. MRI is superior in its ability to provide tissue characterization and differentiation. CT is only superior in its sensitivity for calcified structures and high spatial resolution undisturbed by flow artifacts. CT density or attenuation measurements (Hounsfield [HU] values) do provide some limited insight into the tissue nature of a mass. Lipomas appear with very low HU values (around 0 HU), whereas cysts have walter-like attenuation values (0–10 HU). CT numbers of intracardiac thrombi usually range from 20–90 HU and show substantial overlap with myocardial structures (around 50 HU). CT is very sensitive to identify thrombi in the left atrial appendage but has limited specificity with a large number of false positives generated by slow contrast inflow in patients with atrial fibrillation or flutter (Hur 2009). The most frequent cardiac tumor, atrial myxoma, is represented by a chamber filling defect on cardiac CT images (Figure 26-13).

26.9 CT Imaging for Left Atrial Electrophysiology Applications

Cardiac CT angiography can assess atrial anatomy, pulmonary venous anatomy and coronary venous anatomy, all with great relevance to left atrial arrhythmias including atrial fibrillation, atypical atrial flutter circuits and focal atrial tachycardia. Catheter-based techniques for ablation of

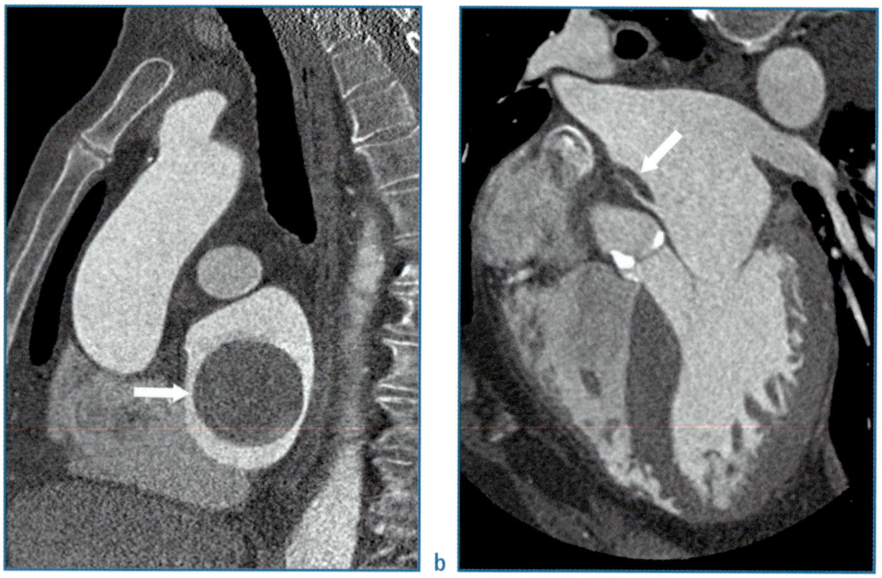

a b

Figure 26-13 Left atrial myxoma becomes apparent on CT images **(a)** as a filling defect (round structure in the left atrium marked with an arrow). Smaller lesions with thrombotic and lipidic components may be easily missed on axial images but are readily apparent on cardiac long-axis views **(b)** (doubling of atrial septum, arrow in **(b)**).

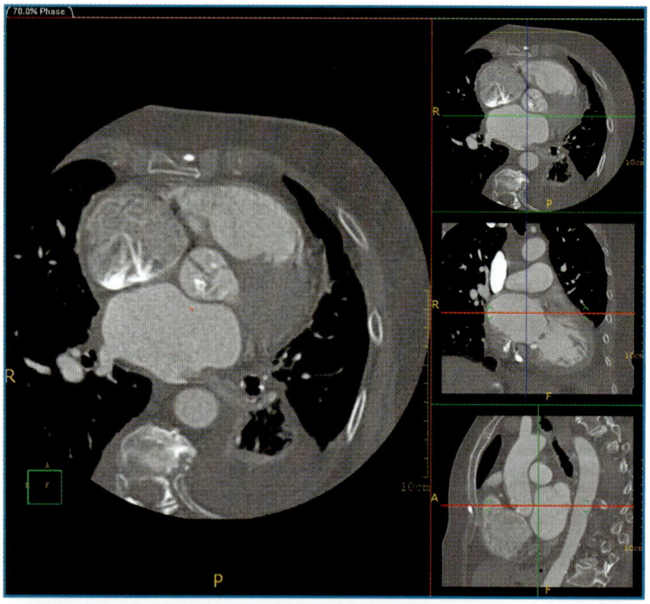

a

Figure 26-14 Cross-sectional CT images **(a)** in transverse (tra), coronal (cor) and sagittal (sag) orientation with the left atrium (LA) in the imaging center. The left atrium is extracted from the cross-sectional dataset and displayed in three-dimensional shape **(b)**. The case sample has four pulmonary vein ostia with the right superior pulmonary vein (RSPV), the right inferior pulmonary vein (RIPV), the left superior pulmonary vein (LSPV) and the left inferior pulmonary vein (LIPV) marked in the volume rendering. The esophagus (purple structure marked with arrows) is in close proximity to the posterior wall of the left atrium **(c)**.

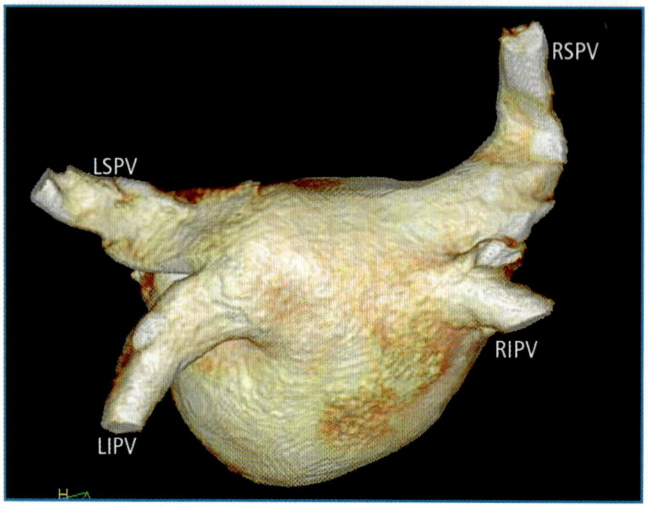

b

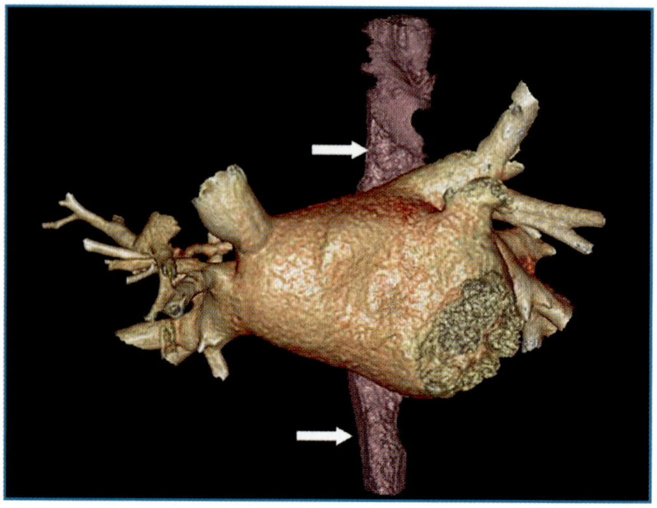

c

atrial fibrillation have focused on ablation of the pulmonary veins with either segmental ablation or complete circumferential electrical isolation of the pulmonary veins. CT imaging can characterize these features through three-dimensional volume rendered and endocardial or endoscopic images (Figure 26-14). The number of veins, the location in the atrium, the vein size and the vein morphology including ostial complexity are easily shown (Blanke 2010). Pre-interventional CT angiography can provide a roadmap of atrial and pulmonary vein structure to guide electrophysiology studies and ablation of atrial fibrillation. The integration of 3D CT images obtained before the procedure (Figure 26-14b) may be realized in a navigation system for real-time catheter positioning (Bertaglia 2009). In addition to the anatomic image generation for intraprocedural orientation, CT imaging of the atrial appendage has been shown to detect thrombus filling defects with a very high sensitivity compared to transesophageal echocardiography.

Pulmonary vein stenosis is a potential complication of atrial fibrillation ablation. CT and MRI have been used to diagnose pulmonary vein stenosis. Pre-operative studies, in addition to providing a roadmap for intervention, can provide a template for follow-up studies assessing the time course of pulmonary venous remodeling and stenosis formation after ostial ablation.

The 3D relationship of the left atrium and the esophagus may have relevance to atrial fibrillation ablation approaches, as left atrial-esophageal fistula have been reported as a fatal complication. There is variability in the course of the esophagus and degree of contact between the posterior left atrial wall and the anterior circumference of the esophagus. This can be visualized by CT imaging (Figure 26-14c).

26.10 Angiography of the Thoracic and Abdominal Aorta

Aortic aneurysms are associated with risk for sudden death due to aortic dissection or rupture. The disease may be induced by connective tissue disorders or acquired cardiovascular atherosclerosis. CT angiography can diagnose aortic aneurysms (Figure 26-15), dissection (Figure 26-16), and wall abnormalities such as penetrating ulcers, intramural hematoma and atherosclerotic plaque rupture in all segments. CT-based angiography of the aorta has emerged as the preferable imaging modality for all aortic emergencies. Whereas recent generations of CT technology were still suffering from pulsation artifacts in the ascending aorta mimicking dissection membranes, this does no longer apply to today's editions with more than 64 detector rows. Accurate delineation of dissection membranes outperforms invasive angiography to visualize the intimal tear and re-entry

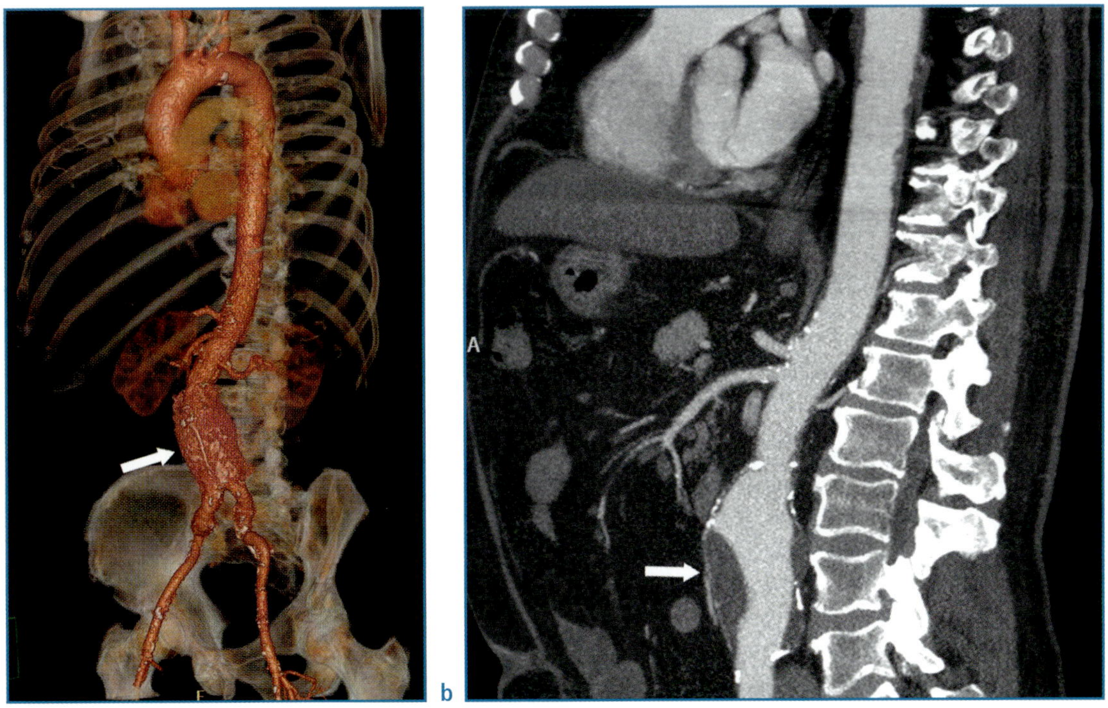

a b

Figure 26-15 CT imaging of the full length of the aorta (a) shows a lumen dilatation of the infrarenal abdominal aorta (arrow). The infrarenal aneurysm shows partial lumen thrombosis as demonstrated in the sagittal section (arrow) (b).

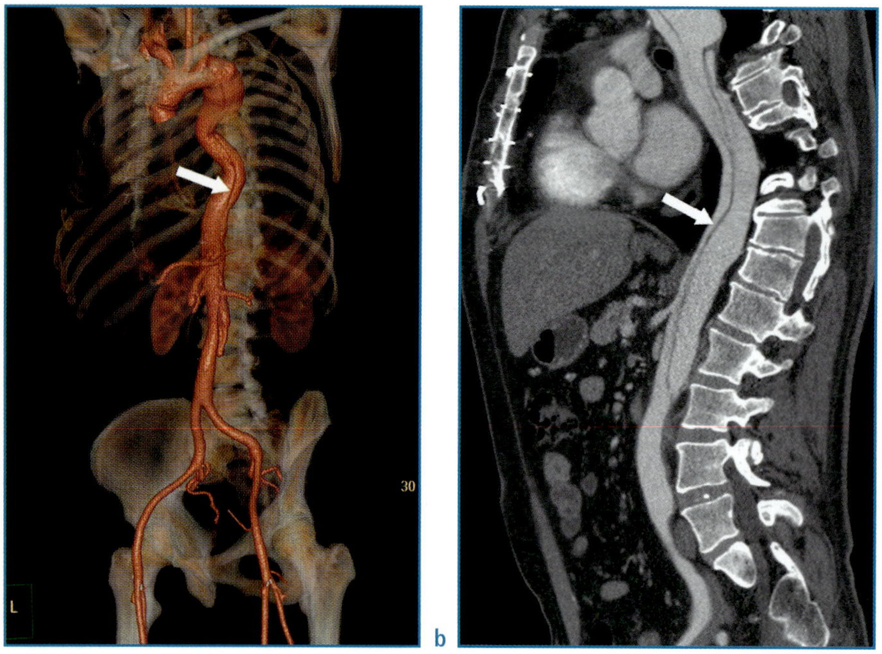

Figure 26-16 A dissection, affecting the descending aorta is visualized on both volume rendering (a) and sagittal cross-section (b). The dissection is related to an aneurysm formation in the proximal descending aorta. The arrows in (a) and (b) mark the dissection membrane extending in full length from the proximal to the distal part of the descending aorta.

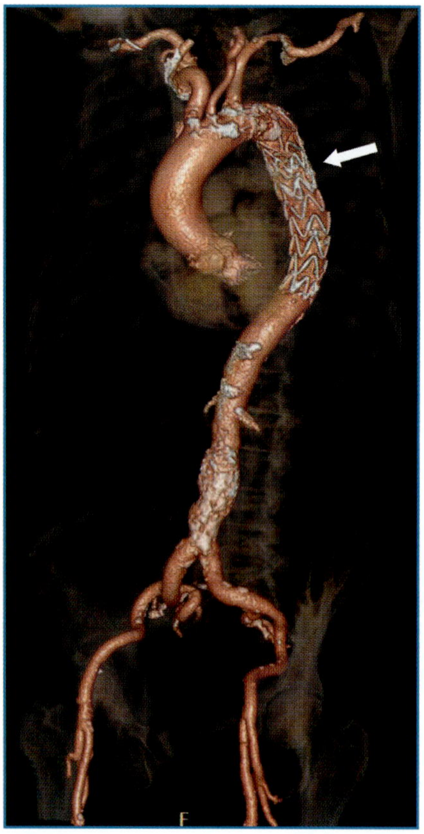

Figure 26-17 Patient with acute traumatic rupture of the proximal descending aorta. The lesion was repaired with endovascular grafting. The endovascular stent graft (arrow) is well visualized both with and without anatomical overlay by CT volume rendering images.

lesions (Figure 26-16). CT imaging is considered the gold standard for the detection of endoleaks after endo-graft occlusion of aneurysm formations. Young patients should be carefully selected for elective CT imaging due to high dose exposure rates associated with the procedure, MRA may be a good alternative in stable or chronic situations. Recent scanner generations have substantially alleviated the problem with dramatic dose reductions realized. As of today the lowest dose for imaging of the thoracic aorta is realized by so-called prospectively ECG-gated image acquisition techniques (Sommer 2010). This phenomenon founds the basis for the combination of pulmonary arterial, thoracic aortic and coronary angiographic imaging in a single ECG-gated chest CT scan, the so-called triple-rule-out protocol. CT imaging of the aorta allows accurate visualization of endovascular stent grafts (Figure 26-17).

26.11 Role of CT for Transcatheter Aortic Valve Implantation (TAVI)

Transcatheter aortic valve implantations have emerged in the last years as an alternative treatment for aortic stenosis. Two first generation devices are available for human implantations today (Grube 2007, Cribier 2009). The native stenotic valve is initially dilated with a valvuloplasty ballon under rapid pacing. Subsequently a bioprosthesis composed of either porcine or bovine pericardium is implanted into the native annular orifice. The bioprosthesis is mounted on a stent frame which serves two purposes: it unfolds the new valve into functional position and pushes the native valve aside into the sinus of Valsalva pouches. The Edwards Sapien valve is ballon mounted and able to cover aortic root sizes up to 26 mm diameter. The device is well-suited for a transapical deployment via a 5 cm left intercostal incision. The Core Valve device is selfexpanding and the method of choice for a percutaneous purely catheter-based approach. It will cover aortic annulus sizes up to 27 mm. The method is considered an alternative treatment for non-surgical candidates only. We can very well predict the durability of surgically implanted devices today but long-term survival and durability data for the transcatheter devices are missing. It will therefore take many more years until the question will be answered: How many surgical candidates can be safely converted for transcatheter approaches?

The critical questions asked during the planning of transcatheter procedures today relate to the size and morphology of the aortic root and the access pathway (transfemoral or transsubclavian or transapical). All these questions pertinent to transcatheter aortic valve replacements can be safely addressed with a supplemental set of diagnostic imaging modalities only. Transthoracic echocardiography is the first line of testing for appropriate annular size and grading of severity of aortic valve stenosis. Invasive angiography is still needed in the majority of cases to rule out or percutaneously treat coronary artery disease. CT coronary angiography would not be appropriate as we are dealing with high pre-test probability populations with a very high propensity for calcifications. But CT is well-suited with its very high sensitivity for calcifications to delineate the distribution of calcium in the aortic root and valvular leaflets. This is the reason why most clinicians today endorse a multi-modality strategy for the assessment of potential TAVI candidates encompassed of echocardiography, invasive coronary angiography and CT angiography for aortic root assessment and peripheral vascular access evaluation.

Multi-slice computed tomography may be the most comprehensive non-invasive imaging modality to evaluate potential candidates for transcatheter aortic valve replacement. This three-dimensional imaging technique provides accurate information on anatomical aspects of the aortic valve, aortic root and surrounding structures (such as the coronary arteries), aorta and peripheral arteries (Figure 26-18). The high accuracy of this technique to measure the aortic valve opening area by planimetry of the stenotic orifice has been shown. Furthermore, with the use of multiphase data sets obtained during ECG gating, motion of the cusps can be evaluated. At the current stage of development the concern of radiation dose exposure associated with the retrospective helical acquisition does not apply in this setting. Most of the patients included for TAVI assessment are octogenerians with little chance to survive long enough for the initiation of radiation induced cancer.

The main application of MDCT imaging is to visualize and quantitatively assess the aortic root. MDCT has a major advantage over MR in this respect. Within a few seconds a complete 4D dataset can be acquired with calcium sensitivity to the benefit of TAVI assessment. The most important lesson learned from a regular application of CT so far concerns the aortic annulus (Schultz 2010). So far a singular diameter was measured mostly utilizing transthoracic echocardiography (TTE). The heart is viewed in the left long parasternal axis and the aortic annulus is measured at the caudal insertion of the valve leaflets. CT measurements were initially carried out in similar fashion measuring a singular diameter in the coronal plane. It was found that the CT derived annular diameters though very accurately calibrated were significantly larger compared to TTE diameters. In order to clarify this discrepancy two-dimensional diameter measurement carried out on a cross-sectional plane were carried out on CT images. The cross-sectional plane corresponding to the aortic annulus was defined by three points. Each point was defined by the three nadirs of the aortic cusp insertion line into the aortic root. It was found that most of the annulus formations were not circular but elliptical. This resulted in a systematic overestimation of aortic annular dimensions in the coronal (used in CT) vs. the sagittal (used in echocardiography) imaging plane. Today's consensus in the TAVI community therefore recommends not to use maximum or singular plane diameters any more. Precise TAVI device planning should rely on either cross-sectional area measurements directly or be based on mean values derived from the maximum and minimum diameters of the annular ellipse (Figure 26-18). The annular diameter may be used for both balloon selection for valvuloplasty and device sizing for the revalving procedure. ECG-gated MDCT will most likely emerge as the standard of reference for acquiring these measurements.

Additional information obtained from the cardiac and vascular CT scan includes individual C-arm angulations and access planning (Figure 26-18). The CT scan reconstructed in a quiescent cardiac phase (either end-systole or mid-diastole) will show the aortic root including the valvular leaflets. In order to position the transcatheter device correctly it is essential to find a fluoroscopy plane perpendicular to the aortic root with all three leaflet structures projected in-line. Other measurements with importance for TAVI planning that can be easily obtained from CT scans are distance of the coronary ostia to the annular plane, width of the sinotubular junction, diameter of the proximal ascending aorta, and extent of calcification present on the leaflet structures.

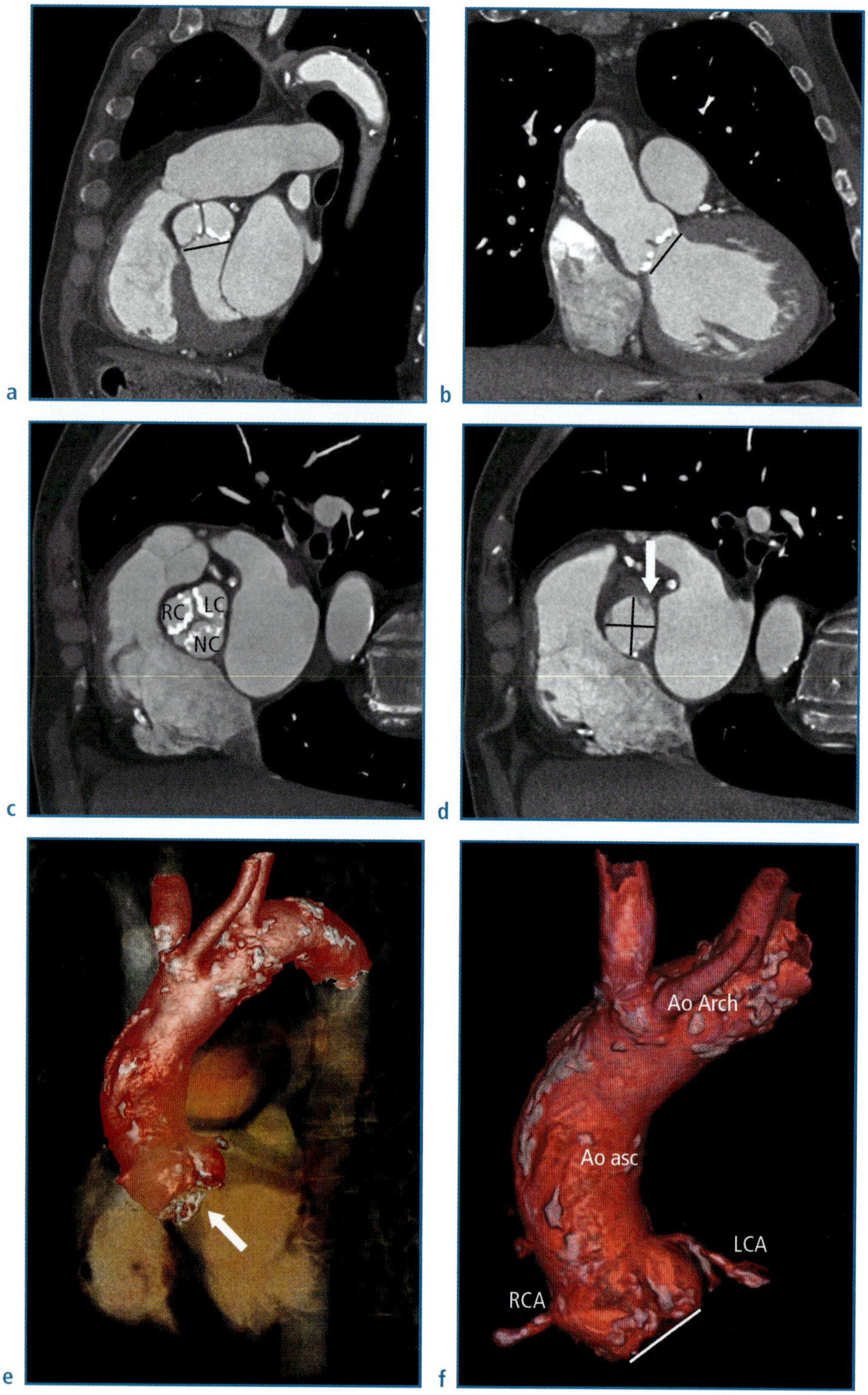

Figure 26-18 Sagittal **(a)** and coronal **(b)** sections at the level of the aortic root demonstrate an aortic valve with calcified leaflets. The aortic annulus is measured in a double oblique plane oriented along the basal attachments of the leaflets (black line in **(a)** and **(b)**). Double oblique plane at the level of the commisures **(c)** shows calcifications of the free edges. Double oblique plane **(d)** oriented along the black line of **(a)** and **(b)**. The basal attachments are visualized as small circular structures (arrow). The annulus is typically elliptical and not circular. The mean value of the largest and smallest diameter is used for sizing the appropriate endovascular device (black lines forming a cross). Volume rendering **(e)** in anteroposterior projection shows the calcified valvular structures at the base of the ascending aorta (arrow). The 3D volume rendering of the isolated aortic root **(f)** can be used to determine the C-arm position for TAVI implantation procedures. In this case the root is rotated in an LAO projection with a cranial tilt. This allows perpendicular viewing of the annulus with all sinuses projection along a singular plane (line in **(f)**). Ao Arch: aortic arch; Ao asc: ascending aorta; LC: left coronary sinus; LCA: left coronary artery; NC: non-coronary sinus; RC: right coronary sinus; RCA: right coronary artery.

The feasibility of a transfemoral approach depends strongly on the size, calcification and tortuosity of the iliofemoral arteries and aorta. Current devices require 18 French introducer sheaths and cross-sectional diameters of < 6 mm would contraindicate a transfemoral approach. Bulky calcifications and angulations of the thoracic aorta may also render a transapical approach the procedure of choice to minimize the risk of vascular complications. Regardless of the vascular access, severe aortic dilatation at the level of the sinotubular junction (> 45 mm) is considered a contraindication for self-expandable stent frames.

26.12 Detection of Pulmonary Embolism

Acute pulmonary embolism (PE) is a potentially life-threatening complication of peripheral deep venous thrombosis (DVT). A certain number of patients with massive pulmonary embolism do not receive any imaging tests because they either die before the diagnosis is suspected or are hemodynamically unstable precluding any transportation for the imaging procedure. In other words patients who are referred for imaging have to be in a sufficiently stable clinical condition. The role of imaging is to confirm or rule out the diagnosis of acute PE; and, if possible, to establish an alternative diagnosis. This is important because 60% of patients have a false positive clinical suspicion of PE. CT angiography is presently the workhorse for the evaluation of stable patients with suspected PE. MDCT-based angiography with more than 4 detector rows is superior to ventilation/perfusion nuclear scanning and is much faster than MRI (Schoepf and Costello 2004). Hence MDCT pulmonary angiography is the first line imaging modality for suspected PE patients. It's accuracy compared to the standard of reference invasive pulmonary angiography is congruent for ruling out PE. To achieve this standard in clinical practice CT imaging equipment with at least 16 detector row technology should be used (Figure 26-19). For latest CT technology the detection rate of subsegmental emboli is even better than for invasive pulmonary angiography. MRI could potentially achieve the same results but for the majority of patients examination and acquisition time are too long.

Direct signs of pulmonary embolism on CT scans are intraluminal filling defects and lack of enhancement of a pulmonary artery. Acute emboli are trapped either at the pulmonary artery bifurcations (riding emboli) or in peripheral arteries that are smaller than the embolus. Complete occlusion of a vessel by a fresh embolus is possible but residual perfusion with a partial occlusion is more common. The typical presentation is a central filling defect with a ring of contrast enhancement representing residual perfusion around it.

The typical chest or cardiac CT angiography protocol has to be modified for PE detection. The ROI for contrast bolus tracking that initiates the scan is placed in the right heart to initiate scanning earlier compared to aortic or coronary CTA.

The **most common factors** leading to either **false positive or false negative results** are:

- Breathing artifacts may occur even with latest cutting edge equipment with a total breath-hold duration for the scan of less than 4 s. Both false positive and false negative results may ensue if the reader is unaware of the artifact.
- Pulsation artifacts predominantely affect the lung parenchyma adjacent to the cardiac structures (namely lingual

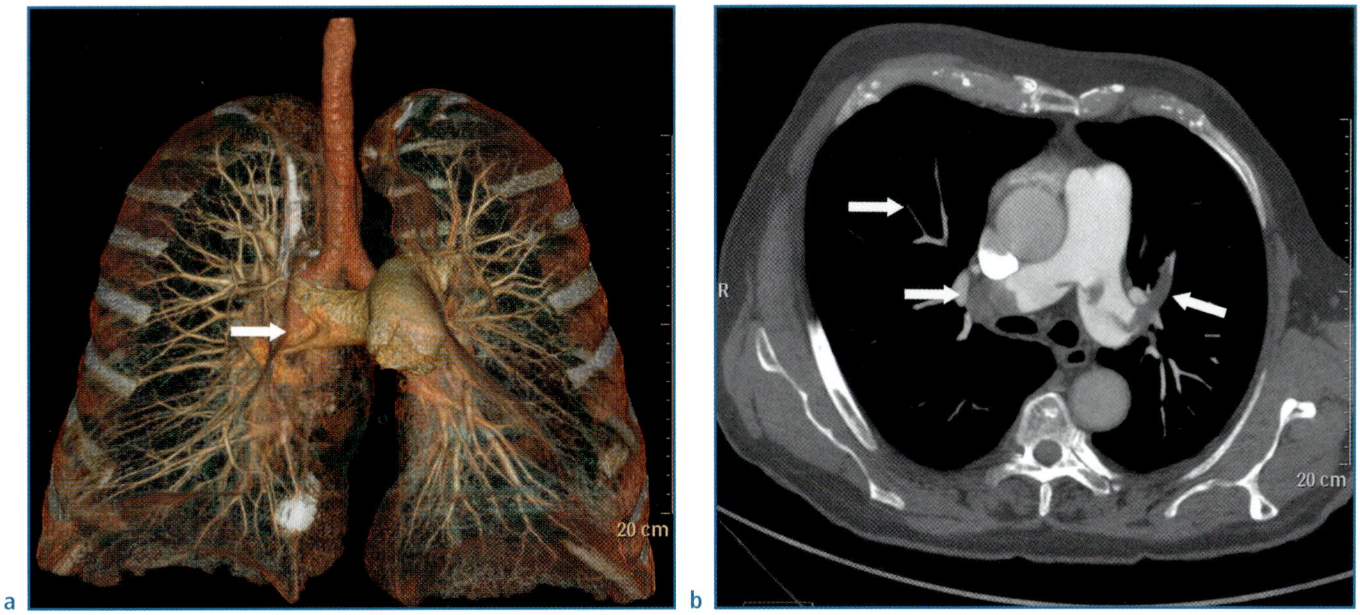

Figure 26-19 Pulmonary embolism: Volume rendering of the lungs with airways and pulmonary vasculature **(a)** shows a large filling defect (arrow) at the right main stem. A single axial slice from the volume stack **(b)** shows additional thrombi on the left side. The right main stem appears completely amputated with total thrombus occlusion (arrow on left side of the image). The segmental artery supplying the lingula is filled with thrombus (right arrow).

and left lower lobe). Both pulsation artifacts and partial volume averaging artifacts are less apparent with newer scanner models used.

- The clinically most important artifact is poor vascular enhancement; insufficient intraluminal contrast enhancement will lead to false negative readings if unrecognized by the reader.
- High contrast artifacts with streaks across the axial images will occur close to densely opacified central veins in the mediastinum.

26.13 Conclusions and Future Perspectives

The rapid evolution of CT technology has been mainly driven by cardiac applications during the past years. The achieved robustness is already satisfying with diagnostic image quality obtained for a large amount of patients. The industry focus has been centered on both temporal resolution and dose exposure. The applicability of CT imaging of the coronaries for the work-up of the cardiac patient has been made possible by the significant reduction in dose exposure. Further evolutionary steps increasing the temporal resolution will occur which in turn will augment robustness of the method to produce diagnostic images for patients with heart rate variability and arrhythmia. A gradual evolutionary increase in spatial resolution is not likely to be provided as spatial resolution utilizing current detector technology is dose limited. But there are revolutionary steps ahead that will be centered on detector technology. All currently available CT scanners work with integrating detectors that disregard the energy level of the individual roentgen ray photon arriving at the detector. Dual energy imaging provides a very first impression of what might be clinically possible with energy discrimination (Bastarrika 2009). Today the major disadvantage of CT imaging is the restricted lumen discrimination adjacent to high density structures like stent struts and calcified plaque.

26.13.1 Basic Principle of Spectral CT

The energy source used for conventional X-ray CT imaging is operating based upon the "bremsstrahlung principle". A continuous spectrum of X-ray photons is emitted and filtered before exposure of the scanned object. After passage through tissue, the energy spectrum of a polychromatic beam of X-rays contains valuable information about the elemental composition of the absorber. Conventional X-ray systems or X-ray computed tomography (CT) systems, equipped with scintillator detectors operate in integrating mode. They are largely insensitive to the spectral information contained in different X-ray photons, since the detector output is proportional to the energy fluence integrated over the whole spectrum.

One first approach to utilize the information contained in the polychromatic beam is to measure two different energy levels separately. This can be achieved with either tube voltage switching or layered detectors (Carmi 2005). The method has great potential for material separation in the high density domain and first clinical results are very encouraging (Johnson 2007). But the application for cardiac purposes is thus far limited by the phase shift inherent in most approaches or hampered by inefficient dose utilization. Another far more sophisticated approach exploiting the full potential of energy dependent imaging is spectral CT (Roessl and Proksa 2007).

The method is based on so-called photon counting detectors. Spectral CT is designed to detect k-edge discontinuities. The k-edges occur in the element specific photoelectric cross-section. X-ray photons are counted by the detector and sorted in energy bins representing pre-selected partial bandwidths of the full spectrum. Material differentiation in the high density domain is fully accomplished by this approach. In order to apply this method for routine clinical imaging completely different detector technology has to be developed. Today's technology provides only low count rates for spectral detectors and it is therefore not realistic to predict clinically usable products within the next 5 yrs.

26.13.2 The Unobscured 3D Luminogram

To achieve a perfect non-invasive 3D luminogram of the coronary tree we would need a visualization unobscured by high density overlay (as e.g. calcium or metal). This may either be achieved by the material separation approaches described for dual energy imaging or be accomplished by acquiring contrast only images. Spectral imaging may be adapted to acquire several images below and above specific k-edges. Subsequent subtraction (or more mathematically correct deconvolution) of images around the k-edge removes all tissue from the dataset except for the element characterized by the k-edge. This allows generating contrast only images for compounds with high z-number. Iodine with a k-edge at 33.2 keV is not suited for such an endeavor. The vast majority of X-ray photons at this energy level is completely absorbed within the human body structure. This renders detection of residual photons on the detector side impossible and only contributes to artifacts as beam hardening and photon starvation. Gadolinium, though originally designed for MRI imaging, is well visualized by conventional

CT and exhibits better attenuation characteristics than iodine. It is not widely used clinically because concentrations much higher than those routinely applied for MRI imaging would be needed. Gadolinium is much better suited for spectral CT with a k-edge discontinuity occurring at 50.2 keV. This is both well inside the energy regime relevant for medical imaging and is sufficiently high enough to render the thorax penetrable for the majority of emitted photons. Other agents that may be considered in the future include gold (k-edge 80.7 keV) and bismuth (k-edge 90.8 keV).

The deconvolution (or simply subtraction) of images adjacent to the k-edge of the contrast agent of interest allows to visualize the lumen without any overlay. This concept has first been shown in simulation studies and subsequently been realized on a prototype scanner. First clinical proof-of-concept papers have shown the feasibility to separate gadolinium from stent struts and calcium in phantom studies (Feuerlein 2008).

The generated images reveal a lot of image noise so far. This is due to a limited count rate of the photon counting detectors, but further technical improvements to address this issue are expected. It may be possible in the near term future to combine higher count rate detectors with a miniaturization that allows to produce very small and efficient detector elements allowing image acquisition at dose exposure levels comparable to conventional CT. The individual detector element would be smaller than the voxel size reconstructed for medical imaging. With such an approach beam hardening is no longer an issue. Partial volume averaging on the other hand prevails, but correction algorithms may utilize the very small individual detector element used for spectral detectors.

Spectral CT could therefore have a major impact on the clinical value of CT coronary angiography. Without beam hardening artifacts in-stent lumina become accessible and with partial volume averaging reduced both vessel lumina adjacent to stent struts and densely calcified plaques are more accurately delineated (Feuerlein 2008).

> Overall, **two new application scenarios** could be feasible:
> - one is the follow-up of patients after percutaneous coronary interventions with stent implantation,
> - the other is the evalution of patients with known CAD or calcified vessels.

Spectral detector technology may promote CT to become the primary tool for CAD imaging (Feuerlein 2008, Roessl and Proksa 2007).

26.13.3 Potential for Plaque Imaging

Conventional integrating CT offers a first step in plaque component visualization and differentiation. Many studies have been published to establish density thresholds for the differentiation of calcified, fibrous and lipidic plaque components. But the discrimination of lipidic and fibrous components failed and in clinical practice only two components are reported: calcified and non-calcified. Initially one study was published that blamed partial volume averaging due to insufficient spatial resolution to be responsible for the failure of soft component differentiation (Cademartiri 2005). But today evidence accumulates that the soft plaque components represent the active plaque structures. The soft structures are vascularized and a rapid wash-in of contrast is thought to be supplied by advential vasa vasorum (Halliburton 2006). This explains why a contrast enhancement-based approach has to fail.

In this context spectral CT could theoretically offer differentiation tools for lipidic and fibrous components. Fat containing structures were found to increase in attenuation with increasing photon energy, this is opposing to higher density structures as e.g. iodine contrast. But a proof-of-concept for the differentiation of lipid vs. fibrous tissue is still lacking.

The more relevant potential of spectral CT technology for the application of plaque imaging is contrast associated. Future applications may utilize two simultaneously injected contrast agents. One with a k-edge of e.g. 50 keV (like gadolinium) is used for luminal opacification, the other with a k-edge of 90 keV (e.g. bismuth) is coupled to a receptor avidly binding to the endothelial surface of a vulnerable plaque. Both contrast agents would be apparent on different deconvolution images of the same dataset and could be secondarily superimposed using colored overlay as available for PET/CT post-processing. The sensitivity of the plaque specific contrast compound will be a couple of orders lower than PET sensitivity. But ease of use and availability may allow a more widespread clinical application at a lower dose exposure.

In summary, the quest for a single modality to serve cardiac imaging in a one-stop shopping fashion has not been successful. Today many modalities with complementary and alternative function serve the field of cardiac medicine. With those modalities firmly located in different medical specialties (namely cardiology, nuclear medicine and radiology) the multi-modality approach will also stimulate a multi-disciplinary approach for diagnostic cardiac imaging.

References

Agatston AS, Janowitz WR, Hildner FJ et al. Quantification of coronary artery calcium using ultrafast computed tomography. J Am Coll Cardiol 1990; 15: 827–32.

Bastarrika G, Lee YS, Huda W et al. CT of coronary artery disease. Radiology 2009; 253: 317–38.

Becker CR, Kleffel T, Crispin A et al. Coronary artery calcium measurement: agreement of multi-row detector and electron beam CT. Am J Roentgenol 2001; 176: 1295–8.

Bertaglia E, Bella PD, Tondo C et al. Image integration increases efficacy of paroxysmal atrial fibrillation catheter ablation: results from the CartoMerge Italian Registry. Europace 2009; 11: 1004–10.

Blanke P, Baumann T, Langer M, Pache G. Imaging of pulmonary vein anatomy using low-dose prospective ECG-triggered dual-source computed tomography. Eur Radiol 2010; 20: 1851–5.

Breen JF. Imaging of the pericardium. J Thorac Imaging 2001; 16: 47–54.

Brenner D, Hall E. Computed tomography – an increasing source of radiation exposure. N Engl J Med 2007; 357: 2277.

Budoff MJ, Achenbach S, Duerinckx A. Clinical utility of computed tomography and magnetic resonance techniques for non-invasive coronary angiography. J Am Coll Cardiol 2003; 42: 1867–78.

Budoff MJ, Dowe D, Jollis JG et al. Diagnostic performance of 64-multi-detector row coronary computed tomographic angiography for evaluation of coronary artery stenosis in individuals without known coronary artery disease: results from the prospective multi-center ACCURACY (Assessment by Coronary Computed Tomographic Angiography of Individuals Undergoing Invasive Coronary Angiography) trial. J Am Coll Cardiol 2008; 52: 1724–32.

Cademartiri F, Mollet N, Runza G et al. Influence of intracoronary attenuation on coronary plaque measurements using multislice computed tomography: observations in an ex vivo model of coronary computed tomography angiography. Eur Radiol 2005; 15: 1426–31.

Carmi R, Naveh G, Altman A. Material separation with dual-layer CT. IEEE Nuclear Science Symposium Conference Record 2005; 4.

Chinnaiyan KM, Raff G, Goldstein J. Cardiac CT in the emergency department. Cardiol Clin 2009; 27: 587–96.

Cribier A, Litzler PY, Eltchaninoff H et al. Technique of transcatheter aortic valve implantation with the Edwards-Sapien heart valve using the transfemoral approach. Herz 2009; 34: 347–56.

Dewey M, Zimmermann E, Deissenrieder F et al. Non-invasive coronary angiography by 320-row computed tomography with lower radiation exposure and maintained diagnostic accuracy: comparison of results with cardiac catheterization in a head-to-head pilot investigation. Circulation 2009; 120: 867–75.

Diamond GA, Forrester JS. Analysis of probability as an aid in the clinical diagnosis of coronary-artery disease. N Engl J Med 1979; 300: 1350–8.

Einstein AJ, Henzlova MJ, Rajagopalan S. Estimating risk of cancer associated with radiation exposure from 64-slice computed tomography coronary angiography. JAMA 2007; 298: 317–23.

Feuerlein S, Roessl E, Proksa R et al. Multi-energy photon-counting k-edge imaging: potential for improved luminal depiction in vascular imaging. Radiology 2008; 249: 1010–6.

Flohr TG, McCollough CH, Bruder H et al. First performance evaluation of a dual-source CT (DSCT) system. Europ Radiol 2006; 16: 256–68.

Garcia M, Lessick J, Hoffmann MH for Investigators CATSCANS. Accuracy of 16-row multi-detector computed tomography for the assessment of coronary artery stenosis. JAMA 2006; 296: 403–11.

George RT, Arbab-Zadeh A, Miller JM et al. Adenosine stress 64- and 256-row detector computed tomography angiography and perfusion imaging: a pilot study evaluating the transmural extent of perfusion abnormalities to predict atherosclerosis causing myocardial ischemia. Circ Cardiovasc Imaging 2009; 2: 174–82.

Greenland P, LaBree L, Azen SP et al. Coronary artery calcium score combined with Framingham score for risk prediction in asymptomatic individuals. JAMA 2004; 291: 210–5.

Grube E, Schuler G, Buellesfeld L et al. Percutaneous aortic valve replacement for severe aortic stenosis in high-risk patients using the second-and current third-generation self-expanding core valve prosthesis device success and 30 d clinical outcome. J Am Coll Cardiol 2007; 50: 69–76.

Halliburton SS, Schoenhagen P, Nair A et al. Contrast enhancement of coronary atherosclerotic plaque: a high-resolution, multi-detector-row computed tomography study of pressure-perfused, human ex-vivo coronary arteries. Coron Artery Dis 2006; 17: 553–60.

Hausleiter J, Meyer T, Hermann F et al. Estimated radiation dose associated with cardiac CT angiography. JAMA 2009; 301: 500–7.

Hecht HS, Budoff MJ, Berman DS et al. Coronary artery calcium scanning: Clinical paradigms for cardiac risk assessment and treatment. Am Heart J 2006; 151: 1139–46.

Hoffmann MH, Shi H, Manzke R et al. Non-invasive coronary angiography with 16-detector row CT: effect of heart rate. Radiology 2005a; 234: 86–97.

Hoffmann MH, Shi H, Schmitz BL et al. Non-invasive coronary angiography with multi-slice computed tomography. JAMA 2005b; 293: 2471–8.

Hounsfield GN. Picture quality of computed tomography. Am J Roentgenol 1976; 127: 3–9.

Hounsfield GN. Computerized transverse axial scanning (tomography). 1. Description of system. Br J Radiol 1973; 46: 1016–22.

Hunold P, Vogt FM, Schmermund A et al. Radiation exposure during cardiac CT: effective doses at multi-detector row CT and electron-beam CT. Radiology 2003; 226: 145–52.

Hur J, Kim YJ, Lee HJ et al. Left atrial appendage thrombi in stroke patients: detection with two-phase cardiac CT angiography versus transesophageal echocardiography. Radiology 2009; 251: 683–90.

Johnson T, Krauß B, Sedlmair M et al. Material differentiation by dual energy CT: initial experience. Eur Radiol 2007; 17: 1510–7.

Kamdar AR, Meadows TA, Roselli EE et al. Multi-detector computed tomographic angiography in planning of reoperative cardiothoracic surgery. Ann Thorac Surg 2008; 85: 1239–45.

Khan NU, Yonan N. Does pre-operative computed tomography reduce the risks associated with re-do cardiac surgery? Interact Cardiovasc Thorac Surg 2009; 9: 119–23.

Khare RK, Courtney DM, Powell ES et al. Sixty-four-slice computed tomography of the coronary arteries: cost-effectiveness analysis of patients presenting to the emergency department with low-risk chest pain. Acad Emerg Med 2008; 15: 623–32.

Klass O, Mutlu S, Hohl K et al. Multi-detector computed tomography coronary angiography: sublingual nitroglycerine improves image quality significantly because of peripheral coronary vasodilatation. J Comp Assist Tomogr 2009; 33: 199–203.

Klass O, Walker M, Siebach A et al. Prospectively gated axial CT coronary angiography: comparison of image quality and effective radiation dose between 64- and 256-slice CT. Eur Radiol 2010; 20: 1124–31.

Kramer SC, Görich J, Aschoff AJ et al. Diagnostic value of spiral-CT angiography in comparison with digital subtraction angiography before and after peripheral vascular intervention. Angiology 1998; 49: 599–606.

Lehman SJ, Schlett CL, Bamberg F et al. Assessment of coronary plaque progression in coronary computed tomography angiography using a semiquantitative score. JACC Cardiovasc Imaging 2009; 2: 1262–70.

Lell M, Hinkmann F, Anders K et al. High-pitch electrocardiogram-triggered computed tomography of the chest: initial results. Invest Radiol 2009; 44: 728–33.

Libby P. Pathophysiology of coronary artery disease. Circulation 2005; 111: 3481–8.

Lipton M, Higgins C, Farmer D, Boyd D. Cardiac imaging with a high-speed cine-CT scanner: preliminary results. Radiology 1984; 152: 579–82.

Lloyd-Jones D, Adams RJ, Brown TM et al. for the American Heart Association Statistics Committee and Stroke Statistics Subcommittee. Heart disease and stroke statistics – 2010 update: a report from the American Heart Association. Circulation 2010; 121 (7): e46–e215.

Maintz D, Burg MC, Seifarth H et al. Update on multi-detector coronary CT angiography of coronary stents: in vitro evaluation of 29 different stent types with dual-source CT. Eur Radiol 2009; 19: 42–9.

Meijboom WB, Meijs MF, Schuijf JD et al. Diagnostic accuracy of 64-slice computed tomography coronary angiography: a prospective, multi-center, multi-vendor study. J Am Coll Cardiol 2008; 52: 2135–44.

Meijboom WB, van Mieghem CA, Mollet N et al. 64-slice computed tomography coronary angiography in patients with high, intermediate, or low pre-test probability of significant coronary artery disease. J Am Coll Cardiol 2007; 50: 1469–75.

Miller J, Rochitte C, Dewey M et al. Diagnostic performance of coronary angiography by 64-row CT. N Engl J Med 2008; 359: 2324.

Nieman K, Shapiro MD, Ferencik M et al. Reperfused myocardial infarction: contrast-enhanced 64-section CT in comparison to MR imaging. Radiology 2008; 247: 49–56.

Ohnesorge B, Flohr T, Becker C et al. Cardiac imaging by means of electrocardiographically gated multi-section spiral CT: initial experience. Radiology 2000; 217: 564–71.

Roessl E, Proksa R. K-edge imaging in X-ray computed tomography using multi-bin photon counting detectors. Phys Med Biol 2007; 52: 4679–96.

Schoepf UJ, Costello P. CT angiography for diagnosis of pulmonary embolism: state of the art. Radiology 2004; 230: 329–37.

Schuijf J, Bax J, Shaw L et al. Meta-analysis of comparative diagnostic performance of magnetic resonance imaging and multi-slice computed tomography for non-invasive coronary angiography. Am Heart J 2006; 151: 404–11.

Schultz CJ, Moelker A, Piazza N et al. Three-dimensional evaluation of the aortic annulus using multi-slice computer tomography: are manufacturer's guidelines for sizing for percutaneous aortic valve replacement helpful? Eur Heart J 2010; 31: 849–56.

Shi H, Aschoff A, Brambs H, Hoffmann M. Multi-slice CT imaging of anomalous coronary arteries. Eur Radiol 2004; 14: 2172–81.

Sommer WH, Schenzle JC, Becker CR et al. Saving dose in triple-rule-out computed tomography examination using a high-pitch dual spiral technique. Invest Radiol 2010; 45: 64–71.

Stanford W, Thompson BH, Burns TL et al. Coronary artery calcium quantification at multi-detector row helical CT versus electron-beam CT. Radiology 2004; 230: 397–402.

van der Vleuten PA, de Jonge GJ, Lubbers DD et al. Evaluation of global left ventricular function assessment by dual-source computed tomography compared with MRI. Eur Radiol 2009; 19: 271–7.

van Werkhoven JM, Schuijf JD, Gaemperli O et al. Prognostic value of multi-slice computed tomography and gated single-photon emission computed tomography in patients with suspected coronary artery disease. J Am Coll Cardiol 2009; 53: 623–32.

Weustink AC, Nieman K, Pugliese F et al. Diagnostic accuracy of computed tomography angiography in patients after bypass grafting: comparison with invasive coronary angiography. JACC Cardiovasc Imaging 2009; 2: 816–24.

White C, Kuo D. Chest pain in the emergency department: role of multi-detector CT. Radiology 2007; 245: 672.

Yamanaka O, Hobbs RE. Coronary artery anomalies in 126,595 patients undergoing coronary arteriography. Cathet Cardiovasc Diagn 1990; 21: 28–40.

Index

Keywords in figures and figure legends are in *italics*.

D

E

F

G

H

I

M

Q

R

S

T

U

V